CARDIOLOGY SECRETS

SECRETS

CARDIOLOGY SECRETS

First South Asia Edition

GLENN N. LEVINE, MD, FACC, FAHA
Professor of Medicine, Baylor College of Medicine;
Director, Cardiac Care Unit,
Michael E. DeBakey VA Medical Center,
Houston, Texas

ELSEVIER

ELSEVIER

RELX India Pvt. Ltd.
Registered Office: 818, Indraprakash Building, 8th Floor, 21, Barakhamba Road, New Delhi - 110001
Corporate Office: 14th Floor, Building No. 10B, DLF Cyber City, Phase II, Gurgaon-122 002, Haryana, India

Cardiology Secrets, 5e, Glenn N. Levine

ISBN: 978-0-323-47870-0

This adapted reprint of Cardiology Secrets, 5e, by Glenn N. Levine was undertaken by RELX India Private Limited and is published by arrangement with Elsevier Inc

Cardiology Secrets, First South Asia Edition, Glenn N. Levine.

Adapted Reprint ISBN: 978-81-312-4906-2

First Adapted Reprinted in India 2017, Reprinted 2019

Notice

Knowledge and best practice in this field are constantly changing. As new research and experience broaden our understanding, changes in research methods, professional practices, or medical treatment may become necessary.

Practitioners and researchers must always rely on their own experience and knowledge in evaluating and using any information, methods, compounds, or experiments described herein. In using such information or methods they should be mindful of their own safety and the safety of others, including parties for whom they have a professional responsibility.

With respect to any drug or pharmaceutical products identified, readers are advised to check the most current information provided (i) on procedures featured or (ii) by the manufacturer of each product to be administered, to verify the recommended dose or formula, the method and duration of administration, and contraindications. It is the responsibility of practitioners, relying on their own experience and knowledge of their patients, to make diagnoses, to determine dosages and the best treatment for each individual patient, and to take all appropriate safety precautions.

To the fullest extent of the law, neither the Publisher nor the authors, contributors, or editors, assume any liability for any injury and/or damage to persons or property as a matter of product liability, negligence or otherwise, or from any use or operation of any methods, products, instructions, or ideas contained in the material herein.

Although all advertising material is expected to conform to ethical (medical) standards, inclusion in this publication does not constitute a guarantee or endorsement of the quality or value of such product or of the claims made of it by its manufacturer.

This publication is licensed for sale in India, Bangladesh, Bhutan, Maldives, Nepal, Pakistan and Sri Lanka only. Circulation of this version outside these territories is unauthorized and illegal.

Content Strategist: Arvind Koul
Content Development Specialist: Supriya Barua Kumar
Project Manager: Karthikeyan Murthy

Printed in India by Rajkamal Electric Press, Kundli, Haryana.

To Lydia, who patiently tolerates my long weekdays and weekends of work. And to Gabby, Sadie, and Coco, who are a little less patient when their morning and evening walks and trips to the park or beach are delayed.

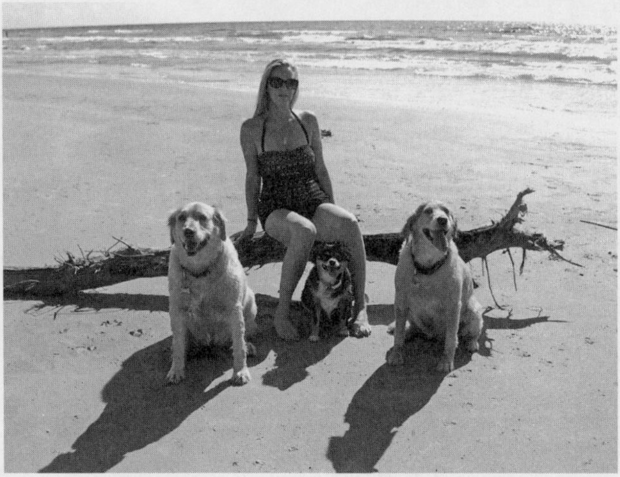

CONTRIBUTORS

Suhny Abbara, MD, FACR, FSCCT
Professor, Department of Radiology
Chief, Cardiothoracic Imaging, UTSW Medical Center
Division of Cardiothoracic Imaging
UT Southwestern Medical Center
Dallas, Texas, USA

David Aguilar, MD
Associate Professor of Medicine
Department of Medicine, Division of Cardiology
Baylor College of Medicine
Houston, Texas, USA

Eric H. Awtry, MD, FACC
Associate Professor of Medicine
Boston University School of Medicine
Associate Chair for Clinical Affairs, Cardiovascular Medicine Section
Boston Medical Center
Boston, Massachusetts, USA

Jose L. Baez-Escudero, MD, FACC, FHRS
Section Head, Cardiac Pacing and Electrophysiology
Robert and Suzanne Tomsich Department of Cardiovascular Medicine
Cleveland Clinic Florida
Weston, FL, USA

Faisal Bakaeen
Staff Surgeon and Professor of Surgery
Department of Thoracic and Cardiovascular Surgery, Heart and Vascular Institute
Cleveland Clinic
Cleveland, Ohio, USA

Gary J. Balady, MD
Director, Non Invasive Cardiovascular Laboratories
Section of Cardiovascular Medicine
Boston Medical Center
Professor of Medicine
Boston University School of Medicine

Dr. Luc M. Beauchesne, MD FRCPC FACC
Director Adult Congenital Heart Disease Program
Division of Cardiology
University of Ottawa Heart Institute
Ottawa, Ontario, Canada

Sheilah A. Bernard, MD, FACC
Associate Program Director, IM Residency Program
Department of Medicine, Section of Cardiology
Boston Medical Center, Boston University School of Medicine
Boston, MA USA

Ozlem Bilen, MD
Cardiology Fellow
Emory School of Medicine, Division of Cardiology
Atlanta, GA

Itamar Birnbaum, MD
Fellow
Department of Medicine, Division of Cardiology
Baylor College of Medicine
Houston, Teaxs, USA

Yochai Birnbaum, MD FACC, FAHA
Professor of Medicine
John S. Dunn Chair in Cardiology Research and Education
The Department of Medicine, Section of Cardiology
Baylor College of Medicine
Houston, TX 77030

Fernando Boccalandro, MD FACC FSCAI CPI
Odessa Heart Institure - ProCare
Vice Chief of Staff
Medical Center Hospital Health Care System
Department of Cardiology
Medical Director
Permian Research Foundation
Assistant Clinical Professor
Department of Internal Medicine
Texas Tech University Health Science Center
Odessa, Texas, USA

Biykem Bozkurt, MD, PhD, FACC, FAHA, FACP, FESC, FHFSA
Professor of Medicine
Medicine Chair (Medical Care Line Executive)
DeBakey VA Medical Center
The Mary and Gordon Cain, Chair
W.A. "Tex" and Deborah Moncrief, Jr., Chair
Vice-Chair of Department of Medicine at Baylor College of Medicine
Associate Director, Cardiovascular Research Institute
Director, Winters Center for Heart Failure Research, Baylor College of Medicine, Houston Texas

Blase Carabello, MD
Professor and Chief, Cardiology
Director, East Carolina Heart Institute
East Carolina University

Jaya Chandrasekhar, MBBS, MRCP, FRACP
Division of Cardiology
Icahn School of Medicine at Mount Sinai
New York, New York, USA

Leslie T. Cooper Jr., M.D.
Professor of Medicine
Chair, Cardiovascular Department
Mayo Clinic in Florida
Jacksonville, FL, USA

Luke Cunningham, MD
Fellow
Cardiovascular Diseases
Baylor College of Medicine
Houston, Texas, USA

Ali E. Denktas, MD, FACC, FSCAI
Director, Cardiac Catheterization Laboratories
Michael E. DeBakey VA Medical Center
Associate Professor of Medicine
Baylor College of Medicine
Houston, Texas, USA

Anita Deswal, MD, MPH
Chief of Cardiology
Director, Heart Failure Program
Michael E. DeBakey VA Medical Center
Professor of Medicine
Baylor College of Medicine
Houston, Texas, USA

Haytham Elgharably, MD
Resident
Thoracic & Cardiovascular Surgery Department
Cleveland Clinic Foundation
Cleveland, Ohio, United States

Lothar Faber, MD, FESC, FACC
Professor
Clinic for Cardiology
Heart and Diabetes Centre NRW, University Clinic of the Ruhr University Bochum
D 32545 Bad Oeynhausen, Germany

Michael E. Farkouh, MD, MSc, FACC, FAHA
Chair and Director
Peter Munk Centre of Excellence in Multinational Clinical Trials
University Health Network
Director, Heart & Stroke Richard Lewar Centre of Excellence in Cardiovascular Research
University of Toronto
Toronto, Canada

Nadeen N. Faza, MD
Cardiovascular Disease Fellow
Department of Cardiology
Baylor College of Medicine
Houston, Texas, USA

Savitri Fedson, MA, MD
Associate Professor
Department of Medicine, Baylor College of Medicine
Michael E. Debakey Medical Center
Associate Professor
Center for Medical Ethics and Health Policy, Baylor College of Medicine
Houston, Texas, USA

G. Michael Felker, MD, MHS, FACC, FAHA, FHFSA
Professor of Medicine
Chief, Heart Failure Section, Division of Cardiology
Duke University School of Medicine
Durham, NC USA

James J. Fenton, MD , FCCP
Clinical Associate Professor
National Jewish Health
Denver, Colorado, USA

Michael E. Field, M.D.
Associate Professor of Medicine
Director of Cardiac Arrhythmia Service
University of Wisconsin School of Medicine & Public Health
600Highland Avenue, MC3248
Madison, WI 53792

Scott D. Flamm, M.D., M.B.A.
Section Head, Cardiovascular Imaging
Imaging, and Heart and Vascular Institutes
Professor of Radiology
Department of Diagnostic Radiology
Cleveland Clinic Lerner College of Medicine of Case Western Reserve University
Cleveland, Ohio, USA

Lee A. Fleisher, MD, FACC, FAHA
Robert D. Dripps Professor and Chair of Anesthesiology
Critical Care Professor of Medicine
Perelman School of Medicine
University of Pennsylvania
Philadelphia, PA

Laura Epstein Flink, MD MS
Assistant Clinical Professor
Division of Cardiology/UCSF
San Francisco VA Medical Center
San Francisco, California

Amy French, MD
Department of Cardiology
Boston Medical Center/Boston University School of Medicine
Boston, MA, USA

Marat Fudim, MD
Department of Medicine, Division of Cardiology
Duke University Medical Center
Durham, NC, USA

Stephen A. Gannon, MD
Teaching Fellow in Medicine
Bio Med Medicine
Brown University
Providence, Rhode Island

Nicholas Governatori, MD
Assistant Residency Program Director
Thomas Jefferson University
Philadelphia, PA 19147

Cindy Grines, MD
Corporate Vice Chief of Academic Affairs
Cardiovascular Medicine
William Beaumont Hospital
Royal Oak, Michigan

Gabriel B. Habib Sr, MS, MD, FACC, FCCP, FAHA
Professor of Medicine
Department of Medicine, Division of Cardiology
Baylor College of Medicine
Houston, Texas, USA

Ihab Hamzeh, MD., FACC
Baylor College of Medicine
Houston, Texas, USA

Tomoya Timothy Hinohara, MD
Resident Physician
Department of Internal Medicine
Duke University Medical Center
Durham, North Carolina, USA

Vu Hoang, MD
Cardiology Fellow
Department of Internal Medicine, Division of Cardiology
Baylor College of Medicine
Houston, Texas, USA

Brian D. Hoit, MD
Professor of Medicine and Physiology and Biophysics
Case Western Reserve University
Harrington Heart & Vascular Institute
University Hospitals Cleveland Medical Center
Cleveland OH 44106

Hani Jneid, MD, FACC, FAHA, FSCAI
Associate Professor of Medicine
Director of Interventional Cardiology Research
Baylor College of Medicine
Director of Interventional Cardiology
The Michael E. DeBakey VA Medical Center
Houston, Texas, USA

Jose A. Joglar, MD, FACC, FAHA, FHRS
Professor of Internal Medicine
Fellowship Program Director, Clinical Cardiac Electrophysiology
Director of Cardiology, Parkland Memorial Hospital
Elizabeth Thaxton Page and Ellis Batten Page Professorship in Clinical Cardiac Electrophysiology Research
UT Southwestern Medical Center
Dallas, Texas, USA

Douglas R. Johnston, MD, FACS
Staff Surgeon
Department of Thoracic and Cardiovascular Surgery
Cleveland Clinic
Cleveland, OH USA

Lee Joseph, MD
Fellow
Internal Medicine, Cardiovascular Medicine
University of Iowa
Iowa City, Iowa, USA

Waleed T. Kayani, MD
Interventional Cardiology Fellow
Department of Medicine, Section of Cardiology
Baylor College of Medicine, Houston, Texas, USA

Thomas A. Kent, MD
Professor and Director of Cerebrovascular Research and Education
Department of Neurology
Baylor College of Medicine
Houston, Texas, USA

Jimmy L. Kerrigan, MD
General Cardiology Fellow
Robert and Suzanne Tomsich Department of Cardiovascular Medicine
Sydell and Arnold Miller Family Heart & Vascular Institute
Cleveland Clinic Foundation
Cleveland, Ohio, USA

Elias Kfoury, MD, RPVI
Division of Vascular Surgery
Cheyenne Regional Medical Center
Cheyenne, WY

Shaden Khalaf, MD
Cardiology Fellow at Baylor College of Medicine
Houston, Texas, USA

Mirza Umair Khalid, MD
Cardiology Fellow
Department of Medicine, Division of Cardiology
Baylor College of Medicine
Houston, Texas, USA

Esther S.H. Kim, MD, MPH
Associate Professor of Medicine
Division of Cardiovascular Medicine
Vanderbilt Heart and Vascular Institute
Nashville, TN

Panos Kougias, MD, FACS
Associate Professor of Surgery
Baylor College of Medicine
Houston, Texas, USA

Amar Krishnaswamy, MD
Program Director, Interventional Cardiology
Department of Cardiovascular Medicine
Heart and Vascular Institute
Cleveland Clinic
Cleveland, OH, USA

Michael H. Kroll, MD
Professor and Chief
Division of Benign Hematology
The University of Texas MD Anderson Cancer Center
Houston, Texas, USA

Nitin Kulkarni, MD
Cardiology Fellow
Division of Cardiology
UT Southwestern Medical Center
Dallas, Texas, USA

Richard A. Lange, MD, MBA
President
Dean, Paul L. Foster School of Medicine
Rick and Ginger Francis Endowed Professor
Texas Tech University Health Sciences Center El Paso
El Paso, Texas, USA

Salvatore Mangione, MD
Associate Professor of Medicine
SKMC of Thomas Jefferson University
1001 Locust Street
Philadelphia, PA 19096

Sharyl R. Martini, MD PhD
Medical Director
VA National Telestroke Program
Department of Veterans Affairs
Assistant Professor
Department of Neurology
Baylor College of Medicine
Houston, Texas, USA

James McCord, MD
Heart and Vascular Institute
Henry Ford Hospital
Wayne State University
Detroit, Michigan, USA

Roxana Mehran, MD, FACC
Professor of Medicine (Cardiology) and Population Health Science and Policy
Director of Interventional Cardiovascular Research and Clinical Trials
The Zena and Michael A. Weiner Cardiovascular Institute
Icahn School of Medicine at Mount Sinai
New York, NY, USA

Geno J. Merli, MD, MACP, FHM, FSVM
Professor of Medicine & Surgery
Senior Vice President, Associate Chief Medical Officer
Co-Director, Jefferson Vascular Center
Thomas Jefferson University Hospital
Philadelphia, PA

Stephanie L. Mick, MD
Cardiac Surgeon, Surgical Director of Transcatheter Aortic Valve Program
Cardiothoracic Surgery, Heart and Vascular Institute
Cleveland Clinic
Cleveland, OH, USA

Curtiss Moore, MD
Clinical Fellow
Residency
University of Texas Southwestern Medical Center
Dallas, Texas, USA

Ajith Nair, MD
Department of Medicine, Division of Cardiology
Baylor College of Medicine
Houston, Texas 77030

Vijay Nambi, MD PhD
Staff Cardiologist and Associate Professor of Medicine
Department of Medicine, Division of Cardiology
Michael E DeBakey Veterans Affairs Hospital and Baylor College of Medicine
Houston, Texas, USA

Heidi Nicewarner, MD, MPH
Cardiology Fellow
Section of Cardiovascular Medicine
Boston Medical Center
Boston, MA, USA

E. Magnus Ohman, MD, FRCPI, FACC
Professor of Medicine
The Kent and Siri Rawson Director, Duke Program for Advanced Coronary Disease
Vice-Chair, Department of Medicine – Development and Innovation
Associate Director, Duke Heart Center
Senior Investigator, Duke Clinical Research Institute
Department of Medicine, Division of Cardiovascular Medicine
Duke University Medical Center
Durham, NC USA

Nicolas Palaskas, MD
Cardiology Fellow
Internal Medicine/Cardiology
Baylor College of Medicine
Houston, Texas, USA

Lavannya M. Pandit, M.D.
Assistant Professor of Medicine
Department of Internal Medicine, Division of Pulmonary, Critical Care, Sleep Medicine Section
Michael E. DeBakey Veterans Affairs Medical Center
Baylor College of Medicine
Houston, Texas. USA

Niraj R. Patel, M.D.
Physician in Nuclear Medicine, Nuclear Cardiology and PET/CT Imaging
Michael E. DeBakey VA Medical Center
Assistant Professor of Radiology
Baylor College of Medicine
Houston, Texas, USA

Lawrence Phillips, MD
Director, Nuclear Cardiology
Division of Cardiology, Department of Medicine
NYU School of Medicine
New York, New York, USA

Andrew Pipe, CM, MD, LLD(Hon), DSc(Hon)
Professor, Faculty of Medicine, University of Ottawa
Chief, Division of Prevention and Rehabilitation, University of Ottawa Heart Institute
Ottawa, Ontario, Canada

Charles V. Pollack Jr., MA, MD, FACEP, FAAEM, FAHA, FESC, FCPP
Professor of Emergency Medicine and Associate Provost
Thomas Jefferson University
Philadelphia, PA USA

Mark Pollet, MD, BSE
Cardiology Fellow
Department of Cardiology
Baylor College of Medicine
Houston, TX, USA

Stuart B. Prenner, MD
Senior Fellow in Cardiovascular Diseases
Division of Cardiology, Department of Medicine
Northwestern University Feinberg School of Medicine
Chicago IL USA

Prabhakar Rajiah, MBBS, MD, FRCR
Associate Professor of Radiology, Cardiothoracic Imaging
Associate Director of Cardiac CT and MRI
UT Southwestern Medical Center
Dallas, Texas, USA

Moises Rodriguez-Manero, MD, PhD
Division of Cardiac Electrophysiology
Cardiology Department
Complejo Hospital Universitario de Santiago
IDIS (Instituto para el Desarrollo e Integración de la Salud)
CIBERCV (Centro de Investigación Biomédica en Red de Enfermedades Cardiovasculares)
Santiago de Compostela (A Coruña)
Spain

Eric E. Roselli, MD, FACS
Director of the Aorta Center
Department of Thoracic and Cardiovascular Surgery
Cleveland Clinic Heart and Vascular Institute
Cleveland, Ohio, USA

Zeenat Safdar, MD, MS
Director of Pulmonary Hypertension Care Center and Clinical Research
Acting Associate Professor, institute of academic medicine
Houston Methodist Hospital
Weill Cornell College of Medicine
Houston, Texas, USA

Catalina Sanchez-Alvarez, MD
Internal Medicine Resident
Department of Internal Medicine
Mayo Clinic Florida
Jacksonville, Florida, USA

Paul Schurmann, MD
Cardiac Electrophysiology
Department Cardiology, Section Electrophysiology
Institution affiliated Houston Methodist/ MEDVAMC
Houston, TX 77025

Nishant R. Shah, MD, MPH, MSc
Assistant Professor of Medicine
Division of Cardiology
Brown University Alpert Medical School
Assistant Professor of Health Services Policy & Practice
Brown University School of Public Health
Providence, RI, USA

Sanjiv J. Shah, MD
Professor of Medicine
Department of Medicine, Division of Cardiology
Northwestern University Feinberg School of Medicine
Chicago, IL, USA

Tina Shah, MD, FACC
Assistant Professor, Baylor College of Medicine
Michael E. DeBakey VA Medical Center
Houston, Texas, USA

Fidaa Shaib, MD, FCCP, FAASM
Associate Professor of Medicine
Department of Medicine, Division of Pulmonary, Critical Care, and Sleep Medicine
Baylor College of Medicine
Houston, Texas, USA

Mandeep S. Sidhu, MD, FACC, FAHA
ISCHEMIA Clinical Coordinating Center Faculty and Investigator
Co-Regional Leader, ISCHEMIA and ISCHEMIA CKD Trials
Associate Professor of Medicine
Assistant Dean for Medical Education and Student Research
Albany Medical College
Division of Cardiology,
Albany Medical Center
Albany, NY
Adjunct Professor of Health Care Management
Clarkson University
Schenectady, NY

Edward G. Soltesz, MD MPH
Staff Surgeon
Department of Thoracic and Cardiovascular Surgery
Cleveland Clinic Foundation
Cleveland, OH, USA

Sarah A. Spinler, PharmD, FCCP, FAHA, FASHP, AACC, BCPS-AQ Cardiology
Professor of Clinical Pharmacy
Department of Pharmacy Practice and Pharmacy Administration
Philadelphia College of Pharmacy
University of the Sciences in Philadelphia
Philadelphia, Pennsylvania, USA

Yamin Sun, MD
Department of Medicine
Baylor College of Medicine
Houston, Texas, USA

Luis A. Tamara, M.D.
Chief of Nuclear Medicine
Nuclear Cardiology and PET CT Imaging
Michael E De Bakey Veterans Administration Medical Center
Associate Professor of Radiology
Baylor College of Medicine
Houston, Texas, USA

Victor Tapson, MD, FCCP, FRCP
Professor of Medicine
Director, Center for Pulmonary Vascular Disease
Duke University Medical Center
Durham, North Carolina

Alisa Thamwiwat, MD
Medical Resident
Baylor College of Medicine
Houston, Texas, USA

Paaladinesh Thavendiranathan, MD, MSc, SM, FRCPC
Assistant Professor of Medicine
Department of Cardiology and Medical Imaging
University Health Network
University of Toronto
Toronto, Ontario
Canada

Rahul Thomas, MD
Cardiovascular Disease
UH Cleveland Medical Center
Cleveland, Ohio. USA

Kara A. Thompson, MD, FACC
Assistant Professor
Department of Cardiology
MD Anderson Cancer Center
Houston, Texas, USA

Megan Titas, MD
Fellow Cardiovascular Medicine
Boston University Medical Center
Boston, MA USA

Michael Zhen-Yu Tong, MD, MBA
Cardiac Surgeon, Surgical director of heart transplantation, Assistant Professor or Surgery
Thoracic and Cardiovascular Surgery, Heart and Vascular Institute
Cleveland Clinic
Cleveland, OH, USA

Miguel Valderrábano, MD
Associate Professor of Medicine, Weill College of Medicine, Cornell University
Adjunct Associate Professor of Medicine, Baylor College of Medicine
Director, Division of Cardiac Electrophysiology, Department of Cardiology
Houston Methodist Hospital
Houston, Texas, USA

Andrew Vekstein, BS
Medical Student
Department of Thoracic and Cardiovascular Surgery
The Cleveland Clinic Cleveland
Case Western Reserve University
School of Medicine
Cleveland, OH

Salim Virani, MD, PhD
Staff Cardiologist/ Associate Professor
Cardiology/ Cardiovascular Research
Michael E. DeBakey VA Medical Center and Baylor College of Medicine
Houston, Texas, USA

Fawad Virk, MD
Resident Physician
Department of Internal Medicine, Division of Cardiology
Henry Ford Health System
Detroit, Michigan, USA

Hercilia Von Schoettler, MD
Medical Center Hospital
Department of Cardiology
Permian Research Foundation
Odessa, Texas, USA

Aaron S. Weinberg, MD MPhil
Fellow in Pulmonary & Critical Care Medicine
Division of Pulmonary & Critical Care/Department of Medicine
Cedars-Sinai Medical Center
Los Angeles, California, USA

Ahmad Zeeshan, MD
Associate Staff Surgeon
Heart and Vascular Institute
Cleveland Clinic
Cleveland, Ohio, United States
Associate Staff Surgeon
Heart and Vascular Institute
Cleveland Clinic Florida
Weston, Florida, USA

FOREWORD

Standard textbooks in cardiology are read by residents and fellows in training to have in-depth knowledge regarding individual cardiovascular diseases. But in daily practice, one is often faced with diagnostic and therapeutic dilemma and need point of care access to knowledge for appropriate care.

Towards this end is the First South Asia edition of Cardiology Secrets edited by Levine and his colleagues. It is written by more than 100 experts in their respective fields and includes approximately 200 tables, flow diagrams and algorithms, for easier understanding and practical application. The book has 71 chapters and covers all aspects of cardiology from physical diagnosis, investigations and therapy. It covers the entire spectrum of adult cardiovascular diseases from Congenital Heart Disease, Valvular Heart Disease, Cardiomyopathies, Coronary Artery Disease, Peripheral Artery Disease and Carotid Artery Disease. It includes cardiovascular disorders secondary to systemic disease, including cardio-oncology.

The format of book is in question and answer form, easy to read, focused, concise, engaging and conforms to recommendations of Professional Bodies (ACC/AHA/ESC etc.). This book, updated in the First South Asia edition with references up to year 2016, fulfills the need of point of care knowledge as it is portable and serves need of many residents and fellows in their daily cardiology practice.

Levine and colleagues should be congratulated for bringing out focused, authentic, point of care knowledge to many aspiring physicians and cardiologists. Elsevier should be appreciated for bringing out the First South Asia edition that reaches out to many trainees in Medicine and Cardiology, to this not so affluent part of the globe.

Dayasagar Rao.V
DM (Cardiology)
FRCP (Canada), FRCP(Edinburgh)
Consultant Cardiologist
Krishna Institute of Medical Sciences,
Hyderabad, Telangana

PREFACE

This book is the first South Asia edition of *Cardiology Secrets* that I have edited and overall the 13th book that I have authored or edited. My hope again is that this book, with its unique format, will serve to educate healthcare providers in a didactic, interactive, interesting, and engaging manner on the optimal evaluation and management of patients with cardiovascular disease. For this edition, we have reorganized the layout of the book and new dedicated sections on peripheral vascular and cerebrovascular disease, venous thromboembolic disease, and the heart in specific populations and conditions. We have added new chapters on hypercoagulability states, specific valvular lesions, sleep apnea and the heart, heart disease in women, cardio-oncology, cardiac arrest, transcatheter aortic valve replacement (TAVR), carotid artery disease, and hemorrhagic stroke. And we have added scores of new figures, illustrations, and flow diagrams.

I am deeply indebted to the more than 100 national and international experts and thought leaders in cardiovascular disease who have taken time from their many academic and clinical responsibilities to contribute to the book. I am similarly indebted to Nicole DiCicco, Elsevier Content Support Manager for the book, and to Jim Merritt, Elsevier Executive Content Strategist, who first recruited me to the *Secrets* series and who I have worked closely with on all the editions of *Cardiology Secrets* that I have edited.

I hope you find this book enjoyable and educational and that it in some small way it serves to improve the care of the patients that entrust their health to us. As always, I welcome comments and suggestions from readers; my email is glevine@bcm.tmc.edu.

Glenn N. Levine, MD, FACC, FAHA

CONTENTS

II Chest Pains, Coronary Artery Disease, and Acute Coronary Syndromes

III Heart Failure and Cardiomyopathies

IV Valvular Heart Disease

TOP 100 SECRETS

These secrets are 100 of the top board alerts. They summarize the concepts, principles, and most salient details of cardiology.

1. Coronary flow reserve (the increase in coronary blood flow in response to agents that lead to microvascular dilation) begins to decrease when a coronary artery stenosis is 50% or more luminal diameter. However, basal coronary flow does not begin to decrease until the lesion is 80% to 90% luminal diameter.
2. Causes of ST segment elevation include acute myocardial infarction (MI) as a result of thrombotic occlusion of a coronary artery, Prinzmetal's angina, cocaine-induced myocardial infarction, pericarditis, left ventricular aneurysm, left bundle branch block (LBBB), left ventricular hypertrophy with repolarization abnormalities, J point elevation, and severe hyperkalemia.
3. The initial electrocardiogram (ECG) manifestation of hyperkalemia is peaked T waves. As the hyperkalemia becomes more profound, there may be loss of visible P waves, QRS widening, and ST segment elevation. The preterminal finding is a sinusoidal pattern on the ECG.
4. Normal cardiac signs and symptoms of pregnancy include hyperventilation (as a result of increased minute ventilation), peripheral edema (from volume retention and vena caval compression by the gravid uterus), dizziness/lightheadedness (from reduced SVR and vena caval compression), and palpitations (normal HR increases by 10 to 15 beats/min). Pathologic cardiac signs and symptoms of pregnancy include the following: anasarca or generalized edema and paroxysmal nocturnal dyspnea, which are not components of normal pregnancy and warrant workup syncope (possibly due to pulmonary embolism, tachy/bradyarrhythmias, pulmonary hypertension, or obstructive valvular pathology); chest pain (possibly due to aortic dissection, pulmonary embolism, angina, or myocardial infarction); and hemoptysis (possibly due to occult mitral stenosis).
5. The major risk factors for coronary artery disease (CAD) are family history of premature coronary artery disease (father, mother, brother, or sister who first developed clinical CAD at age younger than 45 to 55 for males and at age younger than 55 to 60 for females), hypercholesterolemia, hypertension, cigarette smoking, and diabetes mellitus.
6. Important causes of chest pain not related to atherosclerotic coronary artery disease include aortic dissection, pneumothorax, pulmonary embolism, pneumonia, hypertensive crisis, Printzmetal's angina, cardiac syndrome X, anomalous origin of the coronary artery, pericarditis, esophageal spasm or esophageal rupture (Boerhaave's syndrome), and shingles.
7. Other causes of elevated cardiac troponin besides acute coronary syndrome and myocardial infarction that should be considered in patients with chest pains include pulmonary embolism, aortic dissection, myopericarditis, severe aortic stenosis, and severe chronic kidney disease.
8. Prinzmetal's angina, also called *variant angina*, is an unusual cause of angina caused by coronary vasospasm. Patients with Prinzmetal's angina are typically younger and often female. Treatment is based primarily on the use of calcium channel blockers and nitrates.
9. Microvascular angina, previously called "Cardiac syndrome X," is a condition in which patients describe typical exertional anginal symptoms, yet are found on cardiac catheterization to have nondiseased, *normal* epicardial coronary arteries. In such patients, microvascular coronary artery constriction or endothelial dysfunction plays a role in leading to ischemia and angina.

10. Numerous cardiovascular medications are associated with drug-induced lupus erythematosus. Those with a definitive causative relationship include procainamide, hydralazine, diltiazem, quinidine, and methyldopa. Those with a probable causative relationship include beta-blockers, captopril, hydrochlorothiazide, amiodarone, and ticlopidine.
11. Findings that suggest a heart murmur is pathologic and requires further evaluation include the presence of symptoms, extra heart sounds, thrills, abnormal ECG or chest radiography, diminished or absent S2, holosystolic (or late systolic) murmur, any diastolic murmur, and all continuous murmurs.
12. The major categories of ischemic stroke are large vessel atherosclerosis (including embolization from carotid to cerebral arteries), small vessel vasculopathy or lacunar type, and cardioembolic. Hemorrhagic strokes are classified by their location: subcortical (associated with uncontrolled hypertension in 60% of cases) versus cortical (more concerning for underlying mass, arteriovenous malformation, or amyloidosis).
13. The mainstay therapy for cardiogenic shock after acute MI is acute reperfusion and prompt revascularization, which has been shown to substantially improve survival. Percutaneous circulatory assist devices (PCADs) have emerged as an important modality to support patients with cardiogenic shock before, during, and after revascularization.
14. Common radiographic signs of congestive heart failure include enlarged cardiac silhouette, left atrial enlargement, hilar fullness, vascular redistribution, linear interstitial opacities (Kerley's lines), bilateral alveolar infiltrates, and pleural effusions (right > left).
15. Classic ECG criteria for the diagnosis of ST-segment–elevation myocardial infarction (STEMI), warranting thrombolytic therapy, are ST segment elevation greater than 0.1 mV in at least two contiguous leads (e.g., leads III and aVF or leads V2 and V3) or new or presumably new left bundle branch block (LBBB).
16. In patients receiving anthracycline therapy for cancer, cardiac function should be reassessed before therapy and at 3, 6, and 9 months during treatment and at 12 and 18 months after initiation of treatment. If the ejection fraction decreases to less than 40%, the anthracycline should be discontinued. Lifelong cardiac monitoring of cardiac function is recommended, as the incidence of cardiac toxicity increases with length of time since treatment, with left ventricular ejection fraction (LVEF) assessment every 1 to 5 years, depending on the total dose of anthracycline administered. More frequent monitoring is recommended in patients who received radiation therapy in addition to anthracyclines.
17. The triad of findings suggestive of right ventricular infarction are hypotension, distended neck veins, and clear lungs.
18. Cessation of cerebral blood flow for as short a period as 6 to 8 seconds can precipitate syncope.
19. The most common causes of syncope in pediatric and young patients are neurocardiogenic syncope (vasovagal syncope, vasodepressor syncope), conversion reactions (psychiatric causes), and primary arrhythmic causes (e.g., long QT syndrome, Wolff–Parkinson–White syndrome). In contrast, elderly patients have a higher frequency of syncope caused by obstructions to cardiac output (e.g., aortic stenosis, pulmonary embolism) and by arrhythmias resulting from underlying heart disease.
20. Smoking cessation is the most important of the modifiable risk factors for cardiovascular disease. The products of tobacco smoke contribute directly, and distinctly, to the development of atherosclerosis and the adverse consequences that follow. A rapid and sustained reduction in the likelihood of cardiac disease or a cardiac event occurs in those who successfully stop smoking; those with established cardiac disease experience a dramatic reduction in the likelihood of recurrence, complication, or death following cessation. Optimal cessation strategies involve (1) the delivery of personally relevant, unambiguous, nonjudgmental advice regarding the fundamental importance of smoking

cessation in the management of cardiac disease and the offer of specific assistance with cessation; (2) the use of pharmacotherapy to eliminate or curb the symptoms of withdrawal and craving that lead to the use of a cigarette; and (3) the provision of strategic, tactical advice regarding the management or avoidance of those circumstances, settings, and situations that typically accompany and stimulate smoking.

21. Preexisting renal disease and diabetes are the two major risk factors for the development of contrast nephropathy. Preprocedure and postprocedure hydration are the most established methods of reducing the risk of contrast nephropathy.

22. Hypertension is the most common cardiotoxicity of targeted chemotherapeutic drugs that inhibit vascular endothelial growth factor (VEGF), with 100% of patients developing an increase in blood pressure and 25% of patients developing frank hypertension. Treatment of hypertension has not been shown to impair oncologic efficiency of VEGF. The hypertension is reversible when the VEGF inhibitor is stopped.

23. All adults aged 20 years or older should undergo fasting lipoprotein profile testing every 4 to 6 years. Testing should include fasting total cholesterol, low-density lipoprotein (LDL) cholesterol, high-density lipoprotein cholesterol (HDL-C), and triglycerides. If an individual is not fasting, then only the total cholesterol and HDL-C can be adequately interpreted.

24. Based on the 2013 ACC/AHA cholesterol guideline, the four groups in whom statin therapy should be considered are (1) individuals with clinical atherosclerotic cardiovascular disease (ASCVD; i.e., acute coronary syndromes, or a history of MI, stable or unstable angina, coronary or other arterial revascularization, stroke, transient ischemic attack, or peripheral artery disease presumed to be of atherosclerotic origin); (2) individuals with primary elevations of LDL-C defined as LDL-C ≥190 mg/dL (i.e., familial hypercholesterolemia); (3) individuals 40 to 75 years of age with diabetes with LDL-C 70 to 189 mg/dL; and (4) individuals without clinical ASCVD or diabetes who are 40 to 75 years of age with LDL-C 70 to 189 mg/dL and an estimated 10-year ASCVD risk of 7.5% or higher.

25. Important *secondary* causes of hyperlipidemia include diabetes, hypothyroidism, obstructive liver disease, chronic renal failure/nephrotic syndrome, and certain drugs (progestins, anabolic steroids, corticosteroids).

26. Components of high-quality CPR include (1) chest compressions at a rate between 100 and 120 times per minute; (2) chest compressions for adults at least 2 inches but not more than 2.4 inches (6 cm), and for children compressions of 2 inches (5 cm), and for infants compressions of 1.5 inches (4 cm); (3) allowing for complete chest recoil after each compression; (4) minimizing interruptions in chest compressions; and (5) avoiding excessive ventilation.

27. Up to 5% of all hypertension cases are *secondary*, meaning that a specific cause can be identified. Causes of secondary hypertension include renal artery stenosis, renal parenchymal disease, primary hyperaldosteronism, pheochromocytoma, Cushing's disease, hyperparathyroidism, aortic coarctation, and sleep apnea.

28. The term *hypertensive crisis* generally is inclusive of two different diagnoses, *hypertensive emergency* and *hypertensive urgency*. Distinguishing between the two is important because they require different intensities of therapy. Clinical syndromes associated with hypertensive emergency include hypertensive encephalopathy, intracerebral hemorrhage, unstable angina/acute myocardial infarction, pulmonary edema, dissecting aortic aneurysm, or eclampsia. Patients with hypertensive emergencies should be treated as inpatients in an intensive care setting, with an initial goal of reducing mean arterial blood pressure by 10% to 15%, but no more than 25%, in the first hour and then, if stable, to a goal of 160/100 to 110 mm Hg within the next 2 to 6 hours.

29. Elderly patients with acute coronary syndrome present less frequently with typical chest pain than younger patients. Symptoms indicative of acute coronary syndrome among the elderly include dyspnea, altered mental status, confusion, fatigue, and syncope. ECG changes are also more likely to be nondiagnostic.

30. Common causes of depressed left ventricular systolic dysfunction and cardiomyopathy include coronary artery disease, hypertension, valvular heart disease, and alcohol abuse. Other causes include cocaine abuse, collagen vascular disease, viral infection, myocarditis, peripartum cardiomyopathy, human immunodeficiency virus/acquired immunodeficiency disease (HIV/AIDS), tachycardia-induced, hypothyroidism, anthracycline toxicity, and Chagas' disease.

31. The classic signs and symptoms of patients with heart failure are dyspnea on exertion (DOE), orthopnea, paroxysmal nocturnal dyspnea (PND), and lower extremity edema.

32. Side effects due to amiodarone treatment are common and include organ toxicity to the lung, thyroid, and liver. Amiodarone can also cause or exacerbate sinus bradycardia. It also can cause bluish discoloration of the skin, photosensitivity, tremor, peripheral neuropathy, ocular deposits, and optic neuropathy. Monitoring of patients while on amiodarone varies by clinician but includes periodic laboratory testing for liver and thyroid dysfunction, as well as chest radiography and pulmonary function testing.

33. Patients with depressed ejection fractions (less than 40%) should be treated with agents that block the renin-angiotensin-aldosterone system, in order to improve symptoms, decrease hospitalizations, and decrease mortality. Angiotensin-converting enzyme (ACE) inhibitors are first-line therapy; alternate or additional agents include angiotensin II receptor blockers (ARBs) and aldosterone receptor blockers. In July 2015 a new agent was approved by the FDA that included a combination of a neprilysin-inhibitor, sacubitril, and an ARB, valsartan. This agent should be started in patients with NYHA class II to IV heart failure symptoms with reduced ejection fraction and who are either not already on an ACE inhibitor/ARB or in substitution for current ACE inhibitor/ARB therapy.

34. The combination of high-dose hydralazine and high-dose isosorbide dinitrate should be used in patients who cannot be given or cannot tolerate ACE inhibitors or ARBs because of renal function impairment or hyperkalemia.

35. Biventricular pacing (BiV) or cardiac resynchronization therapy (CRT) should be considered for patients in sinus rhythm with NYHA class II to IV symptoms, LVEF less than 35%, and QRS greater than 150 ms.

36. High-risk features in patients hospitalized with acute decompensated heart failure (ADHF) include low systolic blood pressure, elevated blood urea nitrogen (BUN), hyponatremia, history of prior heart failure hospitalization, elevated brain natriuretic peptide (BNP), and elevated troponin I or T.

37. Atrioventricular node reentry tachycardia (AVNRT) accounts for 65% to 70% of paroxysmal supraventricuclar tachycardias (SVTs).

38. Implantable cardioverter defibrillators (ICDs) should be considered for primary prevention of sudden cardiac death in patients whose left ventricular ejection fractions remain less than 30% to 35%, despite optimal medical therapy or revascularization, and who have good-quality life expectancy of at least 1 year.

39. Atrial fibrillation is the most common arrhythmia among the elderly, occurring in up to 9% of individuals older than 80 years of age. Symptoms are typically subtle (e.g., fatigue or generalized lack of energy) or even absent. A rate control strategy is the preferred initial therapy rather than rhythm control, due to diminished clearance of antiarrhythmic medications, resulting in a higher likelihood of adverse effects including bradyarrhythmias. Rate control is typically achieved with beta-blockers or nondihydropyridine calcium channel blockers. Caution must be taken when initiating therapy, as the elderly are more susceptible to bradycardia and orthostatic hypotension.

40. The three primary factors that promote venous thrombosis (known together as *Virchow's triad*) are (1) venous blood stasis; (2) injury to the intimal layer of the venous vasculature; and (3) abnormalities in coagulation or fibrinolysis.

41. Clinical diagnosis of heart failure with preserved ejection fraction (HFpEF) depends on the presence of signs and symptoms of HF and documentation of LVEF (≥50%). Echocardiography with Doppler examination offers a noninvasive method of evaluating diastolic function. The cornerstones of treatment of acute decompensated HFpEF are blood pressure control, volume management, and treatment of exacerbating factors. Nonpharmacologic therapy for HFpEF is the same as therapy for HFrEF, including daily home monitoring of weight, compliance with medical treatment, dietary sodium restriction (2 to 3 g sodium daily), and close medical follow-up. Clinical trials conducted on patients with HFpEF have failed to demonstrate the mortality and morbidity benefit of ACE inhibitors and angiotensin receptor blockers (ARBs) seen in trials of heart failure with reduced systolic function (HFrEF). A subgroup analysis of one trial of spironolactone suggests that this agent could be used in selected patients with HFpEF, who can also be monitored closely for changes in potassium and creatinine levels.

42. The four conditions identified as having the highest risk of adverse outcome from endocarditis for which prophylaxis with dental procedures is still recommended by the American Heart Association are prosthetic cardiac valve, previous infective endocarditis, certain cases of congenital heart disease, and cardiac transplantation recipients who develop cardiac valvulopathy.

43. Findings that should raise the suspicion for endocarditis include bacteremia/sepsis of unknown cause, fever, constitutional symptoms, hematuria/glomerulonephritis/suspected renal infarction, embolic event of unknown origin, new heart murmurs, unexplained new atrioventricular (AV) nodal conduction abnormality, multifocal or rapid changing pulmonic infiltrates, peripheral abscesses, certain cutaneous lesions (Osler nodes, Janeway lesions), and specific ophthalmic manifestations (Roth spots).

44. Transthoracic echo (TTE) has a sensitivity of 60% to 75% in the detection of native valve endocarditis. In cases where the suspicion of endocarditis is higher, a negative TTE should be followed by a transesophageal echo (TEE), which has a sensitivity of 88% to 100% and a specificity of 91% to 100% for native valves.

45. The most common cause of culture-negative endocarditis is prior use of antibiotics. Other causes include fastidious organisms (HACEK group, *Legionella*, *Chlamydia*, *Brucella*, certain fungal infections) and noninfectious causes.

46. Indications for surgery in cases of endocarditis include acute aortic insufficiency or mitral regurgitation leading to congestive heart failure, cardiac abscess formation/perivalvular extension, persistence of infection despite adequate antibiotic treatment, recurrent peripheral emboli, cerebral emboli, infection caused by microorganisms with a poor response to antibiotic treatment (e.g., fungi), prosthetic valve endocarditis (particularly if hemodynamic compromise exists), "mitral kissing infection," and large (greater than 10 mm) mobile vegetations.

47. The main echocardiographic criteria for severe mitral stenosis are mean transvalvular gradient greater than 10 mm Hg, mitral valve area less than 1 cm^2, and pulmonary artery (PA) systolic pressure greater than 50 mm Hg.

48. The symptoms associated with obstructive sleep apnea (OSA) include snoring, excessive daytime sleepiness, and sudden arousals with choking/gasping and are important clues indicative of the diagnosis. Ventricular pauses, second-degree atrioventricular (AV) block, premature ventricular contractions (PVCs), and nonsustained ventricular tachycardia occur more frequently in patients with sleep apnea. Prolonged pauses up to 15 seconds have been reported during OSA in patients in whom electrophysiological evaluation did not reveal significant intrinsic sinus or AV nodal disease. Cardiovascular sequelae of OSA include systemic hypertension, coronary artery disease, congestive heart failure, and pulmonary hypertension. OSA is a frequent cause of uncontrolled hypertension. Continuous positive airway pressure (CPAP) significantly decreases systolic and diastolic BP, more notably in those with resistant hypertension.

49. Coronary artery disease is the leading cause of death for both women and men. The term *Yentl syndrome* refers to the observed gender bias in the management of coronary heart disease. Women receive less guideline-directed management than men, including stress testing, cardiac catheterization and revascularization, antiplatelet therapy, beta-blockers, and lipid-lowering therapies. Although women derive the same treatment benefit from beta-blockers, statins, and antiplatelet therapy, they are underprescribed acute care therapies as well as treatments for secondary prevention compared to men. Women have a higher rate of death within 1 year of their first myocardial infarction (MI) and a higher rate of recurrent MI within 5 years of their first MI than men.

50. Hypertrophic cardiomyopathy (HCM) is a primary cardiac disorder characterized by myocardial hypertrophy and a nondilated left ventricle (LV) in the absence of an accountable increase in cardiac afterload (i.e., aortic stenosis or systemic hypertension). HCM is inherited as an autosomal dominant trait, and first-degree relatives of patients with HCM should be screened. Risk factors for SCD in patients with HCM include prior cardiac arrest or sustained ventricular tachycardia (VT), family history of SCD, unexplained syncope, hypotensive blood pressure response to exercise, nonsustained VT on ambulatory (Holter) monitoring, and identification of a high-risk mutant gene and massive LVH with a wall thickness 30 mm or greater. ICD is indicated for high-risk patients, defined as having two or more of the previously listed major risk factors for SCD.

51. The classic auscultatory findings in mitral valve prolapse (MVP) are a midsystolic click and late systolic murmur, although the click may actually vary somewhat within systole, depending on changes in left ventricular dimension, and there may actually be multiple clicks. The clicks are believed to result from the sudden tensing of the mitral valve apparatus as the leaflets prolapse into the left atrium during systole.

52. In patients with pericardial effusions, echocardiography findings that indicate elevated intrapericardial pressure and tamponade physiology include diastolic indentation or collapse of the right ventricle (RV), compression of the right atrium (RA) for more than one-third of the cardiac cycle, lack of inferior vena cava (IVC) collapsibility with deep inspiration, 25% or more variation in mitral or aortic Doppler flows, and 50% or greater variation of tricuspid or pulmonic valve flows with inspiration.

53. The causes of pulseless electrical activity (PEA) can be broken down to the *H*s and *T*s of PEA, which are hypovolemia, hypoxemia, hydrogen ion (acidosis), hyperkalemia/hypokalemia, hypoglycemia, hypothermia, toxins, tamponade (cardiac), tension pneumothorax, thrombosis (coronary and pulmonary), and trauma.

54. A hypercoagulable state should be suspected in patients with idiopathic thrombosis at any age, family history of venous thromboembolism, thrombosis at unusual sites (such as cerebral, hepatic, mesenteric, renal, or portal veins), recurrent unprovoked/unexplained thromboses, recurrent unexplained fetal loss, warfarin-induced skin necrosis, purpura fulminans, or recurrent superficial thrombophlebitis.

55. The common inherited hypercoagulable states are factor V Leiden and prothrombin G20210A, which are due to mutations in the genes for factor V and prothrombin. Less common inherited hypercoagulable states are due to deficiencies of the natural anticoagulant proteins antithrombin, protein C, and protein S. The antiphospholipid syndrome is the most important cause of acquired hypercoagulability. Other acquired hypercoagulable states are heparin-induced thrombocytopenia, myeloproliferative neoplasms, paroxysmal nocturnal hemoglobinuria, and cancer.

56. Hemodynamically significant atrial septal defects (ASDs) have a shunt ratio greater than 1.5, are usually 10 mm or larger in diameter, and are usually associated with right ventricular enlargement.

57. Findings suggestive of a hemodynamically significant coarctation include small diameter (less than 10 mm or less than 50% of reference normal descending aorta at the diaphragm), presence of collateral blood vessels, and a gradient across the coarctation of more than 20 to 30 mm Hg.

58. Tetralogy of Fallot (TOF) consists of four features: right ventricular outflow tract (RVOT) obstruction, a large ventricular septal defect (VSD), an overriding ascending aorta, and right ventricular hypertrophy.

59. The three *D*s of Ebstein's anomaly are an apically *displaced* tricuspid valve that is *dysplastic*, with a right ventricle that may be *dysfunctional*.

60. The CHA_2DS_2-VASc score is now used to assess the risk of stroke in patients with atrial fibrillation, replacing the CHADS2 score. Factors used to sum the score include CHF, hypertension, diabetes, CVA/TIA, vascular disease, female gender, and older age. In those with a score of 2 or greater, anticoagulation is recommended. US guidelines recommend either aspirin or anticoagulation for those with a score of 1.

61. Echocardiographic findings suggestive of severe mitral regurgitation include enlarged left atrium or left ventricle, the color Doppler mitral regurgitation jet occupying a large proportion (more than 40%) of the left atrium, a regurgitant volume 60 mL or more, a regurgitant fraction 50% or greater, a regurgitant orifice 0.40 cm^2 or greater, and a Doppler vena contracta width 0.7 cm or greater.

62. Pericardial effusions occur in up to 21% of patients with cancer. Malignancies commonly associated with pericardial effusions include lung cancer, leukemia, lymphoma, and breast cancer. Unfortunately, overall 1-year survival for patients with malignant cells in the pericardial fluid is only 12%.

63. Peripartum cardiomyopathy refers to dilated cardiomyopathy and heart failure in postpartum women, commonly presenting within 3 months of delivery. It can be difficult to recognize, since it may be masked by the symptoms of pregnancy; thus diagnosis may be missed or delayed. Risk factors include high maternal age at pregnancy, hypertension in pregnancy, multiparity, and multifetal pregnancy.

64. Active cardiac conditions for which the patient should undergo evaluation and treatment before noncardiac surgery include unstable or severe angina, recent MI, decompensated heart failure, high-grade AV block, symptomatic ventricular arrhythmias, symptomatic bradycardia, severe aortic stenosis, and severe mitral stenosis.

65. Transcatheter aortic valve replacement (TAVR), alternately known as transcatheter aortic valve implantation (TAVI), is a procedure in which a diseased aortic valve is replaced via an endovascular or transapical approach, using an expandable valve delivered with a catheter. The decision on surgical aortic valve replacement (SAVR) versus TAVR should be based upon an individual risk-benefit analysis, performed for each patient by the heart valve team.

66. Myocarditis is most commonly caused by a viral infection. Other causes include nonviral infections (bacterial, fungal, protozoal, parasitic), cardiac toxins, hypersensitivity reactions, and systemic disease (usually autoimmune). Giant cell myocarditis is an uncommon but often fulminant form of myocarditis characterized by multinucleated giant cells and myocyte destruction.

67. Initial therapy for patients with non–ST-segment elevation acute coronary syndrome (NSTE-ACS) should include antiplatelet therapy with aspirin and with clopidogrel, ticagrelor, or a glycoprotein IIb/IIIa inhibitor and antithrombin therapy with unfractionated heparin, enoxaparin, fondaparinux, or bivalirudin (depending on the clinical scenario).

68. Important complications in heart transplant recipients include infection, rejection, vasculopathy (diffuse coronary artery narrowing), arrhythmias, hypertension, renal impairment, malignancy (especially skin cancer and lymphoproliferative disorders), and osteoporosis (caused by steroid use).

69. The classic symptoms of aortic stenosis are angina, syncope, and those of heart failure (dyspnea, orthopnea, paroxysmal nocturnal dyspnea, edema, etc.). Once any of these symptoms occur, the average survival without surgical intervention is 5, 3, or 2 years, respectively.

70. Class I indications for aortic valve replacement (AVR) include (1) development of symptoms in patients with severe aortic stenosis; (2) a left ventricular ejection fraction of less than 50% in the setting of severe aortic stenosis; and (3) the presence of severe aortic stenosis in patients undergoing coronary artery bypass grafting, other heart valve surgery, or thoracic aortic surgery.

71. The major risk factors for venous thromboembolism (VTE) include previous thromboembolism, immobility, cancer and other causes of hypercoagulable state (protein C or S deficiency, factor V Leiden, antithrombin deficiency), advanced age, major surgery, trauma, and acute medical illness.

72. The Wells Score in cases of suspected pulmonary embolism includes deep vein thrombosis (DVT) symptoms and signs (3 points); pulmonary embolism (PE) as likely as or more likely than alternative diagnosis (3 points); heart rate greater than 100 beats/min (1.5 point); immobilization or surgery in previous 4 weeks (1.5 point); previous DVT or PE (1.5 point); hemoptysis (1 point); and cancer (1 point).

73. The main symptoms of aortic regurgitation (AR) are dyspnea and fatigue. Occasionally patients experience angina because reduced diastolic aortic pressure reduces coronary perfusion pressure, impairing coronary blood flow. Reduced diastolic systemic pressure may also cause syncope or presyncope.

74. The physical findings of aortic regurgitation (AR) include widened pulse pressure, a palpable dynamic left ventricular apical beat that is displaced downward and to the left, a diastolic blowing murmur heard best along the left sternal border with the patient sitting upward and leaning forward, and a low-pitched diastolic rumble heard to the left ventricular (LV) apex (*Austin Flint* murmur).

75. Class I indications for aortic valve replacement in patients with aortic regurgitation (AR) include (1) the presence of symptoms in patients with severe AR, irrespective of left ventricular systolic function; (2) chronic severe AR with left ventricular systolic dysfunction (ejection fraction 50% or less), even if asymptomatic; and (3) chronic, severe AR in patients undergoing coronary artery bypass grafting (CABG), other heart valve surgery, or thoracic aortic surgery.

76. Cardiogenic shock is a state of end-organ hypoperfusion caused by cardiac failure characterized by persistent hypotension with severe reduction in cardiac index (less than 1.8 L/min per m^2) in the presence of adequate or elevated filling pressure (left ventricular end-diastolic pressure 18 mm Hg or higher or right ventricular end-diastolic pressure 10 to 15 mm Hg or higher).

77. The rate of ischemic stroke in patients with nonvalvular atrial fibrillation (AF) is about 2 to 7 times that of persons without AF, and the risk increases dramatically as patients age. Both paroxysmal and chronic AF carry the same risk of thromboembolism.

78. The most common cause of carotid artery stenosis (CAS) is atherosclerosis. Fibromuscular dysplasia, dissection, radiation arteritis, and vasculitis are other causes of carotid artery disease. Atherosclerotic lesions frequently occur at the bifurcation of CCA into ECA and ICA and at the branch ostia. As with other cardiovascular diseases, modifiable risk factors for atherosclerotic CAS are tobacco use, diabetes mellitus, hypertension, and hyperlipidemia. Carotid revascularization options include carotid artery endarterectomy (CEA) and carotid artery stenting (CAS). Presence of cerebral ischemic symptoms, severity of stenosis, surgical or procedural risk, age, sex, life expectancy, and carotid anatomy are the factors that influence the decision regarding whether to pursue carotid revascularization or to opt for CEA or CAS. CEA is indicated in symptomatic patients who suffered stroke or TIA within the previous 6 months, have ipsilateral carotid stenosis (>70% by noninvasive imaging or >50% by catheter angiography), and have average or low surgical risk (<6% perioperative mortality or stroke risk). For these patients, CAS is a reasonable alternate option, especially if the arterial anatomy is unfavorable for CEA, if the surgical risk is high, in cases of radiation-induced stenosis, or in whom a repeat CEA is being considered. For patients without contraindications, CEA should be performed within 2 weeks of the index event.

79. The main organ systems that need to be monitored with long-term amiodarone therapy are the lungs, the liver, and the thyroid gland. A chest radiograph should be obtained every 6 to 12 months, and liver function tests (LFTs) and thyroid function tests (thyroid-stimulating hormone [TSH] and free T4) should be checked every 6 months.
80. The target international normalized ratio (INR) for warfarin therapy in most cases of cardiovascular disease is 2.5, with a range of 2.0 to 3.0. In certain patients with mechanical heart valves (e.g., older valves, mitral position), the target is 3.0, with a range of 2.5 to 3.5.
81. A bicuspid aortic valve is present in 0.5% to 1% of the population. The main complications are progressive aortic stenosis, aortic regurgitation, or a combination of both (Fig. 3). Other complications include aortopathy and endocarditis. Although infrequent (<10%), aortic coarctation is also a well-described association and must be ruled out in these patients.
82. The major complications of percutaneous coronary intervention (PCI) include periprocedural MI, acute stent thrombosis, coronary artery perforation, contrast nephropathy, access site complications (e.g., retroperitoneal bleed, pseudoaneurysm, arteriovenous fistula), stroke, and a very rare need for emergency CABG.
83. Anticoagulation improves survival in patients with acute symptomatic pulmonary embolism (PE). In patients with acute PE, a therapeutic level of anticoagulation should ideally be achieved within 24 hours, because this reduces the risk of recurrence. In stable patients, direct oral anticoagulants (DOACs; such as rivaroxaban, epixaban, and dabigatran) can now be considered as initial treatment modalities without the need for parenteral or subcutaneous therapies. Anticoagulation treatment duration depends greatly on whether the PE was provoked (by a clear transient risk factor that has now resolved) versus unprovoked (without a clear cause). Provoked PEs with transient risk factors are typically treated for 3 months but can be extended up to 6 or 12 months. Patients may qualify for indefinite therapy in the event of an unprovoked PE or the presence of ongoing risk factors such as an active malignancy, immobility, or an inherited prothrombotic condition.
84. The widely accepted hemodynamic definition of pulmonary arterial hypertension (PAH) is a mean pulmonary arterial pressure of ≥25 mm Hg. Because the earliest symptoms in patients with PH are manifest with exercise, PH can have an insidious presentation but usually includes dyspnea with exertion. With the onset of right ventricular failure, lower extremity edema or complaints of abdominal distention or early satiety secondary to venous congestion are characteristic. Angina is also common, likely reflecting demand ischemia from impaired coronary blood flow to a markedly hypertrophied right ventricle (RVH). As cardiac output becomes fixed and eventually falls, patients may have episodes of syncope or near-syncope.
85. Conventional therapy for patients with pulmonary hypertension includes supplemental oxygen as needed to maintain an oxygen saturation of at least 91%; treatment of underlying conditions, including obstructive sleep apnea, emphysema, heart failure, and autoimmune diseases; diuretics if the patient has clinically significant edema or ascites; anticoagulation in the absence of contraindications for some GROUP I and all GROUP IV patients; and pulmonary vasodilators if indicated by RHC vasoreactivity testing. Digoxin is occasionally used to improve RV function.
86. Although restrictive cardiomyopathy is a rather uncommon cause of heart failure in North America and Europe, it is a relatively common cause of heart failure and death worldwide due to a much higher incidence of endomyocardial fibrosis in tropical regions, including parts of Africa, Central and South America, India, and other parts of Asia. In the United States, the most common identifiable cause is myocardial infiltration from amyloidosis. Other infiltrative diseases include sarcoidosis, Gaucher's disease, and Hurler's disease. Storage diseases include hemochromatosis, glycogen storage disease, and Fabry's disease. Secondary restrictive physiology develops in

the advanced stages of all forms of heart disease, including dilated, hypertensive, and ischemic cardiomyopathy. One should be sure to distinguish "restrictive cardiomyopathy" from "restrictive physiology" (as may be reported in an echocardiogram report).

87. Acute pericarditis is a syndrome of pericardial inflammation characterized by typical chest pain, a pathognomonic pericardial friction rub, and specific electrocardiographic changes (PR depression, diffuse ST segment elevation).

88. General criteria for surgical intervention in cases of thoracic aortic aneurysm are, for the ascending thoracic aorta, aneurysmal diameter of 5.5 cm (5.0 cm in patients with Marfan syndrome) and for the descending thoracic aorta, aneurysmal diameter of 6.5 cm (6 cm in patients with Marfan syndrome).

89. Cardiac complications of advanced AIDS in untreated patients include myocarditis/cardiomyopathy (systolic and diastolic dysfunction), pericardial effusion/tamponade, marantic (thrombotic) or infectious endocarditis, cardiac tumors (Kaposi's sarcoma, lymphoma), and right ventricular dysfunction from pulmonary hypertension or opportunistic infections. Complications with modern antiretroviral therapy (ART) include dyslipidemias, insulin resistance, lipodystrophy, atherosclerosis, and arrhythmias.

90. The ankle-brachial index (ABI) is the ankle systolic pressure (as determined by Doppler examination) divided by the brachial systolic pressure. An abnormal index is less than 0.90. The sensitivity is approximately 90% for diagnosis of peripheral vascular disease (PVD). An ABI of 0.41 to 0.90 is interpreted as mild to moderate peripheral arterial disease; an ABI of 0.00 to 0.40 is interpreted as severe PAD.

91. Approximately 90% of cases of renal artery stenosis are due to atherosclerosis. Fibromuscular dysplasia (FMD) is the next most common cause and is often seen in women.

92. An acutely ill medical patient admitted to the hospital with congestive heart failure or severe respiratory disease, or who is confined to bed and has one or more additional risk factors, including active cancer, previous venous thromboembolism, sepsis, acute neurologic disease, or inflammatory bowel disease, should receive DVT prophylaxis with unfractionated heparin, a low-molecular-weight heparin, or fondaparinux.

93. The incidence of detected AAA in studies of older men, smokers, and those with family history of AAA is 5.5%. Screening for AAA with ultrasound examination in older (>65 years) men has been shown to decrease AAA-related mortality. In the European guidelines, screening for AAA is recommended in all men greater than 65 years of age and may be considered in women greater than 65 years of age with history of current or past smoking. In the US guidelines, screening is recommended in men ≥60 years of age who are either the siblings or offspring of patients with AAA and in men age 65 to 75 who have ever smoked.

94. Second-degree heart block is divided into two types: *Mobitz type I (Wenckebach)* exhibits progressive prolongation of the PR interval before an atrial impulse (P wave) is not conducted, whereas *Mobitz type II* exhibits no prolongation of the PR interval before an atrial impulse is not conducted.

95. Temporary or permanent pacing is indicated in the setting of acute MI, with or without symptoms, for (1) A complete third-degree block or advanced second-degree block that is associated with a blockage in the His-Purkinje system (wide complex ventricular rhythm) and (2) a transient advanced (second-degree or third-degree) AV block with a new bundle branch block.

96. Whereas the left internal mammary artery (LIMA), when anastomosed to the left anterior descending artery (LAD), has a 90% patency at 10 years, for saphenous vein grafts (SVGs), early graft stenosis or occlusion of up to 15% can occur by 1 year, with 10-year patency traditionally cited at only 50% to 60%.

97. Myocardial contusion is a common, reversible injury that is the consequence of a nonpenetrating trauma to the myocardium. It is detected by elevations of specific cardiac enzymes with no evidence of coronary occlusion and by reversible wall motion abnormalities detected by echocardiography.

98. Classical signs for cardiac tamponade include Beck's triad of (1) hypotension caused by decreased stroke volume, (2) jugulovenous distention caused by impaired venous return to the heart, and (3) muffled heart sounds caused by fluid inside the pericardial sac, as well as pulsus paradoxus and general signs of shock such as tachycardia, tachypnea, and decreasing level of consciousness.

99. The most common tumors that spread to the heart are lung (bronchogenic) cancer, breast cancer, melanoma, thyroid cancer, esophageal cancer, lymphoma, and leukemia.

100. Patients with cocaine-induced chest pain should be treated with intravenous benzodiazepines, which can have beneficial hemodynamic effects and relieve chest pain, and aspirin therapy, as well as nitrate therapy if the patient remains hypertensive. Beta-blockers (including labetolol) should not be administered in the acute setting of cocaine-induced chest pain.

I

Diagnostic Examinations and Procedures

CARDIOVASCULAR PHYSICAL EXAMINATION

Salvatore Mangione

CHAPTER 1

Editor's Note to Readers: *For an excellent and more detailed discussion of the cardiovascular physical examination, read* Physical Diagnosis Secrets, *2nd edition, by Salvatore Mangione.*

1. **What is the meaning of a slow rate of rise of the carotid arterial pulse?**
   A carotid arterial pulse that is reduced *(parvus)* and delayed *(tardus)* suggests the presence of *aortic valvular stenosis.* Occasionally this also may be accompanied by a palpable thrill. If ventricular function is good, a slower upstroke correlates with a higher transvalvular gradient. In left ventricular failure, however, parvus and tardus may occur even with mild aortic stenosis (AS).

2. **What is the significance of a brisk carotid arterial upstroke?**
   It depends on whether it is associated with *normal* or *widened* pulse pressure. If associated with *normal pulse pressure,* a brisk carotid upstroke usually indicates two conditions:
   - *Simultaneous emptying of the left ventricle into a high-pressure bed (the aorta) and a lower pressure bed*: The latter can be the right ventricle (in patients with ventricular septal defect [VSD]) or the left atrium (in patients with mitral regurgitation [MR]). Both will allow a rapid left ventricular emptying, which in turn generates a brisk arterial upstroke. The pulse pressure, however, remains normal.
   - *Hypertrophic cardiomyopathy (HCM)*: Despite its association with left ventricular obstruction, this disease is characterized by a brisk and bifid pulse, due to the hypertrophic ventricle and its delayed obstruction. An example of the carotid pulsation in HCM and other conditions is given in Fig. 1.1.

   If associated with *widened pulse pressure,* a brisk upstroke usually indicates aortic regurgitation (AR). In contrast to MR, VSD, or HCM, the AR pulse has rapid upstroke *and* collapse.

3. **In addition to aortic regurgitation, which other processes cause rapid upstroke and widened pulse pressure?**
   The most common are the hyperkinetic heart syndromes (high-output states). These include anemia, fever, exercise, thyrotoxicosis, pregnancy, cirrhosis, beriberi, Paget disease, arteriovenous fistulas, patent ductus arteriosus, AR, and anxiety—all typically associated with rapid ventricular contraction and low peripheral vascular resistance.

   Examples of the carotid pulse waveform and its correlation to heart sounds are provided in Fig. 1.2.

4. **What is pulsus paradoxus?**
   Pulsus paradoxus is an exaggerated fall in systolic blood pressure during quiet inspiration. In contrast to evaluation of arterial contour and amplitude, it is best detected in a peripheral vessel, such as the radial artery. Although palpable at times, optimal detection of the pulsus paradoxus typically requires a sphygmomanometer. Pulsus paradoxus can occur in cardiac tamponade and other conditions.

5. **What is pulsus alternans?**
   Pulsus alternans is the alternation of strong and weak arterial pulses despite *regular rate and rhythm.* First described by Ludwig Traube in 1872, pulsus alternans is often associated with alternation of strong and feeble heart sounds (auscultatory alternans). Both indicate severe left ventricular dysfunction (from ischemia, hypertension, or valvular cardiomyopathy), with worse ejection fraction and higher pulmonary capillary pressure. Hence, they are often associated with an S_3 gallop. A tracing indicating pulses alternans is given in Fig. 1.3.

6. **What is the Duroziez double murmur?**
   The *Duroziez murmur* is a to-and-fro double murmur over a large central artery—usually the femoral but also the brachial. It is elicited by applying gradual but *firm* compression with the stethoscope's

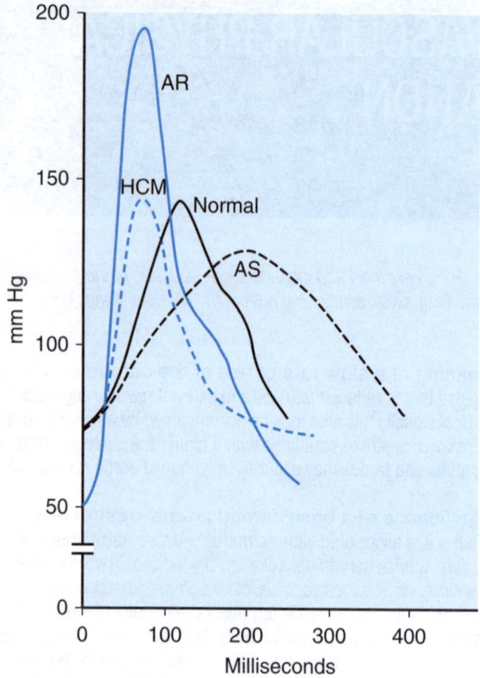

Fig. 1.1. The carotid pulsation. The waveform of the carotid pulse is characterized by the rate of rise of the carotid upstroke. In aortic regurgitation (AR), the upstroke is rapid and followed by abrupt diastolic "collapse." In hypertrophic cardiomyopathy (HCM), the upstroke is also rapid and the pulse has a jerky character. In aortic stenosis (AS), the upstroke is slow with a plateau. *(Adapted from Timmis, A. D., & Archbold, A. [2012]. Cardiovascular system. In M. Glynn & S. M. Drake [Eds.],* Hutchison's clinical methods: an integrated approach to clinical practice *[23rd ed.]. St. Louis, MO: Elsevier.)*

diaphragm. This produces not only a systolic murmur (which is normal) but also a *diastolic* one (which is pathologic and typical of AR). The Duroziez murmur has 58% to 100% sensitivity *and* specificity for AR.

7. What is the carotid shudder?

Carotid shudder is a palpable thrill felt at the peak of the carotid pulse in patients with AS, AR, or both. It represents the transmission of the murmur to the artery and is a relatively specific but rather insensitive sign of aortic valvular disease.

8. What is the Corrigan pulse?

The *Corrigan pulse* is one of the various names for the bounding and quickly collapsing pulse of AR, which is both visible *and* palpable. Other common terms for this condition include *water hammer, cannonball, collapsing,* or *pistol-shot pulse.* It is best felt for by elevating the patient's arm while at the same time feeling the radial artery at the *wrist.* Raising the arm higher than the heart reduces the intraradial diastolic pressure, collapses the vessel, and thus facilitates the palpability of the subsequent systolic thrust.

9. How do you auscultate for carotid bruits?

To auscultate for *carotid bruits,* place your bell on the patient's neck in a quiet room; the patient should be completely relaxed. Auscultate from just behind the upper end of the thyroid cartilage to immediately below the angle of the jaw.

10. What is the correlation between symptomatic carotid bruit and high-grade stenosis?

This correlation is very strong. In fact, bruits presenting with transient ischemic attacks (TIAs) or minor strokes in the anterior circulation should be evaluated aggressively for the presence of high-grade

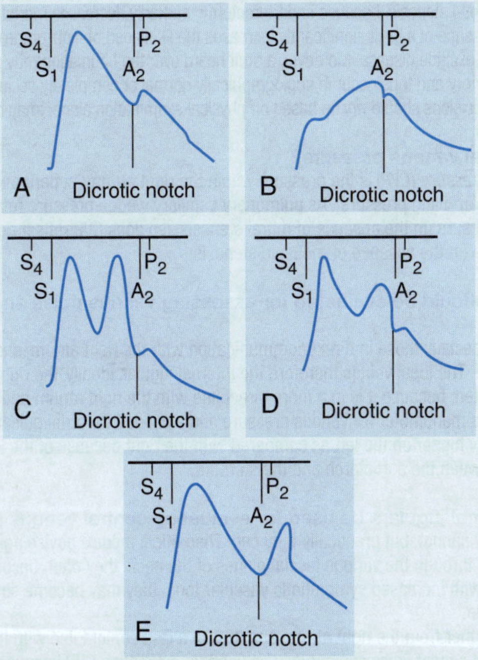

Fig. 1.2. Carotid pulse waveforms and heart sounds. **A,** Normal. **B,** Aortic stenosis: anacrotic pulse with slow upstroke and peak near S_2. **C,** Severe AR: bifid pulse with two systolic peaks. **D,** Hypertrophic obstructive cardiomyopathy (HOCM): bifid pulse with two systolic peaks. The second peak (tidal or reflected wave) is of lower amplitude than the initial percussion wave. **E,** Bifid pulse with systolic and diastolic peaks as may occur with sepsis or intra-aortic balloon counterpulsation. A_2 = aortic component of S_2; P_2 = pulmonic component of S_2. (**A-D,** *From Chatterjee, K. [1991]. Bedside evaluation of the heart: the physical examination. In K. Chatterjee & W. Parmley [Eds.]. Cardiology: an illustrated text/reference. Philadelphia, PA: JB Lippincott, pp. 3.11–3.51;* **E,** *Braunwald, E. [2003]. The clinical examination. In E. Braunwald & L. Goldman [Eds.]. Primary cardiology [2nd ed.]. Philadelphia, PA: WB Saunders, p. 36.)*

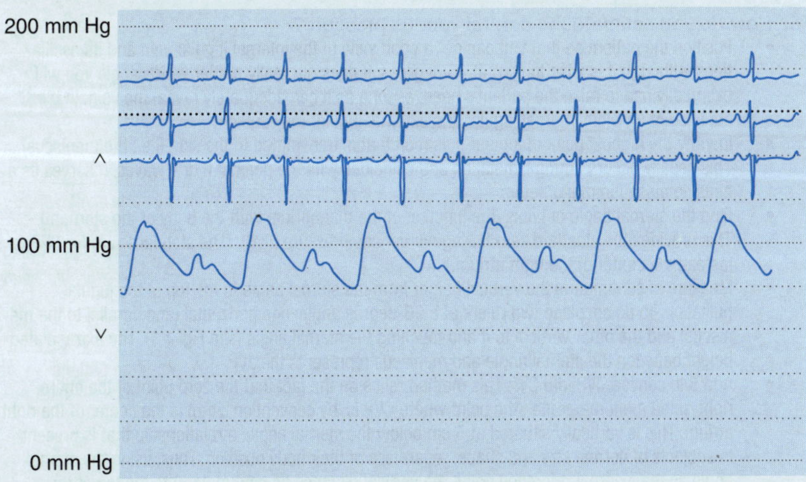

Fig. 1.3. Pulsus alternans in a patient with severe left ventricular systolic dysfunction. The systolic pressure varies from beat to beat, independent of the respiratory cycle. The rhythm is sinus throughout.

(70% to 99%) carotid stenosis, because endarterectomy markedly decreases mortality and stroke rates. Still, although presence of a bruit significantly increases the likelihood of high-grade carotid stenosis, its absence does not exclude disease. Moreover, a bruit heard over the bifurcation may reflect a narrowed *external* carotid artery and thus occur in angiographically normal or completely occluded *internal* carotids. Hence, surgical decisions should *not* be based on physical examination alone; imaging is mandatory.

11. What is central venous pressure?

Central venous pressure (CVP) is the pressure within the right atrium–superior vena cava system (i.e., the right ventricular filling pressure). As pulmonary capillary wedge pressure reflects left ventricular end-diastolic pressure (in the absence of mitral stenosis), so does CVP reflect right ventricular end-diastolic pressure (in the absence of tricuspid stenosis).

12. Which veins should be evaluated for assessing venous pulse and central venous pressure?

Central veins, especially those in direct communication with the right atrium, should be evaluated as much as possible. The ideal vein is therefore the internal jugular. Ideally, the right internal jugular vein should be inspected, because it is in a more direct line with the right atrium and thus better suited to function as both a manometer for venous pressure and a conduit for atrial pulsations. Moreover, CVP may be spuriously higher on the left as compared with the right because of the left innominate vein's compression between the aortic arch and the sternum.

13. Can the external jugulars be used for evaluating central venous pressure?

Theoretically they cannot, but practically they can. Theoretical models advise against this because:

- While going through the various fascial planes of the neck, they often become compressed.
- In patients with increased sympathetic vascular tone, they may become so constricted as to be barely visible.
- They are farther from the right atrium and thus in a less straight line with it. Yet, both internal *and* external jugular veins can actually be used for estimating CVP because they yield comparable estimates.

Hence, if the only visible vein is the external jugular, do what Yogi Berra recommends you should do when coming to a fork in the road: take it.

14. What is a cannon a wave?

A *cannon a wave* is the hallmark of atrioventricular dissociation (i.e., the atrium contracts against a closed tricuspid valve). It is different from the other prominent outward wave (i.e., the presystolic giant a wave) insofar as it begins just after S_1, because it represents atrial contraction against a closed tricuspid valve.

15. How do you estimate the central venous pressure?

- Position the patient so that you can get a good view of the internal jugular vein and its oscillations. Although it is wise to start at 45 degrees, it does not really matter which angle you will eventually use to raise the patient's head, as long as it can adequately reveal the vein. In the absence of a visible internal jugular, the external jugular may suffice.
- Identify the highest point of jugular pulsation that is transmitted to the skin (i.e., the meniscus). This usually occurs during exhalation and coincides with the peak of a or v waves. It serves as a bedside pulsation manometer.
- Find the sternal angle of Louis (the junction of the manubrium with the body of the sternum). This provides the standard zero for jugular venous pressure (JVP). (The standard zero for CVP is instead the center of the right atrium.)
- Measure in centimeters the vertical height from the sternal angle to the top of the jugular pulsation. To do so, place two rulers at a 90-degree angle: one horizontal (and parallel to the meniscus) and the other vertical to it and touching the sternal angle (see Fig. 1.1). The extrapolated height between the sternal angle and meniscus represents the JVP.
- Add 5 to convert JVP into CVP. This method relies on the fact that the zero point of the entire right-sided manometer (i.e., the point where CVP is, by convention, zero) is the center of the right atrium. This is vertically situated at 5 cm below the sternal angle, a relationship that is present in subjects of normal size and shape, regardless of their body position. Thus, using the sternal angle as the external reference point, the vertical distance (in centimeters) to the top of the column of blood in the jugular vein will provide the JVP. Adding 5 to the JVP will yield the CVP. Measurement of the JVP is illustrated in Fig. 1.4.

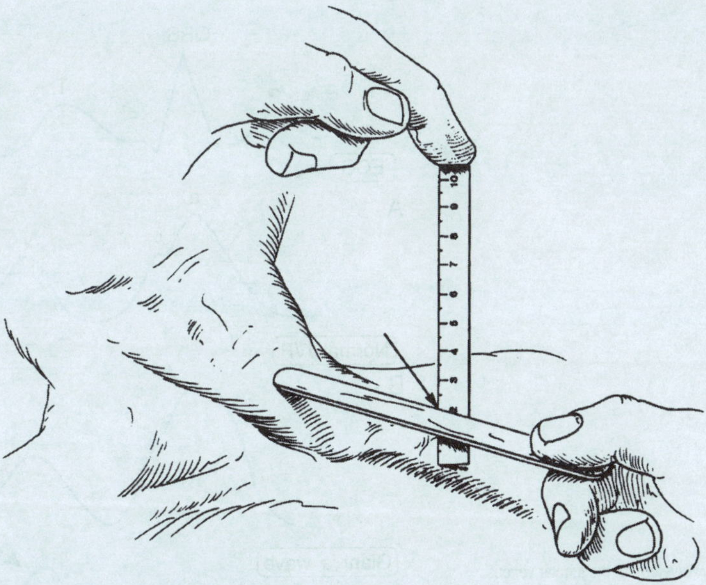

Fig. 1.4. Measurement of jugular venous pressure.

16. Can the jugular vein examination be used to diagnose cardiac pathology?

Yes. The jugular venous examination can suggest stenosed tricuspid valve, noncompliant hypertrophied right ventricle, AV dissociation (heart block, ventricular tachycardia), tricuspid regurgitation, constrictive pericarditis, and other conditions. Examples of the jugular venous examination in pathologic conditions are shown in Fig. 1.5.

17. What is the significance of leg swelling without increased central venous pressure?

It reflects either bilateral venous insufficiency or noncardiac edema (usually hepatic or renal). This is because any cardiac (or pulmonary) disease resulting in right ventricular failure would manifest itself through an increase in CVP. Leg edema *plus ascites* in the absence of increased CVP argues in favor of a hepatic or renal cause (patients with cirrhosis *do not* have high CVP). Conversely, a high CVP in patients with ascites and edema suggests the presence of an underlying cardiac etiology.

18. What is the Kussmaul sign?

The *Kussmaul sign* (Fig. 1.6) is the paradoxical increase in JVP that occurs during inspiration. JVP normally *decreases* during inspiration because the inspiratory fall in intrathoracic pressure creates a "sucking effect" on venous return. Thus, the Kussmaul sign is a true physiologic paradox. This can be explained by the inability of the right side of the heart to handle an increased venous return.

Disease processes associated with a positive Kussmaul sign are those that interfere with venous return and right ventricular filling. The original description was in a patient with constrictive pericarditis. (The Kussmaul sign is still seen in one-third of patients with severe and advanced cases, in whom it is often associated with a positive abdominojugular reflux.) Nowadays, however, the most common cause is severe heart failure, independent of etiology. Other causes include cor pulmonale (acute or chronic), constrictive pericarditis, restrictive cardiomyopathy (such as sarcoidosis, hemochromatosis, and amyloidosis), tricuspid stenosis, and right ventricular infarction.

19. What is the "venous hum"?

Venous hum is a *functional* murmur produced by turbulent flow in the internal jugular vein. It is *continuous* (albeit louder in diastole) and at times strong enough to be associated with a palpable thrill. It is best heard on the right side of the neck, just above the clavicle, but sometimes it can become audible over the sternal and/or parasternal areas, both right and left. This may lead to

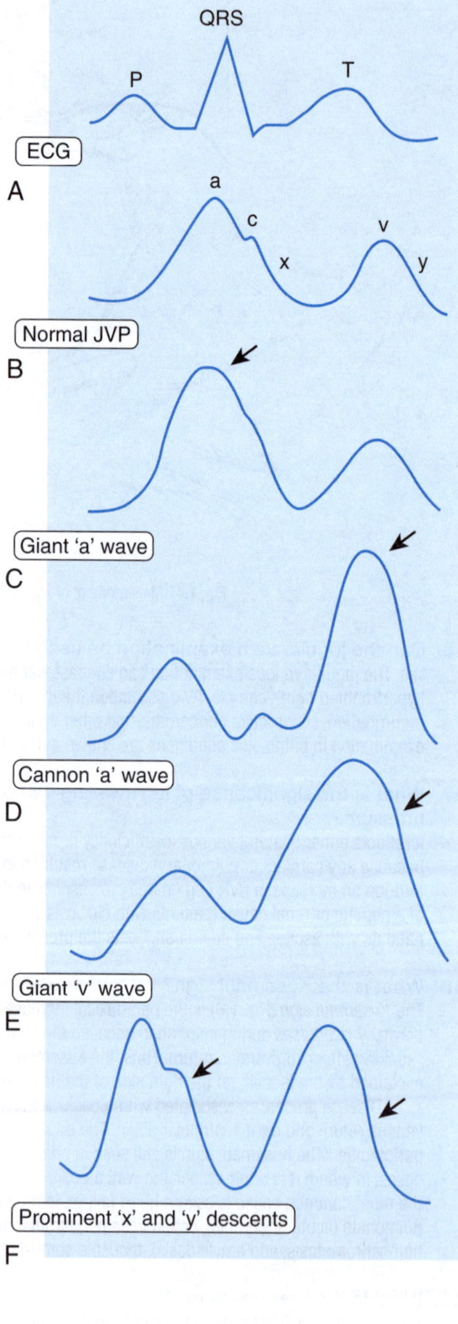

Fig. 1.5. Waveform of the jugular venous pulse. **A,** The ECG is portrayed at the top of the illustration. Note how electrical events precede mechanical events in the cardiac cycle. Thus the P wave (atrial depolarization) and the QRS complex (ventricular depolarization) precede the a and v waves, respectively, of the JVP. **B,** Normal JVP. The a wave produced by atrial systole is the most prominent deflection. It is followed by the *x* descent, interrupted by the small c wave marking tricuspid valve closure. Atrial pressure then rises again (v wave) as the atrium fills passively during ventricular systole. The decline in atrial pressure as the tricuspid valve opens precedes the *y* descent. **C,** Giant a wave. Forceful atrial contraction against a stenosed tricuspid valve or a noncompliant hypertrophied right ventricle produces an unusually prominent a wave. **D,** Cannon a wave. This is caused by an atrial systole against a closed tricuspid valve. It occurs when atrial and ventricular rhythms are dissociated (complete heart block, ventricular tachycardia) and marks coincident atrial and ventricular systole. **E,** Giant v wave. This is an important sign of tricuspid regurgitation. The regurgitant jet produces pulsatile systolic waves in the JVP. **F,** Prominent *x* and *y* descents. These occur in the constructive pericarditis and give the JVP an unusually dynamic appearance. In tamponade, only *x* descent is unusually exaggerated. *(From Glynn, M., & Drake, S. M. [2012].* Hutchison's clinical methods: an integrated approach to clinical practice *[23rd ed.]. St. Louis, MO: Elsevier.)*

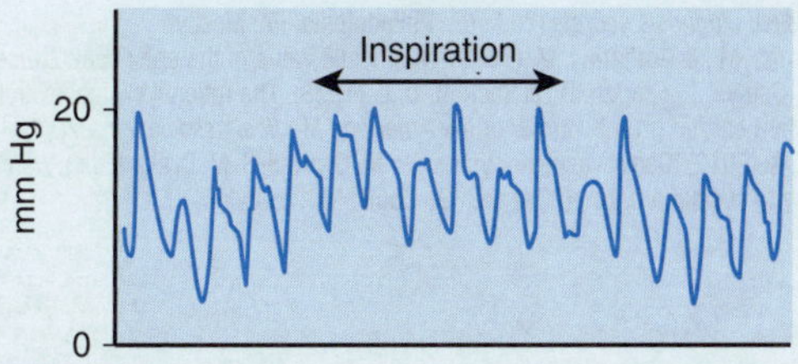

Fig. 1.6. Kussmaul sign. *(From Glynn, M., & Drake, S. M. [2012].* Hutchison's clinical methods: an integrated approach to clinical practice *[23rd ed.]. St. Louis, MO: Elsevier.)*

misdiagnoses of carotid disease, patent ductus arteriosus, AR, or AS. The mechanism of the venous hum is a mild compression of the internal jugular vein by the transverse process of the atlas in subjects with strong cardiac output and increased venous flow; hence it is common in young adults or patients with a high-output state. A venous hum can be heard in 31% to 66% of normal children and 25% of young adults. It also is encountered in 2.3% to 27% of adult outpatients. It is especially common in situations of arteriovenous fistula, being present in 56% to 88% of patients undergoing dialysis and 34% of those *between* sessions.

20. Which characteristics of the apical impulse should be analyzed?

- *Location*: Apical impulse normally occurs over the fifth left interspace midclavicular line, which usually (but not always) corresponds to the area just below the nipple. *Volume loads* to the left ventricle (such as aortic or MR) tend to displace the apical impulse downward and laterally. Conversely, *pressure loads* (such as AS or hypertension) tend to displace the impulse more upward and medially—at least initially. Still, a failing and decompensated ventricle, independent of its etiology, will typically present with a downward and lateral shift in point of maximal impulse (PMI). Although not too sensitive, this finding is very specific for cardiomegaly, low ejection fraction, and high pulmonary capillary wedge pressure. Correlation of the PMI with anatomic landmarks (such as the left anterior axillary line) can be used to better characterize the displaced impulse.
- *Size*: As measured in left lateral decubitus, the normal apical impulse is the size of a dime. Anything larger (a nickel or a quarter) should be considered pathologic. A diameter greater than 4 cm is quite specific for cardiomegaly.
- *Duration and timing*: This is probably one of the most important characteristics. A normal apical duration is brief and never passes midsystole. Thus, a *sustained impulse* (i.e., one that continues into S_2 and beyond—often referred to as a "heave") should be considered pathologic until proven otherwise and is usually indicative of pressure load, volume load, or cardiomyopathy.
- *Amplitude*: This is not the length of the impulse but its *force.* A *hyperdynamic* impulse (often referred to as a "thrust") that is forceful enough to lift the examiner's finger can be encountered in situations of volume overload and increased output (such as AR and VSD) but may also be felt in normal subjects with very thin chests. Similarly, a *hypodynamic* impulse can be due to simple obesity but also to congestive cardiomyopathy. In addition to being hypodynamic, the precordial impulse of these patients is large, somewhat sustained, and displaced downward and/or laterally.
- *Contour*: A normal apical impulse is single. Double or triple impulses are clearly pathologic.

Hence, a normal apical impulse consists of a single, dime-sized, brief (barely beyond S_1), early systolic, and nonsustained impulse, localized over the fifth interspace midclavicular line.

21. What is a thrill?

A *thrill* is a palpable vibration associated with an audible murmur. It automatically qualifies the murmur as being more than 4/6 in intensity and thus pathologic.

Bibliography and Suggested Readings

Davison, R., & Cannon, R. (1974). Estimation of central venous pressure by examination of the jugular veins. *American Heart Journal, 87*, 279–282.

Ellen, S. D., Crawford, M. H., & O'Rourke, R. A. (1983). Accuracy of precordial palpation for detecting increased left ventricular volume. *Annals of Internal Medicine, 99*, 628–630.

Mangione, S. (2008). *Physical diagnosis secrets* (2nd ed.). Philadelphia, PA: Mosby.
O'Neill, T. W., Barry, M., Smith, M., & Graham, I. M. (1989). Diagnostic value of the apex beat. *Lancet, 1*, 410–411.
Sauvé, J. S., Laupacis, A., Ostbye, T., Feagan, B., & Sackett, D. L. (1993). The rational clinical examination. Does this patient have a clinically important carotid bruit? *Journal of the American Medical Association, 270*, 2843–2845.
Timmis, A. D., & Archbold, A. (2012). Cardiovascular system. In M. Glynn & S. M. Drake (Eds.), *Hutchison's clinical methods: an integrated approach to clinical practice* (23rd ed.). St. Louis, MO: Elsevier.

CHAPTER 2

HEART MURMURS AND SOUNDS

*Salvatore Mangione**

1. **What are the auscultatory areas of murmurs?**
Auscultation typically starts in the aortic area, continuing in clockwise fashion: first over the pulmonic, then the mitral (or apical), and finally the tricuspid areas (Fig. 2.1). Because murmurs may radiate widely, they often become audible in areas outside those historically assigned to them. Hence, "inching" the stethoscope (i.e., slowly dragging it from site to site) can be the best way to avoid missing important findings. The typical sequence of auscultation of the heart is illustrated in Fig. 2.2.

2. **What is the Levine system for grading the intensity of murmurs?**
The intensity or loudness of a murmur is traditionally graded by the Levine system (no relation to this book's editor) from 1/6 to 6/6. Everything else being equal, increased intensity usually reflects increased flow turbulence. Thus, a louder murmur is more likely to be pathologic and severe. The grading system is summarized in Table 2.1.

3. **What are the causes of a systolic murmur?**
   - **Ejection:** Increased "forward" flow over the aortic or pulmonic valve. This can be
     - **Physiologic:** Normal valve but flow high enough to cause turbulence (anemia, exercise, fever, and other hyperkinetic heart syndromes)
     - **Pathologic:** Abnormal valve with or without outflow obstruction (i.e., aortic stenosis [AS] vs. aortic sclerosis)

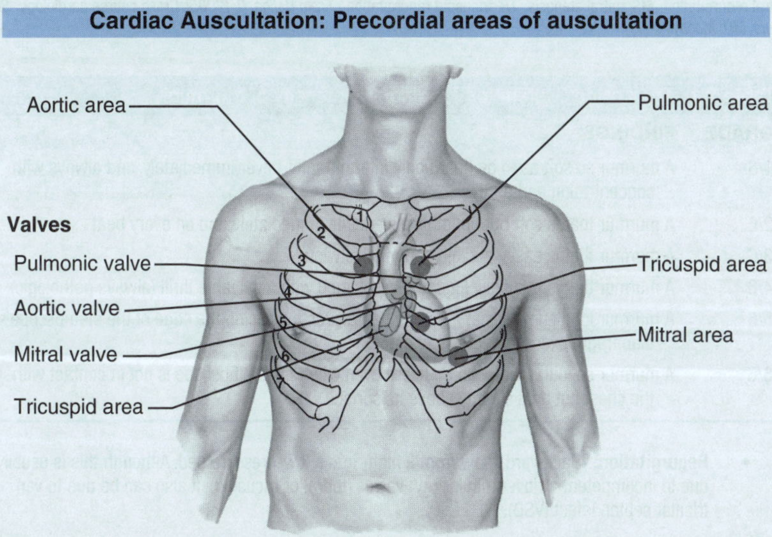

Fig. 2.1. Auscultation for heart murmurs. Illustrated are the areas of the chest where heart murmurs for specific valves are most commonly auscultated. *(Image from Runge, M. S., Ohman, E. M., & Stouffer, G. A. [2010]. The history and physical examination. In M. S. Runge, G. A. Stouffer, & C. Patterson [Eds.],* Netter's cardiology *[2nd ed.]. London: Elsevier.)*

*Editor's Note to Readers: *For an excellent and more detailed discussion of heart murmurs, read* Physical Diagnosis Secrets, *ed 2, by Salvatore Mangione.*)

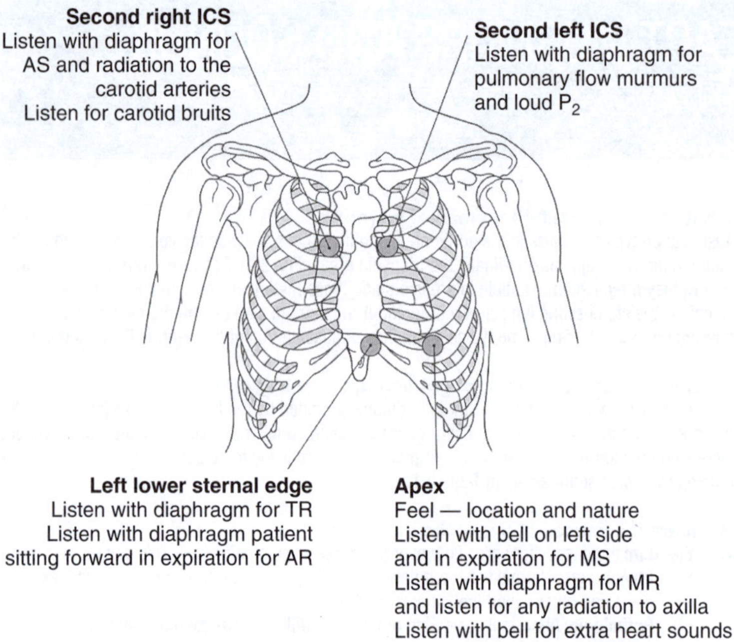

Fig. 2.2. Sequence of auscultation of the heart. *AR,* Aortic regurgitation; *AS,* aortic stenosis; *ICS,* intercostal space; *MR,* mitral regurgitation; *MS,* mitral stenosis; *TR,* tricuspid regurgitation. *(From Baliga, R. [2005].* Crash course cardiology. *St. Louis, MO: Mosby.)*

Table 2.1. The Levine System for Grading the Intensity of Murmurs

GRADE	FINDINGS
1/6	A murmur so soft as to be heard only intermittently, never immediately, and always with concentration and effort
2/6	A murmur that is soft but nonetheless audible immediately and on every beat
3/6	A murmur that is easily audible and relatively loud
4/6	A murmur that is relatively loud and associated with a palpable thrill (always pathologic)
5/6	A murmur loud enough that it can be heard even by placing the edge of the stethoscope's diaphragm over the patient's chest
6/6	A murmur so loud that it can be heard even when the stethoscope is not in contact with the chest but held slightly above its surface

- **Regurgitation:** "Backward" flow from a high- into a low-pressure bed. Although this is usually due to incompetent atrioventricular (AV) valves (mitral or tricuspid), it also can be due to ventricular septal defect (VSD).

4. What are common causes of systolic, diastolic, and continuous murmurs?

- Common causes of systolic murmurs include mitral regurgitation (MR), AS, tricuspid regurgitation, hypertrophic cardiomyopathy (HCM), VSD, and "functional" murmurs.
- Causes of diastolic murmurs include aortic regurgitation (AR), pulmonic regurgitation, mitral stenosis (MS), and tricuspid stenosis.
- Continuous murmurs can be caused by patent ductus arteriosus (PDA), coronary arteriovenous (AV) fistula, ruptured sinus of Valsalva aneurysm, and other etiologies.

Causes of systolic, diastolic, and continuous murmurs are given in Table 2.2.

Table 2.2. Principal Causes of Heart Murmurs

Systolic Murmurs

Early Systolic
- Mitral—acute MR
- VSD
  - Muscular
  - Nonrestrictive with pulmonary hypertension
- Tricuspid—TR with normal pulmonary artery pressure

Midsystolic
- Aortic
  - Obstructive
    - Supravalvular—supravalvular aortic stenosis, coarctation of the aorta
    - Valvular—aortic stenosis and sclerosis
    - Subvalvular—discrete, tunnel, or hypertrophic cardiomyopathy (HCM)
  - Increased flow, hyperkinetic states, AR, complete heart block
  - Dilation of ascending aorta, atheroma, aortitis
- Pulmonary
  - Obstructive
    - Supravalvular—pulmonary artery stenosis
    - Valvular—pulmonic valve stenosis
    - Subvalvular—infundibular stenosis (dynamic)
  - Increased flow, hyperkinetic states, left-to-right shunt (e.g., ASD)
  - Dilation of pulmonary artery

Late Systolic
- Mitral—MVP, acute myocardial ischemia
- Tricuspid—tricuspid valve prolapsed

Holosystolic
- Atrioventricular valve regurgitation (MR, TR)
- Left-to-right shunt at ventricular level (VSD)

Diastolic Murmurs

Early Diastolic
- Aortic regurgitation
  - Valvular—congenital (bicuspid valve), rheumatic deformity, endocarditis, prolapse, trauma, postvalvulotomy
  - Dilation of valve annulus—aortic dissection, annuloaortic ectasia, cystic medial degeneration, hypertension, ankylosing spondylitis
  - Widening of commissures—syphilis
- Pulmonic regurgitation
  - Valvular—postvalvulotomy, endocarditis, rheumatic fever, carcinoid
  - Dilation of valve annulus—pulmonary hypertension, Marfan syndrome
  - Congenital—isolated or associated with tetralogy of Fallot, VSD, pulmonic stenosis

Middiastolic
- Mitral
  - MS
  - Carey Coombs murmur (middiastolic apical murmur in acute rheumatic fever)
  - Increased flow across nonstenotic mitral valve (e.g., MR, VSD, PDA, high-output states, complete heart block)
- Tricuspid
  - Tricuspid stenosis
  - Increased flow across nonstenotic tricuspid valve (e.g., TR, ASD, anomalous pulmonary venous return)
- Left and right atrial tumors (myxoma)
- Severe or eccentric AR (Austin Flint murmur)

Continued on following page

Table 2.2. Principal Causes of Heart Murmurs *(Continued)*

Late Diastolic
• Presystolic accentuation of MS murmur
• Austin Flint murmur of severe or eccentric AR
Continuous Murmurs
• PDA
• AV fistula
• Ruptured sinus of Valsalva aneurysm
• Aortic septal defect
• Cervical venous hum
• Anomalous left coronary artery
• Proximal coronary artery stenosis
• Mammary souffle of pregnancy
• Pulmonary artery branch stenosis
• Bronchial collateral circulation
• Small (restrictive) ASD with MS
• Intercostal arteriovenous fistula

AR, Aortic regurgitation; *ASD*, atrial septal defect; *AV*, arteriovenous; *MS*, mitral stenosis; *MR*, mitral regurgitation; *MVP*, mitral valve prolapse; *PDA*, patent ductus arteriosus; *TR*, tricuspid regurgitation; *VSD*, ventricular septal defect.

From Braunwald, E., & Perloff, J. K. (2005). Physical examination of the heart and circulation. In D. P. Zipes, P. Libby, R. O. Bonow, & E. Braunwald (Eds.), Braunwald's heart disease: a textbook of cardiovascular medicine *(7th ed., pp. 77–106). Philadelphia, PA: Saunders; Norton, P. J., & O'Rourke, R. A. (2003). Approach to the patient with a heart murmur. In E. Braunwald & L. Goldman (Eds.),* Primary cardiology *(2nd ed., pp. 151–168). Philadelphia, PA: Elsevier.*

5. What are functional murmurs?

They are benign findings caused by turbulent ejection into the great vessels. Functional murmurs have no clinical relevance other than getting into the differential diagnosis of a systolic murmur.

6. What is the most common systolic ejection murmur of the elderly?

The murmur of aortic sclerosis is common in the elderly. This early-peaking systolic murmur is extremely age-related, affecting 21% to 26% of persons 65 years of age and 55% to 75% of octogenarians. (Conversely, the prevalence of AS in these age groups is 2% and 2.6%, respectively.) The murmur of aortic sclerosis may be due to either a degenerative change of the aortic valve or abnormalities of the aortic root. Senile degeneration of the aortic valve includes thickening, fibrosis, and occasionally calcification. This can stiffen the valve and yet not cause a transvalvular pressure gradient. In fact, commissural fusion is typically absent in aortic sclerosis. Abnormalities of the aortic root may be diffuse (such as a tortuous and dilated aorta) or localized (like a calcific spur or an atherosclerotic plaque that protrudes into the lumen, creating a turbulent bloodstream).

7. How can physical examination help differentiate functional from pathologic murmurs?

There are two golden and three silver rules, as follows:

- The first golden rule is to always judge (systolic) murmurs like people—by the company they keep. Hence murmurs that keep bad company (like symptoms; extra sounds; thrill; and abnormal arterial or venous pulse or abnormal electrocardiogram/chest radiograph) should be considered pathologic until proven otherwise. These murmurs should receive extensive evaluation, including technology-based assessment.
- The second golden rule is that a diminished or absent S_2 usually indicates a poorly moving and abnormal semilunar (aortic or pulmonic) valve. This is the hallmark of pathology. On the flip side, functional systolic murmurs are always accompanied by a well-preserved S_2, with normal split.

  The three silver rules are these:
- All holosystolic (or late systolic) murmurs are pathologic.
- All diastolic murmurs are pathologic.
- All continuous murmurs are pathologic.

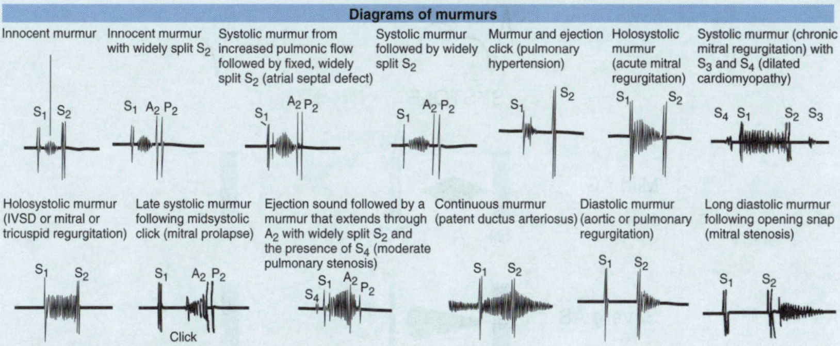

Fig. 2.3. Innocent (functional) and pathologic murmurs. Interventricular septal defect (IVSD). *(Image from Runge, M. S., Ohman, E. M., & Stouffer, G. A. [2010]. The history and physical examination. In M. S. Runge, G. A. Stouffer, & C. Patterson [Eds.],* Netter's cardiology *[2nd ed.]. London: Elsevier.)*

Thus functional murmurs should be systolic, short, soft (typically less than 3/6), early peaking (never passing midsystole), predominantly circumscribed to the base, and associated with a well-preserved and normally split-second sound. They should be part of an otherwise normal cardiovascular examination and often disappear with sitting, standing, or straining (as, e.g., following a Valsalva maneuver).

Fig. 2.3 diagrams innocent (functional) and pathologic heart murmurs.

8. How much reduction in valvular area is necessary for the aortic stenosis murmur to become audible?

Valvular area must be reduced by at least 50% (the minimum for creating a pressure gradient at rest) for the AS murmur to become audible. Mild disease may produce loud murmurs too, but usually significant hemodynamic compromise (along with symptoms) does not occur until there is a 60% to 70% reduction in the valvular area. This means that early to mild AS may be subtle at rest. Exercise, however, may intensify the murmur by increasing the output and gradient.

9. What factors may suggest severe aortic stenosis?

Factors that may suggest severe AS include

- Murmur intensity and timing (the louder and later peaking the murmur, the worse the disease)
- A single S_2
- Delayed upstroke and reduced amplitude of the carotid pulse (pulsus tardus et parvus)

Fig. 2.4 illustrates the auscultatory findings in mild and severe AS.

10. What is a thrill?

It is a palpable vibratory sensation, often compared with the purring of a cat, and typical of murmurs caused by very high pressure gradients. These, in turn, lead to great turbulence and loudness. Hence thrills are present only in pathologic murmurs whose intensity is greater than 4/6.

11. What is isometric hand grip, and what does it do to aortic stenosis and mitral regurgitation murmurs?

Isometric hand grip is carried out by asking the patient to lock the cupped fingers of both hands into a grip and then trying to pull them apart. The resulting increase in peripheral vascular resistance intensifies MR (and VSD), whereas it softens AS (and aortic sclerosis). Hence a louder murmur with hand grip argues strongly in favor of MR.

12. What is the Gallavardin phenomenon?

The Gallavardin phenomenon is noticed in some patients with AS who may exhibit a dissociation of their systolic murmur into two components:

- A typical AS-like murmur (medium- to low-pitched, harsh, right parasternal, typically radiated to the neck, and caused by high-velocity jets into the ascending aorta)

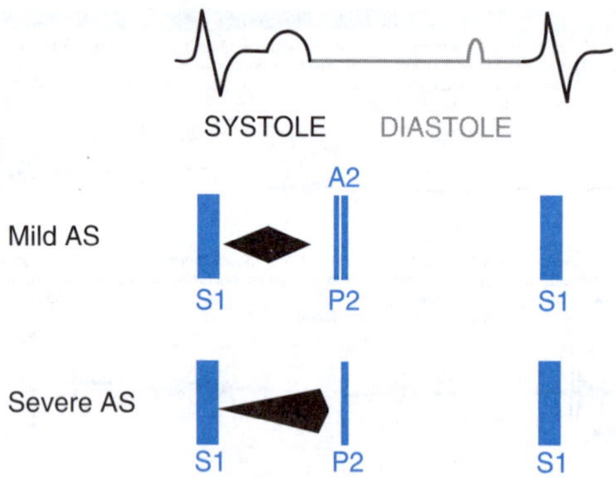

Fig. 2.4. The auscultatory findings for a patient with mild *(upper panel)* and severe *(lower panel)* AS are shown. As the disease severity worsens, the systolic ejection murmur peaks progressively later in systole and the A2 component of the second heart sound is often lost. *AS,* Aortic stenosis. *(Image adapted from Ursula, P., & Wolfgang, D. [2011]. Asymptomatic aortic stenosis—prognosis, risk stratification and follow-up. In M. Hirota [Ed.],* Aortic stenosis—etiology, pathophysiology and treatment. *Croatia: InTech. <http://Intechweb.org>.)*

- A murmur that instead mimics MR (high-pitched, musical, and best heard at the apex)

This phenomenon reflects the different transmission of AS: its medium frequencies to the base and its higher frequencies to the apex. The latter may become so prominent as to be misinterpreted as a separate apical "cooing" of MR.

13. Where is the murmur of hypertrophic cardiomyopathy best heard?

It depends. When septal hypertrophy obstructs not only left but also right ventricular outflow, the murmur may be louder at the left lower sternal border. More commonly, however, the HCM murmur is louder at the apex. This can often cause a differential diagnosis dilemma with the murmur of MR.

14. What are the characteristics of a ventricular septal defect murmur?

VSD murmurs may be holosystolic, crescendo-decrescendo, crescendo, or decrescendo. A crescendo-decrescendo murmur usually indicates a defect in the muscular part of the septum. Ventricular contraction closes the hole toward the end of systole, thus causing the decrescendo phase of the murmur. Conversely, a defect in the membranous septum will enjoy no systolic reduction in flow and thus produce a murmur that remains constant and holosystolic. VSD murmurs are best heard along the left lower sternal border, often radiating left to right across the chest. VSD murmurs always start immediately after S_1.

15. What is a systolic regurgitant murmur?

One characterized by a pressure gradient that causes a retrograde blood flow across an abnormal opening. This can be (1) a VSD, (2) an incompetent mitral valve, (3) an incompetent tricuspid valve, or (4) a fistulous communication between a high-pressure and a low-pressure vascular bed (such as a PDA).

16. What are the auscultatory characteristics of systolic regurgitant murmurs?

They tend to start immediately after S_1, often extending into S_2. They also may have a musical quality, variously described as a "honk" or "whoop." This is usually caused by vibrating vegetations (endocarditis) or chordae tendineae (mitral valve prolapse [MVP], dilated cardiomyopathy) and may help to separate the more musical murmurs of AV valve regurgitation from the harsher sounds of semilunar stenosis. Note that in contrast to systolic ejection murmurs like AS or VSD, systolic regurgitant murmurs do not increase in intensity after a long diastole.

17. What are the characteristics of the mitral regurgitation murmur?

It is loudest at the apex, radiated to the left axilla or interscapular area, high-pitched, plateau, and extending all the way into S_2 (holosystolic). S_2 is normal in intensity but often widely split. If the gradient is high (and the flow is low), the MR murmur is high-pitched. Conversely, if the gradient is low (and the flow is high), the murmur is low-pitched. In general the louder (and longer) the MR murmur, the worse the regurgitation.

18. What are the characteristics of the acute mitral regurgitation murmur?
The acute MR murmur tends to be very short and even absent, because the left atrium and ventricle often behave like a common chamber, with no pressure gradient between them. Hence, in contrast to that of chronic MR (which is either holosystolic or late systolic), the acute MR murmur is often early systolic (exclusively so in 40% of cases) and is associated with an S_4 in 80% of the patients.

19. What are the characteristics of the mitral valve prolapse murmur?
It is an MR murmur—hence loudest at the apex, mid- to late-systolic in onset (immediately following the click), and usually extending all the way into the second sound (A_2). In fact, it often has a crescendo shape that peaks at S_2. It is usually not too loud (never greater than 3/6), with some musical features that have been variously described as whoops or honks (as in the honking of a goose). Indeed, musical murmurs of this kind are almost always due to MVP.

20. How are diastolic murmurs classified?
Diastolic murmurs are classified by their timing. Hence the most important division is between murmurs that start just after S_2 (i.e., early diastolic—reflecting aortic or pulmonic regurgitation) versus those that start a little later (i.e., mid- to late-diastolic, often with a presystolic accentuation—reflecting mitral or tricuspid valve stenosis).

21. What is the best strategy to detect the mitral stenosis murmur?
The best strategy consists of listening over the apex, with the patient in the left lateral decubitus position, at the end of exhalation, and after a short period of exercise. Finally, applying the bell with very light pressure also may help. (Strong pressure will instead completely eliminate the low frequencies of MS.)

22. What are the typical auscultatory findings of aortic regurgitation?
Depending on severity, there may be up to three murmurs (one in systole and two in diastole) plus an ejection click. Of course the typical auscultatory finding is the diastolic tapering murmur, which, together with the brisk pulse and the enlarged and/or displaced point of maximal impulse (PMI), constitutes the bedside diagnostic triad of AR. The diastolic tapering murmur is usually best heard over the Erb point (third or fourth interspace, left parasternal line) but at times also over the aortic area, especially when a tortuous and dilated root pushes the ascending aorta anteriorly and to the right. The decrescendo diastolic murmur of AR is best heard by having the patient sit up and lean forward while holding his or her breath in exhalation. Using the diaphragm and pressing hard on the stethoscope also may help because this murmur is rich in high frequencies. Finally, increasing peripheral vascular resistances (by having the patient squat) will also intensify the murmur. A typical, characteristic early diastolic murmur argues very strongly in favor of the diagnosis of AR.

An accompanying systolic murmur may be due to concomitant AS but most commonly indicates severe regurgitation, followed by an increased systolic flow across the valve. Hence this accompanying systolic murmur is often referred to as *comitans* (Latin for "companion"). It provides an important clue to the severity of regurgitation. A second diastolic murmur can be due to the rumbling diastolic murmur of Austin Flint (i.e., functional MS). The Austin Flint murmur is an MS-like diastolic rumble, best heard at the apex, and results from the regurgitant aortic stream, which prevents full opening of the anterior mitral leaflet.

Auscultatory findings in regurgitant and stenotic cardiac valvular lesions are summarized in Fig. 2.5.

23. What is a mammary souffle?
A mammary souffle is not a fancy French dish but a systolic-diastolic murmur heard over one or both breasts in late pregnancy and typically disappearing at the end of lactation. It is caused by increased flow along the mammary arteries, which explains why its systolic component starts just a little after S_1. It can be obliterated by pressing (with finger or stethoscope) over the area of maximal intensity.

24. Which murmurs require further evaluation?
As discussed in this chapter, factors of a murmur that determine whether further evaluation with echocardiography or other procedures is indicated include grade, timing of the systolic murmur, any continuous murmur, other physical findings (such as carotid upstroke), presence of symptoms, or other signs of cardiac disease. A strategy for determining if a murmur requires further evaluation is given in Fig. 2.6. Indications for echocardiography in evaluating a murmur is are listed in Table 2.3.

Phonocardiogram (inspiration unless noted) | **Description**

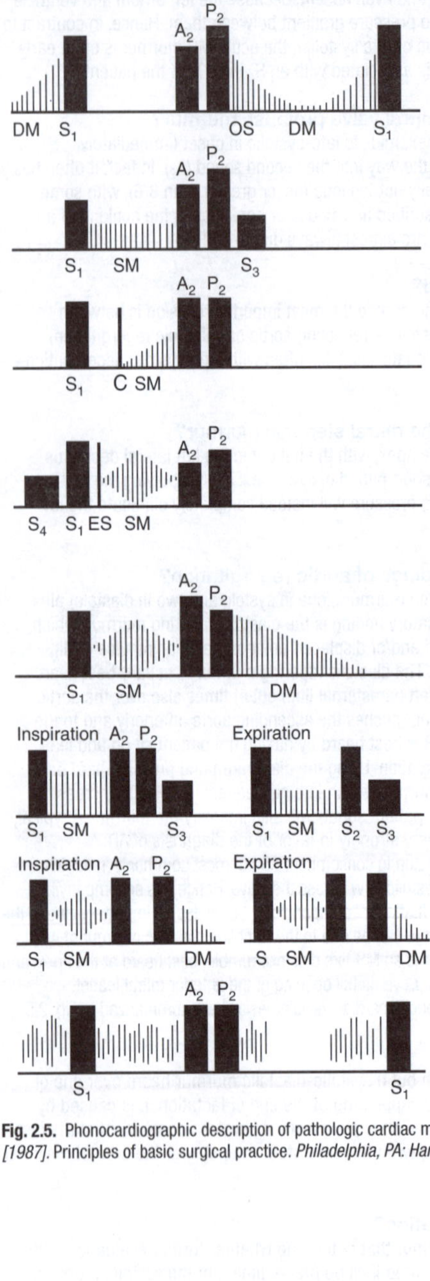

Mitral Stenosis

Precordium—Tapping apex beat; diastolic thrill at apex; parasternal lift.
Auscultation—Loud S_1, P_2; diastolic opening snap followed by rumble with presystolic accentuation.
Atrial fibrillation may be pulse pattern. Cold extremities.

Mitral Regurgitation

Precordium—Apical systolic thrill; apex displaced to left.
Auscultation—Apical systolic regurgitant murmur following a decreased S_1; radiating to axilla; often hear S_3 due to increased left ventricular end diastolic volume.

Mitral Valve Prolapse

Most common in women younger than 30.
Auscultation—A mid- or late systolic click 0.14 seconds or more after S_1. Often followed by a high-pitched systolic murmur; squatting may cause murmur to decrease.

Aortic Stenosis

Precordium—Basal systolic thrill; apex displaced anteriorly and laterally.
Carotids—Slow upstroke to a delayed peak.
Auscultation—A_2 diminished or paradoxically ejection systolic murmur radiating to carotids. Cold extremities.

Aortic Regurgitation

Often associated with Marfan's syndrome, rheumatoid spondylitis.
Precordium—Apex displaced laterally and anteriorly; thrill often palpable along left sternal border and in the jugular notch.
Carotids—Double systolic wave.
Auscultation—Decrescendo diastolic murmur along left sternal border; M_1 and A_2 are increased.

Tricuspid Regurgitation

Usually secondary to pathology elsewhere in heart.
Precordium—Right ventricular parasternal lift; systolic thrill at tricuspid area.
Auscultation—Holosystolic murmur increasing with inspiration; other: V wave in jugular venous pulse; systolic liver pulsation.

Atrial Septal Defect

Normal pulse; break parasternal life; lift over pulmonary artery; normal jugular pulse; systolic ejection murmur in pulmonic area; low-pitched diastolic rumble over tricuspid area (at times); persistent wide splitting of S_2.

Pericarditis

Tachycardia; friction rub; diminished heart sounds and enlarged heart to percussion (with effusion); pulsus paradoxus; neck vein distention, narrow pulse pressure and hypotension (with tamponade).

Fig. 2.5. Phonocardiographic description of pathologic cardiac murmurs. *(From James, E. C., Corry, R. J., & Perry, J. F. [1987]. Principles of basic surgical practice. Philadelphia, PA: Hanley & Belfus.)*

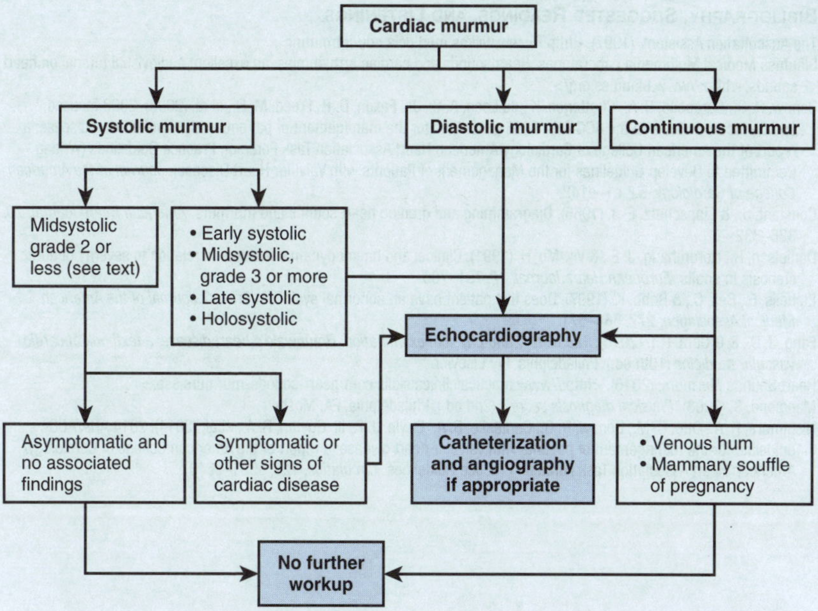

Fig. 2.6. Strategy for evaluating heart murmurs. *(Reproduced from Bonow, R. O., Carabello, B. A., Chatterjee, K., de Leon, A. C., Jr., Faxon, D. P., Freed, M. D., et al. (2008). 2008 focused update incorporated into the ACC/AHA 2006 guidelines for the management of patients with valvular heart disease: a report of the American College of Cardiology/American Heart Association Task Force on Practice Guidelines (Writing Committee to Develop Guidelines for the Management of Patients with Valvular Heart Disease).* Journal of the American College of Cardiology, 52, *e1–e142.)*

Table 2.3. Recommendations for Echocardiography in the Evaluation of Cardiac Murmurs

Class I

1. Echocardiography is recommended for asymptomatic patients with diastolic murmurs, continuous murmurs, holosystolic murmurs, late systolic murmurs, murmurs associated with ejection clicks, or murmurs that radiate to the neck or back.
2. Echocardiography is recommended for patients with heart murmurs and symptoms or signs of heart failure, myocardial ischemia/infarction, syncope, thromboembolism, infective endocarditis, or other clinical evidence of structural heart disease.
3. Echocardiography is recommended for asymptomatic patients who have grade 3 or louder mid-peaking systolic murmurs.

Class IIa

1. Echocardiography can be useful for the evaluation of asymptomatic patients with murmurs associated with other abnormal cardiac physical findings or murmurs associated with an abnormal ECG or chest x-ray.
2. Echocardiography can be useful for patients whose symptoms and/or signs are likely noncardiac in origin but in whom a cardiac basis cannot be excluded by standard evaluation.

Class III

Echocardiography is not recommended for patients who have a grade 2 or softer midsystolic murmur identified as innocent or functional by an experienced observer.

Reproduced from Bonow, R. O., Carabello, B. A., Chatterjee, K., de Leon, A. C., Jr., Faxon, D. P., Freed, M. D., et al. (2008). 2008 focused update incorporated into the ACC/AHA 2006 guidelines for the management of patients with valvular heart disease: a report of the American College of Cardiology/American Heart Association Task Force on Practice Guidelines (Writing Committee to Develop Guidelines for the Management of Patients with Valvular Heart Disease). Journal of the American College of Cardiology, 2008;52:e1–142.

Bibliography, Suggested Readings, and Listenings

The Auscultation Assistant. (1997). <http://www.wilkes.med.ucla.edu/intro.html>.

Blaufuss Medical Multimedia Laboratories. Heart sounds and cardiac arrhythmias, an excellent audiovisual tutorial on heart sounds. <http://www.blaufuss.org/>.

Bonow, R. O., Carabello, B. A., Chatterjee, K., de Leon, A. C., Jr., Faxon, D. P., Freed, M. D., et al. (2008). 2008 focused update incorporated into the ACC/AHA 2006 guidelines for the management of patients with valvular heart disease: a report of the American College of Cardiology/American Heart Association Task Force on Practice Guidelines (Writing Committee to Develop Guidelines for the Management of Patients with Valvular Heart Disease). *Journal of the American College of Cardiology*, *52*, e1–e142.

Constant, J., & Lippschutz, E. J. (1965). Diagramming and grading heart sounds and murmurs. *American Heart Journal*, *70*, 326–332.

Danielsen, R., Nordrehaug, J. E., & Vik-Mo, H. (1991). Clinical and haemodynamic features in relation to severity of aortic stenosis in adults. *European Heart Journal*, *12*, 791–795.

Etchells, E., Bell, C., & Robb, K. (1997). Does this patient have an abnormal systolic murmur? *Journal of the American Medical Association*, *277*, 564–571.

Fang, J. C., & O'Gara, P. T. (2015). *The history and physical examination. Braunwald's heart disease: a textbook of cardiovascular medicine* (10th ed.). Philadelphia, PA: Elsevier.

Heart Sounds Murmurs. (2016). <http://www.practicalclinicalskills.com/heart-sounds-murmurs.aspx>.

Mangione, S. (2008). *Physical diagnosis secrets* (2nd ed.). Philadelphia, PA: Mosby.

Nishimura, R. A., Otto, C. M., Bonow, R. O., Carabello, B. A., Erwin, J. P., III, Guyton, R. A., et al. (2014). 2014 AHA/ACC guideline for the management of patients with valvular heart disease: a report of the American College of Cardiology/American Heart Association Task Force on Practice Guidelines. *Circulation*, *129*, e521–e643.

CHAPTER 3

ELECTROCARDIOGRAPHY

Itamar Birnbaum, Yochai Birnbaum, Glenn N. Levine

1. What are the most commonly used voltage criteria to diagnose left ventricular hypertrophy?

Numerous criteria have been established for the electrocardiographic diagnosis of left ventricular hypertrophy (LVH). Below are listed the two most frequently used:

- R wave in V5-V6 plus S wave in V1-V2 greater than 35 mm
- R wave in lead I plus S wave in lead III greater than 25 mm

2. What are common nonvoltage electrocardiographic findings that suggest left ventricular hypertrophy?

- Left atrial enlargement (LAE) (see below)
- Widened QRS complex greater than 90 ms
- Repolarization abnormality (ST-segment and T-wave abnormalities)
- Left axis deviation
- R-wave peak time greater than 50 ms (also known as delayed intrinsicoid deflection)

3. What are the most commonly used criteria to diagnose right ventricular hypertrophy?

- R wave in V1 ≥ 7 mm
- R/S wave ratio in V1 greater than 1

4. What criteria are used to diagnose left atrial enlargement?

- P wave total width greater than 0.12 seconds (three small boxes) in the inferior leads, usually with a double-peaked P wave
- Terminal portion of the P wave in lead V1 ≥ 0.04 seconds (one small box) wide and ≥1 mm (one small box) deep.

5. What electrocardiogram finding suggests right atrial enlargement?

- P-wave height in the inferior leads (II, III, and aVF) ≥ 2.5 to 3 mm (2.5 to 3 small boxes) (Fig. 3.1).

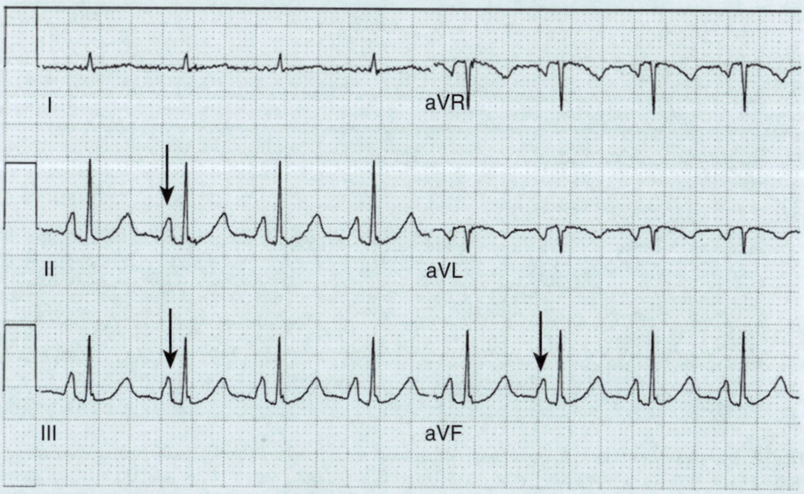

Fig. 3.1. Right atrial enlargement. The tall P waves in the inferior leads (II, III, and avF) are more than 2.5 to 3 mm high.

6. What is the normal rate of a junctional rhythm?

The normal rate is 40 to 60 beats per minute (bpm). Rates of 61 to 99 bpm are referred to as accelerated junctional rhythms, and rates of 100 bpm or higher are referred to as junctional tachycardia.

7. How can one distinguish a junctional escape rhythm from a ventricular escape rhythm in a patient with complete heart block?

Junctional escape rhythms usually occur at a rate of 40 to 60 bpm and will usually be narrow complex (unless the patient has a baseline bundle branch block), whereas ventricular escape rhythms will usually occur at a rate of 30 to 40 bpm and will be wide complex.

8. Describe the three types of heart blocks.

- **First-degree heart block:** The PR interval is a fixed duration of more than 0.20 seconds.
- **Second-degree heart block:** In Mobitz type I (Wenckebach), the PR interval increases until a P wave is nonconducted (Fig. 3.2A). The cycle then resets and starts again. Mobitz type I second-degree heart block is sometimes due to increased vagal tone and is usually a relatively benign finding. In Mobitz type II, the PR interval is fixed and occasional P waves are nonconducted (see Fig. 3.2B). Mobitz type II second-degree heart block usually indicates structural disease in the atrioventricular (AV) node or His-Purkinje system and is an indication for pacemaker implantation.
- **Third-degree heart block:** All P waves are nonconducted, and there is either a junctional or ventricular escape rhythm (see Fig. 3.2C). To call a rhythm third-degree or complete heart block, the atrial rate (as evidenced by the P waves) should be faster than the ventricular escape rate (the QRS complexes). Third-degree heart block is almost always an indication for a permanent pacemaker.

9. What are the causes of ST-segment elevation?

In addition to ST-segment–elevation myocardial infarction (STEMI), there are numerous other causes of ST-segment elevation that must be considered in patients who are found to have ST-elevation on the electrocardiogram (ECG). The differential diagnosis of ST-segment elevation includes the following:

- Acute myocardial infarction (MI) due to thrombotic occlusion of a coronary artery

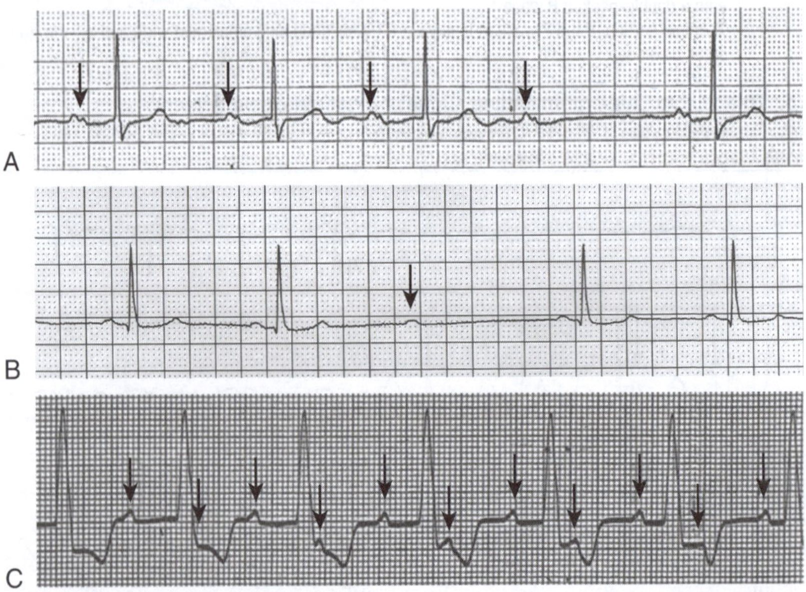

Fig. 3.2. Examples of heart block. **A,** Wenckebach (Mobitz type I second-degree AV block). The PR interval progressively increases until there is a nonconducted P wave *(fourth arrow)*. **B,** Mobitz type II second-degree heart block. The PR interval is constant, but a P wave *(arrow)* is nonconducted. **C,** Complete heart block with P waves *(arrows)* that are not associated with QRS impulses.

- Prinzmetal angina (variant angina), in which there is vasospasm of a coronary artery
- Cocaine-induced MI, in which there is vasospasm of a coronary artery, with or without additional thrombotic occlusion
- Takotsubo (stress) cardiomyopathy
- Brugada syndrome
- Pericarditis, in which there is usually diffuse ST-segment elevation
- Left ventricular aneurysm
- Left bundle branch block (LBBB)
- LVH with repolarization abnormalities
- J-point elevation, a condition classically seen in young African American patients but that can be seen in any patient, which is felt to be due to "early repolarization"
- Severe hyperkalemia

10. What are the electrocardiographic findings of hyperkalemia?

Initially a "peaking" of the T waves is seen (Fig. 3.3). As the hyperkalemia becomes more profound, "loss" of the P waves, QRS widening, and ST-segment elevation may occur. The preterminal finding is a sinusoidal pattern on the ECG (Fig. 3.4).

11. What are the electrocardiographic findings in pericarditis?

The first findings are believed to be PR-segment depression (Fig. 3.5A), possibly caused by repolarization abnormalities of the atria. This may be fairly transient and is often not present by the time the patient is seen for evaluation. Either concurrent with PR-segment depression or shortly following PR-segment depression, diffuse ST-segment elevation occurs (see Fig. 3.5B). At a later time, diffuse T-wave inversions may develop.

12. What is electrical alternans?

In the presence of large pericardial effusions, the heart may "swing" within the large pericardial effusion, resulting in an alteration of the amplitude of the QRS complex (Fig. 3.6).

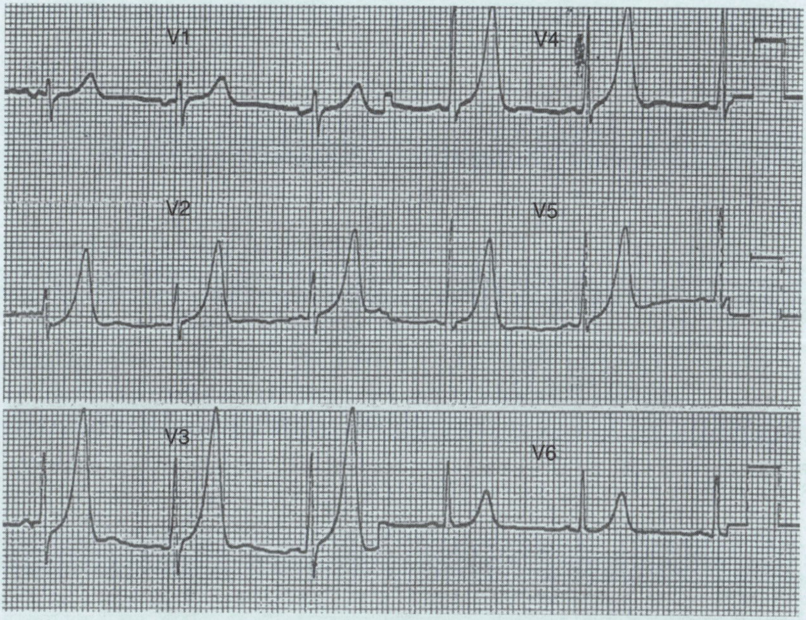

Fig. 3.3. Hyperkalemia. Peaked T waves are seen in many of the precordial leads. *(Adapted with permission from Levine, G. N., & Podrid, P. J. [1995].* The ECG workbook: a review and discussion of ECG findings and abnormalities *[p. 405]. New York, NY: Futura Publishing Company.)*

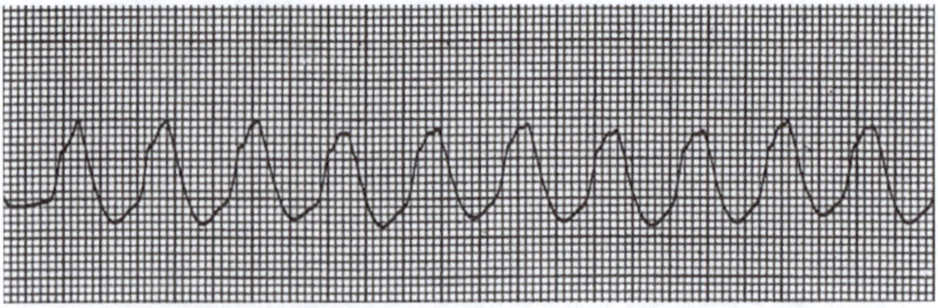

Fig. 3.4. Severe hyperkalemia. The rhythm strip demonstrates the preterminal rhythm sinusoidal wave seen in cases of severe hyperkalemia. *(Adapted with permission from Levine, G. N., & Podrid, P. J. [1995].* The ECG workbook: a review and discussion of ECG findings and abnormalities *[p. 503]. New York, NY: Futura Publishing Company.)*

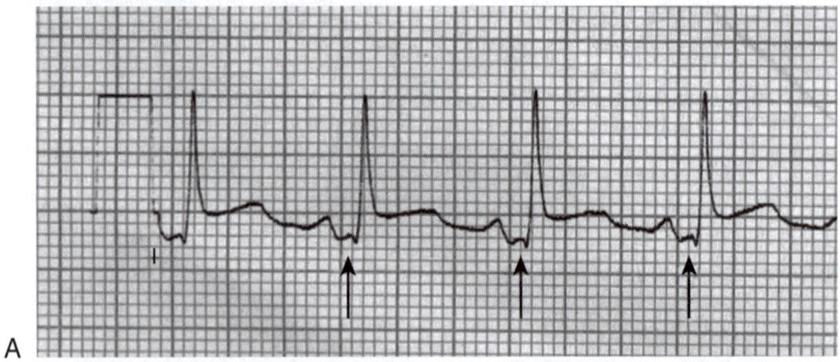

Fig. 3.5. Electrocardiographic findings in pericarditis. **A,** PR depression (arrows) seen early in pericarditis. **B,** Diffuse ST-segment elevation in pericarditis.

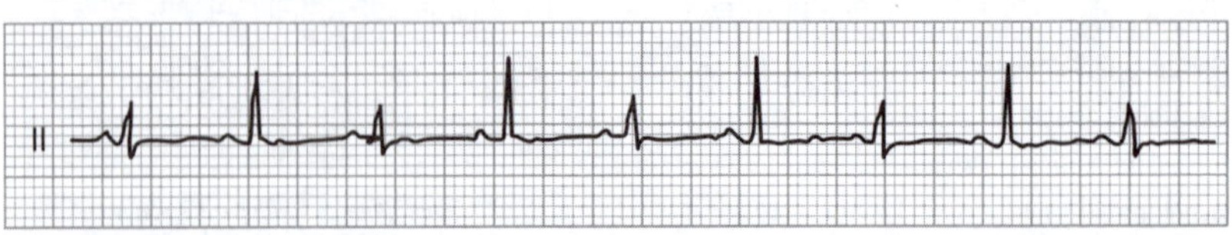

Fig. 3.6. Electrical alternans in a patient with a large pericardial effusion. Note the alternating amplitude of the QRS complexes. *(From Manning, W. J. [2008]. Pericardial disease. In L. Goldman [Ed.],* Cecil medicine *[23rd ed.]. Philadelphia, PA: Saunders.)*

13. What are the main electrocardiographic findings in hyper- and hypocalcemia?

With hypercalcemia, the QT interval shortens. With hypocalcemia, prolongation of the QT interval occurs as a result of delayed repolarization (Fig. 3.7).

14. What electrocardiographic findings may be present with a pulmonary embolus?

The most common ECG finding in pulmonary embolus is the nonspecific finding of sinus tachycardia. However, other findings should raise the suspicion of pulmonary embolus as the cause of a patient's chest pain or shortness of breath. These include the following:

- Sinus tachycardia (the most common ECG finding)
- Right atrial enlargement (P pulmonale)—tall P waves in the inferior leads
- Right axis deviation
- T-wave inversions in leads V1-V2
- Incomplete right bundle branch block (IRBBB)
- S1Q3T3 pattern—an S wave in lead I, a Q wave in lead III, and an inverted T wave in lead III (Although this last is only occasionally seen with pulmonary embolus, it is said to be quite suggestive that a pulmonary embolus has occurred.)

15. How is the QT interval calculated, and what are the causes of short-QT and long-QT intervals?

The QT interval is measured from the beginning of the QRS complex to the end of the T wave. The corrected QT interval (QT_c) takes into account the heart rate, because the QT interval increases at slower heart rates. The formula is

$$QT_C = \frac{\text{measured QT}}{\sqrt{\text{RR interval}}}$$

Causes of short-QT interval include hypercalcemia, congenital short-QT syndrome, and digoxin therapy. Numerous drugs, metabolic abnormalities, and other conditions can cause a prolonged QT interval (Table 3.1). QT_c values greater than 440 to 460 ms are considered prolonged, though the risk of arrhythmia is generally ascribed to be more common at QT_c values greater than 500 ms.

16. What is torsades de pointes?

Torsades de pointes is a ventricular arrhythmia that occurs in the setting of QT prolongation, usually when drugs that prolong the QT interval have been administered. It may also occur in the setting of congenital

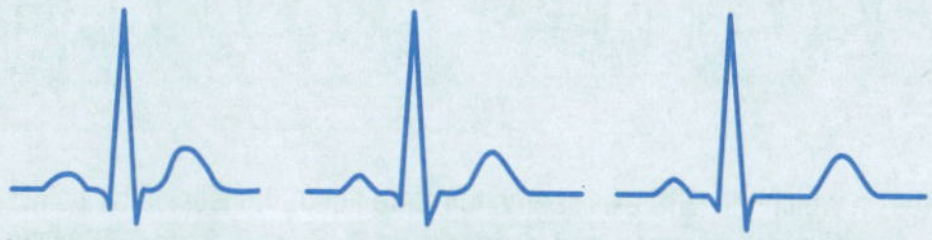

Fig. 3.7. Electrocardiographic findings of hyper- and hypocalcemia. With hypercalcemia, the QT interval shortens. With hypocalcemia, there is prolongation of the QT interval due to delayed repolarization. *(From Park, M. K., & Guntheroth, W. G. [2006].* How to read pediatric ECGs *[4th ed.]. Philadelphia, PA: Mosby.)*

Table 3.1. Causes of Prolonged QT Interval
Antiarrhythmic drugs (e.g., amiodarone, sotalol, quinidine, procainamide, ibutilide, dofetilide, flecainide)
Psychiatric medications, particularly overdoses (tricyclic antidepressants, antipsychotic agents)
Certain antibiotics (e.g., macrolides, fluoroquinolones, antifungals, antimalarials)
Certain antihistamines (e.g., diphenhydramine, astemizole, loratadine, terfenadine)
Electrolyte abnormalities (e.g., hypocalcemia, hypokalemia, hypomagnesemia)
Raised intracranial pressure ("cerebral t waves")
Hypothermia
Hypothyroidism
Congenital long-QT syndrome

prolonged QT syndrome and other conditions. The term was reportedly coined by Dessertenne to describe the arrhythmia, in which the QRS axis appears to twist around the isoelectric line (Fig. 3.8). It is usually a hemodynamically unstable rhythm that can further degenerate and lead to hemodynamic collapse. Although it is commonly taught and present in algorithms that the treatment of this arrhythmia is magnesium, such an infusion usually takes at least minutes or longer to administer. Given that these patients are almost always hemodynamically unstable or pulseless, prompt defibrillation is usually indicated.

17. **What are cerebral T waves?**
Cerebral T waves are strikingly deep and inverted T waves, most prominently seen in the precordial leads, that occur with central nervous system diseases, most notably subarachnoid and intracerebral hemorrhages. They are believed to be due to prolonged and abnormal repolarization of the left ventricle, presumably as a result of autonomic imbalance. They should not be mistaken for evidence of active cardiac ischemia (Fig. 3.9).

18. **What are Osborne waves?**
Osborne waves are upward deflections that occur at the J point of the QRS complex in the setting of hypothermia (Fig. 3.10). They are believed to result from hypothermia-induced repolarization abnormalities of the ventricle.

19. **What findings help distinguish ventricular tachycardia from supraventricular tachycardia with aberrancy?**
The Brugada criteria help to distinguish between ventricular tachycardia (VT) and supraventricular tachycardia (SVT) with aberrancy. If one or more of the criteria below exist, then the rhythm is more likely to be VT.
- AV dissociation (especially if more QRS complexes than P waves are present)
- No R waves in precordial leads (V1-V6)
- Initiation of R wave to peak of S wave duration greater than 100 ms

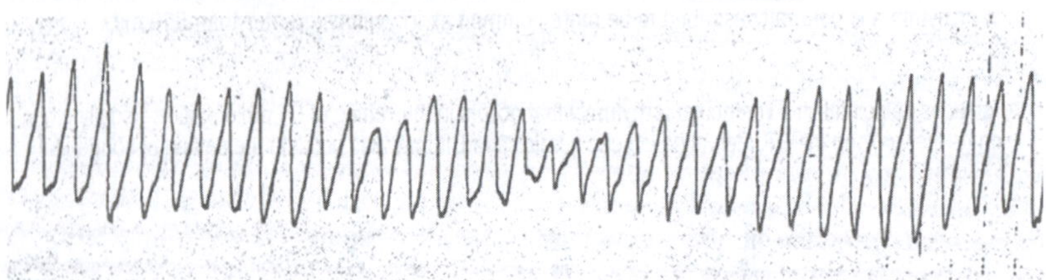

Fig. 3.8. Torsades de pointes, in which the QRS axis seems to rotate about the isoelectric point. *(From Olgin, J. E., & Zipes, D. P. [2008]. Specific arrhythmias: diagnosis and treatment. In P. Libby, R. Bonow, D. Mann, & D. Zipes [Eds.],* Braunwald's heart disease: a textbook of cardiovascular medicine *[8th ed.]. Philadelphia, PA: Saunders.)*

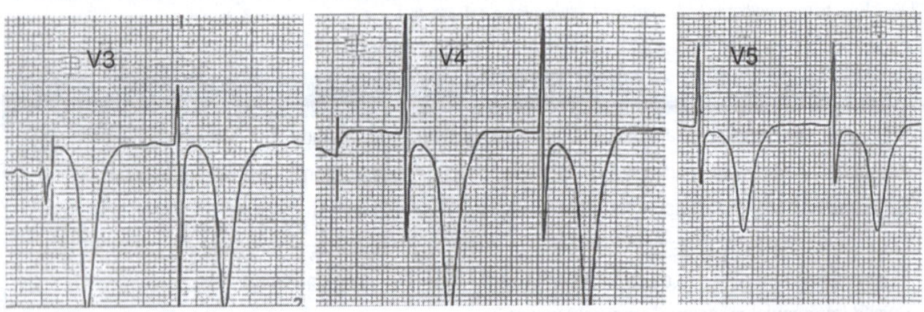

Fig. 3.9. Cerebral T waves. The markedly deep and inverted T waves are seen with central nervous system disease, particularly subarachnoid and intracerebral hemorrhages. *(Reproduced with permission from Levine, G. N., & Podrid, P. J. [1995].* The ECG workbook: a review and discussion of ECG findings and abnormalities *[p. 437]. New York, NY: Futura Publishing Company.)*

20. In a patient presenting with angina and left bundle branch block, what features help determine if there is an ST-segment–elevation myocardial infarction?

LBBB inherently has ST abnormalities and may mask a STEMI. The Sgarbossa criteria (Fig. 3.11) were developed to help clinicians identify STEMI in these patients. They are as follows:

- Concordant ST-segment elevations greater than 1 mm in leads with a positive QRS complex
- Concordant ST-segment depressions greater than 1 mm in leads with a negative QRS complex (usually V1-V3)
- Discordant ST-segment elevations greater than 5 mm or greater than 0.25× of the S wave

Concordance occurs when both the QRS complex and the ST segment have a positive or negative axis. Discordance occurs when the axis of the QRS differs from that of the ST segment.

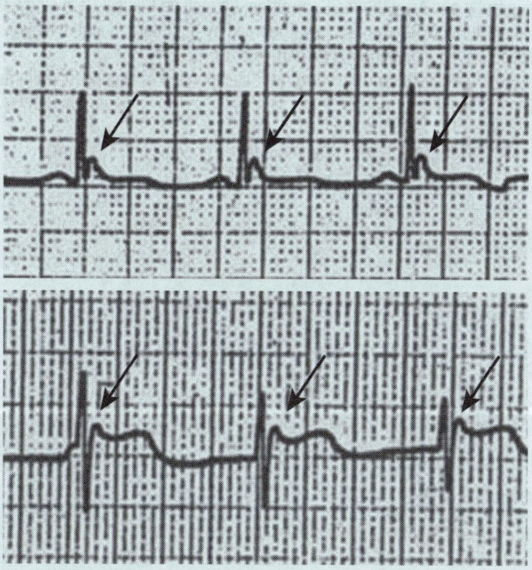

Fig. 3.10. Osborne waves (arrows) seen in hypothermia. *(Modified with permission from Levine, G. N., & Podrid, P. J. [1995].* The ECG workbook: a review and discussion of ECG findings and abnormalities *[p. 417]. New York, NY: Futura Publishing Company.)*

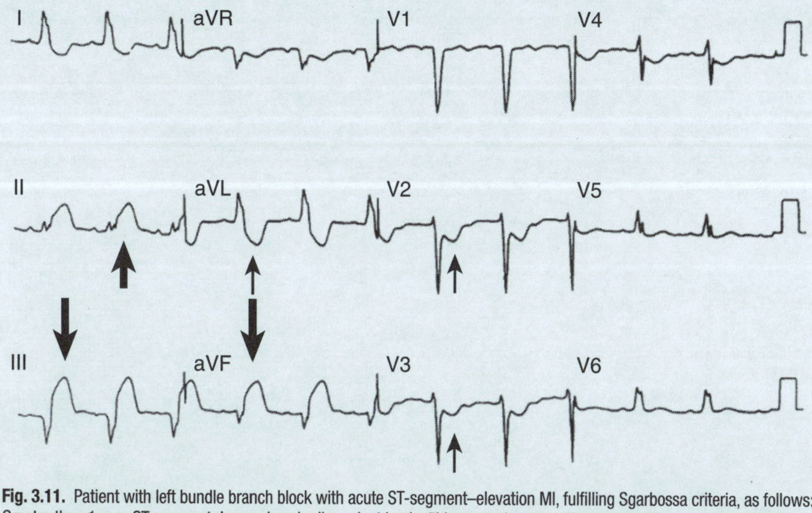

Fig. 3.11. Patient with left bundle branch block with acute ST-segment–elevation MI, fulfilling Sgarbossa criteria, as follows: Greater than 1-mm ST-segment depressions in discordant leads *(thin arrows)*, greater than 5-mm ST-segment elevations in discordant leads *(thick arrows)*, and greater than 1-mm ST-segment elevations in concordant leads *(thick arrowhead)*.

Bibliography and Suggested Readings

Brugada, P., Brugada, J., Mont, L., Smeets, J., & Andries, E. W. (1991). A new approach to the differential diagnosis of a regular tachycardia with a wide QRS complex. *Circulation, 83*(5), 1649–1659.

Dublin, D. (2000). *Rapid interpretation of EKGs.* Tampa, FL: Cover Publishing.

ECG Library. < http://www.ecglibrary.com/ecghome.html >.

ECG Tutorial. < http://www.uptodate.com >.

Electrocardiogram Rhythm Tutor. < http://www.coldbacon.com/mdtruth/more/ekg.html >.

Electrocardiography: An On-Line Tutorial. < http://www.drsegal.com/medstud/ecg/ >.

Levine, G. N. (1998). *Diagnosing (and treating) arrhythmias made easy.* St. Louis, MO: Quality Medical Publishers.

Levine, G. N., & Podrid, P. J. (1995). *The ECG workbook.* Armonk, NY: Futura Publishing.

Mason, J. W., Hancock, E. W., & Gettes, L. S. (2007). Recommendations for the standardization and interpretation of the electrocardiogram: part II: electrocardiography diagnostic statement list, a scientific statement from the American Heart Association Electrocardiography and Arrhythmias Committee, Council on Clinical Cardiology; the American College of Cardiology Foundation; and the Heart Rhythm Society Endorsed by the International Society for Computerized Electrocardiology. *Journal of the American College of Cardiology, 49*(10), 1128–1135.

Wagner, G. S. (2008). *Marriot's practical electrocardiography.* Philadelphia, PA: Lippincott Williams & Wilkins.

CHAPTER 4

CHEST X-RAY

James J. Fenton, Glenn N. Levine

1. Describe a systematic approach to interpreting a chest radiograph (chest x-ray)

Common recommendations are to:

1. Begin with general characteristics such as the age, gender, size, and position of the patient.
2. Next examine the periphery of the film, including the bones, soft tissue, and pleura. Look for rib fractures, rib notching, bony metastases, shoulder dislocation, soft tissue masses, and pleural thickening.
3. Then evaluate the lung, looking for infiltrates, pulmonary nodules, and pleural effusions.
4. Finally, concentrate on the heart size and contour, mediastinal structures, hilum, and great vessels. Also note the presence of pacemakers and sternal wires.

2. Identify the major cardiovascular structures that form the silhouette of the mediastinum.

The major cardiovascular structures that form the silhouette of the mediastinum are shown in Figs. 4.1 and 4.2.

- **Right side:** Ascending aorta, right pulmonary artery, right atrium, right ventricle
- **Left side:** Aortic knob, left pulmonary artery, left atrial appendage, left ventricle

3. What is the most anterior cardiac structure on the lateral chest x-ray?

The right ventricle.

4. How is heart size measured on a chest radiograph?

Identification of cardiomegaly on a chest x-ray (CXR) is subjective, but if the heart size is equal to or greater than twice the size of the hemithorax, then it is enlarged. Remember that a film taken during expiration, in a supine position, or by a portable anteroposterior (AP) technique will make the heart appear larger.

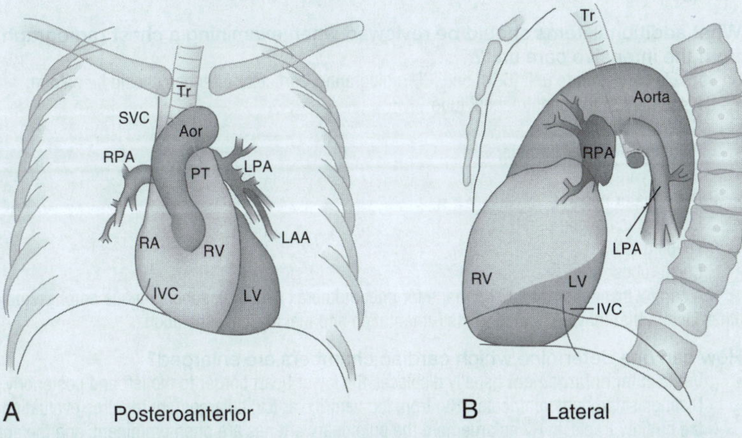

Fig. 4.1. Diagrammatic representations of the anatomy of the chest radiograph. *Aor,* Aorta; *IVC,* inferior vena cava; *LAA,* left atrial appendage; *LPA,* left pulmonary artery; *LV,* left ventricle; *PT,* pulmonary trunk; *RA,* right atrium; *RPA,* right pulmonary artery; *RV,* right ventricle; *SVC,* superior vena cava; *Tr,* trachea. *(From Inaba, A. S. [2006]. Cardiac disorders. In J. Marx, R. Hockberger, & R. Walls [Eds.],* Rosen's emergency medicine: concepts and clinical practice. *[6th ed.]. Philadelphia, PA: Mosby.)*

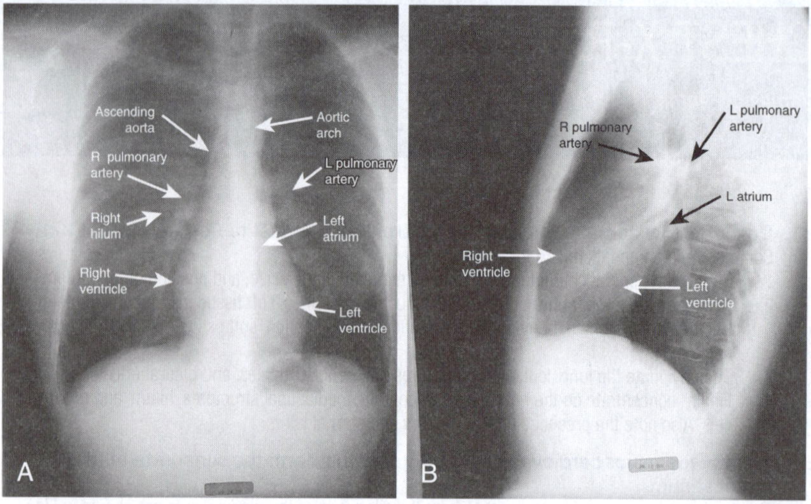

Fig. 4.2. Normal posterioranterior **(A)** and lateral **(B)** chest radiograph with the major cardiovascular structures noted.

5. What factors can affect heart size on the chest radiograph?

Factors that can affect heart size on the chest radiograph include:

- **Size of the patient:** Obesity decreases lung volumes and enlarges the appearance of the heart.
- **Degree of inspiration:** Poor inspiration can make the heart appear larger.
- **Emphysema:** Hyperinflation changes the configuration of the heart, making it appear smaller.
- **Contractility:** Systole or diastole can make up to a 1.5-cm difference in heart size. In addition, low heart rate and increased cardiac output lead to increased ventricular filling.
- **Chest configuration:** Pectus excavatum can compress the heart and make it appear larger.
- **Patient positioning:** The heart appears larger if the film is taken in a supine position.
- **Type of examination:** On an AP projection, the heart is farther away from the film and closer to the camera. This creates greater beam divergence and the appearance of an increased heart size.

6. What additional items should be reviewed when examining a chest radiograph from the intensive care unit?

On portable cardiac care unit (CCU) and ICU radiographs, particular attention should be paid to:

- Placement of the endotracheal tube
- Central lines
- Pulmonary arterial catheter
- Pacing wires
- Defibrillator pads
- Intra-aortic balloon pump
- Feeding tubes
- Chest tubes

A careful inspection should be made for pneumothorax (Fig. 4.3), subcutaneous emphysema, and other factors that may be related to instrumentation and mechanical ventilation.

7. How can one determine which cardiac chambers are enlarged?

- **Ventricular enlargement** usually displaces the lower heart border to the left and posteriorly. Distinguishing right ventricular (RV) from left ventricular (LV) enlargement requires evaluation of the outflow tracts. In RV enlargement the pulmonary arteries are often prominent, and the aorta is diminutive. In LV enlargement the aorta is prominent and the pulmonary arteries are normal.
- **Left atrial (LA) enlargement** creates a convexity between the left pulmonary artery and the left ventricle on the frontal view. Also, a *double density* may be seen inferior to the carina. On the lateral view, LA enlargement displaces the descending left lower lobe bronchus posteriorly.
- **Right atrial enlargement** causes the lower right heart border to bulge outward to the right.

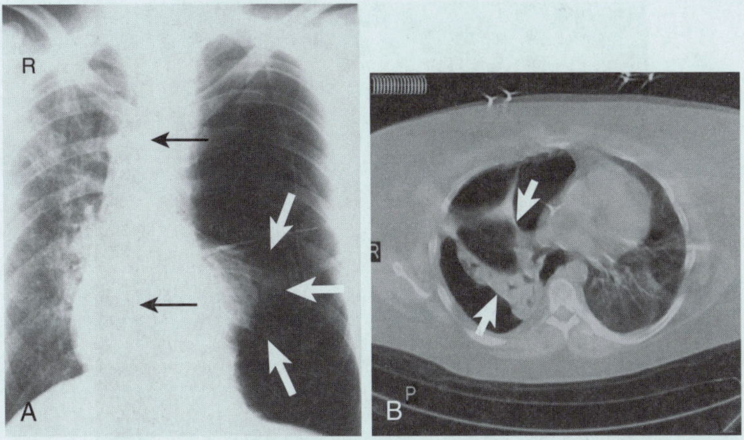

Fig. 4.3. Tension pneumothorax. On a posteroanterior chest radiograph **(A)** the left hemithorax is very dark or lucent because the left lung has collapsed completely *(white arrows)*. The tension pneumothorax can be identified because the mediastinal contents, including the heart, are shifted toward the right, and the left hemidiaphragm is flattened and depressed. **B,** A computed tomography scan done on a different patient with a tension pneumothorax shows a completely collapsed right lung *(arrows)* and shift of the mediastinal contents to the left. *(From Mettler, F. A. [2014].* Essentials of radiology *[2nd ed.]. Philadelphia, PA: Saunders.)*

8. What are some of the common causes of chest pain that can be identified on a chest radiograph?

- Aortic dissection
- Pneumonia
- Pneumothorax (see Fig. 4.3)
- Pulmonary embolism
- Subcutaneous emphysema
- Pericarditis (if a large pericardial effusion is suggested by the radiograph)
- Esophageal rupture
- Hiatal hernia

All patients with chest pain should undergo a CXR even if the cause of the chest pain is suspected myocardial ischemia.

9. What are the causes of a widened mediastinum?

There are multiple potential causes of a widened mediastinum (Fig. 4.4). Some of the most concerning causes of mediastinal widening include aortic dissection/rupture and mediastinal bleeding from chest trauma or misplaced central venous catheters. One of the most common causes of mediastinal widening is thoracic lipomatosis in an obese patient. Tumors should also be considered as a cause of a widened mediastinum—especially germ cell tumors, lymphoma, and thymomas. The mediastinum may also appear wider on a portable AP film compared with a standard posteroanterior/lateral chest radiograph.

10. What are the common radiographic signs of congestive heart failure?

Common radiographic signs of congestive heart failure include:

- Enlarged cardiac silhouette (with heart failure with reduced ejection fraction [HFrEF])
- Left atrial enlargement
- Hilar fullness
- Vascular redistribution
- Linear interstitial opacities (Kerley's lines)
- Bilateral alveolar infiltrates
- Pleural effusions (right greater than left)

11. What is vascular redistribution? When does it occur in congestive heart failure?

Vascular redistribution occurs when the upper-lobe pulmonary arteries and veins become larger than the vessels in the lower lobes. The sign is most accurate if the upper lobe vessels are increased

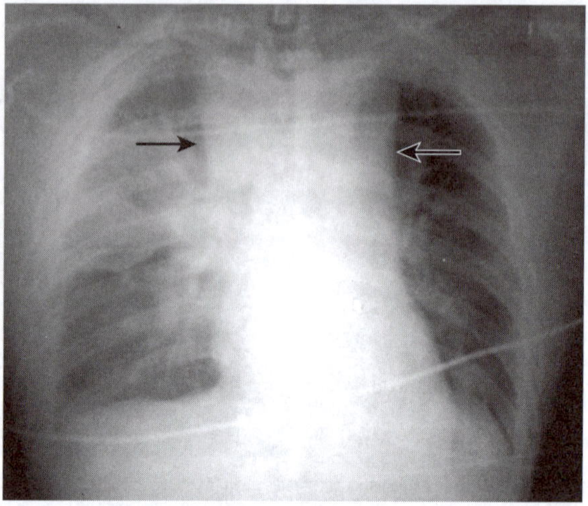

Fig. 4.4. Widened mediastinum *(arrows). (From Marx, J., Hockberger, R., & Walls, R. [2006].* Rosen's emergency medicine: concepts and clinical practice *[6th ed.]. Philadelphia, PA: Mosby.)*

in diameter greater than 3 mm in the first intercostal interspace. It usually occurs at a pulmonary capillary occlusion pressure of 12 to 19 mm Hg. As the pulmonary capillary occlusion pressure rises above 19 mm Hg, interstitial edema develops with bronchial cuffing, Kerley's B lines, and thickening of the lung fissures. Vascular redistribution to the upper lobes is probably most consistently seen in patients with chronic pulmonary venous hypertension (mitral valve disease, left ventricular dysfunction) because of the body's attempt to maintain more normal blood flow and oxygenation in this area. Some authors believe that vascular redistribution is a cardinal feature of congestive heart failure, but it may be a particularly unhelpful sign in the ICU patient with acute congestive failure. In these patients, all the pulmonary arteries look enlarged, making it difficult to assess upper and lower vessel size. In addition, the film is often taken supine, which can enlarge the upper lobe pulmonary vessels because of stasis of blood flow and not true redistribution.

12. How do left ventricular dysfunction and right ventricular dysfunction lead to pleural effusions?

- LV dysfunction causes increased hydrostatic pressures, which lead to interstitial edema and pleural effusions. Right pleural effusions are more common than left pleural effusions, but the majority is bilateral.
- RV dysfunction leads to system venous hypertension, which inhibits normal reabsorption of pleural fluid into the parietal pleural lymphatics.

13. How helpful is the chest radiograph at identifying and characterizing a pericardial effusion?

The CXR is not sensitive for the detection of a pericardial effusion, and it may not be helpful in determining the extent of an effusion. Smaller pericardial effusions are difficult to detect on a CXR but can still cause tamponade physiology if fluid accumulation is rapid. A large cardiac silhouette with a "water bottle" appearance (Fig. 4.5), however, may suggest a large pericardial effusion. Distinguishing pericardial fluid from chamber enlargement is often difficult.

14. What are the characteristic radiographic findings of significant pulmonary hypertension?

Enlargement of the central pulmonary arteries with rapid tapering of the vessels is a characteristic finding in patients with pulmonary hypertension (Fig. 4.6). If the right descending pulmonary artery is greater than 17 mm in transverse diameter, it is considered enlarged. Other findings of pulmonary hypertension include cardiac enlargement (particularly the right ventricle) and calcification of the pulmonary arteries. Pulmonary arterial calcification follows atheroma formation in the artery and represents a rare but specific radiographic finding of severe pulmonary hypertension.

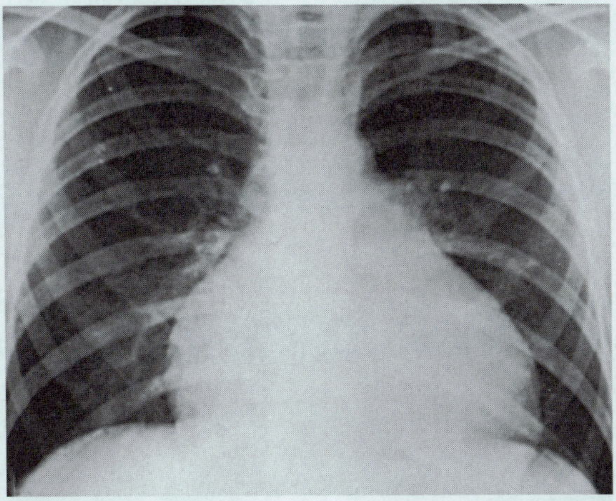

Fig. 4.5. The *water bottle* configuration that can be seen with a large pericardial effusion. *(From Kliegman, R. M., Behrman, R. E., Jenson, H. B., & Stanton, B. F. [2007].* Nelson textbook of pediatrics *[18th ed.]. Philadelphia, PA: Saunders.)*

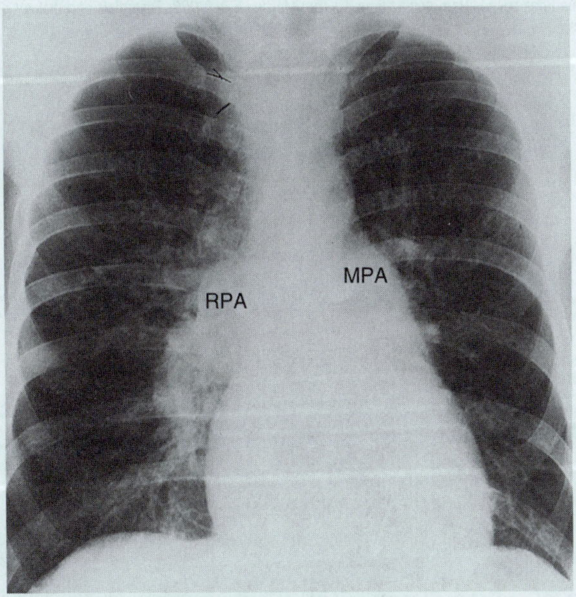

Fig. 4.6. Pulmonary arterial hypertension. Marked dilation of the main pulmonary artery (MPA) and right pulmonary artery (RPA) is noted. Rapid tapering of the arteries as they proceed peripherally is suggestive of pulmonary hypertension and is sometimes referred to as *pruning. (From Mettler, F. A. [2005].* Essentials of radiology *[2nd ed.]. Philadelphia, PA: Saunders.)*

15. What is Westermark's sign and Hampton's hump?

Westermark's sign is seen in patients with pulmonary embolism and represents an area of oligemia beyond the occluded pulmonary vessel. If pulmonary infarction results, a wedge-shaped infiltrate ("Hampton's hump") may be visible (Fig. 4.7).

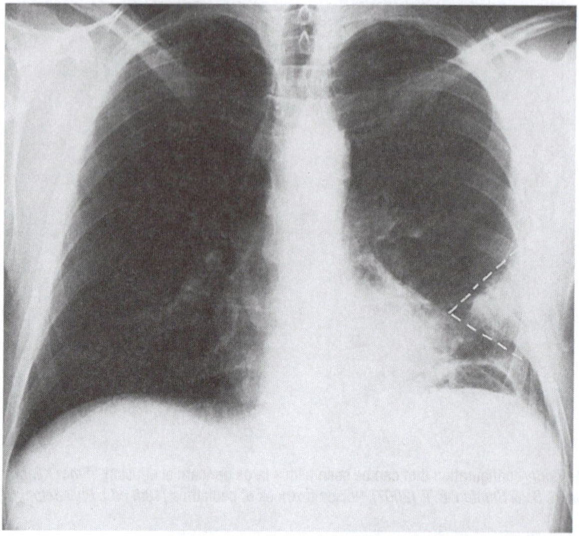

Fig. 4.7. A peripheral wedge-shaped infiltrate *(white dashed lines)* seen after a pulmonary embolism has led to infarction. This finding is sometimes called "Hampton's hump." *(From Mettler, F. A. [2005].* Essentials of radiology *[2nd ed.]. Philadelphia, PA: Saunders.)*

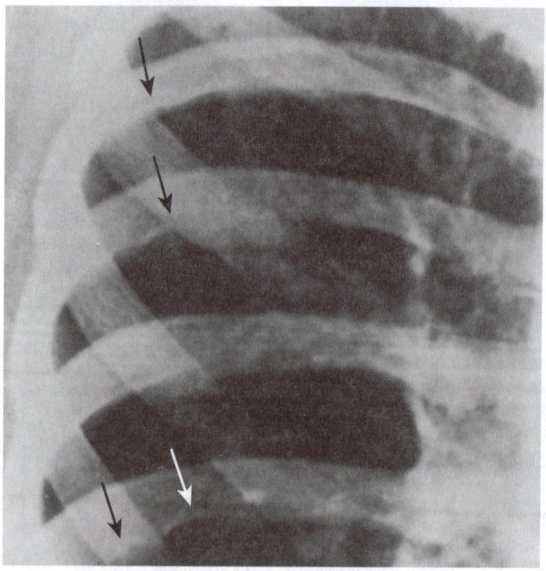

Fig. 4.8. Rib notching in a patient with coarctation of the aorta. *(From Park, M. K. [2008].* Pediatric cardiology for practitioners *[5th ed.]. Philadelphia, PA: Mosby.)*

16. What is rib notching?

Rib notching is erosion of the inferior aspects of the ribs (Fig. 4.8). It can be seen in some patients with coarctation of the aorta and results from a compensatory enlargement of the intercostal arteries as a means of increasing distal circulation. It is most commonly seen between the fourth and eighth ribs. It is important to recognize this life-saving finding because aortic coarctation is treatable with percutaneous or open surgical intervention.

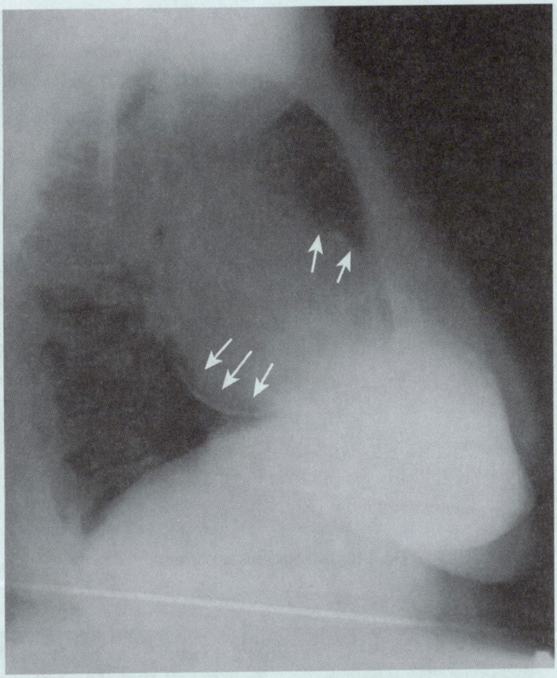

Fig. 4.9. Pericardial calcification *(arrows)*. In a patient with signs and symptoms of heart failure, these findings would strongly suggest the diagnosis of constrictive pericarditis. *(From Libby, P., Bonow, R. O., Mann, D. L., & Zipes, D. P. [Eds.] [2008].* Braunwald's heart disease *[8th ed.]. Philadelphia, PA: Saunders.)*

17. What does the finding in Fig. 4.9 suggest?

The important finding in this figure is pericardial calcification. This can occur in diseases that affect the pericardium, such as tuberculosis. In a patient with signs and symptoms of heart failure, this finding would be highly suggestive of the diagnosis of constrictive pericarditis.

18. What is subcutaneous emphysema?

Subcutaneous emphysema (Fig. 4.10) is the accumulation of air in the subcutaneous tissue, often tracking along tissue plains. Subcutaneous emphysema in the chest can be caused by numerous conditions, including pneumothorax, ruptured bronchus, ruptured esophagus, blunt trauma, stabbing or gunshot wound, or invasive procedure (endoscopy, bronchoscopy, central line placement, intubation). The finding of subcutaneous emphysema almost always is associated with a serious medical condition or complication. The example of subcutaneous emphysema in Fig. 4.9 emphasizes the importance of examining the entire CXR.

19. What is pneumopericardium?

Pneumopericardium, as the name implies, is air in the pericardial space (Fig. 4.11). Pneumopericardium is extremely rare. Causes can include blunt trauma, penetrating injury, infectious pericarditis with a gas-forming organism, fistula between the pericardium and adjacent air-containing structure, and iatrogenic complication.

20. What is a pericardial cyst?

A pericardial cyst (Fig. 4.12) is a fluid-filled structure that can be either congenital or acquired. Pericardial cysts are most commonly seen at the right cardiodiaphragmatic angle but can also be located at the left cardiodiaphragmatic angle, as well as more superiorly. They are usually an incidental finding on either CXR or echocardiography; the diagnosis is most often confirmed by chest CT. Calcification of cyst suggests a bronchogenic cyst, teratoma, or echinococcal cyst.

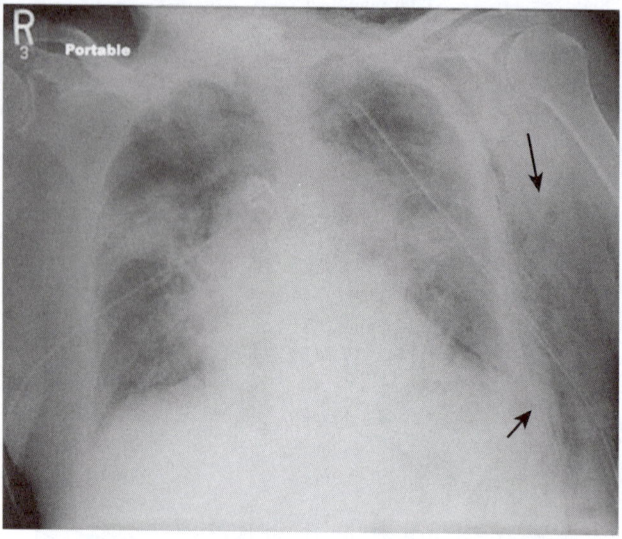

Fig. 4.10. Subcutaneous emphysema.

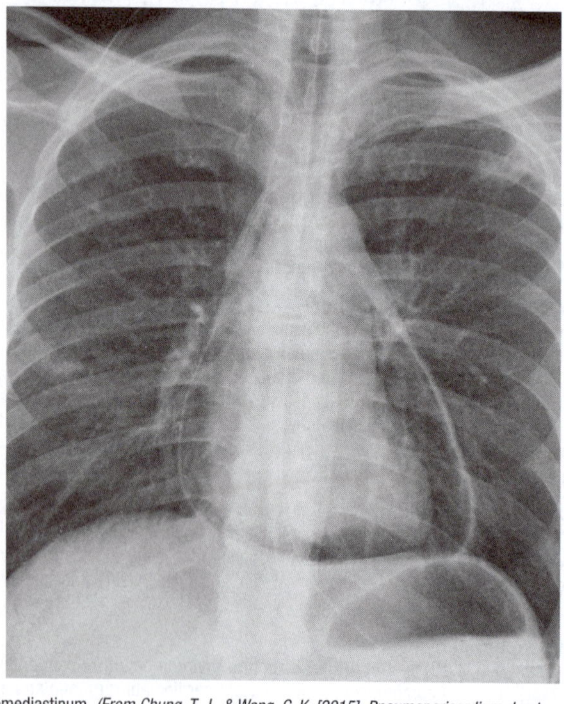

Fig. 4.11. Pneumomediastinum. *(From Chung, T. J., & Wang, C. K. [2015]. Pneumopericardium due to mediastinum metastatic lymph nodes.* Heart, Lung and Circulation, *24[12], e222–e223.)*

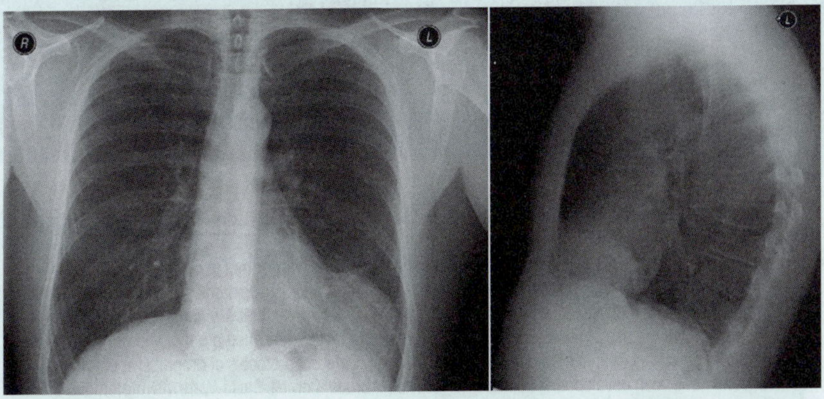

Fig. 4.12. Pericardial cyst. The pericardial cyst is seen at the left cardiophrenic angle. *(From Hutchinson S. J. [2012]. Radiographic findings by diagnosis: pericardial and pleural diseases.* Principles of cardiovascular radiology *[chapter 16, pp. 217–256]. Philadelphia, PA: Saunders.)*

Bibliography and Suggested Readings

Baron, M. G. (1999). Plain film diagnosis of common cardiac anomalies in the adult. *Radiologic Clinics of North America, 37*, 401–420.

Chung, T. J., & Wang, C. K. (2015). Pneumopericardium due to mediastinum metastatic lymph nodes. *Heart, Lung and Circulation, 24*(12), e222–e223.

Hutchison, S. J. (2012). Radiographic findings by diagnosis: pericardial and pleural diseases. In *Principles of cardiovascular radiology* (chapter 16, pp. 217–256). Philadelphia, PA: Saunders.

MacDonald, S. L. S., & Padley, S. (2008). The mediastinum, including the pericardium. In A. Adam & A. K. Dixon (Eds.), *Grainger & Allsion's diagnostic radiology* (5th ed.). Philadelphia, PA: Churchill Livingstone.

Meholic, A. (1996). *Fundamentals of chest radiology*. Philadelphia, PA: Saunders.

Mettler, F. A. (2005). Cardiovascular system. In F. A. Mettler (Ed.), *Essentials of radiology* (2nd ed.). Philadelphia, PA: Saunders.

Newell, J. (1990). Diseases of the thoracic aorta: a symposium. *Journal of Thoracic Imaging, 5*, 1–48.

CHAPTER 5

EXERCISE STRESS TESTING

Fernando Boccalandro, Hercilia Von Schoettler

1. What is the purpose of exercise stress testing, and how can a patient exercise during stress testing?

Exercise stress testing (EST) using electrocardiography is routinely performed to diagnose myocardial ischemia, estimate prognosis, evaluate the outcome of therapy, and assess cardiopulmonary reserve. Exercise is used as a physiologic stress to detect cardiac abnormalities that are not present at rest. The test may involve the use of a treadmill, bicycle ergometer, or rarely an arm ergometer, and may include ventilatory gas analysis (in a cardiopulmonary stress test). Different protocols of progressive cardiovascular workload have been developed specifically for EST (e.g., Bruce, Cornell, Balke-Ware, Asymptomatic Cardiac Ischemia Pilot (ACIP), modified-ACIP (mACIP), Naughton, Weber). Bicycle ergometers are less expensive and smaller than treadmills and produce less motion of the upper body, but early fatigue of the lower extremities is a common problem that limits reaching maximal exercise capacity. As a result, treadmills are more commonly used for EST in the United States. Much of the reported data are based on the multistage Bruce Protocol, which is performed on a treadmill and has become the most common protocol used in clinical practice. Exercise stress tests may involve only electrocardiographic (ECG) monitoring or may be combined with other imaging modalities (i.e., nuclear imaging, echocardiography).

2. What is the difference between a maximal and submaximal exercise stress test?

- *Maximal EST or symptoms-limited EST* is the preferred means to perform an exercise stress test; it attempts to achieve the maximal exercise workload tolerated by the patient. It is terminated based on patient symptoms (e.g., fatigue, angina, shortness of breath); an abnormal ECG (e.g., significant ST-segment depression or elevation, arrhythmias); or an abnormal hemodynamic response (e.g., abnormal blood pressure response). The goal of maximal EST is to achieve a heart rate response of at least 85% of the maximal predicted heart rate (see Question 9).
- *Submaximal EST* is performed when the goal is lower than the individual maximal exercise capacity. Reasonable targets are 70% of the maximal predicted heart rate, 120 beats per minute, or 5 to 6 metabolic equivalents (METs) of exercise capacity (see Question 12). Submaximal EST is used early after myocardial infarction (MI) (see Question 8).

3. How helpful is an exercise stress test in the diagnosis of coronary artery disease?

Multiple studies have compared the accuracy of EST with coronary angiography. However, different criteria have been used to define a significant coronary stenosis, and this lack of standardization—in addition to the variable prevalence of coronary artery disease (CAD) in different populations—complicates the interpretation of the available data. A meta-analysis of 24,074 patients reported a mean sensitivity of 68% and a mean specificity of 77%. The sensitivity increases to 81%, and the specificity decreases to 66% for multivessel disease and to 86% and 53%, respectively, for left main disease or three-vessel CAD. The diagnostic accuracy of EST can be improved by combining other imaging techniques, such as echocardiography or myocardial perfusion imaging, with EST.

The PROMISE trial randomized 10,003 symptomatic patients with suspected CAD to anatomic or functional noninvasive testing. Anatomic testing consisted of coronary computed tomography (CT) angiography (CTA), and functional testing included EST (used in 10% of subjects), stress echocardiography (22%), or nuclear stress testing (68%). The study found no difference in a composite of all-cause mortality, MI, hospitalization for unstable angina, and major complications from cardiovascular procedures between CTA and the various modalities of functional testing, thus supporting EST (which has the lowest cost and no radiation exposure) as the preferred testing strategy for the vast majority of patients with a moderate pretest likelihood of underlying CAD.

4. What are the risks associated with exercise stress testing?

When supervised by an adequately trained physician, the risks are very low. In the general population, the morbidity is less than 0.05%, and the mortality is less than 0.01%. A survey of 151,944 patients 4 weeks after an MI showed slightly increased mortality and morbidity of 0.03% and 0.09%, respectively. According to the national survey of EST facilities, MI and death can be expected in 1 per 2500 tests.

Box 5.1. Indications for Exercise Stress Testing

- To diagnose suspected obstructive CAD based on age, gender, and clinical presentation, including those with right bundle branch block and less than 1 mm of resting ST depression
- For risk stratification, functional class assessment, and prognosis in patients with suspected or known CAD based on age, gender, and clinical presentation
- To evaluate patients with known CAD who have noticed a significant change in their clinical status
- To evaluate patients with vasospastic angina
- To evaluate patients with low- or intermediate-risk unstable angina after they had been stabilized and who had been free of active ischemic symptoms or heart failure
- After MI for prognosis assessment, physical activity prescription, or evaluation of current medical treatment before discharge with a submaximal stress test 4 to 6 days after MI or after discharge with a symptoms-limited EST at least 14 to 21 days after MI
- To detect myocardial ischemia in patients considered for revascularization
- After discharge for physical activity prescription and counseling after revascularization as part of a cardiac rehabilitation program
- In patients with selected valvular abnormalities to assess functional capacity and symptomatic responses in those with a history of equivocal symptoms
- To evaluate the proper settings in patients who have received rate-responsive pacemakers
- To investigate patients with known or suspected exercise-induced arrhythmias

CAD, Coronary artery disease; *MI*, myocardial infarction.

5. What are the indications for exercise stress testing?

The most common indications for EST, according to the current American College of Cardiology (ACC) and American Heart Association (AHA) guidelines, are summarized in Box 5.1. When ordering an EST, three fundamental variables must be considered to achieve an optimal diagnostic test:

- Appropriate indication for EST
- Normal baseline ECG ST-T segments
- Ability to complete the planned exercise protocol

6. Should asymptomatic patients undergo exercise stress tests?

In general, EST for asymptomatic patients is discouraged because the pretest probability of CAD in this population is low, leading to a significant number of false-positive results and requiring unnecessary follow-up tests and expenses without a well-documented benefit. There are no data from randomized studies that support the use of routine screening EST in asymptomatic patients to reduce the risk of cardiovascular events. Nevertheless, selected asymptomatic patients may be considered for EST under specific clinical circumstances if clinically appropriate (e.g., diabetic patients planning to enroll in a vigorous exercise program, certain high-risk occupations, positive calcium score, family history).

7. What are contraindications for exercise stress testing?

Absolute contraindications include MI within 2 days, decompensated heart failure, uncontrolled cardiac arrhythmia or advanced heart block, severe symptomatic aortic stenosis, severe hypertrophic cardiomyopathy, and acute myocarditis. The contraindications and relative contraindications for EST according to the ACC/AHA guidelines are summarized in Box 5.2.

8. What parameters are monitored during an exercise stress test?

During EST, the following three parameters are monitored and reported:

- The patient's clinical response to exercise (e.g., shortness of breath, dizziness, chest pain, angina pectoris, Borg Scale score, functional capacity, etc.)
- The patient's hemodynamic response (e.g., heart rate, blood pressure response, etc.)
- The ECG changes that occur during exercise and the recovery phase of EST

9. What is an adequate heart rate to elicit an ischemic response?

It is essential to reach the target heart rate in EST. It is accepted that a heart rate of 85% of the maximal predicted heart rate for patient's age is sufficient to elicit an ischemic response in the presence of a hemodynamically significant coronary stenosis and is considered an adequate heart rate for a diagnostic exercise stress test. Reaching only 70% compared with 85% of the maximum age-predicted heart rate results in a decrease of stress-related myocardial perfusion defects from 100% to 47% using nuclear imaging and a reduction in anginal symptoms from 84% to 26%.

Box 5.2. Contraindications for Exercise Stress Testing

Absolute Contraindications

- Acute MI within 2 days
- High-risk unstable angina
- Uncontrolled cardiac arrhythmias causing symptoms or hemodynamic compromise
- Severe hypertrophic obstructive cardiomyopathy
- Severe symptomatic aortic stenosis
- Acute aortic dissection
- Acute pulmonary embolism or infarction
- Decompensated heart failure
- Acute myocarditis or pericarditis
- Active endocarditis
- Acute noncardiac disorder that may affect exercise performance or be aggravated by exercise (e.g., infection, renal failure, thyrotoxicosis)

Relative Contraindications

- Left main coronary stenosis
- Moderate aortic stenosis
- Electrolyte abnormalities
- Uncontrolled hypertension
- Advanced atrioventricular block
- Arrhythmias
- Moderate hypertrophic cardiomyopathy and other forms of left ventricular outflow obstruction
- Mental or physical impairment leading to inability to exercise adequately

MI, Myocardial infarction.

10. How do I calculate the predicted maximal heart rate?

The maximal predicted heart rate is estimated with the following formula:

$$\text{Maximal predicted heart rate} = 220 - \text{age}$$

11. What is the Borg Scale?

The Borg Scale is a numeric scale of perceived patient exertion; it is commonly used during EST. Values of 7 to 9 reflect light work and 13 to 17 hard work; a value above 18 is close to the maximal exercise capacity. Readings of 14 to 16 reach the anaerobic threshold. The Borg Scale is particularly useful in evaluating the patient's functional capacity during EST.

12. What is a metabolic equivalent?

METs are defined as the caloric consumption of an active individual compared with the basal metabolic rate at rest. They are used during EST as an estimate of functional capacity. One MET is defined as 1 kilocalorie per kilogram per hour and is the caloric consumption of a person while at complete rest (i.e., 2 METs will correspond to an activity that is twice the resting metabolic rate). Activities of 2 to 4 METs (light walking, doing household chores, etc.) are considered light, whereas running or climbing can yield 10 or more METs. A functional capacity below 5 METs during treadmill EST is associated with a worse prognosis, whereas higher METs during exercise are associated with better outcomes. Patients who can perform more than 10 METs during EST usually have a good prognosis regardless of their coronary anatomy, with very low rates of cardiac death, nonfatal MI, and coronary revascularization. Exercise capacity has been associated as a stronger predictor of mortality than nuclear imaging perfusion defects. These associations remain even in the setting of ischemic ST-segment depression during EST.

13. What is considered a hypertensive response to exercise?

The current ACC/AHA guidelines for EST suggest that a hypertensive response to exercise is one in which systolic blood pressure rises to more than 250 mm Hg or diastolic blood pressure rises to more than 115 mm Hg. This is considered a relative indication to terminate an EST.

14. Can I order an exercise stress test for a patient taking beta-blockers?

ESTs in patients taking beta-blockers may have reduced diagnostic and prognostic value because of an inadequate heart rate response. Nonetheless, according to the current ACC/AHA guidelines

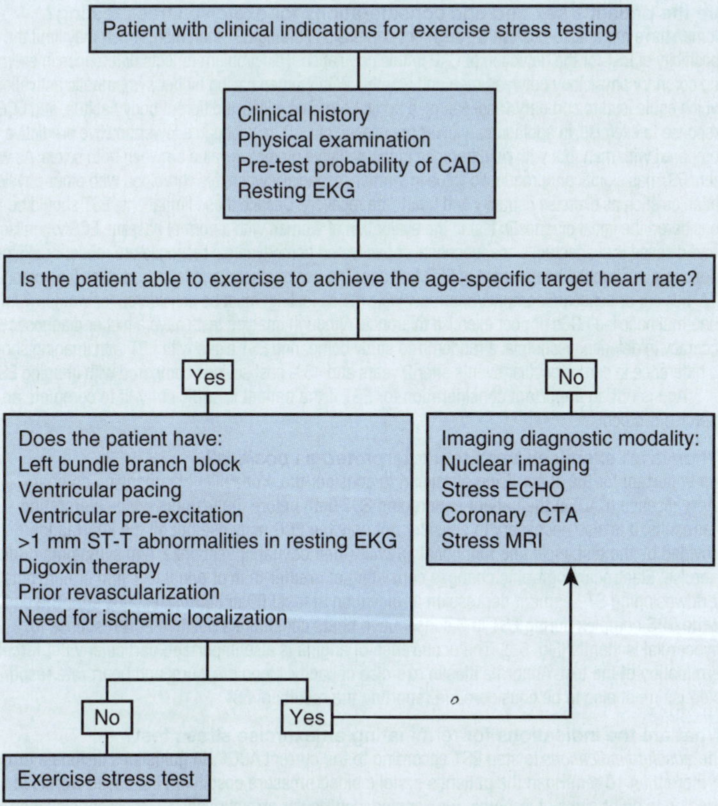

Fig. 5.1. Algorithm of variables to consider when ordering an exercise stress test.

for exercise testing, stopping beta-blockers before EST is discouraged so as to avoid "rebound" hypertension or anginal symptoms.

15. What baseline electrocardiographic findings interfere with the interpretation of an exercise stress test?

Patients with left bundle branch block (LBBB), ventricular pacing, more than 1-mm baseline ST-segment depression (i.e., left ventricular hypertrophy), and those with preexcitation syndromes (Wolff-Parkinson-White syndrome) should be considered for a different diagnostic modality because their baseline ECG abnormalities prevent an adequate ECG interpretation during exercise. Right bundle branch block does not significantly reduce the accuracy of the EST for the diagnosis of ischemia. Digoxin may also cause false-positive ST-segment depressions during exercise and is also an indication to consider an imaging modality to assess for ischemia. Fig. 5.1 presents an algorithm for selecting the appropriate stress test in different settings.

16. When can an exercise stress test be performed after an acute myocardial infarction?

Submaximal EST is occasionally recommended as early as 4 days after the acute event. This can be followed by later (3 to 6 weeks) symptom-limited EST. EST in this circumstance assists in formulating a prognosis, determining activity levels, assessing medical therapy, and planning cardiac rehabilitation. It is unclear whether asymptomatic patients who have had an acute MI with a consequent revascularization procedure benefit from follow-up EST, although it is not generally recommended if the patient is clinically stable.

17. Are the patient's sex and age considerations for exercise stress testing?

Women have more false-positive ST-segment depressions during EST than men, which may limit the specificity of EST for the detection of CAD in this population. This problem reflects differences in exercise and coronary physiology between men and women. With women having higher sympathetic activation (which could lead to coronary vasospasm), a cyclic hormonal milieu, a different body habitus, and ECG response to exercise, in addition to a lower prevalence of CAD, resulting in a lower positive predictive value compared with men; but with no difference in the negative predictive value between both sexes. As with men, EST has significant prognostic value in women, especially when it is combined with other physiologic variables such as exercise capacity and heart rate recovery. Despite these limitations, EST should be considered the initial diagnostic test in the evaluation of women with a normal baseline ECG when ischemic heart disease is suspected, since functional capacity and hemodynamic response are robust predictors of cardiovascular events independent of ECG findings. The use of other diagnostic modalities (i.e., coronary CTA, nuclear or echocardiographic/pharmacologic stress testing) must be considered for women with abnormal baseline ECGs or poor exercise tolerance. Although imaging tests have a higher diagnostic accuracy in detecting ischemia, a randomized study comparing EST alone with EST with imaging showed no difference in cardiovascular events after 2 years and 48% cost savings compared with imaging EST.

Age is not an important consideration for EST if the patient is sufficiently fit to complete an exercise protocol.

18. When is an exercise stress test interpreted as *positive*?

It is important for the supervising physician to consider the probability of underlying coronary artery disease (CAD) in the patient undergoing EST both before the test and while interpreting the results. It is also necessary to consider not only the ECG response but all the information provided by the test, including functional capacity, hemodynamic response, and symptoms during exercise. Electrocardiographic changes consisting of greater than or equal to 1 mm of horizontal or downsloping ST-segment depression or elevation at least 60 to 80 milliseconds after the end of the QRS complex during EST in 3 consecutive beats constitute a positive ECG response for myocardial ischemia (Fig. 5.2). The occurrence of angina is also important, particularly if it forces early termination of the test. Abnormalities in exercise capacity, blood pressure, and heart rate response to exercise must also to be considered in reporting the results of EST.

19. What are the indications for terminating an exercise stress test?

The *absolute indications* to stop EST according to the current ACC/AHA guidelines include a drop of more than 10 mm Hg in the patient's systolic blood pressure despite an increased workload in addition to other signs of ischemia (i.e., angina, ventricular arrhythmias), ST-segment elevation of more than 1 mm in leads without diagnostic Q waves (other than V1 and aVR), moderate to severe angina, neurologic symptoms (i.e., ataxia, dizziness, near syncope), signs of poor tissue perfusion (cyanosis or pallor), difficulties monitoring the ECG or blood pressure, sustained ventricular tachycardia, and the patient's request to stop the test.

Relative indications include a drop of more than 10 mm Hg in the patient's systolic blood pressure despite an increased workload in the absence of other evidence of ischemia; excessive ST-segment depression (more than 2 mm of horizontal or downsloping ST-segment depression) or marked QRS axis shift; arrhythmias other than sustained ventricular tachycardia; fatigue, shortness of breath, wheezing, leg cramps, or claudication; development of bundle branch block or intraventricular conduction delay that cannot be distinguished from ventricular tachycardia; hypertensive response to exercise; and increasing nonanginal chest pain.

20. What is a cardiopulmonary exercise stress test, and what are the indications of this diagnostic test?

During a cardiopulmonary EST the patient's ventilatory gas exchange is monitored in a closed circuit, and measurements of gas exchange are obtained during exercise (i.e., oxygen uptake, carbon dioxide output, anaerobic threshold) in addition to the information provided during routine EST. Cardiopulmonary EST is indicated to differentiate cardiac versus pulmonary causes of exercise-induced dyspnea or impaired exercise capacity. It is also used in the follow-up of patients with heart failure or those being considered for heart transplantation.

21. On the basis of the electrocardiogram obtained during exercise stress testing, can I localize which coronary artery is affected?

The ability of an ECG to localize an ischemic coronary territory during EST depends on the type of ST-segment change noted during exercise. Exercise-induced ST-segment depression is a nonspecific

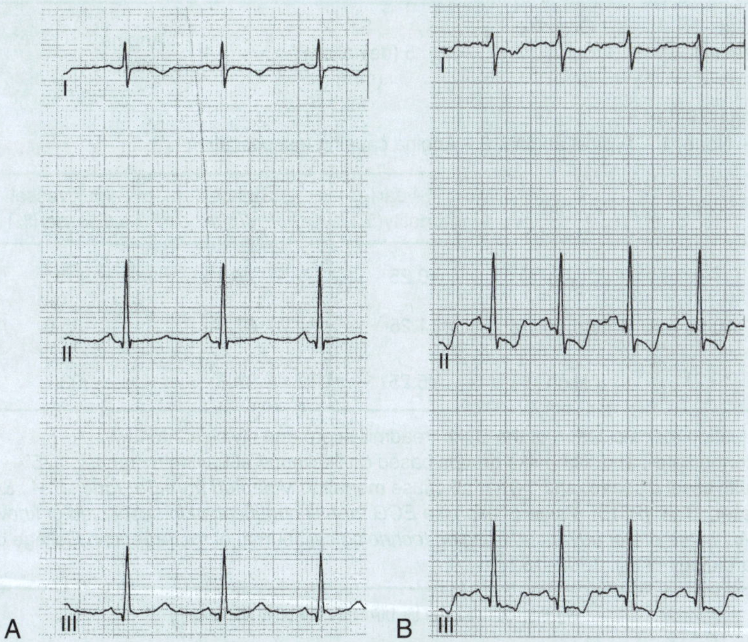

Fig. 5.2. Abnormal ECG response to exercise in a patient found to have severe stenosis of the right coronary artery. **A,** Normal baseline ECG. **B,** Abnormal ECG response at peak exercise with marked downsloping ST-segment depression and T-wave inversion.

ischemic change and cannot be used to localize any given coronary territory. Conversely, ST-segment elevation in a lead with no prior Q waves in a patient with no history of prior MI is consistent with transmural ischemia and can be used to localize the coronary territory affected.

22. **If a patient cannot exercise, can he or she still undergo stress testing?**
If the patient is unable to exercise, pharmacologic methods can detect ischemia by employing imaging modalities such as echocardiography, myocardial nuclear perfusion imaging, computed tomography, or magnetic resonance imaging. Imaging methods can increase the accuracy of detection of CAD at a relatively higher cost compared with EST alone, but they cannot predict functional capacity.

23. **How often should a stress test be repeated?**
Repeating an EST without a specific clinical indication at any interval has not been shown to improve risk stratification or prognosis in patients with or without known CAD and is discouraged. EST can be repeated when a significant change in the patient's cardiovascular status is suspected or according to the appropriate indications as noted in Box 5.1. In patients who have had prior revascularization, stress imaging studies are preferred, since they provide better information regarding the coronary distribution and severity of myocardial ischemia compared with EST.

24. **Is the 12-lead electrocardiogram obtained during an exercise stress test the same as a regular 12-lead electrocardiogram?**
To avoid motion during exercise, the conventional 12-lead ECG position requires that the extremity electrodes move close to the torso. This alternate lead position is called the Mason-Likar modification and requires placing the arm electrodes in the lateral aspect of the infraclavicular fossa and the leg electrodes between the iliac crest and below the rib cage. This change causes a right axis deviation and increased voltage in the inferior leads, which can obscure inferior Q waves and create new Q waves in aVL. Thus the ECG tracing obtained during an EST should not be used to interpret a diagnostic 12-lead ECG.

$$\text{Duke treadmill score} = \text{Exercise duration (min)} - 5\,\text{ST (deviation) (mm)} - 4\,(\text{Angina index})$$

Angina index:
0 – None, 1 – Typical angina, 2 – Angina causing test cessation

Score	Risk group	1-year mortality(%)	Stenosis >75%	Multivessel disease (%)
≥5	Low	0.25	40.1	23.7
–10 to 4	Intermediate	1.25	67.3	55.0
≤–11	High	5.25	99.6	93.7

Equation for calculation of the Duke treadmill score and division into low-, intermediate-, and high-risks groups based on likelihood of having a stenosis ≥75%, multivessel disease, and 1-year all-cause mortality. *(Adapted from Bourque, J. M., & Beller, G. A. [2015]. Value of exercise ECG for risk stratification in suspected or known CAD in the era of advanced imaging technologies.* Journal of the American College of Cardiology 8(11), *1309–1321.)*

Fig. 5.3. Calculation of the Duke treadmill score and its utility.

25. What is the Duke treadmill score?

It is a validated ECG treadmill score created at Duke University and based on data from 2758 patients who had chest pain and underwent EST and coronary angiography. The goal of the Duke score was to estimate the prognosis after EST more effectively. This treadmill score used three exercise-derived parameters. It adds independent prognostic information to that provided by clinical information, left ventricular function, or coronary anatomy and can be used to identify patients in the moderate- to high-risk group who may benefit from further risk stratification (Fig. 5.3).

26. How can I estimate the pretest probability of coronary artery disease?

Because an optimal diagnostic strategy depends on the pretest probability, improving the estimate of the pretest probability is helpful in selecting the best diagnostic modality for a particular patient and deciding on further management based on the results of such tests. The Diamond and Forrester model or the Duke clinical score can be used to estimate the pretest probability of CAD in patients presenting with stable chest pain. However, these models tend to overestimate the pretest probability of CAD in contemporary patients. Therefore more recently the CAD consortium calculator was developed and validated based on more than 5500 patients who underwent either coronary CTA, invasive coronary angiography, or both.

Bibliography and Suggested Readings

Arena, R., & Sietsema, K. E. (2011). Cardiopulmonary exercise testing in the clinical evaluation of patients with heart and lung disease. *Circulation, 123*(6), 668–680.

Bourque, J. M., & Beller, G. A. (2015). Value of exercise ECG for risk stratification in suspected or known CAD in the era of advanced imaging technologies. *JACC: Cardiovascular Imaging, 8*(11), 1309–1321.

Chou, R., Arora, B., Dana, T., Fu, R., Walker, M., & Humphrey, L. (2011). Screening asymptomatic adults with resting or exercise electrocardiography: a review of the evidence for the U.S. Preventive Services Task Force. *Annals of Internal Medicine, 155*(6), 375–385.

Douglas, P. S., Hoffmann, U., Patel, M. R., Mark, D. B., Al-Khalidi, H. R., Cavanaugh, B., et al. (2015). Outcomes of anatomical versus functional testing for coronary artery disease. *New England Journal of Medicine, 372*, 1291–1300.

Fordyce, C. B., Newby, D. E., & Douglas, P. S. (2016). Diagnostic strategies for the evaluation of chest pain. Clinical implications from SCOT-HEART and PROMISE. *Journal of the American College of Cardiology, 67*(7), 843–852.

Gibbons, R. J., Balady, G. J., Beasley, J. W., Bricker, J. T., Chaitman, B. R., Fletcher, G. F., et al. (2002). ACC/AHA 2002 guideline update for exercise testing. Summary article. A report of the American College of Cardiology/American Heart Association Task Force on Practice Guidelines. *Circulation, 106*(14), 1883–1892. <http://circ.ahajournals.org/cgi/content/full/106/14/1883>.

Hendel, R. C., Berman, D. S., Di Carli, M. F., Heidenreich, P. A., Henkin, R. E., Pellikka, P. A., et al. (2009). ACCF/ASNC/ACR/AHA/ASE/SCCT/SCMR/SNM 2009 Appropriate use criteria for cardiac radionuclide imaging. *Journal of the American College of Cardiology, 53*(23), 2201–2229. <http://www.asnc.org/imageuploads/AUCCardiacRadionuclideImaging2009.pdf>.

Lauer, M., Froelicher, E. S., Williams, M., & Kligfield, P. (2005). AHA scientific statement: exercise testing in asymptomatic adults. *Circulation.* <http://dx.doi.org/10.1161/CIRCULATIONAHA.105.166543.> <http://circ.ahajournals.org/cgi/content/full/112/5/771>. Accessed 13.09.16.

Lee, T. H., & Boucher, C. A. (2001). Noninvasive tests in patients with stable coronary artery disease. *New England Journal of Medicine, 344*, 1840–1845.

Mayo Clinic Cardiovascular Working Group on Stress Testing. (1996). Cardiovascular stress testing: a description of the various types of stress tests and indications for their use. *Mayo Clinic Proceedings, 71*, 43–52.

Miller, T. D. (2011). Stress testing: the case for the standard treadmill test. *Current Opinion in Cardiology, 26*(5), 363–369.

Mudrick, D. W., Cowper, P. A., Shah, B. R., Patel, M. R., Jensen, N. C., Peterson, E. D., et al. (2012). Downstream procedures and outcome after stress testing for chest pain without known coronary artery disease in the United States. *American Heart Journal, 163*, 454–461.

CHAPTER 6

AMBULATORY ELECTROCARDIOGRAM MONITORING

Mark Pollet, Glenn N. Levine

1. **What are the major indications for ambulatory electrocardiogram monitoring?**
   Ambulatory electrocardiogram (AECG) monitoring allows the noninvasive evaluation of a suspected arrhythmia during normal daily activities. It aids in the diagnosis, documentation of frequency, severity, and correlation of an arrhythmia with symptoms such as palpitations, lightheadedness, or overt syncope. AECG monitoring can be extremely helpful in excluding an arrhythmia as a cause for a patient's symptoms if there is no associated event during monitoring. AECG can also be used to assess antiarrhythmic drug response in patients with defined arrhythmias. Occasionally AECG is also used in other situations. The current major indications for AECG monitoring are given in Box 6.1.

2. **What are the different types of ambulatory electrocardiogram monitoring available?**
   The major types of AECG monitoring include Holter monitoring, event monitoring, ambulatory telemetry, patch monitoring, and monitoring with an implantable loop recorder (ILR) (Fig 6.1). The type and duration of monitoring depend on the frequency and severity of symptoms. Most modern devices

Box 6.1. Summary of the American College of Cardiology/American Heart Association Guidelines for Ambulatory Electrocardiography and Indications for Ambulatory Electrocardiogram Monitoring

Class I (Recommended)

- Patients with unexplained syncope, near syncope, or episodic dizziness in whom the cause is not obvious
- Patients with unexplained recurrent palpitations
- To assess antiarrhythmic drug response in individuals with well-characterized arrhythmias
- To aid in the evaluation of pacemaker and ICD function and guide pharmacologic therapy in patients receiving frequent ICD therapy

Class IIa (Weight of Evidence/Opinion Is in Favor of Usefulness/Efficacy)

- To detect proarrhythmic responses in patients receiving antiarrhythmic therapy
- Patients with suspected variant angina

Class IIb (Usefulness/Efficacy Is Less Well Established by Evidence/Opinion)

- Patients with episodic shortness of breath, chest pain, or fatigue that is not otherwise explained
- Patients with symptoms such as syncope, near syncope, episodic dizziness, or palpitation in whom a probable cause other than an arrhythmia has been identified but in whom symptoms persist despite treatment
- To assess rate control during atrial fibrillation
- Evaluation of patients with chest pain who cannot exercise
- Preoperative evaluation for vascular surgery of patients who cannot exercise
- Patients with known coronary artery disease and atypical chest pain syndrome
- To assess risk in asymptomatic patients who have heart failure or idiopathic hypertrophic cardiomyopathy or in post–myocardial infarction patients with ejection fraction less than 40%
- Patients with neurologic events when transient atrial fibrillation or flutter is suspected

ICD, Implantable cardioverter defibrillator.

are capable of the transtelephonic transmission of ECG data during or after a detected arrhythmia. Each system has advantages and disadvantages; selection must be tailored to the individual. With any system, however, patients must record in some fashion (e.g., diary, electronically) symptoms and activities during the monitored period.

- **Holter monitors:** A Holter monitor constantly monitors and records 2 to 3 channels of ECG data for 24 to 48 hours. It is ideal for patients with episodes that occur daily.
- **Event monitors:** An event monitor constantly monitors 2 to 3 channels of ECG data for 30 to 60 days. However, it will record events only when the patient experiences a symptom and presses a button that triggers the event monitor to store ECG data 1 to 4 minutes before and 1 to 2 minutes after the event. Some event monitors will also store arrhythmias detected by the monitor itself, based on preprogrammed parameters. An event monitor is appropriate for patients with episodes that occur weekly or monthly.
- **Ambulatory real-time cardiac monitors:** Ambulatory real-time cardiac monitoring has various names. It has been called ambulatory telemetry, real-time continuous cardiac monitoring, and mobile cardiac telemetry (MCOT). Ambulatory telemetry is a monitoring system that continuously records a 1- to 3-lead strip for 14 to 30 days. Depending on the vendor, the ECG data are either stored for offline interpretation or instantaneously transmitted for interpretation by a monitoring technician. In cases where the rhythm is monitored by a technician in real time, the patient or physician can be contacted immediately after an arrhythmia has been detected, thus minimizing delays in treatment. No patient action is necessary for an arrhythmia to be stored and patient compliance can easily be assessed. These features facilitate the detection of silent or asymptomatic arrhythmias.
- **Adhesive patch electrocardiographic monitors:** Adhesive patch monitors self-adhere to the chest wall and are worn continuously for several weeks. Advantages include the patient's ability to wear the device continuously and not have to connect and disconnect wire leads. Currently available devices provide only a single ECG channel.
- **Implantable loop recorders:** An ILR is an invasive monitoring device that allows long-term monitoring and recording of a single ECG channel for over a year. Like an event monitor, it records events based on the patient's symptoms or automatically based on heart rate. It is best reserved for patients with more infrequent episodes occurring more than 1 month apart.

3. How does an implantable loop recorder work?

An ILR is placed subcutaneously below the left shoulder or overlying the fourth anterior intercostal spaces. Previous devices required a small surgical incision for placement. The more recent, smaller version of the device is placed via an incision smaller than 1 cm and a syringe-like device. As discussed above, it monitors bipolar ECG signals continuously for up to a year or more. The patient can use a magnetic activator held over the device to trigger an event at the time of symptoms. In addition, the device automatically records episodes of bradycardia and tachycardia. The older device is then interrogated with an external programmer and recorded events reviewed in a similar manner to a permanent pacemaker. The newer device wirelessly connects to a patient monitor. After a diagnosis is obtained, the device is surgically extracted. In patients with unexplained syncope, an ILR yields a diagnosis in more than 90% of cases after 1 year. An example of an older and a newer ILR is shown in Fig. 6.2. A representative printout of ILR interrogation is shown in Fig. 6.3.

4. Do patients with pacemakers or implantable cardioverter defibrillators require Holter monitors for the detection atrial arrhythmias?

Most modern pacemakers or implantable cardioverter defibrillators (ICDs) will detect and store arrhythmias. The number and types of arrhythmias detected depend on the number of leads, device type, and programming, as well as manufacturing specifications. Detected arrhythmias can be reviewed upon device interrogation.

5. Is every "abnormality" detected during monitoring a cause for concern?

No. It is not uncommon to identify several arrhythmias during AECG that are not necessarily pathologic. These include sinus bradycardia during rest or sleep, sinus arrhythmia with pauses less than 3 seconds, sinoatrial exit block, Wenckebach atrioventricular (AV) block (type I second-degree AV

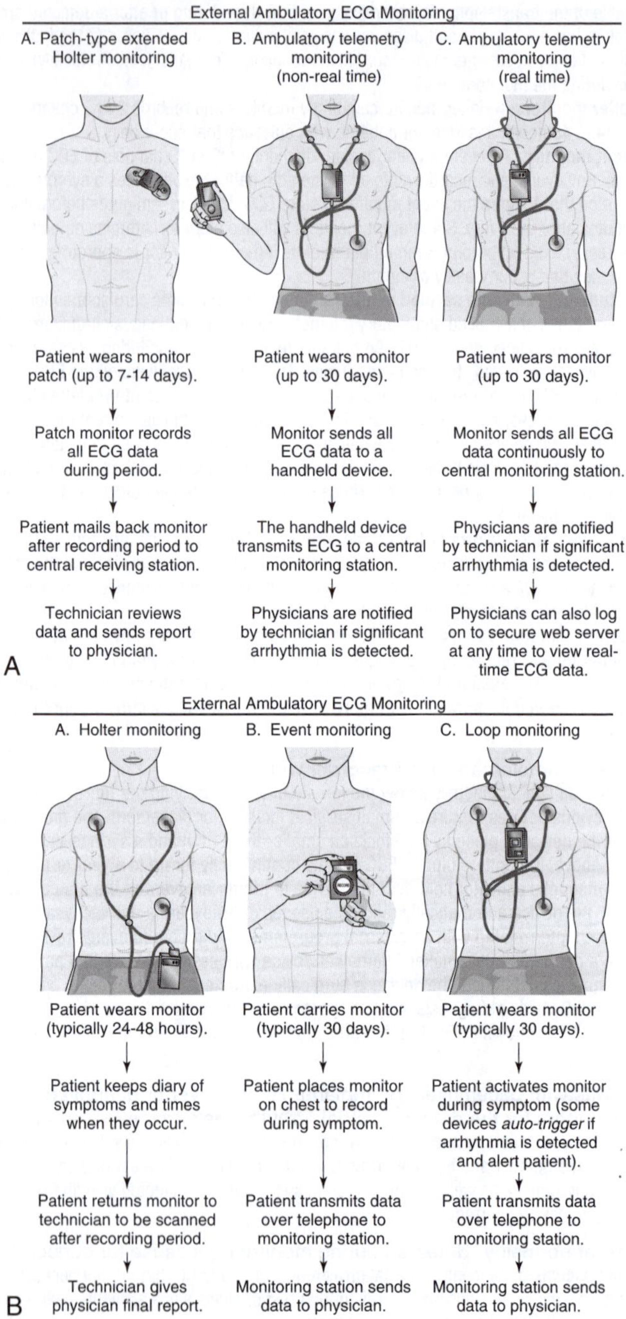

Fig. 6.1. **(A)** Types of AECG monitors currently available in clinical practice. **(B)** Types of AECG monitors currently available in clinical practice. *AECG,* Ambulatory external electrocardiogram; *ECG,* electrocardiogram. *(Figure illustrated by Craig Skaggs.)*

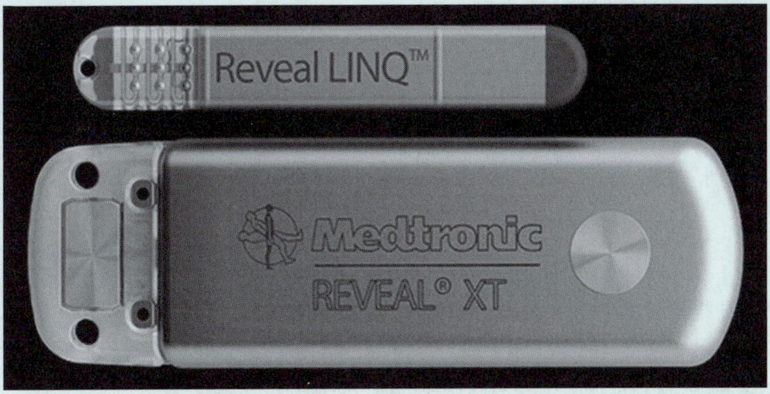

Fig. 6.2. Example of an older (lower image) and a more recent (upper image) generation implantable loop recorder (ILR). Note the more compact size of the newer ILR.

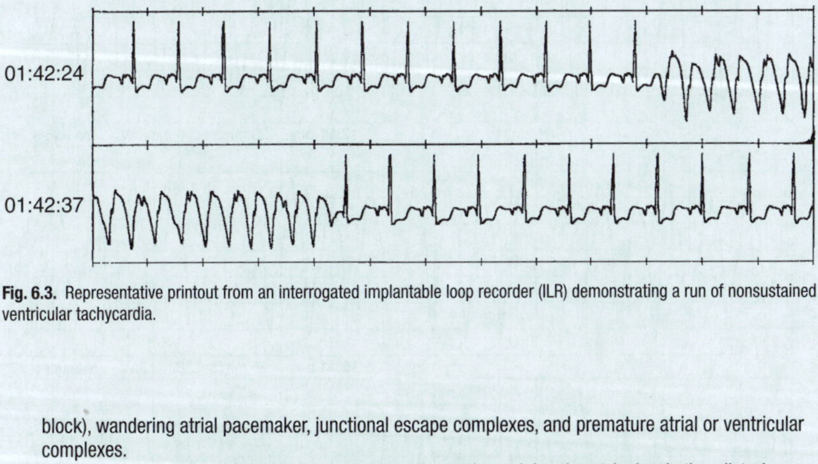

Fig. 6.3. Representative printout from an interrogated implantable loop recorder (ILR) demonstrating a run of nonsustained ventricular tachycardia.

block), wandering atrial pacemaker, junctional escape complexes, and premature atrial or ventricular complexes.

In contrast, often of concern are frequent and complex atrial and ventricular rhythm disturbances that are less commonly observed in normal subjects, including second-degree AV block type II, third-degree AV block, sinus pauses longer than 3 seconds (Fig. 6.4), marked bradycardia during waking hours, and tachyarrhythmias (Fig. 6.5). One of the most important factors for any documented arrhythmia is the correlation with symptoms. In some situations, even some "benign" rhythms may warrant treatment if there are associated symptoms.

6. What is the diagnostic yield of Holter monitors, event monitors, and implantable loop recorders in palpitations and syncope?

Choosing a Holter monitor, an event monitor or patch recorder, or an ILR depends on the frequency of symptoms. In patients with palpitations the highest diagnostic yield occurs in the first week, with 80% of patients receiving a diagnosis. During the next 3 weeks, only an additional 3.4% of patients receive a diagnosis. In patients with recurrent but infrequent palpitations (<1 episode per month lasting >1 minute), ILR resulted in a diagnosis in 73% of patients. In contrast to palpitations, syncope usually requires a longer monitoring period to achieve a diagnosis, with the highest yield coming from the implantation of an ILR.

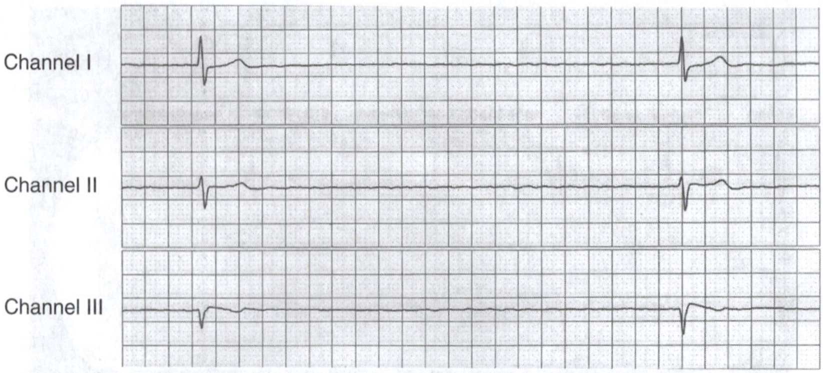

Fig. 6.4. A 4-second pause detected by a 3-channel ambulatory ECG monitor. The patient was being monitored for episodes of sudden presyncope.

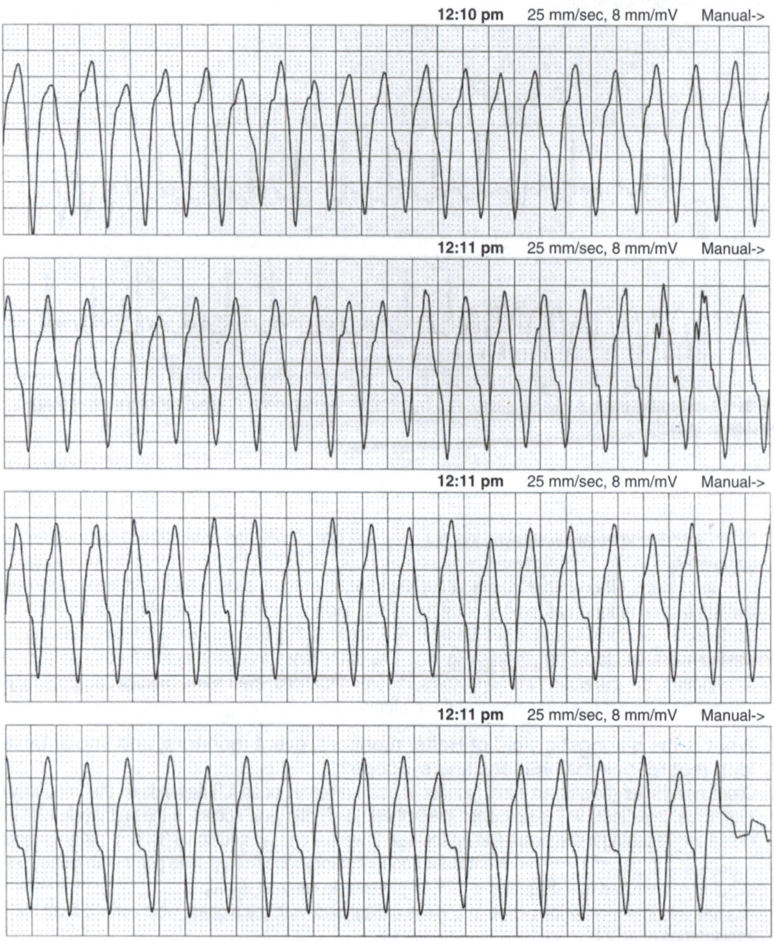

Fig. 6.5. Sustained ventricular tachycardia detected by a Holter monitor in a patient with daily episodes of palpitations and lightheadedness.

7. How often are ventricular arrhythmias identified in apparently healthy subjects during ambulatory electrocardiogram monitoring?

Ventricular arrhythmias are found in 40% to 75% of normal persons as assessed by 24- to 48-hour Holter monitoring. The incidence and frequency of ventricular ectopy increases with age, but this has no impact on long-term prognosis in apparently healthy subjects.

8. What is the significance of frequent premature ventricular contractions detected by ambulatory monitoring?

Frequent premature ventricular contractions (PVCs) can result in a potentially reverse form of cardiomyopathy. The PVC burden is the percentage of heartbeats throughout the course of a day that are PVCs rather than normal sinus beats. When the burden surpasses 24%, a reduction in left ventricular (LV) ejection fraction is significantly more likely to occur. Ablation of these PVCs can improve the LV ejection fraction by an average of 12% and can eliminate the indications for an automatic implantable cardioverter defibrillator (AICD) for this cardiomyopathy in 64% to 92% of patients.

9. What is the role of ambulatory electrocardiogram monitoring in patients with known ischemic heart disease?

Although ejection fraction after myocardial infarction is one of the strongest predictors of survival, AECG monitoring can be helpful in further risk stratification. Ventricular arrhythmias occur in 2% to 5% of patients in long-term follow-up after transmural infarction. In the post–myocardial infarction patient, the occurrence of frequent PVCs (more than 10 per hour) and nonsustained ventricular tachycardia (VT) by 24-hour monitoring is associated with a 1.5- to 2.0-fold increase in death during the 2- to 5-year follow-up independent of LV function.

10. Can Holter monitors assist in the diagnosis of suspected ischemic heart disease?

Yes. Transient ST-segment depression 0.1 mV or greater for more than 30 seconds is rare in normal subjects and correlates strongly with myocardial perfusion scans that show regional ischemia. Although some monitors can detect and quantify ST-segment changes, in current clinical practice Holter monitors are rarely used for this purpose.

11. What have Holter monitors demonstrated about angina and its pattern of occurrence?

Holter monitoring has shown that the majority of ischemic episodes that occur during normal daily activities are silent (asymptomatic) and that symptomatic and silent episodes of ST-segment depression exhibit a circadian rhythm, with ischemic ST changes more common in the morning. Studies have also shown that nocturnal ST-segment changes are a strong indicator of significant coronary artery disease.

12. What is the role of ambulatory monitoring in stroke?

Approximately 25% of stroke remains unexplained after a thorough clinical evaluation and is labeled as cryptogenic. Asymptomatic paroxysmal atrial fibrillation may not occur during telemetry monitoring during hospitalization. Occult atrial fibrillation is identified by ambulatory monitoring in approximately, 3% to 8% of patients with cryptogenic stroke in whom atrial fibrillation is not detected during their hospitalization. Implantation of a loop recorder can increase the rate of detection to 30% over the 3 years following a stroke.

Bibliography and Suggested Readings

Assar, M. D., Krahn, A. D., Klein, G. J., Yee, R., & Skanes, A. C. (2003). Optimal duration of monitoring in patients with unexplained syncope. *American Journal of Cardiology*, *92*, 1231–1233.

Baman, T., Bogun, F., Lange, D. C., Ilg, K. J., Gupta, S. K., Liu, T. Y., et al. (2010). Relationship between burden of premature ventricular complexes and left ventricular function. *Heart Rhythm*, *7*(7), 865–869.

Crawford, M. H., Bernstein, S. J., Deedwania, P. C., DiMarco, J. P., Ferrick, K. J., Garson, A., Jr., et al. (1999). ACC/AHA guidelines for ambulatory electrocardiography: executive summary and recommendations: a report of the American College of Cardiology/American Heart Association Task Force on Practice Guidelines (Committee to revise the guidelines for ambulatory electrocardiography). *Circulation*, *100*, 886–893.

Dixit, S., & Marchlinski, F. E. (2011). Role of continuous monitoring for optimizing management strategies in patients with early arrhythmia recurrences after atrial fibrillation ablation. *Circulation. Arrhythmia and Electrophysiology*, *4*(6), 791–793.

Enseleit, F., & Duru, F. (2006). Long-term continuous external electrocardiographic recording: a review. *Europace*, *8*, 255–266. http://dx.doi.org/10.1093/europace/euj054.

Kadish, A. H., Reiffel, J. A., Clauser, J., Prater, S., Menard, M., & Kopelman, H. (2010). Frequency of serious arrhythmias detected with ambulatory cardiac telemetry. *American Journal of Cardiology, 105*(9), 1313–1316.

Mittal, S., Movsowitz, C., & Steinberg, J. S. (2011). Ambulatory external electrocardiographic monitoring. *Journal of the American College of Cardiology, 58*(17), 1741–1749.

Wimmer, N. J., Scirica, B. M., & Stone, P. H. (2013). The clinical significance of continuous ECG (ambulatory ECG or Holter) monitoring of the ST-segment to evaluate ischemia: a review. *Progress in Cardiovascular Diseases, 56*(2), 195–202.

Zimetbaum, P., & Goldman, A. (2010). Ambulatory arrhythmia monitoring: choosing the right device. *Circulation, 122*(16), 1629–1636.

ECHOCARDIOGRAPHY

Nicolas Palaskas, Glenn N. Levine

1. **How does echocardiography work?**
Echocardiography uses transthoracic and transesophageal probes that emit ultrasound directed at cardiac structures. Ultrasound is a mechanical vibration that is reflected and refracted, and its velocity or speed is determined by the medium through which it passes, where velocity equals frequency multiplied by wavelength. Returning ultrasound signals are received by the probe, and the computer in the ultrasound machine uses algorithms to reconstruct images of the heart. The time it takes for the ultrasound to return to the probe determines the depth of the structures relative to the probe because the speed of sound in soft tissue is relatively constant (1540 ms). The amplitude (intensity) of the returning signal determines the density and size of the structures with which the ultrasound comes in contact.

The probes also perform Doppler, which measures the frequency shift of the returning ultrasound signal to determine the speed and direction of moving blood through heart structures (e.g., through the aortic valve) or in the myocardium itself (tissue Doppler imaging).

Appropriateness criteria for obtaining an echocardiogram are given in Box 7.1.

Box 7.1. Appropriateness Criteria for Echocardiography

Appropriate indications include but are not limited to:

- Symptoms possibly related to cardiac etiology, such as dyspnea, shortness of breath, lightheadedness, syncope, cerebrovascular events
- Initial evaluation of left-sided ventricular function after acute myocardial infarction
- Evaluation of cardiac murmur in suspected valve disease
- Sustained ventricular tachycardia or supraventricular tachycardia
- Evaluation of suspected pulmonary artery hypertension
- Evaluation of acute chest pain with nondiagnostic laboratory markers and electrocardiogram
- Evaluation of known native or prosthetic valve disease in a patient with change of clinical status

Uncertain indications for echocardiography include:

- Cardiovascular source of embolic event in a patient who has normal transthoracic echocardiogram (TTE) and electrocardiogram findings and no history of atrial fibrillation or flutter

Inappropriate indications for echocardiography include:

- Routine monitoring of known conditions, such as heart failure, mild valvular disease, hypertensive cardiomyopathy, repair of congenital heart disease, or monitoring of an artificial valve, when the patient is clinically stable
- Echocardiography is also not the test of choice in the initial evaluation for pulmonary embolus and should not be routinely used to screen asymptomatic hypertensive patients for heart disease.

Appropriate indications for transesophageal echocardiography (TEE) as the initial test instead of TTE include:

- Evaluation of suspected aortic pathology including dissection
- Guidance during percutaneous cardiac procedures including ablation and mitral valvuloplasty
- To determine the mechanism of regurgitation and suitability of valve repair
- To diagnose or manage endocarditis in patients with moderate to high probability of endocarditis
- Persistent fever in a patient with an intracardiac device
- TEE is ***not*** appropriate in evaluation for a left atrial thrombus in the setting of atrial fibrillation when it has already been decided to treat the patient with anticoagulant drugs.

Modified from Douglas, P. S., Khandheria, B., Stainback, R. F., Weissman, N. J., Brindis R. G., Patel M. R., et al. (2007). ACCF/ASE/ACEP/ASNC/SCAI/SCCT/SCMR 2007 appropriateness criteria for transthoracic and transesophageal echocardiography. *Journal of the American College of Cardiology*, 50, 187–204.

2. What is the difference between echocardiography and Doppler?

Echocardiography usually refers to two-dimensional (2D) ultrasound interrogation of the heart in which the brightness mode (B-mode) is utilized to image cardiac structures based on their density and location relative to the chest wall. 2D echocardiography is particularly useful for identifying cardiac anatomy and morphology, such as identifying a pericardial effusion, left ventricular aneurysm, or cardiac mass. It provides excellent spatial resolution but lesser temporal resolution than M-mode (discussed later).

Also included in the majority of echocardiographic studies is M-mode (Fig. 7.1) which was the first ultrasound imaging technique. M-mode differs from 2D echocardiography in that only a single line of ultrasound beam is transmitted and received by the probe. This provides better temporal resolution but worse spatial resolution.

Doppler refers to interrogation of the movement of blood in and around the heart, based on the shift in frequency *(Doppler shift)* that ultrasound undergoes when it comes in contact with a moving object (usually red blood cells). Doppler has three modes:

1. Pulsed Doppler (Fig. 7.2A), which can localize the site of flow acceleration but is prone to aliasing
2. Continuous-wave Doppler (see Fig. 7.2B), which cannot localize the level of flow acceleration but can identify very high velocities without aliasing
3. Color Doppler (Fig. 7.3), which utilizes different colors (usually red and blue) to identify flow toward and away from the transducer, respectively, and identify flow acceleration qualitatively by showing a mix of color to represent high velocity or aliased flow, thus creating a map of velocities on a 2D image.

Doppler is particularly useful for assessing the hemodynamic significance of cardiac structural disease, such as the severity of aortic stenosis, degree of mitral regurgitation, flow velocity across a ventricular septal defect, or severity of pulmonary hypertension.

A large majority of echocardiograms are ordered as *echocardiography with Doppler* to answer cardiac morphologic and hemodynamic questions in one study (e.g., a mitral stenosis murmur); 2D echo to identify the restricted, thickened, and calcified mitral valve; and Doppler to analyze its severity based on transvalvular flow velocities and gradients.

3. How is systolic function assessed using echocardiography?

The most commonly used measurement of left ventricular (LV) systolic function is left ventricular ejection fraction (LVEF), which is defined by:

$$\text{LVEF} = \frac{(\text{End-diastolic volume} - \text{end-systolic volume})}{\text{End-diastolic volume}}$$

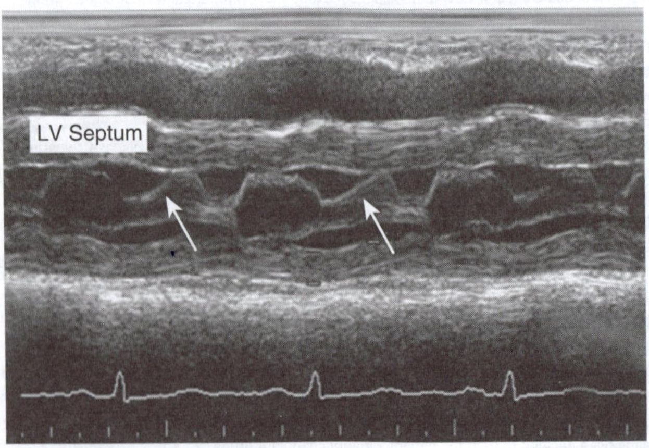

Fig. 7.1. M-mode echocardiography showing an example of systolic anterior motion of the mitral valve *(arrows)* in a patient with hypertrophic obstructive cardiomyopathy and thickened septal wall. M-mode is one linear beam of ultrasound seen through time. This allows for better temporal resolution, such as in this case to see the anterior mitral leaflet opening during systole in which it should be closed.

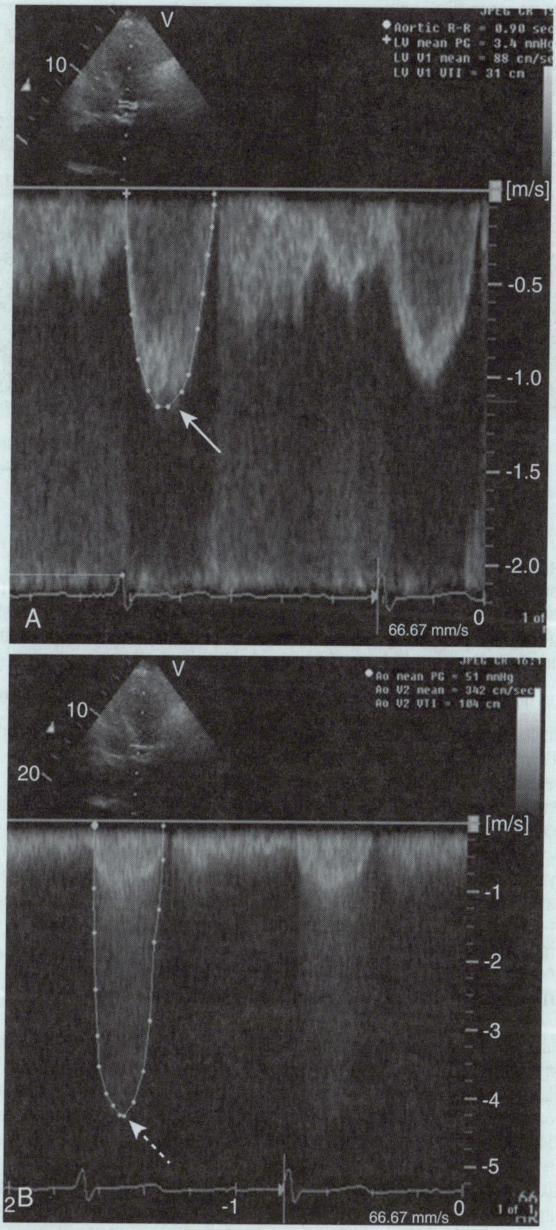

Fig. 7.2. Doppler assessment used in patients with aortic stenosis. **A,** Pulsed Doppler in the left ventricular outflow tract in a patient with aortic stenosis. The peak velocity of the spectral tracing *(solid arrow)* is 1.2 ms, indicating normal flow velocity proximal to the aortic valve. **B,** Continuous Doppler across the aortic valve revealing a peak velocity of 4.5 ms *(dashed arrow)*. Therefore, the blood flow velocity nearly quadrupled across the stenotic aortic valve, consistent with severe aortic stenosis.

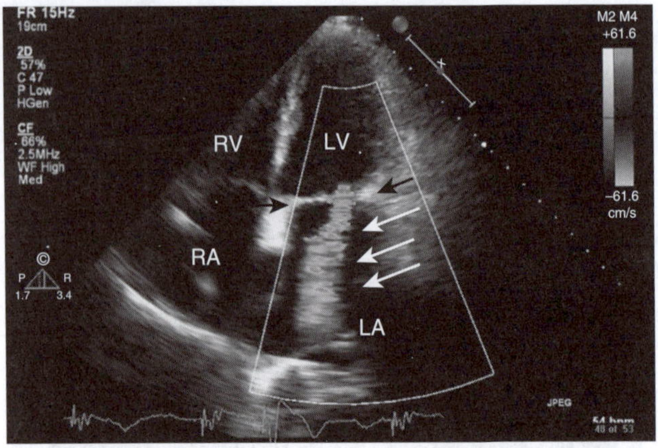

Fig. 7.3. Mitral regurgitation. Apical four-chamber view with color Doppler revealing severe mitral regurgitation *(white arrows). Black arrows* point to the mitral valve. Note that, in actuality, the regurgitant jet is displayed in color, corresponding to the flow of blood. *LA,* Left atrium; *LV,* left ventricle; *RA,* right atrium; *RV,* right ventricle.

There are several methods by which left ventricular function is assessed:

- Simpson's method (method of disks), in which the LV endocardial border of multiple *slices* of the left ventricle is traced in systole and diastole, and the end-diastolic and end-systolic volumes are computed from these tracings, which is one of the most common methods of calculating LVEF.
- The Teicholz method, in which the shortening fraction

  (LV end-diastolic dimension – LV end-systolic dimension)/LV end-diastolic dimension

  is multiplied by 1.7 and can also be used to estimate LVEF, although this method is inaccurate in patients with regional wall motion abnormalities.
- Visual estimation of LVEF by expert echocardiography readers is also commonly used.
- Increasingly, state-of-the-art full volume acquisition using three-dimensional echocardiography can be used to provide accurate LVEF.
- Systolic dysfunction in the presence of preserved LVEF (more than 50%)—such as in patients with hypertrophic hearts, ischemic heart disease, or infiltrative cardiomyopathies—can be identified by other methods such as longitudinal strain imaging, which assesses the longitudinal motion of the myocardium, as opposed to the previously given methods, which mainly assess radial myocardial movement.

4. What is an echocardiographic diastolic assessment? What information can it provide?

A diastolic assessment does two things: identifies LV relaxation and estimates LV filling pressures. LV relaxation is described as the time it takes for the LV to relax in diastole to accept blood from the left atrium (LA) through an open mitral valve. A normal heart is very elastic *(lussitropic)* and readily accepts blood during LV filling. When relaxation is impaired, the LV cannot easily accept increased volume, and this increased LV preload results in increases in LA pressure, which in turn results in pulmonary edema.

LV relaxation is usually best determined using tissue Doppler imaging, which assesses early diastolic filling velocity (Ea) of the LV myocardium. Tissue Doppler is similar to Doppler of the blood flow but changes the settings to allow the transducer to measure velocities that are over 100-fold slower than blood velocity. Normal hearts have Ea of 10 cm/s or greater on the lateral wall and Ea of 8 cm/s or greater on the septal wall; impaired relaxation is present when Ea is less than 10 cm/s or 8 cm/s for the lateral and septal wall, respectively.

An indicator of LV preload is peak transmitral early diastolic filling velocity (E), which measures the velocity of blood flow across the mitral valve. An estimate of the LV filling pressure can be made using the ratio of blood flow velocity across the mitral valve (E) to the velocity of myocardial tissue during early diastole (referred to as the E/Ea ratio). A high E/Ea ratio (e.g., E/Ea >13 averaged between septal and lateral walls) indicates elevated LV filling pressure (LA pressure >15 mm Hg); a lower ratio (e.g., E/Ea <8 averaged between septal and lateral walls) indicates normal LV filling pressure (LA pressure <15 mm Hg). Anything in between is generally considered indeterminate, although there are other specific measurements such as left atrial volume, isovolumetric relaxation time, pulmonary artery systolic pressure, and change in E/A ratio with Valsalva that may suggest elevated or normal filling pressures.

5. How can echocardiography with Doppler be used to answer cardiac hemodynamic questions?

- Doppler echocardiography can be used to estimate stroke volumes, valvular gradients, and pulmonary arterial pressure, as well as to assess hemodynamics in cases of suspected cardiac tamponade or constrictive pericarditis.
- Stroke volume and cardiac output can be calculated by using measurements of the LV outflow tract and time-velocity integral (TVI) of blood through the LV outflow tract. The LV outflow tract area times the TVI equals blood flow through the LV outflow tract.
- Doppler evaluation of right ventricular outflow tract diameter and TVI similarly allow calculation of right ventricular output.
- Tricuspid regurgitation peak velocity gradient is used to estimate the pressure gradient across the tricuspid valve. When added to an estimate of right atrial pressure, this provides an estimation of pulmonary artery systolic pressure.
- Mitral inflow velocities, deceleration time, pulmonary venous parameters, and tissue Doppler imaging of the mitral annulus can give accurate assessment of LV diastolic function, including LV filling pressures.
- Measurement of TVI and valve annular diameters can be used to assess intracardiac shunts (QP/QS) and regurgitant flow volumes.
- Pressure gradients across native and prosthetic valves and across cardiac shunts can be used to assess hemodynamic severity of valve stenosis, regurgitation, or shunt severity, respectively.
- Respiratory variation in valvular flow can aid in the diagnosis of cardiac tamponade or constrictive pericarditis.

6. How is echocardiography used to evaluate valvular disease?

2D echocardiography can provide accurate visualization of valve structure to assess morphologic abnormalities (calcification, prolapse, flail, rheumatic disease, and endocarditis). Fig. 7.4 demonstrates the restricted movement of the mitral valve in a patient with mitral stenosis. Three-dimensional echocardiography is being used more often now to better characterize valvular disorders prior to surgical or percutaneous intervention. It allows for the valve to be seen from a surgical view (Fig. 7.5).

Color Doppler can provide semiquantitative assessment of the degree of valve regurgitation (mild, moderate, severe) for any of the four cardiac valves (aortic, mitral, pulmonic, tricuspid). Pulsed Doppler can help pinpoint the location of a valvular abnormality (e.g., subaortic versus aortic versus supraaortic stenosis). It can also be used to quantitate regurgitant volumes and fractions using the continuity equation. Continuous-wave Doppler is useful for determining the hemodynamic severity of stenotic lesions, such as aortic or mitral stenosis.

7. How can echocardiography help diagnose and manage patients with suspected pericardial disease?

Echocardiography can diagnose pericardial effusions (Fig. 7.6) as fluid in the pericardial space readily transmits ultrasound (appears black on echo). 2D echocardiography and Doppler are pivotal in determining the hemodynamic impact of pericardial fluid—that is, whether the patient has elevated intrapericardial pressure or frank cardiac tamponade.

The following are indicators of elevated intrapericardial pressure in the setting of pericardial effusion:

- Diastolic indentation or collapse of the right ventricle (RV)
- Compression of the right atrium (RA) for more than one-third of the cardiac cycle
- Lack of inferior vena cava (IVC) collapse (<50%) with deep inspiration
- 25% or greater variation in mitral or aortic Doppler flows
- 50% or greater variation of tricuspid or pulmonic valve flows with inspiration

Echocardiographic signs of constrictive pericarditis include thickened or calcified pericardium, diastolic *bounce* of the interventricular septum, restrictive mitral filling pattern with 25% or greater respiratory variation in peak velocities, and lack of inspiratory collapsibility of the IVC.

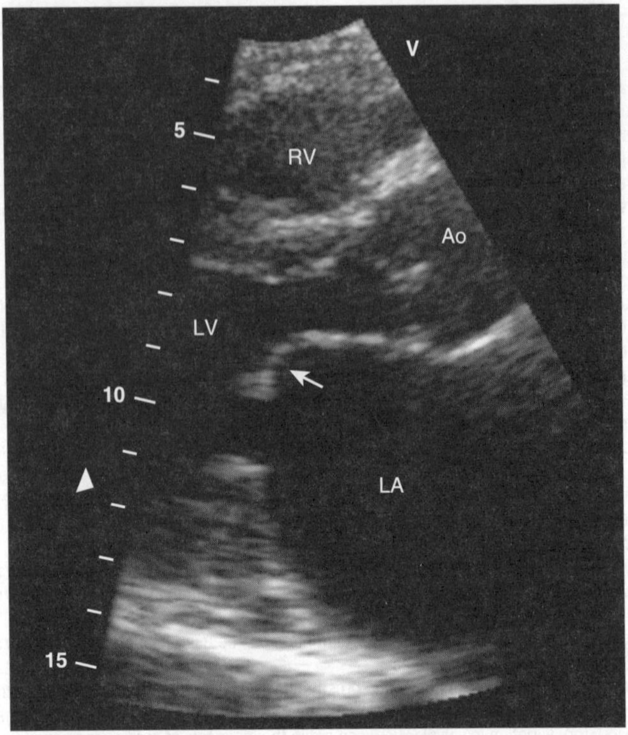

Fig. 7.4. Parasternal long-axis view showing typical *hockey stick* appearance of the mitral valve *(arrow)* in rheumatic mitral stenosis. *Ao,* Aortic valve; *LA,* left atrium; *LV,* left ventricle; *RV,* right ventricle.

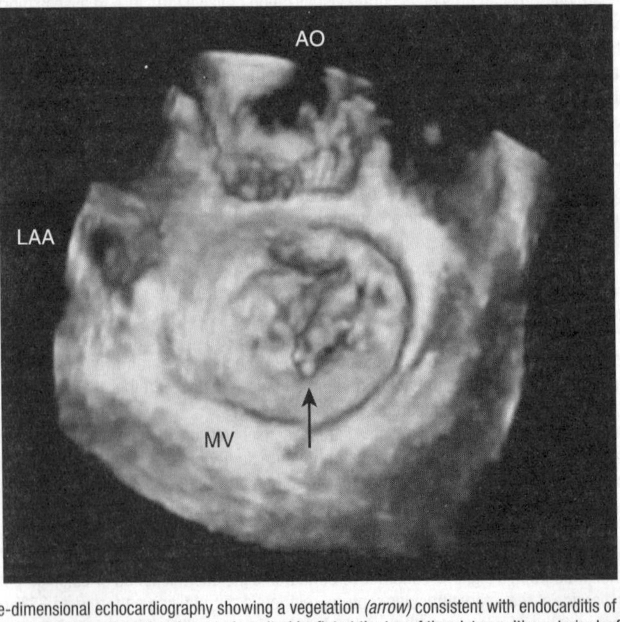

Fig. 7.5. Three-dimensional echocardiography showing a vegetation *(arrow)* consistent with endocarditis of the mitral valve. This is the surgical view depicting the anterior mitral leaflet at the top of the picture with posterior leaflet at the bottom. The annulus, relationship of the two leaflets, and vegetation can clearly be seen in relation to one another. *Ao,* Aortic valve; *LAA,* left atrial appendage; *MV,* mitral valve. *(Image reproduced with permission from Levine, G. N. [Ed.] [2015].* Color atlas of cardiovascular disease. *New Delhi: Jaypee Brothers Medical Publishers.)*

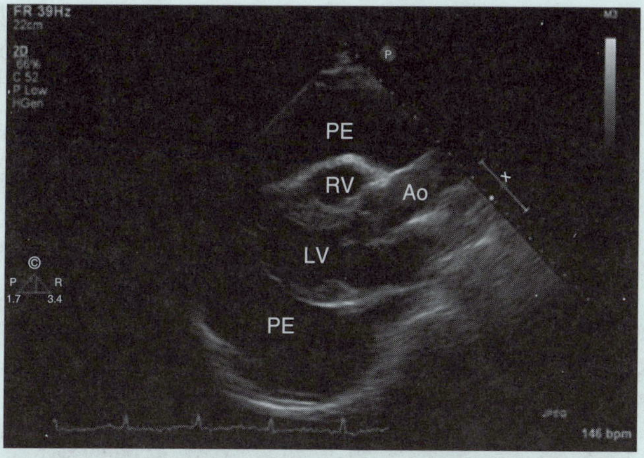

Fig. 7.6. Parasternal long-axis view showing a large pericardial effusion (PE) surrounding the heart. *LV,* Left ventricle; *RV,* right ventricle. *(From Kabbani, S. S., & LeWinter, M. [2001]. Cardiac constriction and restriction. In M. H. Crawford & J. P. DiMarco [Eds.].* Cardiology. *St. Louis, MO: Mosby.)*

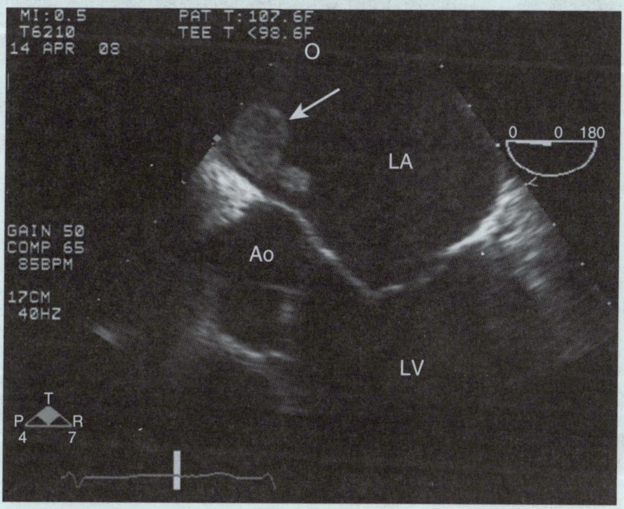

Fig. 7.7. Transesophageal echocardiography showing a left atrial thrombus *(arrow). Ao,* Aortic valve; *LA,* left atrium; *LV,* left ventricle.

Echocardiography is additionally useful for guiding percutaneous needle pericardiocentesis by identifying the transthoracic or subcostal window with the largest fluid *cushion,* monitoring decrease of fluid during pericardiocentesis, and in follow-up studies, assessing for reaccumulation of fluid.

8. What is the role of echocardiography in patients with ischemic stroke?

The following are echocardiographic findings that may be associated with a cardiac embolic cause in patients with stroke:

- Depressed LV ejection fraction, generally less than 40%
- Left atrial or left ventricular clot (Figs. 7.7 and 7.8)

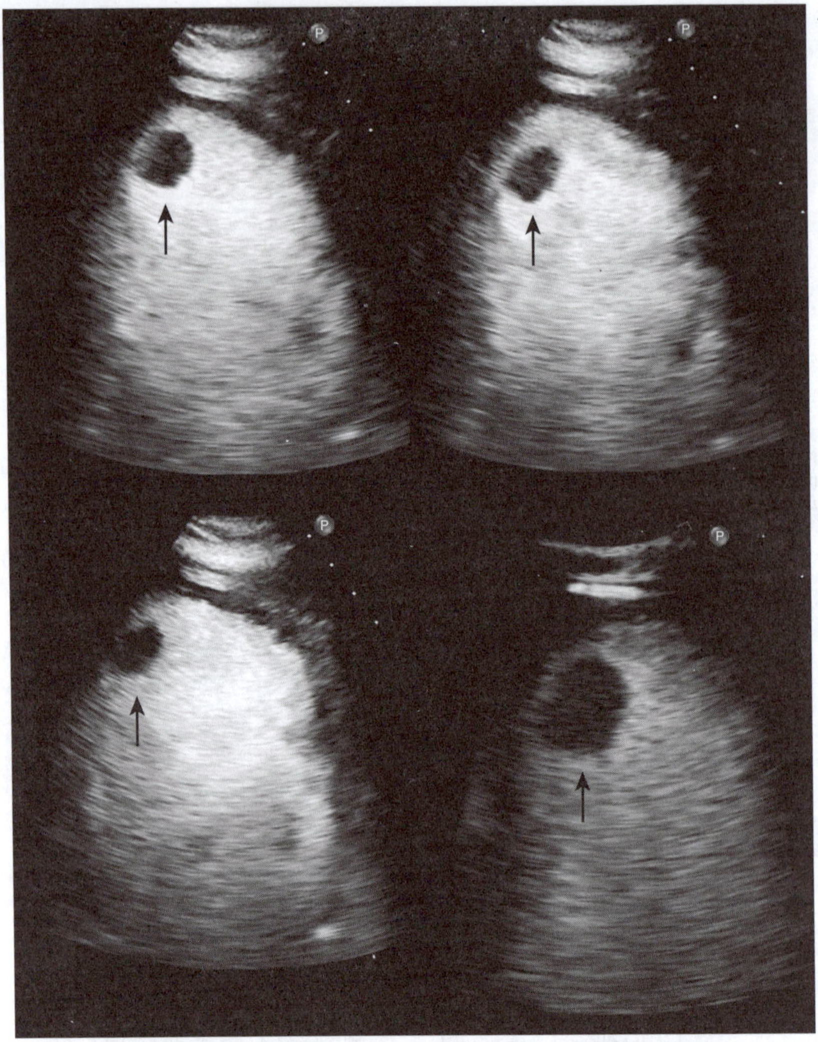

Fig. 7.8. Contrast echocardiography using perflutren showing a mobile left ventricular thrombus *(arrow)* in the apex of the left ventricle. *(Image reproduced with permission from Levine, G. N. [Ed.]. [2015].* Color atlas of cardiovascular disease. *New Delhi: Jaypee Brothers Medical Publishers.)*

- Intracardiac mass such as tumor or endocarditis
- Mitral stenosis (especially with a history of atrial fibrillation)
- Prosthetic valve in the mitral or aortic position
- Significant atherosclerotic disease in the aortic root, ascending aorta, or aortic arch
- Saline contrast study indicating a significant right to left intracardiac shunt, such as atrial septal defect (Fig. 7.9)

A normal transthoracic echocardiogram in a patient without atrial fibrillation generally excludes a cardiac embolic source of clot and generally obviates the need for transesophageal echocardiography (TEE).

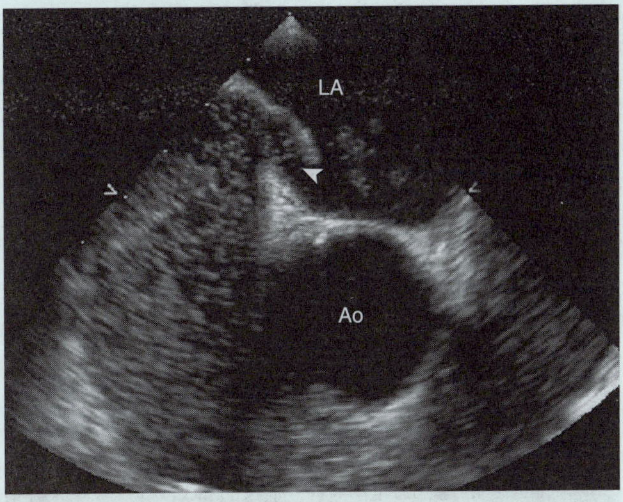

Fig. 7.9. Bubble study showing opacification of the right atrium with bubble and 2D echocardiography showing a patent foramen ovale *(arrow)* with some crossing of bubble to the left atrium. *Ao,* Aortic valve; *LA,* left atrium.

9. What are the echocardiographic findings in hypertrophic cardiomyopathy?

Hypertrophic cardiomyopathy (HCM) is a genetic disorder with numerous phenotypical presentations. The classic finding is asymmetric septal hypertrophy with septal wall thickness greater than 1.5 cm in diameter (measured at end diastole). However, in addition to this well-known form of HCM, other forms of HCM exist, including concentric HCM and apical HCM (Yamaguchi's hypertrophy).

The presence of systolic anterior motion (SAM) of the mitral valve can be seen in some cases of HCM, particularly in patients with asymmetric septal hypertrophy (Fig. 7.10). The increased flow velocity of blood at the area of dynamic obstruction creates a Venturi effect, which "sucks" the anterior mitral leaflet toward the left ventricular outflow tract, worsening the dynamic obstruction and additionally leading to mitral regurgitation.

10. What are the common indications for transesophageal echocardiography?

TEE allows better visualization of cardiac structures, as the probe is positioned in the esophagus immediately adjacent to the heart. TEE is most commonly used for the evaluation of suspected endocarditis, for assessment of valvular regurgitation etiology and severity, and to exclude left atrial appendage thrombus. Indications for TEE include:

- Significant clinical suspicion of endocarditis in patients with suboptimal transthoracic windows
- Significant clinical suspicion of endocarditis in patients with prosthetic heart valve
- Suspected aortic dissection (Fig. 7.11)
- Suspected atrial septal defect (ASD) or patent foramen ovale in patients with cryptogenic embolic stroke
- Embolic stroke with nondiagnostic transthoracic echo
- Endocarditis with suspected valvular complications (abscess, fistula, pseudoaneurysm)
- Evaluation of the mitral valve in cases of possible surgical mitral valve
- Intracardiac shunt in which the location is not well seen on transthoracic echocardiography
- Assessment of the left atria and left atrial appendage for the presence of thrombus (clot) (see Fig. 7.7) prior to planned cardioversion

11. What is contrast echocardiography?

Contrast echocardiography involves injection of either saline contrast or synthetic microbubbles (perflutren bubbles) into a systemic vein and then imaging the heart using ultrasound. Saline contrast, because of its relatively large size, does not cross the pulmonary capillary bed, and it therefore is confined to the right heart. Therefore, rapid appearance of saline contrast in the left heart indicates an intracardiac shunt.

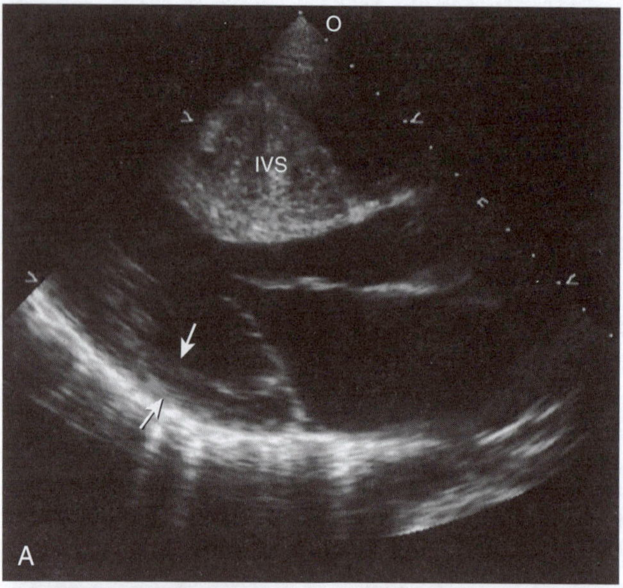

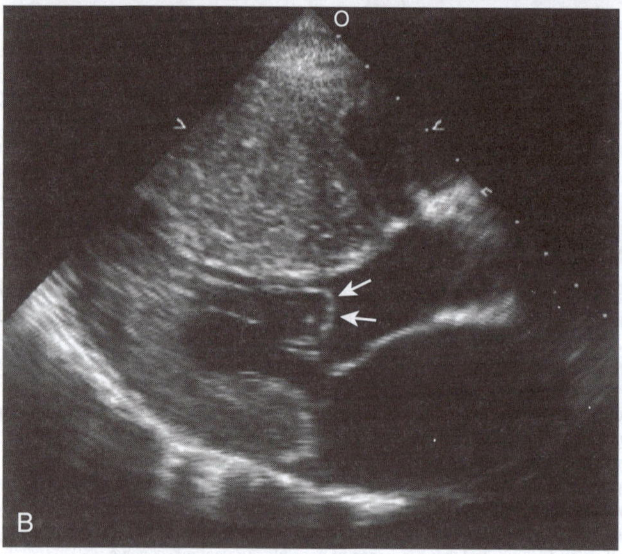

Fig. 7.10. Echocardiographic findings in hypertrophic cardiomyopathy. **A,** Parasternal long axis image during diastole demonstrating massive thickening of the interventricular septum (IVS) when compared to the thickness of the posterior wall *(white arrows)*. **B,** During systole echocardiography demonstrates systolic anterior motion (SAM) of the mitral valve, with the leaflets actually bowing in to the left ventricular outflow tract *(white arrows)*.

Because synthetic microbubbles are smaller than saline bubbles, they cross the pulmonary capillaries and are used to image left heart structures. Most commonly, synthetic microbubbles are used to achieve better endocardial border definition in patients with suboptimal echocardiographic windows. Contrast is also used to better visualize structures such as possible LV thrombus or masses (see Fig. 7.8).

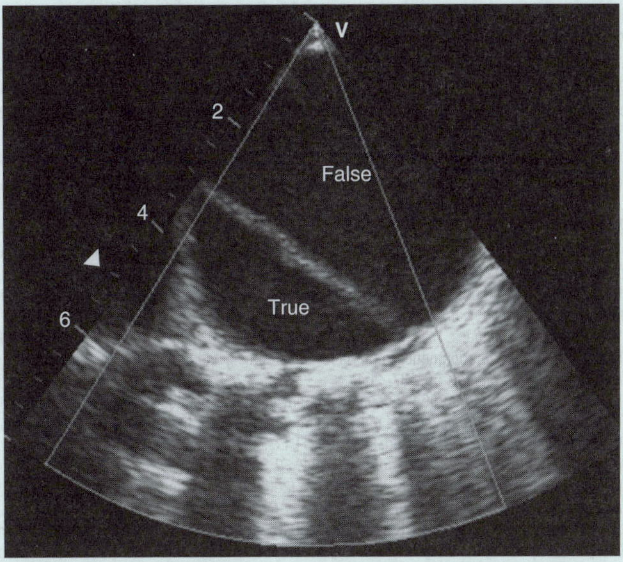

Fig. 7.11. Transesophageal echocardiography revealing dissection of the descending thoracic aorta. The true aortic lumen *(true)* is seen separated from the false lumen *(false)* by the dissection.

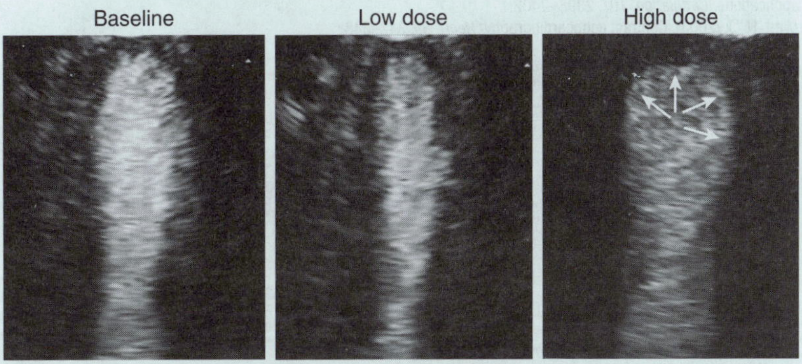

Fig. 7.12. An example of contrast-enhanced dobutamine stress echocardiography. The contrast agent is used to better visualize wall motion. Images during systole are shown. At low-dose dobutamine infusion there is increased contractility. At high-dose dobutamine infusion there is decreased contractility in the distal anterior wall and apex *(arrows)*, suggesting a hemodynamically significant stenosis in the mid left anterior descending artery. *(Image reproduced with permission from Levine, G. N. [Ed.] [2015].* Color atlas of cardiovascular disease. *New Delhi: Jaypee Brothers Medical Publishers.)*

Both synthetic and saline contrast can be used to augment Doppler signals, for example, in patients with pulmonary hypertension in whom a tricuspid regurgitation jet is needed to estimate pulmonary artery pressure.

12. What is stress echocardiography?

Stress echocardiography involves imaging the heart first at rest and subsequently during either exercise (treadmill or bike) or pharmacologic (usually dobutamine) stress to identify LV wall motion abnormalities resulting from the presence of flow-limiting coronary artery disease (Fig. 7.12). Generally it is performed with contrast to better delineate wall motion abnormalities.

Other uses of stress echocardiography include:

- Assessment of mitral or aortic valve disease in patients who have moderate disease at rest but significant symptoms with exercise
- Assessment of patients with suspected exercise-induced diastolic dysfunction
- Assessment of viability in patients with depressed ejection fractions. Improvement in left ventricular function with infusion of low-dose dobutamine (<10 μg/kg per min) suggests viable myocardium.
- Distinguishing between true aortic stenosis and *pseudo*–aortic stenosis in patients with mild to moderate aortic stenosis at rest and depressed ejection fraction with low cardiac output

Bibliography and Suggested Readings

Abraham, T. P., Dimaano, V. L., & Liang, H. Y. (2007). Role of tissue Doppler and strain echocardiography in current clinical practice. *Circulation, 116*, 2597–2609.

Armstrong, W. F., & Zoghbi, W. A. (2005). Stress echocardiography: current methodology and clinical applications. *Journal of the American College of Cardiology, 45*, 1739–1747.

Douglas, P. S., Khandheria, B., Stainback, R. F., Weissman, N. J., Brindis, R. G., Patel, M. R., et al. (2007). ACCF/ASE/ACEP/ASNC/SCAI/SCCT/SCMR 2007 appropriateness criteria for transthoracic and transesophageal echocardiography. *Journal of the American College of Cardiology, 50*, 187–204.

Evangelista, A., & Gonzalez-Alujas, M. T. (2004). Echocardiography in infective endocarditis. *Heart, 90*, 614–617.

Grayburn, P. A. (2008). How to measure severity of mitral regurgitation: valvular heart disease. *Heart, 94*, 376–383.

Kirkpatrick, J. N., Vannan, M. A., Narula, J., & Lang, R. M. (2007). Echocardiography in heart failure: applications, utility, and new horizons. *Journal of the American College of Cardiology, 50*, 381–396.

Lang, R. M., Mor-Avi, V., Sugeng, L., Nieman, P. S., & Sahn, D. J. (2006). Three-dimensional echocardiography: the benefits of the additional dimension. *Journal of the American College of Cardiology, 48*, 2053–2069.

Lester, S. J., Tajik, A. J., Nishimura, R. A., Oh, J. K., Khandheria, B. K., & Seward, J. B. (2008). Unlocking the mysteries of diastolic function: deciphering the Rosetta Stone 10 years later. *Journal of the American College of Cardiology, 51*, 679–689.

Otto, C. M. (2006). Valvular aortic stenosis: disease severity and timing of intervention. *Journal of the American College of Cardiology, 47*, 2141–2151.

Peterson, G. E., Brickner, M. E., & Reimold, S. C. (2003). Transesophageal echocardiography: clinical indications and applications. *Circulation, 107*, 2398–2402.

Stewart, M. J. (2003). Contrast echocardiography. *Heart, 89*, 342–348.

CHAPTER 8

NUCLEAR CARDIOLOGY

Laura Flink, Lawrence Phillips

1. What is nuclear cardiology?

Nuclear cardiology is a field of cardiology that includes cardiac radionuclide imaging, using radioisotopes to assess myocardial perfusion and myocardial function in different clinical settings, as well as radionuclide angiography, metabolic and receptor imaging, and positron emission tomography.

2. What is myocardial perfusion imaging?

Myocardial perfusion imaging (MPI) is a noninvasive method that utilizes radioisotopes to assess regional myocardial blood flow, function, and viability. MPI is used to identify ischemic or infarcted regions by detecting differences in blood flow during stress compared with rest.

During the stress portion of the test, exercise causes an increase in myocardial demand, or a pharmacologic agent is used to produce vasodilation in the coronary vascular bed. A normal vessel vasodilates and can increase coronary blood flow up to four times its baseline in response to stress. However, a markedly diseased or stenotic vessel cannot increase blood flow to the myocardium. The radiotracer is delivered to the myocardium via the blood vessel, so the inability to vasodilate results in less radiotracer uptake. The areas of myocardium supplied by diseased blood vessels will therefore take up less radiotracer than the areas supplied by normal blood vessels because of relatively less blood flow. This heterogeneous radiotracer uptake is seen as a perfusion defect.

3. What are the uses of myocardial perfusion imaging?

- To diagnose coronary artery disease (CAD) in patients with intermediate risk for CAD who present with symptoms concerning for CAD
- To localize and quantify ischemia in patients with known CAD to help guide medical decision making
- To determine infarct size in patients with known CAD
- For risk stratification in those with elevated coronary calcium score on computed tomography (CT) imaging
- To determine areas of residual ischemia or areas of myocardium at risk after revascularization
- To assess the presence of viability of myocardium for consideration of revascularization

4. What is a perfusion defect, and how can a fixed and reversible defect be differentiated?

A perfusion defect is an area of reduced radiotracer uptake in the myocardium. If the perfusion defect occurs during both stress and rest, it is termed a *fixed* defect. Generally, a fixed defect suggests the presence of scar (Fig. 8.1). However, in certain settings a fixed defect may not be scar. Instead, a fixed defect may represent viable tissue that is hibernating due to chronic significant or severe stenosis. Myocardium that is hibernating is able to decrease its metabolism in order to conserve energy. Therefore, it will appear underperfused at both rest and post stress and have hypokinetic or akinetic contractile function. A fixed defect can also be an artifact whereby the diaphragm or the breast, for example, interferes with the nuclear camera's detection of the presence of radiotracer resulting in the image appearing to have a perfusion defect. This can be differentiated by looking at wall motion, because if a fixed defect is truly a scar, there should be some associated wall motion abnormality.

If the perfusion defect occurs during stress and improves or normalizes during rest, it is termed *reversible* (Fig. 8.2). Under basal (rest) conditions, the stenotic coronary artery is still able to supply needed blood flow to the myocardium. There is no difference in radiotracer uptake between segments of myocardium supplied by stenotic and nonstenotic coronary artery segments. However, under stress, the stenotic or diseased vessel cannot vasodilate as much as the healthy vessels, resulting in heterogeneous tracer uptake. When compared to rest images, the stress images have decreased radiotracer uptake in the segments of the myocardium provided by the diseased blood vessels and the perfusion defect is noted to be reversible. Generally, a reversible perfusion defect suggests the presence of ischemia. Defects are categorized as mild, moderate, or severe, depending on the severity

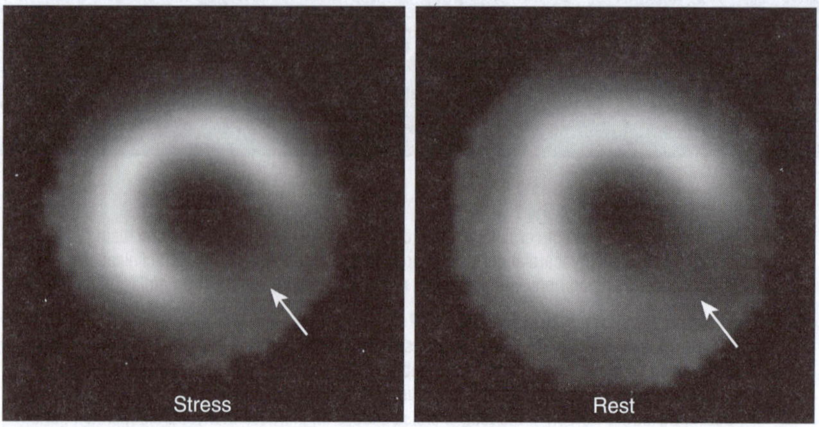

Fig. 8.1. Nuclear stress test showing a fixed inferolateral perfusion defect *(arrows)*, suggestive of prior transmural myocardial infarction. The arrows show that the filling defect is present on both stress and rest imaging.

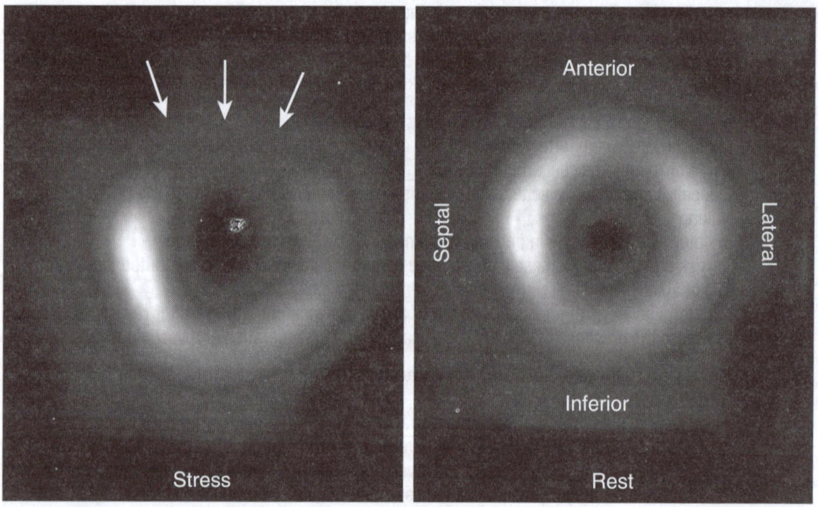

Fig. 8.2. Nuclear testing short-axis view demonstrating a reversible perfusion defect. Normal myocardial perfusion occurred during resting images *(right panel)*, but a large anterior wall perfusion defect *(arrows)* was seen during previous stress imaging *(left panel)*. (Modified from Texas Heart Institute Website: Nuclear stress test. Available at http://www.textsheartinstitute.org/HIC/Topics/Diag/dinuc.cfm. Accessed 1/5/17.

of perfusion defect. They are categorized as small, medium, or large in size, depending on how many myocardial segments are involved. The size and severity of the defect allow the clinician to determine the risk of the defect and aids in clinical decision making.

Semiquantitative analysis of perfusion defects aids in description of the severity of the defect, increases reproducibility of the measurement of the degree of abnormality, and provides prognostic information. Using a 17-segment model (Fig. 8.3), scores from 0 to 4 are assigned to each segment to delineate the severity of perfusion defect. A score of 0 is for normal count, 1 is mildly reduced, 2 is moderately reduced, 3 is severely reduced, and 4 is absent uptake. A summed rest score (SRS) and summed stress score (SSS) can be calculated. The difference between these two scores is called the sum difference score (SDS). The SDS is the amount of ischemia present. An SDS of less than 4 is consistent with no/equivocal ischemia, 4 to 6 mild

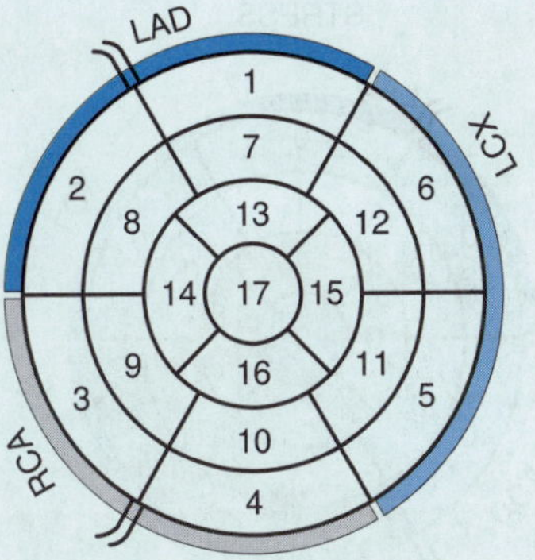

1 – basal anterior	7 – mid anterior	13 – apical anterior
2 – basal anteroseptal	8 – mid anteroseptal	14 – apical septal
3 – basal inferoseptal	9 – mid inferoseptal	15 – apical lateral
4 – basal inferior	10 – mid inferior	16 – apical inferior
5 – basal inferolateral	11 – mid inferolateral	17 – apical
6 – basal anterolateral	12 – mid anterolateral	

Fig. 8.3. The 17-segment left ventricle model. LAD, Left anterior descending artery; LCX, Left circumflex artery; RCA, Right coronary artery.

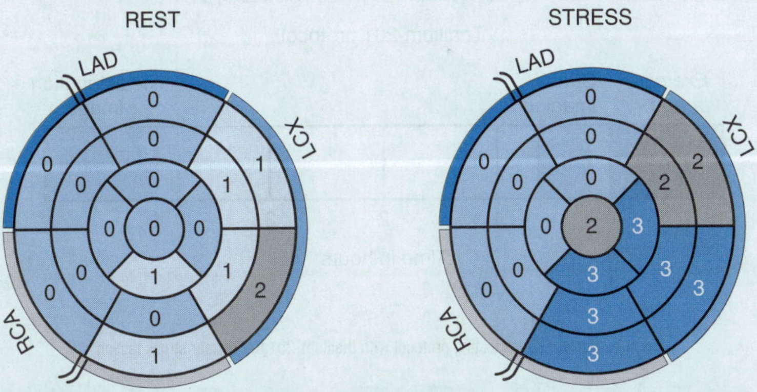

Fig. 8.4. Semi-quantitative evaluation of myocardial ischemia. The summed rest score (SRS) is 7, and the summed stress score (SSS) is 24. The sum difference score (SDS), which represents the amount of ischemia present, is 17 (SSS minus SRS), corresponding to severe ischemia. LAD, Left anterior descending artery; LCX, Left circumflex artery; RCA, Right coronary artery.

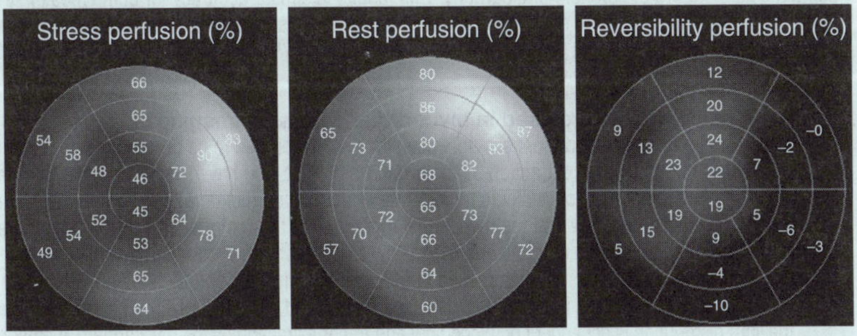

Fig. 8.5. Nuclear stress test results, displayed in the "bull's-eye" 17-segment model, demonstrating anterior and anteroseptal wall ischemia.

ischemia, 7 to 10 moderate ischemia, and greater than 11 severe ischemia. Fig. 8.4 shows an example using this method of a large area of inferolateral ischemia. Fig. 8.5 shows an example of anterior and anteroseptal wall ischemia. Fig. 8.6 shows an example of a patient with a myocardial scar.

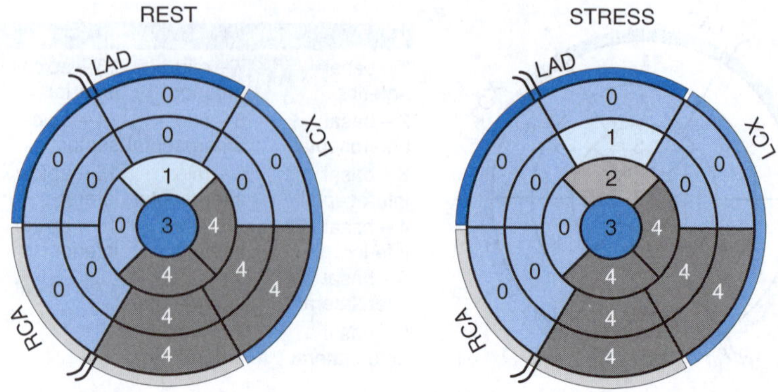

Fig. 8.6. Nuclear stress test results, displayed in the "bull's-eye" 17-segment model. The SRS score is 28, and the SSS score is 30, and thus the SDS score is 2. These findings indicate inferolateral infarct with a small amount of peri-infarct ischemia. LAD, Left anterior descending artery; LCX, Left circumflex artery; RCA, Right coronary artery.

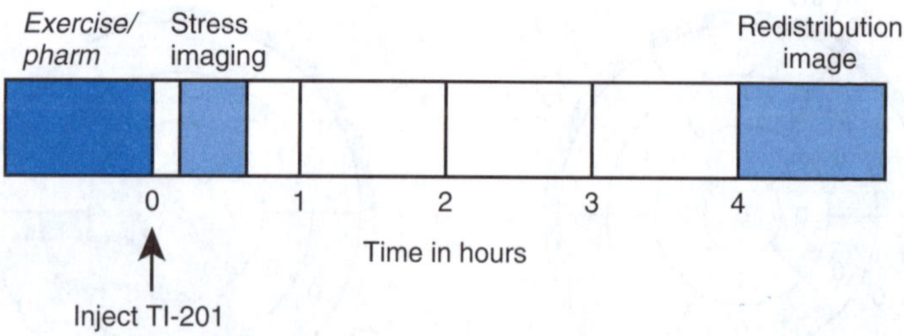

Fig. 8.7. Nuclear stress testing protocol with thallium-201 for nuclear stress testing.

5. **What are the sensitivity and specificity of myocardial perfusion imaging for diagnosing coronary artery disease?**

The sensitivity of an MPI for detecting ischemia or infarction is slightly better than stress echocardiography (85% vs. 75%, respectively), and the specificity is slightly worse (79% vs. 88%) using a gold standard of coronary angiography. This results in similar accuracy for both types of stress tests. Both modalities are more sensitive and specific than exercise electrocardiography testing alone, which has a sensitivity of about 68% and a specificity of about 77% and is thought to less sensitive and specific in women than in men.

6. **What perfusion agents are used in myocardial perfusion imaging?**

For an agent to be an effective radiopharmaceutical, its distribution has to be proportional to regional blood flow, have a high level of extraction by the organ of interest, and have rapid clearance from the blood. The two most important physiologic factors that affect myocardial uptake of a radiotracer are variations in regional blood flow and the myocardial extraction of the radiotracer. There will be more uptake of a radiotracer in areas of increased blood flow and less in areas supplied by diseased or stenosed vessels. The two types of agents used in MPI are thallium-201 and technetium-99m.

- **Thallium-201** (Tl-201) is a potassium analog used for MPI and has a half-life of 73 hours. First-pass thallium distribution is dependent on blood flow and tracer extraction by the myocardium. It enters the myocardium by active transport of membrane-bound Na^+K^+ ATPase. However, one of the most important characteristics of Tl-201 is its myocardial redistribution. Starting soon after initial myocardial uptake (post injection), a washout will occur from the myocardium as well as uptake by viable myocardium. This phenomenon results in normalization or reversibility in areas that are ischemic, and over additional time, improvement or normalization can occur in areas that are viable but appear as a fixed defect (scar) during initial imaging. Because of these isotope characteristics, thallium is often used for assessing myocardial viability. A protocol for stress testing using thallium is seen in Fig. 8.7.

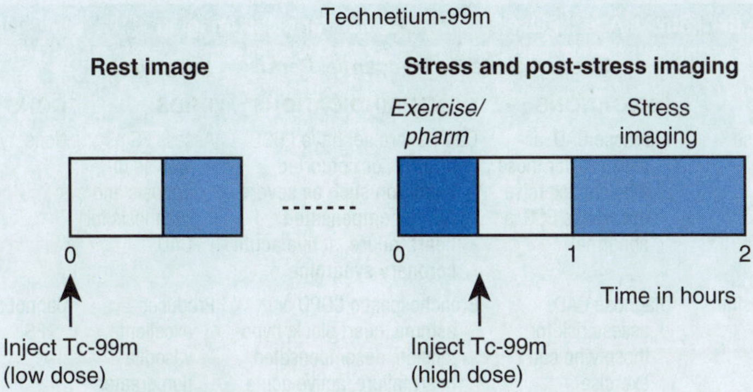

Fig. 8.8. Nuclear stress testing protocol with technetium-99m.

- **Technetium-99m** (Tc-99m) is the most commonly used of the MPI perfusion agents. There are several agents based on the binding agent linked to the isotope. This includes Tc-99m sestamibi, Tc-99m teboroxime (not used clinically at present), and Tc-99m tetrofosmin. The benefit of technetium is its short half-life of 6 hours, which reduces radiation exposure to the patient. MPI with technetium requires an injection at rest and a second injection of a higher dose at peak stress and comparison of the images obtained. **Tc-99m sestamibi** (or MIBI or Cardiolite) was the first of the Tc-99m agents to be approved for commercial use. It contains a hydrophilic cation and an isonitrile hydrophobic portion that allows for the necessary interactions with the cell membrane for uptake into the myocardium. The uptake of MIBI is dependent on mitochondrial-derived membrane electrochemical gradient, cellular pH, and intact energy production. **Tc-99m tetrofosmin** (Myoview) has properties that are similar to MIBI. Studies have shown a more rapid clearance from the liver, allowing for faster imaging times. A protocol for stress testing using technetium is seen in Fig. 8.8.

Unlike Tl-201, Tc-99m does not possess a strong redistribution quality. The reason for this is that the clearance of Tc-99m is slow due to irreversible binding, even though continued uptake occurs during the rest phase of a study. Therefore, there may be some improvement in 2 to 3 hours between stress and rest, but the degree of redistribution is slower and less complete than Tl-201. Importantly, however, only viable tissue can extract and uptake MIBI.

Myocardial extraction is an active process with regard to thallium-201 and a mitochondrial-dependent process with regard to the technetium-99m agents. Uptake can only occur if the cells in that region are viable.

7. What are the different stress modalities for myocardial perfusion imaging?

Stress can be produced in different ways. The goal of MPI is to produce coronary artery vasodilation in order to assess the presence of diseased or stenosed vessels, which will vasodilate to a lesser extent than healthy vessels. Forms of stress are either exercise-induced or pharmacologic (Table 8.1). Of note, there is a small risk of inducing ischemia, including risk of arrhythmia and myocardial infarction, which are known rare complications of stress testing.

Exercise increases myocardial blood flow and metabolic demand. Forms of exercise for stress testing include the treadmill, supine or erect bicycle, dynamic arm, or isometric handgrip. If there are no contraindications to exercising, exercise is preferred for MPI testing. Treadmill stress testing is the most commonly used exercise modality. Functional capacity can also be determined during treadmill exercise testing, and prognosis for cardiac events can be determined using the Duke treadmill score when using the Bruce protocol. The Duke treadmill score takes into account the amount the exercise time, the presence and grade of chest pain (0 indicating no chest pain; 1 indicating nonlimiting chest pain; and 2 indicating limiting chest pain), and the degree of ST-segment deviation during exercise (measured in mm). The Duke treadmill score categorizes patients into low-, medium-, or high-risk categories and predicts risk of death.

When patients are unable to exercise or unable to achieve at least 85% of maximal predicted heart rate by exercise (defined as 85% of the calculation, “220-age”), there are a

Table 8.1. Stress Agents Used for Myocardial Perfusion Imaging

Stress Agents for Myocardial Perfusion Imaging				
	INDICATIONS	**CONTRAINDICATIONS**	**PROS**	**CONS**
Exercise	Diagnose CAD, assess risk for those who can exercise but whose ECG is abnormal	Can't exercise, have LBBB on ECG, or comorbid condition such as severe AS, decompensated heart failure, active acute coronary syndrome	Assess FS as well as diagnosis and prognosis for CAD	None
Adenosine	Diagnose CAD, assess risk for those who can't exercise	Bronchospastic COPD or asthma, heart block, hypotension, decompensated heart failure, active acute coronary syndrome	Produces excellent vasodilation greater than that of exercise	Cannot assess FS
Dipyridamole	Diagnose CAD, assess risk for those who can't exercise	Bronchospastic COPD or asthma, heart block, hypotension, decompensated heart failure, active acute coronary syndrome	Produces excellent vasodilation greater than that of exercise	Cannot assess FS
Regadenoson	Diagnose CAD, assess risk for those who can't exercise	Severe bronchospastic COPD or asthma with active wheeze, heart block, hypotension, decompensated heart failure, active acute coronary syndrome	Produces excellent vasodilation equal to that of exercise	Cannot assess FS
Dobutamine	Diagnose CAD, assess risk for those who can't exercise	Tachyarrhythmias, uncontrolled hypertension, severe AS, decompensated heart failure, active acute coronary syndrome	Reserved for those who need pharmacologic MPI but who have severe bronchospastic disease with active wheeze	Does not produce good vasodilation and cannot assess FS

AS, Aortic stenosis; *CAD*, coronary artery disease; *COPD*, chronic obstructive pulmonary disease; *ECG*, electrocardiogram; *FS*, functional status; *LBBB*, left bundle branch block; *MPI*, myocardial perfusion imaging.

number of pharmacologic agents that can be used. Pharmacologic studies are also preferred if the patient has a left bundle branch block or paces the ventricle due to septal perfusion defects that can occur as a result of abnormal septal activation. These defects can obscure accuracy of MPI findings. Pharmacologic agents include dobutamine, dipyridamole, adenosine, and regadenoson.

Dipyridamole, adenosine, and regadenoson are all vasodilators. They purely produce vasodilation by acting on the adenosine receptors and result in a 3.5- to 5-fold increase in myocardial blood flow. Dipyridamole does this by increasing the endogenous levels of adenosine by preventing its breakdown, whereas adenosine and regadenoson are given exogenously to increase levels. Regadenoson is a specific A_{2a} adenosine receptor agonist rather than a nonspecific adenosine agonist when administering pure adenosine. Adenosine is nonspecific so it can

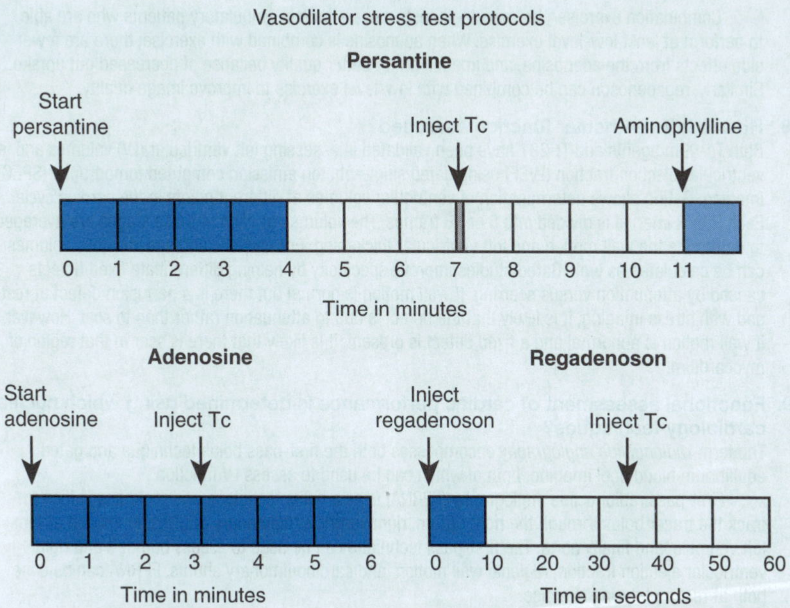

Fig. 8.9. Nuclear stress testing protocol with coronary vasodilators.

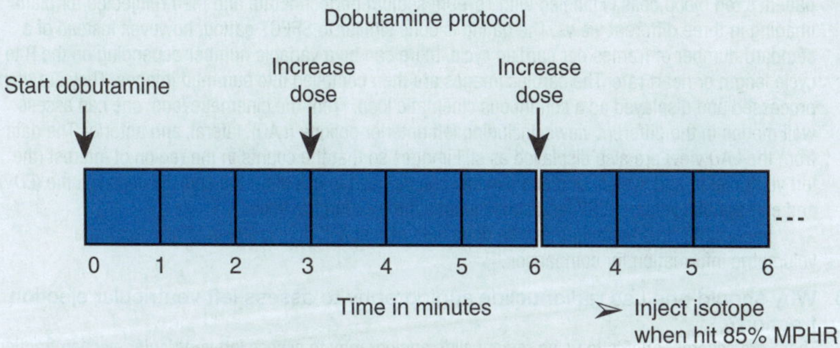

Fig. 8.10. Nuclear stress testing protocol with dobutamine.

cause atrioventricular block, peripheral vasodilation, and bronchospasm through activity on the non-A_{2A} adenosine receptors. They do not affect myocardial metabolic demand. Common side effects of vasodilators include flushing, headache, nausea, and shortness of breath. Vasodilators are contraindicated if the patient has severe chronic obstructive pulmonary disease (COPD) or is actively wheezing, but recent research has shown that using regadenoson in patients with mild and moderate COPD is safe. Fig. 8.9 shows protocols for using these vasodilators in stress testing.

Dobutamine results in both β-1 and β-2 stimulation, which causes an increase in heart rate, blood pressure, and contractility and thus increased metabolic demand. This increased demand indirectly increases myocardial blood flow. Dobutamine can result in the development of arrhythmias, dyspnea, flushing, and headache. This agent is used for nuclear stress MPI when vasodilators are contraindicated, such as in severe bronchospastic lung disease, bradycardia, and heart block. Fig. 8.10 shows a protocol for using dobutamine in stress testing.

Combination exercise/pharmacologic tests can be done in ambulatory patients who are able to perform at least low-level exercise. When adenosine is combined with exercise, there are fewer side effects from the adenosine, and images are of better quality because of decreased gut uptake. Similarly, regadenoson can be combined with low-level exercise to improve image quality.

8. How is left ventricular function assessed?

Both Tc-99m agents and Tl-201 have been validated in assessing left ventricular (LV) volumes and left ventricular ejection fraction (LVEF) using gated single-photon emission computed tomography (SPECT) imaging. Gating allows determination of ventricular volumes at different points in the cardiac cycle. Each R to R interval is divided into 8 or 16 frames. The volumes at each of those stages are averaged to determine the wall motion and left ventricular thickening. End-systolic and end-diastolic volumes can be calculated as well. Gated studies improve specificity by helping differentiate fixed defects caused by attenuation versus scarring. If wall motion is normal but there is a perfusion defect at rest and with stress imaging, it is likely that the defect is due to attenuation rather than to scar. However, if wall motion is abnormal and a fixed defect is present, it is likely that there is scar in that region of myocardium.

9. Functional assessment of cardiac performance is determined using which nuclear cardiology techniques?

The term *radionuclide angiography* encompasses both the first-pass bolus technique and gated equilibrium blood pool imaging, both of which can be used to assess LV function.

First-pass radionuclide angiography (FPRNA) uses a bolus technique and rapid acquisition to track the tracer bolus through the right atrium, right ventricle, pulmonary arteries, lungs, left atrium, left ventricle, and finally aorta. The first-pass technique can be used to assess both left and right ventricular ejection fraction, regional wall motion, and cardiopulmonary shunts. FPRNA can be done both at rest and during exercise.

Gated equilibrium blood pool imaging or multiple gated acquisition (MUGA) can also be used to assess left ventricular function and ejection fraction. The right ventricle is not easily assessed with this technique because of overlap of cardiac structures. The technique is performed after a sample of the patient's red blood cells is labeled with Tc-99m sodium pertechnetate and then reinjected for planar imaging in three different views. The gating is done similar to SPECT gating; however, instead of a standard number of frames per cardiac cycle, there can be a variable number depending on the R to R cycle length or heart rate. The cardiac images are then compiled into summed images. They are then processed and displayed as a continuous cinematic loop. From the cinematic loop, one can assess wall motion in the different views, including left anterior oblique (LAO), lateral, and anterior. The data from the LAO view are also displayed as still images so that the counts in the region of interest (the left ventricle) at end systole and end diastole can be used to calculate the end-diastolic volume (EDV) and end systolic volume (ESV) and subsequently the ejection fraction.

Importantly, this technique can be done both at rest and during stress to give accurate volumetric information for comparison.

10. Why should one use radionuclide angiography to assess left ventricular ejection fraction?

There are several benefits to using radionuclide angiography to assess left ventricular ejection fraction:

1. Radionuclide angiography is a precise and accurate measure of LVEF that is reproducible, especially during serial studies to look for changes in LVEF caused by cardiotoxic agents, valvular heart disease and new therapeutic agents in clinical trials.
2. It is less expensive and more available than magnetic resonance imaging for evaluation of LVEF.
3. Radionuclide angiography can be used to assess LVEF when other methods are not possible because of poor images as a result of body habitus, lung disease, or chest wall deformities.
4. LVEF is an independent predictor of cardiac events and given that it serves as a valid prognostic index in many clinical settings, accurate assessment is important.

11. How much radiation is a patient exposed to?

Radiation exposure depends on the radiotracer used as well as the selected protocol. Exposure can vary from about 3 mSv to upward of 30 mSv. Table 8.2 summarizes radiation exposure from various tests. The goal is to use a protocol that will result in radiation exposure that is as low as reasonably achievable (ALARA) for each patient, because excessive radiation is associated with the development of malignancy. To reduce exposure, it is important to use the minimum radiation dose; weight-based dosing can be used as can imaging strategies that employ a stress-first strategy, and rest images are only obtained if there is a significant abnormality on the stress images. Use of isotopes, such as

Table 8.2. Average Radiation Exposure from Common Cardiac Tests

DIAGNOSTIC TEST	RADIATION EXPOSURE (MSV)
PA chest film	0.02
CT coronary angiography	2–30
CT of the chest	6–7
Nuclear SPECT: Tc-99m MIBI (standard 10/30-mCi dose)	11–12
Nuclear SPECT: Tl-201 (standard 3.5-mCi dose)	15
Coronary artery calcium score	1–5
Invasive coronary angiography	2–20

CT, Computed tomography; *mCi*, milliCurie; *mSv*, milliSievert; *PA*, posteroanterior; *SPECT*, single-photon emission computed tomography.
Adapted from publications listed in the bibliography.

technetium, which has a short half-life, also decreases radiation exposure. Physicians should discuss risks and benefits of radiation exposure for the nuclear test with patients prior to the exam.

The American Society of Nuclear Cardiology has put out a consensus statement recommending that greater than 50% of nuclear stress tests should have a radiation exposure of less than 9 mSv.

Bibliography and Suggested Readings

Arbab-Zadeh, A. (2012). Stress testing and non-invasive coronary angiography in patients with suspected coronary artery disease. *Heart International, 7*(1), e2.

Cabrera, R., Husain, Z., Palani, G., Karthikeyan, A. S., Choudhry, Z., Dhanalakota, S., et al. (2013). Comparison of hemodynamic and stress testing variables in patients undergoing regadenoson stress myocardial perfusion imaging to regadenoson with adjunctive low-level exercise myocardial perfusion imaging. *Journal of Nuclear Cardiology, 20*, 336–343.

Cerqueira, M. D., Weissman, N. J., Dilsizian, V., Jacobs, A. K., Kaul, S., Laskey, W. K., et al. (2002). Standardized myocardial segmentation and nomenclature for tomographic imaging of the heart: a statement for healthcare professionals from the Cardiac Imaging Committee on the Council of Clinical Cardiology of the American Heart Association. *Circulation, 105*, 539–542.

Einstein, A. J., Berman, D. S., Min, J. K., Hendel, R. C., Gerber, T. C., Carr, J. J., et al. (2014). Patient-centered imaging: shared decision making for cardiac imaging procedures with exposure to ionizing radiation. *Journal of the American College of Cardiology, 63*, 1480–1489.

Ghimire, G., Hage, F. G., Heo, J., & Iskandrian, A. (2013). Regadenoson: a focused update. *Journal of Nuclear Cardiology, 20*, 284–288.

Hachamovitch, R., & Berman, D. S. (2005). The use of nuclear cardiology in clinical decision making. *Seminars in Nuclear Medicine, 35*, 62–72.

Hendel, R. C., Berman, D. S., Di Carli, M. F., Heidenreich, P. A., Henkin, R. E., Pellikka, P. A., et al. (2009). ACCF/ASNC/ACR/AHA/ASE/SCCT/SCMR/SNM 2009 appropriate use criteria for cardiac radionuclide imaging. *Journal of the American College of Cardiology, 53*, 2201–2229.

Henzlova MJ, Duvall WL, Einstein AJ, Travin MI, Verberne HJ. (2016). "https://www.ncbi.nlm.nih.gov/pubmed/26914678" ASNC imaging guidelines for SPECT nuclear cardiology procedures: Stress, protocols, and tracers. *Journal of Nuclear Cardiology*, 23, 606–39.

McCollough, C. H., Bushberg, J. T., Fletcher, J. G., & Eckel, L. J. (2015). Answers to common questions about the use and safety of CT scans. *Mayo Clinic Proceedings, 90*, 647–648.

Metz, L. D., Beattie, M., Hom, R., Redberg, R. F., Grady, D., & Fleischmann, K. E. (2007). The prognostic value of normal exercise myocardial perfusion imaging and exercise echocardiography. *Journal of the American College of Cardiology, 49*, 227–237.

Shaw, L. J., Berman, D. S., Maron, D. J., Mancini, G. B., Hayes, S. W., Hartigan, P. M., et al. (2008). Optimal medical therapy with or without percutaneous coronary intervention to reduce ischemic burden: results from the Clinical Outcomes Utilizing Revascularization and Aggressive Drug Evaluation (COURAGE) trial nuclear substudy. *Circulation, 117*, 1283–1291.

Thomas, G. S., Thompson, R. C., Miyamoto, M. I., Ip, T. K., Rice, D. L., Milikien, D., et al. (2009). The RegEx trial: a randomized, double-blind, placebo- and active-controlled pilot study combining regadenoson, a selective a(2a) adenosine agonist, with low-level exercise, in patients undergoing myocardial perfusion imaging. *Journal of Nuclear Cardiology, 16*, 63–72.

Thompson, R. C. (2012). Regadenoson stress in patients with asthma and COPD: a breath of fresh air. *Journal of Nuclear Cardiology, 19*, 647–648.

Travin, M. I., & Bergman, S. R. (2005). Assessment of myocardial viability. *Seminars in Nuclear Medicine, 35*, 2–16.

CHAPTER 9

CARDIAC POSITRON EMISSION TOMOGRAPHY

Niraj R. Patel, Luis A. Tamara

1. What is positron emission tomography?

A positron, as its name implies, is a positively charged particle that is ejected from the nucleus of an unstable atom. It is identical in mass to an electron. Strictly speaking, it is "antimatter," and very shortly after leaving the nucleus, it collides with an electron in what is called an annihilation reaction. This reaction generates two 511-keV gamma photons that are emitted almost diametrically opposite from each other. The energy of these photons is captured by a positron emission tomography (PET) scanner, and through a sophisticated network of electronics as well as computer software and hardware transformed into an image.

2. Which are the two most common positron emission tomography radiopharmaceuticals used for myocardial perfusion imaging?

Rubidium-82 (Rb-82) and Nitrogen-13 (N-13) ammonia.

3. What are the characteristics of rubidium-82?

Rubidium-82 is a monovalent cation analog of potassium. It is commercially available as a strontium-82 generator. Its physical half-life is 75 seconds. It is extracted with high efficiency by myocardial cells through the Na/K/ATPase pump. The adult radiation dose from a Rb-82 myocardial perfusion scan (MPS) varies from 1.75 to 7.5 mSv. An example of a PET study using Rb-82 is shown in Fig. 9.1.

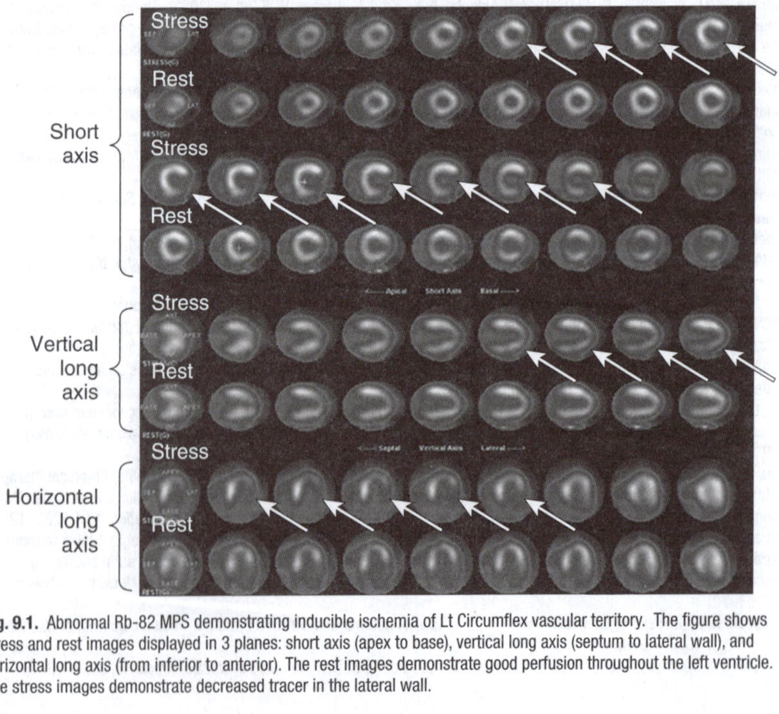

Fig. 9.1. Abnormal Rb-82 MPS demonstrating inducible ischemia of Lt Circumflex vascular territory. The figure shows stress and rest images displayed in 3 planes: short axis (apex to base), vertical long axis (septum to lateral wall), and horizontal long axis (from inferior to anterior). The rest images demonstrate good perfusion throughout the left ventricle. The stress images demonstrate decreased tracer in the lateral wall.

4. What are the characteristics of N-13 ammonia?

N-13 ammonia is an extractable myocardial perfusion tracer that due to its 10-minute half-life requires an on-site cyclotron. It is retained in myocardial tissue as N-13 glutamine by the action of glutamine synthetase. The adult radiation dose from an N-13 ammonia MPS is approximately 1.4 mSv.

5. What are the advantages of positron emission tomography myocardial perfusion imaging over single-photon emission computed tomography?

- It is more sensitive and specific (93% and 92%, respectively).
- It is cost effective. This is primarily due to a reduction in unnecessary coronary angiographies.
- It results in lower radiation dose to the patient.
- It allows for absolute quantification in myocardial blood flow (MBF) in mL/min/g of tissue.

6. My patient's positron emission tomography myocardial perfusion study was reported as demonstrating severe ischemia, but the coronary angiogram showed only nonobstructive coronary artery disease. How can this be?

This can happen because the correlation between stenosis severity and coronary flow reserve (CFR) is weak and nonlinear. Therefore angiographically mild stenoses can cause severe derangement of CFR, whereas severe coronary atherosclerosis can result in little to no alteration in myocardial perfusion.

7. How is coronary flow reserve determined on a positron emission tomography scan?

CFR is a ratio calculated by dividing maximum MBF by baseline MBF at rest in a given coronary artery. The maximum and resting MBF (measured in mL/min/g) is derived by processing radionuclide activity-based data collected on vasodilator stress and resting PET scans, respectively.

8. What is the relationship between fractional flow reserve and coronary flow reserve?

Fractional flow reserve (FFR) is the invasive physiologic gold standard for assessing the clinical significance of coronary arterial stenosis, while CFR (also known as myocardial flow reserve, or MFR) is the noninvasive gold standard for assessing the clinical significance of a given coronary stenosis. FFR and CFR generally have a positive association, such that low CRF correlates with low FFR. However, the two are *not* directly comparable. This is mainly because FFR measures a pressure gradient across a single stenosis, whereas MFR measures a change in flow across the entire vascular bed including both the epicardial (conductance) vessel and the downstream (resistance) microcirculation.

9. Can coronary flow reserve (or myocardial flow reserve) be incorporated into routine clinical decision making?

Yes it can. CFR or MFR adds robust diagnostic and prognostic information to myocardial perfusion PET scan images, which reflect relative differences in MBF. CFR, on the other hand, conveys an absolute (in mL/min/g of tissue) and objective measure of MBF. See the algorithm provided in Fig. 9.2.

10. What is the radiopharmaceutical used in cardiac positron emission tomography for the assessment of myocardial viability?

F-18 fluorodeoxyglucose (FDG).

11. What is meant by "glucose loading" when a viability F-18 fluorodeoxyglucose cardiac positron emission tomography is being performed?

Under fasting nonischemic conditions the myocardium preferentially oxidizes fatty acids. Under ischemic conditions the myocardium switches to oxidation of glucose, as it can do this with a lower oxygen requirement. In order to promote accumulation of F-18 FDG (a glucose analog) within viable myocardial tissue, an oral or intravenous "glucose load" is administered to the patient prior to the injection of F-18 FDG. Under fasting conditions, the relative abundance of circulating glucose will cause the myocardium to switch to glucose oxidation and thus enhance the uptake of F-18 FDG into viable hibernating myocardial tissue.

12. What is the most common approach to preparing a nondiabetic patient for a fluorodeoxyglucose myocardial viability positron emission tomography/computed tomography scan according to the American Society of Nuclear Cardiology, and what is the basis for this?

Ask the patient to fast 6 to 12 hours prior to the scheduled time of the scan. Then give the patient 25 to 100 g of oral glucose to ingest, followed by supplemental IV insulin as needed. Glucose loading induces the pancreas to release endogenous insulin, which signals the myocardium to switch from free fatty acid to glucose utilization. Exogenous insulin ensures an optimal insulin level to maximize

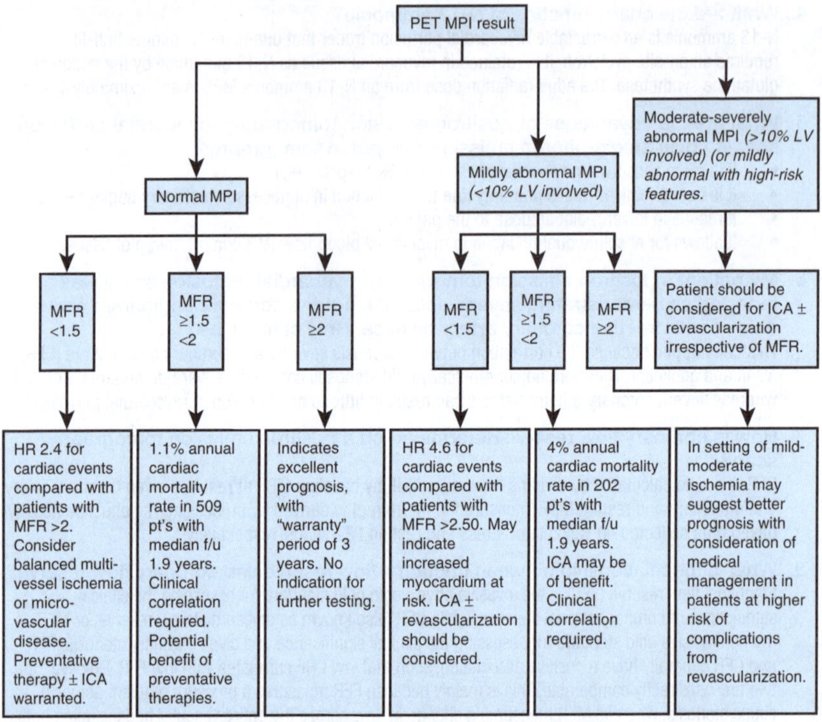

Fig. 9.2. Clinical algorithm proposed by Dr. R. S. Beanlands and his team at the National Cardiac PET Centre at the University of Ottawa Heart Institute for how to interpret myocardial perfusion PET scan findings based on MFR (or CFR) values derived from the PET scan. *PET* = Positron emission tomography; *MPI* = myocardial perfusion imaging; *MFR* = myocardial perfusion reserve; *ICA* = invasive coronary angiogram.

myocardial glucose utilization and by proxy FDG uptake in the setting of relative insulin insensitivity (as detected by blood glucose levels remaining relatively high after glucose loading).

13. **What are common approaches to preparing a patient with diabetes for fluorodeoxyglucose myocardial viability positron emission tomography/computed tomography scan according to the American Society of Nuclear Cardiology?**
In diabetic patients, other approaches are used because the body's response to elevated blood glucose is deranged secondary to impaired insulin production and/or sensitivity. One approach is to use the oral glucose loading protocol for nondiabetics, or IV dextrose loading (13 to 25 g), followed by supplemental IV insulin. Delayed PET scanning is recommended with this approach to ensure sufficient FDG uptake. A second approach is euglycemic hyperinsulinemic clamping, which is time consuming and intensive, requiring a nurse and close monitoring prior and during PET scanning but yields excellent images. A third approach is administering the nicotinic acid derivative acipimox. Note this is commonly used in Europe but is not FDA approved in the United States.

14. **What is meant by perfusion/metabolism "mismatch" on cardiac positron emission tomography viability imaging?**
A perfusion/metabolic mismatch would be present if the area of decreased perfusion demonstrates normal or increased FDG uptake (Fig. 9.3). This finding would be consistent with an area of viable hibernating myocardium.

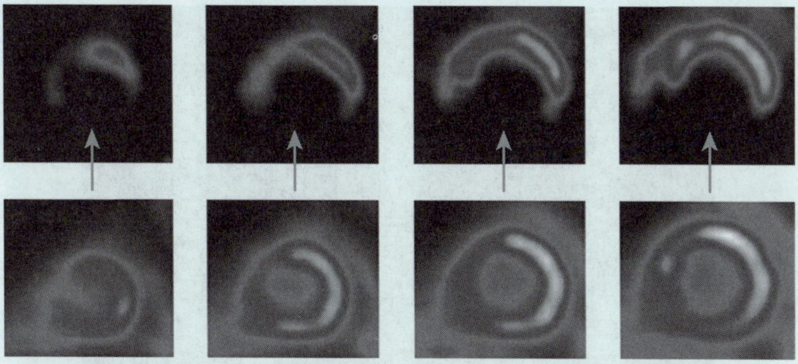

Fig. 9.3. Viability study showing 4 short axis slices of the left ventricle. The top row of images display perfusion with rubidium-82, demonstrating markedly decreased perfusion of the inferior wall *(arrow)*. The bottom row of images display FDG-18 uptake in the inferior wall, indicating that the poorly perfused inferior wall still consists of viable, hibernating, myocardium. *(From Mc Ardle, B., Dowsley, T. F., Cocker, M. S., Ohira, H., deKemp, R. A., DaSilva, J., et al. [2013]. Cardiac PET: metabolic and functional imaging of the myocardium.* Seminars in Nuclear Medicine, 43, *434–448.)*

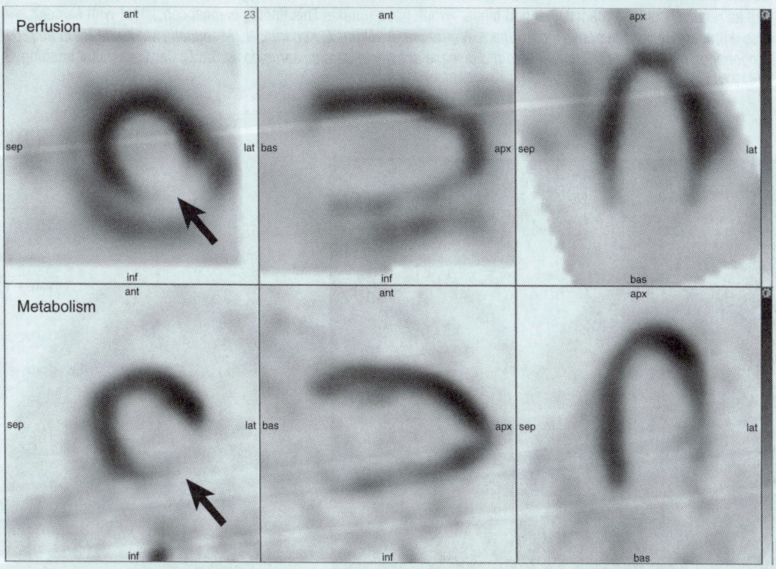

Fig. 9.4. Viability study showing slices from short, vertical long and horizontal long axes of the left ventricle. The top row of images display resting perfusion with Tc-99m sestamibi, demonstrating markedly decreased perfusion of the inferior and inferolateral wall *(arrows)*. The bottom row of images display markedly decreased FDG-18 uptake in the same region *(arrows)*, indicating non-viable myocardial scar.

15. What is meant by perfusion/metabolism "match" on cardiac positron emission tomography viability imaging?

A perfusion/metabolism match is present when there is markedly decreased FDG uptake that corresponds with the area of decreased perfusion (Fig. 9.4). This finding would be consistent with a myocardial scar.

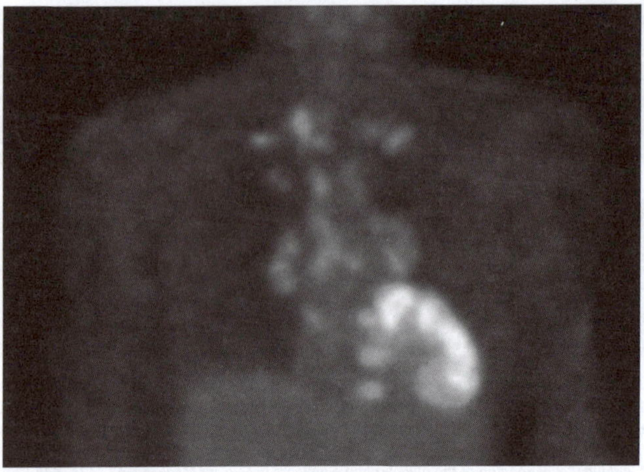

Fig. 9.5. FDG PET scan showing PET MIP (maximum intensity projection) image of the neck to mid-abdomen in anterior projection. The image shows significant FDG uptake in the left ventricle, particularly the anterior and apical myocardium as well as relatively diffuse mediastinal and bihilar lymph node uptake. This finding is most consistent with sarcoid disease with cardiac involvement. *(From Tahara, N., Tahara, A., Nitta, Y., Kodama, N., Mizoguchi, M., Kaida H., et al. [2010]. Heterogeneous myocardial FDG uptake and the disease activity in cardiac sarcoidosis.* JACC: Cardiovascular Imaging, 3, *1219–1228.)*

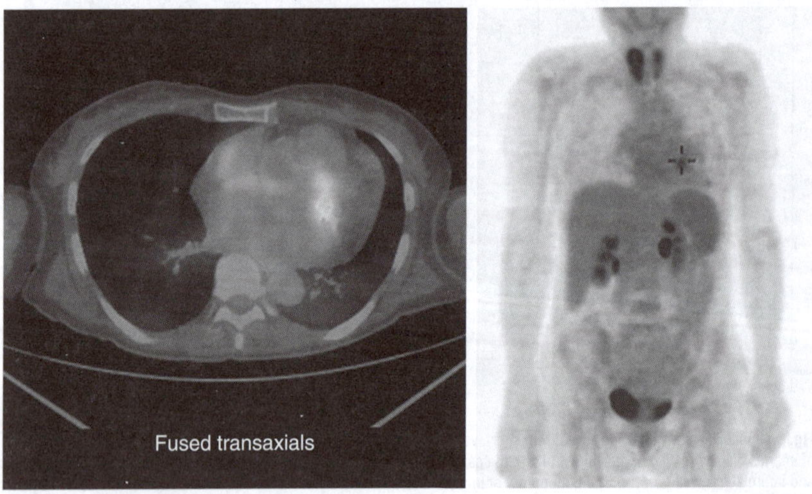

Fig. 9.6. FDG PET/CT scan showing fused PET/CT transaxial image at the level of the mitral valve and a PET MIP (maximum intensity projection) image of the base of skull to thigh in anterior projection. The left image shows increased FDG uptake at the mitral valve. The right image shows crossbar annotation over the increased FDG uptake in the same region. This finding is most consistent with endocarditis, which was confirmed by pathological exam after surgery. *(From Thuny, F., Grisoli, D., Collart, F., Habib, G.,& Raoult, D. [2012]. Management of infective endocarditis: challenges and perspectives.* The Lancet, 379*[9819], 965–975.)*

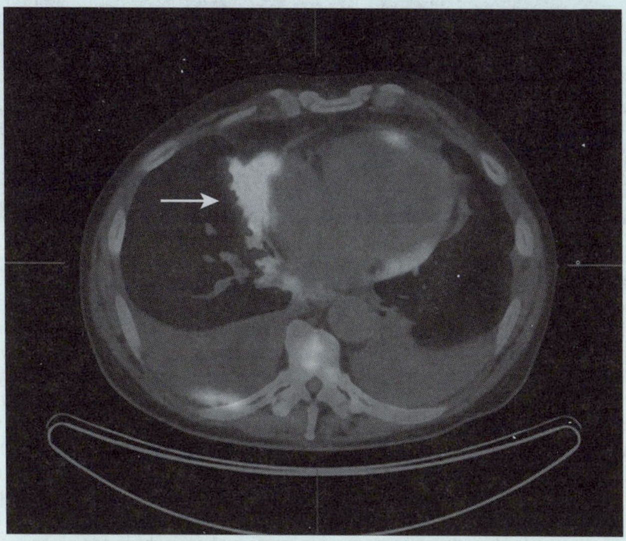

Fig. 9.7. FDG PET/CT scan showing fused PET/CT transaxial image at the level of the 4-chamber heart. The image shows metastatic involvement of the pericardium adjacent to the right atrium from lung cancer.

16. **Are there any other tracers that can be used for positron emission tomography cardiac imaging?**

    Yes. There are many other useful radiopharmaceuticals that can be used to interrogate different aspects of myocardial metabolism, innervation, and adenosine triphosphate (ATP) generation. Some of these include:
    - C-11 acetate (Krebs cycle)
    - C-11 palmitate (fatty acid metabolism)
    - C-11 lactate (myocardial lactate utilization)
    - C-11 phenylephrine (presynaptic catecholamine uptake and metabolism)
    - F-18 fluorodopamine (presynaptic sympathetic function)

    Additionally there are several tracers currently under development for imaging of alpha and beta cardiac receptors.

17. **Aside from myocardial perfusion and viability, are there other applications for cardiac positron emission tomography/computed tomography?**

    Yes. Cardiac PET/computed tomography (CT) can be useful for evaluating cardiac sarcoidosis for both initial diagnosis and response to treatment (Fig. 9.5), endocarditis with large vegetations 5 mm or greater (Fig. 9.6), and cardiac masses or metastases (Fig. 9.7).

Bibliography, Suggested Readings, and Websites

American Society of Nuclear Cardiology. (2009). PET myocardial perfusion and glucose metabolism imaging, Guidelines from the American Society of Nuclear Cardiology. www.asnc.org Accessed Nov 2016.

Bengel, F., & Schwaiger, M. (2006). PET metabolism, innervations and receptors. In V. Dilsizian, & G. M. Pohost (Eds.), *Cardiac CT, PET and MR (1st ed.)*. Malden, MA: Blackwell Futura.

Di Carli, M. F. (2006). PET assessment of myocardial perfusion. In V. Dilsizian, & G. M. Pohost (Eds.), *Cardiac CT, PET and MR (1st ed.)*. Malden, MA: Blackwell Futura.

Dilsizian, V., Bacharach, S. L., Beanlands, R. S., Bergmann, S. R., Delbeke, D., Gropler, R. J., et al. (2009). PET myocardial perfusion and metabolism clinical imaging. *Journal of Nuclear Cardiology*, *16*(4), 651–681.

Gould, K. L. (1991). PET perfusion imaging and nuclear cardiology. *Journal of Nuclear Medicine*, *32*, 579–606.

Gould, K. L. (2009). Does coronary flow trump coronary anatomy? *JACC: Cardiovascular Imaging*, *2*(8), 1009–1023.

Machac, J. (2005). Cardiac positron emission tomography imaging. *Seminars in Nuclear Medicine*, *35*(1), 17–36.

Mc Ardle, B., Dowsley, T. F., Cocker, M. S., Ohira, H., deKemp, R. A., DaSilva, J., et al. (2013). Cardiac PET: metabolic and functional imaging of the myocardium. *Seminars in Nuclear Medicine*, *43*, 434–448.

CHAPTER 10

CARDIAC MAGNETIC RESONANCE IMAGING

Paaladinesh Thavendiranathan, Scott D. Flamm

1. **How does cardiac magnetic resonance imaging produce images?**
CMR uses a strong magnet, 1.5 to 3.0 Tesla (equivalent to 30,000 to 60,000 times the strength of the earth's magnetic field), radiofrequency pulses, and gradient magnetic fields to obtain images of the heart. When placed in the bore of a magnet, positively charged protons, mainly from water, are aligned in the direction of the magnetic field, creating a net magnetization. Radiofrequency pulses are used to tilt these protons away from their alignment, shifting them to a higher energy state. These protons then return to their equilibrium state through the process of relaxation and emit a signal. The relaxation consists of two components—T1 and T2 relaxation. Magnetic gradients are applied across the tissue of interest to localize these signals. The signals are then collected using a receiver coil and placed in a data space referred to as "k-space," which is then used to create an image. CMR uses differences in relaxation properties between and among different tissues, fluids, and blood, and changes that occur due to pathologic processes to create contrast in the image.

2. **What is unique about cardiac magnetic resonance?**
Similar to echocardiography, CMR allows the generation of images of the heart without exposure to ionizing radiation. Although the spatial resolution of CMR is comparable to echocardiography (~1 mm), the contrast-to-noise and signal-to-noise ratios are far superior (Fig. 10.1). The latter allows easier delineation of borders between tissues and in particular between blood pool and myocardium. The contrast between blood pool and myocardium is generated using differences in signal properties of the different tissues without the use of contrast agents. CMR is also not limited by "acoustic windows" that may hinder echocardiography, and images can be obtained in any tomographic plane. Finally, CMR can provide information about tissue characteristics using differences in T1 and T2 signals, with the addition of contrast agents.

3. **What are the limitations of cardiac magnetic resonance?**
The major limitation of CMR is availability. Given the cost, the special construction necessary to host a CMR system, and the technical expertise and support necessary, CMR is not widely available at all centers. CMR is limited with respect to portability, unlike echocardiography where imaging can be performed at the patient's bedside. There are also a set of contraindications (listed later) that limit the use of this technology in selected patient populations. Image acquisition can be challenging in patients with an irregular cardiac rhythm or difficulty breath-holding, though real-time techniques provide an opportunity to overcome these barriers (Fig. 10.2). Finally, since patients have to lie still in a long hollow tube for up to an hour during imaging, claustrophobia may be an important limiting factor.

4. **What are the common imaging pulse sequences used in cardiac magnetic resonance?**
Pulse sequences are orchestrated actions of turning on and off various coils, gradients, and radiofrequency pulses to produce a CMR image. In simple terms, the pulse sequences are based on either gradient echo or spin echo sequences. The most common sequences used are bright blood gradient echo sequences (where the blood pool is bright), dark blood spin echo sequences (where the blood pool is dark), steady-state free precession sequences (also a type of gradient echo sequence, and most commonly used for function or cine images), and inversion recovery sequences (e.g., delayed enhancement imaging used to assess myocardial scar).

5. **What are the appropriate uses of cardiac magnetic resonance?**
Although echocardiography is usually the first-line imaging modality for questions of left ventricular (LV) function and assessment of valvular disease, cardiac MRI still has many important indications. The following questions and answers pertain to the appropriate use of cardiac MRI in the clinical setting as recommended in the multi-society appropriateness criteria of 2006, and in stable ischemic disease as recommended in the multi-society appropriateness criteria of 2014. Appropriate uses of CMR are summarized in Table 10.1.

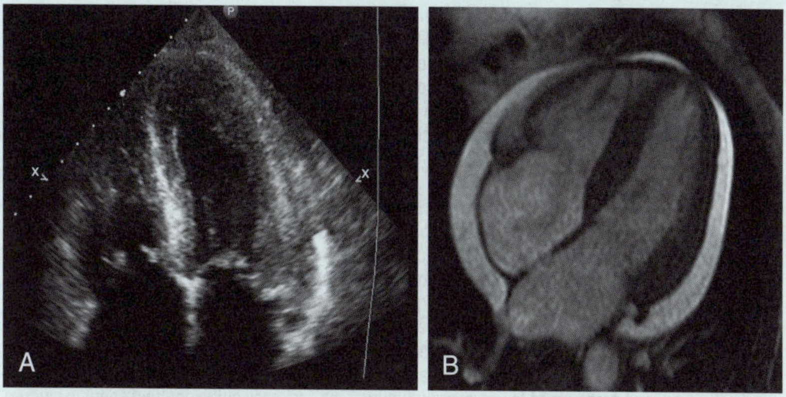

Fig. 10.1. Comparison of an echocardiographic and cardiac magnetic resonance imaging (MRI) cine image of a four-chamber view of the same patient. The superior contrast-to-noise and signal-to-noise ratios are clearly evident in the cardiac magnetic resonance (CMR) image, with clear delineation of the endocardial and epicardial borders of both ventricles.

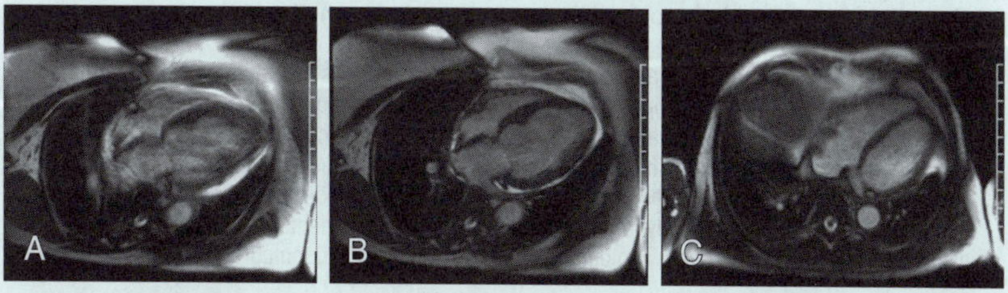

Fig. 10.2. A, Four-chamber view in a patient with difficulty breath-holding *(blurry)*. **B,** The same patient who was able to breath-hold after the acquisition period was shortened. **C,** Another patient with a real-time acquisition with the patient breathing freely.

Table 10.1. Appropriate Indications for Cardiac Magnetic Resonance

- Evaluation of chest pain syndrome in patients with intermediate pretest probability of CAD
- Evaluation of suspected coronary anomalies
- Evaluation of LV function after myocardial infarction *or* in patients with heart failure in patients with technically limited or indeterminate echocardiograms
- Evaluation of extent of myocardial necrosis and microvascular obstruction ("no reflow")
- Evaluation of myocardial viability
- Evaluation of myocarditis
- Evaluation of specific cardiomyopathies (e.g., infiltrative cardiomyopathies, HCM)
- Characterization of native and prosthetic cardiac valve dysfunction in patients with technically limited images from echocardiogram or TEE
- Evaluation of suspected constrictive pericarditis
- Evaluation of cardiac and pericardial masses
- Evaluation of pulmonary veins before pulmonary vein isolation for atrial fibrillation
- Assessment of congenital heart disease
- Evaluation for aortic dissection

CAD, Coronary artery disease; *HCM*, hypertrophic cardiomyopathy; *LV*, left ventricular; TEE, transesophageal echocardiogram.

6. What is late gadolinium enhancement cardiac magnetic resonance imaging?

One of the unique aspects of CMR is the ability to identify myocardial scar/fibrosis. This is most commonly performed using late gadolinium enhancement (LGE) imaging (and also known as delayed enhancement imaging). Gadolinium-based contrast agents are first administered; then after waiting approximately 10 minutes and allowing time for the contrast to distribute into areas of scar/fibrosis, an inversion recovery gradient echo sequence is performed. This sequence nulls normal myocardium (making it black), and anything that is bright within the myocardium is most likely myocardial scar/fibrosis (Fig. 10.3).

7. Does cardiac magnetic resonance have a role in the evaluation of chest pain?

In patients with chest pain, syndrome cardiac MRI stress testing can be performed to assess flow-limiting coronary stenosis. This is most appropriate in patients with intermediate pretest probability of coronary artery disease (CAD) with uninterpretable electrocardiogram (ECG) or who are unable to exercise. The two stress methods used are vasodilator perfusion CMR or dobutamine stress function CMR. Vasodilator stress testing is performed identical to nuclear stress testing with the use of adenosine or comparable agents. With peak coronary vasodilation, a gadolinium contrast agent is administered, and perfusion of the myocardium during the first pass of the contrast agent is captured. Areas of perfusion abnormality can be detected as dark areas (Fig. 10.4). Resting perfusion is also commonly performed, mainly to differentiate imaging artifacts from a true perfusion defect. This is then followed by late gadolinium enhancement imaging to assess for myocardial scar. Alternatively, graded doses of dobutamine can be administered to provide a sympathetic stress with cine imaging to identify regions of the wall motion abnormality similar to echocardiography.

8. Can cardiac magnetic resonance coronary angiography be used to assess chest pain?

Use of coronary angiography for assessment of coronary stenosis is not commonly performed in clinical settings. However, it is appropriate to use coronary magnetic resonance angiography (MRA) to assess the origin, branching pattern, and proximal course of the coronary arteries to assess for coronary anomalies (Fig. 10.5). This can be performed without the use of contrast agents, though the acquisition may require a substantial amount of time and is susceptible to artifacts. The use of this technique may be particularly important, however, in young patients, thereby avoiding radiation exposure from invasive coronary angiography or coronary computed tomographic (CT) angiography.

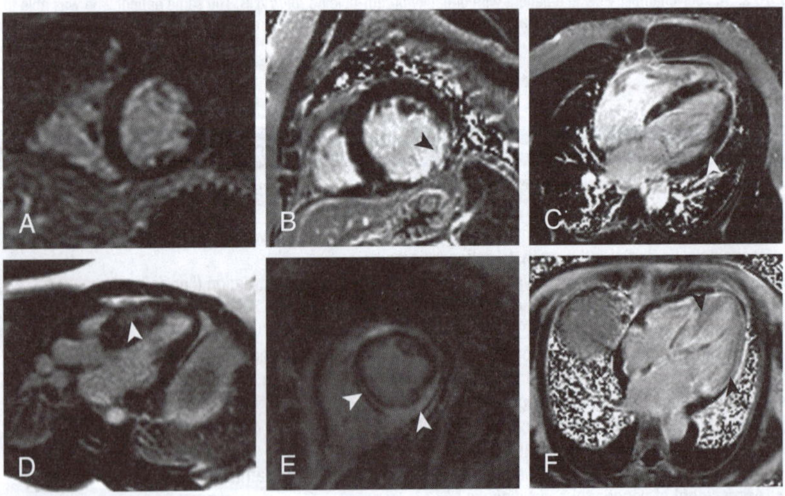

Fig. 10.3. Late gadolinium enhancement patterns. **A,** Normal short-axis late gadolinium enhancement image. **B,** Transmural scar in the circumflex territory. **C,** Cardiomyopathy secondary to sarcoidosis. **D,** Hypertrophic obstructive cardiomyopathy with basal anterioseptal mid-myocardial late gadolinium enhancement (LGE). **E,** Myocarditis with both mid-myocardial and epicardial LGE. **F,** Cardiac amyloidosis with diffuse enhancement of the entire left ventricle.

9. What is the role of cardiac magnetic resonance in the assessment of ventricular function?

CMR is considered the reference standard for the assessment of ventricular volumes, ejection fraction, and ventricular mass of both the left and right ventricles, as a result of the excellent accuracy and reproducibility of this technique for these measurements. The most appropriate use of CMR is in the evaluation of LV function after myocardial infarction or in heart failure patients with technically limited echocardiographic images. In other patient populations CMR can be used to assess LV function when there is discordant information from prior tests.

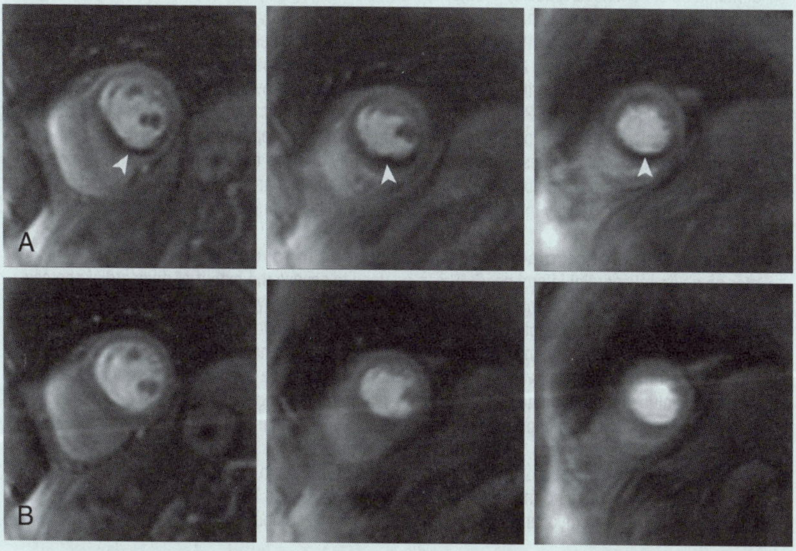

Fig. 10.4. Adenosine perfusion imaging. **A,** Peak stress short-axis and four-chamber perfusion images showing ischemia *(dark area)* in the basal to apical inferior and inferior septal segments consistent with ischemia in the right coronary artery (RCA) territory. **B,** Rest images in panel B illustrate normal perfusion.

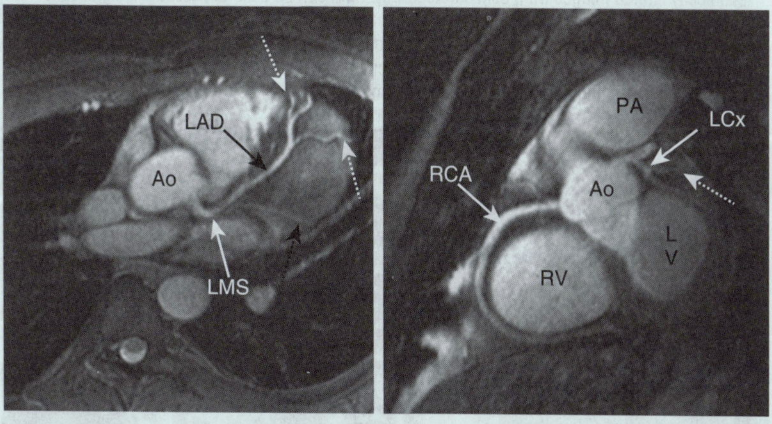

Fig. 10.5. Coronary magnetic resonance angiography. Coronary CMR at 3 Tesla. *Left panel,* Left coronary artery and branches *(dotted arrows). Right panel,* Right coronary artery. *Ao,* Aorta; *LAD,* left anterior descending artery; *LCx,* left circumflex artery; *LMS,* left main stem; *LV,* left ventricle; *PA,* pulmonary artery; *RV,* right ventricle. *(From Stuber, M., Botnar, R. M., Fischer, S. E., Lamerichs, R., Smink, J., Harvey, P., et al. [2002]. Preliminary report on in vivo coronary MRA at 3 Tesla in humans.* Magnetic Resonance in Medicine, *48[3]:425–429. Reprinted with permission of Wiley-Liss, Inc., a subsidiary of John Wiley & Sons, Inc.)*

10. Does cardiac magnetic resonance have a role in the assessment of cardiomyopathies?

CMR has an important role in the evaluation of specific cardiomyopathies, particularly in infiltrative diseases (e.g., amyloid, sarcoid), hypertrophic cardiomyopathy, and cardiomyopathies due to cardiotoxic therapies. Although CMR-based ventricular morphology and functional images can provide certain clues to the etiology of the underlying cardiomyopathy, the most important CMR technique in the assessment of cardiomyopathies is late gadolinium enhancement imaging. Certain late gadolinium enhancement patterns have been associated with particular cardiomyopathies and can be easily identified by experienced readers. Another specific cardiomyopathy that can be assessed by CMR is arrhythmogenic right ventricular cardiomyopathy (ARVC). CMR may be particularly useful in patients presenting with syncope or ventricular arrhythmias to provide excellent assessment of right ventricular (RV) function, RV dilation, focal aneurysms, and also myocardial scarring using late gadolinium enhancement imaging both in the LV and RV. There has been a growing interest in using myocardial mapping techniques (T1 and T2 mapping) in the assessment of cardiomyopathy. Instead of depending on signal intensity differences on T1- or T2-weighted images, mapping sequences provide direct quantification of T1 or T2 values. These can subsequently be used to identify pathologic myocardial changes such as edema and fibrosis. However, these sequences are not routinely used today due to limited experience, variability in the pulse sequences, and lack of universally accepted normal values.

11. What is the role of cardiac magnetic resonance in myocardial infarction?

After an acute myocardial infarction, CMR can be used to assess the extent of myocardial necrosis (see Fig. 10.3B) and areas of microvascular obstruction ("no reflow regions") (Fig. 10.6) via late gadolinium enhancement imaging. In addition, the presence of myocardial hemorrhage can be identified using T2-weighted and T2* imaging. Both the extent of necrosis and the presence of microvascular obstruction as well as myocardial hemorrhage have been shown to have adverse prognostic value. In addition late gadolinium enhancement imaging can be used to determine the likelihood of recovery of function with revascularization (surgical or percutaneous) or medical therapy. Segments of myocardium with >50% transmural scarring are less likely to recover or improve function with revascularization. Another important use of CMR is in patients who present with a positive troponin but have normal coronary angiography. CMR can help identify myocarditis (see Fig. 10.3E) or even myocardial infarction with re-canalized coronary artery.

12. Can valvular disease be assessed by cardiac magnetic resonance?

Echocardiography remains the most commonly used method for assessment of stenotic and regurgitant lesions of both native and prosthetic valves. The role of CMR is mainly in patients with technically limited images from echocardiography. CMR can be used to assess the significance of the valve lesions using several techniques. First an *en face* image of the valvular lesion can be obtained for visual assessment and planimetry of the stenotic or regurgitant orifices. However, the most useful CMR techniques are in the quantitative assessment of valvular stenosis obtained by transvalvular gradients or regurgitant lesions obtained by volumes and flow measurements. The latter is often

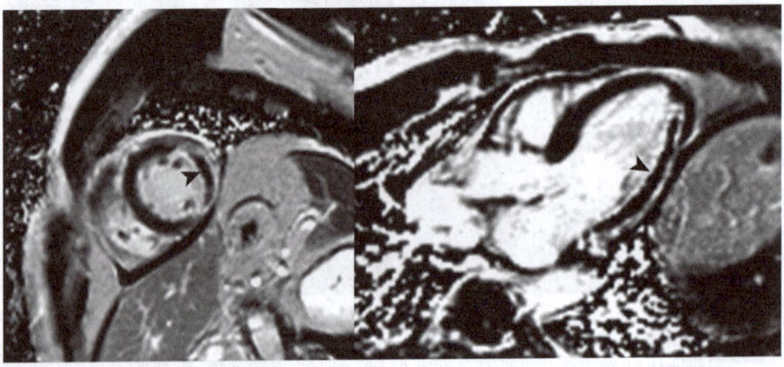

Fig. 10.6. Microvascular obstruction post infarction. A short-axis and long-axis image of microvascular obstruction *(arrows)* seen on late gadolinium enhancement imaging. Both images are from the same patient.

obtained using a combination of stroke volumes by the disk-summation technique of the ventricles, and flow volumes of the great vessels by phase contrast imaging (analogous to Doppler imaging in echocardiography) (Fig. 10.7).

13. **Can cardiac magnetic resonance be used in the assessment of congenital heart disease?**

Among imaging tools, CMR is frequently considered the best modality for the assessment of congenital heart disease (Fig. 10.8). The ability to assess the heart and its relationship to the arterial and venous circulation in 3-dimensional space and obtain hemodynamic data in the same study is unique to CMR. Images can be obtained in any preferred plane, and this is often essential in patients with complex congenital heart disease or with complex repairs. Also, important parameters such as LV and RV volumes and function, which are used to make important clinical decisions, can be measured in an accurate and reproducible manner. Furthermore, as these patients are typically young and require multiple imaging studies throughout their lives, CMR provides excellent assessment without ionizing radiation exposure. The major limitation of CMR in this population is the susceptibility to artifacts from previous surgeries involving surgical clips, valves, and coils.

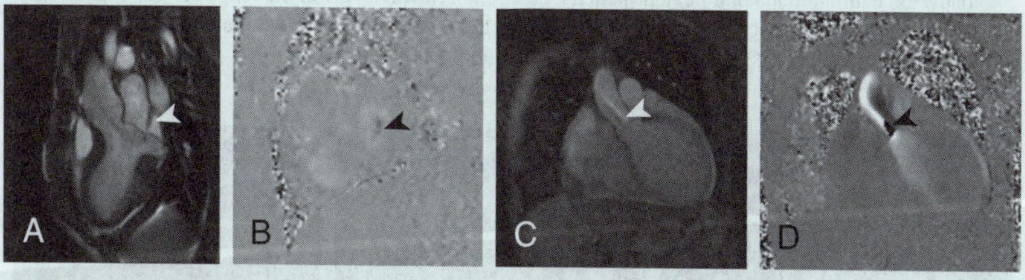

Fig. 10.7. Valvular disease assessment. **A,** Three-chamber steady-state free precession (SSFP) image showing bi-leaflet mitral valve prolapse and a jet of mitral regurgitation *(arrow)*. **B,** Short-axis phase-contrast image of the mitral valve during systole showing the mitral regurgitant orifice *(arrow)*. **C and D,** Coronal magnitude and phase images, respectively, of the aortic valve showing flow acceleration at and beyond the aortic valve of aortic stenosis *(arrow)*.

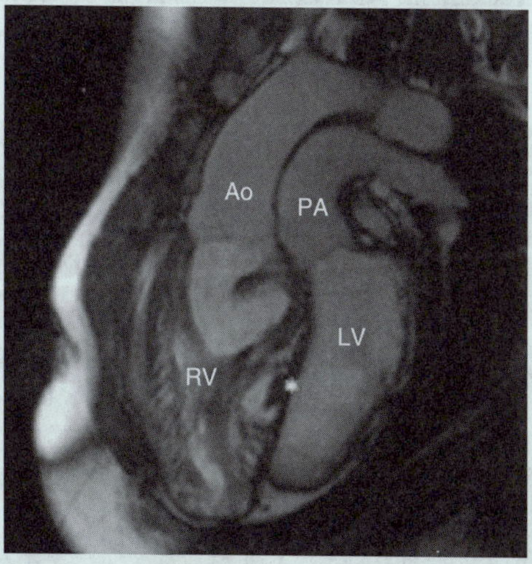

Fig. 10.8. Transposition of the great arteries (TGA) after atrial switch operation with Mustard procedure. The aorta (Ao) is positioned anteriorly and arises from the hypertrophied, morphologic right ventricle (RV). The pulmonary artery (PA) is positioned posteriorly and arises from the left ventricle (LV). *(Image from Steinmetz, M., Preuss, H. C., & Lotz, J. [2012]. Non-invasive imaging for congential heart disease—recent progress in cardiac MRI.* Journal of Clinical & Experimental Cardiology, *S8, 008. doi:10.4172/2155-9880.)*

14. Can cardiac magnetic resonance be used to assess cardiac masses?

Cardiac MRI is a good modality for the assessment of tumors (Fig. 10.9), as tissue characterization using various sequences may provide insights into the differential diagnosis of an identified mass. However, the initial hopes that CMR could definitively characterize tumor tissue (e.g., a noninvasive biopsy) have not quite come to fruition. However, CMR can still help narrow the differential diagnosis and provide information about whether the tumor has characteristics suggestive of malignancy. However, small tumors, and those with high-frequency motion, may not be appropriately assessed using CMR.

15. What are some of the other clinical uses of cardiac magnetic resonance?

Some other appropriate uses of CMR include the assessment of pericardial conditions such as pericardial mass and constrictive pericarditis. Specifically, in constrictive pericarditis, CMR can help assess the thickness of the pericardium, predict the presence of pericardial enhancement suggestive of recent pericardial inflammation or neovascularization, and assess some of the physiologic changes seen.

CMR can also be used to assess the pulmonary vein anatomy prior to ablation for atrial fibrillation. The number, size, and orientation of the pulmonary veins can be assessed, and information about the left atrium can also be provided.

CMR is also used for the assessment of aortic dissection (Fig. 10.10) and is often used in follow-up examinations and postsurgical assessments. However, given the length of the examination and difficulty monitoring the patient closely during the examination, CMR is generally not considered the first modality for dissection assessment in the acute setting.

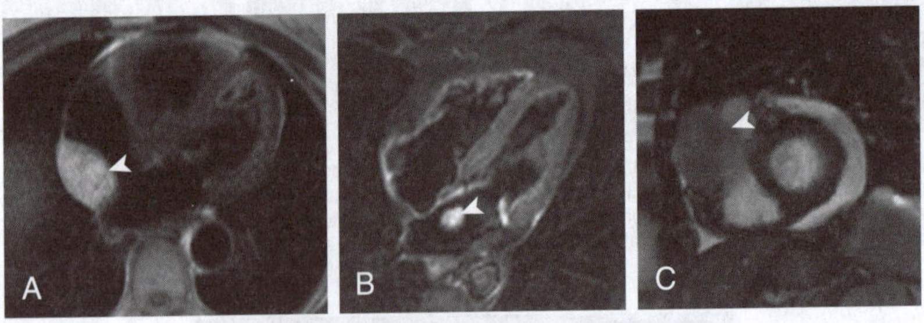

Fig. 10.9. Cardiac masses. Three cardiac masses *(arrows)* are illustrated using three different CMR sequences: **(A)** lipoma, **(B)** left atrial myxoma, **(C)** metastatic melanoma.

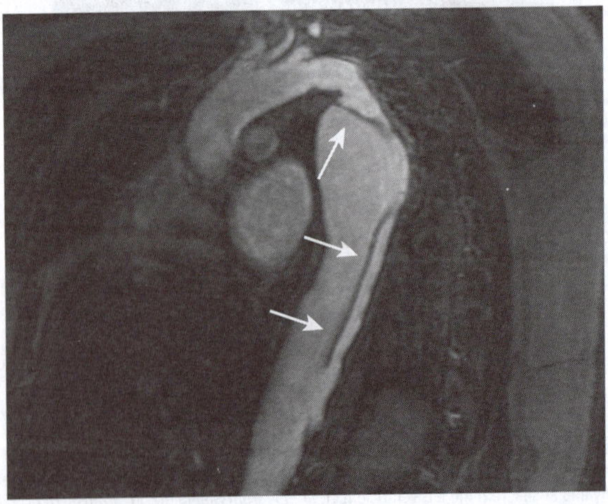

Fig. 10.10. MRI demonstrating aortic dissection. The dissection flaps *(arrows)* are clearly delineated. *(Image courtesy of Dr. Lars Grenacher.)*

16. What are the contraindications to cardiac magnetic resonance?

Some of the most common contraindications to CMR are ferromagnetic objects, such as certain metallic implants and implanted devices. All devices should be checked for MRI compatibility prior to taking the patient into the MRI room. An important reference website for checking the compatibility of a device is www.mrisafety.com. Alternatively, the manufacturer of the device should be contacted to check for compatibility. Table 10.2 lists some of the most important contraindications.

17. Can cardiac magnetic resonance be performed in patients with implanted cardiovascular devices?

Most implanted cardiovascular devices are nonferromagnetic or only weakly ferromagnetic. This includes most commonly used coronary stents, peripheral vascular stents, inferior vena cava (IVC) filters, prosthetic heart valves, cardiac closure devices, aortic stent grafts, and embolization coils. A statement on the safety of scanning patients with cardiovascular devices was published by the American Heart Association, giving guidelines of the timing and safety of device scanning.

Pacemakers and implantable cardioverter defibrillators have been strong relative contraindications to MRI scanning, and scanning of such patients should be performed only under specific conditions in centers with expertise in performing these studies. However, given the widespread use of pacemakers, concerns about not being able to perform MRI for even noncardiac indications have encouraged manufacturers to make multiple MRI safe pacemakers. The first such device is the Revo MRI SureScan system, which was approved by the FDA for use in 2011 as an MRI-conditional device. And in 2015 the Evera MRI implantable cardioverter-defibrillator (ICD) became the first ICD approved by the FDA as an MRI-conditional device. The conditional designation still necessitates specific patient and MRI protocols to be followed to ensure safety. Nonetheless, these advances in pacemaker and ICD design have made it possible to perform both cardiac and noncardiac MRI imaging in patients with these selected devices. However, the artifacts that are generated by the pacemaker lead or the generator itself can affect interpretation of large segments of the cardiac anatomy. Therefore the purpose of a cardiac MRI study in a patient with a pacing or ICD system should be carefully considered before proceeding.

18. What is nephrogenic systemic fibrosis?

Nephrogenic systemic fibrosis (NSF) is a fibrosing condition involving skin, joints, muscles including cardiac myocytes, and other internal organs. Although NSF was first identified in 1997, the association of this entity with gadolinium-based contrast agents was only described in 2006. The most important risk factors for the development of NSF with gadolinium-based contrast agents are advanced renal disease, recent vascular surgical procedures, dialysis, acute renal failure, and higher doses of contrast agent (>0.1 mmol/kg). On average, the time interval between administration of gadolinium-based contrast agent (GBCA) and NSF is 60 to 90 days. As a consequence of the concerns associated with NSF, the FDA issued a black box warning on the use of gadolinium-based contrast agents, restricting its use in patients with reduced renal function. However, since this black box warning, centers have adopted methods to carefully screen patients for renal function and other risk factors prior to gadolinium-based contrast agent administration. This has resulted in the virtual eradication of new cases of NSF over the past 8 years.

Table 10.2. Common Contraindications to Cardiac Magnetic Resonance
• Ocular foreign body (e.g., metal in eye) • Central nervous system aneurysm clips • Implanted neural stimulator • Cochlear implant • Implanted cardiac pacemaker or defibrillator (see the text for caveats) • Other implanted medical devices (drug infusion ports, insulin pump) • Swan-Ganz catheters • Metal shrapnel or bullet • Pregnant women

In patients with advanced renal disease (GFR <30 mL/min), the risks and benefits of gadolinium-enhanced MRI scans should be carefully weighed, and alternate imaging modalities should first be considered. If a contrast-based CMR study is absolutely necessary, then the risks, benefits, and methods to avoid NSF should be discussed with imaging staff, nephrology service, and the patient prior to the study, and the patient should be carefully monitored after the CMR.

Bibliography, Suggested Readings, and Websites

Cummings, K. W., Bhalla, S., Javidan-Nejad, C., Bierhals, A. J., Gutierrez, F. R., & Woodard, P. K. (2009). A pattern-based approach to assessment of delayed enhancement in non-ischemic cardiomyopathy at MR imaging. *RadioGraphics*, *29*, 89–103.

Gold, M. R., Sommer, T., Schwitter, J., Al Fagih, A., Albert, T., Merkely, B., et al. (2015). Full-body MRI in patients with an implantable cardioverter-defibrillator: primary results of a randomized study. *Journal of the American College of Cardiology*, *65*(24), 2581–2588.

Kanal, E., Broome, D. R., Martin, D. R., & Thomsen, H. S. (2008). Response to the FDA's May 23, 2007, nephrogenic systemic fibrosis update. *Radiology*, *246*, 11–14.

Kim, R. J., Wu, E., Rafael, A., Chen, E. L., Parker, M. A., Simonetti, O., et al. (2000). The use of contrast-enhanced magnetic resonance imaging to identify reversible myocardial dysfunction. *New England Journal of Medicine*, *343*(20), 1445–1453.

Kramer, C. M., Barkhausen, J., Flamm, S. D., Kim, R. J., Nagel, E., Society for Cardiovascular Magnetic Resonance Board of Trustees Task Force on Standardized Protocols. (2013). Standardized cardiovascular magnetic resonance (CMR) protocols 2013 update. *Journal of Cardiovascular Magnetic Resonance*, *15*, 91.

Levine, G. N., Gomes, A. S., Arai, A. E., Bluemke, D. A., Flamm, S. D., Kanal, E., et al. (2007). Safety of magnetic resonance imaging in patients with cardiovascular devices: an American Heart Association scientific statement from the Committee on Diagnostic and Interventional Cardiac Catheterization, Council on Clinical Cardiology, and the Council on Cardiovascular Radiology and Intervention: endorsed by the American College of Cardiology Foundation, the North American Society for Cardiac Imaging, and the Society for Cardiovascular Magnetic Resonance. *Circulation*, *116*(24), 2878–2891.

Lin, D., & Kramer, C. (2008). Late gadolinium-enhanced cardiac magnetic resonance. *Current Cardiology Reports*, *10*(1), 72–78.

Hendel, R. C., Patel, M. R., Kramer, C. M., Poon, M., Carr, J. C., & Gerstad, N. C. (2006). ACCF/ACR/SCCT/SCMR/ASNC/NASCI/SCAI/SIR 2006 appropriateness criteria for cardiac computed tomography and cardiac magnetic resonance imaging. *Journal of the American College of Cardiology*, *48*(7), 1476–1497.

Shinbane, J. S., Colletti, P. M., & Shellock, F. G. (2011). Magnetic resonance imaging in patients with cardiac pacemakers: era of "MR Conditional" designs. *Journal of Cardiovascular Magnetic Resonance*, *13*(1), 63.

US Food and Drug Administration. (2013). *Information for healthcare professionals: gadolinium-based contrast agents for magnetic resonance imaging (marketed as Magnevist, MultiHance, Omniscan, OptiMARK, ProHance)*. < http://www.fda.gov/Drugs/DrugSafety/PostmarketDrugSafetyInformationforPatientsandProviders/ucm142884.htm. > Accessed Aug 2016.

Wolk, M. J., Bailey, S. R., Doherty, J. U., Douglas, P. S., Hendel, R. C., Kramer, C. M., et al. (2014). ACCF/AHA/ASE/ASNC/HFSA/HRS/SCAI/SCCT/SCMR/STS 2013 multimodality appropriate use criteria for the detection and risk assessment of stable ischemic heart disease. (2014). *Journal of the American College of Cardiology*, *63*(4), 380–406.

Zou, Z., Zhang, H. L., Roditi, G. H., Leiner, T., Kucharczyk, W., & Prince, M. R. (2011). Nephrogenic systemic fibrosis review of 370 biopsy-confirmed cases. *JACC: cardiovascular Imaging*, *4*(11), 206–216.

Useful Websites

1. www.mrisafety.com.
2. www.scmr.org.
3. www.imaios.com/en/e-Courses/e-MRI.

CARDIAC COMPUTED TOMOGRAPHY

Prabhakar Rajiah, Suhny Abbara

CHAPTER 11

1. **What are the contraindications for cardiac computed tomography?**
   An inability to remain still, hold one's breath, or follow instructions are contraindications to coronary computed tomography angiography (CTA). Anaphylactic reaction to intravenous iodinated contrast is considered an absolute contraindication, though less severe allergic reactions may be acceptable if the patient has been adequately premedicated, usually with a combination of intravenous (IV) or oral diphenhydramine and corticosteroids.

2. **What is the difference between prospective triggering and retrospective gating?**
   Prospective triggering is an axial (step-and-shoot) imaging technique that acquires images of the heart in a predetermined phase of the cardiac cycle—for example, 75% of the R-R interval. During the remainder of the cardiac cycle, the CT tube current is turned off. This is in contrast to retrospective gating, which is a spiral acquisition where the CT tube current remains on during the entire R-R interval. To reduce radiation, the tube current may be decreased during systole (electrocardiogram [ECG]-based tube current modulation). However, there is a significant reduction in radiation dose when prospective triggering is used (Fig. 11.1).

3. **When might retrospective gating be used rather than prospective triggering?**
   Retrospective gating is needed when cardiac function measurements are needed. Because images are acquired throughout the cardiac cycle, volume measurements of the right and left ventricles can be obtained in end-systole and end-diastole, allowing the calculation of stroke volume, ejection fraction, and cardiac output. Retrospective gating is also helpful in patients with irregular heart rhythms to help ensure that diagnostic images of the coronary arteries are acquired. In contrast to

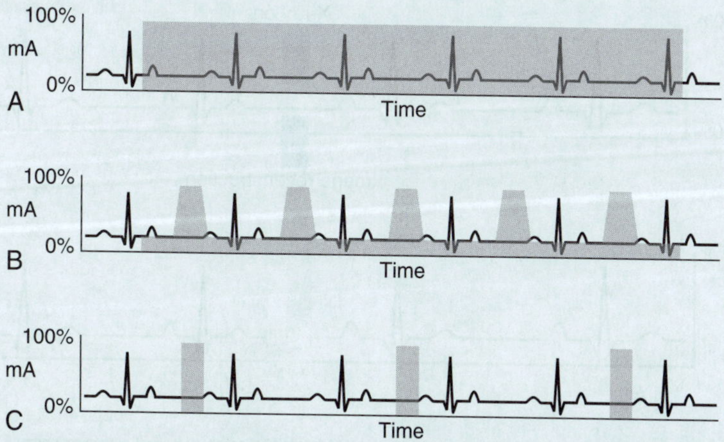

Fig. 11.1. Schematic drawings of retrospective gating *(top)* and prospective triggering *(bottom)* techniques. Retrospective gating without tube current modulation **(A)** utilizes full tube current throughout the cardiac cycle. With tube current modulation applied **(B)**, the full current is delivered only during a specified portion of the R-R interval (usually late diastole). In this case, the remainder of the cardiac cycle receives only 20% of the full tube current. Prospective triggering **(C)** utilizes full tube current only through a specified portion of the R-R interval. Every other heartbeat is imaged in prospective triggering to allow time for table movement.

prospective triggering, retrospective gating allows the user to employ ECG editing to remove artifacts related to premature ventricular contractions or dropped beats.

4. Is it possible to scan the entire heart in a single heartbeat?

With the use of modern CT scanners, it is possible to scan the entire heart within a single heartbeat. Single-heartbeat scanning is associated with significantly lower motion artifacts. This can be done by using either wide-array/volume scanners or high-pitch spiral scanning. Wide-array scanners have multiple rows of detectors (256 or 320 rows). With such scanners, a larger volume of the patient can be scanned in a single rotation of the x-ray tube, making it possible to scan the entire heart in one heartbeat.

Another technique that is available only in a second- or third-generation dual-source CT scanner is a prospective ECG-triggered "high-pitch spiral" mode. With this mode, images of the heart can be obtained within a single R-R interval owing to the use of high pitch, up to 3.4. The use of higher pitch also decreases the radiation dose (Fig. 11.2).

5. What is the radiation dose of a standard cardiac computed tomography examination?

The radiation dose of a standard cardiac CTA depends on a multitude of factors and can range from less than 1 mSv to as high as 30 mSv with older high-dose techniques and scanners. The median dose in an older registry study showed the cardiac CT dose to be just below 10 mSv. Since that study, however, several new scanners and associated hardware have been developed as well as new dose-reduction strategies. In several more recent reports, the median reported dose ranges from 3 to 5 mSv.

To put things in perspective, the average dose from a nuclear perfusion stress test is 6 to 25 mSv (or as high as 40 mSv or more in thallium stress/rest tests), and the average dose from a simple diagnostic coronary angiogram is 5 to 7 mSv.

Factors affecting the radiation dose of a cardiac CT include the type of scanner (single-source vs. dual-source), the number of detectors, the patient's body habitus, the selection of kVp and mAs, and the scan mode (prospective triggering vs. retrospective gating with or without tube current modulation). General measures to reduce the radiation dose to the patient should be used whenever possible according to the "as low as reasonably achievable (ALARA)" principle. Unless a specific reason prohibits its use, tube modulation should be applied routinely if retrospective gating is selected.

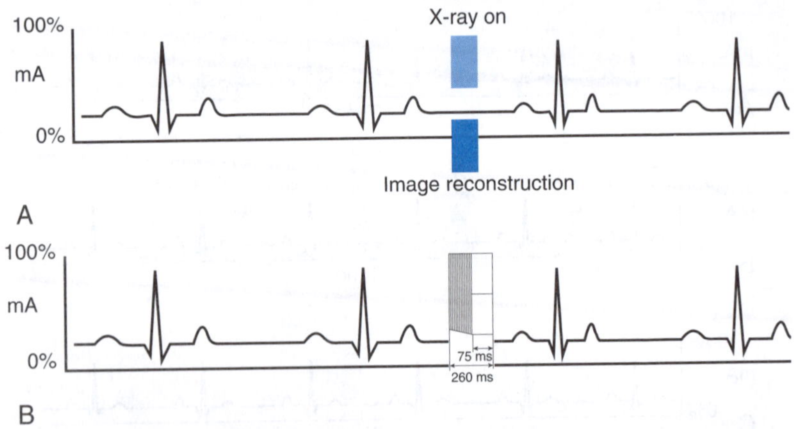

Fig. 11.2. Schematic drawings of wide-detector-array *(top)* and high-pitch helical *(bottom)* dual-source scanners. **A,** Illustration demonstrating prospective ECG-triggered axial acquisition using a wide-array scanner. With wide-array scanners such as 256- and 320-slice scanners, the longitudinal axis coverage is significantly increased, which enables acquisition of the entire heart within one R-R interval. **B,** Using dual-source detectors and a helical acquisition, sampling gaps of the first x-ray system are filled with data from the second x-ray system such that the pitch values with helical acquisition are higher than normal. Thus the entire heart can be imaged within the diastolic phase of one R-R interval. Radiation dose is also reduced because of the higher pitch.

6. What is blooming and what techniques can be done to reduce it?

Blooming is an artifact created when material of very high attenuation is being imaged. The borders of a high-attenuation material will "bleed" into adjacent structures. In the case of coronary CTA, blooming from calcified plaque can lead to overestimation of the degree of coronary stenosis. For this reason, coronary CT scans in patients with heavily calcified coronary arteries may yield nonevaluable coronary artery segments. An example of a heavily calcified coronary artery with blooming effect is shown in Fig. 11.3.

7. Are beta-blockers necessary for coronary computed tomography angiography?

The ability of a scanner to "freeze" cardiac motion depends on the gantry's rotation speed, the technique used, and the patient's heart rate. Most currently available 64-slice scanners have gantry rotation speeds in the range of 150 to 210 ms for a half-gantry rotation (only a 180-degree rotation is needed to reconstruct an image). With these scanners, a target heart rate of 60 bpm or below is required for optimal image quality free of motion artifact. A slower heart rate and regular rhythm are also generally required for prospective triggering, which allows a significant reduction in the radiation dose.

Newer scanners such as the 256-slice CT scanner have half-gantry rotation speeds as fast as 135 ms. Third-generation dual-source CT scanners have two x-ray tubes oriented 90 degrees apart housed within the same gantry. Rather than a 180-degree gantry rotation, only 90 degrees is required to generate an image, resulting in a temporal resolution of approximately 66 ms. This allows images to be acquired without the use of beta-blockers in a greater proportion of patients.

8. What is a coronary calcium score?

A calcium score examination is a specialized type of cardiac CT (Fig. 11.4) without contrast that is processed with software to quantify the amount of coronary calcium. Based on this scan and a standardized scoring protocol, a "coronary calcium score" can be generated. This number, also called the Agatston score, is used as a surrogate for the total amount of coronary plaque and is correlated with patients of the same age and gender. It is most useful in patients at unclear or intermediate risk for coronary artery disease (CAD) to guide decision making, such as whether or not to initiate statin therapy or proceed with additional evaluation of the patient's symptoms.

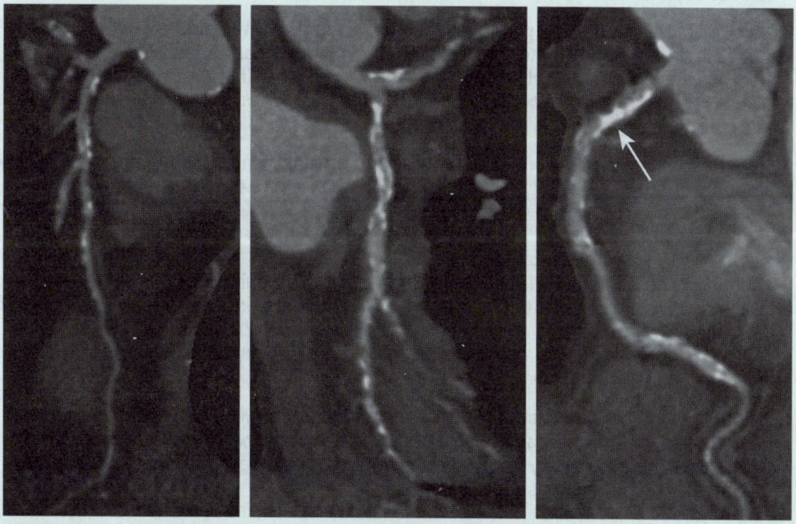

Fig. 11.3. Curved multiplanar reconstructions of the left anterior descending (LAD) *(left)*, left circumflex (LCX) *(middle)*, and right coronary artery (RCA) *(right)* demonstrate substantial calcification with blooming artifact. Evaluation of the degree of stenosis is limited in areas of extensive calcification—for example, in the proximal RCA *(arrow)*. This patient had a calcium score of 867.

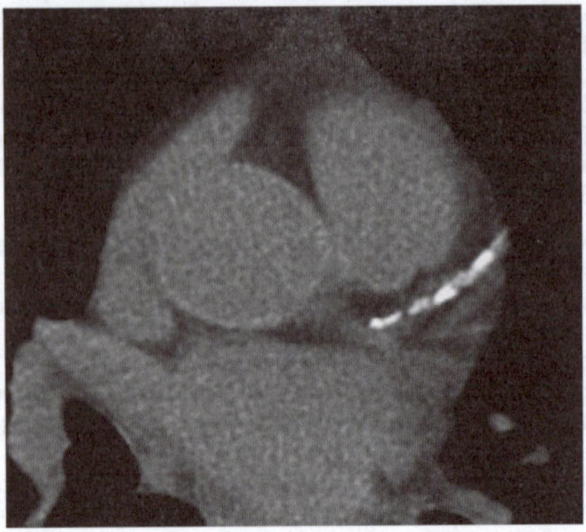

Fig. 11.4. Example of image obtained to calculate the coronary calcium score. Calcification in these images appears white. Note the heavy and diffuse calcification of the left anterior descending (LAD) artery. *(Image adopted from Dey, D., Nakazato, R., Pimentel, R., Paz, W., Hayes, S. W., Friedman, J. D., et al. [2012]. Low radiation coronary calcium scoring by dual-source CT with tube current optimization based on patient body size.* Journal of Cardiovascular Computed Tomography, 6*[2], 113–120. doi:http://dx.doi.org/10.1016/j.jcct.2011.12.008.)*

9. **What is the value of a negative calcium score in a patient with low to intermediate risk?**
   A negative calcium score in a low-risk patient is associated with a very low likelihood of coronary events. The "warranty period" for patients with a calcium score of 0 and low CAD risk is approximately 4 years. For patients with a 0 calcium score and low to intermediate risk, the negative predictive value for detecting obstructive CAD is between 95% and 99%. However, calcium scoring is not recommended in the setting of acute chest pain, whereas coronary CTA may be a consideration and provide actual 2D and 3D images of the coronary arteries (Fig. 11.5).

10. **Is calcium scoring an appropriate test in a patient of low coronary heart disease risk but with a family history of premature coronary heart disease?**
    Patients with a family history of premature coronary heart disease (CHD) have been shown to have detectable coronary artery calcium despite a low Framingham risk estimation. Thus calcium scoring is an appropriate test to evaluate for subclinical coronary atherosclerosis in this population.

11. **In which patients is coronary computed tomography angiography appropriate and inappropriate?**
    Coronary CTA is appropriate in patients with nonacute symptoms potentially representing an ischemic equivalent and low or intermediate pretest probability of CAD. It is also appropriate in patients presenting acutely with suspected acute coronary syndrome (ACS) who have low or intermediate pretest probability of CAD and normal, nondiagnostic, or uninterpretable ECG or cardiac biomarkers. Coronary CTA is not appropriate in patients with definite myocardial infarction (MI) and is inappropriate or of uncertain appropriateness in patients with a high pretest probability of CAD (depending on the setting). Flow diagrams of the appropriateness of coronary CTA in patients with nonacute or acute symptoms suggestive of coronary ischemia are given in Fig. 11.6.

12. **A 49-year-old man with severe osteoarthritis presents with nonacute chest pain. You determine that he has an intermediate pretest probability of coronary artery disease. Would coronary computed tomography angiography be an appropriate first test to evaluate for such disease?**
    Coronary CTA is an appropriate first test in patients who are unable to exercise and who have either a low or intermediate probability of CAD. Coronary CTA has been shown to be a highly sensitive test for the detection of CAD, with negative predictive values approaching 97% to 99%. Patients who are able to exercise with intermediate pretest probability are also appropriate candidates for coronary CTA. CTA in this patient revealed a focal, severe stenosis in the middle of the left anterior descending (LAD) artery (see Fig. 11.7).

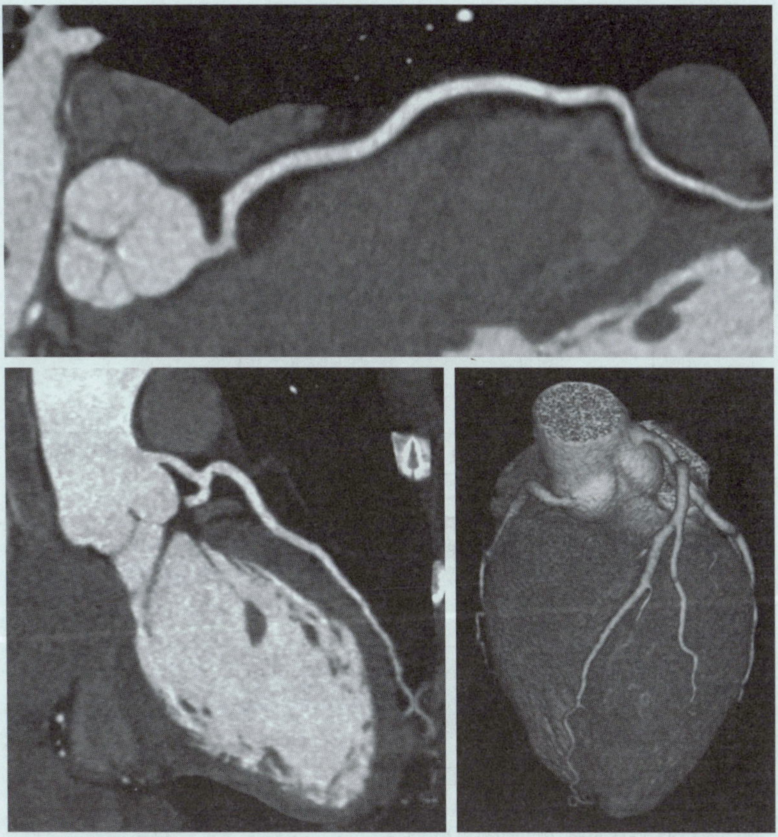

Fig. 11.5. Curved multiplanar reconstructions of the right coronary artery (RCA) *(top)* and left anterior descending (LAD) *(bottom left)* and volume-rendered 3D reconstruction *(bottom right)* show absence of coronary plaque or stenosis. A negative CT with good image quality has a very high negative predictive value and may spare the patient a diagnostic invasive angiogram. This study was done with a total radiation dose of 2.4 mSv.

13. A 59-year-old woman with a low to intermediate pretest probability of coronary artery disease presents with acute chest pain. Despite a negative electrocardiogram and cardiac biomarkers, you still suspect acute coronary syndrome. Is coronary computed tomography angiography an appropriate test to evaluate for coronary artery disease?

Yes, patients with low to intermediate pretest probability of CAD and a normal/equivocal ECG and biomarkers are appropriate for evaluation by coronary CTA. The Rule Out Myocardial Infarction Using Computer Assisted Tomography (ROMICAT) trials demonstrated that patients with no evidence of CAD by coronary CTA have essentially 0% chance of a major adverse cardiovascular event for at least 2 years, and subsequent trials have confirmed a close to zero event rate in this setting. Subsequent trials such as ROMICAT-II, CT-STAT (Coronary Computed Tomographic Angiography for Systematic Triage of Acute Chest Pain), and ACRIN-PA (American College of Radiology Imaging Network/Pennsylvania Department of Health) have shown that CTA is safe modality to triage patients with acute chest pain and consistently reduces the length of hospital stay, thus reducing the cost compared to a standard in-hospital workup.

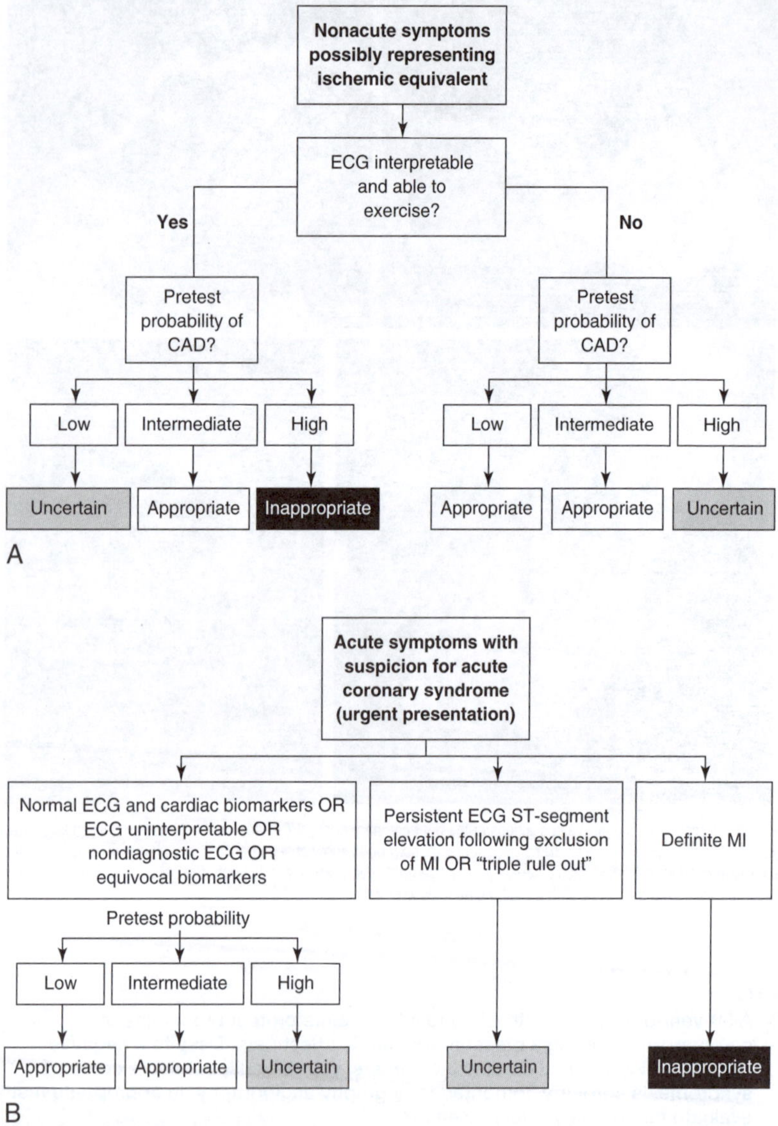

Fig. 11.6. Flow diagrams of the appropriateness of coronary CTA in patients with **(A)** nonacute and **(B)** acute symptoms suggestive of coronary ischemia are given in this figure and Fig. 11.5. *CAD*, Coronary artery disease; *ECG*, electrocardiogram; *MI*, myocardial infarction. *(Reproduced with permission from Taylor, A. J., Cerqueira, M., Hodgson, J. M., Mark, D., Min, J., O'Gara, P. J., et al. [2010]. ACCF/SCCT/ACR/AHA/ASE/ASNC/NASCI/SCAI/SCMR 2010 Appropriate Use Criteria for Cardiac Computed Tomography. A Report of the American College of Cardiology Foundation Appropriate Use Criteria Task Force, the Society of Cardiovascular Computed Tomography, the American College of Radiology, the American Heart Association, the American Society of Echocardiography, the American Society of Nuclear Cardiology, the North American Society for Cardiovascular Imaging, the Society for Cardiovascular Angiography and Interventions, and the Society for Cardiovascular Magnetic Resonance.* Journal of Cardiovascular Computed Tomography, 4*[6], 407.e1–407.e33.)*

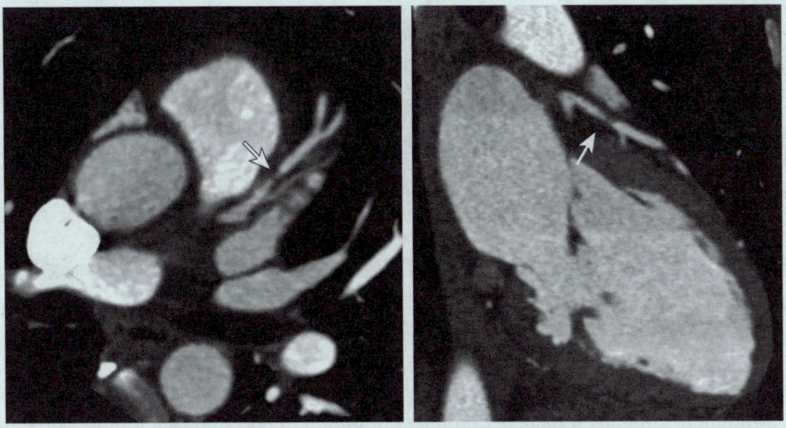

Fig. 11.7. Multiplanar reformatted images demonstrate focal, severe stenosis *(arrows)* of the mid-left anterior descending (LAD) artery.

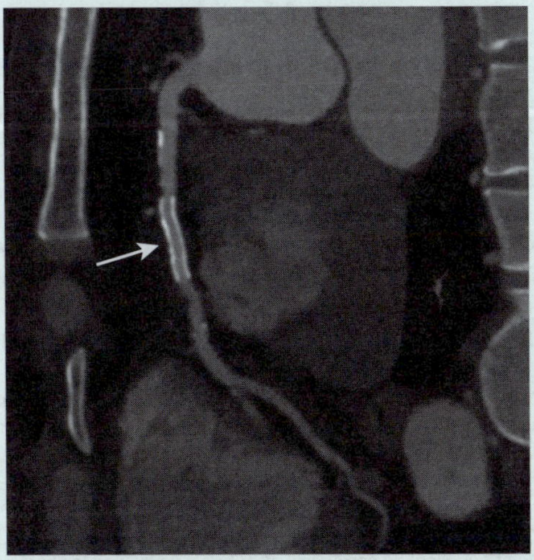

Fig. 11.8. Curved multiplanar reconstruction of the RCA showing a patent stent in the mid-RCA *(arrow)*. Note contrast opacification within the stent and distal to the stent. A sharp reconstruction kernel and thin slices were used for the reconstructions. This stent was 3.5 mm in diameter.

14. A 61-year-old woman presents to your office with nonacute chest pain. She has a history of prior stent placement in the right coronary artery. The stent is 2.5 mm in diameter. Is coronary computed tomography angiography a useful test for detecting in-stent restenosis in this patient?

Accurate assessment of in-stent restenosis is based on a number of factors including the diameter of the stent, material used, and size of the struts as well as the capabilities of the CT scanner. Based on recent appropriateness criteria, stents less than 3 mm in diameter are not appropriate for evaluation by coronary CTA.

A stent is considered occluded if the lumen is unopacified and there is absent distal runoff. The presence of distal contrast opacification alone is not an adequate sign of stent patency because of the potential for retrograde filling from collateral vessels.

Fig. 11.8 shows a patent stent in a different patient with larger (3.5 mm) stent diameter.

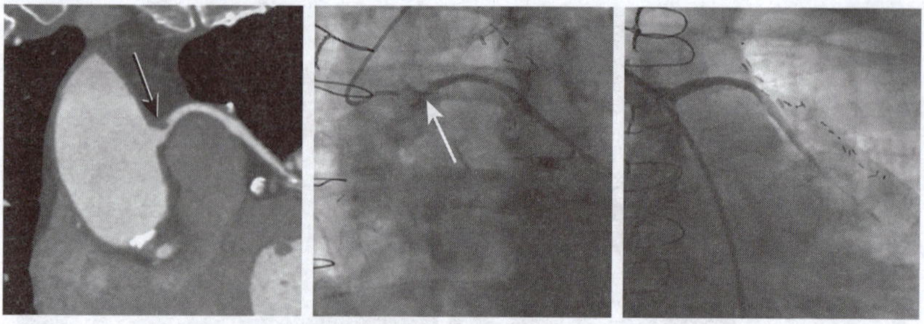

Fig. 11.9. Curved multiplanar reconstruction *(left image)* of a saphenous vein graft demonstrates focal proximal stenosis of the graft *(black arrow)*. A conventional angiogram *(right image)* confirms the high-grade stenosis *(white arrow)*.

15. A 69-year-old man with a history of prior coronary artery bypass graft presents with nonacute chest pain. Is coronary computed tomography angiography useful for detecting graft stenosis in this patient?

Coronary CTA is indicated for symptomatic patients with prior coronary artery bypass grafts (CABGs) to evaluate for graft patency. It is also an excellent method for evaluating graft thrombosis, malposition, aneurysms, and pseudoaneurysms. Inclusion of the entire chest is helpful in postoperative patients for also evaluating pericardial or pleural effusions, mediastinal or wound infection, and the integrity of the sternotomy. An example of CTA in a patient several years post CABG is shown in Fig. 11.9.

16. What is the role of cardiac computed tomography in patients presenting for noncoronary cardiac surgery?

Coronary CTA in this setting is useful for the assessment of coronary arteries for obstructive disease in young and middle-aged patients presenting for noncoronary cardiac surgery such as valve repair, resection of cardiac masses, and aortic surgery. Older patients, however, tend to have a higher calcium score, and up to 10% to 25% of studies in octogenarians may not allow definitive exclusion of obstructive coronary artery disease because of one or more nonevaluable segments. In older patients, coronary angiography is generally preferred.

17. What are the diagnostic accuracy and clinical utility of plaque characterization by cardiac computed tomography?

Cardiac CT is excellent for detection and quantification of calcified portions of coronary plaque (Agatston score) and for the differentiation of calcified, mixed, and noncalcified plaques. However, when compared with the gold standard of intravascular ultrasound (IVUS), CT is only modestly accurate in the detection and quantification of the volume of noncalcified plaques (those that are stable fibrous or potentially vulnerable lipid-rich), and differentiation of the two subtypes is not reliably possible. However, emerging data suggest that high-risk features found on CTA (including positive remodeling and low attenuation) do correlate with future events. Plaque characterization by CTA remains a work in progress, and currently there is no demonstrable utility of plaque characterization for directing medical or interventional therapy.

18. Is cardiac computed tomography safe and useful in patients presenting with newly diagnosed heart failure and reduced left ventricular ejection fraction?

Coronary CTA is an appropriate test for patients with low or intermediate pretest probability of CAD and new-onset or newly diagnosed clinical heart failure with reduced left ventricular ejection fraction. The objective is to exclude CAD as a cause of heart failure.

19. Can cardiac computed tomography be used to differentiate between a subacute and an old myocardial infarction?

Characteristic morphologic changes in the myocardium can be detected by cardiac CT in patients who have a remote history of MI. Patients usually develop wall thinning in relation to normal adjacent myocardium. In some instances, fatty metaplasia or calcification may develop. If retrospective gating is used, a regional wall motion abnormality is usually seen. Delayed enhancement imaging reveals an area of hyperenhancement in the appropriate coronary territory. In contrast, an acute MI will appear as a hypoperfused, akinetic area of myocardium with normal wall thickness. Examples of chronic and acute MI are shown in Fig. 11.10.

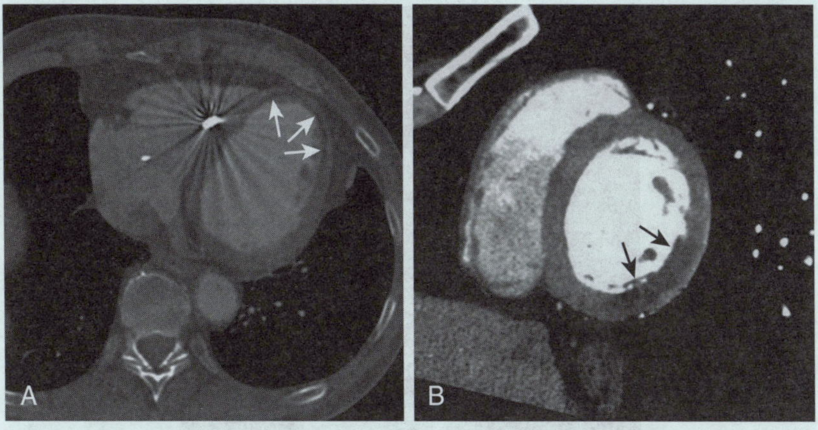

Fig. 11.10. Examples of chronic and acute MI detected by cardiac CT. **A,** Cardiac gated axial CT shows apical myocardial thinning and deposition of subendocardial low-attenuation material *(white arrows)* measuring −15 Hounsfield units (HU), indicating fatty metaplasia in a patient with remote LAD myocardial infarction. **B,** Cardiac gated CT in left ventricular short axis shows inferolateral subendocardial hypoenhancement that measures 35 HU *(black arrows)* and normal myocardial wall thickness, representing a perfusion defect in a patient with acute left circumflex MI.

20. Should noncoronary structures be reviewed and reported on during a cardiac computed tomography examination?

The current consensus and standard of care is to include in the final report all significant findings noted in the acquired dataset, using a wide field of view. Everything that is part of the originally acquired dataset should be reviewed and reported on if potentially significant.

21. Summarize the appropriate uses of cardiac computed tomography in regard to the evaluation of cardiac structure and function.

Cardiac CT is an excellent test for the evaluation of coronary anomalies and assessment of adult congenital heart disease. It is appropriate for evaluating LV function after MI or in patients with heart failure when other imaging modalities are inadequate, and it is useful for evaluating right ventricular morphology and function, including in cases of suspected arrhythmogenic right ventricular dysplasia (ARVD). When other imaging modalities are inadequate or incomplete, it is useful for evaluating native or prosthetic cardiac valves in the setting of valvular dysfunction and for evaluating cardiac masses. Prior to invasive procedures, cardiac CT is useful for pulmonary vein mapping, coronary vein mapping, and for localizing bypass grafts and other retrosternal anatomy. Finally, cardiac CT is an appropriate test for evaluation of the pericardium.

22. Would cardiac CT be an appropriate first modality in the assessment of a 29-year-old woman with suspected Turner syndrome presenting with symptoms of dyspnea, murmur, and hypertension?

Patients with suspected Turner syndrome may have multiple congenital anomalies, including a bicuspid aortic valve, coarctation of the aorta, elongation of the transverse aortic arch, atrial or ventricular septal defect, and partial anomalous pulmonary venous return. Cardiac CT is a reasonable choice as the first modality in assessing all of these congenital anomalies in a single study. Abnormal cardiac CT findings in this patient are illustrated in Figs. 11.11 and 11.12.

23. A 56-year-old woman is being evaluated for syncope. Coronary angiography was not able to image the left circumflex coronary artery. Is coronary computed tomography angiography an appropriate next test?

Coronary CTA is an excellent test for imaging anomalous coronary arteries (Fig. 11.13). Cardiac CT allows for the assessment of artery origin and course, which is critical in assessing the potential clinical significance of the aberrant coronary artery and necessary to determine whether surgical correction is indicated.

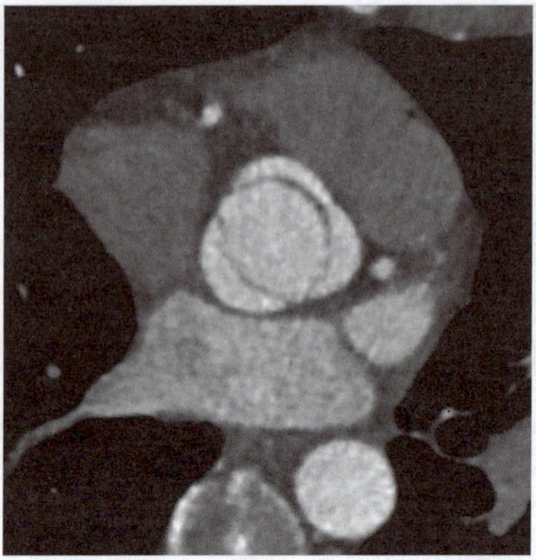

Fig. 11.11. Bicuspid aortic valve. Systolic frame of retrospectively ECG-gated CT in the short-axis plane of the aortic valve shows an open bicuspid aortic valve. There is congenital fusion of the right and left coronary cusps.

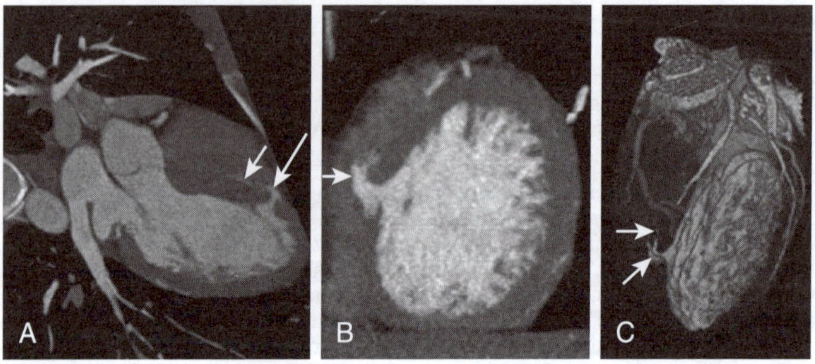

Fig. 11.12. Ventricular septal defect. ECG-gated CT angiogram in **(A)** LV long-axis and **(B)** short-axis views shows a defect in the ventricular septum with contrast spilling from the opacified left ventricular (LV) cavity across the septum into the otherwise unopacified right ventricle *(arrows)*. **C,** The volume-rendered image shows the contrast within the LV cavity and the small shunt volume *(arrow)* crossing into the unopacified right ventricle.

24. A 45-year-old woman is having computed tomography of the pulmonary veins prior to radiofrequency ablation for atrial fibrillation. What is the purpose of pulmonary vein mapping? What is the most common anatomic variant of the pulmonary veins?

Intraoperative pulmonary vein mapping with conventional angiography can be time-consuming, and significant time savings can be realized by mapping the pulmonary veins with CT (Fig. 11.14). DICOM image datasets can be uploaded into cardiac imaging software for direct correlation and fusion with electroanatomic maps during the pulmonary vein isolation procedure. Preoperative mapping is also useful for detecting variant anatomy, which can be fairly common; the most common anatomic variant is a separate ostium for the right middle pulmonary vein. Measurement of the pulmonary vein ostia may be important for the proper catheter selection and for future comparison if there is a question of pulmonary vein stenosis.

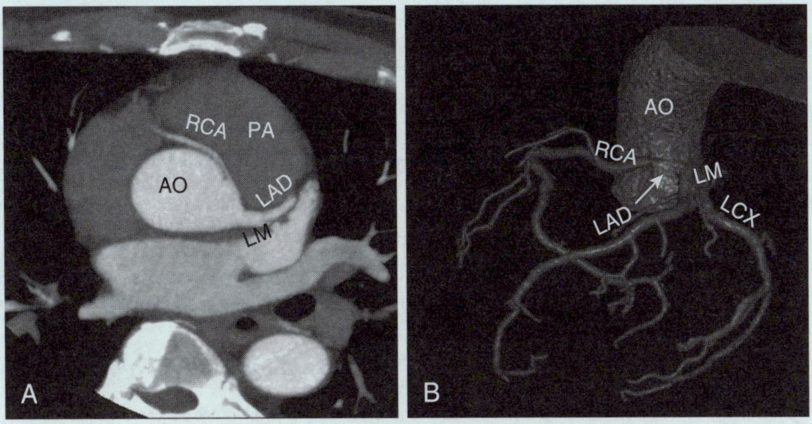

Fig. 11.13. Coronary artery anomaly. Reconstructed axial image **(A)** and volume rendered **(B)** CT images show anomalous origin of the right coronary artery (RCA) from the left aortic sinus and subsequent interarterial course between the aorta (AO) and the main pulmonary artery (PA). There is a short intramural segment *(arrow)* as well. The left main artery (LM) originates normally from the left aortic sinus and divides into LAD and LCX.

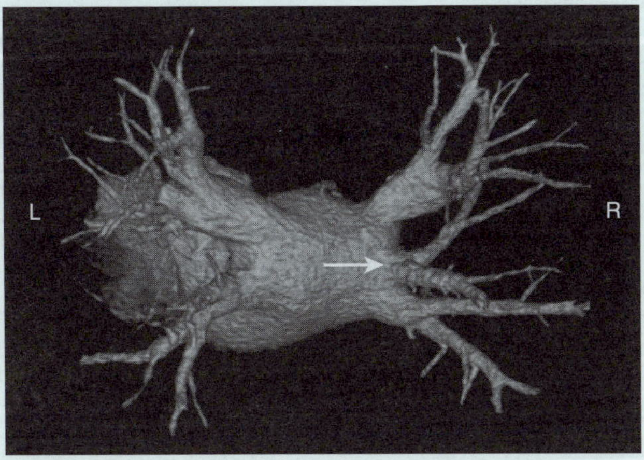

Fig. 11.14. Volume-rendered CTA 3D reconstruction of the left atrium and pulmonary veins. The study was done for pulmonary vein mapping prior to pulmonary vein isolation. Note the presence of a right middle pulmonary vein *(arrow)*.

25. Can cardiac computed tomography be used to measure fractional flow reserve? What are the situations in which it may be helpful?

Revascularization based on fractional flow reserve (FFR) measured using a pressure wire in catheter angiography has been shown to improve event-free survival compared to management based on severity of luminal stenosis. With the recent advances in technology, FFR can be obtained noninvasively from a routine cardiac CTA. Data from cardiac CT are used to generate advanced 3D computer models of coronary arteries and myocardial mass, and FFR is derived by computational fluid dynamic analysis (Fig. 11.15). Several trials such as DISCOVER-FLOW (Diagnosis of Ischemia-Causing Stenoses Obtained Via Non Invasive FFR), DeFACTO (Diagnostic Accuracy of Fractional Flow Reserve from Anatomic CTA), and NXT (Analysis of Coronary Blood flow using CTA: Next Steps) have shown improvement in diagnostic accuracy for CT-FFR

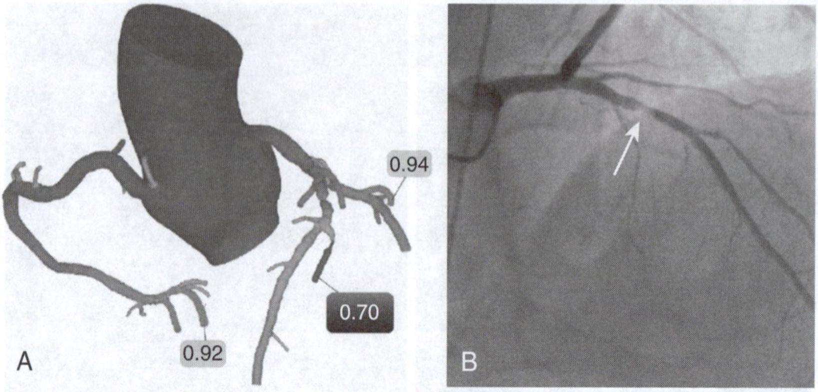

Fig. 11.15. A, CT-FFR showing abnormal FFR in the left anterior descending (LAD) artery and diagonal branch. **B,** Coronary angiogram in the same patient shows severe stenosis in the mid LAD *(arrow)*.

compared with coronary CTA for identifying lesion-specific ischemia. This ability to assess the hemodynamic significance is particularly valuable for intermediate stenotic lesions in coronary CTA, thus reducing the false-positive rate and limiting the use of invasive coronary angiography to interventional procedures.

26. An 85-year-old woman with severe aortic stenosis is being evaluated for transcutaneous aortic valve replacement. Should she undergo computed tomography examination prior to the procedure?

CT plays an important role in the evaluation of patients who are candidates for transcatheter aortic valve replacement (TAVR). CT provides several measurements that are important for planning the procedure, particularly the dimensions of the aortic annulus, aortic root, and sinotubular junction, which are essential for prosthetic sizing. Other measurements include length of leaflets, height of sinus of Valsalva, and distance between the annulus and coronary ostia (Fig. 11.16). CT also helps in predicting the appropriate fluoroscopic projections, which are oriented orthogonal to the aortic valve plane. CTA of the access vessels is performed to measure the minimal luminal diameters and evaluate their suitability for accommodating the large sheaths used in prosthesis delivery systems. Vascular calcification and tortuosity are also measured. The entire aorta is evaluated for kinking, dissection, and thrombi.

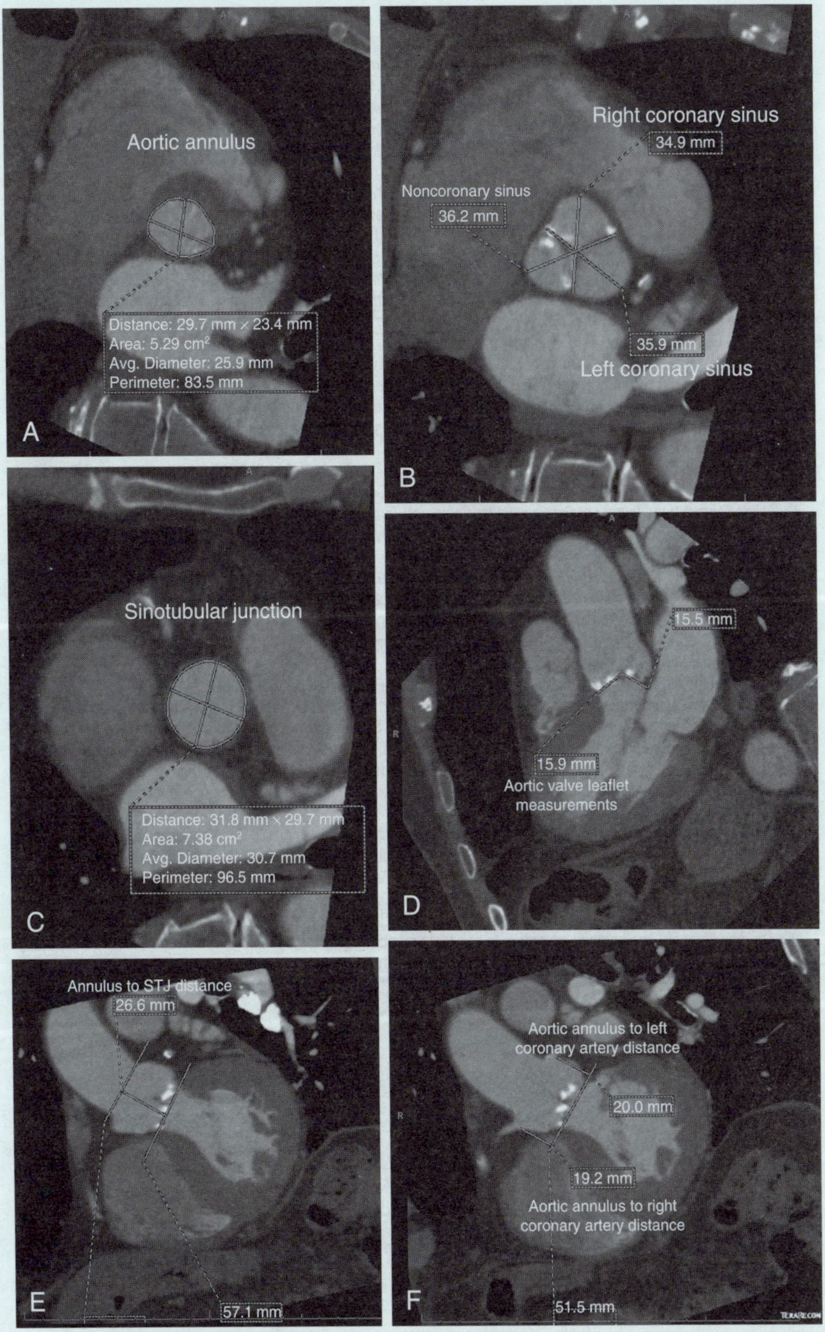

Fig. 11.16. Multiple CT images through the aortic valve and the ascending aorta demonstrate several CT measurements in a patient being evaluated for TAVR. This includes the aortic annulus **(A)**, aortic root **(B)**, sinotubular junction **(C)**, leaflet lengths **(D)**, height of sinuses **(E)**, and distance between aortic annulus and coronary artery ostia **(F)**.

Bibliography and Suggested Readings

Abbara, S. (2013). *Diagnostic imaging: cardiovascular.* Salt Lake City, UT: Amirsys.

Abbara, S., & Kalva, S. (2012). *Problem solving in cardiovascular imaging.* Philadelphia, PA: Elsevier.

Achenbach, S., Delgado, V., Hausleiter, J., Schoenhagen, P., Min, J. K., & Leipsic, J. A. (2012). SCCT expert consensus document on computed tomography imaging before transcatheter aortic valve implantation (TAVI)/transcatheter aortic valve replacement (TAVR). *Journal of Cardiovascular Computed Tomography, 6*(6), 366–380.

Budoff, M., & Shinbane, J. S. (2016). *Cardiac CT imaging: diagnosis of cardiovascular disease* (3rd ed.). New York, NY: Springer.

Cury, R. C., Kitt, T. M., Feaheny, K., Blankstein, R., Ghoshhajra, B. B., Budoff, M. J., et al. (2015). A randomized, multicenter, multivendor study of myocardial perfusion imaging with regadenoson CT perfusion vs single photon emission CT. *Journal of Cardiovascular Computed Tomography, 9*(2), 103–112.

Flohr, T. G., De Cecco, C. N., Schmidt, B., Wang, R., Schoepf, U. J., & Meinel, F. G. (2015). Computed tomographic assessment of coronary artery disease: state-of-the art. *Radiologic Clinics of North America, 53*(2), 271–285.

Fordyce, C. B., Newby, D. E., & Douglas, P. S. (2016). Diagnostic strategies for the evaluation of chest pain: clinical implications from SCOT-HEART and PROMISE. *Journal of the American College of Cardiology, 67*(7), 843–852.

Hoffmann, U., Bamberg, F., Chae, C. U., Nichols, J. H., Rogers, I. S., Seneviratne, S. K., et al. (2009). Coronary computed tomography angiography for early triage of patients with acute chest pain—the ROMICAT (Rule Out Myocardial Infarction Using Computer Assisted Tomography) Trial. *Journal of the American College of Cardiology, 53*(18), 1642–1650.

Hulten, E., Pickett, C., & Bittencourt, M. S. (2013). Outcomes after coronary computed tomography angiography in the emergency department; a systematic review and meta-analysis of randomized, controlled trials. *Journal of the American College of Cardiology, 61*, 880–892.

Leipsic, J., Abbara, S., Achenbach, S., Cury, R., Earls, J. P., Mancini, G. J., et al. (2014). SCCT guidelines for the interpretation and reporting of coronary CT angiography: a report of the Society of Cardiovascular Computed Tomography Guidelines committee. *Journal of Cardiovascular Computed Tomography, 8*(5), 342–358.

Lu, M., Chen, J. J., Awan, O., & White, C. S. (2010). Evaluation of bypass grafts and stents. *Radiologic Clinics of North America, 48*, 757–770.

Precious, B., Blanke, P., Norgaard, B. L., Min, J. K., & Leipsic, J. (2015). Fractional flow reserve modeled from resting coronary CT angiography: state of the science. *American Journal of Roentgenology, 204*, W243–W248.

Schoepf, U. J. (2008). *CT of the heart: principles and applications* (2nd ed.). Totowa, NJ: Humana Press.

Stojanovska, J., & Cronin, P. (2008). Computed tomography imaging of left atrium and pulmonary veins for radiofrequency ablation of atrial fibrillation. *Seminars in Roentgenology, 43*(2), 154–166.

Taylor, A. J., Cerqueira, M., Hodgson, J., Mark, D., Min, J., O'Gara, P., et al. (2010). ACCF/SCCT/ACR/AHA/ASE/ASNC/NASCI/SCAI/SCMR 2010 appropriate use criteria for cardiac computed tomography: a report of the American College of Cardiology Foundation Appropriate Use Criteria Task Force, the Society of Cardiovascular Computed Tomography, the American College of Radiology, the American Heart Association, the American Society of Echocardiography, the American Society of Nuclear Cardiology, the North American Society for Cardiovascular Imaging, the Society for Cardiovascular Angiography and Interventions, and the Society for Cardiovascular Magnetic Resonance. *Journal of the American College of Cardiology, 56*(22), 1864–1894.

Thompson, A. G., Raju, R., Blanke, P., Yang, T. H., Mancini, G. B., Budoff, M. J., et al. (2015). Diagnostic accuracy and discrimination of ischemia by fractional flow reserve CT using a clinical use rule: results from the Determination of Fractional Flow Reserve by Anatomic Computed Tomographic Angiography study. *Journal of Cardiovascular Computed Tomography, 9*(2), 120–128.

Zadeh, A. A., Miller, J. M., Rochitte, C. E., Dewey, M., Niinuma, H., Gottlieb, I., et al. (2012). Diagnostic accuracy of computed tomography coronary angiography according to pre-test probability of coronary artery disease and severity of coronary arterial calcification—the CORE-64 International Multicenter Study. *Journal of the American College of Cardiology, 59*(4), 379–387.

SWAN-GANZ CATHETERS AND CARDIAC HEMODYNAMICS

Ajith Nair

CHAPTER 12

1. **What is a Swan-Ganz catheter?**
   A Swan-Ganz catheter (also called a pulmonary artery [PA] catheter) is a soft, flexible catheter with an inflatable balloon at its tip that is used in right-sided heart catheterization. The balloon tip allows the catheter to float with the flow of blood from the great veins through the right-sided heart chambers and into the PA before wedging in a distal branch of the PA.

2. **How is a Swan-Ganz catheter constructed?**
   The most common Swan-Ganz catheter in current clinical use has four lumens. One is connected to the distal port of the catheter, allowing for measurement of PA pressure when the balloon is deflated and pulmonary artery wedge pressure (PAWP) when the balloon is inflated. The second lumen is attached to a temperature-sensing thermocouple 5 cm proximal to the catheter tip and is used for measurement of cardiac output (CO) by thermodilution. The third lumen is connected to a port 15 cm proximal to the catheter tip, allowing for measurement of pressure in the right atrium (RA) and for infusion of drugs or fluids into the central circulation. The fourth lumen is used to inflate the balloon with air when initially floating the catheter into position and later to reinflate the balloon for intermittent measurement of PAWP. Many catheters contain an additional proximal port for infusion of fluids and drugs. Some catheters have an additional lumen through which a temporary pacing electrode can be passed into the apex of the right ventricle for internal cardiac pacing.

3. **What information can be gained from a Swan-Ganz catheter?**
   Direct measurements obtained from the catheter include vascular pressures and oxygen saturations within the cardiac chambers, CO, and systemic venous oxygen saturation (SvO_2). These hemodynamic measurements can be used to calculate other hemodynamic parameters, such as systemic vascular resistance and pulmonary vascular resistance.

4. **How is a Swan-Ganz catheter inserted?**
   At the bedside, venous access is usually obtained by introducing an 8 French sheath into the internal jugular or subclavian vein using the Seldinger technique. The right internal jugular or left subclavian veins are preferred sites because the natural curve of the catheter will allow easier flotation into the PA. The antecubital or femoral veins are less commonly used.

   Next, a 7.5 French Swan-Ganz catheter is passed through the introducer sheath and advanced approximately 15 cm to exit the sheath into the central vein. The balloon is then inflated with 1.5 cc air, and the catheter is advanced slowly, allowing the balloon to float through the RA, right ventricle, and PA, and finally achieving a wedge position in a distal branch of the PA that is smaller in diameter than the balloon itself. The wedge position is usually achieved when the catheter has advanced a total of 35 to 55 cm, depending on which central vein is cannulated and the size of the heart.

5. **Describe the normal pressure waveforms along the path of an advancing Swan-Ganz catheter.**
   The *a wave* is produced by atrial contraction and follows the electrical P wave on electrocardiogram (ECG). The *x descent* reflects atrial relaxation. The *c wave* is produced at the beginning of ventricular systole as the closed tricuspid valve bulges into the RA. The *x' descent* is thought to be the result of the descent of the atrioventricular ring during ventricular contraction and continued atrial relaxation. The *v wave* is caused by venous filling of the atrium during ventricular systole, when the tricuspid valve is closed. This should correspond with the electrical *T wave*. However, at the bedside, because of a lag in pressure transmission, the *a wave* will align with the QRS complex, and the *v wave* will

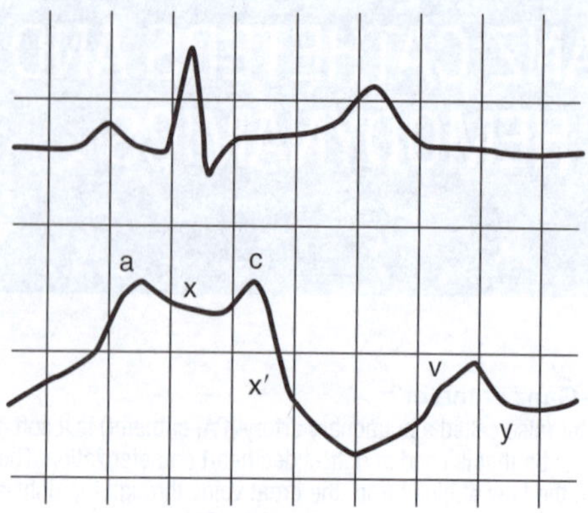

Fig. 12.1. Atrial pressure tracing. See the text for label descriptions.

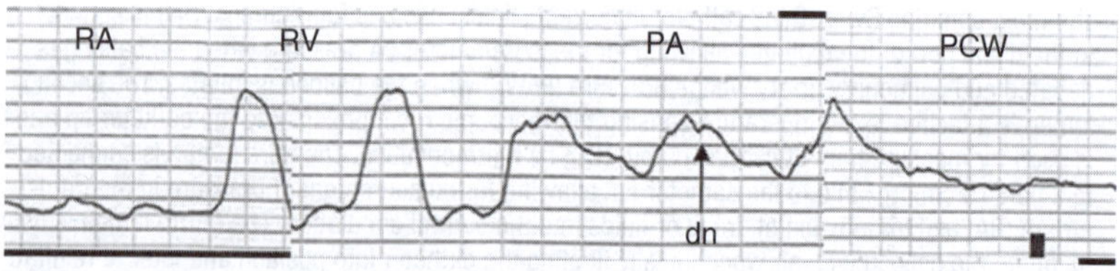

Fig. 12.2. Pressure tracings as the catheter is advanced through the right-sided chambers. As the catheter moves from the RA to the right ventricle, a ventricular waveform is seen representing isovolumic contraction, ejection, and diastole. When the catheter passes into the PA, the diastolic pressure rises. The dicrotic notch *(dn)* is produced by the closure of the pulmonic valve. If the catheter is advanced farther, it attains the wedge position. *dn,* Dicrotic notch; *PA,* pulmonary artery; *RA,* right atrium; RV, right ventricular.

follow the *T wave.* Finally, the *y descent* is produced by rapid atrial emptying, when the tricuspid valve opens at the onset of diastole (Figs.12.1 and 12.2).

6. **How do we know that the catheter is in the true wedge position?**

There are three ways to confirm that the catheter is in the wedge position. At the bedside, an atrial tracing (reflecting left atrial pressure) will be seen when the catheter is in the wedge position. Second, if the catheter is withdrawn from the wedge position, the mean arterial pressure should be observed to rise from the wedge pressure (reflecting a physiologic gradient between the mean PA and mean wedge pressure). Gentle aspiration of blood from the distal port should reveal highly oxygenated blood if the catheter is truly wedged.

Additionally, in the catheterization laboratory, fluoroscopy can be used to determine that the catheter is in a distal pulmonary arteriole, immobile in the wedge position.

7. **What does the pulmonary artery wedge pressure signify?**

When the catheter is in the wedge position (Fig. 12.3), proximal blood flow is occluded and a static column of blood is created between the catheter tip and the distal cardiac chambers. With the balloon shielding the catheter tip from the pressure in the PA proximally, the pressure transducer measures pressure distally in the pulmonary arterioles. This pressure closely approximates left atrial pressure. When the mitral valve is open at end diastole, left ventricular (LV) end-diastolic pressure is measured, assuming that there is no obstruction between the catheter tip and the left ventricle (i.e., mitral stenosis). The PAWP can be used to approximate LV preload.

8. **How is cardiac output determined?**

CO can be determined either by the measured thermodilution method or calculated via the Fick method.

With **thermodilution,** 10 mL of normal saline is injected rapidly via the proximal port into the RA. The injectate mixes completely with blood and causes a drop in temperature that is measured continuously by a thermocouple near the catheter tip. The area under the curve (AUC) is calculated and is inversely related to CO (Fig. 12.4). This method of measurement is not reliable in patients with

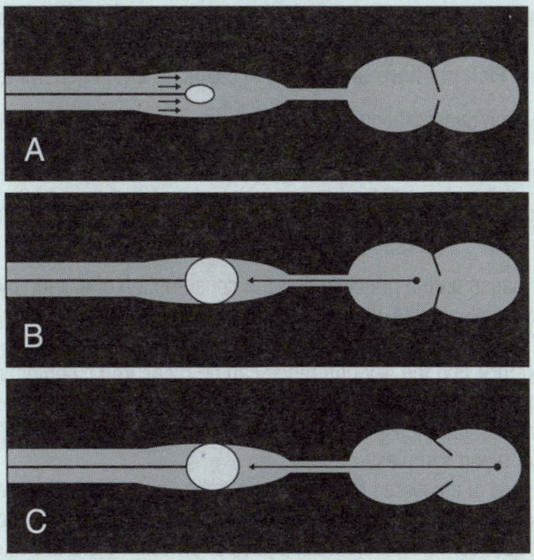

Fig. 12.3. A, With the balloon tip deflated, the pressure transducer at the catheter tip measures pressure in the proximal pulmonary artery (PA). **B**, With the balloon tip inflated, proximal blood flow is occluded, and a static column of blood is created between the catheter tip and the distal cardiac chamber. With the mitral valve closed, left atrial pressure is approximated. **C,** With the mitral valve open at end diastole, left ventricular (LV) end-diastolic pressure can be measured, assuming there is no significant mitral stenosis.

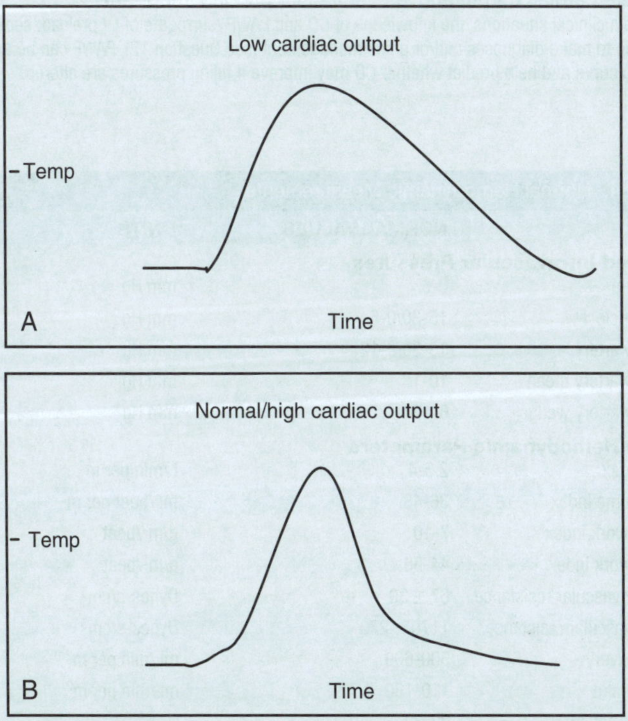

Fig. 12.4. Area under the curve (AUC) is inversely proportional to cardiac output (CO). **A**, The illustration depicts a larger AUC in a patient with low CO. **B**, Temperature equilibrates faster in a patient with a higher CO, resulting in a smaller AUC.

low CO or significant tricuspid regurgitation. In a low-cardiac-output state, blood is rewarmed by the walls of the cardiac chambers and surrounding tissue, resulting in an overestimation of CO.

Alternatively, the **Fick method** can be used to calculate CO. In general terms, the formula is

$$\text{Cardiac output} = \text{Oxygen consumption (mL/min)/Arteriovenous } O_2 \text{ difference} \times \text{Blood } O_2 \text{ capacity}$$

The exact formula is

$$\text{Cardiac output} = \text{Measured oxygen consumption (mL/min)/A} - \text{V difference} \times \text{Hgb (g \%)} \times 1.36 \text{ (mL } O_2\text{/g of Hb)} \times 10$$

This method is based on the principle that the consumption of oxygen by any organ is determined by the arteriovenous (A-V) difference of oxygen and the blood flow (CO) to that organ. The consumption of oxygen by a patient can be measured using a covered hood in the cardiac catheterization laboratory, and the A-V difference can be measured by obtaining blood gases from a systemic artery and from the PA. This method is more accurate than the thermodilution method in patients with atrial fibrillation, tricuspid regurgitation, and low CO. Common sources of error include improper collection of blood samples.

At the bedside, use of a covered hood can be cumbersome and impractical. For this reason, some laboratories assume that resting oxygen consumption is 125 mL/m^2 and calculate CO based on an assumed Fick equation. However, studies have shown that there is wide variability in resting oxygen consumption among patients, particularly in those patients who are critically ill. In such patients, the thermodilution method can be used to confirm the accuracy of the Fick measurement.

9. What are normal values for intravascular pressures and hemodynamic parameters?

The normal values for intravascular pressures and hemodynamics are provided in Table 12.1.

10. Why are cardiac output and left ventricular preload important?

In certain clinical situations, the knowledge of CO and PAWP (surrogate of LV preload; see Question 8) can help to make diagnoses and/or guide management (see Question 12). PAWP can be applied to the Starling curve and help predict whether CO may improve if filling pressures are altered.

Table 12.1. Normal Hemodynamic Measurements

	NORMAL VALUES	UNITS
Measured Intravascular Pressures		
Right atrium	0-6	mm Hg
Right ventricle	15-30/0-6	mm Hg
Pulmonary artery	15-30/6-12	mm Hg
Pulmonary artery mean	10-18	mm Hg
Pulmonary artery wedge	6-12	mm Hg
Derived Hemodynamic Parameters		
Cardiac index	2.5-4	L/min per m^2
Stroke volume Index	36-48	mL/beat per m^2
RV stroke work index	7-10	g/m^2/beat
LV stroke work index	44-56	g/m^2/beat
Pulmonary vascular resistance	67 ± 30	Dynes-s/cm^5
Systemic vascular resistance	1170 ± 270	Dynes-s/cm^5
Oxygen delivery	500-600	mL/min per m^2
Oxygen uptake	110-160	mL/min per m^2
Oxygen extraction	22-32	—

LV, Left ventricle; *RV*, right ventricle.

11. What are possible uses of a Swan-Ganz catheter in patients with heart failure or shock?

- To differentiate between cardiogenic and noncardiogenic pulmonary edema when a trial of diuretic and/or vasodilator therapy has failed. It is *not* indicated for the routine management of pulmonary edema.
- To differentiate causes of shock and guide management when a trial of intravascular volume expansion has failed
- To determine whether pericardial tamponade is present when clinical assessment is inconclusive and echocardiography is unavailable
- Assessment of valvular heart disease
- To determine pulmonary vascular resistance and assess vasoreactivity in patients being considered for heart transplantation
- Management of cardiogenic shock, particularly in the setting of end-organ compromise (e.g., renal dysfunction) and guiding management of percutaneous circulatory support (e.g., intra-aortic balloon pump)
- Management of congestive heart failure refractory to standard medical therapy, especially in the setting of acute myocardial infarction (MI). Of note, a major randomized trial, Evaluation Study of Congestive Heart Failure and Pulmonary Artery Catheterization Effectiveness (ESCAPE), showed no significant difference in endpoints of mortality and days out of hospital at 6 months in this category of patients.

12. What are possible uses of a Swan-Ganz catheter in patients with acute myocardial infarction?

The American College of Cardiology/American Heart Association (ACC/AHA) guidelines state that Swan-Ganz catheters should be used in those patients who have progressive hypotension unresponsive to fluids and in patients with suspected mechanical complications of ST-elevation MI if an echocardiogram has not been performed (class I). However, mortality benefit has not been demonstrated in a randomized trial.

The use of Swan-Ganz catheters can also be considered in the following situations:

- Diagnosis of mechanical complications of MI (i.e., mitral regurgitation, ventricular septal defect)
- Diagnosis of intracardiac shunts and to establish their severity before surgical correction
- Guidance of management of cardiogenic shock with pharmacologic or mechanical support
- Guidance of management of right ventricular (RV) infarction with hypotension or signs of low CO not responding to intravascular volume expansion or low doses of inotropic drugs
- Short-term guidance of pharmacologic or mechanical management of acute mitral regurgitation before surgical correction

13. What are possible perioperative uses of a Swan-Ganz catheter?

A 2003 randomized trial in high-risk surgical patients showed no significant difference in mortality with the use of Swan-Ganz catheters. Although the routine use of Swan-Ganz catheters perioperatively remains of unclear benefit, it should be considered in the following situations:

- In patients undergoing cardiac surgery, to differentiate between causes of low CO or to differentiate between right and LV dysfunction, when clinical assessment and echocardiography is inadequate
- In guidance of perioperative management in selected patients with decompensated heart failure undergoing intermediate or high-risk noncardiac surgery

14. What are possible uses of a Swan-Ganz catheter in patients with pulmonary hypertension?

- Exclusion of post-capillary causes of pulmonary hypertension (elevated PAWP)
- To establish diagnosis and assess severity of pulmonary arterial hypertension (normal PAWP)
- Selection and establishment of safety and efficacy of long-term vasodilator therapy based on acute hemodynamic response

15. What are possible uses of a Swan-Ganz catheter in intensive care units?

Studies have shown that clinical data predict PAWP and CO poorly and that insertion of the catheter often changes patient management. However, despite widespread use of these devices in intensive care units, only a few observational studies have shown their use to decrease mortality. A 2005 meta-analysis of several randomized trials showed that the use of Swan-Ganz catheters was associated with neither benefit nor increased mortality. Current thinking is reflected in a 1997 PA consensus

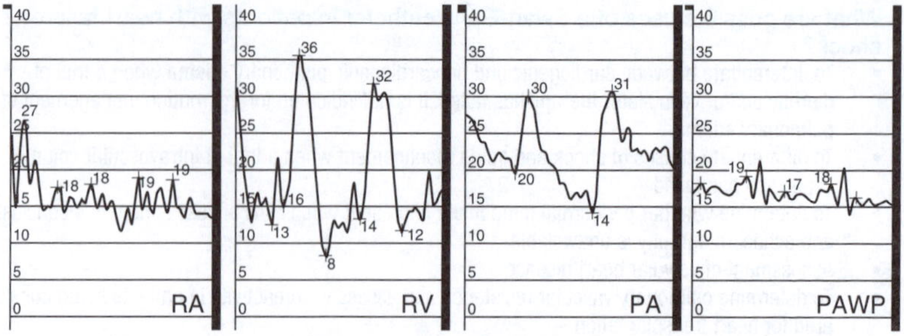

Fig. 12.5. Pressure tracings in cardiac tamponade. *PA,* Pulmonary artery; *PAWP,* pulmonary artery wedge pressure; *RA,* right atrium; *RV,* right ventricular. Note that there is equalization of RA, RV diastolic, PA diastolic, and PAWP pressures. Absent is a notable *y descent* in the RA and PAWP waveforms.

statement recommending that the decision to insert a Swan-Ganz catheter be made on an individual basis, such that the potential risks and benefits are considered in each case.

16. What are absolute and relative contraindications to placement of a Swan-Ganz catheter?

Absolute contraindications include:

- Right-sided endocarditis
- Mechanical tricuspid or pulmonic valve prosthesis
- Presence of thrombus or tumor in a right-sided heart chamber

Relative contraindications include:

- Coagulopathy
- Recent implantation of a permanent pacemaker or cardioverter defibrillator
- Left bundle branch block
- Bioprosthetic tricuspid or pulmonic valve

17. What diagnoses can the catheter help make?

The characteristic waveform of the Swan-Ganz catheter is altered in several disease states.

- In pericardial tamponade, equalization of diastolic pressures across all chambers is seen (Fig. 12.5).
- In atrial fibrillation, the *a wave* disappears from the right atrial pressure tracing, whereas in atrial flutter, mechanical flutter waves occur at a rate of 300/minute.
- *Cannon a waves* occur when the atria contract against closed valves due to atrioventricular dissociation. Irregular *cannon a waves* during a wide-complex tachycardia strongly suggest ventricular tachycardia.
- Complications of MI can be detected on the PAWP tracing, such as giant *v waves* seen with acute mitral insufficiency and the *dip and plateau* pattern of the RV pressure tracing seen with RV infarction.

18. How can causes of shock be differentiated by Swan-Ganz catheterization?

Table 12.2 illustrates hemodynamic parameters in different etiologies of shock.

19. How can left-to-right intracardiac shunts be diagnosed by Swan-Ganz catheterization?

An intracardiac shunt results in flow of blood from left-sided to right-sided cardiac chambers or vice versa. With ventricular septal defects, flow is often left to right as a result of higher left-sided pressures. Atrial septal defects can result in a shunt in either direction. Because of the flow of oxygenated blood into right-sided chambers, a sudden increase in oxygen saturation in right-sided chambers is observed. A step-up in mean oxygen saturation of 7% between the caval chambers and the RA is diagnostic of an atrial septal defect. A step-up of 5% between the RA and right ventricle is diagnostic for a ventricular septal defect.

Mixed venous saturation is calculated using the following equation, which weights oxygen saturation in the superior vena cava (SVC) more than oxygen saturation in the inferior vena cava (IVC).

$$\text{Mixed venous saturation} = 3 \times (\text{SVC } O_2 \text{ content}) + (\text{IVC } O_2 \text{ content})/4$$

Table 12.2. Hemodynamic Parameters in Different Etiologies of Shock

ETIOLOGY	RIGHT ATRIUM	RIGHT VENTRICLE	PULMONARY ARTERY	PULMONARY CAPILLARY WEDGE PRESSURE	CARDIAC OUTPUT	SYSTEMIC VASCULAR RESISTANCE
Hypovolemic	↓	↓	↓	↓	↓	↑
Cardiogenic	↑↑	↑↑	↑↑	↑↑	↓	↑
Septic (Distributive)	↔	↔	↔	↔	↑	↓

The Qp/Qs ratio, which indicates the degree of left-to-right shunting, is calculated using the following formula:

$$Qp/Qs = (SAO_2 - MVO_2)/(PVO_2 - PAO_2)$$

20. What complications are associated with use of a Swan-Ganz catheter?

Complications of Swan-Ganz catheters include:

- All complications of central venous cannulation, including bleeding and infection
  - Local infection rates range from 18% to 63% in patients with catheter in place for an average of 3 days.
  - Bloodstream infection has been reported in up to 5% of patients.
- Transient right bundle branch block
- Complete heart block (particularly in patients with preexisting left bundle branch block)
- Ventricular tachyarrhythmias
  - Clinically insignificant ventricular arrhythmias can occur in up to 30% to 60% of patients.
  - Sustained arrhythmias usually occur in patients with myocardial ischemia or infarction.
- Pulmonary infarction (incidence 0% to 1.3%)
- PA rupture
  - Risk factors include pulmonary hypertension and recent cardiopulmonary bypass.
- Thrombophlebitis
- Venous or intracardiac thrombus formation
- Endocarditis
- Catheter knotting

21. How can complications be minimized?

- The use of fluoroscopy should be considered for placement of the catheter, particularly if access is obtained from a nontraditional site or if the patient has a dilated right ventricle.
- Consideration should be given to removing the catheter after the first set of data is obtained.
- The duration the catheter is kept in place should be minimized because infectious and thrombotic complications increase significantly after 3 to 4 days.
- Use of the introducer side arm for infusion of medications should be minimized.
- Manipulation of the catheter should only be performed by trained personnel.
- Daily chest radiographs should be obtained to verify proper positioning.

22. The wedge tracing is abnormal. What should I do?

- Check a chest radiograph for proper catheter position. The tip should lie in lung zone 3, below the level of the left atrium.
- Aspirate and flush the catheter to remove clots and bubbles.
- Check all connecting lines and stopcocks.
- Confirm that the pressure transducers are zeroed to the level of the RA.
- Check that the balloon is not overinflated; try letting out the air and refilling it slowly.
- Consider the possibility that the tracing really is a wedge tracing with a *giant v wave*, as is seen in acute mitral insufficiency and several other conditions.

23. The cardiac output does not make sense. What is wrong?

- Check that at least three values were averaged and that the range of these values is no greater than 20% of the mean.
- Check the chest radiograph: Is the distal tip of the catheter in the PA and the proximal port in the RA?
- Check to see if the computer is calibrated to the proper temperatures.
- If the computer can display the time versus temperature curve, check that the curve is shaped properly.

Bibliography and Suggested Readings

Baim, D. S. (2013). *Grossman's cardiac catheterization, angiography, and intervention.* Philadelphia, PA: Lippincott Williams & Wilkins.

Binanay, C., Califf, R. M., Hasselblad, V., O'Connor, C. M., Shah, M. R., Sopko, G., et al. (2005). Evaluation study of congestive heart failure and pulmonary artery catheterization effectiveness: the ESCAPE trial. *Journal of the American Medical Association, 294*, 1625–1633.

Leatherman, J. W., & Marini, J. J. (1998). Clinical use of the pulmonary artery catheter. In J. B. Hall, G. A. Schmidt, & L. D. H. Wood (Eds.), *Principles of critical care* (2nd ed.). New York, NY: McGraw-Hill.

Mann, D., Zipes, D. P., Libby, P., & Bonow, R. O. (Eds.). (2014). *Braunwald's heart disease.* Philadelphia, PA: Elsevier Saunders.

Mueller, H. S., Chatterjee, K., Davis, K. B., Fifer, M. A., Franklin, C., Greenberg, M. A., et al. (1998). American College of Cardiology consensus statement. Present use of bedside right heart catheterization in patients with cardiac disease. *Journal of the American College of Cardiology, 32*, 840–864.

Nishimura, R., & Carabello, B. (2012). Hemodynamics in the cardiac catheterization laboratory of the 21st century. *Circulation, 125*, 2138–2150.

Pulmonary Artery Catheter Consensus Conference Participants. (1997). Pulmonary artery catheter consensus conference: consensus statement. *Critical Care Medicine, 25*(6), 910–925.

Robin, E. D. (1985). The cult of the Swan-Ganz catheter. *Annals of Internal Medicine, 103*, 445–449.

Sandham, J. D., Hull, R. D., Brant, R. F., Knox, L., Pineo, G. F., Doig, C. J., et al. (2003). A randomized, controlled trial of the use of pulmonary-artery catheters in high-risk surgical patients. *New England Journal of Medicine, 348*, 5–14.

Shah, M. R., Hasselblad, V., Stevenson, L. W., Binanay, C., O'Connor, C. M., Sopko, G., et al. (2005). Impact of the pulmonary artery catheter in critically ill patients: meta-analysis of randomized clinical trials. *Journal of the American Medical Association, 294*, 1664–1670.

Sharkey, S. W. (1987). Beyond the wedge: clinical physiology and the Swan Ganz catheter. *American Journal of Medicine, 83*, 111–122.

Sise, M. J., Hollingsworth, P., Brimm, J. E., Peters, R. M., Virgilio, R. W., & Shackford, S. R. (1981). Complications of the flow-directed pulmonary-artery catheter: a prospective analysis of 219 patients. *Critical Care Medicine, 9*, 315–318.

Walston, A., & Kendall, M. E. (1973). Comparison of pulmonary wedge and left atrial pressure in man. *American Heart Journal, 86*, 159–164.

CORONARY ANGIOGRAPHY AND INTRACORONARY IMAGING AND PHYSIOLOGIC ASSESSMENT

CHAPTER 13

Waleed T. Kayani, Glenn N. Levine

1. What are generally accepted indications for cardiac catheterization?

Although recommendations are consistently evolving, those listed here are generally accepted as reasonable indications for cardiac catheterization (Table 13.1). Cardiac catheterization is a relatively safe procedure; however, life-threatening complications can rarely occur, so there needs to be a clearly thought-out and documented indication for catheterization and a plan for how to use the information obtained during catheterization for patient management. In most cases, coronary angiography is best reserved for patients who are amenable to and candidates for coronary revascularization and when findings are likely to result in changes to therapy.

Generally accepted indications for cardiac catheterization include:

- Class III-IV angina despite medical treatment or intolerance of medical therapy in patients who are candidates for coronary revascularization
- High-risk results on noninvasive stress testing (rest- or exercise-induced left ventricular ejection fraction [LVEF] <35%, moderate to large area of vasodilator-induced ischemia, or findings suggestive of multivessel disease, hypotension, or 1- to 2-mm ST depressions and decreased exercise capacity on standard exercise treadmill test)
- Patients with suspected symptomatic coronary artery disease (CAD) who cannot undergo diagnostic stress testing or have indeterminate or nondiagnostic stress test results
- Sustained (>30 seconds) monomorphic ventricular tachycardia or nonsustained (<30 seconds) polymorphic ventricular tachycardia
- Sudden cardiac death survivors
- Most patients with non–ST-segment elevation acute coronary syndrome (NSTE-ACS) who have high-risk features and no contraindications to early cardiac catheterization and revascularization
- Systolic dysfunction and stress testing results suggesting multivessel disease and potential benefit from revascularization
- Recurrent typical angina within 9 months of percutaneous coronary revascularization
- Recurrent typical angina within 12 months of coronary artery bypass grafting (CABG)
- As part of primary percutaneous coronary intervention (PCI) for ST-segment elevation myocardial infarction (STEMI)
- Patients status post STEMI treated with thrombolytic therapy
- Patients with STEMI who within 36 hours of presentation develop cardiogenic shock
- Middle-aged and older patients who are to undergo valve replacement/repair
- In assessment and management of patients with congenital heart disease and cardiac transplant recipients
- For assessment of valvular dysfunction or other hemodynamic assessment when the results of echocardiography are indeterminate

2. What findings on noninvasive testing prompt performance of cardiac catheterization?

High-risk results on noninvasive stress testing that prompt cardiac catheterization include:

- Stress-induced decrease in left ventricular (LV) systolic function
- Stress-induced left ventricular dilation (transient ischemic dilation)

Table 13.1. Generally Accepted Indications for Diagnostic Cardiac Catheterization

Diagnosis of Stable Ischemic Heart Disease
• Follow-up of high-risk findings on noninvasive stress testing
• Patients with unacceptable ischemic symptoms despite optimum medical therapy and who are amenable to and candidates for coronary revascularization
• Patients with suspected symptomatic CAD who cannot undergo diagnostic stress testing or have indeterminate or nondiagnostic stress test results
• Unexplained left ventricular systolic dysfunction
• Stress testing results suggesting multivessel disease and potential survival benefit from revascularization
Acute Coronary Syndromes
• As part of primary PCI for STEMI
• As part of early invasive strategy in patients with NSTE-ACS who have moderate- to high-risk features and no contraindications
• Patients status post STEMI treated with thrombolytic therapy
• Patients with STEMI who within 36 h of presentation develop cardiogenic shock
Post-revascularization
• Recurrent angina within 9 months of percutaneous coronary revascularization
• Recurrent angina within 12 months of coronary artery bypass grafting
• Select patients in special professions, such as pilots, due to regulatory issues
Ventricular Arrhythmias
• Survivors of sudden cardiac death
• Sustained (>30 s) monomorphic ventricular tachycardia or nonsustained (<30 s) polymorphic ventricular tachycardia
Valvular Heart Disease
• Hemodynamic assessment when the results of echocardiography are indeterminate
• Preoperative to assess for presence and extent of CAD in middle-aged and older patients who are to undergo open surgical valve replacement/repair
• Preprocedure to assess for presence and extent of CAD in patients undergoing TAVR
Other Conditions
• Suspected Prinzmetal variant angina
• Hemodynamic assessment of shunts in patients with congenital heart disease or acquired shunts
• Survey assessments in cardiac transplants for coronary vasculopathy

CAD, Coronary artery disease; *NSTE-ACS*, non–ST-segment elevation acute coronary syndrome; *PCI*, percutaneous coronary intervention; *STEMI*, ST-segment elevation myocardial infarction; *TAVR*, transcatheter aortic valve replacement.

- Large area or areas of induced ischemia
- Findings suggestive of multivessel disease
- Hypotension
- ≥2-mm ST depressions, ST depression in numerous leads, and/or ST depression lasting well into recovery
- Sustained ventricular tachycardia.

3. What are the risks of cardiac catheterization?

The risks of cardiac catheterization will depend to some extent on the individual patient. For "all comers," the risk of death is approximately 1 in 1000, with the risk of myocardial infarction or stroke rarer than 1 in 1000. The risk of any major complication in "all comers" is less than 1%. Factors that increase the risks of complication include older age, vascular disease, and chronic kidney disease. These risks are summarized in Table 13.2.

4. How are coronary lesions assessed?

Coronary lesions are most commonly assessed in day-to-day practice based on subjective visual impression (Fig. 13.1). Lesions are subjectively given a percent stenosis, ideally based on ocular

Table 13.2. Complication and Risk During Diagnostic Cardiac Catheterization

COMPLICATION	RISK (%)
Mortality	0.11
Myocardial infarction	0.05
Cerebrovascular accident	0.07
Arrhythmia	0.38
Vascular complications	0.43
Contrast reaction	0.37
Hemodynamic complications	0.26
Perforation of heart chamber	0.03
Other complications	0.28
Total of major complications	1.70

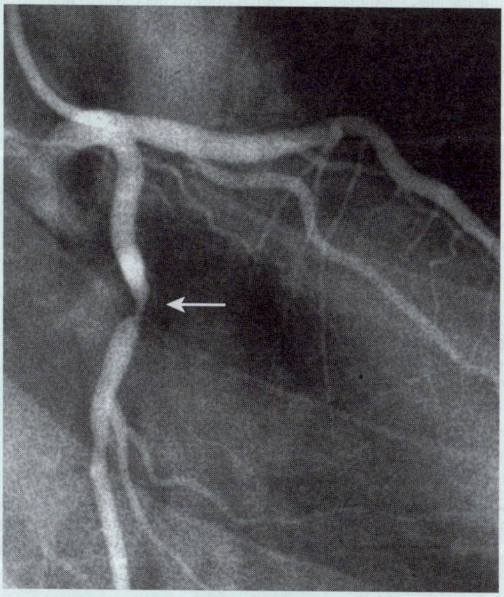

Fig. 13.1. Coronary angiography of the left coronary artery demonstrates an approximate 90% lesion *(arrow)* in the left coronary artery.

assessment of at least two orthogonal images of the lesion. Studies have shown interobserver and intraobserver variability in judging coronary stenosis from as little as 7% to as much as 50%.

Quantitative coronary angiography (QCA) more objectively assesses the lesion severity than "ocular judgment" but is not commonly used in day-to-day practice. QCA generally grades lesions as less severe than subjective ocular judgment of a lesion's severity. Fractional flow reserve (FFR) is increasingly being used to measure the functional or physiologic severity of a lesion. Intravascular ultrasound (IVUS) and optical coherence tomography (OCT) provide a more complete and accurate anatomic assessment of total plaque burden and lesion severity than that obtained with angiography.

5. What is considered a "significant" stenosis?

The classification of significant stenosis depends on the clinical context and what one considers "significant." Coronary flow reserve (the increase in coronary blood flow in response to agents that lead to microvascular dilation) begins to decrease when a coronary artery stenosis is 50% or more of the luminal diameter. However, basal coronary flow does not begin to decrease until the lesion is 80% to 90% of the luminal diameter. The hemodynamic significance of a given stenosis does not merely rely on the reduction in luminal diameter, because numerous additional factors such as stenosis length, shape, and eccentricity affect the flow dynamics and thus the physiologic significance. Therefore, techniques like FFR, OCT, and IVUS are gaining popularity in the assessment of lesion significance, especially if the stenosis appears between 40% and 60% or intermediate visually.

6. What are the major vascular complications associated with cardiac catheterization?

In general, major vascular complications are uncommon with diagnostic cardiac catheterization and more common with percutaneous coronary intervention, which may require larger sheath placement, venous sheath placement, and more intense or prolonged anticoagulation. Nevertheless, practitioners and patients should be aware of the following potential vascular complications:

- *Retroperitoneal hematoma*: This should be suspected in cases of flank, abdominal, or back pain, with unexplained hypotension, or with a marked decrease in hematocrit. Diagnosis is by computed tomography (CT) scan.
- *Pseudoaneurysm*: A pseudoaneurysm results from the failure of the puncture site to seal properly. Pseudoaneurysm is a communication between the femoral artery and the overlying fibromuscular tissue, resulting in a blood-filled cavity. Pseudoaneurysm is suggested by the finding of groin tenderness, palpable pulsatile mass, or new bruit in the groin area. Pseudoaneurysm is diagnosed by Doppler flow imaging.
- *Arteriovenous (AV) fistula*: An AV fistula can result from sheath-mediated communication between the femoral artery and the femoral vein. AV fistula is suggested by the presence of a systolic and diastolic bruit in the groin area. Diagnosis is confirmed by Doppler ultrasound.
- *Stroke*: Periprocedural stroke is a rare but morbid complication of cardiac catheterization and is often associated with unfavorable neurologic outcome. A proportion of strokes may be due to disruption and embolization of atherosclerotic material from the aorta during the procedure.
- *Cholesterol embolus syndrome*: This is a rare and potentially catastrophic complication that results from plaque disruption in the aorta, with distal embolization in the kidneys, lower extremities, and other organs.

7. What is fractional flow reserve?

Physiologic assessment of blood flow through a stenotic lesion can be safely and reliably performed in the catheterization laboratory using a coronary wire with a pressure sensor at its tip. The wire is advanced across the lesion of interest, and the ratio of distal coronary pressure to proximal aortic pressure is assessed after maximal hyperemia is achieved (Fig. 13.2). This ratio is called FFR. Normal values are close to 1, and a ratio less than 0.75 to 0.80 is taken as indicating a "physiologically significant stenosis." Adenosine is typically used as a pharmacologic agent to achieve maximal hyperemia.

8. How is fractional flow reserve used to guide coronary stenting?

In patients with angina, if the "culprit" lesion is visually estimated to be intermediate (40% to 60% stenosis) in severity, FFR may be used to guide management in determining if the lesion is physiologically significant. When evaluating whether a lesion warrants revascularization, use of FFR has been shown to be a clinically useful tool. Although initial studies used FFR to guide revascularization decisions in intermediate lesions, more recent studies have shown that FFR is of use to evaluate lesions that visually appear more stenotic than 40% to 60%. Revascularization may be safely deferred for lesions with FFR greater than 0.75 to 0.80. If the FFR is less than 0.75, revascularization with PCI or CABG is appropriate if clinically indicated. An FFR-guided revascularization approach has been shown in studies to significantly reduce overall costs, the number of stents placed, and the need for urgent revascularization.

9. During cardiac catheterization, how is aortic or mitral regurgitation graded?

For aortic regurgitation, an aortogram is performed in the ascending thoracic aorta above the aortic valve, and the amount of contrast that regurgitates into the left ventricle (LV) is

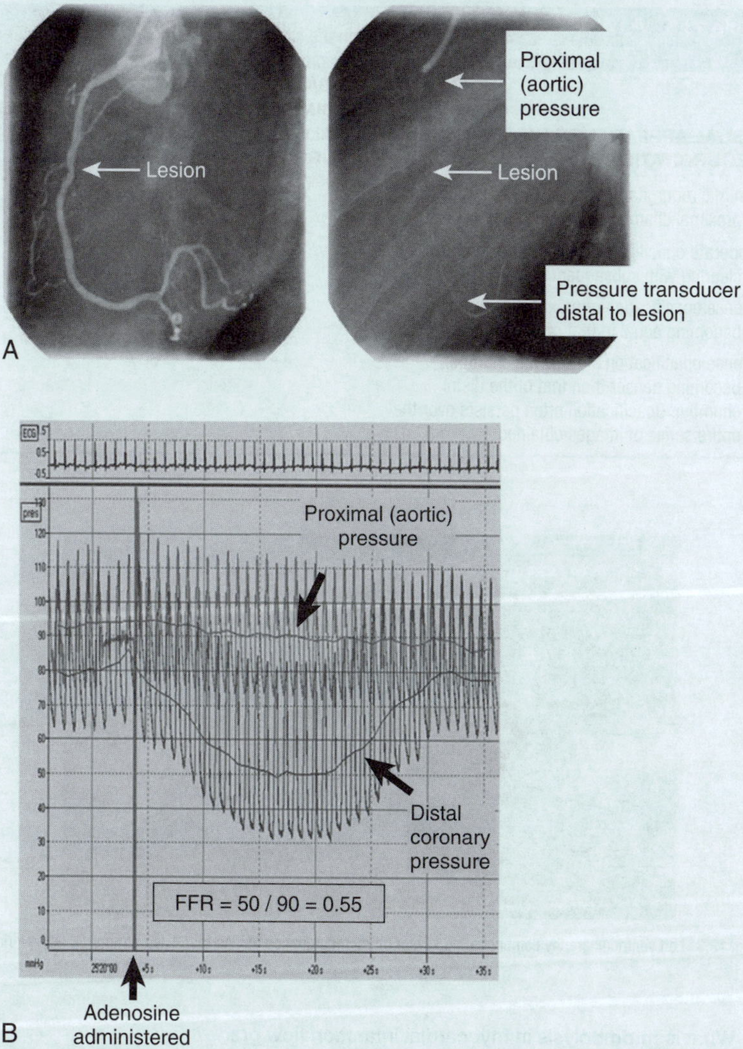

Fig. 13.2. Fractional flow reserve (FFR). **A**, shows the coronary lesion in question, where the proximal pressure is assessed, and where the distal pressure transducer is. **B**, shows the acquired pressure tracings during the study. Note that at baseline there is already a modest drop in pressure distal to the lesion. With adenosine administration, there is a marked drop in pressure, with a calculated FFR of 0.55, which is considered significant.

noted. For mitral regurgitation, a left ventriculogram is performed, and the amount of contrast that regurgitates into the left atrium (LA) is noted. The systems used to grade the degree of regurgitation are similar for the two valvular abnormalities and based on a 1+ to 4+ system, where 1+ is little if any regurgitation and 4+ is profound or severe regurgitation. Regurgitation of 3+ or 4+ is often considered "surgical" regurgitation, although the criteria for surgery are more complex than this. Table 13.3 summarizes the grading of regurgitant lesions as assessed by cardiac catheterization and "ballpark" regurgitant fractions for each degree of regurgitation (Fig. 13.3).

Table 13.3. Visual Assessment of Valvular Regurgitation and Approximate Corresponding Regurgitant Fraction

VISUAL APPEARANCE OF REGURGITATION	DESIGNATED GRADING/SEVERITY OF VALVULAR REGURGITATION	APPROXIMATE CORRESPONDING REGURGITANT FRACTION
Minimal regurgitant jet seen. Clears rapidly from proximal chamber with each beat	1+	<20%
Moderate opacification of proximal chamber, clearing with subsequent beats	2+	21-40%
Intense opacification of proximal chamber, becoming equal to that of the distal chamber	3+	41-60%
Intense opacification of proximal chamber, becoming denser than that of the distal chamber. Opacification often persists over the entire series of images obtained.	4+	>60%

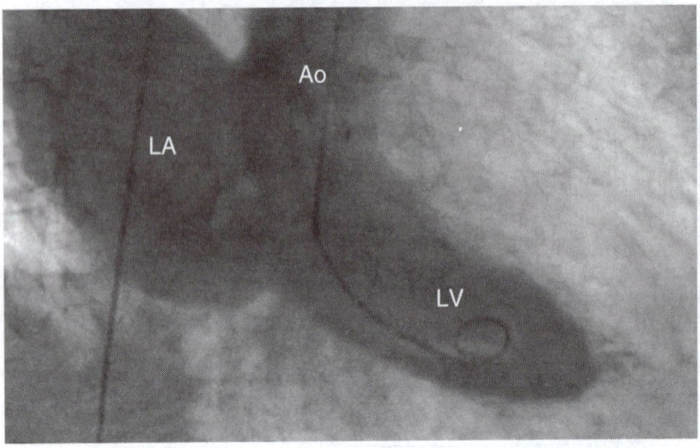

Fig. 13.3. Left ventriculography demonstrating severe mitral regurgitation. *Ao*, Aorta; *LA*, left atrium; *LV*, left ventricle.

10. What is thrombolysis in myocardial infarction flow grade?

Thrombolysis in myocardial infarction (TIMI) flow grade is a system for qualitatively describing blood flow in a coronary artery. It was originally derived to describe blood flow down the infarct-related artery in patients with STEMI. Reportedly, the initial concept was originally written down on a napkin or the back of an envelope during an airplane flight. The grades are based on observing contrast flow down the coronary artery after injection of the contrast, given as follows:

- TIMI grade 3: normal contrast (blood) flow down the entire artery
- TIMI grade 2: contrast (blood) flows through the entire artery but at a delayed rate compared with flow in a normal (TIMI grade 3 flow) artery
- TIMI grade 1: contrast (blood) flows beyond the area of vessel occlusion but without perfusion of the distal coronary artery and coronary bed
- TIMI grade 0: complete occlusion of the infarct-related artery

11. What is intravascular ultrasound?

IVUS is the direct assessment of the coronary arterial wall using a flexible catheter with a miniature ultrasound probe at its tip. Upon insertion into the coronary artery, IVUS provides true cross-sectional

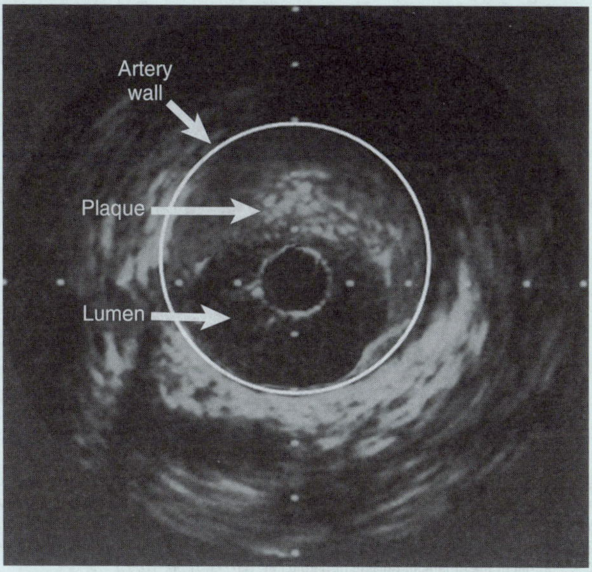

Fig. 13.4. Intravascular ultrasound (IVUS).

images of the vessel, delineating the three layers of the vessel wall (Fig. 13.4). IVUS may aid in the assessment of coronary stenosis, optimal stent expansion, and plaque morphology when angiographic imaging is inadequate or indeterminate.

12. What is optical coherence tomography?

Optical coherence tomography (OCT) is a relatively newer method of assessing arterial anatomy using an imaging catheter. Instead of sound waves, as used in IVUS, OCT uses near-infrared light to image arterial anatomy. OCT-based images have a much higher resolution compared to IVUS (Fig. 13.5); however, this is at the cost of a decrease in the depth of imaging (from 10 mm with IVUS to 1 to 2.5 mm with OCT). OCT is especially useful in evaluation of plaque morphology, identifying thrombus and optimal stent expansion, and also aids in coronary stenosis when angiographic imaging is inadequate or indeterminate.

13. What are the different methods of describing the aortic transvalvular gradient in a patient undergoing cardiac catheterization for the evaluation of aortic stenosis?

Three terms used to describe the gradient (Fig. 13.6) are:

- Peak instantaneous gradient: The maximal pressure difference between the left ventricular pressure and aortic pressure assessed at the exact same time
- Peak-to-peak gradient: The difference between the maximal left ventricular pressure and the maximal aortic pressure
- Mean gradient: The integral of the pressure difference between the LV and the aorta during systole.

14. Which patients should be premedicated to prevent allergic reactions to iodine-based contrast?

In patients with a history of prior true allergic reaction (e.g., hives, urticaria, bronchoconstriction) to iodine-based contrast, the risk of repeat anaphylactoid reaction to contrast agents is reported to be 17% to 35%. Such patients should be premedicated before angiography. A common regimen is 60 mg orally (PO) of prednisone the night before and morning of the procedure and 50 mg oral diphenhydramine the morning of the procedure. The 2011 ACCF/AHA/SCAI guidelines do not consider allergy to fish or shellfish an indication for steroid pretreatment.

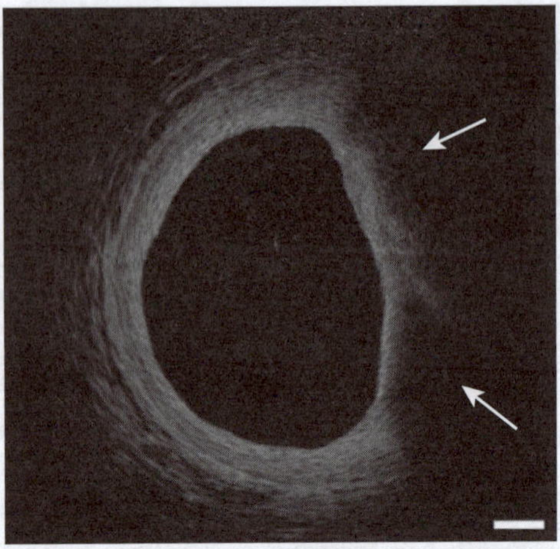

Fig. 13.5. Optical coherence tomography (OCT) showing a thin-capped lipid-rich plaque *(arrows)*. The lipid-rich plaque and thin cap (best appreciated in the lower right quadrant) make this plaque more likely to lead to future plaque rupture and acute coronary syndrome. *(Image adapted from Tearney, G. J., Regar, E., Akasaka, T., Adriaenssens, T., Barlis, P., Bezerra, H. G., et al. [2012]. Consensus standards for acquisition, measurement, and reporting of intravascular optical coherence tomography studies.* Journal of the American College of Cardiology, 59*(12), 1058–1072.)*

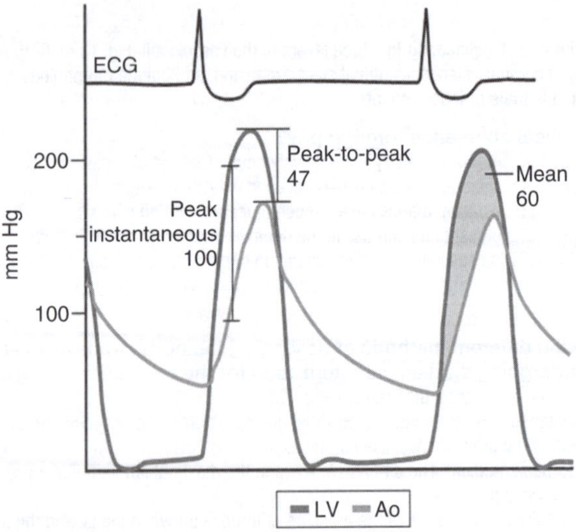

Fig. 13.6. Various methods of describing the aortic transvalvular gradient. *ECG*, Electrocardiogram.

15. What are the major risk factors for contrast nephropathy?

Preexisting renal disease and diabetes are the two major risk factors for the development of contrast nephropathy. The risk of contrast nephropathy is also related to the amount of iodine-based contrast used during the catheterization procedure. Preprocedure and postprocedure hydration is the most established method of reducing the risk of contrast nephropathy. The 2011 ACCF/AHA/SCAI PCI guidelines suggest a regimen of isotonic crystalloid (e.g., normal saline) 1.0 to 1.5 mL/kg per hour for 3 to 12 hours before the procedure and continuing for 6 to 24 hours after the procedure. Those same guidelines conclude that treatment with *N*-acetylcysteine does not reduce the risk of contrast nephropathy and is not indicated. Measures of other treatments to decrease the risk of contrast nephropathy, such as sodium bicarbonate infusion or ultrafiltration, have produced heterogeneous and conflicting data.

16. What are vascular closure devices?

Vascular closure devices are hemostatic devices that obviate the need for prolonged compression at the arterial access site following angiography. These devices decrease the duration of bed rest and afford earlier mobility after the procedure. Vascular closure devices have not been convincingly demonstrated to decrease the risk of vascular complications, including bleeding.

17. What is the difference between radial and femoral access in cardiac catheterization?

Left heart catheterization and coronary angiography are commonly performed using catheters inserted through either the femoral or radial arteries. Radial access is associated with a lower incidence of vascular complications such as bleeding.

18. What is intracardiac echo?

Intracardiac echo (ICE) is the direct imaging of cardiac structures via transvenous insertion of a miniaturized echo probe. Most commonly, the device is inserted via the femoral vein and threaded up to the right atrium. ICE is used to visualize the interatrial septum and fossa ovalis, aiding with transseptal puncture, percutaneous treatment of atrial septal defect (ASD), or patent foramen ovale (PFO), and during electrophysiologic procedures, imaging the fossa ovalis and pulmonary veins.

19. How are coronary angiographic projections named?

Coronary angiography utilizes multiple orthogonal views to evaluate coronary anatomy to decrease the risk of missing an eccentric but significant stenosis. By convention, angiographic views are named according to position of the image intensifier (located above the patient) and degree of angulation denoted. Anteroposterior projection (AP) signifies the position of the image intensifier directly above the patient. Left anterior oblique (LAO) 30-degree angulation means the position of the image intensifier is at 30 degrees to the left of the patient, whereas right anterior oblique (RAO) implies position of the image intensifier to the right of the patient. Cranial angulation denotes position of the image intensifier to the head of the patient and vice versa. Native coronary arteries are usually engaged in LAO 30-degree angulation.

20. What are the standard angiographic views to image the left coronary system?

In general, caudal projections are best for viewing the left main coronary artery and proximal segments of left anterior descending (LAD) and left circumflex (LCx) arteries. Specifically, the left main coronary artery is best visualized in the AP projection with slight (10 to 20 degrees) caudal angulation. The best angiographic views for assessing the course of LAD are cranially angulated LAO, AP, and RAO views. The RAO caudal and LAO caudal projections are best for visualization of the proximal and middle LCx and obtuse marginal branches. Standard views of the left coronary system are shown in (Fig. 13.7).

21. What are the standard angiographic views to image right coronary artery?

The right coronary artery (RCA) is initially imaged in the LAO 30-degree view, which displays the proximal and distal RCA well, and the artery appears as the letter C. To evaluate the right posterior descending artery (rPDA) and posterior lateral branches (rPL), RAO 0-degree, cranial 30-degree view is utilized. Standard views of the RCA are shown in (Fig. 13.8).

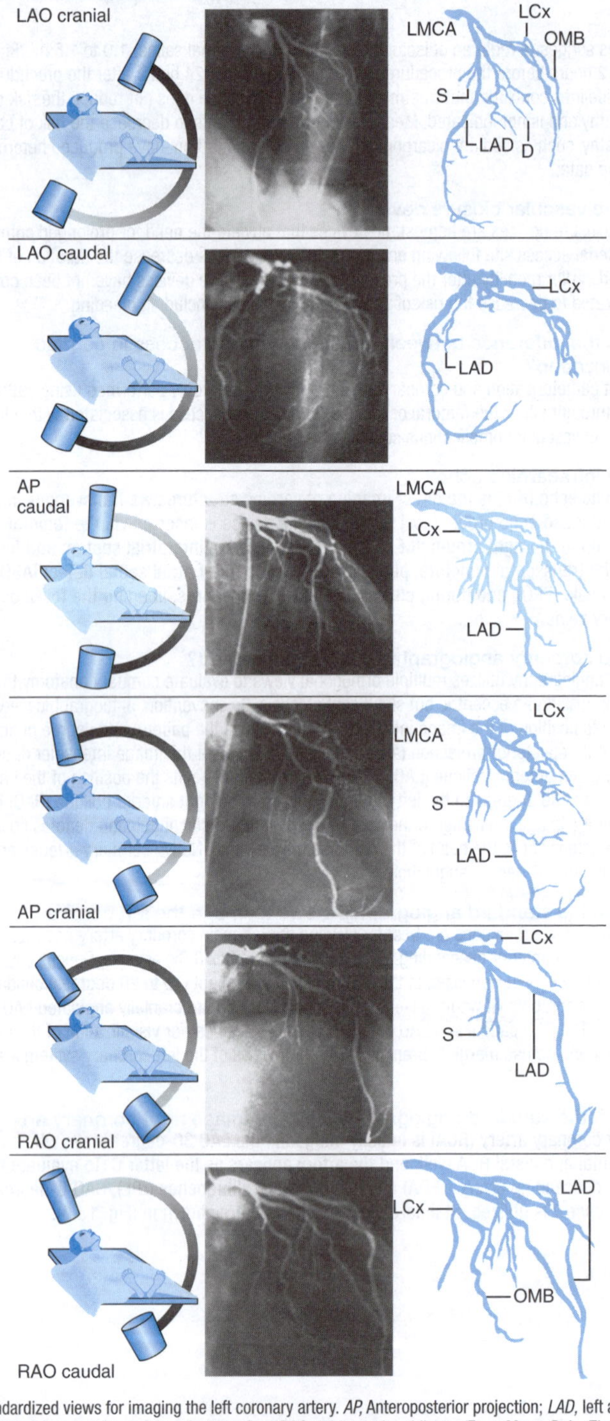

Fig. 13.7. Standardized views for imaging the left coronary artery. *AP,* Anteroposterior projection; *LAD,* left anterior descending; *LAO,* left anterior oblique; *LCx,* left circumflex; *RAO,* right anterior oblique. *(From Mann, D. L., Zipes, D. P., Libby, P., & Bonow, R. O. [2015].* Braunwald's heart disease *[10th ed.]. Philadelphia, PA: Elsevier, Fig. 20.7.)*

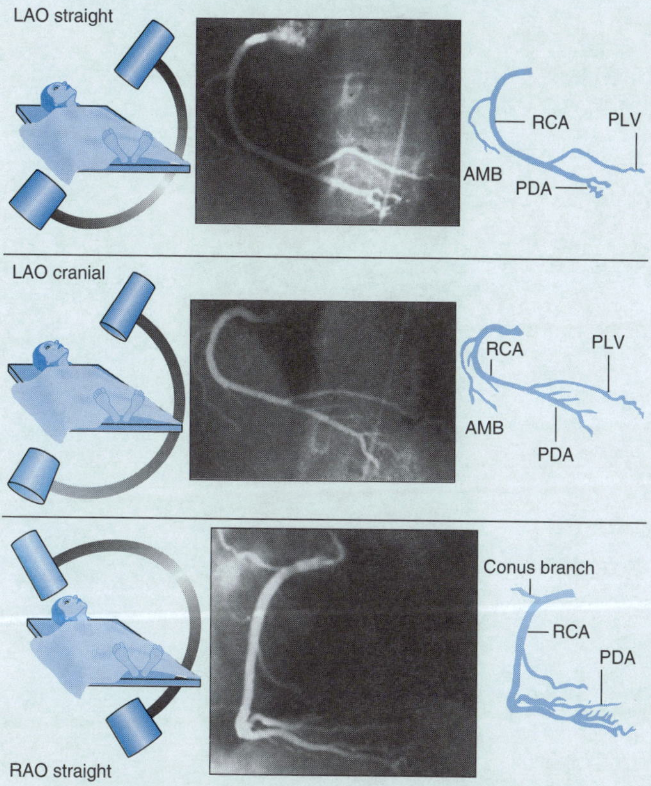

Fig. 13.8. Standardized views for imaging the left right coronary artery. *AMB,* acute marginal branch; *AP,* Anteroposterior projection; *PDA,* posterior descending artery; *PLV,* posterior left ventricular branch; *RCA,* right coronary artery. *(From Mann, D. L., Zipes, D. P., Libby, P., & Bonow, R. O. [2015].* Braunwald's heart disease *[10th ed.]. Philadelphia, PA: Elsevier, Fig. 20.7.)*

Bibliography and Suggested Readings

Fihn, S. D., Blankenship, J. C., Alexander, K. P., Bittl, J. A., Byrne, J. G., Fletcher, B. J., et al. (2014). 2014 ACC/AHA/AATS/PCNA/SCAI/STS focused update of the guideline for the diagnosis and management of patients with stable ischemic heart disease. *Journal of the American College of Cardiology, 64*(18), 1929–1949.

Kern, M. J. (2011). *The cardiac catheterization handbook* (4th ed.). St. Louis, MO: Mosby.

Levine, G. N. (chair), Bates, E. R., Blankenship, J. C., Bailey, S. T., Bittl, J. A., Cercek, B., et al. (2011). 2011 ACCF/AHA/SCAI Guideline for Percutaneous Coronary Intervention: executive summary. A report of the American College of Cardiology Foundation/American Heart Association Task Force on Practice Guidelines and the Society for Cardiovascular Angiography and Interventions. *Circulation, 124*(23), 2574–2609.

Levine, G. N., Kern, M. J., Berger, P. B., Brown, D. L., Klein, L. W., Kereiakes, D. J., et al. (2003). Management of patients undergoing percutaneous coronary revascularization. *Annals of Internal Medicine, 139*, 123–136.

Scanlon, P. J., Faxon, D. P., Audet, A. M., Carabello, B., Dehmer, G. J., Eagle, K. A., et al. (1999). ACC/AHA guidelines for coronary angiography. *Journal of the American College of Cardiology, 33*(6), 1756–1824.

II

Chest Pains, Coronary Artery Disease, and Acute Coronary Syndromes

CHEST PAINS AND ANGINA

Alisa Thamwiwat, Glenn N. Levine

CHAPTER 14

1. **Are most emergency room visits for chest pain caused by acute coronary syndromes?**
No. Acute coronary syndromes (e.g., unstable angina, myocardial infarction) account for only a small percentage of emergency room (ER) visits for chest pain. Depending on the study, only a small percentage of patients (1% to 11%) are diagnosed as having chest pains caused by coronary artery disease (CAD) or acute coronary syndrome (ACS). *ACS* is the term used to describe the continuum of syndromes that include *unstable angina* and *myocardial infarction* (MI).

2. **What are the other important causes of chest pains besides chronic stable angina and acute coronary syndrome?**
It is important to quickly recognize and exclude the life-threatening causes of chest pain, which include ACS, aortic dissection, pneumothorax, pulmonary embolism (PE), and esophageal rupture.
The differential diagnosis for chest pains includes cardiovascular, pulmonary, gastrointestinal, musculoskeletal, psychiatric, and dermatologic causes. Cardiovascular causes include ACSs (unstable angina, non–ST-segment elevation ACS and ST-segment elevation myocardial infarction [STEMI]), aortic dissection, hypertensive crisis, severe aortic stenosis, coronary artery spasm (Prinzmetal angina, cocaine abuse), and cardiac syndrome X (microvascular disease). Pulmonary causes include pneumonia, pneumothorax, PE, and pleuritis. Gastrointestinal causes include esophageal spasms, esophageal reflux and esophagitis, esophageal rupture (Boerhaave syndrome), peptic ulcer disease, gallbladder disease, and pancreatitis. Musculoskeletal causes include costrochondritis and rib fractures. Other causes include cervical radiculopathies, shingles, and somatiform disorders. Table 14.1 summarizes the clinical descriptions and presenting features of the different causes of chest pain.

3. **Why is prompt diagnosis of acute aortic dissection so important?**
In aortic dissection, the mortality rate increases by approximately 1% every hour from presentation to diagnosis and treatment. Additionally, the treatment of aortic dissection is dramatically different from the treatment of ACS, because anticoagulation is contraindicated with aortic dissection.

4. **What is angina?**
Angina is the term used to denote the discomfort associated with myocardial ischemia or MI. Angina occurs when myocardial oxygen demand exceeds myocardial oxygen supply, usually as a result of a severely stenotic or occluded coronary artery. Patients with angina most commonly describe a sensation of *chest pain, chest pressure*, or *chest tightness*. They may also use words such as *heaviness, discomfort, squeezing*, or *suffocating*. The discomfort is more commonly over a region the size of a fist or a larger sized region—that is, larger than just a pinpoint area (although this distinction is not enough in itself to confidently distinguish angina from nonanginal pain). The discomfort classically occurs over the left precordium but may manifest as right-sided chest discomfort, retrosternal discomfort, or discomfort in other areas of the chest. Some people may experience the discomfort only in the upper back, in the arm or arms, or in the neck or jaw. Angina can also manifest as epigastric pain or discomfort and thus is often misdiagnosed as indigestion.
Typical angina is described as having three characteristics: (1) substernal chest discomfort (with the typical sensations noted above), (2) discomfort provoked by exertion or emotional stress, and (3) discomfort relieved by rest or nitroglycerin within minutes.
Table 14.2 summarizes specific details of the chest pain history that are likely to be helpful in distinguishing anginal chest pain from pain of noncardiac causes.

5. **Who first described angina and when?**
The association between chest pain (angina pectoris) and heart disease was first noted by William Heberden in 1772. He described this as a *strangling sensation in the chest* in his manuscript entitled "Some Account of a Disorder of the Breast."

Table 14.1. Common Causes of Acute Chest Pain

SYNDROME	CLINICAL DESCRIPTION	PRESENTING FEATURES
Cardiovascular		
Stable angina	Retrosternal pressure, heaviness, burning; may radiate to arms, neck, jaw	Provoked by physical or emotional stress
Unstable angina	Same as stable angina but usually more severe and prolonged	Occurs at rest or with minimal exertion
Acute MI	Same as angina but usually more severe	Usually >30-min duration; associated symptoms include dyspnea, weakness, diaphoresis
Aortic dissection	Sudden severe pain, may radiate to back	Commonly associated with hypertension or connective tissue disease
Pericarditis	Pleuritic pain, worse in supine position	Fever, pericardial friction rub
Pulmonary		
PE	Sudden onset of pain and dyspnea; pain may be pleuritic with pulmonary infarction	Dyspnea, tachypnea, tachycardia
Pneumonia	May be associated with localized pleuritic pain	Cough, fever, crackles
Spontaneous pneumothorax	Unilateral pleuritic pain associated with dyspnea	Sudden onset of symptoms
Gastrointestinal		
Esophageal reflux	Burning retrosternal and epigastric discomfort	Aggravated by large meals and postprandial recumbency
Peptic ulcer	Prolonged epigastric or retrosternal burning	Relieved by antacid or food
Biliary disease	Right upper quadrant pain	Unprovoked or following meal
Pancreatitis	Intense epigastric and retrosternal pain	Associated with alcoholism, elevated triglycerides
Musculoskeletal		
Costochondritis	Fleeting localized pain, may be intense	May be reproducible by pressure to affected site
Cervical disk disease	Sudden fleeting pain	May be reproduced by movement of neck
Psychological		
Somatoform disorders, sudden fleeting pain, may be produced by movement of neck	Symptoms are atypical for any organ system	Symptoms may persist despite negative evaluations of multiple organ systems

MI, Myocardial infarction; *PE*, pulmonary embolism.

From Lee T. H. & Cannon C. P. (2008). Approach to the patient with chest pain. In R. O. Bonow, P. Libby, D. L. Mann, D. P. Zipes (Eds.), Braunwald's heart disease: a textbook of cardiovascular medicine *(8th ed., Chapter 49).*

6. **What is the difference between stable and unstable angina?**

Angina is typically further classified into *stable* and *unstable* types. Stable angina occurs in situations of increased myocardial oxygen demand, such as exercise. Unstable angina occurs at rest. It may have a new onset within 2 months of initial presentation or can increase in frequency, intensity, or duration. Unstable angina can occur at any time and falls within the spectrum of ACSs.

Table 14.2. Specific Details of the Chest Pain History Helpful in Distinguishing Anginal Chest Pain Due to Myocardial Infarction from Pain of Noncardiac Causation

ELEMENT	QUESTION	COMMENTS
Chest Pain Characteristics		
Quality	In your own words, how would you describe the pain? What adjectives would you use?	Pay attention to language and cultural considerations; use interpreter if necessary.
Location	Point with your finger to where you are feeling the pain.	Can elicit size of chest pain area with the same question.
Radiation	If the pain moves out of your chest, trace where it travels with your finger.	Patient may need to point to examiner's scapula or back.
Size of area or distribution	With your finger, trace the area on your chest where the pain occurs.	Focus on distinguishing between a small coin-sized area and a larger distribution.
Severity	If 10 is the most severe pain you have ever had, on this 10-point scale, how severe was this pain?	Patient may need to be coached in this: pain of fetal delivery, kidney stone, bony fracture are good references for 10.
Time of onset and is it continuing	Is the pain still present? Has it gotten better or worse since it began? When did it begin?	Ongoing pain a concern: it is worthwhile to obtain an initial ECG while pain is present.
Duration	Does the pain typically last seconds, minutes, or hours? Roughly, how long is a typical episode?	Focus on the most recent (especially if ongoing) and the most severe episode; be precise: if the patient says "seconds," tap out 4 seconds.
First occurrence	When is the first time you ever had this pain?	Interest should focus on this recent episode—that is, the past few days or weeks.
Frequency	How many times per hour or per day has it been occurring?	Relevant only for recurring pain: a single index episode is not uncommon.
Similar to previous cardiac ischemic episodes	If you have had a heart attack or angina in the past, is this pain similar to the pain you had then? Is it more or less severe?	Follow-up questions elicit how the diagnosis of CAD was confirmed and whether any intervention occurred.
Precipitating or Aggravating Factors		
Pleuritic	Is the pain worse if you take a deep breath or cough?	Distinguish between whether these maneuvers only partially or completely reproduce the pain and if it reproduces the pain only some or all of the time.
Positional	Is the pain made better or worse by your changing body position? If so, what position makes the pain better or worse?	Distinguish between whether these maneuvers only partially or completely reproduce the pain: on physical examination, turn the chest wall, shoulder, and back.

Continued on following page

Table 14.2. Specific Details of the Chest Pain History Helpful in Distinguishing Anginal Chest Pain Due to Myocardial Infarction from Pain of Noncardiac Causation *(Continued)*

ELEMENT	QUESTION	COMMENTS
Palpable	If I press on your chest wall, does that reproduce the pain?	Distinguish between whether these maneuvers only partially or completely reproduce the pain: ask the patient to lead you to the area of pain; then palpate.
Exercise	Does the pain come back or get worse if you walk quickly, climb stairs, or exert yourself?	Helpful to quantify a change in pattern (e.g., the number of stairs or distance walked before the pain began).
Emotional stress	Does becoming upset affect the pain?	Are there other stress-related symptoms (e.g., acroparesthesias)?
Relieving factors	Are there any things that you can do to relieve the pain once it has begun?	In particular, ask about response to nitrates, antacids, ceasing strenuous activity.
Associated symptoms	Do you typically get other symptoms when you get this chest pain?	After asking question in open-ended way, ask specifically about nausea or vomiting and about sweating.

CAD, Coronary artery disease; ECG, electrocardiogram.
Modified from Swap, C. J., & Nagurney, J. T. (2005). Value and limitations of chest pain history in the evaluation of patients with suspected acute coronary syndromes. Journal of American Medical Association, 294, 2623–2629.

7. What are the associated symptoms that people with angina may experience in addition to chest discomfort?

Patients with angina may experience one or more of the following symptoms along with chest discomfort:

- Shortness of breath
- Diaphoresis
- Nausea
- Fatigue, particularly in the elderly and in women
- Radiating pains

Patients may describe pains or discomfort that *radiates* to the back (typically the midscapula), neck, jaw, or down one or both arms. They may also describe a sensation of *numbness* in the arm.

Some patients do not experience classic chest discomfort but instead manifest only one or more of these associated symptoms. In such cases, the symptom is referred to as an "angina equivalent." New or increased dyspnea on exertion is the most common angina equivalent.

8. What are the major risk factors for coronary artery disease?

- Age above 45 years for men and above 55 years for women
- Gender: Males are at higher risk of developing CAD earlier in life, although late-life CAD is common in both men and women.
- Family history of premature CAD: This is traditionally defined as a first-degree male relative (i.e., father, brother) who first developed clinical CAD at an age younger than 55 years or first-degree female relative (i.e., mother, sister) at an age younger than 65 years.
- Hypercholesterolemia
- Hypertension
- Cigarette smoking
- Diabetes mellitus

Other factors that have been associated with an increased risk of CAD include inactivity (lack of regular exercise), obesity (specifically excessive abdominal girth), end-stage renal disease, chronic inflammatory diseases, human immunodeficiency virus (HIV) infection and acquired immunodeficiency syndrome (AIDS), mental stress, depression, elevated C-reactive protein, and elevated homocysteine.

The American College of Cardiology/American Heart Association (ACC/AHA) Cardiovascular Risk Calculator (the app of which can be downloaded onto a smartphone) can be used to estimate a patient's 10-year cardiovascular risk. This score takes into consideration age, gender, race, total cholesterol, high-density lipoprotein (HDL) cholesterol, systolic blood pressure and treatment status, diabetes, and smoking status.

9. What symptoms and findings make it more (or less) likely that the patient's chest pains are due to angina or that the patient has acute coronary syndrome?

The answer to this question is given below. Tables 14.1 and 14.2) are taken from an excellent review article on this subject in the *Journal of the American Medical Association* and summarize many of the relevant questions and the value of the chest pain characteristics in distinguishing angina and ACS/MI pain from other causes. It is important to remember, no single element of chest pain history is a powerful enough predictor in itself to rule out ACS.

- **Quality and characteristics of chest discomfort:** Patients who describe chest *tightness* or *pressure* are more likely to have angina. Pain that is stabbing, pleuritic, positional, or reproducible is less likely to be angina; this is often categorized as *atypical chest pain,* although the presence of such symptoms does not absolutely rule out the possibility that the pain may be due to CAD. Pleuritic chest pain, pain exacerbated by deep breaths, is often associated with pulmonary causes, pericarditis, or musculoskeletal causes. Pain that improves when the patient leans forward and gets worse when supine is consistent with pericarditis. Although it is generally accepted that a more diffuse area of discomfort is suggestive of angina whereas a coin-sized, very focal area of discomfort is more likely to have a noncardiac cause, this distinction in itself is not enough to confidently dismiss very focal pain as noncardiac. The severity of the pain or discomfort is not helpful in distinguishing angina from other causes of chest pain. Chest pain that is sudden in onset and of maximal intensity at onset is suggestive of aortic dissection, PE, or pneumothorax, as opposed to pain that reaches its peak intensity only gradually in those with ischemic chest pain due to ACS. Patients with aortic dissection may describe the pain as *tearing* or *ripping* and as radiating to the back. The Levine sign (pronounced La-Vine and has no relationship to this book's editor) occurs when the patient spontaneously clenches his or her fist and puts it over the chest while describing the chest discomfort; this is often said to be characteristic of ischemic chest pain.
- **Duration of the discomfort:** Angina usually lasts on the order of minutes, not seconds; hours (unless the patient is suffering a MI); or days. Typically, patients will describe stable anginal pain as lasting approximately 2 to 10 minutes and subsiding after the patient ceases the activity causing an increase in myocardial oxygen demand. Unstable anginal pain may last 10 to 30 minutes. Pain that truly lasts just several seconds or greater than 30 minutes is usually not angina unless the patient is having an acute MI. One has to be careful because some patients will initially describe the pain as lasting seconds when, on further questioning, it becomes clear it has really lasted minutes. Pain that lasts continuously (not off and on) for a day or days is usually not angina.
- **Precipitating factors:** Because angina results from a mismatch between myocardial oxygen demand and supply, activities that increase myocardial oxygen demand or decrease supply may cause angina. Discomfort that is brought on by exercise or exertion is highly suggestive of angina. Mental stress or anger may not only increase heart rate and blood pressure but can also lead to coronary artery vasoconstriction, precipitating angina. However, one must be careful not to rule out angina as the cause of the chest discomfort in patients who experience chest discomfort at rest without precipitation, as this may be due to ACS. The problem in this case is primarily thrombus formation in the coronary artery, leading to decreased myocardial oxygen supply.
- **Relieving factors**
    - **Relief with sublingual nitroglycerin (SL NTG) or rest:** Nitroglycerin is a coronary artery vasodilator. Although there are some recent studies to the contrary, typically patients who report partial or complete relief of their chest discomfort within 2 to 5 minutes of taking SL NTG are more likely to be experiencing angina as the cause of their chest discomfort. Patients must be questioned carefully because some will report that the SL NTG decreased their discomfort, but

on further questioning, it becomes clear that the discomfort decreased only 30 to 60 minutes after the SL NTG was taken. Because SL NTG exerts its effect within minutes, this does not necessarily imply that the chest discomfort was *relieved* by the SL NTG. However, in patients experiencing MI caused by an occluded coronary artery, the fact that the chest discomfort is not relieved with SL NTG does not necessarily make it less likely that the pain is due to CAD. Of note, nitroglycerin is a smooth muscle relaxant; thus it can relieve pain cause by esophageal and biliary spasms as well. Patients are more likely to have angina if they say that their chest discomfort resolved after sitting or resting for a few minutes.

  - **Relief with a "GI cocktail,"** as with antacids or viscous lidocaine, does not rule out ischemic chest pain.

- **Probability of having angina or ACS:** In patients with multiple risk factors for CAD or with known CAD, the occurrence of chest pain is more likely to be due to angina or ACS.
- **Associated symptoms:** The presence of one or more associated symptoms, such as shortness of breath, diaphoresis, nausea, or radiating pain increases the likelihood that the discomfort is due to angina.
- **Electrocardiographic (ECG) abnormalities:** ST-segment depressions or elevations or T-wave inversions increase the likelihood that the discomfort is due to angina or ACS. However, the lack of these findings should not rule out angina as a cause of the chest discomfort. The initial ECG has a sensitivity of only 20% to 60% for MI, let alone merely the presence of CAD.
- **Troponin elevation:** The finding of an elevated troponin level significantly increases the likelihood that the discomfort is due to angina and CAD. However, the lack of an elevated troponin does not rule out angina and CAD as a cause of the discomfort. Further, as discussed earlier, other conditions besides angina can cause an elevated troponin (discussed below).

Table 14.3 summarizes the value of specific components of the chest pain history for the diagnosis of acute myocardial infarction (AMI).

Table 14.3. Value of Specific Components of the Chest Pain History for the Diagnosis of Acute Myocardial Infarction

PAIN DESCRIPTOR	POSITIVE LIKELIHOOD RATIO (95% CI)
Increased Likelihood of AMI	
Radiation to right arm or shoulder	4.7 (1.9-12)
Radiation to both arms or shoulders	4.1 (2.5-6.5)
Associated with exertion	2.4 (1.5-3.8)
Radiation to left arm	2.3 (1.7-3.1)
Associated with diaphoresis	2.0 (1.9-2.2)
Associated with nausea or vomiting	1.9 (1.7-2.3)
Worse than previous angina or similar to previous MI	1.8 (1.6-2.0)
Described as pressure	1.3 (1.2-1.5)
Decreased Likelihood of AMI	
Described as pleuritic	0.2 (0.1-0.3)
Described as positional	0.3 (0.2-0.5)
Described as sharp	0.3 (0.2-0.5)
Reproducible with palpation	0.3 (0.2-0.4)
Inframammary location	0.8 (0.7-0.9)
Not associated with exertion	0.8 (0.6-0.9)

AMI, Acute myocardial infarction; CI, confidence interval.

Modified from Swap, C. J., & Nagurney, J. T. (2005). Value and limitations of chest pain history in the evaluation of patients with suspected acute coronary syndromes. Journal of American Medical Association, 294, 2623–2629.

10. What physical exam findings make the chest pain more or less likely to be due to angina?

The physical exam in a patient with angina is often unremarkable or nonspecific. However, some findings can suggest other causes of the chest pain. A rub heard on auscultation can be due to pericardial or pleural disease. Different palpated pulse volumes and a difference in systolic blood pressure of 15 mm Hg or more between both arms as well as an aortic regurgitation murmur all support aortic dissection. A systolic murmur at the right upper sternal border radiating to the carotid arteries is consistent with aortic stenosis. Differential breath sounds are consistent with pneumothorax. Asymmetric swelling of an extremity can suggest deep vein thrombosis (DVT) that has resulted in a PE. Reproduction of the chest pain with palpation of the chest is likely due to musculoskeletal or dermatologic causes. Physical exam findings of associated risk factors for CAD are also helpful. Diminished peripheral pulses, carotid or renal bruits, or a palpable abdominal aneurysm suggests peripheral vascular disease, which increases the likelihood that the patient has significant CAD. Xanthomas suggest hyperlipidemia. Acanthosis nigricans suggests the possibility of diabetes mellitus.

11. How is an electrocardiogram helpful in distinguishing the causes of chest pain?

Although the ECG is often normal, it can show ST-segment depressions or T-wave inversions in the setting of ischemia due to unstable angina. There can be transient ST-segment elevation in patients with Prinzmetal angina. In pericarditis, there are diffuse concave ST-segment elevation (as opposed to the convex ST-segment elevation seen in ST-segment elevation MI [STEMI]) and PR depression. The classic ECG findings in a patient with a large PE are a prominent S wave in lead I, a Q wave in lead III, and T-wave inversion in lead III ($S_1Q_3T_3$) (granted this is not sensitive or specific for PE) as well as a right-axis deviation and right bundle branch block. Most commonly, though, sinus tachycardia is seen with PE. ST-segment elevation can be seen in aortic dissection if the dissection involves the origin of a coronary artery.

12. What is the initial workup of patients presenting with chest pain?

Patients presenting with chest pain should have an ECG, as noted above. A chest x-ray should also be performed, although it is typically unremarkable in those with ACS. That said, the x-ray can detect other life-threatening causes of chest pain. A chest x-ray can identify pulmonary causes, including pneumothorax, pneumonia, and pleural effusion. It can also show a widened mediastinum, supportive of aortic dissection. Mediastinal emphysema suggests esophageal rupture. In addition, musculoskeletal pain due to rib fractures can be detected. Further testing will be tailored depending on the likelihood and pretest probability of the suspected diagnosis. If ACS is being considered, cardiac biomarkers—including troponin, CK, and CK-MB—should be obtained. Depending on the probability of PE, a D-dimer test or computed tomography (CT) angiogram should be performed. If aortic dissection is suspected, CT angiography or transesophageal echocardiography (TEE) can diagnose it.

A comprehensive approach to the patient with chest pain is given in Fig. 14.1.

13. If one is still in doubt as to the diagnosis of coronary artery disease, should a stress test be obtained?

Yes. Stress testing for diagnostic purposes is best implemented in patients who, after initial evaluation, have an intermediate probability of having CAD. For example, in a patient with a pretest probability of having CAD of 50%, a *positive* exercise stress test makes the posttest probability of CAD 85%, whereas a *negative* exercise stress test makes the posttest probability of CAD just 15%. Stress testing can also be used for prognostic purposes. Stress testing is discussed in greater detail in the chapters on exercise stress testing (Chapter 5), nuclear cardiology (Chapter 8), echocardiography (Chapter 7), and magnetic resonance imaging (Chapter 10). Coronary (CT) angiography is an emerging alternate form for diagnosis and is discussed in Chapter 13.

14. Are there exceptions to the classic presentations of anginal pain?

Yes. It is well known that women often do not present with *typical* anginal symptoms (e.g., substernal exertional pain relieved by rest or SL NTG). In fact, women are often misdiagnosed because of a lower suspicion by doctors that they have CAD and the fact that they often experience discomfort that is not *classic* for angina. In the Women's Ischemia Syndrome Evaluation study, over half the women (65%) with ischemia presented with atypical symptoms. Older patients may have difficulty in remembering or describing their chest discomfort and so also may not describe *classic* anginal symptoms.

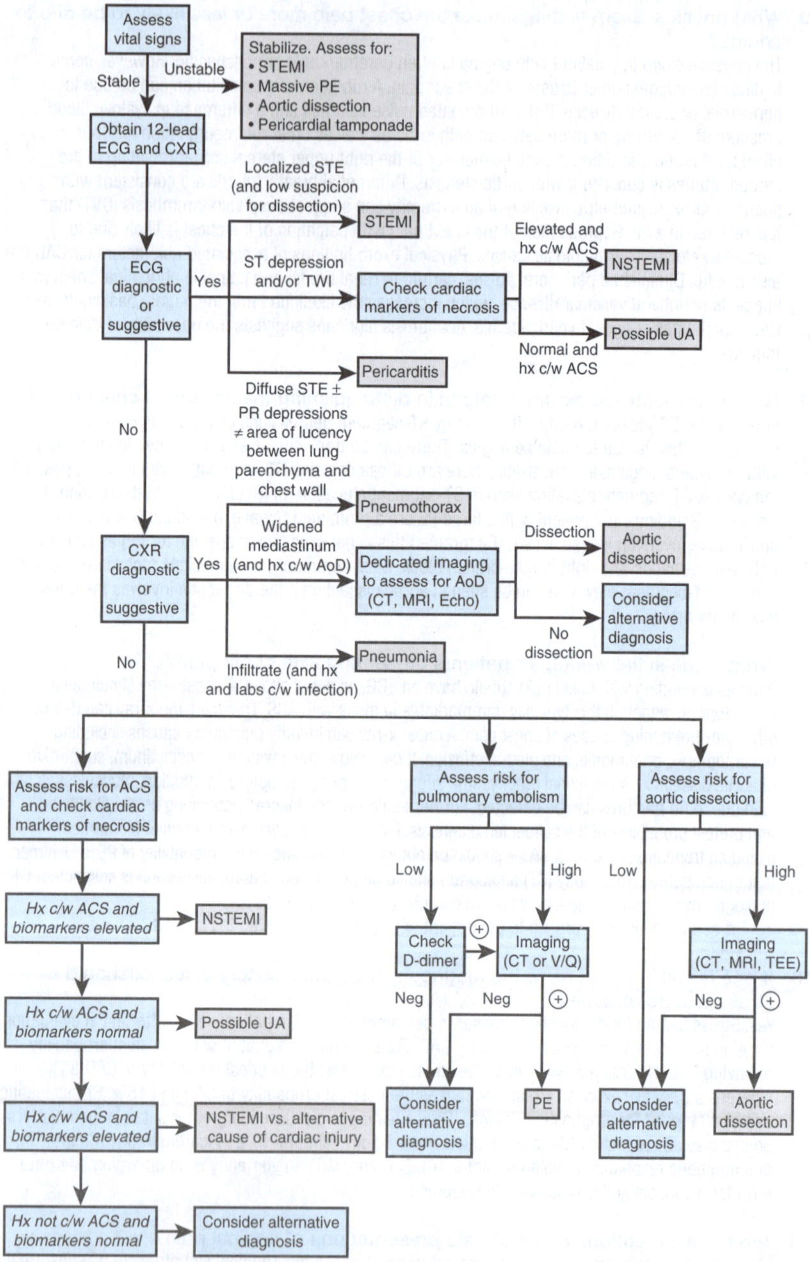

Fig. 14.1. A comprehensive approach to the patient with chest pain. *ACS,* Acute coronary syndrome; *CT,* computed tomography; *CXR,* chest x-ray; *ECG,* electrocardiogram; *MRI,* magnetic resonance imaging; *NSTEMI,* non-ST-elevation myocardial infarction; *PE,* pulmonary embolism; ST is a segment of the ECG and is not defined; *STE,* ST elevation; *STEMI,* ST elevation myocardial infarction; *TEE,* transesophagael echocardiogram; *TWI,* T wave inversion; *UA,* unstable angina; *V/Q,* ventilation/perfusion. *(Reproduced from Sabatine, M. S., & Cannon, C. P. (2012). Approach to the patient with chest pain. In D. L. Mann, D. P. Zipes, P. Libby, R. O. Bonow (Eds.),* Braunwald's heart disease: a textbook of cardiovascular medicine *(10th ed., 1057–1067, Chapter 50). Philadelphia: Saunders.)*

Some diabetic patients appear to have an impaired sensation of chest discomfort when the heart experiences myocardial ischemia. Thus some diabetic patients may not report chest discomfort but rather only one or more associated symptoms, such as shortness of breath or diaphoresis. Cardiac transplant patients do not experience ischemic chest pain owing to denervation of the transplanted heart.

15. What is Prinzmetal angina?

Prinzmetal angina, also called *variant angina*, is an uncommon type of angina caused by coronary vasospasm. The coronary artery is believed to spasm, thus severely reducing myocardial oxygen supply to the affected myocardium. Although the spasm can occur in either a *normal* or a diseased coronary artery, it most commonly occurs within 1 cm of an atherosclerotic plaque. Most commonly, the right coronary artery (RCA) is involved, followed by the left anterior descending (LAD). Patients with Prinzmetal angina are typically younger, often female. Smoking, chronic alcohol use, and cocaine increase the risk of coronary artery spasm. Prinzmetal angina usually does not occur with physical exertion or stress but rather during rest, most typically between midnight and 8 am. The pain can be severe. If an ECG is obtained during an episode, it may demonstrate transient ST-segment elevations during the episode, as opposed to a STEMI, where the ST-segment elevations are persistent. Coronary angiography is recommended in patients with suspected Prinzmetal angina to rule out severe fixed obstruction. Provocative testing can be performed, primarily using acetylcholine and methacholine, during coronary angiography when this diagnosis is suspected. But provocative testing is rarely done owing to the risk of coronary spasm refractory to nitroglycerin and other vasodilators, resulting in prolonged ischemia, MI, and even death. Treatment of Prinzmetal angina is based primarily on the use of calcium channel blockers and nitrates, which are first-line therapies.

16. What is cardiac syndrome X and microvascular angina?

Cardiac syndrome X is an entity in which patients describe exertional anginal symptoms yet are found on cardiac catheterization to have nonobstructive epicardial CAD. Patients may also have ST-segment depressions on exercise stress testing, perfusion defects, or wall motion abnormalities with imaging-based stress testing, and abnormal coronary flow reserve on invasive testing or positron emission tomography (PET). Unlike Prinzmetal angina, they do not have spontaneous coronary spasm and do not have provocable coronary spasm. Although there are likely multiple causes and explanations for cardiac syndrome X, it does appear that, at least in some patients, microvascular coronary artery constriction or dysfunction plays a role. Because of this, the term *cardiac syndrome X* is being abandoned in preference for the term *microvascular angina*. The recommended initial treatment for microvascular angina is beta-blockers, which can reduce or modulate myocardial oxygen demand. Other antianginal agents—including calcium channel blockers, nitrates, and ranolizine—can subsequently or additionally be considered. Treatment is usually individually tailored to the patient and sometimes includes cognitive behavioral therapy and imipramine, which is used in chronic pain syndromes. No one standardized approach will fit all patients.

17. Does an elevated troponin level confirm the diagnosis acute coronary syndrome?

Not necessarily. To make the clinical diagnosis of ACS, troponin elevation has to be accompanied by angina or angina equivalent, ECG changes, and/or new wall motion abnormalities on echocardiography. Additionally, there is a typical rise-and-fall pattern of the troponin level with an MI as opposed to an unvaried mild elevation of troponin levels. Although troponin elevations are fairly sensitive and specific for myocardial necrosis, numerous other conditions can also be associated with elevations in cardiac troponins. In fact, up to 45% of elevated troponins in acutely ill, hospitalized patients are not due to CAD. Any condition that results in a demand/supply mismatch (e.g., sepsis, hypotension, severe hypoxia, severe anemia, severe hypertension, tachyarrhythmias, and cocaine use) can cause an elevation in troponin. Myocardial strain in heart failure exacerbation can cause troponin release. Importantly, troponin elevation can occur with PE and is, in fact, associated with a worse prognosis in cases of PE with elevated troponins. Myopericarditis (inflammation of the myocardium and pericardium) can also cause elevated troponin levels. In addition, aortic dissection that involves the RCA can lead to secondary MI. Further, troponins can be modestly chronically elevated in patients with severe chronic kidney disease. Troponin elevation has also been noted in patients with acute stroke.

Bibliography and Suggested Readings

Amsterdam, E. A., Kirk, J. D., Bluemke, D. A., Diercks, D., Farkouh, M. E., Garvey, J. L., et al. (2010). Testing of low-risk patients presenting to the emergency department with chest pain: a scientific statement from the American Heart Association. *Circulation, 122*(17), 1756–1776.

Amsterdam, E. A., Wenger, N. K., Brindis, R. G., Casey, D. E., Jr., Ganiats, T. G., Holmes, D. R., Jr., et al. (2014). 2014 AHA/ACC guideline for the management of patients with non-ST-elevation acute coronary syndromes: a report of the American College of Cardiology/American Heart Association Task Force on practice guidelines. *Journal of the American College of Cardiology, 64*(24), 2713–2714.

Anderson, J. L. (2011). 2011 ACCF/AHA focused update incorporated into the ACC/AHA 2007 guidelines for the management of patients with unstable angina/non-ST elevation myocardial infarction: a report of the American College of Cardiology Foundation/American Heart Association Task Force on practice guidelines. *Circulation, 123*, e426–e579.

Boudi, F. B. (2016). *Risk factors for coronary artery disease.* < http://emedicine.medscape.com/article/164163-overview> Accessed 24.01.16.

Cohn, J. K., & Cohn, P. F. (2002). Chest pain. *Circulation, 106*, 530.

Fihn, S. D., Gardin, J. M., Abrams, J., Berra, K., Blankenship, J. C., Dallas, A. P., et al. (2012). 2012 ACCF/AHA/ACP/AATS/PCNA/SCAI/STS guideline for the diagnosis and management of patients with stable ischemic heart disease: a report of the American College of Cardiology Foundation/American Heart Association task force on practice guidelines, and the American College of Physicians, American Association for Thoracic Surgery, Preventative Cardiovascular Nurses Association, Society for Cardiovascular Angiography and Interventions, and Society of Thoracic Surgeons. *Journal of the American College of Cardiology, 60*(24), e44–e164.

Hanna, E. (2009). Note about Prinzmetal's angina = variant angina = chronic vasospastic angina. In E. B. Hanna, R. E. Quintal, & N. Jain (Eds.), *Cardiology: handbook for clinicians* (p. 47). Arlington, VA: Scrub Hill Press, Inc.

Hanna, E. (2009). Elevated cardiac troponin without an acute coronary event (nonthrombotic troponin elevations). In E. B. Hanna, R. E. Quintal, & N. Jain (Eds.), *Cardiology: handbook for clinicians* (pp. 51–54). Arlington, VA: Scrub Hill Press, Inc.

Haro, L. H., Decker, W. W., Boie, E. T., & Wright, R. S. (2006). Initial approach to the patient who has chest pain. *Cardiology Clinics, 24*(1), 1–17.

Hollander, J. E., & Chase, M. (2016). *Evaluation of the adult with chest pain in the emergency department.* < http://www.uptodate.com/contents/evaluation-of-the-adult-with-chest-pain-in-the-emergency-department?source=search_result&search=chest+pain&selectedTitle=8%7E150> Accessed 23.01.16.

Lanza, G. A. (2007). Cardiac syndrome X: a critical overview and future perspectives. *Heart, 93*, 159–166.

Mayer, S., & Hillis, L. D. (1998). Prinzmetal's variant angina. *Clinical Cardiology, 21*, 243–246.

Meisel, J. L. (2016). *Diagnostic approach to chest pain in adults.* < http://www.uptodate.com/contents/diagnostic-approach-to-chest-pain-in-adults> Accessed 29.01.2016.

National Heart, Lung, and Blood Institute. (2013). *Who is at risk for coronary heart disease?.* < http://www.nhlbi.nih.gov/health/health-topics/topics/cad/atrisk> Accessed 25.01.2016.

Ringstrom, E., & Freedman, J. (2006). Approach to undifferentiated chest pain in the emergency department: a review of recent medical literature and published practice guidelines. *The Mount Sinai Journal of Medicine, 73*(2), 499–505.

Swap, C. J., & Nagurney, J. T. (2005). Value and limitations of chest pain history in the evaluation of patients with suspected acute coronary syndromes. *Journal of the American Medical Association, 294*(20), 2623–2629.

CHRONIC STABLE ANGINA

Richard A. Lange

CHAPTER 15

1. **Can a patient with new-onset chest pain have chronic stable angina?**
   The term *chronic stable angina* refers to angina that has been stable in frequency and severity for at least 2 months and with which the episodes are provoked by exertion or stress of similar intensity. Chronic stable angina is the initial manifestation of coronary artery disease (CAD) in about 50% of patients; the other half initially experience unstable angina, myocardial infarction (MI), or sudden death.

2. **What causes chronic stable angina?**
   Angina occurs when myocardial oxygen supply is inadequate to meet the metabolic demands of the heart, thereby causing myocardial ischemia. This is usually caused by increased oxygen demands (i.e., increase in heart rate, blood pressure, or myocardial contractility) that cannot be met by a concomitant increase in coronary arterial blood flow, due to narrowing or occlusion of one or more coronary arteries (Fig. 15.1).

3. **How is chronic stable angina classified or graded?**
   The most commonly used system is the Canadian Cardiovascular Society system, in which angina is graded on a scale of I to IV. These grades and this system are described in Table 15.1. This grading system is useful for evaluating functional limitation, treatment efficacy, and stability of symptoms over time.

4. **What tests should be obtained in the patient with newly diagnosed angina?**
   After a careful history (Hx) and physical examination, the laboratory tests for the patient with suspected angina should include a measurement of hemoglobin, hemoglobin A1c, fasting lipids (i.e., serum concentrations of total cholesterol, high density lipoprotein (HDL) cholesterol, triglycerides, calculated low density lipoprotein (LDL) cholesterol), and a 12-lead electrocardiogram (ECG).

5. **What are the goals of treatment in the patient with chronic stable angina?**
   - Ameliorate angina.
   - Prevent major cardiovascular (CV) events, such as heart attack or cardiac death.
   - Identify high-risk patients who would benefit from revascularization.

6. **What therapies improve symptoms?**
   - Beta-blockers
   - Nitrates
   - Calcium-channel blockers
   - Ranolazine

7. **What is the initial approach to the patient with chronic stable angina?**
   The initial approach should be focused upon eliminating unhealthy behaviors such as smoking and effectively promoting lifestyle changes that reduce CV risk such as maintaining a healthy weight, engaging in physical activity, and adopting a healthy diet. In addition, annual influenza vaccination reduces mortality (by ~35%) and morbidity in patients with underlying CAD. Tight glycemic control was thought to be important in the diabetic, but this approach actually increases the risk of CV death and complications.

8. **What is first-line drug therapy for the treatment of stable angina?**
   When considering medications, beta-blockers decrease myocardial oxygen demands by reducing heart rate, myocardial contractility, and blood pressure. They are first-line therapy in the treatment of chronic CAD, as they delay the onset of angina and increase exercise capacity in subjects with stable angina. Although many guidelines recommend combination therapy in different drug classes (i.e., beta-blockers, calcium-channel blockers, or long-acting nitrates), studies have not shown that combination therapy is more effective for reducing ischemia or anginal symptoms than beta-blocker monotherapy. Aspirin and a statin should also be prescribed (see below), as they reduce the risk of MI and CV death in patients with chronic stable angina.

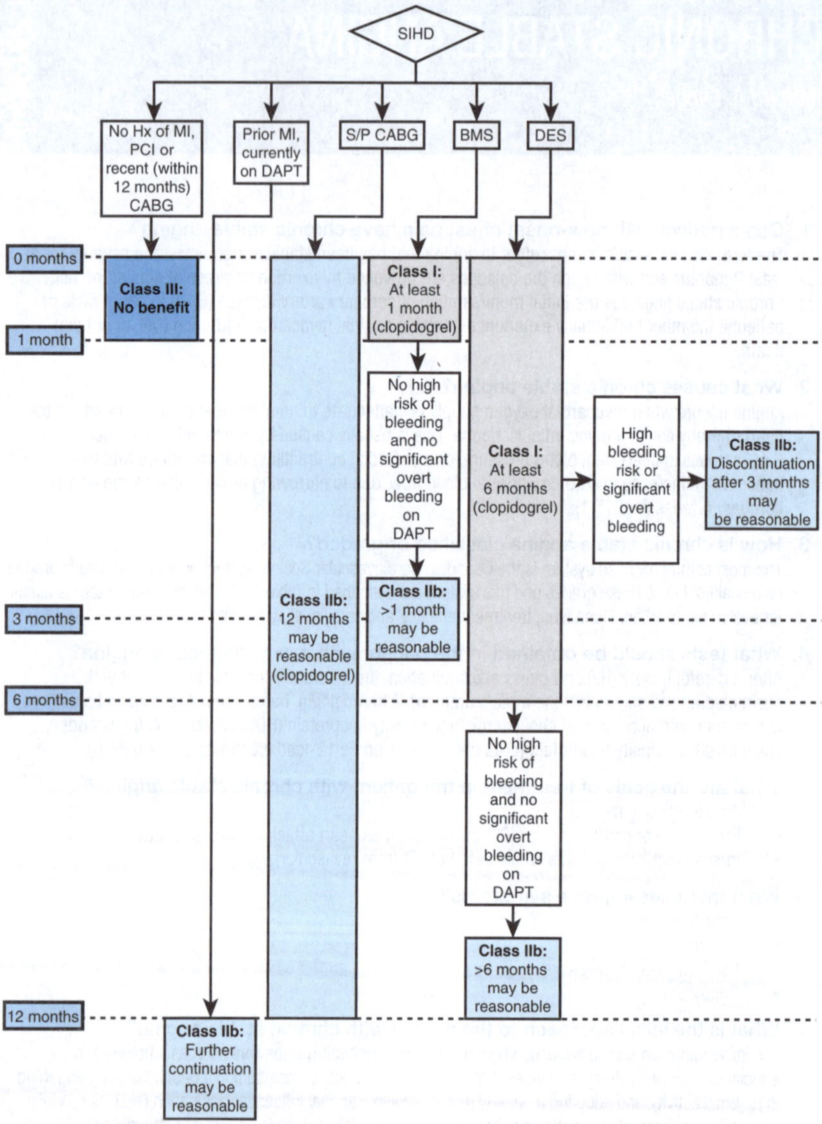

Fig. 15.1. Treatment algorithm for duration of P2Y12 inhibitor therapy in patients with SIHD. Patients with a Hx of ACS greater than 1 year prior who have since remained free of recurrent ACS are considered to have transitioned to SIHD. Arrows at the bottom of the figure denote that the optimal duration of prolonged DAPT is not established. Clopidogrel is the only currently used P2Y12 inhibitor studied in patients with SIHD undergoing PCI. Aspirin therapy is almost always continued indefinitely in patients with coronary artery disease (CAD). *High bleeding risk denotes those who have or develop a high risk of bleeding (e.g., treatment with oral anticoagulant therapy) or are at increased risk of severe bleeding complication (e.g., major intracranial surgery). *ACS,* Acute coronary syndrome; *BMS,* bare metal stent; *CABG,* coronary artery bypass graft surgery; *DAPT,* dual antiplatelet therapy; *DES,* drug-eluting stent; *Hx,* history; *MI,* myocardial infarction; *PCI,* percutaneous coronary intervention; *SIHD,* stable ischemic heart disease (chronic stable angina); *S/P,* status post. *(Reproduced from Levine, G. N., Bates, E. R., Bittl, J. A., Brindis, R. G., Fihn, S. D., Fleisher, L.A., et al. [2016]. 2016 ACC/AHA Guideline Focused Update on Duration of Dual Antiplatelet Therapy in Patients With Coronary Artery Disease,* Journal of the American College of Cardiology, 68, *1082–1115.)*

Table 15.1. Grading of Angina by the Canadian Cardiovascular Society Classification System

Class I
- Ordinary physical activity, such as walking and climbing stairs, does not cause angina.
- Angina occurs with strenuous, rapid, or prolonged exertion at work or recreation.

Class II
- Slight limitation of ordinary activity
- Angina occurs while walking or climbing stairs rapidly, while walking uphill, while walking or climbing stairs after meals in cold or in wind, while under emotional stress, or only during the first several hours after waking.
- Angina occurs while walking more than 2 blocks on level grade and climbing more than 1 flight of ordinary stairs at a normal pace and in normal conditions.

Class III
- Marked limitations of ordinary physical activity
- Angina occurs while walking 1 or 2 blocks on level grade and climbing 1 flight of stairs in normal conditions and at a normal pace.

Class IV
- Inability to engage in any physical activity without discomfort
- Angina may be present at rest.

9. Is any beta-blocker better than the others?

Although the various beta-blockers have different properties (i.e., cardioselectivity, vasodilating actions, concomitant alpha-adrenergic inhibition, and partial beta-agonist activity; Table 15.2), they appear to have similar efficacy in patients with chronic stable angina. Beta-blockers prevent reinfarction and improve survival in survivors of MI, but such benefits have not been demonstrated in patients with chronic CAD without previous MI.

10. What is the proper dosage for a beta-blocker?

The dosage of a beta-blocker is titrated to achieve a resting heart rate of 55 to 60 beats/minute and an increase in heart rate during exercise that does not exceed 75% of the heart rate response associated with the onset of ischemia. Beta-blockers are contraindicated in the presence of severe bradycardia, high-degree atrioventricular block, sinus node dysfunction, and uncompensated heart failure. They are also contraindicated in the patient with vasospastic angina, in whom they may worsen angina as a result of unopposed alpha-adrenergic stimulation; calcium-channel blockers are preferred in these patients.

11. Which is more effective: calcium-channel blockers or beta-blockers?

Calcium-channel blockers and beta-blockers are similarly effective at relieving angina and improving exercise time to the onset of angina or ischemia. Calcium-channel blockers can be used as monotherapy in patients with chronic stable angina, although combination therapy with a beta-blocker or nitrate relieves angina more effectively than their use alone. In this regard, beta-blockers may be particularly useful in blunting the reflex tachycardia that occurs with dihydropyridine calcium-channel blocker use.

12. When should a peripherally acting calcium-channel blocker (i.e., dihydropyridine, such as amlodipine or felodipine) be used versus one that has effects on both the heart and the periphery (i.e., verapamil, diltiazem)?

Amlodipine and felodipine are used primarily as second- or third-line antianginal agents in patients already on beta-blockers (and, often, long-acting nitrates). They act mainly as vasodilators, lowering blood pressure and likely having some coronary vasodilating effects. Verapamil and diltiazem, in addition to having vasodilating effects, have negative chronotropic and inotropic effects. Thus they are used in patients with contraindications or intolerance to beta-blockers. They are typically avoided in patients with an ejection fraction less than 40% or on a beta-blocker because of their negative inotropic effects.

Table 15.2. Antianginal Classes, Effects, Side Effects, and Contraindications

CLASS	EFFECTS	SIDE EFFECTS	CONTRAINDICATIONS
Beta-blockers	Negative chronotropy Negative inotropy	Extreme bradycardia AV node block and PR prolongation Exacerbation of acute heart failure Bronchospasm Blood pressure reduction	Resting bradycardia Prolonged PR interval (>220-240 ms) Acute decompensated heart failure Severe reactive airway disease Baseline hypotension
Long-acting nitrates	Coronary vasodilation Venodilation	Headache Venous pooling	Use of erectile dysfunction medication
Calcium-channel blockers: verapamil and diltiazem	Peripheral vasodilation Coronary vasodilation Negative chronotropy Negative inotropy	Extreme bradycardia AV node block and PR prolongation Blood pressure reduction Exacerbation of chronic and acute heart failure	Resting bradycardia Prolonged PR interval (>220-240 ms) Baseline low blood pressure Acute decompensated heart failure Ejection fraction <40% Usually patients already on beta-blockers
Calcium-channel blockers: amlodipine and felodipine	Peripheral vasodilation Coronary vasodilation Coronary vasodilation No net negative chronotropic or inotropic effects	Blood pressure reduction Peripheral edema	Baseline low blood pressure

AV, Atrioventricular.

13. Should sublingual nitroglycerin (or nitroglycerin spray) be prescribed to all chronic stable angina patients?

Yes. This is the standard of care. Patients should be instructed on how to use sublingual nitroglycerin or spray—generally one tablet (or spray) every 5 minutes up to a maximum of three tablets (or sprays). They should be instructed to call 911 and seek immediate medical attention if their angina is not relieved after three tablets (or sprays) or 15 minutes.

14. When is a long-acting nitrate prescribed?

Long-acting nitrates are often prescribed along with beta-blockers or nondihydropyridine calcium-channel blockers (i.e., verapamil or diltiazem) in patients with chronic stable angina. Continuous exposure to nitroglycerin can result in tolerance to its vasodilating effects. Nitrate tolerance can be avoided by providing the patient with a "nitrate-free" period for 4 to 6 hours/day.

15. When is ranolazine added?

The use of ranolazine is reserved for individuals with angina that is refractory to maximal doses of other antianginal medications. Ranolazine targets the underlying derangements in sodium and calcium that occur during myocardial ischemia; it does not affect resting heart rate or blood pressure. Its antianginal efficacy is not related to its effect on heart rate, the hemodynamic state, the inotropic state, or coronary blood flow, as with currently available agents.

In randomized trials, ranolazine increased exercise tolerance, decreased anginal frequency, and decreased sublingual nitroglycerin use when used as monotherapy or in combination with beta-blockers or calcium-channel blockers in subjects with chronic stable angina. Randomized long-term trials evaluating its impact on mortality in stable CAD have not been performed.

Since ranolazine prolongs the QTc interval, it should not be used in patients with baseline QT prolongation or those on other medications that can prolong the QT interval. Furthermore, patients initiated on this drug should have their QT duration monitored periodically with 12-lead ECGs.

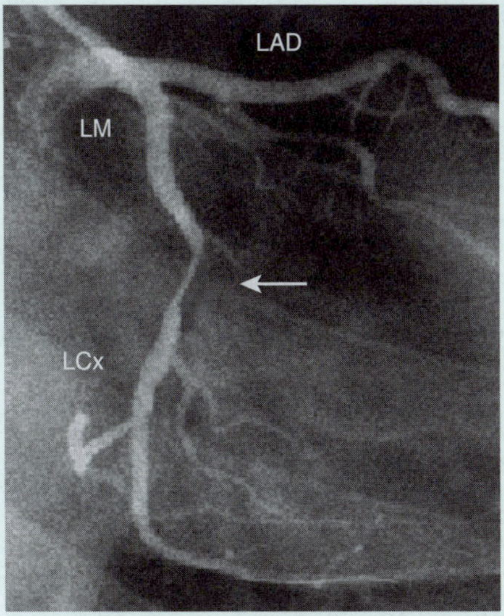

Fig. 15.2. Coronary angiogram demonstrating a significant stenosis *(arrow)* in the LCx artery. *LAD,* Left anterior descending artery; *LCx,* left circumflex; *LM,* left main coronary artery.

16. What medications prevent myocardial infarction or death in patients with stable chronic angina?

- Antiplatelet agents
- Angiotensin converting enzyme (ACE) inhibitors (in selected patients)
- Lipid-lowering therapy

17. What is the proper dose of aspirin?

An aspirin dose of 75 to 162 mg daily is equally as effective as 325 mg, but with a lower risk of bleeding. Doses less than 75 mg have less proven benefit. In patients with chronic CAD, aspirin treatment is associated with a 33% reduction in the risk of vascular events (nonfatal MI, nonfatal stroke, and vascular death). Over the course of a couple of years of treatment, aspirin would be expected to prevent about 10 to 15 vascular events for every 1000 people treated.

18. How should patients with chronic stable angina and aspirin allergy be treated?

Clopidogrel is a reasonable alternative in the patient with stable CAD who is allergic to or cannot tolerate aspirin.

19. Which patients with chronic stable angina should be treated with both clopidogrel and a P2Y12 receptor blocker?

The three P2Y12 receptor blockers are clopidogrel, prasugrel, and ticagrelor. In patients with an MI 1 to 3 years prior who are now stable and have tolerated dual antiplatelet therapy (DAPT) without bleeding complications, continuation of DAPT may be reasonable.

Patients with chronic stable angina treated with coronary stent implantation are treated for at least 6 months of DAPT. Continuation of DAPT for more than 6 months may be reasonable. On the other hand, for those at high risk of bleeding, only 3 months of DAPT may be reasonable.

Modest data suggest that DAPT for 1 year after coronary artery bypass grafting (CABG) may increase saphenous vein graft patency rates. Treatment of such patients with DAPT after CABG may be reasonable.

In patients with stable CAD without Hx of MI, percutaneous coronary intervention (PCI) or recent CABG, DAPT is not recommended.

Recommendations on the use and duration of DAPT in patients with chronic stable angina are given in Fig. 15.2.

20. Should patients with chronic stable angina be treated with an ACE inhibitor?

The addition of an ACE inhibitor to standard therapy does not reduce the risk of CV events in low-risk stable CAD patients (i.e., those with normal ejection fraction in whom CV risk factors are well controlled and revascularization has been performed). Conversely, in high-risk patients, ACE inhibitors reduce the incidence of MI, stroke, or CV death by ~20%. Thus, ACE inhibitors may be started and continued indefinitely in all patients with left ventricular ejection fraction (LVEF) ≤40% and in those with hypertension, diabetes, or chronic kidney disease, unless contraindicated.

21. What is the proper statin dose for the patients with chronic stable angina?

Previously, the dose of statin was gradually increased until a target serum LDL cholesterol concentration was achieved. However, recent guidelines recommend treating chronic stable angina patients who are younger than 75 years old with a high-intensity statin (Table 15.3) regardless of serum LDC cholesterol concentration. Individuals greater than 75 years of age or with safety concerns may be treated with a moderate intensity statin.

22. Which patients with chronic stable angina should be referred for stress testing?

The two purposes of stress testing are *diagnosis* of CAD and *prognosis* in patients with presumed or known CAD. Stress testing performed for diagnostic purposes is usually performed with the patient off antianginal therapy, whereas stress testing performed for prognostic purposes may sometimes be performed with the patient on antianginal agents.

An estimation of the pretest probability of CAD—based on an assessment of the patient's chest pain and his or her risk factors for atherosclerosis—is essential in determining if further testing is warranted. In general, diagnostic testing is appropriate for the patient with an intermediate pretest probability of CAD, but it is not recommended for those with a low (≤10% pretest probability) or high (≥90% pretest probability) risk.

For example, an abnormal exercise test in a 35-year-old woman with atypical chest pain and no risk factors for atherosclerosis (pretest probability of clinically significant CAD <5%) is likely to be falsely positive, thereby prompting the use of unnecessary medications or invasive diagnostic testing; a negative test would simply support a low clinical suspicion of CAD. Similarly, testing of high-risk patients is unlikely to provide information that will alter the diagnosis of CAD. A positive exercise test will only confirm the high clinical suspicion of CAD; a negative result would only lower the estimate of likelihood of CAD into the moderate range and would not exclude the diagnosis.

The results of noninvasive diagnostic testing are most likely to influence subsequent decisions when the pretest probability of CAD is in the intermediate range. For example, a positive exercise test in a 55-year-old man with atypical chest pain and no risk factors for atherosclerosis (pretest probability of clinically significant CAD, approximately 50%) substantially increases the likelihood of clinically important coronary heart disease (CHD) (posttest probability, 85%), whereas a negative exercise test dramatically reduces the likelihood (posttest probability, 15%).

The chronic stable angina guidelines advocate obtaining a stress test for prognostic reasons in many cases—if the stress test reveals low-risk findings, then the patient can be managed medically,

Table 15.3. Statin Recommendations for Stable Angina Patients

HIGH-INTENSITY STATIN THERAPY	MODERATE-INTENSITY STATIN THERAPY
Daily dose lowers serum LDL cholesterol on average ~50%	Daily dose lowers serum LDL cholesterol on average ~30% to 50%
Atorvastatin 40-80 mg	Atorvastatin 10-20 mg
Rosuvastatin 20-40 mg	Rosuvastatin 5-10 mg
	Simvastatin 20-40 mg
	Pravastatin 40-80 mg
	Lovastatin 40 mg
	Fluvastatin XL 80 mg
	Pitavastatin 2-4 mg

LDL, Low-density lipoprotein.

whereas if the stress test reveals high-risk findings, the patient is usually referred for cardiac catheterization.

23. Which patients with chronic stable angina should have a cardiac catheterization?

- High-risk findings on stress testing
- Symptoms not adequately controlled with antianginal medications
- Depressed ejection fraction
- Unstable symptoms develop

24. Which patients with chronic stable angina should be referred for revascularization?

In most individuals, survival with optimal medical therapy is similar to that observed following revascularization. In the patient with stable angina and preserved ejection fraction receiving optimal medical therapy, PCI does not reduce the incidence of subsequent MI or cardiac death. Although PCI-treated patients initially may experience a greater improvement in symptom control and quality of life, these salutary effects largely disappear within 24 months. Hence intensive medical therapy and lifestyle intervention are appropriate as initial therapy for most patients with chronic stable angina.

Revascularization should be reserved for those with (1) symptoms that interfere with the patient's lifestyle despite optimal medical therapy or (2) coronary anatomic findings that indicate that revascularization would provide a survival benefit, including

- Left main CAD
- Three-vessel CAD and depressed ejection fraction (<50%)
- Multivessel CAD with stenosis of the proximal left anterior descending (LAD) artery

The optimal method of revascularization—CABG or PCI—is selected based on the coronary angiographic findings, the likelihood of success (or complications) of each procedure, and the subject's preferences. Ideally, both an interventional cardiologist and cardiac surgeon should review the patient's data (including the angiogram) and reach agreement on which procedure(s) should be offered, after which the patient is presented with the advantages and disadvantages of each and allowed to choose between them. Among subjects with left main CAD (or in those with extensive two- or three-vessel CAD), either procedure could be considered, but the weight of published evidence supports the more durable benefit afforded by CABG (mortality reduction and lower incidence of repeat revascularization).

25. Is there an easy way to remember how to manage the patient with chronic stable angina?

Consider the "ABCDEs" of treatment for patients with chronic stable angina:

- **A** = Aspirin and antianginal therapy: ACE inhibitors in patients not considered low risk
- **B** = Beta-blocker and blood pressure control
- **C** = Cigarette smoking and cholesterol
- **D** = Diet and diabetes
- **E** = Education and exercise

Bibliography and Suggested Readings

Antithrombotic Trialists' Collaboration. (2002). Collaborative meta-analysis of randomised trials of antiplatelet therapy for prevention of death, myocardial infarction, and stroke in high risk patients. *British Medical Journal, 324*, 71–86.

Bhatt, D. L., Fox, K. A., Hacke, W., Berger, P. B., Black, H. R., Boden, W. E., et al. (2006). Clopidogrel and aspirin versus aspirin alone for the prevention of atherothrombotic events. *New England Journal of Medicine, 354*, 1706–1717.

Boden, W. E., O'Rourke, R. A., Teo, K. K., Hartigan, P. M., Maron, D. J., Kostuk, W. J., et al. (2007). Optimal medical therapy with or without PCI for stable coronary disease. *New England Journal of Medicine, 356*, 1503–1516.

Braunwald, E., Domanski, M. J., Fowler, S. E., Geller, N. L., Gersh, B. J., Hsia, J., et al. (2004). Angiotensin-converting-enzyme inhibition in stable coronary artery disease. *New England Journal of Medicine, 351*, 2058–2068.

Fihn, S. D., Blankenship, J. C., Alexander, K. P., Bittl, J. A., Byrne, J. G., Fletcher, B. J., et al. (2014). 2014 ACC/AHA/AATS/PCNA/SCAI/STS focused update of the guideline for the diagnosis and management of patients with stable ischemic heart disease: a report of the American College of Cardiology/American Heart Association Task Force on Practice Guidelines, and the American Association for Thoracic Surgery, Preventive Cardiovascular Nurses Association, Society for Cardiovascular Angiography and Interventions, and Society of Thoracic Surgeons. *Journal of the American College of Cardiology, 64*, 1929–1949.

Fox, K. M. (2003). Efficacy of perindopril in reduction of cardiovascular events among patients with stable coronary artery disease: randomised, double-blind, placebo-controlled, multicentre trial (the EUROPA study). *Lancet, 362*, 782–788.

Gerstein, H. C., Miller, M. E., Genuth, S., Ismail-Beigi, F., Buse, J. B., Goff, D. C., Jr., et al. (2011). Long-term effects of intensive glucose lowering on cardiovascular outcomes. *New England Journal of Medicine, 364*, 818–828.

Hillis, L. D., Smith, P. K., Anderson, J. L., Bittl, J. A., Bridges, C. R., Byrne, J. G., et al. (2011). 2011 ACCF/AHA Guideline for coronary artery bypass graft surgery: executive summary. A report of the American College of Cardiology Foundation/ American Heart Association Task Force on Practice Guidelines. *Journal of the American College of Cardiology*, *58*, 2584–2614.

Levine, G. N., Bates, E. R., Bittl, J. A., Brindis, R. G., Fihn, S. D., Fleisher, L. A., et al. (2016). 2016 ACC/AHA guideline focused update on duration of dual antiplatelet therapy in patients with coronary artery disease. *Journal of the American College of Cardiology*, *68*, 1082–1115. http://dx.doi.org/10.1016/j.jacc.2016.03.513.

Levine, G. N., Bates, E. R., Blankenship, J. C., Bailey, S. R., Bittl, J. A., Cercek, B., et al. (2011). 2011 ACCF/AHA/SCAI Guideline for percutaneous intervention: executive summary. A report of the American College of Cardiology Foundation/ American Heart Association Task Force on Practice Guidelines. *Journal of the American College of Cardiology*, *58*, 2550–2583.

Ohman, M. E. (2016). Chronic stable angina. *New England Journal of Medicine*, *374*, 1167–1176.

Serruys, P. W., Morice, M. C., Kappetein, A. P., Colombo, A., Holmes, D. R., Mack, M. J., et al. (2009). Percutaneous coronary intervention versus coronary-artery bypass grafting for severe coronary artery disease. *New England Journal of Medicine*, *360*, 961–972.

Trikalinos, T. A., Alsheikh-Ali, A. A., Tatsioni, A., Nallamothu, B. K., & Kent, D. M. (2009). Percutaneous coronary interventions for non-acute coronary artery disease: a quantitative 20-year synopsis and a network meta-analysis. *Lancet*, *373*, 911–918.

Weintraub, W. S., Spertus, J. A., Kolm, P., Maron, D. J., Zhang, Z., Jurkovitz, C., et al. (2008). Effect of PCI on quality of life in patients with stable coronary disease. *New England Journal of Medicine*, *359*, 677–687.

CHAPTER 16

NON–ST-ELEVATION ACUTE CORONARY SYNDROME

Glenn N. Levine

1. What is non–ST-elevation acute coronary syndrome?

It is now recognized that unstable angina, non–Q-wave myocardial infarction (MI), non–ST-segment elevation MI, and ST-segment elevation myocardial infarction (STEMI) are all part of a continuum of the pathophysiologic process in which a coronary plaque ruptures, thrombus formation occurs, and partial or complete transient or more sustained vessel occlusion may occur (Fig. 16.1). This process is deemed acute coronary syndrome (ACS) when it is clinically recognized and causes symptoms. ACSs can be subdivided for treatment purposes into non–ST-elevation acute coronary syndrome (NSTE-ACS) and ST-segment elevation acute coronary syndrome (STE-ACS).

2. What is the current definition of a myocardial infarction?

According to the "universal definition of MI," the term *MI* should be used when there is evidence of myocardial necrosis in a clinical setting consistent with myocardial ischemia. For patients with ACSs, this includes detection of the rise or fall of cardiac biomarkers (preferably troponin) with at least one value above the 99th percentile of the upper reference limit and evidence of myocardial ischemia with at least one of the following:

- Symptoms of ischemia
- Electrocardiogram (ECG) changes indicative of new ischemia (new ST-T changes or new left bundle branch block)
- Development of pathologic Q waves in the ECG
- Imaging evidence of new loss of viable myocardium or new regional wall motion abnormalities
- Identification of an intracoronary thrombus by angiography or autopsy

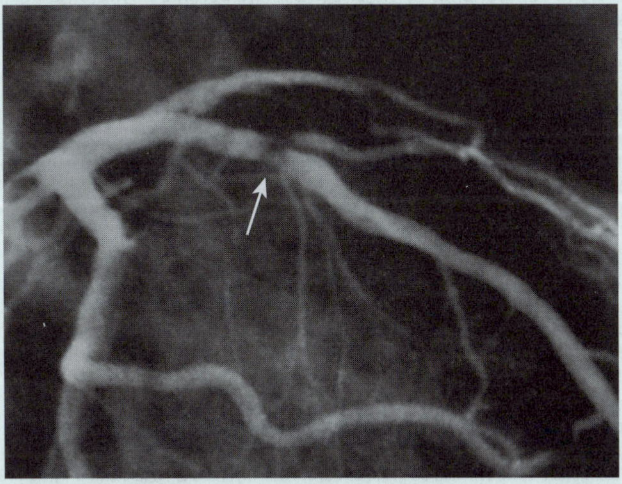

Fig. 16.1. Plaque rupture in the proximal left anterior descending (LAD) has led to thrombus formation *(arrow)* and partial occlusion of the vessel. *(Reproduced with permission from Cannon, C. P., & Braunwald, E. [2008]. Unstable angina and non–ST elevation myocardial infarction. In P. P. Libby, R. O. Bonow, D. L. Mann, D. P. Zipes (Eds.),* Braunwald's heart disease: a textbook of cardiovascular medicine *[8th ed.]. Philadelphia, PA: Saunders.)*

Note that using this definition, patients admitted with anginal chest pains and troponin elevations of as little as 0.04 to 0.08 ng/mL may now be diagnosed as having MI, depending on locally established 99th percentile ranges of troponin values.

3. What other conditions besides epicardial coronary artery disease and acute coronary syndrome can cause elevations in troponin?

Although troponins have extremely high myocardial tissue specificity and sensitivity with new assay, numerous conditions besides epicardial coronary artery disease (CAD) and ACSs *may cause* elevations of troponins. Such conditions include noncoronary cardiac disease (myocarditis, acute CHF exacerbation, cardiac contusion, tachyarrhythmias, takotsubo, stress cardiomyopathy), acute vascular pathology (hypertensive crisis, aortic dissection, pulmonary embolus), infiltrative diseases (amyloidosis, sarcoidosis), and systemic illnesses (anemia, chronic kidney disease (CKD), hypothyroidism, hypoxemia). Conditions that have been associated with elevation of troponin levels are given in Table 16.1.

4. What are the factors that make up the thrombolysis in myocardial infarction risk score?

The seven factors that make up the thrombolysis in myocardial infarction (TIMI) risk score are given below. Each factor counts as 1 point. A total score of 0 to 2 is a low TIMI risk score and is associated with a 4.7% to 8.3% 2-week risk of adverse cardiac events; a total score of 3 to 5 is an intermediate TIMI risk score and is associated with a 13.2% to 26.2% 2-week risk of adverse cardiac events; and a total score of 6 to 7 is a high TIMI risk score and is associated with a 40.9% risk of adverse cardiac events.

- Age greater than 65 years
- Three or more risk factors for CAD
- Prior catheterization demonstrating CAD
- ST-segment deviation
- Two or more anginal events within 24 hours
- Acetylsalicylic acid (ASA) use within 7 days
- Elevated cardiac markers

Importantly, although the TIMI risk score can give one a statistical likelihood of risk and prognosis, individual patient management decisions should still be based on clinical evaluation of the patient, integrating history (recurrent or ongoing angina-like chest discomfort), ECG findings, biomarker elevation, and other factors (such as the TIMI risk score).

5. What are the components of the GRACE acute coronary syndrome risk model (at the time of admission)?

The components of the Global Registry of Acute Coronary Events (GRACE) ACS risk model at the time of admission consist of

- Age
- Heart rate (HR)
- Systolic blood pressure (SBP)
- Creatinine
- Congestive heart failure Killip class
- Cardiac arrest at admission (yes/no)
- ST-segment deviation (yes/no)
- Elevated cardiac enzymes/markers

Scores are calculated based on established criteria. Calculation algorithms are easily downloadable to computers and handheld devices. A low-risk score is considered 108 or less and is associated with a less than 1% risk of in-hospital death. An intermediate score is 109 to 140 and is associated with a 1% to 3% risk of in-hospital death. A high-risk score is greater than 140 and associated with a more than 3% risk of in-hospital death.

6. What other biomarkers and measured blood levels have been shown to correlate with increased risk of adverse cardiovascular outcome?

Multiple biomarkers can be measured in the blood, but it is important to understand what they represent. The most common are creatine kinase-MB (CK-MB) and troponin T and I levels, which are related to myocardial injury and are independent predictors of adverse cardiovascular outcomes. Troponin measurements are more sensitive and specific than CK-MB measurements and have supplanted the use of CK-MB measurements in clinical decision making. In current American College of Cardiology/American Heart Association (ACC/AHA) guidelines, measurements of CK-MB are no longer considered necessary and are not recommended.

Table 16.1. Conditions Other Than Coronary Artery Diseases Associated with Elevation in Cardiac Troponin

SYSTEM	CAUSES OF TROPONIN ELEVATION
Cardiovascular	Acute aortic dissection Arrhythmia Medical ICU patients Hypotension Heart failure Apical ballooning syndrome Cardiac inflammation • Endocarditis, myocarditis, pericarditis Hypertension Infiltrative disease • Amyloidosis, sarcoidosis, hemochromatosis, scleroderma Left ventricular hypertrophy
Myocardial injury	Blunt chest trauma Cardiac surgeries Cardiac procedures • Ablation, cardioversion, percutaneous intervention Chemotherapy Hypersensitivity drug reactions Envenomation
Respiratory	Acute pulmonary embolism
Infectious/immune	Sepsis/SIRS Viral illness Thrombotic thrombocytopenic purpura
Gastrointestinal	Severe GI bleeding
Nervous	Acute stroke • Ischemic stroke • Hemorrhagic stroke Head trauma
Renal	Chronic kidney disease
Endocrine	Diabetes Hypothyroidism
Musculoskeletal	Rhabdomyolysis
Integumentary	Extensive skin burns
Inherited	Neurofibromatosis Duchenne muscular dystrophy Klippel-Feil syndrome
Others	Endurance exercise Environmental exposure • Carbon monoxide, hydrogen sulfide

ARDS, Acute respiratory distress syndrome; *GI*, gastrointestinal; *ICU*, intensive care unit; *PE*, pulmonary embolism; *SIRS*, systemic inflammatory response syndrome.

Reproduced with permission from Januzzi, J. L., Jr. (2010). Causes of non–ACS related troponin elevations. <http://www.cardiosource.org>. Accessed 16.02.13.

Common inflammatory biomarkers like C-reactive protein (CRP), matrix metalloproteinase (MMP-9), myeloperoxidase (MPO), B-type natriuretic peptide (BNP), and ischemia modified albumin (IMA) have been shown to be independent predictors of adverse cardiovascular outcomes. How these findings should be used in clinical practice is subject to continued investigation and debate, and routine use of any of these markers is not mandated in current guidelines.

Table 16.2. Characteristics of the Three Oral Antiplatelet Agents Used in the Treatment of Patients with Non–ST-Elevation Acute Coronary Syndrome

	CLOPIDOGREL	PRASUGREL	TICAGRELOR
Class	$P2Y_{12}$, thienopyridine	$P2Y_{12}$ thienopyridine	$P2Y_{12}$ triazolopyrimidine
Reversibility	Irreversible	Irreversible	Reversible
Activation	Prodrug	Prodrug	Active drug
Onset of action	2-4 h	30 min	30 min
Duration	3-10 days	5-10 days	3-4 days
Withdrawal before CABG	5 days	7 days	5 days

CABG, Coronary artery bypass graft.
Reproduced with permission from Hamm, C. W., Bassand, J. P., Agewall, S., Bax, J., Boersma, E., & Bueno, H. (2011). ESC Guidelines for the management of acute coronary syndromes in patients presenting without persistent ST-segment elevation. European Heart Journal, 32, 2999-3054.

7. What are the three currently used $P2Y_{12}$ receptor inhibitors?

Dual antiplatelet therapy (DAPT) refers to the combination of aspirin and a second oral antiplatelet agent that blocks the $P2Y_{12}$ platelet receptor (a receptor on the platelet member that leads to platelet activation). The three $P2Y_{12}$ receptors used in current practice are clopidogrel, prasugrel, and ticagrelor. Compared to clopidogrel, prasugrel and ticagrelor lead to quicker platelet inhibition, more reliable platelet inhibition, and a greater degree of platelet inhibition. Prasugrel and ticagrelor have been studied in large clinical trials of patients with ACSs treated with medical therapy alone or with medical therapy plus coronary revascularization (primarily coronary stent implantation). Compared to treatment with clopidogrel, treatment with prasugrel or ticagrelor leads to lower rates of ischemic complications and stent thrombosis at the expense of a higher risk of bleeding.

Like clopidogrel, prasugrel irreversibly inhibits the platelet. Although ticagrelor does not irreversibly inhibit the platelet, there nevertheless is effective platelet inhibition for days following discontinuation of ticagrelor.

Prasugrel is approved for use in patients with ACSs who undergo coronary stent implantation. Ticagrelor is approved for use in patients with ACSs treated with either medical therapy alone or with coronary stent implantation.

The characteristics of these three agents are summarized in Table 16.2.

8. What antiplatelet agents are recommended in patients with non–ST-elevation acute coronary syndrome?

Aspirin should be administered as soon as possible and in patients with true aspirin allergies or aspirin contraindications; clopidogrel should be administered as a substitute for aspirin.

The ACC/AHA recommends up-front therapy with either the oral antiplatelet agents clopidogrel or ticagrelor. Administration of intravenous glycoprotein inhibitors (eptifibatide or tirofiban) is now less enthusiastically endorsed and is now a class IIb recommendation ("may be considered") in patients treated with an early invasive strategy and with intermediate or high-risk features.

Based on the results of the Platelet Inhibition and Patient Outcomes (PLATO) study, both American and European guidelines suggest preferential use of ticagrelor over clopidogrel. Antiplatelet recommendations are summarized in (Table 16.3).

9. What are the differences between the intravenous antiplatelet agents?

Eptifibatide and tirofiban are small-molecule GP IIb/IIIa inhibitors that are both used for "up-front" treatment of NSTE-ACS and during percutaneous coronary intervention (PCI). Abciximab is an antibody fragment that is used at the time of PCI. Eptifibatide and tirofiban lead to reversible platelet inhibition, while abciximab leads to irreversible platelet inhibition. All three agents lead to a high degree of platelet inhibition, are associated with a small but real increased risk of major bleeding, and are associated with a small (1% to 4%) incidence of thrombocytopenia. Thrombocytopenia can occur rapidly and be profound, and careful monitoring of platelet counts is warranted when these agents are begun. Due to increased concerns about bleeding complications and their consequences, and the disappointing results of the most recent trial of eptifibatide in patients with NSTE-ACS, the use of eptifibatide and tirofiban as part of up-front therapy has decreased over the past decade.

Table 16.3. American College of Cardiology/American Heart Association Guidelines for Antiplatelet Therapies in Patients With Non–ST-Elevation Acute Coronary Syndrome

RECOMMENDATIONS	DOSING AND SPECIAL CONSIDERATIONS	COR	LOE
Aspirin: Non–enteric-coated aspirin to all patients promptly after presentation	162-325 mg	I	A
Aspirin maintenance dose continued indefinitely	81 mg daily	I	A
$P2Y_{12}$ inhibitors: Clopidogrel loading dose followed by daily maintenance dose in patients unable to take aspirin	300-600 mg loading dose, then 75 mg/daily	I	B
$P2Y_{12}$ inhibitor, in addition to aspirin for up to 12 months for patients treated initially with either an early invasive or initial ischemia-guided strategy: • Clopidogrel • Ticagrelor	300-mg or 600-mg loading dose, then 75 mg/daily 180-mg loading dose, then 90 mg BID	I	B
P2Y Inhibitor therapy (clopidogrel, prasugrel, or ticagrelor) continued for at least 12 month in post-PCI patients treated with coronary stents	N/A	I	B
Ticagrelor in preference to clopidogrel for patients treated with an early invasive or ischemia-guided strategy	N/A	IIa	B
GP IIb/IIa inhibitors: GP IIb/IIa inhibitor in patients treated with an early invasive strategy and DAPT with intermediate/high-risk features (e.g., positive troponin)	Preferred options are eptifibatide or tirofiban	IIb	B
Parenteral anticoagulant and fibrinolytic therapy: SC enoxaparin for duration of hospitalization or until PCI is performed	1 mg/kg SC every 12 h (reduce dose to 1 mg/kg/d SC in patients with CrCl <30 mL/min) Initial 30 mg IV loading dose in selected patients	I	A
Bivalirudin until diagnosis angiography or PCI is performed in patients with early invasive strategy only	Loading dose 0.10 mg/kg loading dose followed by 0.25 mg/kg/daily Only provisional use of GP IIb/IIa inhibitor in patients also treated with DAPT	I	B
SC fondaparinux for the duration of hospitalization or until PCI is performed	2.5 mg SC daily	I	B
Administer additional anticoagulant with anti-IIa activity if PCI is performed while patient is on fondaparinux	N/A	I	B
IV UFH for 48 h or until PCI is performed	Initial loading dose 60 IU/kg (max 4000 IU) with initial	—	—
IV fibrinolytic treatment not recommended in patients with NSTE-ACS	N/A	III: Harm	A

DAPT, Dual antiplatelet therapy; *N/A*, not applicable; *NSTE-ACS*, non–ST-elevation acute coronary syndrome; *PCI*, percutaneous coronary intervention; *UFH*, unfractionated heparin.

Adapted from Amsterdam, E. A., Wenger, N. K., Brindis, R. G., Casey, D. E., Jr., Ganiats, T. G., Holmes, D. R., Jr., et al. (2014). 2014 AHA/ACC guideline for the management of patients with non–ST-elevation acute coronary syndromes: a report of the American College of Cardiology/American Heart Association Task Force on Practice Guidelines. Journal of the American College of Cardiology, 64, *e139-e228*.

Table 16.4. American College of Cardiology/American Heart Association Guidelines for Parenteral Anticoagulant and Fibrinolytic Therapy in Patients with Non–ST-Elevation Acute Coronary Syndrome

PARENTERAL ANTICOAGULANT AND FIBRINOLYTIC THERAPY		COR	LOE
SC enoxaparin for duration of hospitalization or until PCI is performed	• 1 mg/kg SC every 12 h (reduce dose to 1 mg/kg/d SC in patients with CrCl <30 mL/min) • Initial 30-mg IV loading dose in selected patients	I	A
Bivalirudin until diagnostic angiography or PCI is performed in patients with early invasive strategy only	• 0.10-mg/kg loading dose followed by 0.25 mg/kg/h • Only provisional use of GP IIb/IIIa inhibitor in patients also treated with DAPT	I	B
SC fondaparinux for the duration of hospitalization or until PCI is performed	2.5 mg SC daily	I	B
Administer additional anticoagulant with anti-IIa activity if PCI is performed while patient is on fondaparinux	N/A	I	B
IV UFH for 48 h or until PCI is performed	• Initial loading dose 60 IU/kg (max 4000 IU) with initial infusion 12 IU/kg/h (max 1000 IU/h) • Adjusted to therapeutic activated partial thromboplastin time (aPTT) range	I	B
IV fibrinolytic treatment not recommended in patients with NSTE-ACS	N/A	—	—

DAPT, Dual antiplatelet therapy; *N/A*, not applicable; *NSTE-ACS*, non–ST-elevation acute coronary syndrome; *PCI*, percutaneous coronary intervention; *UFH*, unfractionated heparin.

Adapted from Amsterdam, E. A., Wenger, N. K., Brindis, R. G., Casey, D. E., Jr., Ganiats, T. G., Holmes, D. R. Jr., et al. (2014). 2014 AHA/ACC guideline for the management of patients with non–ST-elevation acute coronary syndromes: a report of the American College of Cardiology/American Heart Association Task Force on Practice Guidelines. Journal of the American College of Cardiology, 64, *e139-e228.*

10. What anticoagulant agents are recommended by the American College of Cardiology/American Heart Association and European Society of Cardiology guidelines?

Parenteral anticoagulant therapy is recommended in all patients with NSTE-ACS. The ACC/AHA guidelines give a Class I recommendation to unfractionated heparin (UFH), enoxaparin, fondaparinux, and bivalirudin. The European Society of Cardiology (ESC) guidelines place a strong emphasis on the prevention of bleeding complications and preferentially recommend fondaparinux, although bivalirudin, enoxaparin, and UFH are also considered to be options.

Anticoagulant agent recommendations and doses in the ACC/AHA NSTE-ACS guidelines are summarized in Table 16.4.

11. Which patients with non–ST-elevation acute coronary syndrome should be treated with a strategy of early catheterization and revascularization?

Studies performed in the 1980s comparing a strategy of early catheterization and revascularization with a strategy of initial medical therapy failed to show benefits of early catheterization and revascularization. More recent studies have demonstrated benefits of early catheterization and revascularization in appropriately selected patients with high-risk features.

An *urgent/immediate invasive strategy* is recommended in patients with NSTE-ACS with refractory angina or hemodynamic or electrical instability.

An *early invasive* strategy (within 24 hours of admission) is recommended in initially stabilized patients with NSTE-ACS who have an elevated risk for clinical events. Criteria for elevated risk for clinical events include recurrent angina/ischemia, elevated troponin, new ST depression,

CHF exacerbation, reduced LV function, high-risk findings on noninvasive testing, hemodynamic instability, sustained ventricular tachycardia (VT), PCI within 6 months, prior coronary artery bypass graft (CABG), and high risk score (TIMI ≥6, GRACE >140).

An early invasive strategy is not recommended in patients with extensive comorbidities such as hepatic or renal failure or cancer, in whom the risks of catheterization and revascularization are likely to outweigh the benefits of such a strategy. An early invasive approach is also not recommended in patients with acute chest pain who are felt to have a low likelihood of ACS and do not have elevated troponin levels—particularly women.

12. Should platelet function testing be used routinely to determine platelet inhibitory response?

No. Currently the routine use of platelet function test in NSTE-ACS is not recommended by the ACC/AHA or ESC. However, it may be considered in selected cases if the results of testing may alter management (Class IIb; level of evidence (LOE) B).

13. Should all patients who present with non–ST-elevation acute coronary syndrome be treated with supplemental oxygen?

No. The benefits of supplemental oxygen in normoxic patients have never been demonstrated. Additionally, routine supplemental oxygen may have unknown side effects, including increased vascular resistance and reduced coronary blood flow. Supplemental oxygen is now only recommended for patients with oxygen saturation less than 90%, respiratory distress, or other high-risk features of hypoxemia.

14. Should nonsteroidal anti-inflammatory drugs or COX-2 inhibitors (other than aspirin) be continued in patients admitted for non–ST-elevation acute coronary syndrome?

No. Recent data suggest potential adverse effects of these agents, and it is now recommended to stop such therapy in patients admitted for NSTE-ACS.

15. Can nitrate therapy be administered to patients currently taking erectile dysfunction agents?

No. Concurrent use of nitrates and currently available erectile dysfunction (ED) agents may lead to profound hypotension because of increased levels of the vasodilator nitric oxide. Patients who have taken an ED agent should not be treated with nitrates for the following periods:

- Sildenafil (Viagra): 24 hours
- Tadalafil (Cialis): 48 hours
- Vardenafil (Levitra): Not established at the time of this writing, but common sense would dictate at least 24 hours and perhaps a little longer

16. Can statin therapy be safely started in patients admitted with acute coronary syndromes?

Yes. Several trials, among them Myocardial Ischemia Reduction with Acute Cholesterol Lowering (MIRACL) and Pravastatin or Atorvastatin Evaluation and Infection Therapy—Thrombolysis in Myocardial Infarction (PROVE IT–TIMI 22) demonstrated a very low incidence of liver function test (LFT) elevation and rhabdomyolysis in appropriately selected patients. These patients presented with ACS and were started on high-dose/high-intensity lipid therapy (e.g., atorvastatin 80 mg). Based on these and other studies, it is now recommended that statin therapy, when appropriate, be initiated or continued in all patients with NSTE-ACS without contraindications to its use.

17. What are the recommendations regarding drug discontinuation in patients who are to undergo coronary artery bypass grafts?

The following recommendations have been made regarding the medications commonly used in patients with NSTE-ACS who are to undergo CABG.

When possible, for elective CABG:

- Wait at least 5 days after the last dose of clopidogrel or ticagrelor before CABG.
- Wait at least 7 days after the last dose of prasugrel before CABG.
- Discontinue eptifibatide or tirofiban at least 2 to 4 hours before CABG; discontinue abciximab at least 12 hours before CABG.
- Discontinue enoxaparin 12 to 24 hours before CABG and dose with UFH.
- Discontinue fondaparinux 24 hours before CABG and dose with UFH.
- Discontinue bivalirudin 3 hours before CABG and dose with UFH.

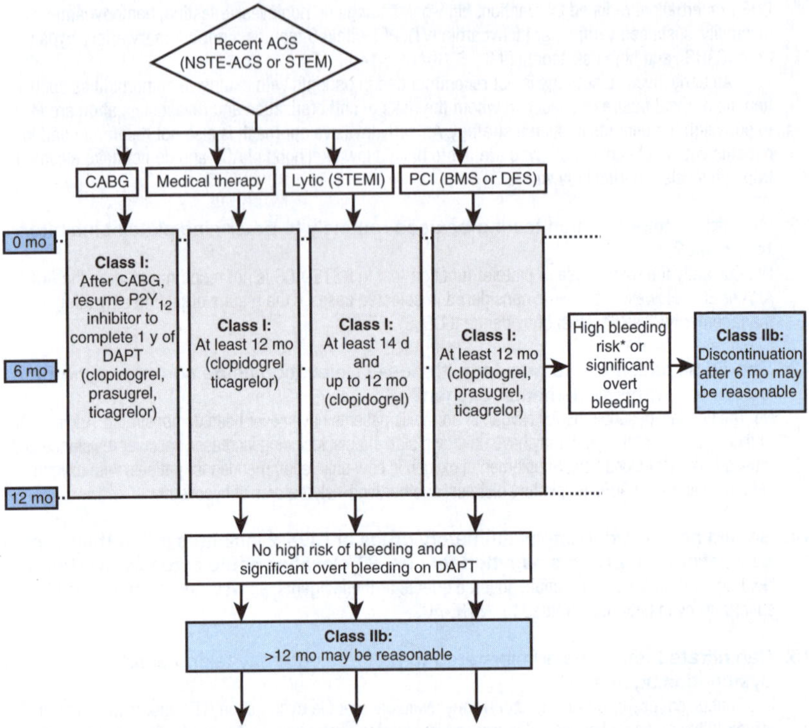

Fig. 16.2. Algorithm for recommended duration of DAPT in patients with acute coronary syndromes, including NSTE-ACS. The algorithm applies to the duration of $P2Y_{12}$ inhibitor therapy; aspirin is almost always continued indefinitely. *BMS,* bare metal stent; *CABG,* Coronary artery bypass graft; *DAPT,* dual antiplatelet therapy; *DES,* drug-eluting stent; *mo,* months; *NSTE-ACS,* non–ST-elevation acute coronary syndrome; *PCI,* percutaneous coronary intervention; *STEMI,* ST-segment elevation myocardial infarction. *(Reproduced from Levine, G. N., Bates, E. R., Bittl, J. A., Brindis, R. G., Fihn, S. D., Fleisher, L. A., et al. (2016). 2016 ACC/AHA guideline focused update on duration of dual antiplatelet therapy in patients with coronary artery disease: a report of the American College of Cardiology/American Heart Association task force on clinical practice guidelines.* Journal of the American College of Cardiology, 68*(10), 1082-1115.)*

For urgent CABG:

- Clopidogrel or ticagrelor should be held a minimum of 24 hours to reduce major bleeding complications.
- It may be reasonable to perform surgery less than 5 days after clopidogrel or ticagrelor has been discontinued and less than 7 days after prasugrel has been discontinued.

18. How long should patients with non–ST-elevation acute coronary syndrome be treated with dual antiplatelet therapy?

DAPT refers to combination oral antiplatelet therapy with aspirin plus a $P2Y_{12}$ inhibitor (clopidogrel, prasugrel, or ticagrelor). Patients with NSTE-ACS should in general be treated with DAPT for at least 12 months, whether they are treated with medical therapy alone, with a drug-eluting stent, or with CABG. In those treated with a drug-eluting stent, a shorter course of 6 months of therapy can be considered in those with high bleeding risk. Treatment with prolonged (>12 months) DAPT may be reasonable in those not with high bleeding risk. The recommended treatment algorithm for duration of DAPT is given in Fig. 16.2.

Bibliography and Suggested Readings

Amsterdam, E. A., Wenger, N. K., Brindis, R. G., Casey, D. E., Jr., Ganiats, T. G., Holmes, D. R., Jr., et al. (2014). 2014 AHA/ACC guideline for the management of patients with non–ST-elevation acute coronary syndromes: a report of the American College of Cardiology/American Heart Association Task Force on Practice Guidelines. *Journal of the American College of Cardiology, 64,* e139–e228.

Cannon, C. P., & Braunwald, E. (2012). Unstable angina and non–ST-elevation myocardial infarction. In R. Bonow, D. Mann, & P. Zipes (Eds.), *Braunwald's heart disease: a textbook of cardiovascular medicine* (9th ed.). Philadelphia, PA: Saunders.

GRACE Risk Calculator. < http://www.outcomesumassmed.org/grace/acs_risk/acs_risk_content.html > Accessed Nov 2016.

Hillis, L. D., Smith, P. K., Anderson, J. L., Bittl, J. A., Bridges, C. R., Byrne, J. G., et al. (2011). 2011 ACCF/AHA guideline for coronary artery bypass graft surgery: a report of the American College of Cardiology Foundation/American Heart Association task force on practice guidelines developed in collaboration with the American Association for Thoracic Surgery, Society of Cardiovascular Anesthesiologists, and Society of Thoracic Surgeons. *Journal of the American College of Cardiology, 58*, e123–e210.

Levine, G. N., Bates, E. R., Bittl, J. A., Brindis, R. G., Fihn, S. D., Fleisher, L. A., et al. (2016). 2016 ACC/AHA guideline focused update on duration of dual antiplatelet therapy in patients with coronary artery disease: a report of the American College of Cardiology/American Heart Association task force on clinical practice guidelines. *Journal of the American College of Cardiology, 68*(10), 1082–1115. http://dx.doi.org/10.1016/j.jacc.2016.03.513.

Roffi, M., Patrono, C., Collet, J. P., Mueller, C., Valgimigli, M., & Andreotti, F. (2015). 2015 ESC Guidelines for the management of acute coronary syndromes in patients presenting without persistent ST-segment elevation. *European Heart Journal, 37*(3), 267-315.

Thygesen, K., Alpert, J. S., Jaffe, A. S., Simoons, M. L., Chaitman, B. R., White, H. D., et al. (2012). Third universal definition of myocardial infarction. *European Heart Journal, 33*(20), 2551–2567. http://dx.doi.org/10.1093/eurheartj/ehs184.

CHAPTER 17

ST-ELEVATION MYOCARDIAL INFARCTION

Glenn N. Levine

1. What are the electrocardiograph criteria for the diagnosis of ST-segment elevation myocardial infarction?

Criteria for the diagnosis of ST-segment elevation myocardial infarction (STEMI) derive from criteria established for the administration of thrombolytic therapy (Fig. 17.1), which evolved in the late 1980s and 1990s. ECG criteria for suspected coronary artery occlusion include the following:

- American College of Cardiology Foundation/American Heart Association (ACCF/AHA) criteria for STEMI consist of ST-segment elevation greater than 0.1 mV (one small box) in at least two contiguous leads (e.g., leads III and aVF, or leads V2 and V3). The European Society of Cardiology (ESC) STEMI guidelines note that ST-segment elevation in acute myocardial infarction (MI), measured at the J point, should be found in two contiguous leads and should typically be greater than 0.25 mV in men below the age of 40 years, greater than 0.2 mV in men over the age of 40 years, or greater than 0.15 mV in women in leads V2–V3 and/or greater than 0.1 mV in other leads.
- New or presumably new left bundle branch block (LBBB)
- In patients with known prior LBBB, the diagnosis of STEMI is difficult. Criteria have been proposed, although in practice are rarely used. Perhaps the most suggestive and useful finding is concordant ST elevation in leads with a positive (upward) QRS complex.

2. In patients who clinically appear to be having an acute myocardial infarction but do not have ST elevation, what else can be done to diagnose an ST-segment elevation myocardial infarction?

Although occlusion of the left anterior descending (LAD) artery and right coronary artery (RCA) typically produces recognizable ST elevation, occlusion of the left circumflex artery or one of its branches often produces modest or no overt ST elevation. The left circumflex artery supplies the lateral and often inferolateral walls of the left ventricle, and thus the standard 12-lead ECG is less sensitive in detecting ST elevation in cases of left circumflex occlusion. United States and ESC guidelines suggest that assessing leads V7–V9 may be reasonable in cases of suspected STEMI without diagnostic ST elevation.

To obtain leads V7–V9, simply move leads V4–V6 to positions on the back directly below the scapula, with lead V7 along the posterior axillary line, V8 midscapular, and V9 paraspinal (Fig. 17.2).

3. Is intracoronary thrombus common in ST-segment elevation myocardial infarction?

Yes. Most STEMIs are a result of plaque rupture, fissure, or disruption, leading to superimposed thrombus formation and vessel occlusion. Angioscopy demonstrates coronary thrombus in more than 90% of patients with STEMI (as opposed to 35% to 75% of patients with non–ST-segment elevation acute coronary syndrome [NSTE-ACS] and 1% of patients with stable angina).

4. What is primary percutaneous coronary intervention?

Primary percutaneous coronary intervention (PCI) refers to the strategy of taking a patient who presents with STEMI directly to the cardiac catheterization laboratory to undergo mechanical revascularization using balloon angioplasty, coronary stents, aspiration thrombectomy, and other measures. Patients are not treated with thrombolytic therapy in the emergency room (or ambulance) but preferentially taken directly to the cardiac catheterization laboratory for primary PCI. Studies have demonstrated that primary PCI is superior to thrombolytic therapy when it can be performed in a timely manner by a skilled interventional cardiologist with a skilled and experienced catheterization laboratory team. An example of primary PCI is shown in Fig. 17.3.

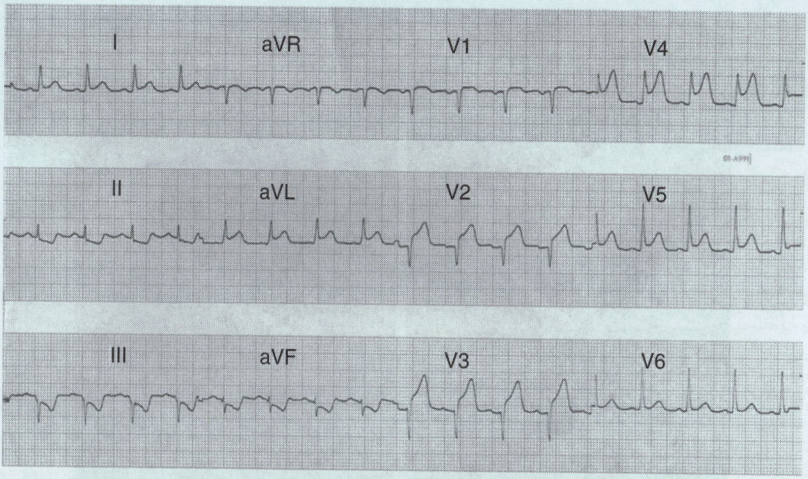

Fig. 17.1. ST elevation in a patient with acute myocardial infarction. There is 3- to 4-mm ST elevation in the anterior leads (V2–V4), with lesser degrees of ST elevation in the lateral leads (I, aVL, V5, V6).

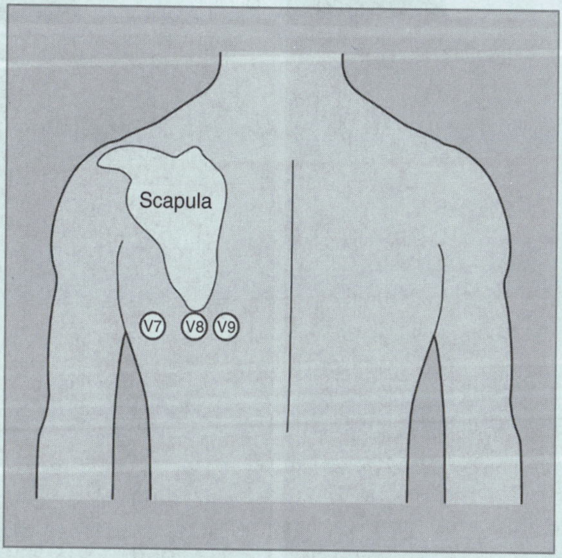

Fig. 17.2. Placement of leads V7–V9 in suspected cases of left circumflex occlusion and lateral or inferolateral MI. *(Image from EMS 12-lead.* <http://www.ems12lead.com/2008/10/17/12-lead-ecg-lead-placement-diagrams/> *Accessed 22.09.16.)*

5. What are considered to be contraindications to thrombolytic therapy?

Several absolute contraindications to thrombolytic therapy and several relative contraindications (or cautions) must be considered in deciding whether to treat a patient with lytic agents. As would be expected, these are based on the risks and consequences of bleeding resulting from thrombolytic therapy. These contraindications and cautions are given in Table 17.1.

6. What is *door-to-balloon time*?

Door-to-balloon time is a phrase that denotes the time between the arrival of a patient with STEMI in the emergency room until the time that a balloon is inflated in the occluded, culprit coronary artery.

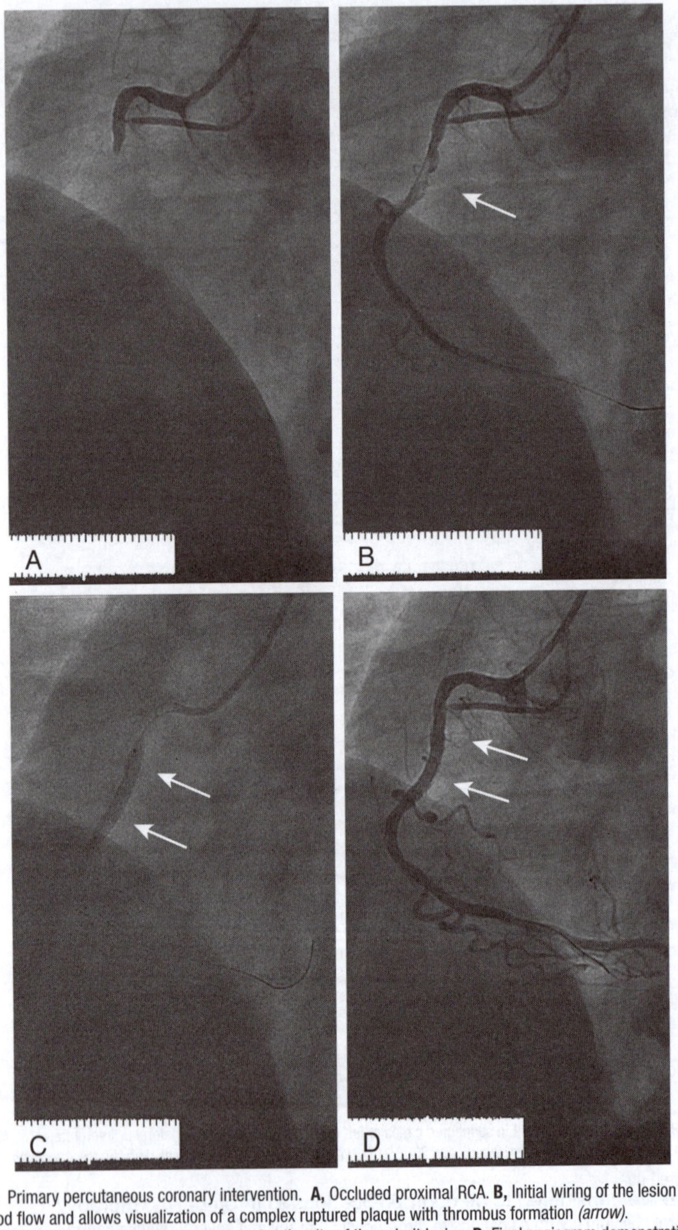

Fig. 17.3. Primary percutaneous coronary intervention. **A,** Occluded proximal RCA. **B,** Initial wiring of the lesion restores some blood flow and allows visualization of a complex ruptured plaque with thrombus formation *(arrow)*. **C,** Balloon dilation and stent deployment *(arrows)* at the site of the culprit lesion. **D,** Final angiogram demonstrating the deployed stent *(arrows)* and restoration of blood flow. *(Reproduced with permission from Levine, G. N. [2014].* Color atlas of cardiovascular disease. *New Delhi, India: Jaypee Brothers Medical Publishers.)*

Table 17.1. Contraindications and Relative Contraindications for Fibrinolytic Therapy

Absolute Contraindications
Any prior ICH
Known structural cerebral vascular lesion (e.g., arteriovenous malformation)
Known malignant intracranial neoplasm (primary or metastatic)
Ischemic stroke within 3 months
EXCEPT acute ischemic stroke within 4.5 h
Suspected aortic dissection
Active bleeding or bleeding diathesis (excluding menses)
Significant closed-head or facial trauma within 3 months
Intracranial or intraspinal surgery within 2 months
Severe uncontrolled hypertension (unresponsive to emergency therapy)
For streptokinase, prior treatment within the previous 6 months
Relative Contraindications*
History of chronic, severe, poorly controlled hypertension
Significant hypertension on presentation (SBP >180 mm Hg or DBP >110 mm Hg)
History of prior ischemic stroke >3 months
Dementia
Known intracranial pathology not covered in absolute contraindications
Traumatic or prolonged (>10 min) CPR
Major surgery (<3 week)
Recent (within 2 to 4 week) internal bleeding
Noncompressible vascular punctures
Pregnancy
Active peptic ulcer
Oral anticoagulant therapy

*Viewed as advisory for clinical decision making and may not be all-inclusive or definitive, *CPR*, cardiopulmonary resuscitation; *DBP*, diastolic blood pressure; *ICH*, intracranial hemorrhage; *SBP*, systolic blood pressure; *STEMI*, ST-segment elevation myocardial infarction.

Adapted from O'Gara, P. T., Kushner, F. G., Ascheim, D. D., Casey, D. E., Chung, M. K., De Lemos, J. A., et al. (2013). 2013 ACCF/AHA guideline for the management of ST-elevation myocardial infarction: a report of the American College of Cardiology Foundation/American Heart Association Task Force on Practice Guidelines. Journal of the American College of Cardiology, 61, *e78–e140. http://dx.doi.org/10.1016/j.jacc.2012.11.019.*

More recently, the concept of *medical contact-to-balloon time* has been emphasized, given that STEMI may first be diagnosed in the transporting ambulance in some cases. Because balloon angioplasty is no longer always the first intervention performed on an occluded artery, the term has further evolved to *medical contact-to-device time.* The generally accepted medical contact-to-device time goal is 90 minutes or less in cases in which the patient presents or is taken directly to a hospital that performs PCI. In cases in which the patient must be transferred from a hospital that does not perform PCI to a hospital that does perform PCI, the goal is a medical contact-to-device time of no more than 120 minutes.

7. What is door-to-needle time?

Door-to-needle time is a phrase that denotes the time between the arrival of a patient with STEMI in the emergency room until the beginning of thrombolytic therapy administration. The generally accepted goal for door-to-needle time is 30 minutes or less.

8. In patients treated with thrombolytic therapy, how long should antithrombin therapy be continued?

Patients who are treated with unfractionated heparin (UFH) should be treated for 48 hours. Studies of low-molecular-weight heparins [Enoxaparin and Thrombolysis Reperfusion for Acute Myocardial Infarction Treatment (EXTRACT), Clinical Trial of Metabolic Modulation in Acute Myocardial Infarction Treatment Evaluation (CREATE)] and of direct thrombin inhibitors [Sixth Organization to Assess Strategies in Acute Ischemic Syndromes (OASIS-6)] have suggested that patients treated with these agents should be treated throughout their hospitalizations, up to 8 days maximum.

Table 17.2. Recommendations from the 2011 American College of Cardiology Foundation/American Heart Association/Society for Cardiovascular Angiography and Interventions Guidelines on Percutaneous Coronary Intervention Regarding Coronary Angiography in Patients with ST-Segment Elevation Myocardial Infarction

INDICATIONS	COR	LOE
Immediate Coronary Angiography		
Candidate for primary PCI	I	A
Severe heart failure or cardiogenic shock (if suitable revascularization candidate)	I	B
Moderate to large area of myocardium at risk and evidence of failed fibrinolysis	IIa	B
Coronary Angiography 3 to 24 H After Fibrinolysis		
Hemodynamically stable patients with evidence of successful fibrinolysis	IIa	A
Coronary Angiography Before Hospital Discharge		
Stable patients	IIb	C
Coronary Angiography at Any Time		
Patients in whom the risks of revascularization are likely to outweigh the benefits or the patient or designee does not want invasive care	III: No benefit	C

ACCF, American College of Cardiology Foundation; *AHA*, American Heart Association; *COR*, class of recommendation; *LOE*, level of evidence; *PCI*, percutaneous coronary intervention; *SCAI*, Society for Cardiovascular Angiography and Interventions; *STEMI*, ST-segment elevation myocardial infarction.

Adapted from Levine, G. N., *Bates*, E. R., *Blankenship*, J. C., *Bailey*, S. R., *Bittl*, J. A., *Cercek*, B., *et al.* (2011). 2011 ACCF/AHA/SCAI *guideline for percutaneous coronary intervention: a report of the American College of Cardiology Foundation/American Heart Association Task Force on Practice Guidelines and the Society for Cardiovascular Angiography and Interventions*. Journal of the American College of Cardiology, 58(24), *e44–e122*.

9. **Which patients with ST-segment elevation myocardial infarction should undergo cardiac catheterization?**
Patients with STEMI who should undergo immediate coronary angiography include those who are candidates for primary PCI, those with severe heart failure or cardiogenic shock (if they are suitable candidates for revascularization), and many of those with moderate to large areas of myocardium at risk and evidence of failed fibrinolysis. Cardiac catheterization is reasonable in hemodynamically stable patients with evidence of successful fibrinolysis. Recommendations from the 2011 ACCF/AHA/Society for Cardiovascular Angiography and Interventions (SCAI) Guidelines on PCI regarding coronary angiography in patients with STEMI are given in Table 17.2.

10. **Which patients with ST-segment elevation myocardial infarction should undergo primary percutaneous coronary intervention?**
Primary PCI should be performed in patients with STEMI who present within 12 hours of symptom onset, in patients with severe heart failure or cardiogenic shock, and in those with contraindications to fibrinolytic therapy. PCI can also be considered in those who have clinical evidence for fibrinolytic failure or infarct artery reocclusion after fibrinolytic failure, as well as those treated with likely successful fibrinolytic therapy. Recommendations from the 2011 ACCF/AHA/SCAI Guidelines on PCI regarding PCI in patients with STEMI are given in Table 17.3.

11. **What is rescue percutaneous coronary intervention?**
Rescue PCI is the performance of PCI after a patient has *failed* thrombolytic therapy. Studies of rescue PCI versus medical management generally have shown a modest benefit with rescue PCI in appropriately selected patients. The problem with rescue PCI is that clinical and electrocardiographic criteria for predicting which patients have actually failed thrombolytic therapy (have not had successful lysis of coronary thrombosis and restoration of coronary perfusion) are imprecise. Thus, some

Table 17.3. Recommendations from the 2011 American College of Cardiology Foundation/American Heart Association/Society for Cardiovascular Angiography and Interventions Guidelines on Percutaneous Coronary Intervention Regarding Percutaneous Coronary Intervention in Patients With ST-Segment Elevation Myocardial Infarction

INDICATIONS	COR	LOE
Primary PCI	I	A
STEMI symptoms within 12 h	I	B
Severe heart failure or cardiogenic shock	I	B
Contraindications to fibrinolytic therapy with ischemic symptoms less than 12 h	I	B
Asymptomatic patient presenting between 12 and 24 h after symptom onset and higher risk	IIB	C
Noninfarct artery PCI at the time of primary PCI in patients without hemodynamic compromise	III: Harm	B
Delayed or elective PCI in patients with STEMI (i.e., nonprimary PCI)		
Clinical evidence for fibrinolytic failure or infarct artery reocclusion	IIA	B
Patent infarct artery 3 to 24 h after fibrinolytic therapy	IIA	B
Ischemia on noninvasive testing	IIA	B
Hemodynamically significant stenosis in a patient infarct artery greater than 24 h after STEMI	IIB	B
Totally occluded infarct artery greater than 24 h after STEMI in a hemodynamically stable asymptomatic patient without evidence of severe ischemia	III: No benefit	B

ACCF, American College of Cardiology Foundation; *AHA*, American Heart Association; *COR*, class of recommendation; *LOE*, level of evidence; *PCI*, percutaneous coronary intervention; *SCAI*, Society for Cardiovascular Angiography and Interventions; *STEMI*, ST-segment elevation myocardial infarction.

Adapted from Levine, G. N., Bates, E. R., Blankenship, J. C., Bailey, S. R., Bittl, J. A., Cercek, B., et al. (2011). 2011 ACCF/AHA/SCAI *guideline for percutaneous coronary intervention: a report of the American College of Cardiology Foundation/American Heart Association Task Force on Practice Guidelines and the Society for Cardiovascular Angiography and Interventions.* Journal of the American College of Cardiology, 58(24), e44–e122.

patients with continued occluded arteries may not be referred for rescue PCI, and some patients with successful reperfusion will be referred for unnecessary cardiac catheterization. As with the term *facilitated PCI*, some have advocated elimination of the term *rescue PCI*.

12. In patients with ST-segment elevation myocardial infarction who present to rural hospitals without percutaneous coronary intervention capability, what is the recommended treatment strategy?

Primary PCI is the generally preferred treatment strategy. In patients who can be transferred to a facility with primary PCI capabilities, and the anticipated first medical contact-to-device activation is less than 120 minutes, this strategy is preferred. If the anticipated delay is greater than 120 minutes, then fibrinolytic therapy is advised, with urgent or elective transfer and angiography within 24 hours.

A newly adopted term is *door-in door-out* (DIDO). This refers to the acceptable time frame in which a patient with STEMI who presents to an emergency room in a hospital without PCI capabilities is diagnosed and transferred to a hospital with PCI capability. The goal for DIDO is less than 30 minutes. Unfortunately, this target time frame is often not met.

13. Which patients should not be treated with beta-blocker therapy?

Beta-blockers have been a mainstay of STEMI therapy for decades. However, in the Clopidogrel and Metoprolol in Myocardial Infarction Trial/Second Chinese Cardiac (COMMIT/CCS-2) study, the potential benefits of beta-blocker therapy were offset by an increased incidence of cardiogenic shock and shock-related death with beta-blocker therapy. Therefore, in patients with signs of heart failure, evidence of a low-output state, or increased risk for cardiogenic shock, beta-blocker therapy should not be initiated. Risk factors for cardiogenic shock include age older than 70 years, systolic blood pressure less than 120 mm Hg, sinus tachycardia greater than 110 beats/min, and heart rate less than 60 beats/min. Other contraindications to initiating beta-blocker therapy include PR interval more than 0.24 seconds, second- or third-degree heart block, active asthma, or severe reactive airway disease.

14. Which patients should be treated with nitrate therapy?

Sublingual (SL) nitroglycerin (0.4 mg) every 5 minutes, up to three doses, should be administered for ongoing ischemic discomfort. Intravenous nitroglycerin is indicated for relief of ongoing ischemic discomfort that responds to nitrate therapy, for control of hypertension, and for management of pulmonary edema. Nitrates should not be administered to patients who have received a phosphodiesterase inhibitor for erectile dysfunction within 24 to 48 hours (depending on the specific agent). Nitrates should also not be administered to those with suspected right ventricular (RV) infarction, systolic blood pressure less than 90 mm Hg (or 30 mm Hg or more below baseline), severe bradycardia (less than 50 beats/min), or tachycardia (more than 100 beats/min).

15. Should patients with ST-segment elevation myocardial infarction be continued on nonselective nonsteroidal anti-inflammatory drugs (other than aspirin) or COX-2 inhibitors?

No. Use of these agents has been associated with increased risk of reinfarction, hypertension, heart failure, myocardial rupture, and death. Therefore, such agents should be discontinued at the time of admission.

16. What are the main mechanical complications of myocardial infarction?

- **Free wall rupture:** Acute free wall rupture is almost always fatal. In some cases of *subacute free wall rupture,* only a small quantity of blood initially reaches the pericardial cavity and begins to cause signs of pericardial tamponade. Emergent echocardiography and immediate surgery are indicated.
- **Ventricular septal rupture:** A ventricular septal defect (VSD) caused by myocardial infarction and septal rupture occurred in 1% to 2% of all patients with infarction in older series, although the incidence in the fibrinolytic age is 0.2% to 0.3%. Patients may complain of a chest pain somewhat different from their MI pain and will usually develop cardiogenic shock. A new systolic murmur may be audible, often along the left sternal border. Mortality without surgery is 54% in the first week and up to 92% within the first year.
- **Papillary muscle rupture:** Papillary muscle rupture leads to acute and severe mitral regurgitation. It occurs in approximately 1% of STEMIs. Because of the abrupt elevation in left atrial pressure, there may not be an audible murmur of mitral regurgitation. Pulmonary edema and cardiogenic shock usually develop. Treatment is urgent/emergent mitral valve replacement (or in rare cases, mitral valve repair).

17. What is the triad of findings suggestive of right ventricular infarction?

The triad of findings suggestive of RV infarction is hypotension, distended neck veins, and clear lungs. Clinical RV infarction occurs in approximately 30% of inferior MIs. Because the infarcted right ventricle is dependent on preload, administration of nitroglycerin (or morphine), which leads to venous pooling and decreased blood return to the right ventricle, may lead to profound hypotension. When such hypotension occurs, patients should be placed in reverse Trendelenburg position (legs above chest and head) and treated with extremely aggressive administration of several liters of fluid through large-bore intravenous needles. Those who do not respond to such therapy may require treatment with such agents as dopamine.

In patients with inferior MI, a *right-sided* ECG should be obtained (Fig. 17.4). The precordial leads are placed over the right side of the chest in a mirror-image pattern to normal. The finding of 1 mm or greater ST elevation in leads RV4–RV6 is highly suggestive of RV infarction (Fig. 17.5), although the absence of this often-transient finding should not be used to dismiss a diagnosis of RV infarction made on clinical grounds.

18. In addition to plaque rupture and thrombotic occlusion, what are other causes of ST-segment elevation myocardial infarction?

Although plaque rupture with subsequent thrombus formation is the most common cause of STEMI, other causes to consider include the following:

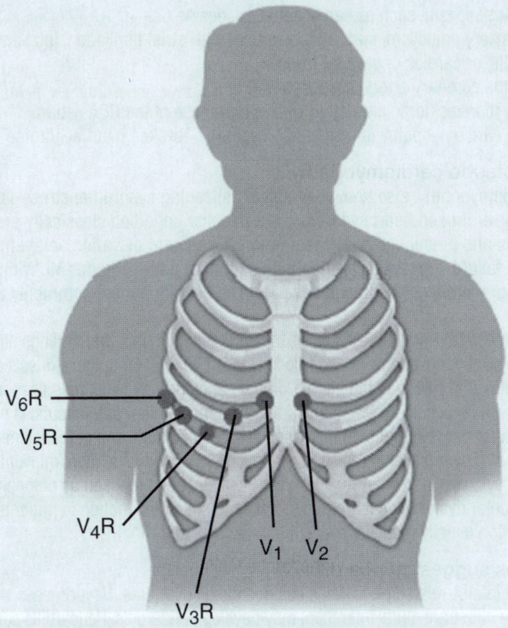

Fig. 17.4. Placement of right-sided ECG leads for the diagnosis of right ventricular infarction. *(Image from Mega, J. L., & Morrow, D. A. ST-elevation myocardial infarction: management. In* Braunwald's heart disease: a textbook of cardiovascular medicine *[10th ed., pp. 1095–1115].)*

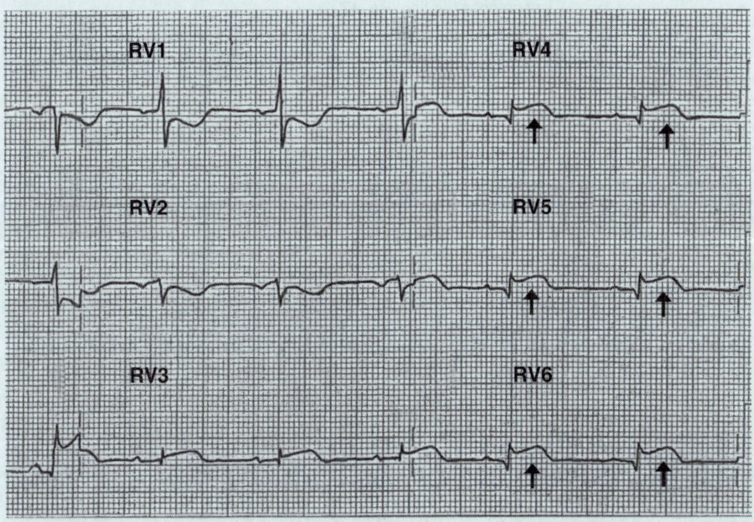

Fig. 17.5. Right-sided leads demonstrating ST-segment elevation *(arrows)* in leads RV4–RV6, highly suggestive of right ventricular infarction.

- Coronary vasospasm, such as can occur with cocaine use
- Coronary artery embolism, such as in a patient with atrial fibrillation, left ventricular thrombus, endocarditis, or cardiac or valvular tumor
- Spontaneous coronary artery dissection
- Ascending thoracic aortic dissection with compromise of the RCA ostium
- Takotsubo cardiomyopathy (stress cardiomyopathy, "broken heart syndrome").

19. What is Takotsubo cardiomyopathy?

Takotsubo cardiomyopathy, also known as apical ballooning syndrome, stress-induced cardiomyopathy, or broken heart syndrome, is a peculiar condition classically precipitated by emotional stress and presenting with chest pain, ST-segment elevation, left ventricular dysfunction, and often heart failure. Presentation often mimics that of acute anterior MI, with a frequent finding of anterior and precordial ST-segment elevation. The condition most commonly affects older women.

The word *takotsubo* in Japanese means a kind of octopus trap, and findings on echocardiography of left ventriculography most commonly demonstrate left ventricular apical akinesis or dyskinesis, with normal contractility of the base of the heart. Coronary angiography usual reveals minimal or no coronary artery disease, with no occluded or "culprit" artery. The mechanism of takotsubo is not well understood, but in some manner may be related to increased sympathetic state and catecholamine release related to the acute stress. Epicardial artery vasospasm, microvascular dysfunction, midventricular outflow obstruction, myocytolysis, and other mechanisms have all been proposed as pathophysiologic causes.

Left ventricular dysfunction is treated similarly to such dysfunction in patients with acute MI. Ventricular function usually recovers over the course of 1 to 2 months.

20. What findings suggest pericarditis?

The incidence of infarct-related pericarditis has decreased over time. Nevertheless, some patients, particularly those with transmural infarction, may develop pericarditis. Pericarditis can develop as early as 1 day and as late as 8 weeks post MI, with later development suggestive of Dressler syndrome (see next question). Factors that suggest pericarditis (and not re-infarction) include the following:

- Pain that is pleuritic
- Pain that is positional (often worse lying down and better sitting up and leaning forward)
- Pain that radiates to the trapezius ridge
- Pain associated with an audible friction rub
- Diffuse (not focal) ST-segment elevation (Fig. 17.6)

Treatment usually includes high-dose aspirin and colchicine. The use of nonsteroidal anti-inflammatory drugs (NSAIDs) is not recommended given concerns that this can adversely impact myocardial healing after MI.

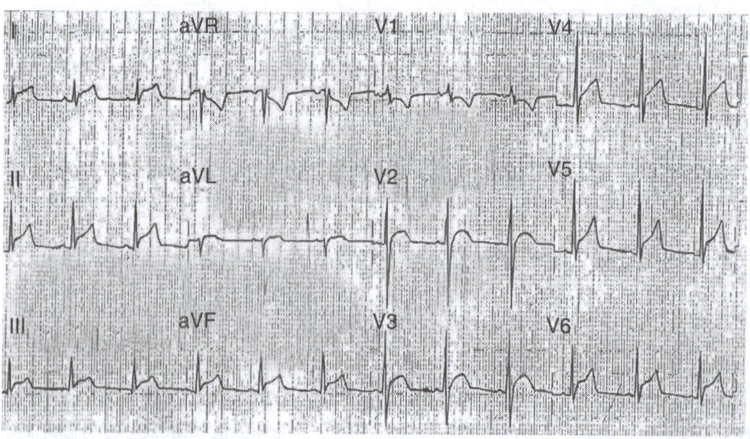

Fig. 17.6. Diffuse ST-segment elevations in a post–myocardial infarction patient who developed pericarditis.

21. What is Dressler syndrome?

Dressler syndrome, also known as post-MI syndrome, includes the development of pericarditis in the week or weeks after MI. When initially described, the incidence was 3% to 4% post infarction, although this has notably decreased in the reperfusion era. The syndrome can additionally include fever, malaise, leukocytosis, and elevated erythrocyte sedimentation rate (ESR). The cause of Dressler syndrome may be immune mediated. First-line therapy is high-dose aspirin. As discussed previously, the use of NSAIDs and steroids should be avoided.

22. Should a prophylactic implantable cardioverter-defibrillator be implanted in ST-segment elevation myocardial infarction patients with depressed ejection fraction before discharge?

The answer is generally no. Patients with an initially reduced left ventricular ejection fraction (LVEF) who are possible candidates for implantable cardioverter-defibrillator (ICD) therapy should undergo reevaluation of LVEF 40 or more days after discharge. This is because an initially low ejection fraction, which may in part be a result of myocardial stunning, may improve over time with successful reperfusion therapy and after appropriate medical therapy (e.g., beta-blockers, angiotensin converting enzyme [ACE] inhibitors).

23. What long-term therapies are indicated in patients with ST-segment elevation myocardial infarction?

Long-term medical therapies are used to reduce cardiac morbidity and mortality.

- Beta-blockers are indicated in all patients without contraindications. In those with depressed ejection fraction (<40%), metoprolol succinate, carvedilol, or bisoprolol are used, because these agents have specifically been shown to be of benefit in such patients.
- ACE inhibitors should be prescribed to all patients with anterior MI, heart failure, or ejection fraction less than 40%, unless contraindicated. ACE inhibitor therapy is considered reasonable in all other patients with STEMI. In those who do not tolerate ACE because of cough, an angiotensin II receptor blocker (ARB) is used.
- An aldosterone antagonist should be prescribed to those on ACE inhibitor and beta-blocker therapy who have LVEF less than 40% and symptomatic heart failure or diabetes, unless contraindicated (e.g., significant chronic kidney disease (CKD), elevated potassium level).
- High-intensity statin therapy is indicated in all patients without contraindication.
- Aspirin should be prescribed to all patients. Dosage of 81 mg is generally preferred in current practice. $P2Y_{12}$ inhibitor therapy is appropriate for most patients. The duration of $P2Y_{12}$ inhibitor therapy is addressed in the following question.

24. What other therapies and interventions should be considered?

Smoking cessation quickly and dramatically reduces the risk of future cardiac events. It is clear that health-care professionals too often provide only "lip service" to this goal. An excellent discussion of the benefits of smoking cessation and actionable plans of treatment are provided in Chapter 44.

Cardiac rehabilitation can increase functional capacity, decrease angina, reduce disability, improve quality of life, modify coronary risk factors, and reduce morbidity and mortality. Referral to a formal cardiac rehabilitation program should be considered in all patients with STEMI.

25. How long should patients with ST-segment elevation myocardial infarction be treated with dual antiplatelet therapy?

As of 2016, new guidelines on duration of dual antiplatelet therapy (DAPT) recommend that patients with STEMI generally be treated with at least 12 months of DAPT regardless of management strategy (PCI, fibrinolytic therapy, coronary artery bypass grafting [CABG], or medical therapy alone) unless they are at high risk of bleeding. In patients who are not at high risk of bleeding or have overt bleeding during the 12 months of therapy, continuation of DAPT may be reasonable. These new recommendations are summarized in Fig. 17.7.

26. What intermediate and long-term complications can result from ST-segment elevation myocardial infarction?

- Dressler syndrome, which includes pericarditis, can occur 1 to 8 weeks post MI.
- Heart failure with reduced ejection fraction (HFrEF) resulting from pump dysfunction and negative remodeling. Heart failure may also result from mechanical complication such as papillary muscle dysfunction or rupture with resultant mitral regurgitation.

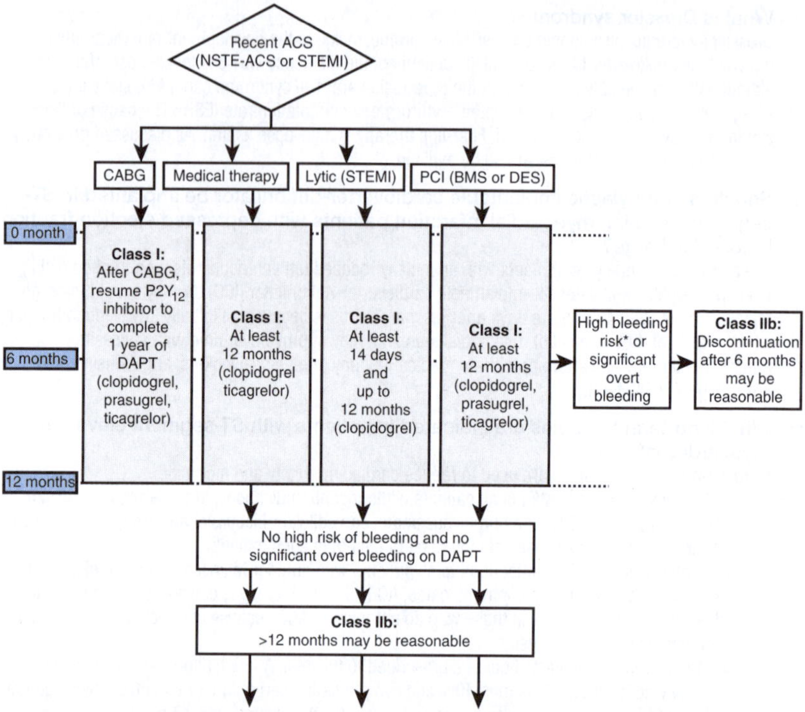

Fig. 17.7. Treatment algorithm for duration of $P2Y_{12}$ inhibitor therapy in a patient with recent ACS (NSTE-ACS or STEMI). *ACS*, Acute coronary syndrome; *CABG*, coronary artery bypass graft; *DAPT*, dual antiplatelet therapy; *NSTE-ACS*, ST-segment elevation acute coronary syndrome; *STEMI*, ST-segment elevation myocardial infarction; *PCI*, percutaneous coronary intervention; *BMS*, bare metal stent; *DES*, drug-eluting stent. *(Reproduced from Levine, G. N., Bates, E. R., Bittl, J. A., Brindis, R. G., Fihn, S. D., Fleisher, L. A., et al. [2016]. 2016 ACC/AHA guideline focused update on duration of dual antiplatelet therapy in patients with coronary artery disease: a report of the American College of Cardiology/American Heart Association Task Force on Clinical Practice Guidelines.* Journal of the American College of Cardiology, 68*(10), 1082–1115.* http://dx.doi.org/10.1016/j.jacc.2016.03.513.*)*

- Ventricular aneurysm
- LV thrombus. LV thrombus occurs most commonly in the first 3 to 6 months post MI in patients with anteroapical akinesis. Prophylactic oral anticoagulation may be considered in such patients, although issues regarding anticoagulation are complicated in the era of DAPT, given the notably increased rate of bleeding in those treated with both DAPT and oral anticoagulant therapy ("triple therapy").
- Ventricular tachycardia, as an area of myocardial fibrosis and ventricular aneurysm, can serve as foci for a reentrant circuit to develop.

Bibliography and Suggested Readings

Levine, G. N., Bates, E. R., Bittl, J. A., Brindis, R. G., Fihn, S. D., Fleisher, L. A., et al. (2016). 2016 ACC/AHA guideline focused update on duration of dual antiplatelet therapy in patients with coronary artery disease: a report of the American College of Cardiology/American Heart Association Task Force on Clinical Practice Guidelines. *Journal of the American College of Cardiology*, *68*(10), 1082–1115. http://dx.doi.org/10.1016/j.jacc.2016.03.513.

Levine, G. N., O'Gara, P. T., Bates, E. R., Blankenship, J. C., Kushner, F. G., Ascheim, D. D., et al. (2016). 2015 ACC/AHA/SCAI focused update on primary percutaneous coronary intervention for patients with ST-elevation myocardial infarction: an update of the 2011 ACCF/AHA/SCAI guideline for percutaneous coronary intervention and the 2013 ACCF/AHA guideline for the management of ST-elevation myocardial infarction: a report of the American College of Cardiology/American Heart Association Task Force on Clinical Practice Guidelines and the Society for Cardiovascular Angiography and Interventions. *Journal of the American College of Cardiology*, *67*, 1235–1250.

Mega, J. L., & Morrow, D. A. (2015). ST-elevation myocardial infarction: management. In D. L. Mann, R. O. Bonow, D. P. Zipes, P. Libby (Eds.), *Braunwald's heart disease: a textbook of cardiovascular medicine*, (10th ed.), (pp. 1095–1115). Philadelphia, PA: Elsevier Saunders.

O'Gara, P. T., Kushner, F. G., Ascheim, D. D., Casey, D. E., Chung, M. K., De Lemos, J. A., et al. (2013). 2013 ACCF/AHA guideline for the management of ST-elevation myocardial infarction: a report of the American College of Cardiology Foundation/American Heart Association Task Force on Practice Guidelines. *Journal of the American College of Cardiology*, *61*, e78–e140. http://dx.doi.org/10.1016/j.jacc.2012.11.019.

Steg, P. G., James, S. K., Atar, D., Badano, L. P., Blömstrom-Lundqvist, C., Borger, M. A., et al. (2012). ESC Guidelines for the management of acute myocardial infarction in patients presenting with ST-segment elevation. *European Heart Journal*, *33*(20), 2569–2619. http://dx.doi.org/10.1093/eurheartj/ehs215.

CHAPTER 18

CARDIOGENIC SHOCK

Hani Jneid

1. **Define cardiogenic shock.**
   Cardiogenic shock is a state of end-organ hypoperfusion due to cardiac failure and the inability of the cardiovascular system to provide adequate blood flow to the extremities and vital organs. In general patients with cardiogenic shock manifest persistent hypotension (systolic blood pressure less than 80 to 90 mm Hg or a mean arterial pressure 30 mm Hg below baseline), with a severe reduction in cardiac index (less than 1.8 L/min per m^2) in the presence of adequate or elevated filling pressure (left ventricular [LV] end-diastolic pressure above 18 mm Hg or right ventricular (RV) end-diastolic pressure above 10 to 15 mm Hg).

2. **What are the various types of shock?**
   Blood flow is determined by three entities: blood volume, vascular resistance, and pump function. There are three main types of shock: (1) hypovolemic, (2) vasogenic or distributive, and (3) cardiogenic. Examples of causes of *hypovolemic shock* include gastrointestinal bleeding, severe hemorrhage, and severe diabetic ketoacidosis (as a result of volume depletion). Examples of *vasogenic shock* include septic shock, anaphylactic shock, neurogenic shock, and shock from pharmacologic causes. There are many causes of *cardiogenic shock*, although acute myocardial infarction (MI) is the most common. Cardiogenic shock can be separated into *true cardiac causes*, such as MI, and *extracardiac causes* stemming from obstruction to inflow (tension pneumothorax, cardiac tamponade) or outflow (pulmonary embolus).

3. **Describe the clinical signs observed in cardiogenic shock and other types of shock.**
   The medical history and clinical examination help in making the diagnosis of cardiogenic shock. Feeling the extremities and examining the jugular veins provide vital clues: warm skin is suggestive of a vasogenic cause; cool, clammy skin reflects enhanced reflex sympathoadrenal discharge leading to cutaneous vasoconstriction, suggesting hypovolemia or cardiogenic shock. Distended jugular veins, rales, and an S3 gallop suggest a cardiogenic cause rather than hypovolemia.

   It is important to note that the clinical examination and chest radiograph may not be reliable predictors of the pulmonary capillary wedge pressure (PCWP). Neither clinically reflects an elevated PCWP in up to 30% of patients with cardiogenic shock. In addition, both cardiac tamponade and massive pulmonary embolism can present as cardiogenic shock without associated pulmonary congestion. Right-sided heart catheterization with intracardiac pressure and cardiac output measurements as well as cardiac imaging (e.g., two-dimensional [2D] echocardiography) are important to confirm the diagnosis of cardiogenic shock.

4. **Do all patients with cardiogenic shock have an increased heart rate?**
   No. Patients with cardiogenic shock related to third-degree heart block or drug overdose (e.g., with beta-blockers and calcium-channel antagonists) can present with bradycardia and require temporary transvenous pacemaker implantation.

5. **What are the determinants of central venous pressure?**
   The normal central venous pressure (CVP) is 5 to 12 cm H_2O. Intravascular volume, intrathoracic pressure, RV function, and venous tone all affect the CVP. To reduce variability caused by intrathoracic pressure, CVP should be measured at the end of expiration.

6. **How can one differentiate cardiogenic from septic shock?**
   In classic septic shock, the systemic vascular resistance (SVR) and PCWP are reduced, and cardiac output is increased. These are usually opposite to the findings in cardiogenic shock. However, a significant decrease in cardiac output may occur in advanced and late stages of sepsis (*cold* septic shock, which carries a very high mortality rate). Many patients with cardiogenic shock may have normal SVR (i.e., relatively low) even while on vasopressor therapy. Patients with cardiogenic shock

may also become *dry* (normal or low PCWP) with overzealous diuresis. Conversely, patients with septic shock may become *wet* (normal or high PCWP) with overzealous volume replacement. It is therefore unwise to depend solely on the aforementioned hemodynamic criteria to differentiate cardiogenic shock from septic shock. The findings in cardiogenic shock are summarized in Table 18.1.

7. What is the most common cause of cardiogenic shock?

Acute MI (Fig. 18.1) remains the leading cause of cardiogenic shock in the United States. In fact, despite its decline in incidence due to the progressive use of timely primary percutaneous intervention (PCI), cardiogenic shock still occurs in 5% to 8% of hospitalized patients with ST-segment elevation myocardial infarction (STEMI). Unlike what is commonly believed, cardiogenic shock may also occur in up to 2% to 3% of patients with non–ST-segment-elevation myocardial infarction (NSTEMI). Overall, 40,000 to 50,000 cases of cardiogenic shock occur annually in the United States.

8. Describe the pathophysiology of cardiogenic shock among patients with acute myocardial infarction.

LV pump failure is the primary insult in most forms of cardiogenic shock. The degree of myocardial dysfunction that initiates cardiogenic shock is often but not always severe. Hypoperfusion causes

Table 18.1. Diagnosis of Cardiogenic Shock

Clinical Signs
• Hypotension
• Oliguria
• Clouded sensorium
• Cool, mottled extremities
Hemodynamic Criteria
• Systolic blood pressure <90 mm Hg for >30 min or mean arterial pressure >30 mm Hg below baseline
• Cardiac index <2.2 L/min per m^2
• Pulmonary artery occlusion pressure >15-18 mm Hg

Adapted from Hollenberg, S. M., & Parrillo, J. E. Cardiogenic shock. In Critical care medicine: principles of diagnosis and management in the adult *[Vol. 22, pp. 325–337.e4]. Philadelphia, PA: Elsevier.*

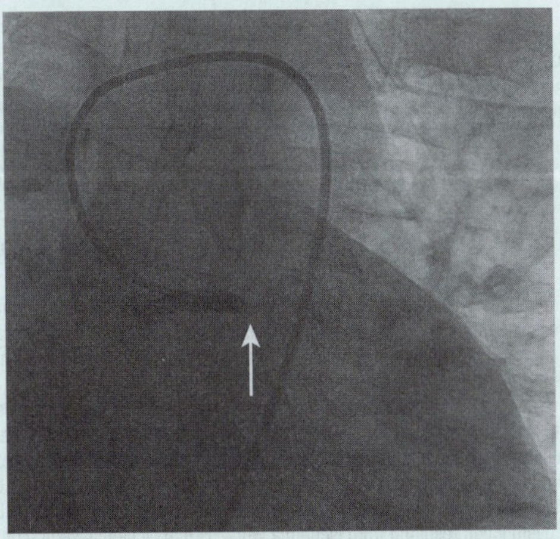

Fig. 18.1. Acute myocardial infarction due to occlusion of the distal left main coronary artery *(arrow)* in a patient with cardiogenic shock. *(Image from Levine, G. N. [2014].* Color atlas of cardiovascular disease. *New Delhi, India: Jaypee Brothers Medical Publishers.)*

the release of catecholamines, which increase contractility and peripheral blood flow; however, this comes at the expense of increased myocardial oxygen demand and its proarrhythmic and cardiotoxic effects. The decrease in cardiac output also triggers the release of vasopressin and angiotensin II, which lead to improvement in coronary and peripheral perfusion at the cost of increased afterload. Neurohormonal activation also promotes salt and water retention, which may improve perfusion but exacerbates pulmonary edema.

The reflex mechanism of increased SVR is in some cases not fully effective, and many patients have normal SVR even while on vasopressor therapy. Systemic inflammation, including the expression of inducible nitric oxide synthase and generation of excess nitric oxide, is believed to contribute to the pathogenesis and inappropriate vasodilation in some cases of cardiogenic shock.

The downward spiral in cardiogenic shock is illustrated in Fig. 18.2.

9. **Describe other mechanisms that cause or contribute to cardiogenic shock after myocardial infarction.**

It is critical to exclude mechanical complications after MI, which may cause or exacerbate cardiogenic shock in some patients. These mechanical complications include ventricular septal rupture, ventricular free wall rupture, and papillary muscle rupture. 2D echocardiography is the preferred diagnostic modality and should be promptly performed when mechanical complications are suspected. Among STEMI patients with suspected mechanical complications in whom a 2D echocardiogram is not available, diagnostic pulmonary artery catheterization should be

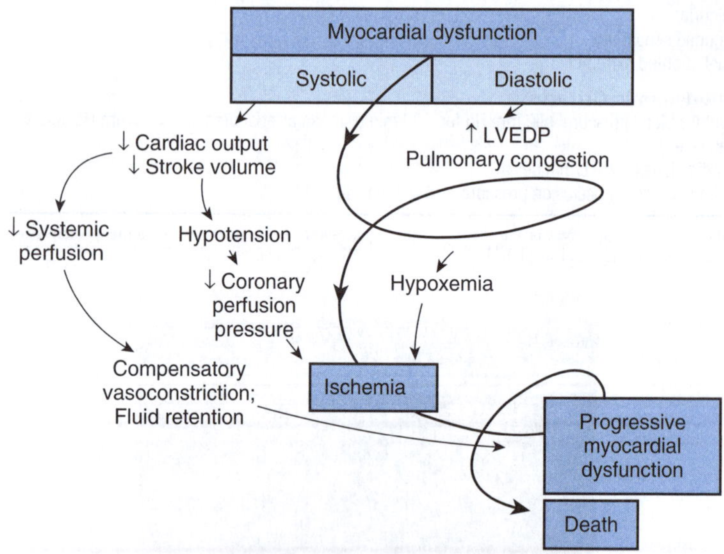

Fig. 18.2. The downward spiral in cardiogenic shock. Cardiac dysfunction is usually initiated by myocardial infarction or ischemia. When a critical mass of left ventricular myocardium fails to pump, stroke volume and cardiac output decrease. Myocardial perfusion is compromised by hypotension and tachycardia, exacerbating ischemia. The increased ventricular diastolic pressures that result from pump failure further reduce coronary perfusion pressure, and the additional wall stress elevates myocardial oxygen requirements, also worsening ischemia. Decreased cardiac output also compromises systemic perfusion, which can lead to lactic acidosis and further compromise of systolic performance. When myocardial function is depressed, several compensatory mechanisms are activated, including sympathetic stimulation to increase heart rate and contractility and renal fluid retention to increase preload. These compensatory mechanisms may become dysfunctional and can actually worsen the situation when cardiogenic shock develops by increasing myocardial oxygen demand and afterload. Thus myocardial dysfunction resulting from ischemia worsens that ischemia, setting up a vicious cycle that must be interrupted to prevent the patient's demise. *LVEDP*, Left ventricular end-diastolic pressure. *(Image and legend from Hollenberg, S. M., & Parrillo, J. E. Cardiogenic shock. In* Critical care medicine: principles of diagnosis and management in the adult *[Vol. 22, pp. 325–337.e4]. Philadelphia, PA: Elsevier.)*

performed. The detection of mechanical complications before coronary angiography may help in dictating the revascularization strategy (surgical revascularization with mechanical repair of the complication rather than primary PCI of the infarct vessel without mechanical repair of the complication).

Additional contributing factors to shock after MI include hemorrhage, infection, and bowel ischemia (the latter may be related to embolization after large anterior MI or persistent hypotension or may be a complication of prolonged intra-aortic balloon pump placement).

10. What is the significance of a loud holosystolic murmur in a patient with shock after acute myocardial infarction?

New loud holosystolic murmurs with MI indicate either acute mitral regurgitation (usually from ischemic papillary muscle dysfunction or papillary muscle/chordal rupture) or an acute ventricular septal defect (VSD) (Fig. 18.3). These two causes may be difficult to distinguish by auscultation alone. Acute VSD usually occurs with an anteroseptal MI and has an associated palpable thrill. Papillary rupture often does not have a thrill and is usually seen in inferior MI. These two entities often cause shock on the basis of reduced forward blood flow. They can be differentiated by echocardiography or pulmonary artery catheterization. Both require the use of percutaneous circulatory assist devices (PCADs) and surgical repair. Note that in some patients, particularly those who develop acute mitral regurgitation, the murmur may be soft or inaudible (as the result of a small pressure gradient between the left ventricle and left atrium [or right ventricle]).

11. Can right ventricular dysfunction result in cardiogenic shock?

RV dysfunction may cause or contribute to cardiogenic shock. Predominant RV shock represents 5% of all cases of cardiogenic shock complicating MI. RV failure may limit LV filling via a decrease in RV output, ventricular interdependence, or both. Treatment of patients with RV dysfunction and shock has traditionally focused on ensuring adequate right-sided filling pressures to maintain cardiac output and adequate LV preload. However, it is important not to overfill the RV and thus compromise LV filling (via ventricular interdependence).

Shock caused by isolated RV dysfunction carries nearly as high a mortality as LV shock and benefits equally from revascularization.

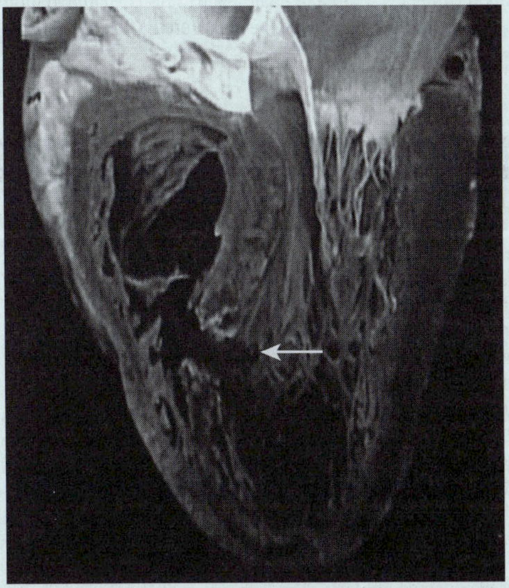

Fig. 18.3. Pathologic example of a ventricular septal defect *(arrows)* following myocardial infarction. *(Image courtesy of William D. Edwards, Mayo Clinic.)*

12. **List the other major causes of cardiogenic shock**
Cardiovascular causes of cardiogenic shock are given in Table 18.2.

13. **What are the mortality and morbidity rates of cardiogenic shock?**
In the modern era, the mortality rate of cardiogenic shock ranges between 30% and 50% depending on its severity (with severe refractory cardiogenic shock having an in-hospital mortality in excess of 50%). In the Should We Emergently Revascularize Occluded Coronaries for Cardiogenic Shock (SHOCK) trial, 3- and 6-year survival rates among patients in the early revascularization group were 41% and 33%, respectively, with persistence of treatment benefits for up to 6 years. Importantly, 83% of 1-year survivors in the SHOCK trial were in New York Heart Association (NYHA) classes I or II, and many of them were enjoying an acceptable quality of life at 6-year follow-up. Therefore cardiogenic shock should be regarded as a very serious but treatable (and possibly preventable) condition that, when treated aggressively and in a timely manner, carries a reasonable chance for full recovery.

14. **What is the mainstay therapy for patients with cardiogenic shock complicating myocardial infarction?**
Acute reperfusion and prompt revascularization for cardiogenic shock improve survival substantially and are considered the mainstays of therapy for cardiogenic shock after acute MI. The SHOCK study was a landmark trial conducted in the 1990s; it enrolled patients with acute MI complicated by cardiogenic shock and randomized them to emergency revascularization or initial medical stabilization. Six-month mortality was lower in the early revascularization group than in the medical therapy group (50% vs. 63%). At 1 year, survival was 47% for patients in the early revascularization group compared with 34% in the initial medical stabilization group. The benefits of early revascularization persisted at long-term follow-up, and the strategy of early revascularization was associated with a 67% relative improvement in 6-year survival compared with initial medical stabilization. Subsequent studies have also demonstrated the benefits of early revascularization in elderly patients.

15. **Which is the best revascularization strategy in patients with cardiogenic shock complicating myocardial infarction?**
Among patients assigned to revascularization in the SHOCK trial, PCI accounted for 64% of initial revascularization attempts and coronary artery bypass grafting (CABG) for 36%. Although those treated with CABG had more diabetes and worse coronary disease, survival rates were similar with both revascularization strategies. Therefore emergency CABG is an important treatment strategy in patients with cardiogenic shock and should be considered a complementary revascularization

Table 18.2. Cardiovascular Causes of Cardiogenic Shock

- Acute myocardial infarction with severe left ventricular dysfunction
- Acute myocardial infarction with mechanical complication (ruptured papillary muscle, ventricular septal defect, free wall rupture)
- Aortic dissection (± acute aortic regurgitation)
- Endocarditis leading to mitral and/or aortic regurgitation
    - Cardiac tamponade
    - Massive pulmonary embolism
    - Chronic congestive cardiomyopathy
    - Takotsubo cardiomyopathy
    - Acute myopericarditis
    - Brady- or tachyarrhythmias
- Critical mitral or aortic stenosis
- Hypertrophic cardiomyopathy
    - Toxins or drugs (negative inotropes, negative chronotropes, vasodilators)
    - Traumatic cardiogenic shock (cardiac penetration with subsequent tamponade, myocardial contusion, or tension pneumothorax)
- Left atrial myxoma

option to PCI in patients with extensive coronary artery disease. Both modalities can be more safely implemented when supported by PCADs.

The American College of Cardiology/American Heart Association (ACC/AHA) guidelines recommend CABG in patients with cardiogenic shock who have multivessel coronary artery disease. However, staged multivessel PCI may be performed if surgery is not an option. Multivessel PCI at the time of primary PCI may be considered if the patient remains in shock after PCI of the infarct-related artery and if there is another vessel (or vessels) with a critical flow-limiting lesion that supplies a large myocardium at risk.

16. Does the timing of revascularization matter in the treatment of cardiogenic shock?

It is essential that revascularization and reperfusion be conducted promptly in patients with STEMI and cardiogenic shock. As with any STEMI, the desired time from first medical contact (FMC) to device activation (FMC-device) is less than 90 minutes. Although fibrinolytic therapy is less effective, it is indicated when timely PCI is unlikely to be implemented and MI and cardiogenic shock occur within a period of 2 to 3 hours. Contrary to common belief, prompt CABG is feasible and safe, especially when supported by PCADs. In the SHOCK trial, patients underwent CABG at a median time of 2.7 hours after randomization. It is also important to emphasize that approximately three-fourths of patients with cardiogenic shock after MI develop shock after hospital admission. Therefore prompt revascularization and early reperfusion after acute MI may serve as a strategy to prevent the occurrence of cardiogenic shock.

17. Describe the common medical therapies for cardiogenic shock.

Antiplatelet and antithrombotic therapies with aspirin and heparin should be administered to all patients with MI. Beta-blockers, calcium-channel inhibitors, and vasodilators (including nitroglycerin) should be avoided. Optimal oxygenation and a low threshold to institute mechanical ventilation should be considered. Antiarrhythmic therapies (intravenous amiodarone) should be instituted when indicated (but not prophylactically).

Pharmacologic support with inotropic and vasopressor agents may be needed for short-term hemodynamic improvement. Although inotropic agents have a central role in the treatment of cardiogenic shock because the initiating event involves contractile failure, these agents increase myocardial adenosine triphosphate (ATP) consumption; hence their short-term hemodynamic benefits occur at the cost of increased oxygen demand. Higher doses of vasopressors have also been associated with poorer survival. Therefore these agents should be used in the lowest possible doses and for the shortest possible time. Norepinephrine is recommended for more severe hypotension because of its high potency and is preferable to dopamine. An inotropic agent, such as dobutamine or milrinone, is often added to vasopressors to improve cardiac output.

18. What are percutaneous circulatory assist devices?

The PCADs have emerged as an important modality to support patients with cardiogenic shock before, during, and after revascularization (Fig. 18.4). Temporary support with PCADs interrupts the vicious cycles of ischemia, hypotension, and myocardial dysfunction and allows the recovery of stunned and hibernating myocardium and reversal of neurohormonal derangements.

In the IABP-SHOCK II (IntraAortic Balloon Pump in Cardiogenic Shock II) trial, the conventional intra-aortic balloon pump device failed to demonstrate a survival benefit in patients with acute MI complicated by cardiogenic shock. Its use has thus been largely abandoned in this patient population.

On the other hand, one of the PCADs, the Impella device (Abiomed Inc., Danvers, Massachusetts), has recently received FDA approval for use in patients with cardiogenic shock. It is an intravascular microaxial blood pump that can be introduced via the femoral artery and placed across the aortic valve into the left ventricle to unload the left ventricle and provide short-term mechanical support for the failing heart. It reduces end-diastolic wall stress, improves diastolic compliance, increases aortic and intracoronary pressure and coronary flow velocity reserve, and stimulates a decrease in coronary microvascular resistance.

Another PCAD, the TandemHeart (CardiacAssist, Inc., Pittsburgh, Pennsylvania), is inserted via the femoral vein and right atrium into the left atrium via a transseptal puncture. The outflow cannula is inserted in either femoral artery and positioned at the level of the aortic bifurcation, providing left heart bypass into the lower abdominal aorta or iliac arteries at a flow rate of 4 L/min.

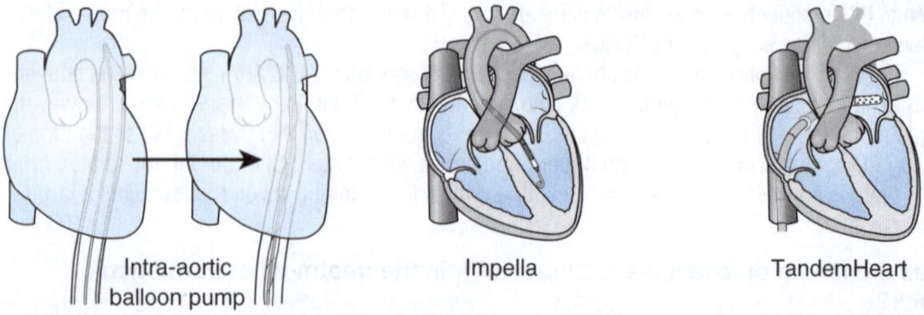

Intra-aortic balloon pump	Impella	TandemHeart
Advantages	**Advantages**	**Advantages**
• Ubiquitous–available in most cardiac catheterization laboratories throughout the world • Ease of percutaneous implantation • Available in 7 Fr, 7.5 Fr, and 8 Fr catheter sizes, minimizing threat of vascular complications • Contemporary systems use fiber-optic technology, negating risks associated with a fluid-filled pressure line • Newer systems calibrate automatically in vivo, accelerating the time to effective diastolic augmentation • Range of balloon sizes available to accommodate patients of all heights • Larger volume balloons displace more blood, providing enhanced diastolic augmentation and systolic unloading	• Can augment cardiac output by 2.5 L/min (Impella 2.5) to 4 L/min (Impella CP™/cVAD) • Can be used to support the circulation for up to 7 days • Does not require a stable cardiac rhythm or native cardiac output/blood pressure signal for optimal functions—the device does, however, require adequate filling of the left ventricle for optimal function	• Can augment native cardiac output by up to 4–5 L/min • Can be used to support the circulation for up to 14 days • Does not require a stable cardiac rhythm or native cardiac output/blood pressure signal for optimal function
Potential disadvantages	**Potential disadvantages**	**Potential disadvantages**
• Can only supplement cardiac output by up to 0.3–0.5 L/min and requires a degree of native cardiac output to function • Relies on synchronization with the cardiac cycle so circulatory support may not be reliable with dysrhythmia • Risk of balloon displacement, rupture, leak, or entrapment • Twisting/kinking of and clot formation in the pressure line or catheter • Small but tangible risk of aortic dissection or rupture • Systemic embolization (e.g., cholesterol, helium) • Stroke • Infection • *Lower limb ischemia + • *Hemolysis + • *Bleeding at insertion site +	• Not universally available • Requires 12–14 Fr catheters for implantation, thus increasing the risk of vascular complications • Non-pulsatile flow • Risk of displacement of inflow from the left ventricle to the aorta • Insufficient flow to the periphery in larger patients (>100 kg body mass) • Systemic embolization • Stroke • Infection • *Lower limb ischemia ++ • *Hemolysis ++ • *Bleeding at insertion site ++	• Not universally available • Requires specific expertise with transseptal punctures for implantation of a 2Fr cannula • Relatively long implantation time • Implantation cannot be performed during cardiopulmonary resuscitation • Relatively complex post-implantation management • Risk of left atrial cannula tip displacement into the right atrium causing profound desaturation • 17 Fr femoral arterial cannula increases risk of vascular complications • Systemic embolization • Stroke • Infection • *Lower limb ischemia +++ • *Hemolysis ++ • *Bleeding at insertion site ++

*Denotes relative grading among all three devices.

Fig. 18.4. Percutaneous circulatory assist devices. *(Image from Myat, A., Patel, N., Tehrani, S., Banning, A. P., Redwood, S. R., & Bhatt, D. L. [2015]. Percutaneous circulatory assist devices for high-risk coronary intervention.* JACC: Cardiovascular Interventions, 8*[2], 229–244.)*

BIBLIOGRAPHY AND SUGGESTED READINGS

Hochman, J. S., Sleeper, L. A., Webb, J. G., Dzavik, V., Buller, C. E., Aylward, P., et al. (2006). Early revascularization and long-term survival in cardiogenic shock complicating acute myocardial infarction. *Journal of the American Medical Association, 295*(21), 2511–2515.

Hochman, J. S., Sleeper, L. A., Webb, J. G., Sanborn, T. A., White, H. D., Talley, J. D., et al. (1999). Early revascularization in acute myocardial infarction complicated by cardiogenic shock. SHOCK Investigators. Should we emergently revascularize occluded coronaries for cardiogenic shock. *New England Journal of Medicine, 341*(9), 625–634.

Hollenberg, S. M., & Parrillo, J. E. Cardiogenic shock. In *Critical care medicine: principles of diagnosis and management in the adult* (Vol. 22, pp. 325–337.e4). Philadelphia, PA: Elsevier.

Kastrati, A., Colleran, R., & Ndrepepa, G. (2016). Cardiogenic shock: how long does the storm last? *Journal of the American College of Cardiology, 67*(7), 748–750.

Levine, G. N., Bates, E. R., Blankenship, J. C., Bailey, S. R., Bittl, J. A., Cercek, B., et al. (2011). 2011 ACCF/AHA/SCAI Guideline for percutaneous coronary intervention: a report of the American College of Cardiology Foundation/American Heart Association Task Force on Practice Guidelines and the Society for Cardiovascular Angiography and Interventions. *Circulation, 124*(23), e574–e651.

Myat, A., Patel, N., Tehrani, S., Banning, A. P., Redwood, S. R., & Bhatt, D. L. (2015). Percutaneous circulatory assist devices for high-risk coronary intervention. *JACC: Cardiovascular Interventions, 8*(2), 229–244.

O'Gara, P. T., Kushner, F. G., Ascheim, D. D., Casey, D. E., Jr., Chung, M. K., de Lemos, J. A., et al. (2013). 2013 ACCF/AHA guideline for the management of ST-elevation myocardial infarction: a report of the American College of Cardiology Foundation/American Heart Association Task Force on Practice Guidelines. *Journal of the American College of Cardiology, 61*, e78–e140. http://dx.doi.org/10.1016/j.jacc.2012.11.019.

Rihal, C. S., Naidu, S. S., Givertz, M. M., Szeto, W. Y., Burke, J. A., Kapur, N. K., et al. (2015). 2015 SCAI/ACC/HFSA/STS clinical expert consensus statement on the use of percutaneous mechanical circulatory support devices in cardiovascular care: endorsed by the American Heart Association, the Cardiological Society of India, and Sociedad Latino Americana de Cardiologia Intervencion; Affirmation of Value by the Canadian Association of Interventional Cardiology-Association Canadienne de Cardiologie d'intervention. *Journal of the American College of Cardiology, 65*, e7–e26.

Rogers, P. A., Daye, J., Huang, H., Blaustein, A., Virani, S., Alam, M., et al. (2014). Revascularization improves mortality in elderly patients with acute myocardial infarction complicated by cardiogenic shock. *International Journal of Cardiology, 172*(1), 239–241.

Steg, P. G., James, S. K., Atar, D., Badano, L. P., Blömstrom-Lundqvist, C., Borger, M. A., et al. (2012). ESC Guidelines for the management of acute myocardial infarction in patients presenting with ST-segment elevation. *European Heart Journal, 33*(20), 2569–2619. http://dx.doi.org/10.1093/eurheartj/ehs215.

Wayangankar, S. A., Bangalore, S., McCoy, L. A., Jneid, H., Latif, F., Karrowni, W., et al. (2016). Temporal trends and outcomes of patients undergoing percutaneous coronary interventions for cardiogenic shock in the setting of acute myocardial infarction: a report from the CathPCI Registry. *JACC: Cardiovascular Interventions, 9*(4), 341–351.

CHAPTER 19

PERCUTANEOUS CORONARY INTERVENTION

Ali E. Denktas, Cindy Grines

1. What does the term *percutaneous coronary intervention* mean?

The first successful balloon angioplasty procedure in humans was performed by Andreas Gruentzig in 1977. Initial coronary interventions involving only balloon angioplasty were referred to as percutaneous transluminal coronary angioplasty (PTCA). Since then, there have been huge advances in the field of interventional cardiology. The development of coronary stents was a major boost to interventional cardiology, addressing many of the complications and limitations associated with balloon angioplasty. Over the past decade the use of drug-eluting stents (DESs) has supplanted the use of older stents, referred to as bare-metal stents (BMSs). Almost all percutaneous coronary interventions (PCI) performed currently involve stent placement. Thus, although the term *percutaneous coronary intervention* refers to any therapeutic coronary intervention, it has become essentially synonymous with coronary stent implantation.

PCI has become one of the most commonly performed medical procedures in the United States, with more than 600,000 procedures performed annually. PCI is performed for coronary revascularization in patients with stable coronary disease as well as, in the appropriate clinical settings, in those with acute coronary syndromes.

The PCI procedure is shown schematically in Fig. 19.1 and angiographically in Fig. 19.2.

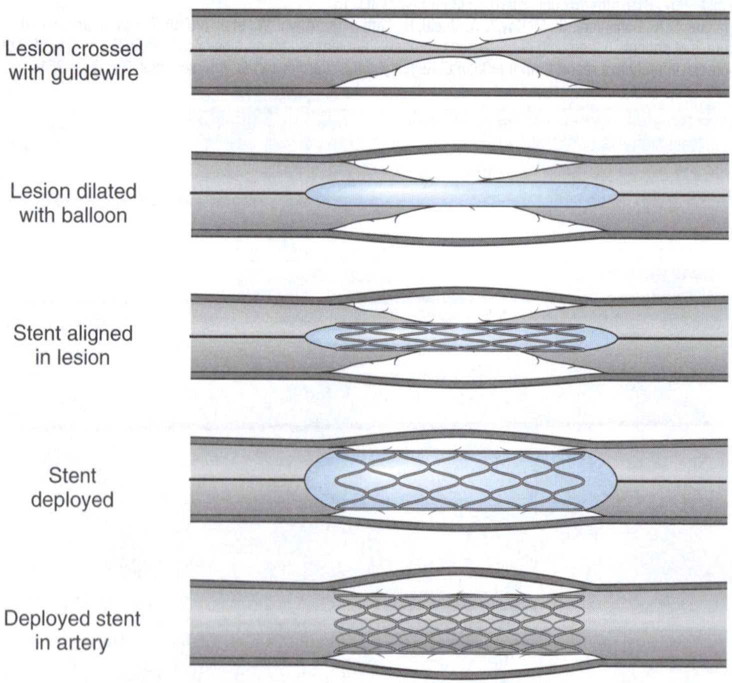

Fig. 19.1. Schematic illustration of a typical percutaneous coronary intervention.

2. Which patients with chronic stable angina benefit from percutaneous coronary intervention?

The goals of treatment in patients with coronary artery disease are to:

1. Relieve symptoms
2. Prevent adverse outcomes such as cardiovascular death, myocardial infarction (MI), left ventricular dysfunctions, and arrhythmias

Multiple clinical trials of PCI plus medical therapy or medical therapy alone involving patients with chronic stable angina over the past two decades have consistently shown improvement in angina, exercise duration, and quality of life with PCI. However, they have not demonstrated any difference in death and MI between treatment with PCI plus medical therapy compared with medical therapy alone. In contrast, the use of PCI in patients with acute coronary syndromes has been shown to decrease recurrent ischemia, nonfatal MI, and death.

In general patients with chronic stable angina in whom PCI should be considered are those with unacceptable angina, one or more significant coronary artery stenoses, a high likelihood of technical success, and a low risk of complications (Guideline Directed Medical Therapy: GDMT). These patients are generally not responsive to two or more classes of antianginals. The goal of PCI in patients with stable coronary artery disease (CAD) is to alleviate the symptoms and not to decrease mortality.

In patients with three-vessel CAD, particularly if they have complex and/or extensive CAD (reflected in a high Synergy between PCI with TAXUS drug-eluting stent and Cardiac Surgery (SYNTAX) score—not an abbreviation but an angiographic grading tool to determine the complexity of CAD), bypass surgery is generally preferred over multivessel PCI. Unprotected left main PCI can be considered in the case of a stenosis that has a high likelihood of procedural success and long-term durability and where the patient is at high risk for surgery (reflected by a high Society of Throacic Surgeons (STS) score). In patients with low SYNTAX scores, the outcomes of bypass surgery and PCI are comparable in terms of mortality. The difference between the two modalities for revascularization lies in the higher risk of stroke in surgery patients and the higher number of repeat procedures in PCI patients.

3. Which patients with non–ST-segment elevation acute coronary syndrome should undergo a strategy of early cardiac catheterization and revascularization?

Two major strategies, conservative (medical therapy without an initial strategy of catheterization and revascularization) and early invasive, are employed in treating patients with non–ST-segment elevation acute coronary syndrome (NSTE-ACS). The early invasive approach involves performing diagnostic angiography with the intent to perform PCI along with the usual anti-ischemic, antiplatelet, and anticoagulant medications. Evidence from clinical trials suggests that an early invasive approach with NSTE-ACS leads to a reduction in adverse cardiovascular outcomes such as death and nonfatal MI, especially in high-risk patients. Several risk assessment tools are available; these assign a score based on the patient's clinical characteristics (e.g., Thrombolysis in Myocardial Infraction [TIMI] and Global Registry of Acute

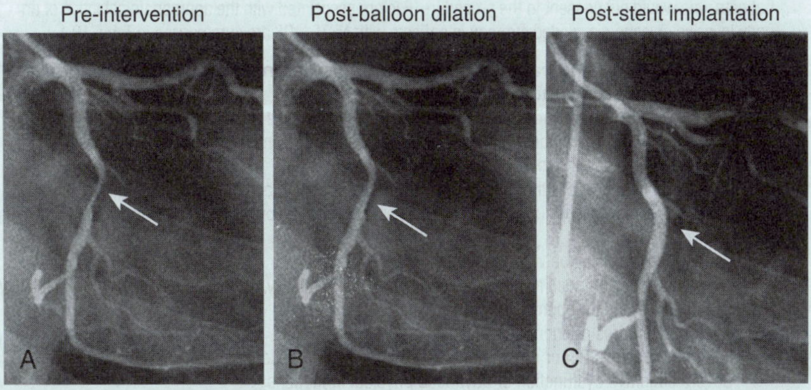

Fig. 19.2. Percutaneous coronary intervention of the left circumflex artery. **A,** Stenosis *(arrow)* in the left circumflex artery. **B,** After balloon angioplasty the degree of stenosis is decreased, but a significant residual lesion remains. **C,** After coronary artery stenting no residual stenosis is visible on angiography. *(Images from Levine, G. N. [2014].* Color atlas of cardiovascular disease. *New Delhi, India: Jaypee Brothers Medical Publishers.)*

Table 19.1. Factors Associated with Appropriate Selection of Early Invasive Strategy or Ischemia-Guided Strategy in Patients with Non–ST-Segment Elevation Acute Coronary Syndrome

Immediate invasive (within 2 h)	Refractory angina Signs and symptoms of HF or new or worsening mitral regurgitation Hemodynamic instability Recurrent angina or ischemia at rest or with low-level activities despite intensive medical therapy Sustained VT or VF
Ischemia-guided strategy	Low risk score (e.g., TIMI [0 or 1], GRACE [<109]) Low-risk Tn-negative female patients Patient or clinician preference in the absence of high-risk features
Early invasive (within 24 h)	None of the above but GRACE risk score >140 Temporal change in Tn (Sections 3 and 4) New or presumably new ST-segment depression
Delayed invasive (within 25-72 h)	None of the above but diabetes mellitus Renal insufficiency (GFR <60 mL/min per 1.73 m^2) Reduced LV systolic function (EF <0.40) Early postinfarction angina PCI within 6 months Prior CABG GRACE risk score 109-140; TIMI score ≥2

EF, Ejection fraction; *GFR*, glomerular filtration rate; *GRACE*, Global Registry of Acute Coronary Events; *HF*, heart failure; *PCI*, percutaneous coronary intervention; *TIMI*, thrombolysis in myocardial infarction.
From Amsterdam, E. A., Wenger, N. K., Brindis, R. G., Casey, D. E., Jr., Ganiats, T. G., Holmes, D. R., Jr., et al. [2014]. 2014 AHA/ACC *guideline for the management of patients with non–ST-elevation acute coronary syndromes: a report of the American College of Cardiology/American Heart Association Task Force on Practice Guidelines*. Journal of American College of Cardiology, 64, *e139–e228*.

Coronary Events [GRACE]). Patients who present with NSTE-ACS should be risk stratified to identify those who would benefit most from an early invasive approach. Factors favoring an invasive approach include recurrent or refractory angina, positive cardiac biomarkers, dynamic ST-segment changes, heart failure, hemodynamic instability, ventricular arrhythmias, and high-risk scores. Initially stabilized patients without such risk factors (low-risk patients) may be treated with an initial conservative (or selective invasive) strategy. An early invasive approach should not be undertaken in patients with extensive comorbidities, organ failure, or advanced cancer, in whom the risk of revascularization is greater than the benefit, or in patients who would not consent to the procedure. Factors associated with the appropriate selection of an early invasive or ischemia-guided strategy in patients with NSTE-ACS are summarized in Table 19.1.

4. What are the contraindications to percutaneous coronary intervention and the predictors of adverse outcomes?

The only absolute contraindication to PCI is lack of vascular access or active untreatable severe bleeding, which precludes the use of anticoagulation and antiplatelet agents. Relative contraindications include the following:

- A bleeding diathesis or other conditions that predispose to bleeding during antiplatelet therapy
- Severe renal insufficiency unless the patient is on hemodialysis or has severe electrolyte abnormalities
- Sepsis
- Poor patient compliance with medications
- A terminal condition, such as advanced or metastatic malignancy, that indicates a short life expectancy
- Other indications for open-heart surgery
- Anatomic features of poor success
- Failure of previous PCI or not amenable to PCI based on previous angiograms
- Severe cognitive dysfunction or advanced physical limitations

Patients generally should not undergo PCI if the following conditions are present:

- Only a very small area of myocardium is at risk.
- There is no objective evidence of ischemia (unless the patient has clear anginal symptoms and has not had a stress test) with either noninvasive or invasive testing (e.g., fractional flow reserve). One should also beware of false-negative stress tests in patients with left main CAD.

- There is a low likelihood of technical success.
- The patient has left main or multivessel CAD with a high SYNTAX score and is a candidate for coronary artery bypass grafting (CABG).
- There is insignificant stenosis (less than 50% luminal narrowing).
- The patient has end-stage cirrhosis with portal hypertension resulting in encephalopathy or visceral bleeding.

Clinical predictors of poor outcomes include older age, an unstable condition (ACS, acute MI, decompensated congestive heart failure, cardiogenic shock), left ventricular (LV) dysfunction, multivessel coronary disease, diabetes mellitus, renal insufficiency, small body size, and peripheral artery disease.

Angiographic predictors of poor outcomes include the presence of thrombus, calcified lesions, a degenerated bypass graft, unprotected left main CAD, long lesions (>20 mm), excessive tortuosity of a proximal segment, extremely angulated lesions (>90 degrees), a bifurcation lesion with involvement of major side branches, or chronic total occlusion.

With the developing hemodynamic support technologies, high-risk patients with high-risk lesions are now still undergoing PCI with hemodynamic support. The classic teaching of high risk is also evolving with the advent of newer PCI methods.

5. What are the major complications related to percutaneous coronary intervention?

The incidence of major complications has constantly decreased over the last two decades as a result of the use of activated clotting time to measure the degree of anticoagulation, better antithrombotic and antiplatelet agents, advanced device technology, more skilled operators, and superior PCI strategies. These factors have particularly lowered the incidence of MI and the need for emergent CABG. Major complications of PCI include the following:

Death: The overall in-hospital mortality rate is 1.27% ranging from 0.65% in elective PCI to 4.81% in ST-Elevation Myocardial Infarction (STEMI) (based on a National Cardiovascular Data Registry (NCDR) CathPCI database of patients undergoing PCI).

MI: The incidence of PCI-related MI is 0.4% to 4.9%; it varies depending on the acuity of symptoms, lesion morphology, the definition of MI, and the frequency with which biomarkers are measured.

Stroke: The incidence of PCI-related stroke is 0.22%. In-hospital mortality in patients with PCI-related stroke is 25% to 30% (based on a contemporary analysis from the NCDR).

Emergency CABG: The need to perform emergency CABG in the stent era is extremely low (between 0.1% and 0.4%).

Vascular complications: The incidence of vascular complications ranges from 2% to 6%. They include access-site hematoma, retroperitoneal hematoma, pseudoaneurysm, arteriovenous fistula, and arterial dissection. In randomized trials, closure devices were beneficial only in reducing time to hemostasis; they did not reduce the incidence of vascular complications.

Complications of radial artery access: There is significant reduction in vascular complications with the use of radial arterial access as compared with femoral artery access. Complications include loss of the radial pulse in less than 5% of cases, which is usually asymptomatic; compartment syndrome; pseudoaneurysm (in less than 0.01%); sterile abscess; and radial artery spasm.

Other complications associated with PCI: These include transient ischemic attack (TIA), renal insufficiency, and anaphylactoid reactions to contrast agents.

6. What laboratory values should be measured in post–percutaneous coronary intervention patients?

The American College of Cardiology/American Heart Association (ACC/AHA) guidelines recommend measuring creatine kinase myocardial-bound (CK-MB) and troponin I or T in all patients who have signs or symptoms suggestive of MI during or after PCI and in those who undergo complicated procedures. Currently there are no compelling data to support routine measurement of cardiac biomarkers for all PCI procedures.

Patients who have received GpIIb-IIIa inhibitors should have a complete blood count (CBC) 4 hours and 24 hours post procedure, since there can be a sudden drop in platelets. Renal function should also be assessed in patients with potential renal failure. However, one must be careful not to select only these patients for the measurement of renal function because ultimately all patients are at risk for renal failure, and measuring only the higher risk ones will falsely increase the institution's renal failure rate.

7. What is abrupt vessel closure?

Abrupt vessel closure occurs when an artery becomes completely occluded within hours of the PCI procedure. This can be due to stent thrombosis, dissection flap, vessel spasm, or side-branch occlusion. The incidence of abrupt vessel closure has decreased to less than 1% in the modern era of stents and antiplatelet therapies.

8. What is stent thrombosis?

Stent thrombosis occurs when there is complete occlusion of the artery due to the formation of thrombus in the stent. This may occur in the first 24 hours after stent deployment (acute stent thrombosis); in the first month after implantation (subacute stent thrombosis); between 1 and 12 months after implantation (late stent thrombosis); or even more than 1 year after implantation, most notably after the implantation of a DES (very late stent thrombosis). Most instances of stent thrombosis occur in the first 30 days after implantation. Beyond 30 days the incidence is 0.2% to 0.6% per year.

Stent thrombosis is a potentially catastrophic event and often presents as STEMI, requiring emergency revascularization. Stent thrombosis carries a mortality rate of 20% to 45%. The primary factors contributing to stent thrombosis are inadequate stent deployment, incomplete stent apposition, residual stenosis, unrecognized dissection impairing blood flow, and noncompliance with dual antiplatelet therapy (DAPT). Noncompliance with DAPT is the most common cause of stent thrombosis. Resistance to aspirin and clopidogrel and hypercoagulable states such as those associated with malignancy are additional less common causes of stent thrombosis.

Stent thrombosis should be differentiated from in-stent stenosis, which is the process whereby gradual hyperplasia of the smooth muscle cells within the implanted stent can lead to the recurrence of stenosis or in some cases complete occlusion of the stent over time.

9. What do the terms *slow flow* and *no reflow* mean?

Slow flow is the term applied when contrast injection of the coronary artery reveals delayed clearing of the contrast down the coronary artery; *no reflow* is the more extreme form, when the contrast does not appear to flow down the coronary artery at all. By definition no reflow is an acute reduction in coronary flow in the absence of dissection, thrombosis, spasm, or high-grade stenosis. These entities are caused by vasospasm, distal embolization, and microvascular plugging resulting in impaired epicardial blood flow, quantified as abnormal TIMI frame rates and myocardial blush scores. It occurs more commonly in the setting of atherectomy, thrombus, or PCI involving degenerated saphenous vein grafts (SVGs). Another form of no reflow is seen when reperfusion in the infarct-related artery is suboptimal. The etiology includes myocardial edema and endothelial injury in addition to vasospasm and embolization. Treatment consists of ruling out the other causes already mentioned and then administering vasodilators such as adenosine, nicardipine, or nitoprusside. If the blood pressure (BP) is low, even intracoronary epinephrine may be required.

10. Are bleeding complications related to percutaneous coronary intervention clinically important?

A bleeding complication is an independent predictor of early and late mortality in patients undergoing elective or urgent PCI. The potential for bleeding complications is always present owing to the routine use of potent antithrombin and antiplatelet agents during PCI. Bleeding can affect a patient adversely because of not only ensuing severe anemia but also the potential for ischemic events when anticoagulation is reversed. Additionally accumulating data suggest a possible direct link between blood transfusion and poor outcome. The proinflammatory and prothrombotic effects of red blood cell transfusion have been demonstrated. Use of a restrictive transfusion policy has been associated with improved outcomes.

Factors contributing to the risk of bleeding include advanced age, low body mass index, renal insufficiency, anemia at baseline, difficult vascular access, site and condition of access vessel, sheath size, and degree of anticoagulation and platelet inhibition. Measures to reduce bleeding complications include using weight-based anticoagulation regimens, frequent assessment of anticoagulation status to prevent excessive anticoagulation, use of bivalirudin, and adjustment of the dosing of certain medications when chronic kidney disease is present. Use of radial access also decreases bleeding complications.

11. What important complications can occur at the access site?

Potential complications of vascular access include retroperitoneal bleeding, pseudoaneurysm, arteriovenous fistula, arterial dissection, thrombosis, distal artery embolization, groin hematoma, infection/abscess, and femoral neuropathy. Risk factors for access site complications include older age, female gender, morbid obesity or low body weight, hypertension, low platelet count, peripheral artery disease, larger sheath size, prolonged sheath time, use of an intra-aortic balloon pump, concomitant venous sheath, excessive anticoagulation, use of thrombolytic therapy, and repeated intervention. Patients with a femoral puncture site above the inferiormost border of the inferior epigastric artery are at increased risk for retroperitoneal bleeding. Conversely, development of pseudoaneurysm and arteriovenous fistula is associated with a puncture site at or below the level of the femoral bifurcation.

Arteriotomy closure devices (vascular closure devices) have emerged as an alternative to mechanical compression for achieving rapid vascular hemostasis. These devices are categorized based on the principal mechanism of hemostasis, which includes biodegradable plug, suture, or staples. Although arteriotomy closure devices offer advantages over mechanical compression (shorter time to hemostasis and patient ambulation, high rate of patient satisfaction, and greater cost effectiveness), no prospective randomized study has been able to show a clear-cut reduction in vascular complications with these devices.

12. What are some treatment options for various vascular complications?

Pseudoaneurysm: For small pseudoaneurysms, observation is recommended. For larger pseudoaneurysms, ultrasound-guided compression or percutaneous thrombin injection under ultrasound guidance is the treatment of choice. For pseudoaneurysms with a large neck, simultaneous balloon inflation to occlude the entry site can be helpful. In cases of thrombin failure, surgical repair should be considered. Endovascular repair with stent graft implantation can also be used in the treatment of pseudoaneurysms.

Arteriovenous fistula: For small arteriovenous fistulas, observation is recommended; most close spontaneously or remain stable. For a large fistula or when significant shunting is present, options include ultrasound-guided compression, covered stent, or surgical repair.

Dissection: If there is no effect on blood flow and retrograde dissection, a conservative approach is indicated. In the presence of flow impairment (distal limb ischemia), angioplasty, stenting, and surgical repair are the treatment options.

Retroperitoneal bleeding: This should always be suspected with unexplained hypotension, a marked decrease in hematocrit, flank/abdominal or back pain, and high arterial sticks. The absence of hematoma does not rule out the diagnosis of retroperitoneal hematoma. Treatment includes intravascular volume replacement, reversal of anticoagulation, blood transfusion, and occasionally vasopressor agents and monitoring in the intensive care unit with serial hemoglobin checks. Endovascular management with covered stents, prolonged balloon inflation, or surgical repair are options but rarely necessary.

13. What is contrast nephropathy?

Contrast-induced nephropathy (CIN) is a worsening in renal function, as assessed by creatinine levels, due to the administration of intravascular iodinated contrast, as is used during cardiac catheterization and PCI. CIN usually first becomes manifest clinically 48 hours after contrast administration and peaks approximately 3 days later. CIN has been associated with increased mortality and morbidity. Several predisposing factors for CIN have been identified, including chronic renal insufficiency (the risk of CIN is directly proportional to the severity of preexisting renal insufficiency), diabetes, congestive heart failure, intravascular volume depletion, multiple myeloma, and the use of a large volume of contrast. The most widely accepted measure to prevent CIN consists of assuring adequate hydration with isotonic saline (such as 1.0 to 1.5 mL/kg per hour for 3 to 12 hours before and continuing for 6 to 24 hours after the procedure). In patients with creatinine clearance of less than 60 mL/minute, contrast volume should be kept to a minimum and adequate intravenous (IV) hydration initiated. Diuretics, nonsteroidal anti-inflammatory agents, and other nephrotoxic drugs should be held before PCI.

Both a meta-analysis and a large randomized trial assessing the efficacy of *N*-acetylcysteine for CIN found no benefit with the administration of *N*-acetylcysteine. Based on these data, the 2011 ACC/AHA guidelines on PCI do not recommend the use of *N*-acetylcysteine for the prevention of CIN, giving it a "class III-no benefit" indication. Studies of the administration of bicarbonate or hemofiltration (ultrafiltration) have produced conflicting results.

14. What is restenosis?

Restenosis means the recurrence of a treated coronary artery stenosis over time. Restenosis usually manifests itself clinically over the 1- to 6-month period following PCI. Patients with restenosis most commonly present with exertional angina and less frequently with unstable angina or MI. The process of restenosis is driven by the following mechanisms:

- Neointimal hyperplasia caused by the migration and proliferation of smooth muscle cells and the production of extracellular matrix
- Platelet deposition and thrombus formation

- Elastic recoil of a vessel after balloon inflation and negative remodeling of the vessel over time

Restenosis occurs more commonly in patients with diabetes, renal insufficiency, ostial bifurcation, or SVG locations, small vessels (<2.5 mm), and long lesions (>40 mm).

Based upon randomized controlled trials, rates of angiographic restenosis after balloon PTCA range from 32% to 42%; approximately half of these patients require clinically driven repeat target lesion revascularization within the first year.

Coronary stents prevent elastic recoil and negative remodeling of vessels and significantly reduce both angiographic and clinical rates of restenosis. The main factor leading to restenosis in coronary arteries treated with a BMS is neointimal hyperplasia as a result of smooth muscle cell proliferation and the production of extracellular matrix. Angiographic restenosis rates with BMSs range from 16% to 32%, with a target lesion revascularization rate of 12% and target vessel revascularization rate of 14% at 1 year. As in the case of PTCA, restenosis after placement of a BMS typically occurs within the first 6 months.

DESs are coated with a polymer that contains an antirestenotic (antiproliferative) medication, which is slowly released over a period of weeks. Restenosis after DES placement ranges from 5% to 10%, depending on the type of DES, stent size, stent length, lesion morphology, and the presence of diabetes. Compared with BMSs, DESs significantly reduce the rates of target lesion revascularization (approximately 6.2% vs. 16.6%), without any effect on all-cause mortality.

Options to treat restenosis include aggressive medical therapy, repeat PCI, and CABG. Patient factors such as compliance with DAPT, the type of intervention (BMS or DES) initially performed, chances of recurrence of restenosis, and appropriateness of CABG should be considered in addressing restenotic lesions.

15. What are the recommendations regarding antiplatelet therapy after percutaneous coronary intervention?

Patients undergoing PCI should receive DAPT with aspirin and a $P2Y_{12}$ inhibitor. The duration of antiplatelet therapy depends upon the type of intervention (PTCA, BMS, or DES) and setting (elective vs. ACS) of the intervention performed.

Recommendations for aspirin:

Patients who are already on aspirin therapy should continue with 81 mg of aspirin daily. Those who are not on aspirin should receive 325 mg of non–enteric-coated aspirin preferably 24 hours prior to PCI, after which aspirin should be continued indefinitely at a dose of 81 mg daily.

Recommendations for $P2Y_{12}$ receptor inhibitors:

- A loading dose of a $P2Y_{12}$ inhibitor should be given prior to PCI with stent placement. The loading doses for the three recommended drugs are clopidogrel 600 mg, prasugrel 60 mg, and ticagrelor 180 mg.
- Following a loading dose of a $P2Y_{12}$ inhibitor, a maintenance dose is continued. The recommendations for dose and duration are as follows:
    - In patients undergoing elective BMS implantation, the duration of $P2Y_{12}$ inhibitor therapy should be a minimum of 1 month.
    - For patient undergoing elective DES implantation (with a second-generation DES) for stable ischemic heart disease, the duration of $P2Y_{12}$ inhibitor therapy should be at least 6 months.
    - For patients undergoing stent BMS or DES implantation in the setting of ACS, clopidogrel 75 mg daily, prasugrel 10 mg daily, or ticagrelor 90 mg twice daily should be continued for at least 12 months. In this setting ticagrelor and prasugrel are preferred over clopidogrel.
    - Shorter duration therapy may be reasonable in patients at high risk for bleeding. Conversely, longer duration therapy may be reasonable in those at higher risk for ischemia but not for bleeding.
    - The recommended duration of DAPT in patients undergoing PCI is summarized in Fig. 19.3.

16. What steps should be taken to prevent premature discontinuation of dual antiplatelet therapy?

Although stent thrombosis most commonly occurs in the first month after stent implantation, numerous cases of late stent thrombosis (1 month to 1 year) or even very late stent thrombosis (after 1 year) have been reported, particularly in patients who have been treated with DES.

Premature discontinuation of antiplatelet therapy markedly increases the risk of stent thrombosis and with this the risk for MI or death. Factors contributing to premature cessation of $P2Y_{12}$ therapy include drug cost, inadequate patient and healthcare provider understanding about the importance of continuing therapy, and requests to discontinue therapy before noncardiac procedures.

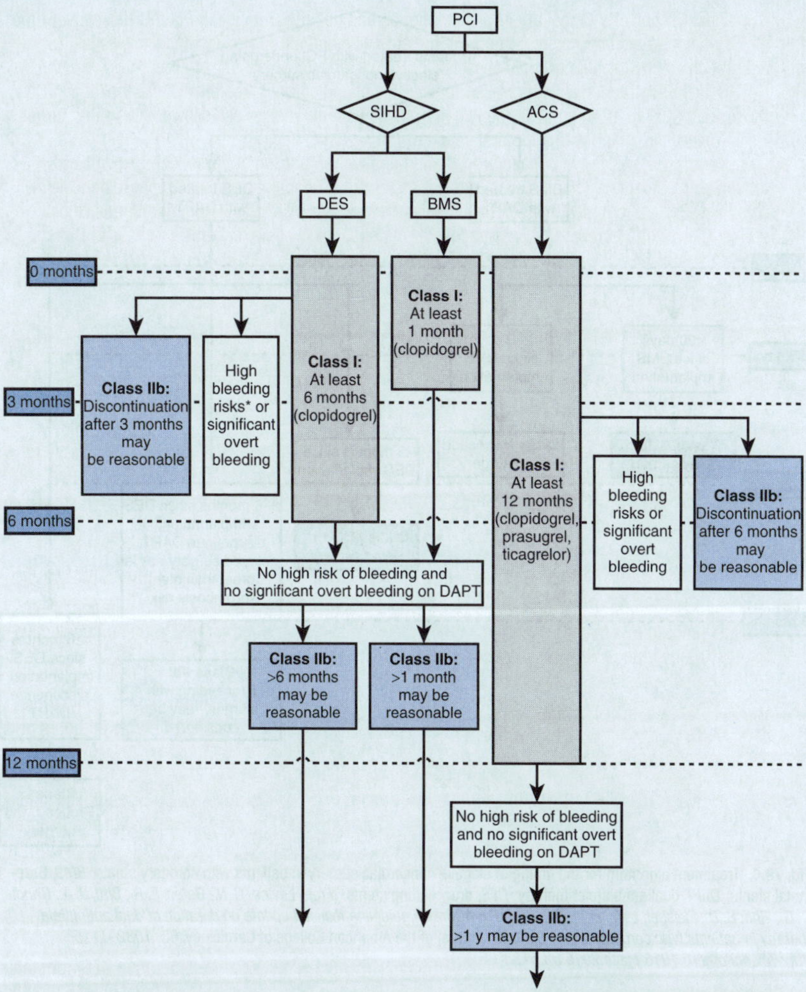

Fig. 19.3. Recommended duration of dual antiplatelet therapy (DAPT) in patients undergoing coronary stent implantation. *ACS,* Acute coronary syndrome; *BMS,* bare-metal stents; *DES,* drug-eluting stents; *PCI,* percutaneous coronary intervention. *(From Levine, G. N., Bates, E. R., Bittl, J. A., Brindis, R. G., Fihn, S. D., Fleisher, L. A., et al. [2016]. 2016 ACC/AHA guideline focused update on duration of dual antiplatelet therapy in patients with coronary artery disease.* Journal of the American College of Cardiology, 68, *1082–1115. http://dx.doi.org/10.1016/j.jacc.2016.03.513.)*

To eliminate premature discontinuation of $P2Y_{12}$ therapy, the following recommendations should be followed:

- Patients should be clearly educated about the rationale for not stopping antiplatelet therapy and the potential consequences of stopping such therapy. They should be instructed to call their cardiologists if bleeding develops or if another physician advised them to stop antiplatelet therapy.
- Healthcare providers who perform invasive or surgical procedures and are concerned about periprocedural bleeding must be made aware of the potentially catastrophic risks of premature discontinuation of $P2Y_{12}$ therapy. Professionals who perform these procedures should contact the patient's cardiologist to discuss the optimal patient management strategy.
- Elective procedures that pose a significant risk of perioperative bleeding should be deferred until patients have completed an appropriate course of $P2Y_{12}$ therapy (12 months after DES implantation if they are not at high risk of bleeding and a minimum of 1 month for BMS implantation).

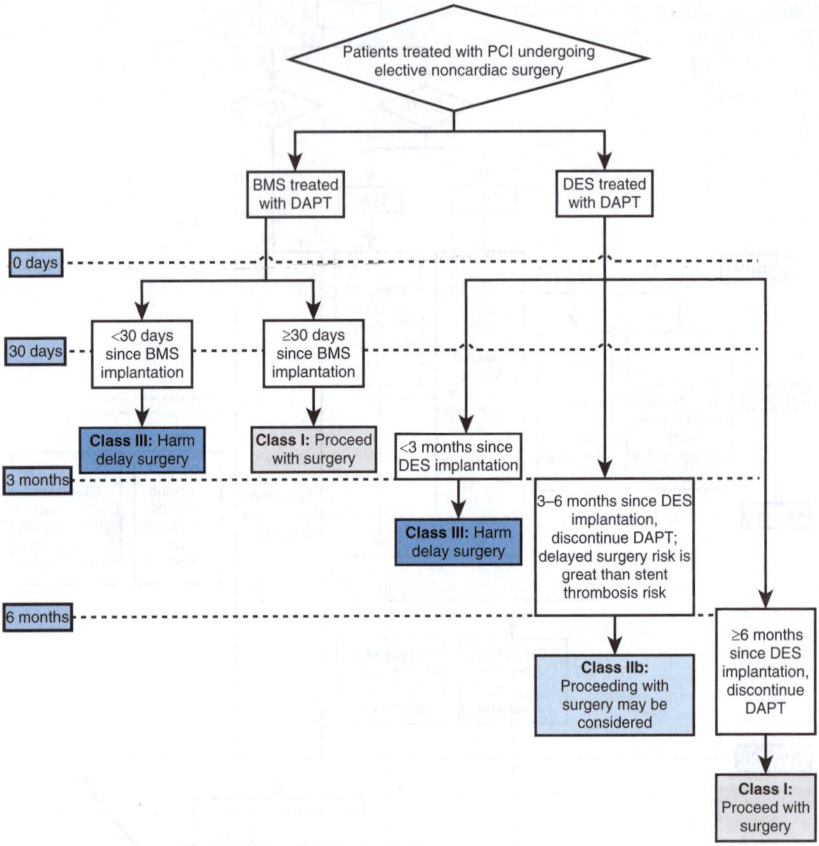

Fig. 19.4. Treatment algorithm for the timing of elective noncardiac surgery in patients with coronary stents. *BMS,* Bare-metal stents; *DAPT,* dual antiplatelet therapy; *DES,* drug-eluting stents. *(From Levine, G. N., Bates, E. R., Bittl, J. A., Brindis, R. G., Fihn, S. D., Fleisher, L. A., et al. [2016]. 2016 ACC/AHA guideline focused update on duration of dual antiplatelet therapy in patients with coronary artery disease.* Journal of the American College of Cardiology, 68, *1082–1115. http://dx.doi.org/10.1016/j.jacc.2016.03.513.)*

- For patients treated with DESs who are to undergo procedures that mandate discontinuation of $P2Y_{12}$ therapy, aspirin should be continued if at all possible and the thienopyridine restarted as soon as possible after the procedure.

17. What should be the management of a patient with a drug-eluting stent who requires urgent noncardiac surgery?

In patients treated with DESs, it is now recommended that elective surgery be deferred for 6 months. For such patients that the $P2Y_{12}$ inhibitor therapy will have to be discontinued temporarily; this may be considered after 3 months if the risk of further delay of surgery is greater than the expected risks of stent thrombosis. Aspirin should not be discontinued if possible. The benefits of "bridging" patients with intravenous antiplatelet or antithrombotic therapy in whom $P2Y_{12}$ therapy is held has not been clearly demonstrated.

In cases where antiplatelet therapy must be held, surgery should ideally be performed in an institution with a 24-hour catheterization laboratory in case of stent thrombosis; emergency PCI is strongly preferred over thrombolysis in cases of stent thrombosis, and thrombolytic therapy is contraindicated in patients who have recently undergone surgery.

A treatment algorithm for the timing of elective noncardiac surgery in patients with coronary stents is given in Fig. 19.4.

Table 19.2. Factors Used to Calculate the Dual Antiplatelet Therapy Score

VARIABLE	POINTS
Age ≥75 years	−2
Age 65 to <75 years	−1
Age <65 years	0
Current cigarette smoker	1
Diabetes mellitus	1
MI at presentation	1
Prior PCI or prior MI	1
Stent diameter <3 mm	1
Paclitaxel-eluting stent	1
CHF or LVEF <30%	2
SVG PCI	2

CGF, *CHF*, Congestive heart failure; *LVEF*, left ventricular ejection fraction; *MI*, myocardial infarction; *PCI*, percutaneous coronary intervention; *SVG*, saphenous vein graft.

Adapted from Yeh, R. W., Secemsky, E. A., Kereiakes, D. J., Normand, S. L., Gershlick, A. H., Cohen, D. J., et al. [2016]. Development and validation of a prediction rule for benefit and harm of dual antiplatelet therapy beyond 1 year after percutaneous coronary intervention. Journal of the American Medical Association, *315, 1735–1749. http://dx.doi.org/10.1001/jama.2016.3775.*

18. What should be discussed with the patient after percutaneous coronary intervention and before discharge?

Compliance with medications, especially adherence to dual antiplatelet therapy, is of utmost importance in these patients. This should be emphasized in a discussion with every patient before discharge, preferably by more than one healthcare provider. Healthy living, diet, exercise, and smoking cessation should also be included in the predischarge discussion. Patients should ideally be enrolled in a comprehensive cardiac rehabilitation program, which can improve their adherence to medications as well as promote exercise and smoking cessation.

19. What is the dual antiplatelet therapy score, and how can we use it?

This is a score derived from an analysis of the results of the DAPT study. After a year of antiplatelet treatment and no bleeding complications, a DAPT score can be calculated using the variables listed in Table 19.2. Patients with high (≥2) DAPT scores may benefit from prolonged dual antiplatelet therapy. Those with low scores do not, at least statistically, benefit from prolonged DAPT.

Bibliography and Suggested Readings

Investigators, A. C. T. (2011). Acetylcysteine for prevention of renal outcomes in patients undergoing coronary and peripheral vascular angiography: Main results (from the randomized Acetylcysteine for Contrast-induced nephropathy Trial (ACT). *Circulation, 124*, 1250–1259.

Amsterdam, E. A., Wenger, N. K., Brindis, R. G., Casey, D. E., Jr., Ganiats, T. G., Holmes, D. R., Jr., et al. (2014). 2014 AHA/ACC guideline for the management of patients with non–ST-elevation acute coronary syndromes: a report of the American College of Cardiology/American Heart Association Task Force on Practice Guidelines. *Journal of the American College of Cardiology, 64*, e139–e228.

Anderson, J. L., Adams, C. D., Antman, E. M., Bridges, C. R., Califf, R. M., Casey, D. E., Jr., et al. (2011). 2011 ACCF/AHA Focused Update Incorporated Into the ACC/AHA 2007 Guidelines for the management of patients with unstable angina/non–ST-elevation myocardial infarction. A Report of the American College of Cardiology Foundation/American Heart Association Task Force on Practice Guidelines. *Circulation, 123*, e426–e579.

Bavry, A. A., Kumbhani, D. J., Rassi, A. N., Bhatt, D. L., & Askari, A. T. (2006). Benefit of early invasive therapy in acute coronary syndromes: a meta-analysis of contemporary randomized clinical trials. *Journal of American College of Cardiology, 48*, 1319–1325.

Boden, W. E., O'Rourke, R. A., Teo, K. K., Hartigan, P. M., Maron, D. J., Kostuk, W. J., et al. (2007). Optimal medical therapy with or without PCI for stable coronary disease. *New England Journal of Medicine, 356*, 1503–1516.

Gonzales, D. A., Norsworthy, K. J., Kern, S. J., Banks, S., Sieving, P. C., Star, R. A., et al. (2007). A meta-analysis of *N*-acetylcysteine in contrast-induced nephrotoxicity: unsupervised clustering to resolve heterogeneity. *BMC Medicine, 5*, 32.

Grines, C. L., Bonow, R. O., Casey, D. E., Gardner, T. J., Lockhart, P. B., Moliterno, D. J., et al. (2007). Prevention of premature discontinuation of dual antiplatelet therapy in patients with coronary artery stents. *Journal of the American College of Cardiology, 49,* 734–739.

Keeley, E. C., Boura, J. A., & Grines, C. L. (2006). Comparison of primary and facilitated percutaneous coronary interventions for ST-elevation myocardial infarction: quantitative review of randomised trials. *Lancet, 367*(9510), 579–588.

Levine, G. N., Bates, E. R., Bittl, J. A., Brindis, R. G., Fihn, S. D., Fleisher, L. A., et al. (2016). 2016 ACC/AHA Guideline focused update on duration of dual antiplatelet therapy in patients with coronary artery disease. *Journal of the American College of Cardiology, 68,* 1082–1115. http://dx.doi.org/10.1016/j.jacc.2016.03.513.

Levine, G. N., Bates, E. R., Blankenship, J. C., Bailey, S. T., Bittl, J. A., Cercek, B., et al. (2011). 2011 ACCF/AHA/SCAI guideline for percutaneous coronary intervention. A report of the American College of Cardiology Foundation/American Heart Association Task Force on Practice Guidelines and the Society for Cardiovascular Angiography and Interventions. *Journal of the American College of Cardiology, 58*(24), e44–e122.

Levine, G. N., Kern, M. J., Berger, P. B., Brown, D. L., Klein, L. W., Kereiakes, D. J., et al. (2003). Management of patients undergoing percutaneous coronary revascularization. *Annals of Internal Medicine, 139,* 123–136.

Patel, M. R., Dehmer, G. J., Hirshfeld, J. W., Smith, P. K., & Spertus, J. A. (2012). ACCF/SCAI/STS/AATS/AHA/ASNC/HFSA/SCCT 2012 Appropriate use criteria for coronary revascularization focused update. *Journal of the American College of Cardiology, 59*(9), 857–881.

Serruys, P. W., Morice, M. C., Kappetein, A. P., Colombo, A., Holmes, D. R., Mack, M. J., et al. (2009). Percutaneous coronary intervention versus coronary-artery bypass grafting for severe coronary artery disease. *New England Journal of Medicine, 360,* 961–972.

Shaw, L. J., Berman, D. S., Maron, D. J., Mancini, G. B., Hayes, S. W., Hartigan, P. M., et al. (2008). Optimal medical therapy with or without percutaneous coronary intervention to reduce ischemic burden results (From the Clinical Outcomes Utilizing Revascularization and AGgressive drug Evaluation (COURAGE) Trial Nuclear Substudy. *Circulation, 117,* 1283–1291.

CORONARY ARTERY BYPASS SURGERY

Faisal Bakaeen, Michael Tong, Stephanie Mick

CHAPTER 20

1. **What are the indications for coronary artery bypass grafting?**
According to the American College of Cardiology/American Heart Association (ACC/AHA) guidelines, class I indications for coronary artery bypass grafting (CABG) include significant left main stenosis and three-vessel coronary artery disease. Class I indications also include two-vessel disease involving the proximal left anterior descending (LAD) artery. CABG should be considered as a reasonable treatment strategy (class IIa) in patients with proximal LAD disease and in 2-vessel disease without proximal LAD disease but with extensive ischemia.
After myocardial infarction (MI), primary surgical revascularization should be considered in patients not suitable for percutaneous coronary intervention (PCI), patients who have failed PCI, or patients with ongoing ischemia or symptoms. After a transmural infarct, mechanical complications such as a postinfarction ventricular septal defect (VSD), acute mitral regurgitation (MR) as a result of papillary rupture, and free-wall pseudoaneurysm should be considered as indications for primary surgical intervention.

2. **How does coronary artery bypass grafting compare with medical management for coronary artery disease?**
Three early prospective randomized trials comparing CABG with medical therapy were conducted in the late 1970s and were reported in the early 1980s. The Veterans' Affairs (VA) cooperative trial, European Coronary Surgery Study (ECSS), and Coronary Artery Surgery Study (CASS) showed long-term superiority of surgery over medical therapy in patients with left main (LM) coronary artery disease, significant coronary artery disease involving the LAD artery, and multivessel disease.

3. **How does coronary artery bypass grafting compare with drug-eluting stents?**
Drug-eluting stents (DES) have reduced the problem of restenosis, but data directly comparing DES with CABG are limited and still relatively short-term. In a registry study from the New York State cardiovascular database, CABG resulted in improved survival at 3 years compared with DES for patients with double- and triple-vessel disease. ARTS II randomized patients to DES or CABG and showed the primary composite outcomes at 1 year were similar.
The international SYNTAX trial, involving 85 centers and 1800 patients with multivessel or left main coronary artery disease, recently published 5-year follow-up data. These showed worse outcomes in the PCI group as compared to the CABG group, with increased composite major adverse cardiac and cerebrovascular events (MACCE: death, stroke, MI, or repeat revascularization). Although there was no significant difference in all-cause mortality and stroke at 5 years, MI and repeat revascularization were both increased in the PCI group. Of note, in patients with three-vessel coronary artery disease (CAD), CABG in comparison with PCI was associated with a significantly reduced rate of MI-related death, which was the leading cause of death after PCI. The study concluded that patients with more complex disease (3VD with intermediate-high SYNTAX scores and LM with high SYNTAX score) have an increased risk of a MACCE event with PCI, and CABG is the preferred treatment option.

4. **What is the syntax score?**
The syntax score is a scoring system developed by the SYNTAX trial investigators to quantify the extent and complexity of CAD based on findings at cardiac catheterization. Scores are divided into terciles: low (0 to 22), intermediate (23 to 32), and high (≥33), with higher scores representing more extensive and complex CAD. The SYNTAX score was found to correlate with PCI risk and outcome but not with CABG risk and outcome. Patients with higher SYNTAX scores generally benefited from a revascularization strategy of CABG in preference to PCI. This is reflected in current guidelines, which state that it is reasonable to choose CABG over PCI as a revascularization strategy in patients with complex three-vessel disease and high SYNTAX score (class IIa recommendation).

5. Which patients benefit most from coronary artery bypass grafting?

The decision for surgery is made based on the comprehensive evaluation of the patient. Anatomic considerations that favor recommendation for CABG include presence of significant LM or proximal LAD CAD, multivessel CAD, and presence of lesions not amenable to stenting. The presence of diabetes also favors surgical revascularization over stenting in operable patients. Depressed ejection fraction has been recognized as an additional indication for CABG.

Although the coronary anatomy may be suitable for bypass, each patient's comorbidities should be considered in the overall risk-benefit analysis. Preoperative renal insufficiency, peripheral vascular disease, recent myocardial infarction, or recent stroke, as well as emergency operation and cardiogenic shock, have been identified as factors that increase mortality. The decision to offer CABG or PCI should be determined by a multidisciplinary heart team that evaluates the appropriate therapy on a case-by-case basis.

6. What is the cardiopulmonary bypass pump, and how is it used?

The "pump" involves temporarily placing a patient on a machine to supply circulation and oxygenation during an operation, so that the heart can be stopped to facilitate the procedure. The bypass circuit consists of the tubing, a collection chamber, oxygenator, heater-cooler machines to control temperature, and the pump. An aortic cannula is placed in the distal ascending aorta, and this is connected to tubing that will be used to bring artificially oxygenated blood from the pump back to the patient's arterial bloodstream. A venous cannula is placed in the right atrium, and advanced down into the inferior vena cava, to collect venous blood and return it toward the pump. Once the venous blood is oxygenated, it is pumped back into the arterial line to the patient's aorta. A perfusionist runs the pump under the direction of the surgeon.

7. Why is heparin required for cardiopulmonary bypass?

The cardiopulmonary bypass circuit is thrombogenic, and systemic anticoagulation is required to prevent clotting and embolization. The standard anticoagulant is heparin (300 U/kg), which is administered to produce a target activated clotting time (ACT) of greater than 480 seconds. In patients with previously documented heparin-induced thrombocytopenia, direct thrombin inhibitors have been used for anticoagulation. Heparin is used in off-pump CABG at partial dose. After termination of CPB and decannulation, heparin-related anticoagulation is reversed with protamine.

8. How is the heart stopped while on cardiopulmonary bypass?

First, a completely occluding cross clamp is placed across the ascending aorta, below the aortic cannula, eliminating arterial blood flow to the coronary arteries. Cardioplegia is then used to induce arrest of the heart and can be given antegrade and/or retrograde. Components of cardioplegia solution are varied in different institutions but include potassium to achieve diastolic arrest. Cardioplegia can be administered in an antegrade fashion via a small cannula, placed in the aorta below the cross clamp, providing cardioplegia to the myocardium via the coronary ostia. Retrograde cardioplegia is also used frequently, by infusing cardioplegia into the coronary sinus with backward filling of the cardiac veins to reach the myocardium, and is especially important in situations where antegrade cardioplegia may not be as effective, such as with severe CAD and aortic valve insufficiency. Most commonly, cold cardioplegia at 4°C is administered intermittently in 15- to 20-minute intervals. Blood can be mixed to the crystalloid component of cardioplegia in a 4:1 mix to provide oxygenated blood to the myocardium and to buffer the pH of the tissue (Fig. 20.1).

9. How is the myocardium protected during cardiac arrest during bypass surgery?

Myocardial ischemia occurs when the aortic cross clamp is applied, at which time the coronary arteries no longer perfuse the myocardium. Strategies to protect the myocardium during this time include cooling the heart, unloading the ventricle, and arresting the heart. Systemic cooling of the heart and the body is accomplished with the cardiopulmonary bypass machine. Direct cooling of the heart is also accomplished with cold cardioplegia and topical ice solution. Unloading the ventricles is accomplished by the cardiopulmonary bypass, which empties the heart. The greatest decrease in oxygen demand (by as much as 80%) occurs with the diastolic arrest of the heart using cardioplegia, which eliminates the electrical and mechanical work of the myocardium.

10. What is the long-term patency of the saphenous vein?

The saphenous vein is readily available and relatively easy to procure, provides multiple graft segments, and is the most common bypass graft used other than the left internal mammary artery (LIMA). The major limitation of the saphenous vein graft (SVG) is its long-term patency. Early attrition of up to 15% can occur by 1 year, with 10-year patency traditionally cited at 60%. Early patency has been shown to be improved by use of aspirin postoperatively. There are only limited and conflicting data on whether dual antiplatelet therapy for up to 1 year postoperatively can improve SVG patency.

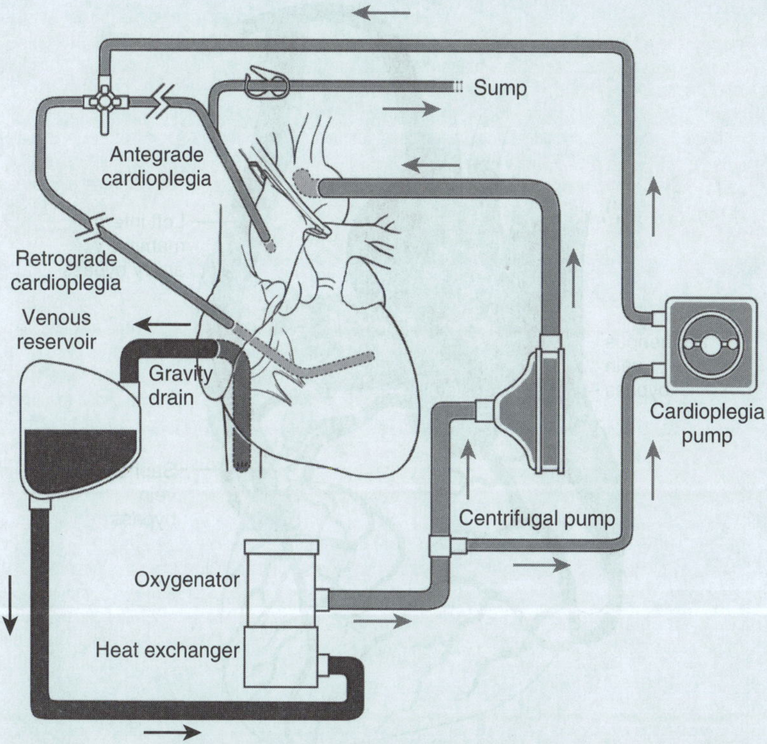

Fig. 20.1. Schematic of total cardiopulmonary bypass circuit. All returning venous blood is siphoned into a venous reservoir and is oxygenated and temperature regulated before being pumped back through a centrifugal pump into arterial circulation. The common site for inflow into the patient is the ascending aorta, but alternate sites include the femoral arteries or the right axillary artery in special circumstances (discussed later). A parallel circuit derives oxygenated blood that is mixed with cold (4°C) cardioplegic solution in the ratio of 4:1 and administered in an antegrade or retrograde fashion to accomplish cardiac arrest. Antegrade cardioplegia is administered into the aortic root and retrograde through the coronary sinus. During the administration of retrograde cardioplegia, the efflux of blood from the coronary ostium is siphoned off via the sump drain. The sump drain, a return parallel circuit connected to the venous reservoir (not shown), also helps keep the heart decompressed during the arrest phase. *(From Townsend, C. M. Jr., Beauchamp, R. D., Evers, B. M., & Mattox, K. L. [2012].* Sabiston textbook of surgery *[19th ed.]. Philadelphia, PA: Saunders.)*

SVG can be harvested using a single long leg incision, multiple short incisions with intervening skin islands, or endoscopic techniques. Early patency has largely been found to be equivalent both clinically and angiographically between open and endoscopic techniques.

11. What are the benefits of using the internal mammary artery for bypass?

Use of the internal mammary artery (IMA) was first described by Kolessov in 1967, but its impact on survival wasn't noted until the mid-1980s. LIMA anastomosed to the LAD artery has an approximately 90% patency at 10 years and offers an advantage in both survival and freedom from reoperation. The current guidelines for CABG include a class I recommendation for use of the LIMA to bypass the LAD artery when bypass of the LAD is indicated (Fig. 20.2).

12. What about other arterial conduits?

The right internal mammary artery (RIMA), radial artery, gastroepiploic artery, and inferior epigastric arteries have also been used as bypass conduits, and some surgeons have favored all-arterial strategies for bypass grafting, with hopes to improve long-term patency over SVG. However, these other arterial grafts have not duplicated the success of the LIMA to the LAD. Experts believe that the clinical benefit of additional arterial grafts manifests after 5 to 10 years of the index operation. The radial artery has been evaluated in several randomized trials, the largest of which is the VA

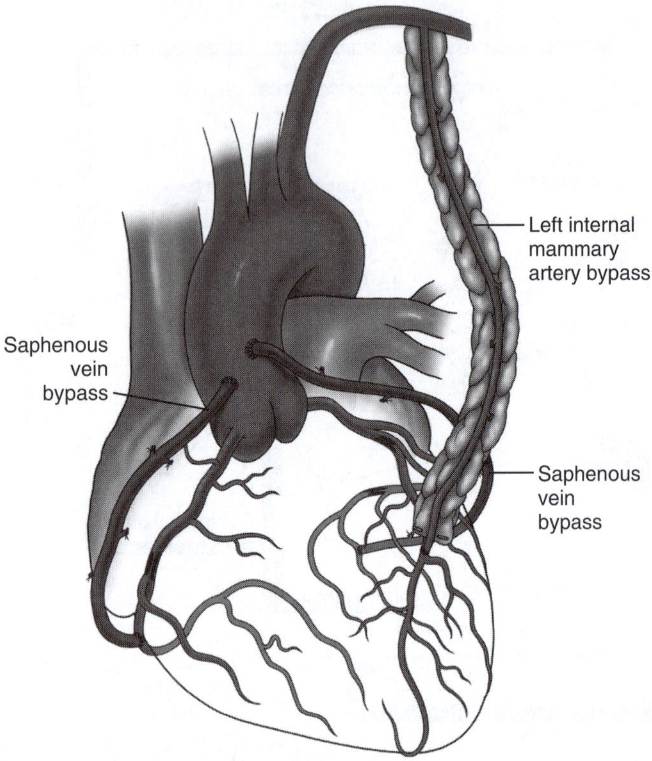

Fig. 20.2. Typical configuration for a three-vessel coronary artery bypass. The left internal mammary artery is anastomosed to the left anterior descending artery. Aortocoronary bypasses are created using the reversed saphenous vein to the distal right coronary artery and an obtuse marginal branch of the circumflex coronary artery. The circumflex coronary artery is usually avoided as a target for bypass because it is located well into the atrioventricular groove and difficult to visualize. *(From Townsend, C. M. Jr., Beauchamp, R. D., Evers, B. M., & Mattox, K. L. [2012].* Sabiston textbook of surgery *[19th ed.]. Philadelphia, PA: Saunders.)*

Table 20.1. The Society of Thoracic Surgeons Clinical Practice Guidelines on Arterial Conduits for Coronary Artery Bypass Grafting

- The IMA should be used to bypass the LAD artery when bypass of the LAD is indicated (COR I, LOE B).
- As an adjunct to LIMA, a second arterial graft (right internal mammary artery or RA) should be considered in appropriate patients (COR IIa, LOE B).
- Use of BIMAs should be considered in patients who do not have an excessive risk of sternal complications (COR IIa, LOE B).

BIMA, Bilateral internal mammary arteries, *COR*, class of recommendation; *LAD*, left anterior descending; *LIMA*, left internal mammary artery; *LOE*, level of evidence; *RA*, radial artery.

cooperative study, which randomized 733 patients to radial versus saphenous vein graft and showed equivalent graft patency at 1 year (89% in each group). Similarly, the Arterial Revascularization Trial (ART) showed no clinical benefit of bilateral mammary grafting over vein at 1 year. More recently, the Radial Artery Patency Study (RAPS) had randomized 510 patients at nine Canadian centers, and at 5 years the radial artery patency (88%) was superior to that of saphenous vein (80.3%). Additional long-term data are needed, but at present experts recommend consideration of multiple arterial grafting because of a wealth of observational data that support their advantage (Table 20.1).

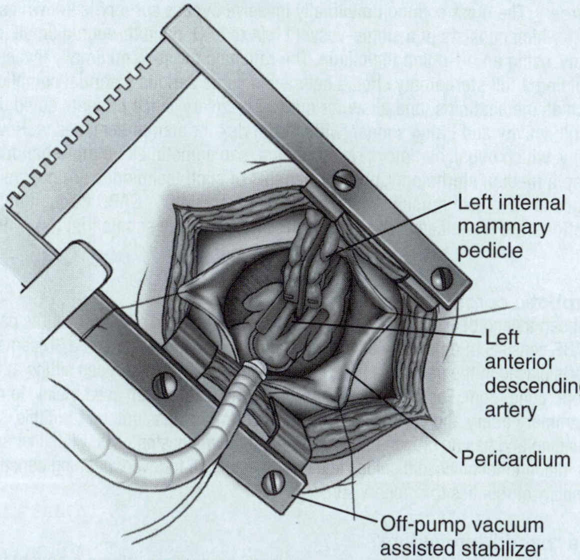

Fig. 20.3. Left thoracotomy approach for performing off-pump left internal mammary to left anterior descending bypass. This is commonly used in the minimally invasive direct coronary artery bypass (MIDCAB) approach. Multiarticulating stabilizers are essential for this technique. *(From Townsend, C. M. Jr., Beauchamp, R. D., Evers, B. M., & Mattox, K. L. [2012]. Sabiston textbook of surgery [19th ed.]. Philadelphia, PA: Saunders.)*

13. What is off-pump coronary artery bypass grafting, and what are the differences between on-pump and off-pump coronary artery bypass grafting?

Off-pump bypass is CABG surgery performed without use of a cardiopulmonary bypass machine. The heart remains beating throughout the procedure, and stabilizers and coronary occlusion and shunts are used to perform the bypass graft to native coronary artery anastomoses. Since off-pump surgery avoids cardiopulmonary bypass, it should lessen the side effects of the extracorporeal circulation, such as activation of inflammatory mediators, coagulopathy, and risk of embolic events. Surgeons have debated the merits of off-pump versus on-pump bypass for many years, and the goal of demonstrating differences between the two techniques in hard endpoints such as mortality, stroke, and renal failure has been elusive. In fact, the literature largely shows equivalency in these major early outcomes. In some studies, slightly shorter lengths of hospital stay and lower transfusion rates have been noted with off-pump surgery.

Surgeons that prefer on-pump bypass surgery argue that the use of cardiopulmonary bypass allows maintenance of hemodynamic stability and aids in complete revascularization. The motionless and bloodless field allows precise and exact anastomoses. Off-pump revascularization on a beating heart is technically more demanding, especially with small or diffusely diseased targets, and the technical difficulty may result in decreased long-term patency of the grafts.

In the largest randomized clinical trial in cardiac surgery ever, 4752 patients were randomized to on-pump versus off-pump CABG. At 1 year, there were no differences in the composite outcome, the rate of repeat revascularization, quality of life, or neurocognitive function.

The technique of off-pump revascularization can be particularly useful in selected cases, such as in patients with a heavily calcified aorta (often called a “porcelain aorta”). In experienced centers, patency rates of the bypass grafts performed on-pump versus off-pump should not differ greatly. Most centers use off-pump selectively. In the United States, currently more than 80% of CABG operations are performed on-pump using cardiopulmonary bypass (Fig. 20.3).

14. What is a “mid-cab” operation?

Minimally invasive CABG involves the use of smaller (<10 cm) incisions, sometimes with videoscopic guidance, and is often referred to by the acronym “MICS” for minimally invasive cardiac surgery. The most common minimally invasive bypass surgery is known as the "MID-CAB," which consists of a single-vessel LIMA to LAD, done through a small left anterior thoracotomy, using an off-pump technique. The rationale for such minimally invasive operations is that avoiding a full sternotomy should help avoid some serious potential complications of CABG, such as mediastinitis, and allow for quicker recovery, since patients could theoretically return to full activity and lifting sooner, without the risk for sternal dehiscence. However, mini-thoracotomy, which usually employs rib spreading, can sometimes be more painful for the patient than a median sternotomy, and the benefits of such techniques are not well established. Some surgeons have also pursued multivessel off-pump "MICS" CABG through mini-thoracotomy, but such efforts are technically very demanding and may have substantial risk without proven benefit.

15. What is robotic coronary artery bypass grafting?

There has been a good deal of fanfare about robotic cardiothoracic surgery over the past decade. Robotic CABG consists of robotically controlled endoscopic instruments and a 3D camera set up through ports placed in the patient's chest, controlled remotely by a surgeon sitting at a console in the same operating room. For CABG, the robotic instruments are often used mainly to mobilize the internal mammary artery and can also be used to perform the anastomoses, but this is technically very challenging and has no proven benefit over hand-sewn anastomoses. High cost and cumbersome setup, in addition to technical difficulties and lack of evidence for overwhelming benefit, have limited the applicability of robotics to coronary surgery.

16. What is a "hybrid" procedure?

Some centers have popularized performing "hybrid" procedures, where a patient will receive a single-vessel CABG with LIMA to LAD, most commonly using a mini-thoracotomy, and other non-LAD coronary lesions will be treated with coronary stents, either at the same or staggered settings. One rationale for this strategy is to attempt to capitalize on the high long-term patency and mortality benefit demonstrated with the LIMA to LAD graft, while avoiding the downside of sternotomy. In the current CABG guidelines, hybrid CABG has a class IIa indication if there are limitations to traditional CABG, such as heavily calcified aorta, poor target vessels, lack of suitable conduit, or unfavorable LAD for PCI. Otherwise, indications for hybrid CABG are deemed class IIb, or a "potentially reasonable alternative," in an attempt to improve the overall risk-benefit ratio. These techniques are used in a minority of CABG procedures performed in the United States.

17. What complications can occur following coronary artery bypass grafting?

Operative mortality is currently approximately 2% overall and less than 1% in low-risk patients. Sentinel complications include stroke, MI, renal failure, respiratory failure, and mediastinitis (see the following question). The incidence of each is approximately 1% to 5% and varies with age and preoperative comorbidities of the patient.

Atrial fibrillation is the most common complication after cardiothoracic surgery, with an incidence of 20% to 40%. The incidence of atrial fibrillation increases with age, duration of cardiopulmonary bypass, presence of chronic obstructive pulmonary disease (COPD), and preexisting heart failure, among other risk factors. The peak incidence of postoperative atrial fibrillation is between 2 and 4 days after surgery, is usually self-limited, and usually resolves over time as the inflammatory state of the heart improves. The use of beta-blockers postoperatively is routine and is useful to decrease the risk of atrial fibrillation. Goals of therapy are rate control and conversion to normal sinus rhythm if possible. Anticoagulation may be advisable if timely conversion cannot be accomplished, or if the arrhythmia recurs intermittently.

18. Who is at risk for mediastinitis?

Mediastinitis is a deep surgical site infection following sternotomy. The infection involves the sternal bone and underlying heart and mediastinum. The organism most commonly recovered is *Staphylococcus,* but gram-negative organisms can also be found. The incidence of mediastinitis has been reported in the past to be 1% to 4%, but a recent Society of Thoracic Surgeons (STS) database study has shown an incidence less than 1%. The incidence of mediastinitis increases with the presence of diabetes, morbid obesity, and COPD and when bilateral mammary harvesting is performed. Perioperative prophylactic antibiotics, proper skin preparation and clipping, and active control of hyperglycemia in the postoperative setting are important measures believed to decrease the incidence of mediastinitis.

19. **What causes strokes during coronary bypass?**
The incidence of stroke (type I neurologic deficit) in the perioperative period after cardiac surgery is 1% to 6% and varies with age. The risk of stroke is dependent on the atherosclerotic burden in the cerebrovascular circulation and in the aorta. Atherosclerotic plaques in the ascending aorta can be the source of atheroemboli during aortic cannulation, cross clamping, or manipulation of the ascending aorta. Microemboli may also be due to fat and to air that can arise during extracorporeal circulation. Regional hypoperfusion can occur in the brain as a result of intracranial and extracranial vascular lesions when there are significant fluctuations in the blood pressure during on-pump or off-pump surgery.

20. **What is a type II neurologic deficit?**
A type II neurologic deficit is a neurocognitive change after CABG, and its true incidence remains controversial. Changes in intellectual abilities, memory, and mood are often based on subjective assessment and often difficult to quantitatively evaluate. Reported incidence ranges widely from 2% to 50%. Studies have shown decreases in neurocognitive functioning after CABG, but in small series similar declines over time have been noted in on-pump, off-pump, PCI, and CAD "control patients" not undergoing intervention.

21. **How should clopidogrel and other antiplatelet agents be managed preoperatively?**
Preoperative clopidogrel use increases blood transfusion during cardiac surgery and increases the risk of reoperation after surgery for mediastinal bleeding. The current recommendation is to avoid clopidogrel and ticagrelor for 5 days before CABG and to avoid prasugrel for 7 days before CABG, unless the need for urgent or emergent revascularization for ongoing ischemia exceeds the risk of bleeding.

22. **Which patients should be on dual antiplatelet therapy after coronary artery bypass grafting?**
All patients post CABG are treated with aspirin postop, as is the case with all patients with coronary artery disease. Per recent guidelines, in patients with ACS (NSTE-ACS or STEMI) being treated with DAPT who undergo CABG, $P2Y_{12}$ inhibitor therapy (clopidogrel, prasugrel, or ticagrelor) should be resumed after CABG to complete 12 months of DAPT therapy after ACS.

As noted previously, there are only limited and conflicting data on whether dual antiplatelet therapy for up to 1 year postoperatively can improve SVG patency. Current guidelines state that in patients with stable ischemic heart disease who undergo CABG, DAPT (with clopidogrel initiated early postoperatively) for 12 months after CABG may be reasonable to improve vein graft patency.

23. **What factors are important in the follow-up of coronary artery bypass grafting patients?**
Secondary prevention and control of atherosclerotic risk factors are important in maintaining the long-term clinical success of the operation. Use of statins, beta-blockers, and aspirin is advised in all post-CABG patients who do not have strong contraindications to those medications. Angiotensin-converting enzyme (ACE) inhibitors are also recommended in patients with depressed left ventricular ejection fraction (<40%). In addition, control of hypertension and diabetes and smoking cessation are also essential aspects of secondary prevention.

24. **What is the incidence of recurrent disease requiring redo coronary artery bypass grafting?**
Reoperation may be required because of progression of native coronary disease or failure of previous grafts. Historically, the incidence of reoperation in studies has been reported to be approximately 10% by 10 years, although aggressive secondary prevention and advances in the use of PCI for the treatment of native and graft disease are decreasing the need for reoperation. Redo CABG is technically more challenging. Scarring of the mediastinum increases the risk of complications, including damage to the LIMA graft. The increased burden of atherosclerosis, difficulty identifying the target vessels, and lack of suitable bypass conduits are potential concerns in patients undergoing redo bypass surgery.

Bibliography and Suggested Readings

Aldea, G. S., Bakaeen, F. G., Pal, J., Fremes, S., Head, S. J., Sabik, J., et al. (2016). The Society of Thoracic Surgeons Clinical Practice Guidelines on arterial conduits for coronary artery bypass grafting. *Annals of Thoracic Surgery, 101*(2), 801–809.

Bakaeen, F. G., Shroyer, A. L., Gammie, J. S., Sabik, J. F., Cornwell, L. D., Coselli, J. S., et al. (2014). Trends in use of off-pump coronary artery bypass grafting: results from the Society of Thoracic Surgeons Adult Cardiac Surgery Database. *Journal of Thoracic and Cardiovascular Surgery, 148*(3), 856–864.

Goldman, S., Sethi, G. K., Holman, W., Thai, H., McFalls, E., Ward, H. B., et al. (2011). Radial artery grafts vs saphenous vein grafts in coronary artery bypass surgery. A randomized trial. *Journal of the American Medical Association, 305*(2), 167–174.

Goldman, S., Zadin, K., Moritz, T., Ovitt, T., Sethi, G., Copeland, J. G., et al. (2004). Long-term patency of saphenous vein and left internal mammary artery grafts after coronary artery bypass surgery: results from a Department of Veterans Affairs cooperative study. *Journal of the American College of Cardiology, 44*, 2149–2156.

Hannan, E. L., Wu, C., Walford, G., Culliford, A. T., Gold, J. P., Smith, C. R., et al. (2008). Drug-eluting stents vs. coronary artery bypass grafting in multivessel coronary disease. *New England Journal of Medicine, 358*, 331–334.

Hillis, L. D., Smith, P. K., Anderson, J. L., Bittl, J. A., Bridges, C. R., Byrne, J. G., et al. (2012). 2011 ACCF/AHA guideline for coronary artery bypass graft surgery: executive summary: a report of the American College of Cardiology Foundation/American Heart Association Task Force on Practice Guidelines. *Journal of Thoracic and Cardiovascular Surgery, 143*, 4–34.

Lamy, A., Devereaux, P. J., Prabhakaran, D., Taggart, D. P., Hu, S., Paolasso, E., et al. (2012). Off-pump or on-pump coronary-artery bypass grafting at 30 days. *New England Journal of Medicine, 366*(16), 1489–1497.

Levine, G. N., Bates, E. R., Bittl, J. A., Brindis, R. G., Fihn, S. D., Fleisher, L. A., et al. (2016). 2016 ACC/AHA guideline focused update on duration of dual antiplatelet therapy in patients with coronary artery disease. *Journal of the American College of Cardiology, 68*, 1082–1115. http://dx.doi.org/10.1016/j.jacc.2016.03.513.

McKhann, G. M., Grega, M. A., Borowicz, L. M., Jr., Bailey, M. M., Barry, S. J., Zeger, S. L., et al. (2005). Is there cognitive decline 1 year after CABG? Comparison with surgical and nonsurgical controls. *Neurology, 65*, 991–999.

Mohr, F. W., Morice, M. C., Kappetein, A. P., Feldman, T. E., Ståhle, E., Colombo, A., et al. (2013). Coronary artery bypass graft surgery versus percutaneous coronary intervention in patients with three-vessel disease and left main coronary disease: 5-year follow-up of the randomised, clinical SYNTAX trial. *Lancet, 381*(9867), 629–638. http://dx.doi.org/10.1016/S0140-6736(13)60141-5.

Shroyer, A. L., Grover, F. L., Hattler, B., Collins, J. F., McDonald, G. O., Kozora, E., et al. (2009). Veterans Affairs randomized on/off bypass (ROOBY) study group. On-pump versus off-pump coronary artery bypass surgery. *New England Journal of Medicine, 361*(19), 1827–1837.

Taggart, D. P., Altman, D. G., Gray, A. M., Lees, B., Nugara, F., Yu, L. M., et al. (2010). Randomized trial to compare bilateral vs. single internal mammary coronary artery bypass grafting: 1-year results of the Arterial Revascularisation Trial (ART). *European Heart Journal, 31*(20), 2470–2819.

III

Heart Failure and Cardiomyopathies

MYOCARDITIS

Catalina Sanchez Alvarez, Leslie T. Cooper

CHAPTER 21

1. **What is myocarditis?**
Myocarditis is an inflammatory disease of the myocardium, often characterized by a viral prodrome with subsequent cardiac signs and symptoms. The cardiac manifestations include acute heart failure, arrhythmias, atrioventricular block, sudden death, and chronic dilated cardiomyopathy.

There are different classifications based on etiologic, histologic, immunologic, and clinicopathologic criteria. The four clinicopathologic forms of myocarditis are

- Fulminant myocarditis
- Acute myocarditis
- Chronic active myocarditis
- Chronic persistent myocarditis

2. **What is the incidence of myocarditis?**
Myocarditis affects 22 per 100,000 people worldwide. The incidence of myocarditis in the community may be greater because this figure is estimated from hospital dismissal diagnosis codes. Fatal cases outside of a hospital and cases misdiagnosed as dilated cardiomyopathy (DCM) would add to the global disease burden. The heterogeneous clinical presentation of this disease and the lack of a highly sensitive and specific noninvasive diagnostic test confound estimation of the true impact of disease.

Myocarditis causes 9% to 16% of the cases of unexplained nonischemic DCM and 4% to 12% of sudden death in young athletes. Myocarditis has been reported in up to 12% of the autopsies performed for unexplained sudden death in Australia.

3. **What is the demographic presentation of myocarditis?**
The prevalence of myocarditis is slightly higher and the severity of disease slightly greater in men. Testosterone exacerbates myocarditis through proinflammatory pathways in the postviral phase in animal models. Myocarditis prevalence as a percent of all heart failure has two peaks, one within the first year of life and the second one between puberty and approximately age 40.

4. **What is the etiology of myocarditis?**
The primary causes of myocarditis are viral infections (Figs. 21.1 and 21.2) and a variety of toxic and noninfectious triggers. Until the 1990s coxsackievirus was the most prevalent virus associated with myocarditis; adenovirus became a common pathogen in the 1990s, and currently parvovirus B19 and human herpesvirus 6 are the most common viruses identified on endomyocardial biopsy (EMB). Other viruses such as human immunodeficiency virus (HIV) and hepatitis C have been linked with myocarditis in specific regions.

Primary bacteria associated with myocarditis include *Borrelia burgdorferi*, the cause of Lyme disease; *Corynebacterium diphtheriae*; and *Streptococcus viridans*. Parasitic infections, particularly Chagas disease, caused by *Trypanosoma cruzi*, is mainly found in central and northern South America.

Hypersensitivity myocarditis is an uncommon and underdiagnosed form of adverse drug reaction. The symptoms typically develop within 8 weeks after the initiation of a new medication but may occur up to 2 years later. Eosinophilia and elevated results on liver function tests are present in a substantial minority of cases. The symptoms usually resolve after withdrawal of the offending medication. Dobutamine has frequently been associated with this. Clozaril, sulfonylureas, and methyldopa are three of the more common medications associated with myocarditis.

Left ventricular (LV) giant cell myocarditis (GCM) is a rare, primarily autoimmune heart disease associated with ventricular arrhythmias and a poor prognosis.

The causes of myocarditis are given in Table 21.1.

5. **What is the pathogenesis of myocarditis?**
Most knowledge about the pathogenesis derives from experiments in susceptible murine strains of autoimmune or enteroviral myocarditis. Acute viral injury progresses to a chronic DCM through three phases: injury, activation of immunity with acute myocardial inflammation, and remodeling to DCM.

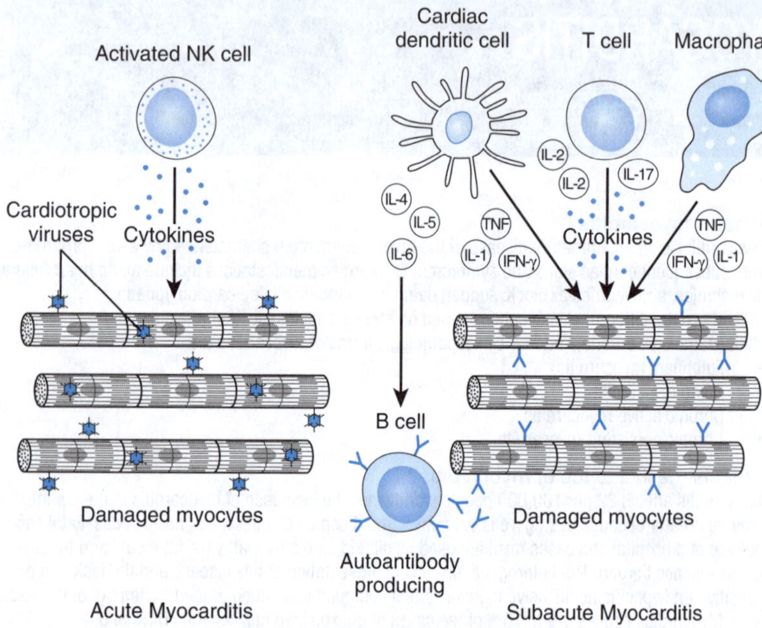

Fig. 21.1. Pathophysiology of viral myocarditis. After viral entry, virus replication leads to acute injury of the myocytes (acute myocarditis) and to activation of the host's immune system (subacute myocarditis). *IFN,* Interferon; *IL,* interleukin; *TNF,* tumor necrosis factor. *(Reproduced from Kindermann, I., Barth, C., Mahfoud, F., Ukena, C., Lenski, M., Yilmaz, A., et al. [2012]. Update on myocarditis.* Journal of the American College of Cardiology, 59*[9], 779–792.).*

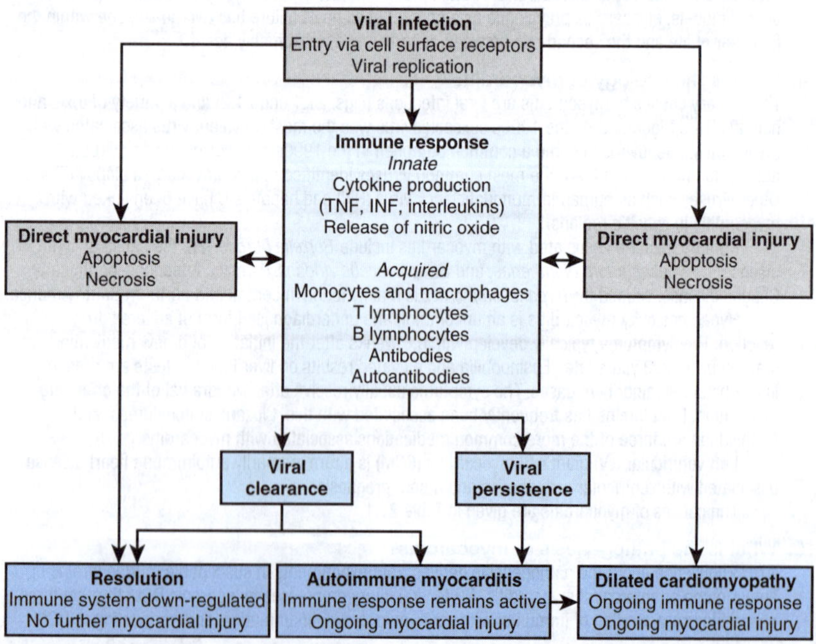

Fig. 21.2. Pathogenesis of viral myocarditis. *(Blauwet, L. A., & Cooper, L. T. [2010]. Myocarditis.* Progress in Cardiovascular Diseases, 52*[4], 274–288.)*

Table 21.1. Causes of Myocarditis

VIRUSES	BACTERIA	CARDIOTOXINS	HYPERSENSITIVITY
Adenovirus*	*Chlamydia*	Ethanol*	Cephalosporins
Coxsackievirus B*	Cholera	Anthracycline drugs*	Clozapine
Cytomegalovirus*	*Mycoplasma*	Arsenic	Diuretics
Epstein-Barr virus	*Neisseria*	Carbon monoxide	Insect bites
Hepatitis C virus	*Salmonella*	Catecholamines	Lithium
Herpes simplex virus	*Staphylococcus*	Cocaine*	Snake bites
HIV*	*Streptococcus*	Heavy metals	Sulfonamides
Influenza virus	Tetanus	Copper	Tetanus toxoid
Mumps	Tuberculosis	Mercury	Tetracycline
Parvovirus B19		Lead	
Poliovirus	**SPIROCHETES**	**PROTOZOA**	**SYSTEMIC DISORDERS**
Rabies	Leptospirosis	Chagas disease	Hypereosinophilia
Rubella	Lyme disease	Leishmaniasis	Kawasaki disease
Varicella zoster virus	Relapsing fever	Malaria	Sarcoidosis
Yellow fever	Syphilis		Wegener granulomatosis

HIV, Human immunodeficiency virus.
*Frequent cause of myocarditis.
From Elamm, C., Fairweather, D., Cooper, L. T. (2012). Pathogenesis and diagnosis of myocarditis. Heart, 98, 835–840.

- *Phase 1 (acute viral injury)*: After viral penetration and proliferation in the myocardium, a direct tissue injury signals damage the innate immune system.
- *Phase 2 (subacute immune)*: The innate immunity signals and forms an adaptive immune response characterized by upregulation of inflammatory mediators and ultimately antigen-specific T- and B-cell responses.
- *Phase 3 (chronic myopathic)*: Fibrosis from the initial injury response with or without chronic inflammation and persistent viral infection triggers ventricular remodeling in susceptible individuals.

The three phases of viral myocarditis are shown in Fig. 21.3. The inflammation and fibrosis in any of the phases can cause ventricular arrhythmias and heart block.

6. What is the clinical presentation?

The clinical presentation varies and often includes a viral prodrome with fever, arthralgia, and myalgias. Chest pain, palpitations, dyspnea, and—in severe cases—ventricular arrhythmias and cardiogenic shock develop. The following presentations form discrete clinical phenotypes:

- Acute coronary syndrome mimic: typical anginal chest pain, ST-segment elevation, elevated cardiac biomarkers, and sometimes impaired ventricular function (coronary artery disease [CAD] and other mechanisms of ischemia should be excluded in suspected cases of myocarditis).
- Myopericarditis
- New-onset or worsening heart failure symptoms, including dyspnea, peripheral edema, and ventricular dysfunction
- Life-threatening arrhythmias and sudden or aborted cardiac death

The clincopathologic classification of myocarditis is summarized in Table 21.2.

7. What is the clinical classification based on the level of diagnostic certainty?

The diagnosis of myocarditis traditionally has required a histologic diagnosis according to the 1986 Dallas criteria or immunohistology. However, owing to limited access to an EMB, myocarditis is significantly underdiagnosed. The following classification was proposed based on the level of certainty of diagnosis:

- *Possible subclinical acute myocarditis*: Patient with a suspected trigger for myocardial injury without cardiac symptoms but with at least one of the following: elevation of cardiac injury biomarkers, an electrocardiographic (ECG) pattern of injury, or new cardiac dysfunction on imaging

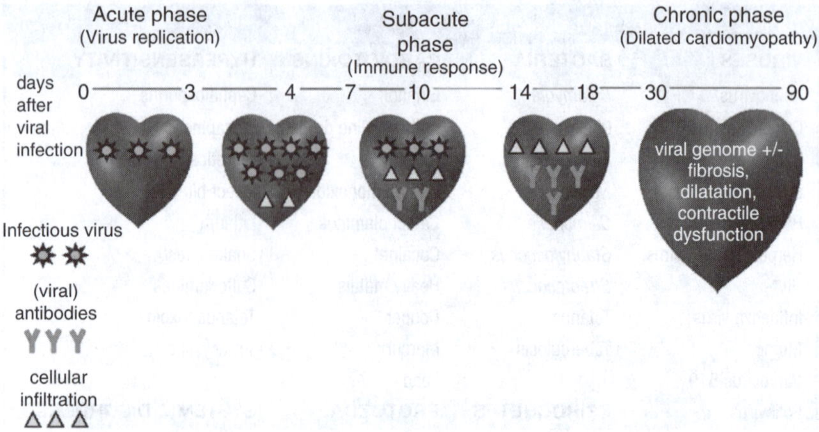

Fig. 21.3. Time course of viral myocarditis in three phases (derived from murine models). The acute phase of myocarditis takes only a few days, whereas the subacute and chronic phases cover a few weeks to several months. *(Modified from Kawai, C. [1999]. From myocarditis to cardiomyopathy: mechanisms of inflammation and cell death: learning from the past for the future.* Circulation, 99, *1091–1100. Image reproduced from Kindermann, I., Barth, C., Mahfoud, F., Ukena, C., Lenski, M., Yilmaz, A., et al. [2012]. Update on myocarditis.* Journal of the American College of Cardiology, 59*[9], 779–792.)*

Table 21.2. Clincopathologic Classification of Myocarditis

PARAMETERS CONSIDERED	FULMINANT	ACUTE	CHRONIC ACTIVE	CHRONIC PERSISTENT
Onset of cardiac symptoms	Abrupt	Insidious	Insidious	Insidious
Initial presentation	Cardiogenic shock	Heart failure with LV dysfunction	Heart failure with LV dysfunction	Asymptomatic and no LV dysfunction
Initial endomyocardial biopsy findings	Multiple foci of active myocarditis	Active or borderline myocarditis	Active or borderline myocarditis	Active or borderline myocarditis
Clinical course	Complete recovery or death	Incomplete recovery or chronic, stable DCM	Progressive end-stage DCM	Mild symptoms with stable LV function
Histologic course	Complete resolution	Complete resolution	Ongoing or resolving myocarditis; fibrosis and giant cells	Persistent inflammation with foci of myocyte necrosis
Response to immunosuppressive therapy	No benefit	Variable	Initial response followed by relapses	No benefit

DCM, Dilated cardiomyopathy; *LV*, left ventricle.

Permission obtained from Elsevier Ltd. Liberman, E. B., Hutchins, G. M., Herskowitz, A., Rose, N. R., & Baughman, K. L. (1991). Clinicopathologic description of myocarditis. Journal of the American College of Cardiology, 18, 1617–1626.

- *Probable acute myocarditis*: Patient with compatible cardiac symptoms and at least one of the following: elevation of cardiac biomarkers, ECG pattern of injury, or new cardiac dysfunction on imaging
- *Definite myocarditis*: Histologic or immunohistologic evidence of myocarditis

8. What blood tests can guide the diagnosis?

Blood tests that can guide the diagnosis include

- *Inflammatory markers*: Erythrocyte sedimentation rate (ESR) and C-reactive protein (CRP) are frequently elevated in myocarditis patients; however, these tests are neither sensitive nor specific.
- *Cardiac biomarkers*: Creatine kinase-MB isoenzyme (CK-MB) and troponin I are elevated in a minority of patients and are not specific for myocarditis. In hospitalized patients with fulminant myocarditis, a CK-MB above 29.5 ng/mL predicts inpatient mortality.

Cardiac troponin should be determined in all patients; however, a negative result should not rule out the diagnosis if there is high clinical suspicion.

9. What noninvasive diagnostic tests are useful in myocarditis?

Noninvasive diagnostic tests are useful in myocarditis

- *EKG* is recommended in the 2013 European Society of cardiology position statement on the management of myocarditis. Despite its low sensitivity (47%), an ECG may suggest a myocardial infarction–like pattern or pericarditis. The presence of atrioventricular (AV) block raises concern for Lyme disease, cardiac sarcoidosis, or GCM. QRS prolongation greater than 120 ms and Q waves are negative predictors of transplant-free survival.
- *Echocardiography*: All patients with suspected myocarditis should have a transthoracic echocardiogram (TTE) to assess ventricular function and exclude valvular and hemodynamic causes of heart failure. Wall motion abnormalities (e.g., basal septal aneurysm) in a noncoronary distribution suggest myocarditis. Right ventricular dysfunction at the time of presentation predicts greater risk of death or transplant. Patients with fulminant myocarditis requiring inotropes or mechanical circulatory support often have normal cardiac chamber dimensions and thickened walls compared with patients with an acute, less fulminant clinical course.
- *Cardiac MRI* is useful to distinguish ischemic from nonischemic cardiomyopathies. Patterns of T1 postgadolinium dynamic glucose-enhanced (DGE) signal abnormality correlated with histologic areas of viral myocarditis. The sensitivity of cardiovascular magnetic resonance (CMR) decreases with time from symptom onset. The Lake Louise Criteria recommend that both T1- and T2-weighted sequences be performed to predict the risk of cardiovascular death and ventricular arrhythmias following myocarditis.

10. Is viral serology useful?

No. Viral serology is limited because most viral infections associated with myocarditis are highly prevalent in the general population, resulting in a low specificity. Antibody levels may wane with time and do not correlate with myocardial viral genomes determined by polymerase chain reaction (PCR). Routine viral serology for the diagnosis of a specific pathogen in suspected acute myocarditis is not recommended.

11. What is giant cell myocarditis?

GCM is a rare and generally progressive cause of acute heart failure that primarily affects young and otherwise healthy patients. It is associated with thymoma and autoimmune diseases such as ulcerative colitis. GCM should be suspected when there is no response to optimal heart failure treatment and/or high-grade atrioventricular block and/or sustained ventricular arrhythmias.

The diagnosis is made by EMB demonstrating diffuse inflammation with T-cell predominance in association with eosinophils, histiocytes, and multinucleated giant cells.

12. What is the role of endomyocardial biopsy?

EMB remains the gold standard for the diagnosis of myocarditis; however, it is not indicated in all patients with this condition. The Dallas pathologic criteria require the first biopsy to have an inflammatory cellular infiltrate (borderline myocarditis) associated with myocyte necrosis (active myocarditis). EMB has a high specificity but a lower sensitivity that is likely due to sampling error. Focal involvement of the myocardium is typical in lymphocytic myocarditis and cardiac sarcoidosis and leads to frequent false-negative results. Biopsies from both the left and right ventricular wall increase the sensitivity, as does the use of electrogram guidance.

EMB should be performed when the results will likely affect management or prognosis. The most common reasons for EMB are clinically suspected GCM, cardiac sarcoidosis, or eosinophilic myocarditis. EMB is also used for the surveillance of allograft rejection following heart transplantation.

13. How is an endomyocardial biopsy performed?

The Stanford-Caves-Schultz and the King bioptomes access the right ventricle (RV) through the right internal jugular vein. A modified Cordis bioptome (B-18110, Medizintechnik Meiners, Monheim, Germany) or similar device with a long sheath is used for access from the right femoral vein. The femoral artery may be used as an access site for left ventricular biopsy. The right ventricular septum is the preferred initial site for EMB to minimize the risk of perforation. Fluoroscopic and/or echocardiographic guidance will be required to localize the site of biopsy. Endocardial voltage mapping has been used to identify biopsy sites in suspected arrhythmogenic right ventricular cardiomyopathy/dysplasia (ARVC/D) and cardiac sarcoidosis. Six to eight samples are generally obtained using the Stanford-Caves device. Up to 10 samples are obtained by investigators who use the Medizintechnik Meiners bioptome with smaller jaws. The sample must be handled carefully to minimize crush artifacts. The biopsy specimen should be transferred from the bioptome to fixative by using a sterile needle and not with forceps.

14. How is the endomyocardial biopsy tissue analyzed?

Specimen preparation depends on the clinical question to be answered. Standard histologic preparation for light microscopy can be used in the diagnosis of transplant rejection and myocarditis; this involves formalin fixation and paraffin wax embedding. Transmission electron microscopy requires glutaraldehyde fixation and can be helpful is the assessment of hydroxychloroquine or anthracycline drug toxicity as well as metabolic and storage disorders. PCR for viral DNA amplification is best performed on unfixed samples. An RNase inhibitor is often used to prevent degradation of RNA viral genomes. Molecular typing of amyloidosis (AL, ATTR, and Familial) is best performed with tandem mass spectroscopy with genotyping for familial transthyretin polymorphisms if indicated.

Examples of myocarditis at the microscopic level are shown in Fig. 21.4.

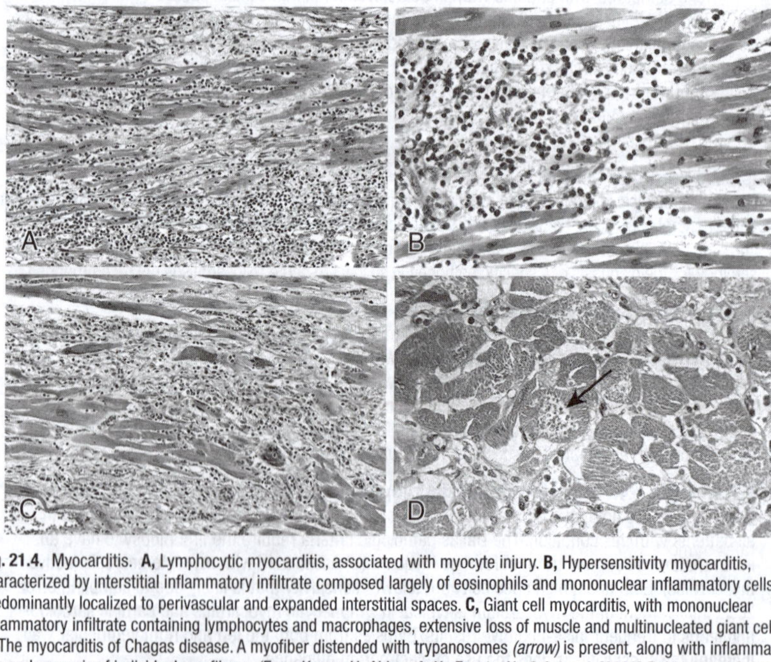

Fig. 21.4. Myocarditis. **A,** Lymphocytic myocarditis, associated with myocyte injury. **B,** Hypersensitivity myocarditis, characterized by interstitial inflammatory infiltrate composed largely of eosinophils and mononuclear inflammatory cells, predominantly localized to perivascular and expanded interstitial spaces. **C,** Giant cell myocarditis, with mononuclear inflammatory infiltrate containing lymphocytes and macrophages, extensive loss of muscle and multinucleated giant cells. **D,** The myocarditis of Chagas disease. A myofiber distended with trypanosomes *(arrow)* is present, along with inflammation and necrosis of individual myofibers. *(From Kumar, V., Abbas, A. K., Fausto, N., & Aster, J. [2009].* Robbins and Cotran pathologic basis of disease, professional edition *[8th ed.]. Philadelphia, PA: Saunders.)*

15. **What are the risks associated with an endomyocardial biopsy?**

Complications associated with the insertion of the sheath and biopsy have been reported in 1% to 6% of the procedures. However, the incidence of serious complications such as ventricular perforation is less than 1% when flexible bioptomes are used and the procedure is performed by experienced operators. Complications include hematoma in the puncture site, transient arrhythmias, tricuspid regurgitation, and less frequently occult pulmonary embolism. The incidence of tricuspid regurgitation is higher in patients who require multiple biopsies, as in transplant surveillance for cardiac rejection. To minimize risks, EMB should be guided by two-dimensional (2D) echocardiography, fluoroscopy, or both. In experienced centers the risk of complication is significantly lower.

16. **When is it appropriate to proceed with an endomyocardial biopsy?**

EMB is indicated only in disorders that cannot be diagnosed by less invasive methods. In 2007 an American College of Cardiology/American Heart Association/European Society of Cardiology (ACC/AHA/ESC) scientific statement outlined 13 clinical scenarios where EMB may be considered (Table 21.3). Only two scenarios received class I recommendations. A 2013 position statement of the European Society of Cardiology Working Group on Myocardial and Pericardial Diseases stated that all patients with clinically suspected myocarditis should be considered for selective coronary angiography and EMB ("should be considered" is class IIa language).

17. **What are the limitations of the endomyocardial biopsy? How can the sensitivity be increased?**

The two main limitations of EMB are limited availability of the procedure and low sensitivity. Postmortem analyses suggest that more than 17 samples are required to achieve a sensitivity of 80% with EMB.

Biopsies from the left ventricle (LV) provide a higher sensitivity in diagnosis than do those from the right ventricle (RV), owing to the more frequent involvement of the LV in myocarditis. The sensitivity can increase from 53% to 97.8% when EMB is done in both the LV and RV and immunoperoxidase stains are used to identify inflammation.

Localizing the inflammation through prior cardiac imaging can also improve the performance of EMB. Intracardiac electrograms have been used to identify areas of inflammation and fibrosis. Biopsy of the myocardium with 1.5- to 5.0-mV amplitude in the electrogram increases the likelihood of obtaining affected tissue.

18. **What is the treatment of myocarditis?**

The main treatment is supportive, guideline-based therapy for ventricular systolic dysfunction. The majority of the patients will improve with the recommended standard heart failure treatment with standard doses of beta-blockers, angiotensin-converting enzyme (ACE) inhibitors, and diuretics. Some patients will require hemodynamic support with inotropes; in selected cases, intra-aortic balloon pump or ventricular assist devices may also be necessary as bridges to recovery or transplantation.

Patients who present with symptomatic heart block or ventricular arrhythmias should be admitted to the hospital for ECG monitoring. In the majority of the patients with viral myocarditis, nonsustained arrhythmias will resolve after several weeks. A temporary external pacemaker or defibrillator vest may be used for short-term management. In the cases involving cardiac sarcoidosis and GCM, an implantable cardiac defibrillator may be considered early owing to the greater rate of ventricular arrhythmias.

Cardiomyopathy following acute viral infection is often diagnosed after the initial infection has been cleared; therefore antiviral therapy is not universally beneficial. In persistent virus-positive cardiomyopathy, beta interferon has been used with a successful response. At this time clinical trial data are not available.

Immunosuppressive therapy is recommended for acute cardiac sarcoidosis, GCM, and probably eosinophilic myocarditis. Routine immunosuppressive therapy of acute lymphocytic myocarditis is not recommended.

Treatment with nonsteroidal anti-inflammatory drugs (NSAIDs) has been associated with higher rates of mortality in animal models and therefore is not recommended.

19. **Should physical exercise be avoided in myocarditis?**

Yes; continuous aerobic exercise increases mortality in animal models of coxsackievirus group B myocarditis and in epidemiologic studies. Sustained aerobic physical activity should be avoided for a minimum of 3 months. The reinitiation of physical exercise depends on the recovery of ventricular dysfunction and absence of ventricular arrhythmias.

Table 21.3. The Role of Endomyocardial Biopsy in 14 Clinical Scenarios

SCENARIO NUMBER	CLINICAL SCENARIO	CLASS OF RECOMMENDATION	LEVEL OF EVIDENCE
1	New-onset heart failure of <2 weeks' duration associated with a normal-sized or dilated LV and hemodynamic compromise	I	B
2	New-onset heart failure of 2 weeks' to 3 months' duration associated with a dilated LV and new ventricular arrhythmias, second- or third-degree heart block, or failure to respond to usual care within 1 to 2 weeks	I	B
3	Heart failure of >3 months' duration associated with a dilated LV and new ventricular arrhythmias, second- or third-degree heart block, or failure to respond to usual care within 1 to 2 weeks	IIa	C
4	Heart failure associated with a DCM of any duration associated with suspected allergic reaction and/or eosinophilia	IIa	C
5	Heart failure associated with suspected anthracycline cardiomyopathy	IIa	C
6	Heart failure associated with unexplained restrictive cardiomyopathy	IIa	C
7	Suspected cardiac tumors	IIa	C
8	Unexplained cardiomyopathy in children	IIa	C
9	New-onset heart failure of 2 weeks' to 3 months' duration associated with a dilated LV, without new ventricular arrhythmias or second- or third-degree heart block, that responds to usual care within 1 to 2 weeks	IIb	B
10	Heart failure of >3 months' duration associated with a dilated LV, without new ventricular arrhythmias or second- or third-degree heart block, that responds to usual care within 1 to 2 weeks	IIb	C
11	Heart failure associated with unexplained HCM	IIb	C
12	Suspected ARVD/C	IIb	C
13	Unexplained ventricular arrhythmias	IIb	C
14	Unexplained atrial fibrillation	III	C

ARVD/C, Arrhythmogenic right ventricular dysplasia/cardiomyopathy; *DCM*, dilated cardiomyopathy; *HCM*, hypertrophic cardiomyopathy; *LV*, left ventricle.

Table from Cooper, L. T., Baughman, K. L., Feldman, A. M., Frustaci, A., Jessup, M., Kuhl, U., et al. (2007). The role of endomyocardial biopsy in the management of cardiovascular disease: a scientific statement from the American Heart Association, the American College of Cardiology, and the European Society of Cardiology. Endorsed by the Heart Failure Society of America and the Heart Failure Association of the European Society of Cardiology. Journal of the American College of Cardiology, 50*(19), 1914–1931.*

20. What are the outcomes, prognoses, and long-term sequelae in myocarditis?

Outcome varies based on the severity of the presentation, the etiology, and the host. The greater the LV end-diastolic diameter, the less likely it is that the ventricle will recover normal systolic function. One-third of patients with DCM due to myocarditis will recover within 1 year, and 25% to 40% will have long-term cardiac dysfunction. The risk of death or transplant is as high as 10% at 1 year.

Predictors of mortality and the need for cardiac transplantation include syncope at the time of presentation, greater ventricular systolic dysfunction, greater pulmonary hypertension, QRS greater than 120 ms, and Q waves in the ECG. Normal ventricular function is a predictor of good outcome. Despite a severe presentation, recovery after a period of hemodynamic support is not uncommon; therefore an implantable cardioverter defibrillator (ICD) is usually not indicated in the acute phase.

Bibliography and Suggested Readings

Blauwet, L. A., & Cooper, L. T. (2010). Myocarditis. *Progress in Cardiovascular Diseases*, *52*(4), 274–288.

Caforio, A. L., Pankuweit, S., Arbustini, E., Basso, C., Gimeno-Blanes, J., Felix, S. B., et al. (2013). Current state of knowledge on aetiology, diagnosis, management, and therapy of myocarditis: a position statement of the European Society of Cardiology Working Group on Myocardial and Pericardial Diseases. *European Heart Journal*, *34*(33), 2636–2648. 2648a–2648d. 10.1093/eurheartj/eht210. [Epub 2013 Jul 3].

Cooper, L., & Knowiton, K. U. (2015). Myocarditis. In *Braunwald's heart disease: a textbook of cardiovascular medicine* (10th ed.) (pp. 1589–1602). St. Louis, MO: Elsevier.

Cooper, L. T. (2009). Myocarditis. *New England Journal of Medicine*, *360*(15), 1526–1538.

Cooper, L. T., Baughman, K. L., Feldman, A. M., Frustaci, A., Jessup, M., Kuhl, U., et al. (2007). The role of endomyocardial biopsy in the management of cardiovascular disease: a scientific statement from the American Heart Association, the American College of Cardiology, and the European Society of Cardiology. Endorsed by the Heart Failure Society of America and the Heart Failure Association of the European Society of Cardiology. *Journal of the American College of Cardiology*, *50*(19), 1914–1931.

Dennert, R., Crijns, H. J., & Heymans, S. (2008). Acute viral myocarditis. *European Heart Journal*, *29*(17), 2073–2082.

Elamm, C., Fairweather, D., & Cooper, L. T. (2012). Pathogenesis and diagnosis of myocarditis. *Heart*, *98*(11), 835–840.

Friedrich, M. G., Sechtem, U., Schulz-Menger, J., Holmvang, G., Alakija, P., Cooper, L. T., et al. (2009). Cardiovascular magnetic resonance in myocarditis: a JACC white paper. *Journal of the American College of Cardiology*, *53*(17), 1475–1487.

From, A. M., Maleszewski, J. J., & Rihal, C. S. (2011). Current status of endomyocardial biopsy. *Mayo Clinic Proceedings*, *86*(11), 1095–1102.

GBD 2013 Mortality and Causes of Death Collaborators (2015). Global, regional, and national age-sex specific all-cause and cause-specific mortality for 240 causes of death, 1990–2013: a systematic analysis for the Global Burden of Disease Study 2013. *Lancet*, *385*(9963), 117–171.

Grün, S., Schumm, J., Greulich, S., Wagner, A., Schneider, S., Bruder, O., et al. (2012). Long-term follow-up of biopsy-proven viral myocarditis: predictors of mortality and incomplete recovery. *Journal of the American College of Cardiology*, *59*(18), 1604–1615.

Kindermann, I., Barth, C., Mahfoud, F., Ukena, C., Lenski, M., Yilmaz, A., et al. (2012). Update on myocarditis. *Journal of the American College of Cardiology*, *59*(9), 779–792.

Monney, P. A., Sekhri, N., Burchell, T., Knight, C., Davies, C., Deaner, A., et al. (2011). Acute myocarditis presenting as acute coronary syndrome: role of early cardiac magnetic resonance in its diagnosis. *Heart*, *97*(16), 1312–1318.

Sagar, S., Liu, P. P., & Cooper, L. T. (2012). Myocarditis. *Lancet*, *379*(9817), 738–747.

CHAPTER 22

DILATED CARDIOMYOPATHY

Shaden Khalaf, Glenn N. Levine, Biykem Bozkurt

1. What is dilated cardiomyopathy?

Dilated cardiomyopathy (DCM) is the unifying term that describes myocardial dysfunction with progressive ventricular wall thinning and dilation with concomitant reduction in function. The condition must occur in the absence of abnormal loading conditions (i.e., hypertension or valvular disease). DCM can be envisioned as the final common pathway for myriad cardiac disorders that damage the heart muscle or, alternatively, disrupt the ability of the myocardium to generate force and subsequently cause chamber dilation.

2. Are nonischemic cardiomyopathy and dilated cardiomyopathy the same?

Previously, DCM and nonischemic cardiomyopathy (NICM) have been used interchangeably. However, this has fallen out of favor. NICM includes myocardial dysfunction and systolic heart failure (HF) related to hypertension or valvular disease.

3. What are the incidence and prevalence of dilated cardiomyopathy?

The annual incidence of newly diagnosed DCM is approximately 5% to 8% per 100,000, with an age-adjusted prevalence of 36 cases per 100,000. In registries and clinical trials, DCM accounts for 30% to 40% of all patients.

DCM is a major cause of sudden death in young adults. The patients who are most frequently referred for heart transplantation are patients with DCM.

4. How does dilated cardiomyopathy present?

The presenting features of DCM are typical of HF and include symptoms of left ventricular (LV) failure including progressive exertional dyspnea, fatigue, reduced exercise tolerance, weakness, orthopnea, paroxysmal nocturnal dyspnea, and nocturnal cough. Physical examination can be notable for elevated jugular vein pressure (JVP), pulmonary congestion, and lower extremity edema. With progression of disease and development of right-sided dysfunction, patients can develop ascites, right-upper-quadrant abdominal pain, early satiety, postprandial fullness, and nausea. In advanced HF, cardiac cachexia may develop. A minority of patients (4% to 13%) with DCM are asymptomatic and diagnosed based on LV dysfunction and LV dilation.

5. What kinds of diagnostic studies should be obtained in patients with suspected dilated cardiomyopathy?

The diagnostic evaluation is similar to the evaluation of patients with ischemic HF and should include routine assessment of serum electrolytes, liver function tests, complete blood cell count, cardiac enzymes, serum natriuretic peptide levels (B-type natriuretic peptide [BNP] or N-terminal pro B-type natriuretic peptide [NT-proBNP]), chest radiograph, electrocardiogram, and assessment of LV function by echocardiography or radionuclide imaging.

Echocardiography typically shows four-chamber dilation, wall thinning, global hypokinesis, and left ventricular ejection fraction (LVEF) less than 35% to 40%. LV apical thrombi can be identified in up to 40% of patients with DCM. Tricuspid and mitral regurgitation may be present as a result of annular dilation and altered LV geometry. Doppler mitral inflow patterns may reveal elevated filling pressures.

Multigated radionuclide angiocardiography (MUGA) may be used to assess LV systolic function in those with poor echocardiographic windows. Compared with echo assessment of LVEF, MUGA may have less interobserver and intertest variability. Thallium-201 myocardial scintigraphy is not a reliable technique for differentiating patients with ischemic cardiomyopathy (ICM) from those with DCM, because patients with DCM may have both reversible and fixed perfusion abnormalities related to the presence of myocardial fibrosis, although a completely normal scan (without reversible or fixed defects) would favor the diagnosis of nonischemic cardiomyopathy.

Cardiac MRI (CMR) is a reasonable diagnostic modality to assess LVEF and volume when alternate studies are inconclusive. CMR is also an option when assessing myocardial infiltration or scar.

Table 22.1. Causes of Dilated Cardiomyopathy*

Genetic (familial)
Toxins (alcohol, cocaine, chemotherapy such as anthracycline, trastuzumab)
Inflammatory disorders (such as collagen vascular disease, hypersensitivity myocarditis)
Nutritional (thiamine and selenium deficiencies)
Peripartum cardiomyopathy
Endocrine (diabetes, hypothyroidism, and hyperthyroidism)
Tachycardia-mediated
Stress induced (takotsubo)
Chagas disease
Viral (post myocarditis, HIV-related)
Hemochromatosis, amyloidosis, sarcoidosis
"Non-DCM" causes of HFrEF (CAD, hypertension, valvular heart disease, congenital heart disease)

CAD, Coronary artery disease; *DCM*, dilated cardiomyopathy; *HFrEF*, heart failure with reduced ejection fraction; *HIV*, human immunodeficiency virus.

*DCM is the unifying term that describes myocardial dysfunction with progressive ventricular wall thinning and dilation with concomitant reduction in function occurring in the absence of abnormal loading conditions. The definition of DCM has evolved over time, and what is and is not considered a "DCM" may vary. Common causes of ventricular dilation and reduced systolic function that are not currently classified as DCM but that often result in similar end pathology include CAD (ischemic cardiomyopathy), hypertension, and valvular heart disease.

Cardiac catheterization may be performed if symptoms suggestive of ischemia are present or if coronary artery disease (CAD) is strongly suspected. Catheterization in DCM generally shows normal coronary arteries or mild, nonobstructive, isolated atherosclerotic lesions that are insufficient to explain the extent of cardiomyopathy.

Endomyocardial biopsy (EMB) may be performed if and only if a specific diagnosis is suspected in which specific therapy may be efficacious upon establishment of diagnosis.

Table 22.1 summarizes American College of Cardiology/American Heart Association (ACC/AHA) recommendations for noninvasive cardiac imaging in patients with HF.

6. What are the common causes of dilated cardiomyopathy?

Causes of DCM include genetic causes (familial cardiomyopathies), toxins (alcohol, cocaine, chemotherapy such as anthracycline, trastuzumab), infection (such as coxsackievirus, influenza virus, human immunodeficiency virus [HIV], *Trypanosoma cruzi*), inflammatory disorders (such as collagen vascular disease, hypersensitivity myocarditis), nutritional disorders (such as thiamine and selenium deficiencies, which may occur in patients with malabsorption disorders), pregnancy (also termed *peripartum* cardiomyopathy [PPCM]), endocrine disorders (such as diabetes, hypothyroidism, and hyperthyroidism), tachycardia, and stress-induced (takotsubo) cardiomyopathy. Causes of DCM are summarized in Table 22.2.

7. What are the features of alcohol-induced cardiomyopathy?

Alcohol-induced cardiomyopathy is said to occur when cardiomyopathy is noted in a heavy drinker in the absence of other causes (i.e., by exclusion). Alcoholic patients consuming more than 90 g of alcohol per day (approximately 7 to 8 standard drinks per day) for more than 5 years are at risk for this condition. Symptoms may develop with continued drinking. Approximately 20% of subjects with excessive drinking may demonstrate clinical HF. The typical patient is a man 30 to 55 years old who has been a heavy alcohol consumer for 10 years. Women may be more susceptible to the cardiodepressive effects of alcohol. Death rates are higher in African Americans (vs. Caucasians). Abstinence may partially or completely reverse the cardiomyopathy. Overall prognosis remains poor, with a mortality of 40% to 50% at 3 to 6 years without abstinence.

8. What are the features of cocaine-induced cardiomyopathy?

Approximately 4% to 18% of cocaine users have depressed LV function. Cardiac catheterization reveals normal or mildly diseased coronary arteries insufficient to explain the extent of myocardial dysfunction. Abstinence may lead to reversal.

Table 22.2. Summary of American College of Cardiology/American Heart Association Heart Failure Guideline Recommendations for Noninvasive Cardiac Imaging in Patients with Heart Failure

RECOMMENDATIONS	CLASS OF RECOMMENDATIONS	LEVEL OF EVIDENCE
Patients with suspected, acute, or new-onset HF should undergo a chest x-ray.	I	C
A two-dimensional echocardiogram with Doppler should be performed for initial evaluation of HF.	I	C
Repeat measurement of EF is useful in patients with HF who have had a significant change in clinical status or received treatment that might affect cardiac function or for consideration of device therapy,	I	C
Noninvasive imaging to detect myocardial ischemia and viability is reasonable in HF and CAD.	IIa	C
Viability assessment is reasonable before revascularization in HF patients with CAD.	IIa	B
Radionuclide ventriculography or MRI can be useful to assess LVEF and volume.	IIa	C
MRI is reasonable when assessing myocardial infiltration or scar.	IIa	B
Routine repeat measurement of LV function assessment should not be performed.	III: No benefit	B

CAD, Coronary artery disease; *EF*, ejection fraction; *HF*, heart failure; *LV*, left ventricular; *LVEF*, left ventricular ejection fraction; *MRI*, magnetic resonance imaging.

Adapted from Yancy, C. W., Jessup, M., Bozkurt, B., Butler, J., Casey, D. E. Jr., Drazner, M. H., et al. (2013). 2013 ACCF/AHA guideline for the management of heart failure: a report of the American College of Cardiology Foundation/American Heart Association Task Force on Practice Guidelines. Journal of the American College of Cardiology, 62, *e147–e239.*

9. What are the features of chemotherapy-induced cardiomyopathy?

Anthracyclines and trastuzumab are among the more prominent chemotherapeutic agents associated with cardiomyopathy. Three major types of anthracycline cardiotoxicities are distinguished: acute, chronic, and late onset, which differ considerably in clinical picture and prognosis. Cardiac failure is rare with acute toxicity. Chronic cardiotoxicity is observed in 0.4% to 23% several weeks or months after chemotherapy. Such anthracycline-induced cardiomyopathy carries a 27% to 61% mortality rate despite aggressive medical treatment. Late cardiotoxicity occurs years after chemotherapy at 5% at 10 years and presents as HF, arrhythmia, or conduction abnormalities.

The primary risk factor for cardiomyopathy is the cumulative dose administered. Toxicity is rare (less than 3%) with cumulative doses below 400 mg/m^2. Other risk factors include extremes of age and coexisting cardiac disease. Elevated cardiac troponin and brain natriuretic peptide after chemotherapy may allow identification of patients who may develop cardiac toxicity. Anthracyclines should not be administered to patients with a baseline LVEF of 30% or less. LV function should be assessed repeatedly before each subsequent dose (or if the initial ejection fraction [EF] is more than 50%, after a cumulative dose of 350 to 500 mg/m^2), and treatment stopped if EF declines by 10% or more or to a value less than 30% (or less than 50% if EF was normal at baseline). Reversibility has been documented anecdotally. The most effective protection is dexrazoxane (an iron chelator), with a twofold to threefold decrease in the risk of cardiomyopathy.

Trastuzumab is a monoclonal antibody that selectively binds human epidermal growth factor receptor-2 (HER2), which is expressed in 25% of cases of breast cancer. In earlier trials in advanced breast cancer, trastuzumab was associated with the development of HF in up to 27% of patients. Most of these patients, however, had received significant cumulative doses of anthracyclines or had preexisting cardiac disease. Risk factors for development of trastuzumab-associated HF include increasing age, lower LVEF, and higher anthracycline dose. Trastuzumab-associated HF responds better to standard therapy than anthracycline-induced HF, with complete recovery usually seen within 6 months of discontinuing trastuzumab.

10. What are the features of human immunodeficiency virus–related cardiomyopathy?

HIV-related cardiomyopathy accounts for up to 4% of DCM. The incidence is higher among patients with a CD4 count of less than 400 cells/mm^3. This diagnosis is less common with the advent of highly active antiretroviral therapy (HAART). Patients with HIV who are diagnosed with cardiomyopathy should be worked up for underlying CAD, nutritional deficiencies, and myocarditis secondary to opportunistic infections.

11. What are the associations between collagen vascular disease and dilated cardiomyopathies?

In systemic lupus erythematosus (SLE), global LV dysfunction has been reported in 5% of patients, segmental LV wall motion abnormalities in 4% of patients, and right ventricular enlargement in 4% of patients, but DCM is rare. In rheumatoid arthritis, symptomatic cardiac disease, including myocarditis, develops in 8% of patients. Progressive systemic sclerosis can rarely lead to HF through myocardial fibrosis, arrhythmia, or intermittent vascular spasm. Dermatomyositis may be associated with cardiomyopathy in some patients.

12. What is peripartum cardiomyopathy?

PPCM is the development of symptomatic HF in the last trimester of pregnancy or within 6 months of parturition. Other causes of DCM must be excluded in such patients before making the PPCM diagnosis. The cause is not well understood. PPCM occurs in 1 per 2289 to 4000 live births. Risk factors may include older age, multiparity, African American race, multiple gestation, toxemia, chronic hypertension, and use of tocolytics. In recent case series, up to 50% of PPCM developed with the first two pregnancies. Fifty percent of women recover baseline cardiac function within 6 months. Although the prognosis in subsequent pregnancies is better if cardiac function recovers, 21% of these patients will develop HF symptoms. The prognosis in subsequent pregnancies is poorer if cardiac function remains abnormal—37% deliver prematurely and 19% die. The Cardiac Disease in Pregnancy (CARPREG) Risk Score can be used to predict chances of cardiac complication in subsequent pregnancies.

Treatment is similar to other patients with cardiomyopathy, although one needs to weigh in on medication selection during pregnancy and lactation (e.g., substituting ACE-I and ARBs with nitrates/hydralazine for afterload reduction).

13. What are the features of tachycardia-induced cardiomyopathy?

Sustained elevated ventricular rates have been shown to cause changes in LV geometry and dilation. This condition should be considered in patients with no other explanation for LV dysfunction and a concomitant tachyarrhythmia. Hyperthyroid-induced sinus tachycardia or atrial fibrillation should be excluded in such patients. Treatment involves restoration of normal sinus rhythm or control of ventricular rate, with which there is typically resolution in as few as 4 to 6 weeks.

14. What are the features of nutritional causes of dilated cardiomyopathy?

Thiamine deficiency causes cardiovascular beriberi, in which the circulation is hyperkinetic and DCM results. Treatment for beriberi should consist of administration of thiamine along with standard HF therapy. DCM as a result of thiamine deficiency may occur with chronic alcoholism, anorexia nervosa, and malabsorption disorders and after gastric bypass.

15. What are the features of cardiomyopathy caused by iron overload?

Iron-overload cardiomyopathy occurs as a result of increased cardiac iron deposition, commonly in disorders such as hereditary hemochromatosis, secondary hemochromatosis (from repeated blood transfusions), and β-thalassemia major. Extracardiac manifestations typically precede symptomatic HF. Initially, the hemodynamic profile represents a restrictive pattern. As cardiomyopathy advances, DCM ensues. The diagnosis of iron overload is suggested by elevated serum ferritin and a ratio of iron to total iron-binding capacity of greater than 50%. The most definitive test for calculation of iron stores is measurement of iron concentration by liver biopsy. Magnetic resonance imaging (MRI) can be used to assess cardiac involvement in patients with hemochromatosis and DCM.

The mainstays of therapy are phlebotomy (in hereditary hemochromatosis) and chelation therapy (in secondary iron overload related to blood transfusions, prophylactically after transfusion of 20 to 30 units of red blood cells (RBCs), or when serum ferritin is more than 2500 ng/mL). Early diagnosis and treatment before tissue damage has occurred are essential, because life span seems to be normal in treated patients but markedly shortened in those who are not treated.

16. **Which patients with heart failure should be considered for endomyocardial biopsy?**
EMB is not commonly indicated in the evaluation of heart disease and should only be performed in specific clinical circumstances in which EMB results may meaningfully modify prognosis or guide treatment. Biopsy results are often nonspecific or unrevealing, and in most cases there is no specific therapy initiated based on the biopsy results. In 2007, a scientific statement by the AHA, ACC, and European Society of Cardiology (ESC) recommended that EMB be used selectively in a limited set of clinical scenarios. These recommendations are summarized in Table 22.3.

17. **What is the natural history of dilated cardiomyopathy?**
The natural history of DCM depends on the underlying cause. Generally, symptomatic patients have a 25% mortality at 1 year and 50% mortality at 5 years. The prognosis in those with asymptomatic LV dysfunction is less clear. Pump failure accounts for approximately 70% of deaths, whereas sudden cardiac death accounts for approximately 30%. Approximately 25% of symptomatic DCM patients will improve spontaneously. Idiopathic DCM has a lower total mortality compared with ischemic cardiomyopathy, although the risk of sudden death may be higher.

18. **What are the prognostic features of dilated cardiomyopathy?**
Many of the prognostic features are similar to those in ischemic cardiomyopathy, including age, LVEF, New York Heart Association (NYHA) class, lack of heart rate variability, elevated levels of neurohormones, and elevated markers of myocardial cell death. However, certain causes of DCM carry

Table 22.3. Summary of Recommendations for Performance of Endomyocardial Biopsy

EMB is recommended for
Unexplained new-onset HF of less than 2 weeks' duration associated with a normal size or DCM in addition to hemodynamic compromise
Unexplained new-onset HF of 2 weeks' to 3 months' duration associated with a dilated left ventricle and new ventricular arrhythmias, Mobitz type II second-degree AV block, third-degree AV block, or failure to respond to usual care within 1 to 2 weeks
EMB is reasonable for
Unexplained HF of more than 3 months' duration associated with a dilated left ventricle and new ventricular arrhythmias, Mobitz type II second-degree AV block, third-degree AV block, or failure to respond to usual care within 1 to 2 weeks
Unexplained HF with a DCM of any duration associated with a suspected allergic reaction in addition to eosinophilia
Unexplained HF associated with suspected anthracycline cardiomyopathy
HF associated with restrictive cardiomyopathy
Suspected cardiac tumors with the exception of typical myxomas
Unexplained cardiomyopathy in children
Unexplained new-onset HF of 2 weeks' to 3 months' duration associated with a DCM without new ventricular arrhythmias or AV block
Unexplained HF of more than 3 months' duration associated with a DCM without new ventricular arrhythmias or AV block that responds to usual care within 1 to 2 weeks
EMB can be considered for
HF associated with unexplained hypertrophic cardiomyopathy
Suspected arrhythmogenic right ventricular cardiomyopathy
Unexplained ventricular arrhythmias

AV, Atrioventricular; *DCM*, dilated cardiomyopathy; *EMB*, endomyocardial biopsy; *HF*, heart failure.
Adapted from Cooper, L. T., Baughman, K., Feldman, A. M., Frustaci, A., Jessup, M., Kuhl, U., et al. (2007). The role of endomyocardial biopsy in the management of cardiovascular disease: a scientific statement from the American Heart Association, the American College of Cardiology, and the European Society of Cardiology. Journal of the American College of Cardiology, 50, *1914–1931*.

a more favorable prognosis and are potentially reversible—for example, cardiomyopathy associated with alcohol, the peripartum state, trastuzumab, or tachycardia. Other causes, such as anthracyclines or HIV, have a worse prognosis.

19. **What are the pharmacologic treatments to be used in dilated cardiomyopathy?**
Similar to therapy for chronic stable HF, standard medical therapy with beta-blockers and angiotensin-converting enzyme (ACE) inhibitors (or angiotensin-receptor blockers) is indicated per current guidelines from the ACC/AHA. Intake of salt should be restricted. Depending on the circumstances, spironolactone, or a combination of isosorbide dinitrate and hydralazine may be added in symptomatic HF, and digoxin may be considered in some patients. Use of spironolactone should entail judicious adjustment of potassium supplements and close laboratory follow-up. Diuretics should be used to manage volume overload symptoms. Antiarrhythmic therapy is reserved for individualized treatment of symptomatic arrhythmias, especially for suppression of ventricular arrhythmias after an implantable cardioverter defibrillator (ICD).

20. **Should dilated cardiomyopathy patients be anticoagulated?**
Patients with DCM have multiple risk factors that predispose to thromboembolic events, with the incidence ranging from 0.8 to 2.5 per 100 patient-years. Pooled data from small, randomized, controlled clinical trials and current guidelines do not support routine anticoagulation in HF with sinus rhythm. The results of the Warfarin versus Aspirin in Reduced Cardiac Ejection Fraction (WARCEF) trial showed that in a large randomized comparison of aspirin versus warfarin in patients with HF and reduced EF (not in atrial fibrillation), there was no overall difference in the combined primary outcome of death, ischemic stroke, or intracranial hemorrhage between treatment groups. Available data do support the use of anticoagulants in the presence of atrial fibrillation, previous stroke or other thromboembolic events, or visible protruding or mobile thrombus on echocardiography.

21. **What is the role of exercise therapy?**
Exercise training should be considered in stable patients with DCM. Training has been shown to decrease symptoms, improve exercise tolerance, and improve quality of life beyond pharmacologic treatment. Long-term outcomes, however, are not entirely known, although small studies have shown reduction in mortality or readmission for HF. The Heart Failure and a Controlled Trial Investigating Outcomes of Exercise Training (HF-ACTION) trial failed to demonstrate a reduction in all-cause mortality or all-cause hospitalization in patients randomized to a structured exercise program when compared to "usual care," although secondary analysis did suggest some benefit.

22. **Should patients with dilated cardiomyopathy be prescribed statin therapy?**
In addition to lipid-lowering effects, statins have favorable effects on inflammation, oxidative stress, vascular performance, and possibly antiarrhythmic effects. However, two large randomized trials failed to demonstrate any benefit in patients with HF with reduced ejection fraction. Therefore, statin therapy is not recommended in patients with HF without CAD or other indications for statin therapy.

23. **When is device therapy (implantable cardioverter defibrillator or cardiac resynchronization therapy) recommended in patients with dilated cardiomyopathy?**
ICD implantation is routine in patients with DCM and prior sustained ventricular arrhythmia or sudden cardiac death. In patients with DCM, ICD implantation for the purposes of primary prevention is recommended (class I) in the following patients:

- Selected patients with LVEF of 35% or less and NYHA class II or III symptoms on chronic guideline-directed medical therapy (GDMT), who are expected to live longer than 1 year
- Selected patients with LVEF of 30% or less and NYHA class I symptoms on chronic GDMT, who are expected to live longer than 1 year

Cardiac resynchronization therapy (CRT), also referred to as biventricular pacing, has been shown to improve ejection fraction, symptoms, and even survival in some patients with DCM. CRT is indicated (class I recommendation) for patients who have LVEF of 35% or less, sinus rhythm, left bundle branch block (LBBB) with a QRS greater than 150 ms, and NYHA class II, III, or ambulatory IV symptoms on GDMT. Numerous class IIa (can be useful) and class IIb (may be considered) recommendations exist for patients who do not meet class I criteria. In general, this includes those with LVEF of less than 30% to 35% and QRS duration of 120 to 149 ms, with or without an LBBB.

Bibliography and Suggested Readings

Cooper, L. T., Baughman, K., Feldman, A. M., Frustaci, A., Jessup, M., Kuhl, U., et al. (2007). The role of endomyocardial biopsy in the management of cardiovascular disease: a scientific statement from the American Heart Association, the American College of Cardiology, and the European Society of Cardiology. *Journal of the American College of Cardiology, 50*, 1914–1931.

Homma, S., & Thompson, J. L. P. (February 3, 2012). *Results of the warfarin versus aspirin in reduced cardiac ejection fraction (WARCEF) trial. International stroke conference 2012.* New Orleans, LA: Abstract LB, 12–4372.

Kumar, S., Stevenson, W. G., & John, R. M. (2015). Arrhythmias in dilated cardiomyopathy. *Cardiac Electrophysiology Clinics, 7*(2), 221–233.

Merlo, M., Pivetta, A., Pinamonti, B., Stolfo, D., Zecchin, M., Barbati, G., et al. (2014). Long-term prognostic impact of therapeutic strategies in patients with idiopathic dilated cardiomyopathy: changing mortality over the last 30 years. *European Journal of Heart Failure, 16*(3), 317–324. http://dx.doi.org/10.1002/ejhf.16.

Rubis, P. (2015). The diagnostic work up of genetic and inflammatory dilated cardiomyopathy. *E-Journal of Cardiology Practice, 13*(19). http://www.escardio.org/Guidelines-&-Education/Journals-and-publications/ESC-journals-family/E-journal-of-Cardiology-Practice/Volume-13/The-diagnostic-work-up-of-genetic-and-inflammatory-dilated-cardiomyopathy.

Yancy, C. W., Jessup, M., Bozkurt, B., Butler, J., Casey, D. E., Jr., Drazner, M. H., et al. (2013). a report of the American College of Cardiology Foundation/American Heart Association Task Force on Practice Guidelines. *Journal of the American College of Cardiology, 62*(16): 1495–1539.

CHAPTER 23

HEART FAILURE WITH PRESERVED EJECTION FRACTION

Umair Khalid, Anita Deswal

1. What is diastolic dysfunction?

Diastolic dysfunction is a mechanical abnormality in the functioning of the myocardium during the diastolic phase of the cardiac cycle. It can occur with or without systolic dysfunction as well as with or without the clinical syndrome of heart failure (HF). Diastolic dysfunction may include abnormalities in left ventricular (LV) stiffness and relaxation that impair filling and/or result in elevated LV filling pressure, thus failing to achieve adequate LV preload (end-diastolic volume) at rest or during physiologic stress.

2. What is diastolic heart failure?

Diastolic HF is a clinical syndrome characterized by the signs and symptoms of HF, a preserved left ventricular ejection fraction (LVEF), and evidence of diastolic dysfunction. Earlier studies of patients with HF with preserved LVEF uniformly referred to this condition as *diastolic HF*, based on the premise that diastolic dysfunction was the sole mechanism for this syndrome. However, more recent studies suggest that a number of other abnormalities, both cardiac and noncardiac, may play important roles in the pathophysiology of HF with normal or near normal LVEF. Therefore the term *heart failure with preserved ejection fraction* (HFpEF) is more commonly used to refer to this clinical syndrome. According to the most recent American Heart Association/American College of Cardiology Foundation (AHA/ACC) HF guidelines of 2013, HF patients are classified as HFpEF if the LVEF is equal to or greater than 50%, and as HF with reduced ejection fraction (HFrEF) when the LVEF is equal to or less than 40%. Those patients with HF symptoms and LVEF between 40% and 50% fall in the intermediate or borderline group.

3. What is the prevalence of heart failure with preserved ejection fraction?

An estimated 5.7 million Americans over 20 years of age have HF based on data from the National Health and Nutrition Examination Survey of 2009–2012. There are some 870,000 new cases of HF annually, and projections suggest that by 2030 more than 8 million US adults will have a diagnosis of HF. Epidemiologic studies of various HF cohorts have documented a prevalence of HFpEF ranging from 40% to 71% (average about 50%). The prevalence of this condition is higher among women, and it is increasing overall as the population ages.

4. What are the morbidity and mortality associated with heart failure with preserved ejection fraction compared with heart failure with reduced ejection fraction?

Compared with age-matched controls without HF, patients with HFpEF have a significantly higher mortality. However, studies examining the risk of death in HF patients have demonstrated a somewhat lower or similar mortality in patients with HFpEF compared to patients with HFrEF. Once patients have been hospitalized for HF, the mortality in those with HFpEF may be as high as 22% to 29% at 1 year and approximately 65% at 5 years. Although survival has significantly improved over time for patients with HFrEF, there has been no similar improvement in survival for HFpEF patients.

In contrast to mortality, both groups have similar morbidity, as reflected by hospital admissions. Although the total or all-cause admissions are similar between these groups, patients with HFpEF have higher non-HF–related admissions, which are driven by the higher prevalence of noncardiac comorbidities in this population.

5. Which patients are at highest risk for developing heart failure with preserved ejection fraction?

Patients with HFpEF are generally elderly and are predominantly women (60% to 70%). The reasons for this female predominance are not entirely clear but may be related to the fact that women have a greater tendency for the left ventricle to hypertrophy in response to load and a lesser predisposition for the ventricle to dilate.

Hypertension is the most common cardiovascular condition associated with HFpEF. Hypertensive heart disease results in LV hypertrophy, with resultant impairment in relaxation and an increase in LV stiffness. Acute myocardial ischemia results in diastolic dysfunction, although its role in chronic diastolic dysfunction and chronic HFpEF remains uncertain. Valvular heart diseases, including regurgitant and stenotic aortic and mitral valve disease, can also result in the development of HFpEF.

Other recognized risk factors associated with HFpEF include obesity, diabetes mellitus, and renal insufficiency. Onset of atrial fibrillation with a rapid ventricular response rate may precipitate decompensation of HFpEF; the presence of diastolic dysfunction in general is a risk factor for the development of this arrhythmia as well.

6. What are the proposed pathophysiologic mechanisms of heart failure with preserved ejection fraction?

Diastolic dysfunction has been thought to be the major mechanism contributing to HFpEF, with abnormalities in active LV relaxation and in LV passive diastolic stiffness. LV relaxation is an active, energy-dependent process that may begin during the ejection phase of systole and continue throughout diastole.

On the other hand, LV stiffness stems from the passive viscoelastic properties that contribute to returning the ventricular myocardium to its resting force and length. These viscoelastic properties depend on both intracellular and extracellular structures. The greater the stiffness of the LV myocardium for any given change in LV volume during diastolic filling, the higher the corresponding diastolic LV filling pressures. In other words, in comparing a left ventricle with normal diastolic function with a left ventricle with diastolic dysfunction for any given left ventricle volume during diastole, LV pressure will be higher in the ventricle with diastolic dysfunction compared with one functioning normally. The net result of these processes is that LV diastolic pressures and thus left atrial (LA) pressures become elevated either at rest or during exercise, with a resultant elevation in pulmonary capillary wedge pressure and pulmonary vascular congestion.

Clinically this manifests as dyspnea at rest or with exertion, paroxysmal nocturnal dyspnea, and orthopnea. Furthermore, these stiffer hearts cannot increase end-diastolic volume and stroke volume via the Frank-Starling mechanism despite significantly elevated LV filling pressure. The resultant failure to increase cardiac output, which normally occurs with exercise, results in reduced exercise tolerance and fatigue.

Chronotropic incompetence with exercise is more commonly seen in the elderly and can contribute to a limitation in cardiac output during exercise, thus resulting in exertional fatigue.

Pulmonary hypertension is common in HFpEF. This may be related to both pulmonary venous and reactive pulmonary arterial hypertension in both HFpEF and HFrEF. Because the right ventricle (RV) is very sensitive to afterload, resting and exercise-induced pulmonary hypertension can contribute to progressive right ventricular dysfunction.

7. What factors can precipitate decompensated heart failure with preserved ejection fraction?

In patients with underlying diastolic dysfunction and other abnormalities detailed in question 6, acute decompensation of HF can be exacerbated by uncontrolled hypertension, atrial fibrillation or flutter (especially with rapid ventricular rates), myocardial ischemia, thyroid disorders, medication noncompliance (especially diuretics and antihypertensives), dietary indiscretion (e.g., high-sodium foods), anemia, and infection. In addition, the clinical manifestations of HFpEF in patients with the associated cardiovascular substrate often become manifest with the onset of chronic kidney disease, which can contribute to neurohormonal alterations as well as salt and water retention.

8. How is the diagnosis of heart failure with preserved ejection fraction made?

The clinical diagnosis of HFpEF depends on the presence of signs and symptoms of HF and documentation of LVEF (≥50%) by echocardiography, radionuclide ventriculography, contrast ventriculography, or cardiac magnetic resonance imaging (MRI).

9. What common tests are useful in the diagnosis of heart failure with preserved ejection fraction, and what do they often reveal?

- Routine laboratory analysis can help to identify renal failure or anemia as factors associated with decompensation, electrolyte abnormalities such as hyponatremia seen with HF, and bilirubin or transaminase elevation due to hepatic congestion. In addition, thyroid function tests can rule out hyperthyroidism (a consideration particularly in patients who develop atrial fibrillation) or hypothyroidism. Studies have shown that B-type natriuretic peptide (BNP) and N-terminal (NT) pro-BNP levels are elevated in HFpEF patients compared with persons without HF. However, BNP and NT-pro-BNP levels in HFpEF patients are usually lower than those of HFrEF patients. It should also be kept in mind that BNP levels increase with age and are higher in women, both of which are common features of HFpEF. Levels of BNP are also higher with worsening renal insufficiency. On the other hand, obesity is associated with lower levels of BNP, making the diagnosis of HFpEF more difficult in this group of patients, especially given the frequent association of obesity and HFpEF.

- The electrocardiogram (ECG) may demonstrate hypertrophy, ischemia, or arrhythmia.
- Chest radiographs may demonstrate cardiomegaly (as a result of hypertrophy), pulmonary venous congestion, pulmonary edema, or pleural effusions.
- Echocardiography can be used to assess ventricular function; atrial and ventricular size; hypertrophy; diastolic function and filling pressures (see Question 11); wall motion abnormalities; and pericardial, valvular, or myocardial (hypertrophic or infiltrative) disease. Echocardiography often demonstrates LV hypertrophy, enlarged left atrium, diastolic dysfunction, and pulmonary hypertension. LV volumes are usually normal or even small in HFpEF. Valvular heart disease such as significant aortic or mitral stenosis/regurgitation (MS/MR) can lead to a presentation of HFpEF but must be differentiated, because management often requires surgical intervention for the valvular pathology.

10. What is the clinical approach to further evaluate patients with heart failure with preserved ejection fraction?

The diagnostic algorithm based on the 2010 Heart Failure Society of America Heart Failure Practice Guidelines provides a systematic approach for the clinical workup and classification of HFpEF (Fig. 23.1). This framework addresses the common clinical conditions presenting as HFpEF, including hypertensive heart disease, hypertrophic cardiomyopathy, ischemic HF, valvular heart disease, infiltrative (restrictive) cardiomyopathy, pericardial constriction, high cardiac output state, and right ventricular dysfunction with cor pulmonale.

11. What tests are available for the evaluation of diastolic function?

Echocardiography with Doppler examination is a noninvasive method of evaluating diastolic function. In addition to the Doppler criteria for diastolic dysfunction, enlargement of the left atrium on two-dimensional (2D) echocardiography suggests the presence of significant diastolic dysfunction (in the absence of significant mitral valvular disease or chronic atrial fibrillation). The degree of LA enlargement estimated either by LA diameter or more accurately by LA volume is a marker of the severity and duration of diastolic dysfunction. Importantly, the lower LA function index, which is a function of LA emptying, portends a poor prognosis in HFpEF patients, which is independent of the severity of diastolic dysfunction and LA volumes.

Doppler measurements of mitral and pulmonary venous flow as well as Doppler tissue imaging (DTI), allow for determination of ventricular and atrial filling patterns and estimation of LV diastolic filling pressures. The normal transmitral filling pattern consists of early rapid filling (E wave) and atrial contraction (A wave). The contribution of each of these stages of diastole is expressed as the E/A ratio. Mitral annular tissue Doppler velocities (which measure tissue velocities rather than the conventional Doppler, which measures blood flow velocities) are relatively independent of preload conditions. Therefore the early diastolic filling annular tissue velocity (E') is a marker of LV relaxation and correlates well with hemodynamic catheter-derived values of tau. The ratio of the transmitral early filling velocity to the annular DTI early filling velocity (E/E') has been shown to estimate mean LA pressure. Using these various echocardiographic parameters, the severity of diastolic dysfunction and of elevated LV diastolic pressures can be assessed. These issues are also discussed in Chapter 7, on echocardiography. An algorithm for the diagnosis of LV diastolic dysfunction in patient with normal LV ejection fraction is presented in Fig. 23.2.

Cardiac catheterization with a high-fidelity pressure manometer allows for precise intracardiac pressure measurements. This information can be used to estimate the rate of LV relaxation by calculation of indices such as peak instantaneous LV pressure decline ($-dP/dt$ max) and the time constant of LV relaxation, tau. Estimation of LV myocardial stiffness requires simultaneous assessment of LV volume and pressure to evaluate the end-diastolic pressure-volume relationship. However, these measurements are invasive and cannot be performed on a routine basis. Therefore noninvasive markers of diastolic dysfunction are more commonly used in clinical practice.

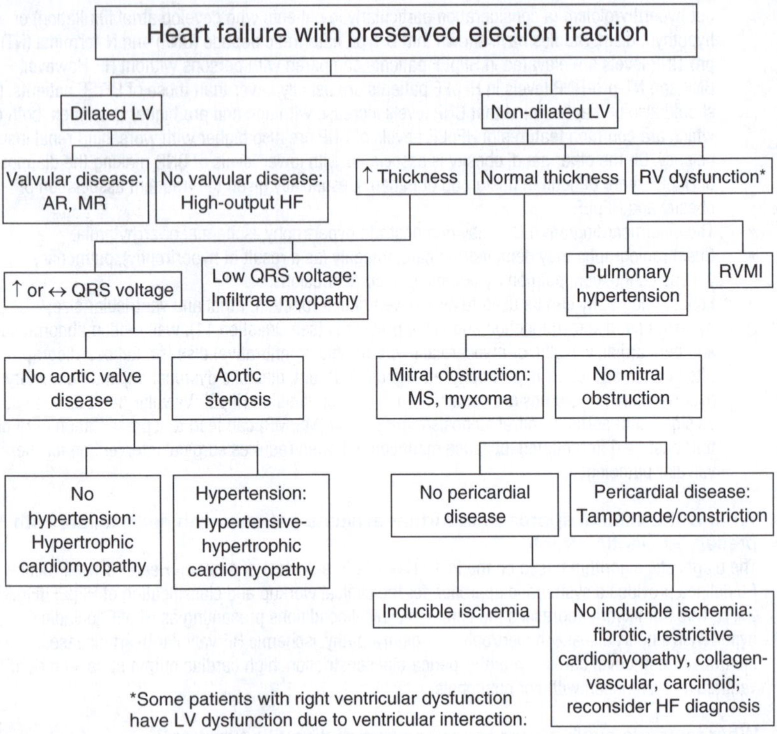

Fig. 23.1. Diagnostic considerations in patients with heart failure with preserved ejection fraction (HFpEF). *AR,* Aortic regurgitation; *HF,* heart failure; *LV,* left ventricle; *MR,* mitral regurgitation; *MS,* mitral stenosis; *RV,* right ventricle. *(Lindenfeld, J., Albert, N. M., Boehmer, J. P., Collins, S. P., Ezekowitz, J. A., Givertz, M. M., et al. [2010]. HFSA 2010 comprehensive heart failure practice guideline.* Journal of Cardiac Failure, 16, *e126–e133.)*

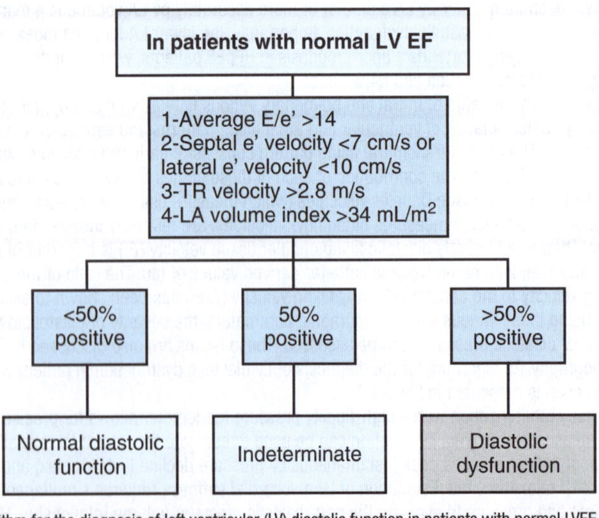

Fig. 23.2. Algorithm for the diagnosis of left ventricular (LV) diastolic function in patients with normal LVEF. *LA,* Left atrial; *LVEF,* left ventricular ejection fraction. *(Image from Nagueh, S. F., Smiseth, O. A., Appleton, C. P., Byrd, B. F. 3rd, Dokainish, H., Edvardsen, T., et al. [2016]. Recommendations for the evaluation of left ventricular diastolic function by echocardiography: an update from the American Society of Echocardiography and the European Association of Cardiovascular Imaging.* Journal of the American Society of Echocardiography, 29*(4), 277–314.)*

Nuclear imaging is another, less commonly used, noninvasive modality for evaluating diastolic dysfunction. Certain diastolic parameters such as peak filling rate (PFR) and time to peak rate (TTPR) can be calculated using this modality.

12. How do you treat acutely decompensated heart failure with preserved ejection fraction?

The cornerstones of treatment of acute decompensated HFpEF are blood pressure control, volume management, and treatment of exacerbating factors. These recommendations are highlighted in the 2013 ACC/AHA HF guidelines.

Systemic blood pressure control is of paramount importance because blood pressure directly affects LV diastolic pressure and thus LA pressures. The goal of blood pressure control is usually a systolic blood pressure less than 140/90 and possibly even less than 130/80 mm Hg.

Volume management in the inpatient setting often requires use of intravenous diuretics. Loop diuretics (e.g., furosemide) are the primary diuretic of choice but may be combined with thiazide-like diuretics (e.g., metolazone and chlorothiazide) for additional effect. Although treatment of pulmonary vascular congestion with diuresis is a primary goal of therapy, rapid or aggressive diuresis in some of these patients who have a combination of severe LV hypertrophy and small LV volume may result in development of hypotension and renal insufficiency. While a patient is undergoing diuresis, it is imperative to monitor electrolytes (particularly potassium, sodium, and magnesium), renal function (serum blood urea nitrogen [BUN] and creatinine), and clinical response (daily weights, meticulous fluid balance, blood pressure) and perform physical examinations (jugular venous distention, lung examination, and peripheral edema) in order to adjust diuretic doses appropriately.

Nitrates are thought to provide symptomatic benefit by reducing preload, leading to a reduction in ventricular filling pressures and pulmonary congestion. In acute decompensated HF, they can be used intravenously and may improve symptoms by reducing filling pressures as well as by controlling systemic hypertension. However, the role of nitrates in chronic HFpEF has been questioned based on recent data, as discussed in question 13.

Patients with significant volume overload and resistance to diuretics may benefit from ultrafiltration. Last, patients with advanced renal failure and volume overload who are refractory to diuretics may require urgent dialysis.

Evaluation and treatment of exacerbating factors form a crucial part of the treatment of acutely decompensated HFpEF. Uncontrolled atrial arrhythmias such as atrial fibrillation or atrial flutter can be detrimental in HFpEF. The combination of the loss of atrial contraction to LV diastolic filling and shortened diastolic filling time with tachycardia can cause marked elevation of mean LA pressure and result in pulmonary edema. Rate control alone with beta-blockers, nondihydropyridine calcium-channel blockers (verapamil or diltiazem), or digoxin, with a target heart rate less than 70 to 90 beats/minute at rest, may improve symptoms. When ventricular rates remain uncontrolled or there is inadequate response to the treatment of HF, direct current cardioversion with restoration of sinus rhythm may be beneficial. In addition to these measures, management of other factors such as myocardial ischemia, anemia, medical noncompliance, and infections is important in the treatment of the patient with HFpEF. It is also important to rule out significant valvular heart disease, which can precipitate decompensation and require surgical intervention, both for acute decompensation and for chronic HFpEF.

13. How do you treat patients with chronic heart failure with preserved ejection fraction?

Nonpharmacologic therapy for HFpEF is the same as therapy for HFrEF, including daily home monitoring of weight, compliance with medical treatment, dietary sodium restriction (2 to 3 g sodium daily), and close medical follow-up. As with HFrEF, structured exercise training improves exercise capacity and may lead to atrial reverse remodeling and improvement in LV diastolic function in HFpEF patients.

The clinical trials of HFpEF have failed to demonstrate the mortality and morbidity benefit of angiotensin-converting enzyme (ACE) inhibitors, and angiotensin receptor blockers (ARBs) seen in trials of HFrEF. This suggests fundamental differences in the pathophysiology underlying HFpEF and HFrEF.

The Treatment of Preserved Cardiac Function Heart Failure with an Aldosterone Antagonist (TOPCAT) trial investigated the effect of spironolactone versus placebo in HFpEF. After a mean follow-up of 3.3 years, there was no difference in primary composite outcome between the two groups, although HF hospitalizations were less frequent in the spironolactone group than in the placebo group. Subsequently a post hoc regional analysis demonstrated a lower rate of primary

Table 23.1. Treatment Recommendations for Patients with Chronic Heart Failure and Preserved Ejection Fraction

- Control of systolic and diastolic hypertension as per published hypertension guidelines
- Control of ventricular rate in atrial fibrillation
- Diuretics to control pulmonary congestion and peripheral edema
- Consider revascularization in patients with significant coronary artery disease and symptoms and/or demonstrable ischemia, where ischemia may be regarded as a contributor to abnormal cardiac function
- Restoration and maintenance of sinus rhythm in certain patients with atrial fibrillation may be useful to control symptoms
- Beta-blockers can be considered for HFpEF with
  - Prior myocardial infarction
  - Hypertension
  - Atrial fibrillation
- ACE inhibitors or ARBs can be considered for HFpEF with
  - Hypertension
  - Diabetes
  - Atherosclerotic vascular disease
- Calcium-channel blockers can be considered for HFpEF with
  - Atrial fibrillation requiring control of ventricular rate in whom blockers have proven inadequate: consider diltiazem or verapamil
  - Symptom-limiting angina
  - Hypertension: Consider amlodipine.
- Digitalis may be considered for rate control in atrial fibrillation if patient is not responsive to other agents listed above.

ARBs, Angiotensin receptor blockers; *HFpEF*, heart failure with preserved ejection fraction.

outcome with spironolactone in the Americas but not in patients enrolled from elsewhere. However, this was a subgroup analysis and, given the overall null results of the trial, can be considered hypothesis-generating. The spironolactone group had twice the rate of hyperkalemia and worse creatinine levels. Given that there are no other proven therapies that improve morbidity and mortality in HFpEF, it has been suggested that spironolactone could be used in selected patients with HFpEF who can also be monitored closely for changes in potassium and creatinine levels.

A recent trial investigated the effect of long-acting nitrates on activity tolerance in patients with chronic HFpEF and found such therapy did not improve quality of life or exercise capacity. The role of beta-blockers in the treatment of HFpEF is still uncertain. Beta-blockers may theoretically help in patients of HFpEF by preventing tachycardia and hence allowing more time for LV filling. They may also help by reducing myocardial oxygen demand and controlling blood pressure. However, a subgroup of HFpEF patients, often elderly, have chronotropic incompetence, which may contribute to exercise intolerance. No large trial with morbidity and mortality endpoints has been performed specifically in HFpEF patients, and the role of beta-blockers in improving morbidity and mortality in this patient group remains unknown.

HFpEF patients usually have several non–HF-related comorbidities. These comorbidities lead to non–HF-related admissions that are even higher than in HF with HFrEF. Overall, the comorbidities in the HFpEF population require aggressive management, as they have a significant impact on overall outcomes. The most common among these is hypertension. Its aggressive management is strongly recommended, especially as hypertension can lead to HFpEF. Also, treatment of atrial fibrillation and coronary artery disease should be performed as indicated by the guidelines. Some benefits have been observed in small trials with treatment of anemia and sleep-disordered breathing. Of course beta-blockers, ACE inhibitors, ARBs, and nitrates should be used as indicated for coexisting morbidities such as angina, atrial fibrillation, and hypertension (Table 23.1).

14. What are current class I recommendations for the treatment of heart failure with preserved ejection fraction?

The paucity of interventions that have clearly been demonstrated to reduce morbidity and mortality in patients with HFpEF is illustrated by the fact that there are only two ACC/AHA class I recommendations for the management of patients with stage C (symptomatic) HFpEF. They are

- Systolic and diastolic blood pressure should be controlled in accordance with published clinical practice guidelines to prevent morbidity.
- Diuretics should be used for relief of symptoms due to volume overload.

Bibliography, Suggested Readings, and Websites

Ahmed, A., Rich, M. W., Fleg, J. L., Zile, M. R., Young, J. B., Kitzman, D. W., et al. (2006). Effects of digoxin on morbidity and mortality in diastolic heart failure: the ancillary digitalis investigation group trial. *Circulation, 114*, 397–403.

Alehagen, U., Benson, L., Edner, M., Dahlström, U., & Lund, L. H. (2015). Association between use of statins and mortality in patients with heart failure and ejection fraction of ≥50. *Circulation: Heart Failure, 8*, 862–870.

Ather, S., Chan, W., Bozkurt, B., Aguilar, D., Ramasubbu, K., Zachariah, A. A., et al. (2012). Impact of non-cardiac comorbidities on morbidity and mortality in a predominantly male population with heart failure and preserved versus reduced ejection fraction. *Journal of the American College of Cardiology, 59*, 998–1006.

Borlaug, B. A., & Paulus, W. J. (2011). Heart failure with preserved ejection fraction: pathophysiology, diagnosis, and treatment. *European Heart Journal, 32*, 670–679.

Deswal, A. (2011). Treatment of heart failure with a positive ejection fraction. In D. L. Mann (Ed.), *Heart failure: a companion to Braunwald's heart disease.* St. Louis, MO: Elsevier Saunders.

Hogg, K., Swedberg, K., & McMurray, J. (2004). Heart failure with preserved left ventricular systolic function; epidemiology, clinical characteristics, and prognosis. *Journal of the American College of Cardiology, 43*, 317–327.

Lindenfeld, J., Albert, N. M., Boehmer, J. P., Collins, S. P., Ezekowitz, J. A., Givertz, M. M., et al. (2010). HFSA 2010 comprehensive heart failure practice guideline. *Journal of Cardiac Failure, 16*, e126–e133.

Mozaffarian, D., Benjamin, E. J., Go, A. S., Arnett, D. K., Blaha, M. J., Cushman, M., et al. (2015). Heart disease and stroke statistics—2015 update: a report from the American Heart Association. *Circulation, 131*(4), e29–e322.

Paulus, W. J., Tschöpe, C., Sanderson, J. E., Rusconi, C., Flachskampf, F. A., Rademakers, F. E., et al. (2007). How to diagnose diastolic heart failure: a consensus statement on the diagnosis of heart failure with normal left ventricular ejection fraction by the Heart Failure and Echocardiography Associations of the European Society of Cardiology. *European Heart Journal, 28*, 2539–2550.

Pitt, B., Pfeffer, M. A., Assmann, S. F., Boineau, R., Anand, I. S., Claggett, B., et al. (2014). Spironolactone for heart failure with preserved ejection fraction. *New England Journal of Medicine, 370*, 1383–1392.

Redfield, M. M., Anstrom, K. J., Levine, J. A., Koepp, G. A., Borlaug, B. A., Chen, H. H., et al. (2015). Isosorbide mononitrate in heart failure with preserved ejection fraction. *New England Journal of Medicine, 373*, 2314–2324.

Yancy, C. W., Jessup, M., Bozkurt, B., Butler, J., Casey, D. E., Jr., Drazner, M. H., et al. (2013). ACCF/AHA guideline for the management of heart failure: a report of the American College of Cardiology Foundation/American Heart Association Task Force on Practice Guidelines. *Journal of the American College of Cardiology, 62*, e147.

Yusuf, S., Pfeffer, M. A., Swedberg, K., Granger, C. B., Held, P., McMurray, J. J., et al. (2003). Effects of candesartan in patients with chronic heart failure and preserved left-ventricular ejection fraction: the CHARM-preserved trial. *Lancet, 362*, 777–781.

Zile, M. R., & Baicu, C. F. (2011). Alterations in ventricular function: diastolic heart failure. In D. L. Mann (Ed.), *Heart failure: a companion to Braunwald's heart disease.* St. Louis, MO: Elsevier Saunders.

CHAPTER 24

HYPERTROPHIC CARDIOMYOPATHY

Lothar Faber

1. What is hypertrophic cardiomyopathy?

Hypertrophic cardiomyopathy (HCM) is a primary cardiac disorder characterized by myocardial hypertrophy and a nondilated left ventricle (LV) in the absence of an accountable increase in cardiac afterload (i.e., aortic stenosis or systemic hypertension). Historically, and due to the fact that two basic phenotypes (i.e., with and without obstruction to outflow, discussed later) exist within the HCM spectrum, there has been a confusing array of names, such as idiopathic hypertrophic subaortic stenosis (IHSS) or muscular subaortic stenosis. Currently, *hypertrophic cardiomyopathy* is the preferred term.

2. What is the prevalence of hypertrophic cardiomyopathy?

The reported prevalence of HCM from epidemiologic studies is about 1:500 in the general population (0.2%). HCM affects men and women equally and occurs in many races and countries.

3. What are the genetic mutations that cause hypertrophic cardiomyopathy, and how are they transmitted?

Thus far, more than 1500 mutations in a wide array of genes have been identified that can cause HCM. These genes encode for cardiac sarcomere proteins that serve contractile, structural, and regulatory functions. HCM has therefore been conceptualized as a "sarcomeric disease." Mutant proteins are cardiac troponin T, cardiac troponin I, myosin regulatory light chain, myosin essential light chain, cardiac myosin binding protein C, alpha- and beta-cardiac myosin heavy chain, cardiac alpha actin, alpha tropomyosin, titin, and muscle LIM protein (MLP). Mutations in cardiac myosin binding protein C, beta-cardiac myosin heavy chain, and the troponin genes are the most common and account for about two-thirds of all mutations. HCM is inherited as an autosomal dominant trait; therefore, patients with HCM have a 50% chance of transmitting the disease to each of their offspring. However, penetrance is incomplete, meaning that not all gene carriers develop the full HCM phenotype. On the other hand, the HCM phenotype may also be caused by other disease entities like storage diseases and mutations in non-sarcomeric proteins.

4. Who should be screened for hypertrophic cardiomyopathy?

Patients with known HCM mutations, but without evidence of disease, and first-degree relatives of patients with HCM should be screened. Screening is performed primarily with history, physical examination, 12-lead ECG, and two-dimensional echocardiography. Traditionally, screening was performed on a 12- to 18-month basis, usually beginning by age 12 until age 18 to 21. However, it is now recognized that development of the HCM phenotype uncommonly can occur later in adulthood. Therefore, the current recommendation is to extend clinical surveillance into adulthood at about 5-year intervals or to undergo genetic testing (Table 24.1).

5. Who should undergo genetic testing?

Genetic testing has become recognized as an important aspect in the evaluation of HCM. It is strongly recommended that a careful family history is taken in patients diagnosed with HCM. A genetics specialist may be involved, in particular in families in whom sudden cardiac deaths have occurred. In an index patient, genetic testing is able to identify the disease-causing abnormality, which can then be used to identify the risk of developing HCM in first-degree family members. First-degree relatives of patients with HCM should undergo the aforementioned clinical screening with or without genetic testing based on genetic counseling. However, genetic testing is not helpful in first-degree family members of an HCM patient without identifiable pathologic mutation, and not all gene carriers develop the phenotype.

Table 24.1. Clinical Screening Strategies for Detection of Hypertrophic Cardiomyopathy in Families*

<12 years old
Optional unless
Malignant family history of premature HCM death or other adverse complications
Competitive athlete in an intense training program
Onset of symptoms
Other clinical suspicion of early LV hypertrophy
18-21 years old
Every 12-18 months
>21 years old
Probably approximately every 5 years or more frequent intervals with a family history of late-onset hypertrophic cardiomyopathy and/or malignant clinical course

HCM, Hypertrophic cardiomyopathy; *LV*, left ventricle.
*In the absence of laboratory-based genetic testing.
From Maron, B. J., Seidman, J. G., & Seidman, C. E. (2004). *Proposal for contemporary screening strategies in families with hypertrophic cardiomyopathy.* Journal of the American College of Cardiology, 44, *2125–2132.*

6. What are the histologic characteristics of hypertrophic cardiomyopathy?

The histology of HCM is characterized by hypertrophy of cardiac myocytes and myocardial fiber disarray. The abnormal myocytes contain bizarre-shaped nuclei and are arranged in disorganized patterns. The volume of the interstitial collagen matrix is greatly increased, and the arrangement of the matrix components is also disorganized. Myocardial disarray is seen in substantial portions of hypertrophied and nonhypertrophied LV myocardium. Almost all HCM patients have some degree of disarray, and in the majority, at least 5% of the myocardium is involved.

7. What are the common types of hypertrophic cardiomyopathies?

The distribution and severity of LV hypertrophy in patients with HCM can vary greatly. Even first-degree relatives with the same genetic mutation may show different patterns of hypertrophy. The most common site of hypertrophy is the anterior interventricular septum, which is seen in more than 80% of HCM patients and is known as asymmetric septal hypertrophy (ASH). Concentric LV hypertrophy, with maximal thickening at the level of the papillary muscles, is seen in 8% to 10%. A variant with primary involvement of the apex (apical HCM) is common in Japan and rare in the United States (less than 2%) and is characterized by spade-like deformity of the LV.

Not only the myocardium is affected in HCM; the mitral valve and its apparatus, including the papillary muscles, may show abnormalities like leaflet enlargement and thickening, atypical chordal attachment, or papillary muscle displacement. Occasionally, the right ventricle may be obstructed as well.

Two basic phenotypes exist within the HCM spectrum:

1. Obstructive HCM (OHCM). In the majority of cases (two-thirds), at rest or during provocation like physical exercise, left ventricular outflow is mechanically impeded due the thickening of the sub-aortic septum interacting with the mitral valve (discussed later) or by the thickened muscle itself.
2. Nonobstructive HCM (NHCM). In a minority of one-third, outflow is unobstructed at all times.

8. What are the most common symptoms in patients with hypertrophic cardiomyopathy?

Most patients with HCM have no or only minor symptoms and often are diagnosed during family screening. The most common symptoms are as follows:

- Dyspnea
  - Present in more than 90% of symptomatic patients
  - Caused mainly by LV diastolic dysfunction with impaired filling resulting from abnormal relaxation and increased chamber stiffness
  - Also caused by dynamic LV outflow tract obstruction leading to elevated intraventricular pressures
- Angina pectoris
  - May occur in both obstructive and nonobstructive HCM
  - Caused by a mismatch of supply and demand in myocardial perfusion
  - Several mechanisms have been proposed, including increased muscle mass and wall stress, decreased coronary perfusion pressure secondary to LV outflow obstruction,

Table 24.2. Clinical Parameters Used to Distinguish Hypertrophic Cardiomyopathy from Athlete's Heart

PARAMETERS	HYPERTROPHIC CARDIOMYOPATHY	ATHLETE'S HEART
LV wall thickness	>16 mm	<16 mm
Pattern of hypertrophy	Asymmetric, symmetric, or apical	Symmetric
LV end-diastolic dimension	<45 mm	>55 mm
Left atrium size	Enlarged	Normal
LV diastolic filling pattern	Impaired relaxation	Normal
Response to deconditioning	None	LV wall thickness decreases
ECG findings	Very high QRS voltage; Q waves; deep negative T waves	Criteria for LVH but without unusual features
Family history of HCM	Present	Absent
Sarcomeric protein mutation	Present	Absent

LV, Left ventricular; *LVH*, left ventricular hypertrophy.
Modified from Elliott, P. M., & McKenna, W. J. (2008). Diagnosis and evaluation of hypertrophic cardiomyopathy. Available from <www.UpToDate.com>. Accessed February 2008.

elevated diastolic filling pressures, systolic compression of large intramural coronary arteries, inadequate capillary density, impaired vasodilatory reserve, and abnormally narrowed small intramural coronary arteries

- Syncope and presyncope
  - Caused by inadequate cardiac output with exertion as a result of left ventricular outflow tract (LVOT) obstruction, small diastolic cavity size, or cardiac arrhythmia
  - Identifies patients at risk for sudden death

9. How is hypertrophic cardiomyopathy differentiated from athlete's heart?

Long-term athletic training can lead to cardiac hypertrophy, known as *athlete's heart.* This clinically benign physiologic condition must be differentiated from HCM, because HCM is the most common cause of sudden death in competitive athletes. Clinical parameters that support the diagnosis of HCM instead of athlete's heart are asymmetric hypertrophy greater than 16 mm, LV end-diastolic dimension less than 45 mm, enlarged left atrium, impaired LV relaxation on Doppler mitral valve inflow parameters and tissue Doppler echocardiography, absent response to deconditioning (e.g., hypertrophy does not regress with absence of exercise), family history of HCM, and sarcomeric protein mutation identified by genetic testing. These parameters are summarized in Table 24.2. In addition, athletes of African origin seem to be particularly prone to LV wall thickening, while women very rarely develop pronounced wall thickening.

10. Describe the classic murmur of obstructive hypertrophic cardiomyopathy and bedside maneuvers that differentiate it from other cardiac abnormalities.

The classic murmur of obstructive HCM is a harsh crescendo–decrescendo systolic murmur, heard best between the left sternal border and apex. It often radiates to the axilla and base but not into the neck vessels. Due to the dynamic nature of obstruction, a variety of provocative maneuvers can augment or suppress the murmur to help differentiate it from other systolic murmurs.

Maneuvers that increase intracardiac blood volume or decrease contractility typically lead to a decrease in murmur intensity, and maneuvers that decrease intracardiac blood volume or increase contractility lead to an increase in murmur intensity (Table 24.3).

11. How does the carotid pulse in obstructive hypertrophic cardiomyopathy differ from that in valvular aortic stenosis?

In patients with obstructive HCM, the carotid pulse has an initial brisk rise, followed by midsystolic decline as a result of LVOT obstruction, and then a second rise *(pulsus bisferiens).* In contrast, as a result of the fixed obstruction in aortic stenosis, the carotid upstroke is diminished in amplitude and delayed *(pulsus parvus and tardus).*

Table 24.3. Effect of Bedside Maneuvers on Systolic Murmurs

MANEUVER	HYPERTROPHIC CARDIOMYOPATHY	AORTIC STENOSIS	MITRAL REGURGITATION	VENTRICULAR SEPTAL DEFECT
Valsalva	↑	↓	↓	↓
Hand grip	↓	↓	↑	↑
Squatting	↓	↑	↑	↑
Amyl nitrite	↑	↑	↓	↓
Leg raise	↓	↑	↑	↑

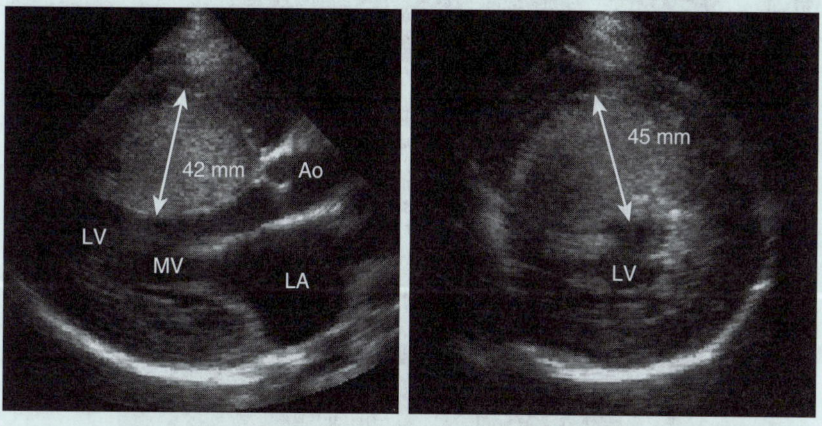

Fig. 24.1. Typical 2D-echo findings in hypertrophic cardiomyopathy with left atrial (LA) dilatation and marked left ventricular (LV) wall thickening, particularly involving the interventricular septum. *Ao*, Ascending aorta; *MV*, mitral valve. *(Reproduced with permission from Levine, G. N. [2014].* Color atlas of cardiovascular disease. *New Delhi, India: Jaypee Brothers Medical Publishers.)*

12. What noninvasive studies are helpful in making the diagnosis of hypertrophic cardiomyopathy?

The ECG is abnormal in the majority of patients with HCM; however, no particular changes are pathognomonic for HCM. The common abnormalities are ST-segment and T-wave changes, voltage criteria for left ventricular hypertrophy (LVH), prominent Q waves in the inferior (II, III, aVF) or precordial (V_2–V_6) leads, left axis deviation, and left atrial enlargement. Apical HCM, seen predominantly in Japanese patients, is characterized by giant negative T waves in the precordial leads.

Echocardiography is the primary and preferred diagnostic modality for HCM (Fig. 24.1). The cardinal feature is LVH with diastolic wall thickness 15 mm or greater. Other findings include a septal-to-posterior wall ratio of 1:3 or more (seen in patients with asymmetric septal hypertrophy), small LV cavity, reduced septal motion and thickening, normal or increased motion of the posterior wall, systolic anterior motion of the mitral leaflets, mitral regurgitation (mid- to late systolic), partial mid-systolic closure of the aortic valve with coarse fluttering of the leaflets in late systole, and features of diastolic LV dysfunction. In the setting of dynamic LVOT obstruction, a resting LVOT gradient may or may not be detected. A significant gradient is defined as a resting gradient more than 30 mm Hg and a provocable gradient more than 50 mm Hg. The LVOT Doppler signal in HCM is typically late peaking and is referred to as *dagger shaped* (Fig. 24.2).

Magnetic resonance imaging (MRI) is becoming a valuable tool to complement echocardiographic findings. It offers high-resolution images, three-dimensional imaging, and tissue characterization. MRI is especially useful to detect LVH in areas that may be difficult to assess by echocardiography or if the technical quality of echocardiographic images is inadequate, and to provide an assessment of cardiac fibrosis (Fig. 24.3).

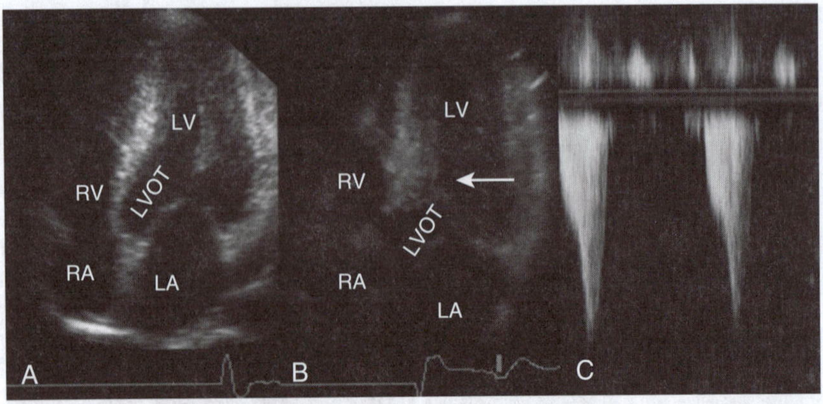

Fig. 24.2. 2D-echo findings in nonobstructive hypertrophic cardiomyopathy. **A,** Predominant thickening of the apical segments and a wide open, unobstructed outflow tract, and in obstructive hypertrophic cardiomyopathy (OHCM). **B,** A protruding subaortic septum making systolic contact with the mitral valve (systolic anterior motion [SAM] phenomenon, *arrow*). **C,** Typical late-peaking continuous-wave (cw)-Doppler LV outflow profile in OHCM indicating to dynamic nature of obstruction involving contracting muscle as opposed to the more symmetric signal of fixed valvular stenosis. The peak pressure gradient equals 4× (peak velocity)^2. *(Reproduced with permission from Levine, G. N. [2014].* Color atlas of cardiovascular disease. *New Delhi, India: Jaypee Brothers Medical Publishers.)*

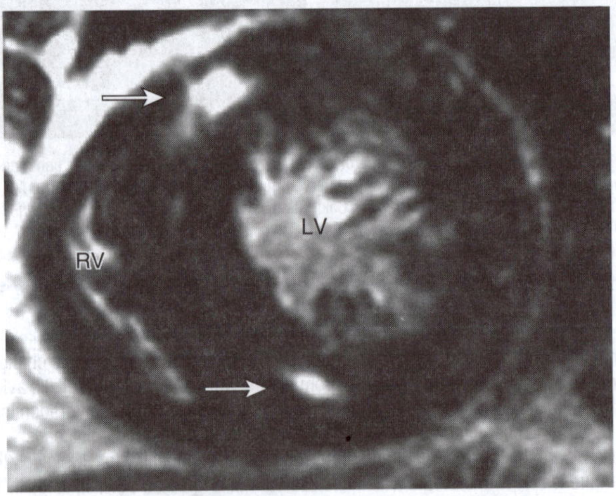

Fig. 24.3. Cardiac magnetic resonance imaging short-axis view in hypertrophic cardiomyopathy with two bright areas of gadolinium late enhancement near the left-right ventricular junction. *RV,* Right ventricle.

13. What is systolic anterior motion, and what causes it?

Systolic anterior motion (SAM) is the abnormal anterior displacement of the anterior mitral leaflet toward the septum during mid-systole (see Fig. 24.1). Several mechanisms have been proposed for SAM:

- The anterior mitral leaflet is drawn toward the septum by a Venturi effect produced by the lower pressure in the LVOT that occurs as blood is accelerated in a narrow outflow tract.
- The anterior mitral leaflet is pushed against the septum by blood flow abnormally attacking the valve from behind, resulting from the curvature of the hypertrophied septum or maloriented papillary muscles.

SAM typically results in a posteriorly directed, eccentric mitral regurgitation jet. Because SAM worsens during the course of systole, the mitral regurgitation also becomes more prominent during mid- to late systole.

14. Describe the mechanism of left ventricular outflow tract obstruction in hypertrophic cardiomyopathy.

LVOT obstruction in HCM is produced by SAM of the anterior mitral leaflet and mid-systolic contact with the hypertrophic ventricular septum (see Fig. 24.1). The magnitude of the subaortic gradient is directly related to the duration of contact between the mitral leaflet and the septum. The subaortic gradient is often dynamic and responds to provocative maneuvers in the same manner as the systolic murmur (see Question 9 and Table 24.3). Obstruction may also occur without SAM at a midcavity or even apical level, between the septum and thickened papillary muscles, or just following the distribution of the thickened wall segments. Occasionally, obstruction may also affect right ventricular outflow.

15. What are the characteristic hemodynamic findings during cardiac catheterization in obstructive hypertrophic cardiomyopathy?

Cardiac catheterization is not required for the diagnosis of HCM, and the diagnosis is usually made using noninvasive tests. Cardiac catheterization is generally reserved for assessment of coronary artery disease and evaluation before interventional or surgical procedures such as septal ablation or myectomy. The typical findings during cardiac catheterization are subaortic or mid-ventricular outflow gradient on catheter pullback, spike-and-dome pattern of aortic pressure tracing, elevated left atrial and LV end-diastolic pressures, elevated pulmonary capillary wedge pressure, increased V wave on wedge tracing (as a result of mitral regurgitation), and elevated pulmonary arterial pressure (Fig. 24.4).

16. What is the Brockenbrough-Braunwald sign?

Normally, following a premature ventricular contraction (PVC), with the subsequent sinus beat there is increased contractility and stroke volume, leading to an increase in the systolic blood pressure and thus an increase in the pulse pressure (the difference between systolic and diastolic pressure). However, in patients with HCM, the increased contractility after a PVC results in increased LVOT obstruction, leading to a decrease in stroke volume and systolic pressure and thus a decrease in pulse pressure. This phenomenon is known as the Brockenbrough-Braunwald sign (see Fig. 24.4).

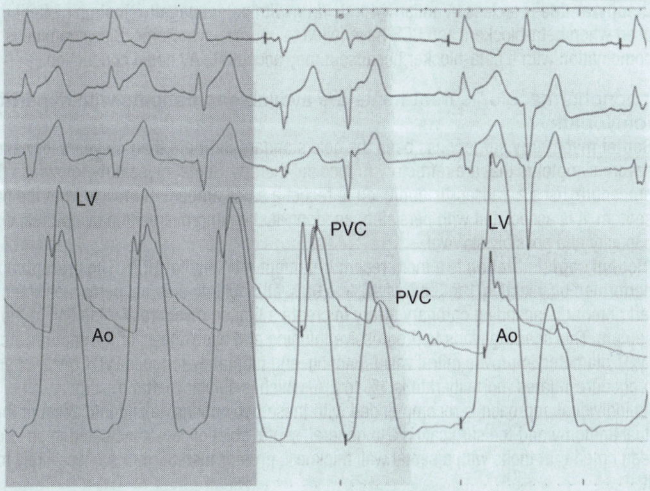

Fig. 24.4. Simultaneous pressure tracing from the left ventricle and the aorta demonstrating the increase of obstruction after a premature ventricular contraction (PVC). Note that the aortic pressure in the beat after the PVC is lower, due to the increased outflow obstruction.

17. What are the risk factors for sudden cardiac death in patients with hypertrophic cardiomyopathy?

Sudden cardiac death (SCD) is the most devastating consequence of HCM and is often the initial clinical manifestation in asymptomatic individuals. The most common cause of SCD in HCM patients is ventricular tachyarrhythmias. Several risk factors for SCD have been identified: prior cardiac arrest or sustained ventricular tachycardia (VT), family history of SCD, unexplained syncope, hypotensive blood pressure response to exercise, nonsustained VT on ambulatory (Holter) monitoring, identification of a high-risk mutant gene, and massive LVH with wall thickness 30 mm or greater. The magnitude of the outflow gradient and of left atrial dilatation has also been identified as being related to SCD risk.

18. What medications should generally be avoided in patients with obstructive hypertrophic cardiomyopathy?

Medications that decrease preload and afterload and increase contractility will worsen LVOT obstruction and therefore should be avoided.

- **Preload-reducing** agents are diuretics and nitroglycerin. Diuretics may be used cautiously in patients with persistent heart failure symptoms and volume overload.
- **Afterload-reducing** agents include dihydropyridine calcium channel blockers (CCB), nitroglycerin, angiotensin-converting enzyme (ACE) inhibitors, and angiotensin II receptor blockers.
- **Increased contractility** is produced by medications such as digoxin, dobutamine, and phosphodiesterase inhibitors (milrinone).

19. What are the pharmacologic therapies for patients with hypertrophic cardiomyopathy?

Pharmacologic therapy is primarily used to alleviate symptoms of heart failure, angina, and syncope in HCM patients. Routine pharmacologic therapy is not recommended in asymptomatic patients.

- **Beta-blockers** are generally considered first-line therapy for HCM. The beneficial effects of beta-blockers are mediated by their negative chronotropic property, which increases ventricular diastolic filling time, and by the negative inotropic property.
- **Nondihydropyridine CCB** is an alternative to beta-blockers in the treatment of HCM. Verapamil has been the most widely used CCB and improves symptoms by increasing LV relaxation and diastolic filling and by decreasing LV contractility. However, because of its vasodilatory effect, verapamil should be used cautiously in particular in patients with marked outflow obstruction. Diltiazem has been used less often but may improve LV diastolic function. Dihydropyridine CCBs should be avoided in patients with HCM because of their predominantly vasodilatory properties, which can result in worsening of the LVOT obstruction.
- **Disopyramide** is a class IA antiarrhythmic drug with potent negative inotropic effect that is used when beta-blockers and CCB have failed to improve symptoms. Disopyramide is used in combination with a beta-blocker because it may accelerate AV nodal conduction.

20. What nonpharmacologic treatments are available to patients with hypertrophic cardiomyopathy?

- **Septal myectomy** surgery has been the gold standard for more than 45 years for patients with severe symptoms that are refractory to medical therapy. Septal myectomy, known as the Morrow procedure, uses a transaortic approach to resect a small amount of muscle from the proximal septum. It is associated with persistent and long-lasting improvement in symptoms, exercise capacity and possibly survival.
- **Alcohol septal ablation** is a more recent treatment modality for HCM. The procedure is performed by injecting 1 to 3 mL of 96% to 98% ethanol into a septal perforator branch of the left anterior descending coronary artery to create a limited myocardial infarction in the proximal septum. This scarring leads to progressive thinning and hypokinesis of the septum, increases LVOT diameter, improves mitral valve function, and ultimately reduces LVOT obstruction. The procedure-related mortality rate is 1% to 2%, which is similar to that of surgery.

An individual approach is recommended with these two options, taking into account the individual anatomy and the surgical risk. In general, septal ablation is not indicated in children. It has also been noted that those with a septal wall thickness greater than 30 mm are less likely to receive benefit.

- **Dual-chamber pacing** was promoted to be an alternative to myectomy to improve symptoms and reduce LVOT obstruction in the early 1990s. However, subsequent randomized studies have shown that subjectively perceived symptomatic improvement was not accompanied by objective evidence of improved exercise capacity and may be due to a placebo effect. Dual-chamber pacing has a limited role in the contemporary management of HCM, mainly in the subgroup of elderly patients who are not candidates for myectomy or alcohol septal ablation (ASA).

21. What are the indications for an implantable cardioverter defibrillator in hypertrophic cardiomyopathy?

An implantable cardioverter defibrillator (ICD) is the preferred therapy for prevention of SCD in HCM patients. The recommended indications are as follows:

- ICD can be used for secondary prevention in survivors of cardiac arrest or sustained VT.
- ICD is indicated for high-risk patients, defined as having two or more of the major risk factors for SCD (see Question 16).
- In patients with one major risk factor, care needs to be individualized. The decision to implant an ICD should take into account the age of the patient, the strength of the risk factor, the level of risk acceptable to the patient and family, and the potential complications.
- ICD can be used in patients with end-stage HCM, characterized by LV systolic dysfunction, LV wall thinning, and chamber dilation.
- A risk calculation algorithm has been proposed by the European Society of Cardiology (http://www.doc2do.com/hcm/webHCM.html).

22. What is the natural history of hypertrophic cardiomyopathy?

The clinical course of patients with HCM is highly variable. Clinical manifestation can present at any age, from birth to age 90 or older. Many patients remain asymptomatic or mildly symptomatic for many years and achieve normal life expectancy. Others develop progressive symptoms of heart failure with exertional dyspnea and functional limitation despite medical therapy. Increase in LVH is predominantly seen in adolescents and young adults. In older adults, LV wall thickness generally remains stable. Approximately 5% to 10% of patients will progress to end-stage HCM as described earlier. Atrial fibrillation occurs in up to 30% of HCM patients and may lead to clinical deterioration. The annual mortality rate in patients with HCM is about 1% in adults and 2% in children.

Bibliography and Suggested Readings

Elliott, P. M., Anastasakis, A., Borger, M. A., Borggrefe, M., Cecchi, F., Charron, P., et al. (2014). 2014 ESC guidelines on diagnosis and management of hypertrophic cardiomyopathy. *European Heart Journal.* http://dx.doi.org/10.1093/eurheartj/ehu284.

Fatkin, D., Seidman, J. G., & Seidman, C. E. (2007). Hypertrophic cardiomyopathy. In J. T. Willerson, J. N. Cohn, H. J. J. Wellens, & D. R. Holmes (Eds.), *Cardiovascular medicine* (3rd ed.). London: Springer.

Gersh, B. J., Maron, B. J., Bonow, R. O., Dearani, J. A., Fifer, M. A., Link, M. S., et al. (2011). 2011 ACCF/AHA guideline for the diagnosis and treatment of hypertrophic cardiomyopathy: a report of the American College of Cardiology Foundation/American Heart Association Task Force on practice guidelines. *Circulation, 124*(24), e783–e831.

Kimmelstiel, C. D., & Maron, B. J. (2004). Role of percutaneous septal ablation in hypertrophic obstructive cardiomyopathy. *Circulation, 109*(4), 452–456.

Maron, B. J. (2002). Hypertrophic cardiomyopathy: a systematic review. *Journal of the American Medical Association, 287*(10), 1308–1320.

Maron, B. J., Zipes, D. P., et al. (2008). *Hypertrophic cardiomyopathy Braunwald's heart disease* (8th ed.), Philadelphia, USA: Elsevier.

Maron, B. J., Dearani, J. A., Ommen, S. R., Maron, M. S., Schaff, H. V., Gersh, B. J., et al. (2004). The case for surgery in obstructive hypertrophic cardiomyopathy. *Journal of the American College of Cardiology, 44*(10), 2044–2053.

Maron, B. J., & Pelliccia, A. (2006). The heart of trained athletes: cardiac remodeling and the risks of sports, including sudden death. *Circulation, 114*, 1633–1644.

Maron, B. J., Seidman, J. G., & Seidman, C. E. (2004). Proposal for contemporary screening strategies in families with hypertrophic cardiomyopathy. *Journal of the American College of Cardiology, 44*, 2125–2132.

Ommen, S. R., Maron, B. J., Olivotto, I., Maron, M. S., Cecchi, F., Betocchi, S., et al. (2005). Long-term effects of surgical septal myectomy on survival in patients with obstructive hypertrophic cardiomyopathy. *Journal of the American College of Cardiology, 46*(3), 470–476.

Richard, P., Charron, P., Carrier, L., Ledeuil, C., Cheav, T., Pichereau, C., et al. (2003). Hypertrophic cardiomyopathy: distribution of disease genes, spectrum of mutations, and implications for a molecular diagnosis strategy. *Circulation, 107*(17), 2227–2232.

Sherrid, M. V., Barac, I., McKenna, W. J., Elliott, P. M., Dickie, S., Chojnowska, L., et al. (2005). Multicenter study of the efficacy and safety of disopyramide in obstructive hypertrophic cardiomyopathy. *Journal of the American College of Cardiology, 45*(8), 1251–1258.

CHAPTER 25

RESTRICTIVE CARDIOMYOPATHY

Stuart B. Prenner, Sanjiv J. Shah

1. **What is the basic pathophysiology in restrictive cardiomyopathy?**
The basic pathophysiology in restrictive cardiomyopathy is increased *stiffness* of the ventricular walls as a result of myocardial disease, leading to impaired diastolic filling of the ventricles. The result is a steep rise in pressure with small increases in volume (preload). Ejection fraction is usually preserved in most cases at least in the early stages but can become severely impaired in end-stage disease, particularly in cardiac amyloidosis. The condition can affect either or both of the ventricles, and they may not be uniformly affected.

2. **What are the main causes of restrictive cardiomyopathy?**
Approximately half the cases of restrictive cardiomyopathy have an identifiable cause. The most common identifiable cause is myocardial infiltration from amyloidosis. Other infiltrative diseases include sarcoidosis, Gaucher's disease, and Hurler's disease. Storage diseases include hemochromatosis, glycogen storage disease, and Fabry's disease. Hydroxychloroquine, which is commonly used to treated connective tissue diseases, can cause cardiotoxicity (typically after prolonged use), which results in a restrictive cardiomyopathy. Myocardial damage from radiation and anthracycline toxicity can lead to restrictive cardiomyopathy, as can endomyocardial involvement from endomyocardial fibrosis. Although restrictive cardiomyopathy is a rather uncommon cause of heart failure in North America and Europe, it is a relatively common cause of heart failure and death worldwide due to a much higher incidence of endomyocardial fibrosis in tropical regions, including parts of Africa, Central and South America, India, and other parts of Asia. Causes of restrictive cardiomyopathy are summarized in Table 25.1.

Secondary restrictive physiology develops in the advanced stages of all forms of heart disease, including dilated, hypertensive, and ischemic cardiomyopathy. While both are associated with elevated left ventricular (LV) filling pressures, one should be sure to distinguish "restrictive cardiomyopathy" from "restrictive physiology" (as may be reported in an echocardiogram report).

3. **What are the usual echocardiographic findings in restrictive cardiomyopathy?**
Echocardiography usually demonstrates normal or near-normal LV ejection fraction, ventricles of normal or decreased volumes, increased ventricular wall thickness, impaired ventricular relaxation and filling (*diastolic dysfunction,* which is typically at an advanced stage), and biatrial enlargement (Fig. 25.1).

Most restrictive cardiomyopathies preferentially affect the subendocardium of the heart. Therefore, on tissue Doppler imaging and speckle-tracking echocardiography, tissue velocities and longitudinal strain, respectively, are severely reduced, reflecting severe longitudinal systolic and diastolic dysfunction of the heart. If an infiltrative process is present, the myocardium may appear brighter than normal, with a sparkling or grainy appearance on echocardiography.

On Doppler echocardiography, one observes accentuated early diastolic filling of the ventricles (prominent E wave), shortened deceleration time, and diminished atrial filling (diminutive A wave), resulting in a high E-to-A wave ratio on the mitral inflow velocities (Fig. 25.2).

4. **How does amyloidosis affect the heart?**
As with other organs, in amyloidosis there may be protein deposition in myocardial tissue. The term *amyloidosis* was reportedly coined by Virchow and means "starch-like." The myocardium is found to be firm, rubbery, and noncompliant. This protein deposition leads to *restrictive physiology*, as well as severely impaired longitudinal systolic function (with eventual reduction in LV ejection fraction in some patients) and possible conduction abnormalities. The most common forms of cardiac amyloidosis include primary immunoglobulin light chain (AL) amyloidosis due to plasma cell dyscrasias; familial amyloid cardiomyopathy due to mutations in the transthyretin (TTR) gene (most commonly the

Table 25.1. Classification of Types of Restrictive Cardiomyopathies According to Cause

Infiltrative
Amyloidosis
Sarcoidosis
Gaucher's disease
Hurler's disease
Storage disease
Hemochromatosis
Fabry disease
Glycogen storage diseases
Endomyocardial
Endomyocardial fibrosis
Prior chest radiation
Hypereosinophilic syndrome (Löffler's endocarditis)
Carcinoid syndrome
Myocardial noninfiltrative
Idiopathic restrictive cardiomyopathy
Diabetic cardiomyopathy
Familial restrictive cardiomyopathy
Hypertrophic cardiomyopathy
Hemochromatosis
Systemic sclerosis*
Transplant rejection
Anthracycline toxicity
Chloroquine and hydroxychloroquine cardiotoxicity

*Note that restrictive cardiomyopathy in patients with systemic sclerosis can mimic an "infiltrative" appearance, but the protein that is causing this appearance is collagen.

Adapted from Falk, R. H., & Hershberger, R. E. (2015). The dilated, restrictive, and infiltrative cardiomyopathies. In D. L. Mann, D. P. Zipes, P. Libby, & R. O. Bonow (Ed.), Braunwald's heart disease: a textbook of cardiovascular medicine *(10th ed.). Philadelphia, PA: Saunders.*

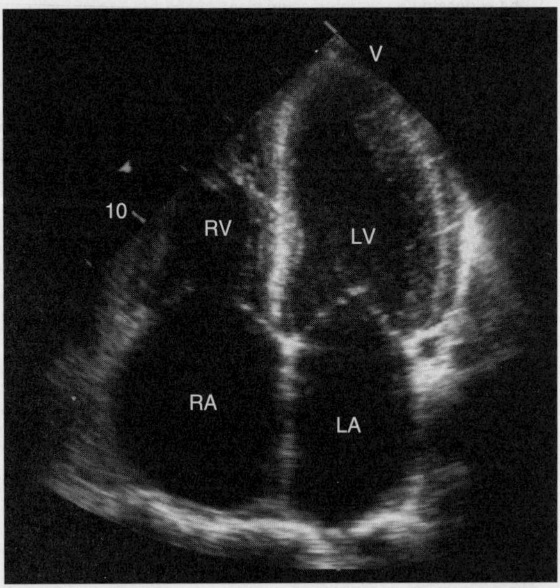

Fig. 25.1. Apical four-chamber view echocardiogram of a patient with restrictive cardiomyopathy demonstrating dilated atria and normal-sized ventricles. *LA*, Left atrium; *LV*, left ventricle; *RA*, right atrium; *RV*, right ventricle.

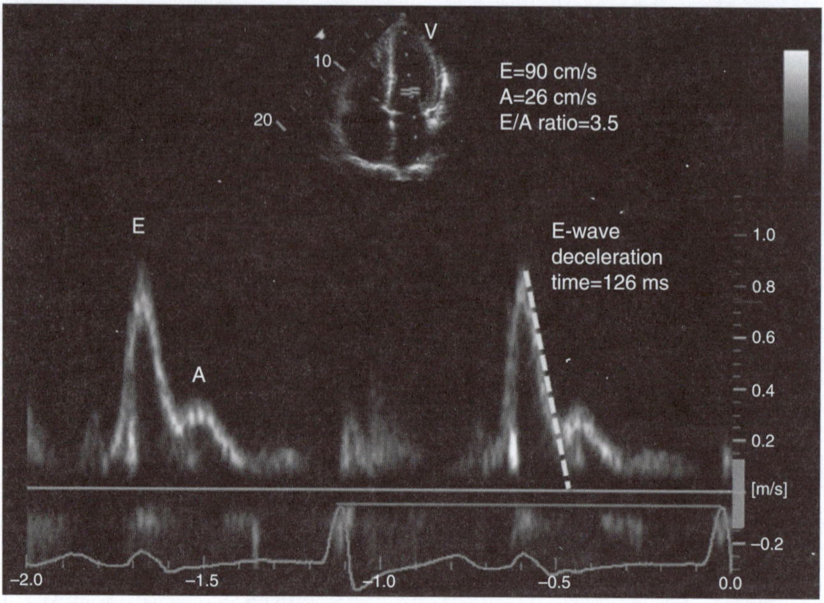

Fig. 25.2. Mitral inflow pattern in a patient with restrictive cardiomyopathy showing augmented early filling E wave (E) with shortened deceleration time and attenuated A waves (A).

V122I mutation, which is present in 3% to 4% of African Americans); and senile (wild-type) cardiac amyloidosis due to excessive deposition of wild-type TTR protein in the heart.

5. **How is cardiac amyloidosis diagnosed?**
If the patient is not otherwise known to have systemic amyloidosis, cardiac amyloidosis may be suggested by symptoms and signs of heart failure as well as an echocardiogram that demonstrates a restrictive filling pattern (grade 3 diastolic dysfunction) and often thickened ventricular walls with a "sparkling" pattern on echocardiography (Fig. 25.3). The classic finding of thickened ventricular walls yet inappropriately normal or even low voltage on the electrocardiogram is common.

On tissue Doppler imaging, s′, a′, and e′ velocities can be severely reduced (Fig. 25.4), which is also associated with the "cherry-on-the-top sign" on the speckle-tracking echocardiography bull's-eye map, reflective of severely reduced longitudinal strain at the LV base with relative preservation of longitudinal strain at the apex (Fig. 25.5).

Cardiac magnetic resonance imaging (MRI) can also reveal diffuse subendocardial hyperenhancement representing infiltration with amyloid protein. The diagnosis is usually confirmed, if necessary, by endomyocardial biopsy or with biopsy of another involved organ and the above cardiac findings.

Radionuclide imaging showing increased cardiac uptake of technetium-99m (^{99m}Tc) pyrophosphate in cardiac amyloidosis can also be used to make the diagnosis and is highly specific for TTR forms of cardiac amyloidosis.

6. **What are the main cardiac manifestations of sarcoidosis?**
Sarcoidosis can lead to non-caseating granulomas infiltrating the myocardium leading to fibrosis and scar formation. Infiltration may be patchy throughout the myocardium, and as a result biopsy yield is often lower than in other infiltrative processes. Cardiac MRI (Fig. 25.6) may reveal delayed hyper-enhancement with a patchy distribution in the subepicardium, with sparing of the subendocardium, and is often more intense on the right ventricular side of the septum. The hyper-enhancement does not conform to the distribution of a coronary artery territory. MRI may also reveal areas of thinned myocardium. However, MRI cannot reliably distinguish between active and inactive ("burned out") sarcoidosis.

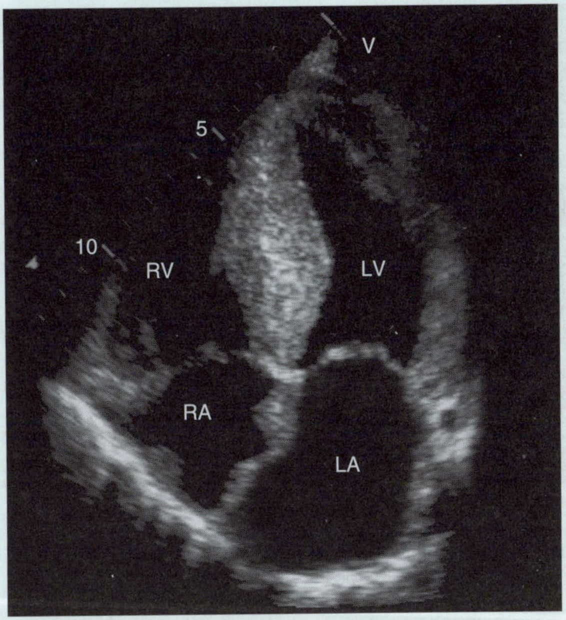

Fig. 25.3. Echocardiogram demonstrating the *sparkling* pattern that can be seen in patients with cardiac amyloidosis. *LA*, Left atrium; *LV*, left ventricle; *RA*, right atrium; *RV*, right ventricle.

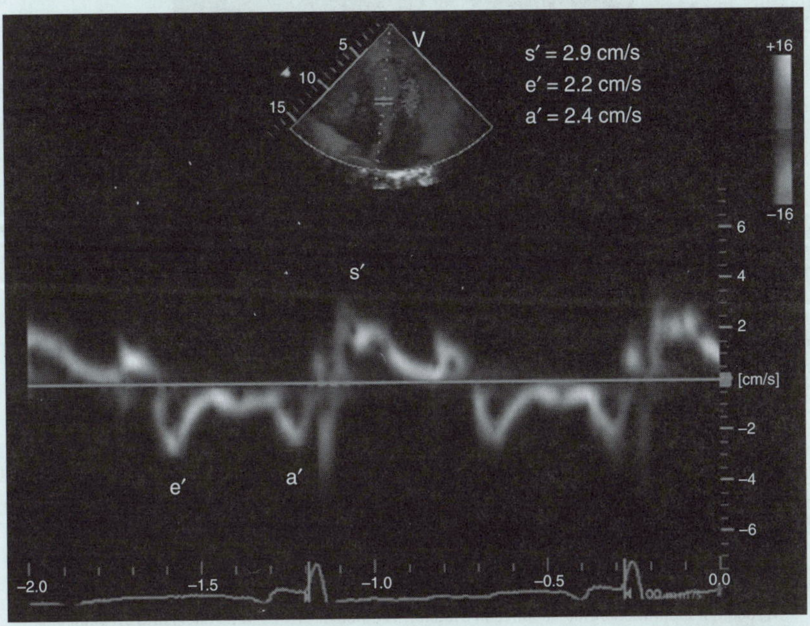

Fig. 25.4. Tissue Doppler imaging demonstrates severely reduced systolic (s′), early diastolic (e′), and late diastolic (a′) longitudinal tissue velocities in cardiac amyloidosis.

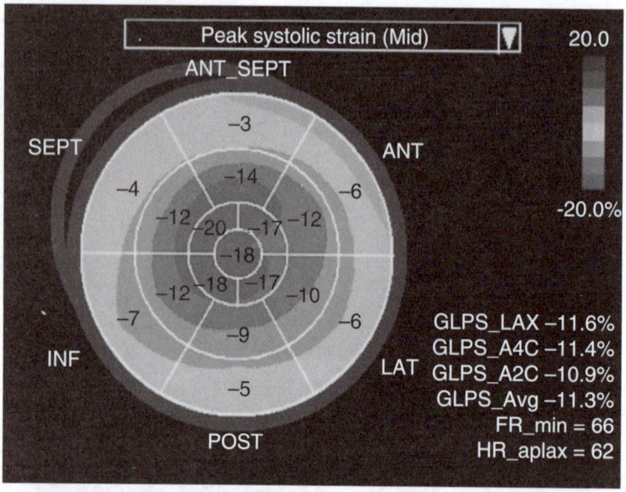

Fig. 25.5. Longitudinal strain analysis bull's-eye map of the left ventricle shows preserved apical strain (center of the bull's-eye) with impaired mid and basal strain (outer portions of the bull's-eye), resulting in the hallmark "cherry on top" pattern in cardiac amyloidosis (when shown in full color, the darker portion in the center of the bulls eye image is typically red while the basal segments are white or light blue).

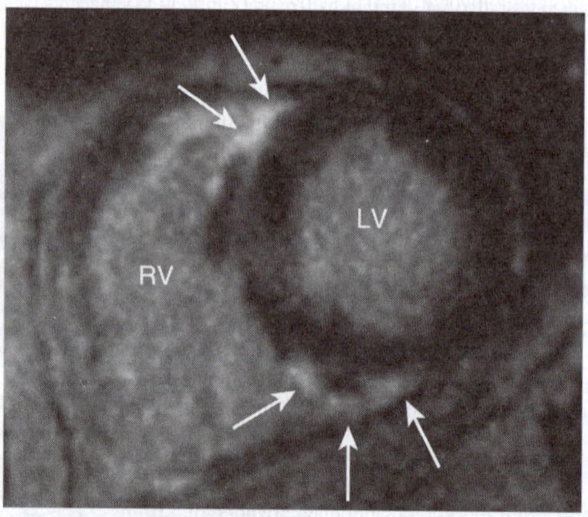

Fig. 25.6. Cardiac MRI in a patient with cardiac sarcoidosis demonstrating patchy delayed hyper-enhancement. In the image the hyper-enhancement appears as bright white areas *(arrows)*. *LV*, Left ventricle; *RV*, right ventricle.

Cardiac 18-fluoro-deoxyglucose positron emission tomography (FDG-PET) scanning is the imaging modality of choice for the identification of active cardiac sarcoidosis. If performed appropriately (i.e., after 24 hours of a very low-glucose, high-fat diet), cardiac FDG-PET will demonstrate patchy abnormal uptake in the affected segments of the myocardium (Fig. 25.7).

Myocardial infiltration in the setting of sarcoidosis can lead to heart block and syncope (as a result of infiltration of the conduction system), ventricular arrhythmias (including syncope and sudden death), as well as heart failure. Polymorphic nonsustained ventricular tachycardia or ventricular premature beats without evidence of myocardial ischemia can be a clue to the presence

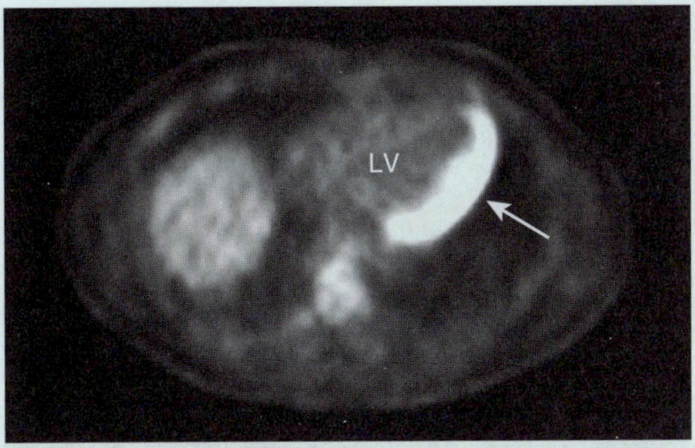

Fig. 25.7. Cardiac FDG-PET imaging showing intense uptake in the lateral wall *(arrow)* of the left ventricle (LV) indicative of active cardiac sarcoidosis.

of sarcoidosis. Pulmonary involvement may lead to pulmonary hypertension and its associated effects on right-sided heart function.

7. **Is endomyocardial biopsy useful in cases of suspected restrictive cardiomyopathy?**
Endomyocardial biopsy is considered *reasonable* in the setting of heart failure associated with unexplained restrictive cardiomyopathy. It is a class IIa, level of evidence C, recommendation in the scientific statement on endomyocardial biopsy by the American College of Cardiology/American Heart Association/European Society of Cardiology (ACC/AHA). Endomyocardial biopsy may reveal specific disorders, such as amyloidosis or hemochromatosis, or myocardial fibrosis and myocyte hypertrophy consistent with idiopathic restrictive cardiomyopathy. Endomyocardial biopsy should not be performed if computed tomography (CT) or MRI suggests the patient instead has constrictive pericarditis or if other less invasive tests and studies can identify a specific cause of the restrictive cardiomyopathy.

8. **Is cardiac computed tomography or cardiac magnetic resonance imaging useful in cases of possible restrictive cardiomyopathy?**
Both cardiac CT and cardiac MRI can be useful in cases of restrictive cardiomyopathy. Both imaging modalities can demonstrate a thickened pericardium, which may suggest constrictive pericarditis rather than restrictive cardiomyopathy. Cardiac MRI, through delayed hyper-enhancement, may demonstrate patterns particular to specific diseases, including sarcoidosis, eosinophilic endomyocardial disease, hemochromatosis, amyloidosis, and other causes of restrictive cardiomyopathy. In some cases, MRI may also be used to guide the utility and location of endomyocardial biopsy.

9. **What are hypereosinophilic syndrome and Loeffler's disease?**
Hypereosinophilic syndrome (HES) and Loeffler's disease are similar (and possibly the same) diseases characterized by persistent marked eosinophilia, absence of a primary cause of eosinophilia (e.g., parasitic, neoplastic, or allergic disease), and eosinophil-mediated end-organ damage. The most common cardiac manifestation of HES is endomyocardial fibrosis, which was first described in the 1930s by Loeffler. Large LV thrombus can form, and thus these conditions are sometimes referred to as "restrictive obliterative cardiomyopathies" (Fig. 25.8). The reader should be aware that there is a confusing and variable use of the terms *HES, Loeffler's disease, Loeffler's endomyocardial fibrosis,* and *endomyocardial fibrosis* throughout the literature, with some authorities believing the syndromes are related and others treating them as distinct entities.

10. **What is Gaucher's disease?**
Gaucher's disease is a disease in which there is deficiency of the enzyme β-glucocerebrosidase, resulting in the accumulation of cerebroside in the heart and other organs.

11. **How does Hurler's syndrome affect the heart?**
Hurler's syndrome leads to the deposition of mucopolysaccharides in the myocardium, cardiac valves, and coronary arteries.

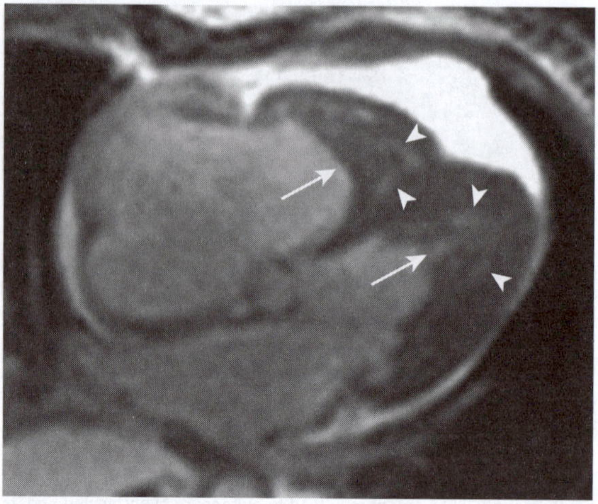

Fig. 25.8. Cardiac MRI demonstrating endomyocardial fibrosis and intracardiac thrombus, partially obliterating the left and right ventricles. The long arrows point to ventricular thrombus; the arrowheads demonstrate areas of endomyocardial fibrosis. *(Adapted with permission from Salanitri, G. C. (2005). Endomyocardial fibrosis and intracardiac thrombus occurring in idiopathic hypereosinophilic syndrome.* American Journal of Roentgenology, 184, *1432–1433.)*

12. What are the clinical features of restrictive cardiomyopathy?

Increased filling pressures cause pulmonary and systemic congestion and symptomatic dyspnea. Reduced LV filling leads to reduced stroke volume, resulting in low cardiac output symptoms such as fatigue and lethargy. Upon physical examination, the pulse may reflect low stroke volume with low amplitude and tachycardia. Jugular venous pulse is often elevated, with prominent y descent consistent with rapid early ventricular filling. Inspiratory rise in jugular venous pressure (Kussmaul sign) may be seen. Upon heart examination, S3 gallop may be heard due to abrupt cessation of rapid ventricular filling. Importantly, S4 is rarely heard with cardiac amyloidosis, despite thickened ventricular walls, due to involvement of the left atrium with reduced left atrial contractility even in the absence of atrial fibrillation.

13. What drugs can cause restrictive cardiomyopathy?

Certain drugs such as serotonin, methysergide, ergotamine, busulfan, and mercurial agents cause fibrous endocarditis, which leads to restrictive cardiomyopathy. In addition, both hydroxychloroquine and chloroquine can cause a restrictive cardiomyopathy characterized by intense vacuolization of cardiomyocytes.

14. What are the hemodynamic findings on cardiac catheterization?

It may be difficult to distinguish restrictive cardiomyopathy from constrictive pericarditis in the catheterization laboratory. The diastolic "dip-and-plateau" or "square-root sign" and prominent y descent in right atrium (RA) pressure are seen in both conditions. Features more consistent with restriction include difference in ventricular diastolic pressure greater than 5 mm Hg, pulmonary artery (PA) systolic pressure greater than 50 mm Hg, and ratio of right ventricle (RV) diastolic to systolic pressure of less than 1:3. Most important, ventricular interdependence with inspiration is not observed with restrictive cardiomyopathy (i.e., the RV and LV pressure tracings will be concordant throughout the respiratory cycle in restrictive cardiomyopathy) (Fig. 25.9).

15. What is the prognosis of idiopathic restrictive cardiomyopathy?

In a series of 94 symptomatic patients, 5-year survival was 64% (vs. 85% in age- and gender-matched controls). Adverse risk factors were male gender, age greater than 70 years, advanced New York Heart Association (NYHA) class, and left atrial diameter greater than 6 cm.

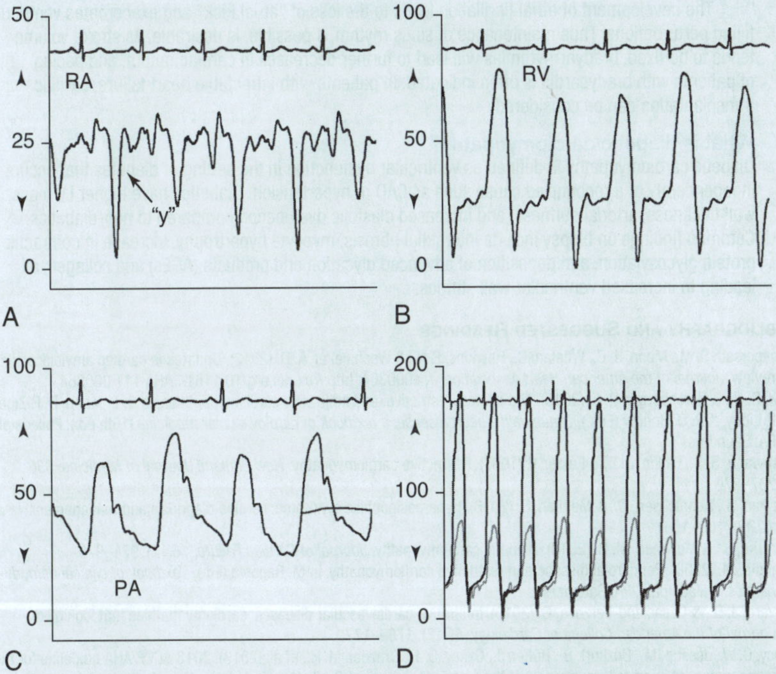

Fig. 25.9. Hemodynamics obtained from right heart catheterization in a patient with restrictive cardiomyopathy. Note **(A)** prominent y descent on the RA waveform, **(B)** "square-root" sign in diastole on the RV waveform, **(C)** PA systolic pressure above 50 mm Hg, **(D)** systolic concordance and lack of ventricular interdependence. *(Modified from Ragosta, M. (2008). Pericardial disease and restrictive cardiomyopathy. In M. Ragosta (Ed.),* Textbook of clinical hemodynamics. *Philadelphia, PA: Saunders.)*

16. What are the treatment options for restrictive cardiomyopathy?

When possible, treatment of the underlying cause of restrictive cardiomyopathy is essential. For patients with primary (AL) cardiac amyloidosis, newer chemotherapy agents and stem cell transplantation have dramatically improved survival. In addition, there are several novel medications currently in development for TTR cardiac amyloidosis.

Symptomatic treatment includes loop diuretics to treat systemic and pulmonary venous congestion. Caution should be exercised since patients are frequently extremely sensitive to alterations in LV volume and may become hypotensive or develop renal dysfunction.

Heart rate–lowering agents such as non-dihydropyridine calcium-channel blockers (diltiazem and verapamil) and beta-blockers should be avoided, as most patients with restrictive cardiomyopathy have fixed stroke volume and are dependent on increased heart rate to maintain cardiac output, though low doses of beta-blockers can be helpful in patients with atrial arrhythmias who have a heart rate greater than 100 bpm.

Angiotensin-converting enzyme (ACE) inhibitors and angiotensin receptor blockers (ARB) can result in worsening hypotension and should generally be avoided unless the patient has systemic hypertension.

Digoxin increases intracellular calcium, thus worsening diastolic function, and may increase the risks of arrhythmias and should be used with caution. There is also evidence that digoxin may bind certain types of amyloid proteins and should therefore be avoided in cardiac amyloidosis.

Many patients with restrictive cardiomyopathies will have debilitating hypotension, which can be orthostatic in nature and can also be associated with significant right heart failure. In these patients, compression stockings, abdominal binders, and midodrine (an alpha-agonist that results in vasoconstriction) can be very helpful in improving quality of life.

The development of atrial fibrillation leads to the loss of "atrial kick" and exacerbates ventricular filling perturbations. Thus maintenance of sinus rhythm, if possible, is desirable. As stroke volume tends to be fixed, bradyarrhythmias will lead to further decreases in cardiac output, and pacing of patients with bradycardia is often indicated. In patients with intractable heart failure, cardiac transplantation can be considered.

17. What is diabetic cardiomyopathy?

Diabetic cardiomyopathy is defined as ventricular dysfunction in the setting of diabetes that occurs independently of a recognized cause such as CAD or hypertension. Diabetics have higher LV mass, wall thickness, arterial stiffness, and increased diastolic dysfunction compared to non-diabetics. Common findings on biopsy include interstitial fibrosis, myocyte hypertrophy, increase in contractile protein glycosylation, and deposition of advanced glycation end products (AGEs) and collagen, all leading to increased ventricular wall stiffness.

Bibliography and Suggested Readings

Banypersad, S. M., Moon, J. C., Whelan, C., Hawkins, P. N., & Wechalekar, A. D. (2012). Updates in cardiac amyloidosis: a review. *Journal of the American Heart Association, 1*, e000364. http://dx.doi.org/10.1161/JAHA.111.000364.

Falk, R. H., & Hershberger, R. E. (2015). The dilated, restrictive, and infiltrative cardiomyopathies. In D. L. Mann, D. P. Zipes, P. Libby, & R. O. Bonow (Eds.), *Braunwald's heart disease: a textbook of cardiovascular medicine* (10th ed.). Philadelphia, PA: Saunders.

Kushwaha, S. S., Fallon, J. T., & Fuster, V. (1997). Restrictive cardiomyopathy. *New England Journal of Medicine, 336*, 267–276.

Mankad, R., Bonnichsen, C., & Mankad, S. (2016). Hypereosinophilic syndrome: cardiac diagnosis and management. *Heart, 102*(2), 100–106.

Murarka, S., & Movahed, M. R. (2010). Diabetic cardiomyopathy. *Journal of Cardiac Failure, 16*(12), 971–979.

Ragosta, M. (2008). Pericardial disease and restrictive cardiomyopathy. In M. Ragosta (Ed.), *Textbook of clinical hemodynamics*. Philadelphia, PA: Saunders.

Seward, J. B., & Casacland-Verzosa, G. (2010). Infiltrative cardiovascular diseases: cardiomyopathies that look alike. *Journal of the American College of Cardiology, 55*(17), 1769–1779.

Yancy, C. W., Jessup, M., Bozkurt, B., Butler, J., Casey, D. E., Drazner, M. H., et al. (2013). 2013 ACCF/AHA guideline for the management of heart failure: a report of the American College of Cardiology Foundation/American Heart Association Task Force on Practice Guidelines. *Journal of the American College of Cardiology, 62*(16), e147–e239.

ACUTE DECOMPENSATED HEART FAILURE

G. Michael Felker, Marat Fudim

1. What is acute decompensated heart failure? Isn't it just a worsening of chronic heart failure?

Acute decompensated heart failure (ADHF) is a clinical syndrome of worsening signs or symptoms of heart failure (HF) requiring hospitalization or other unscheduled medical care. For many years, ADHF was viewed as simply an exacerbation of chronic HF as a result of volume overload, with few implications beyond a short-term need to intensify diuretic therapy (a similar paradigm to exacerbations of chronic asthma). Recent decades have seen an explosion of research into the epidemiology, pathophysiology, outcomes, and treatment of ADHF. Although some controversy persists, multiple lines of evidence now support the concept that ADHF is a unique clinical syndrome with its own epidemiology and underlying mechanisms and that there is a need for specific therapies. This viewpoint suggests that ADHF is not just a worsening of chronic HF any more than an acute myocardial infarction (MI) is just a worsening of chronic angina.

Outcome data from a variety of studies now support the concept that hospitalization for ADHF can often signal a dramatic change in the natural history of the HF syndrome. Rates of rehospitalization or death are as high as 50% within 6 months of the initial ADHF event, which is a much higher event rate than is seen with acute MI.

A schematic representation of the pathophysiology of acute HF is given in Fig. 26.1.

2. Are there clinically important subcategories of acute decompensated heart failure?

There is great interest in developing a framework for understanding ADHF that would assist in stratifying patients, guiding therapy, and developing new treatments, similar to the basic framework developed for acute coronary syndromes (i.e., ST-segment elevation myocardial infarction [STEMI], non–ST-segment elevation myocardial infarction [NSTEMI], and unstable angina). Although this area is rapidly evolving, a few general clinical *phenotypes* of ADHF have emerged.

- **Hypertensive acute heart failure:** Data from large registries such as ADHERE and OPTIMIZE have shown that a substantial portion of ADHF patients are hypertensive on initial presentation to the emergency department. Such patients often have relatively little volume overload (see discussion of volume redistribution later) and preserved or only mildly reduced ventricular function and are more likely to be older and female. Symptoms often develop quickly (minutes to hours), and many such patients have little or no history of chronic HF. Hypertensive urgency or emergency with acute pulmonary edema represents an extreme form of this phenotype.
- **Decompensated heart failure:** This describes patients with a background of significant chronic HF who develop symptoms of volume overload and congestion over a period of days to weeks. These patients typically have significant left ventricular dysfunction and chronic HF at baseline. Although specific triggers are poorly understood, episodes are often triggered by noncompliance with diet or medical therapy.
- **Cardiogenic shock/advanced heart failure:** Although patients with advanced forms of HF are often seen in tertiary care centers, they are relatively uncommon in the broader population (probably fewer than 10% of ADHF hospitalizations). These patients may present with so-called low-output symptoms that may make diagnosis challenging, including confusion, fatigue, abdominal pain, or anorexia. Hypotension (systolic blood pressure [SBP] less than 90 mm Hg) and significant end-organ dysfunction (especially renal dysfunction) are common features. Many of these patients have concomitant evidence of significant right ventricular dysfunction, with ascites or generalized anasarca.

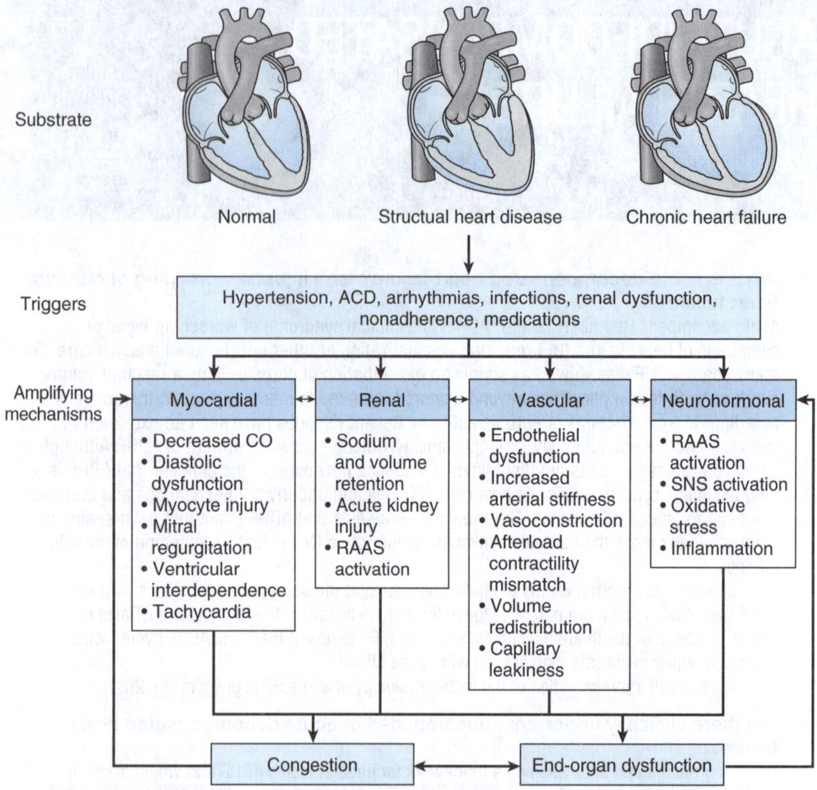

Fig. 26.1. A schematic representation of the pathophysiology of acute heart failure. *ACS*, Acute coronary syndrome; *CO*, cardiac output; *RAAS*, renin-angiotensin-aldosterone system; *SNS*, sympathetic nervous system. *(Image from Felker, G. M., & Teerlink, J. R. [2016]. Diagnosis and management of acute heart failure. In* Braunwald's heart disease: a textbook of cardiovascular medicine *[10th ed., Vol. 24, pp. 484–511]. Philadelphia, PA: Elsevier.)*

3. Is heart failure simply a problem of too much extra fluid?

The classic teaching of HF pathophysiology emphasizes the mechanism of poor forward flow (i.e., low cardiac output), resulting in neurohumoral upregulation and poor end-organ function. There is increasing recognition of the central role of systemic congestion as both the consequence and a driver of HF progression. Registry data demonstrate that only about 50% of patients presenting with ADHF gain greater than 2 pounds in weight prior to admission. The transition from chronic HF to ADHF is associated with a progressive increase in cardiac filling pressures. Right-sided cardiac filling pressures begin to increase within 5 days preceding an admission for ADHF, often preceding measurable weight gain or the onset of symptoms. This suggests an internal volume redistribution as a component of ADHF. The largest storage compartment for intravascular volume and likely source of internal volume redistribution is the splanchnic vascular bed. Chronic HF results in splanchnic vascular congestion due to poor cardiac function and a poor vascular capacity due to an increased sympathetic tone, reducing the buffering ability of the abdominal compartment. Specific therapies to address this form of congestion associated with "vascular redistribution" have yet to be developed.

4. What is the role of biomarkers like b-type natriuretic peptides in the diagnosis of acute decompensated heart failure?

Although the clinical symptoms (dyspnea, paroxysmal nocturnal dyspnea [PND], orthopnea, fatigue) and signs (elevated jugular venous pressure, pulmonary rales, edema) of ADHF are well

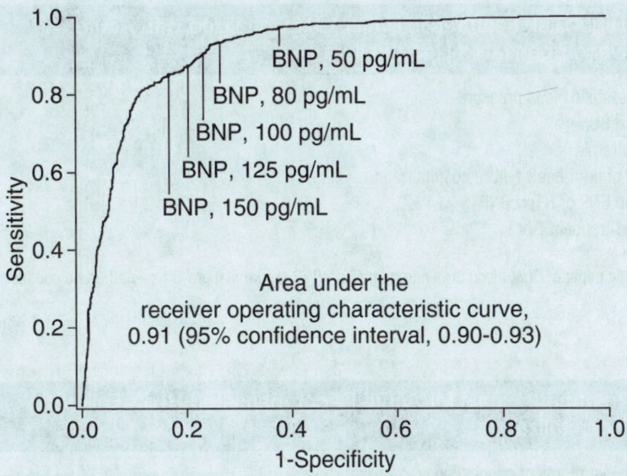

Fig. 26.2. Receiver operator curve for use of BNP in making diagnosis of ADHF in patients with acute unexplained dyspnea. *(Adapted from Maisel, A. S., Krishnaswamy, P., Nowak, R. M., McCord, J., Hollander, J. E., Duc, P., et al. [2002]. Rapid measurement of B-type natriuretic peptide in the emergency diagnosis of heart failure.* New England Journal of Medicine, *347[3], 161–167.)*

known, the diagnosis can often be challenging in patients presenting to acute care settings. This is especially true in the elderly and patients with significant comorbid conditions such as chronic obstructive pulmonary disease (COPD). The development of natriuretic peptides as a diagnostic tool has been a major advance in ADHF diagnosis. The clinically available natriuretic peptides for ADHF diagnosis include b-type natriuretic peptide (BNP) and its biologically inert amino-terminal fragment, N-terminal pro-B-type natriuretic peptide (NTproBNP). Despite some subtle differences between these two biomarkers, they provide similar diagnostic information when used in patients presenting to the emergency department with unexplained dyspnea, although the range of values is significantly different (in general, NT-proBNP levels are approximately 5 to 10 times greater than BNP levels in the same patient). The landmark Breathing Not Properly Study measured BNP levels in 1586 patients presenting to the emergency department with unexplained dyspnea. In this study, treating physicians were blinded to BNP values, and a panel of cardiologists adjudicated whether hospitalizations were due to ADHF or other causes (based on all clinical data other than the BNP values). As shown in Fig. 26.2, a cutoff of 100 pg/mL of BNP had a positive predictive value of 79% and a negative predictive value of 89% for the diagnosis of ADHF. The area under the receiver operating curve (ROC) was 0.91, suggesting a very high degree of accuracy for establishing the diagnosis of ADHF. Subsequent studies have demonstrated similar findings for NTproBNP, although optimal diagnostic cutoffs are different (450 pg/mL for patients younger than 50 years and 900 pg/mL for patients older than 50 years). The use of natriuretic peptide has now become standard of care in the diagnosis of patients with dyspnea presenting to acute care settings and has a class I indication ("should be done") in clinical practice guidelines. A potentially important new development in the interpretation of natriuretic peptides is the recent approval of valsartan/sacubitril (Entresto) for chronic HF. This medication increases BNP levels (presumably due to inhibition of neprilysin, which catalyzes the degradation of BNP) but decreases NT-proBNP levels (reflecting an improved hemodynamic state).

5. What features suggest patients who are particularly high risk?

Analysis of large datasets from both clinical trials and registries of ADHF patients have identified a few features that consistently suggest a high risk of short-term morbidity and mortality in patients hospitalized with ADHF (Box 26.1). Across studies, the most consistent of these are blood urea nitrogen (BUN), serum creatinine, SBP, and hyponatremia. Interestingly, BUN has consistently proved to be a stronger predictor of outcomes than creatinine (see Fig. 26.2). One potential explanation of this finding is that BUN may integrate both renal function and

Box 26.1. High-Risk Features in Patients Hospitalized with Acute Decompensated Heart Failure

- Lower systolic blood pressure
- Elevated BUN
- Hyponatremia
- History of prior heart failure hospitalization
- Elevated BNP or NTproBNP
- Elevated troponin T or I

BNP, b-type natriuretic peptide; *BUN*, blood urea nitrogen; *NTproBNP*, N-terminal pro-B type natriuretic peptide.

Box 26.2. Treatment Goals for Acute Decompensated Heart Failure Hospitalization

- Improve symptoms of congestion.
- Optimize volume status.
- Identify and address triggers for decompensation.
- Optimize chronic oral therapy.
- Minimize side effects.
- Identify patients who might benefit from revascularization.
- Educate patients concerning medications and disease management.

hemodynamic information. Unlike the situation in many other cardiovascular conditions, *higher* blood pressure has consistently been associated with *lower* risk. Hyponatremia appears to be associated with lower output and greater neurohormonal activation, and risk appears to be increased with even mild forms of hyponatremia. A variety of biomarkers also appear to have strong prognostic implications in ADHF, in particular the natriuretic peptides (BNP or NTproBNP) and troponin.

6. **What are the goals of therapy in acute decompensated heart failure?**
Specific therapies for ADHF should be assessed in the context of the overall goals of therapy. A summary of suggested goals of therapy based on current guidelines is shown in Box 26.2.

7. **What is the role of noninvasive cardiac imaging and invasive cardiac monitoring?**
Despite advances in imaging technology and increasing access, a detailed history and a good physical exam continue to be the foundation in the assessment of patients with HF. The history provides evidence for the etiology of the cardiomyopathy as well as severity of the disease and offers clues for possible interventions. The physical examination evaluates the volume status and severity of the disease.

Beyond a history and physical, it is recommended to obtain a chest x-ray to evaluate heart size, pulmonary congestion, and alternative cardiac causes of the presentation, such as pulmonary disease. Noninvasive imaging such as nuclear single photon emission computed tomography (SPECT), stress echocardiography, or magnetic resonance imaging (MRI) can be used to establish the etiology of HF and evaluate possible benefit from invasive therapies. Detection of myocardial ischemia and remaining viability is reasonable in patients presenting with de novo HF, who have known CAD and no angina, unless the patient is not eligible for revascularization of any kind.

A two-dimensional echocardiogram can become very useful in the evaluation of acute HF. It not only provides useful diagnostic information but also prognostic information. It is of great use in cardiogenic shock and refractory pulmonary edema when the underlying etiology is unclear, as well as for suspected mechanical complications of MI. An echocardiogram provides very useful information on ventricular size and function, wall thickness, and wall motion. Consequently it is very useful to assess the extent of myocardial ischemia in acute ischemia and infarction. Further, it provides a good assessment of the valvular function. Thus an echocardiogram should be used to evaluate new cardiac murmurs, which could help unmask significant valvular lesions that not uncommonly contribute to ADHF.

The routine use of invasive hemodynamic monitoring (such as with pulmonary artery catheters) is not indicated in patients with ADHF. This recommendation is based primarily on the results of the ESCAPE study, which demonstrated no advantage in terms of days alive and free from hospitalization when patients hospitalized with advanced HF were randomized to pulmonary artery catheter-guided therapy versus usual care. Invasive hemodynamic monitoring may be indicated to guide therapy in selected patients who are refractory to initial therapy, particularly those with hypotension or worsening renal function.

8. **How should we give diuretics in acute decompensated heart failure?**

Because most episodes of ADHF are associated with some degree of congestion or volume overload, intravenous (IV) loop diuretics remain a cornerstone of ADHF therapy. Because many symptoms in ADHF (in particular dyspnea) appear to be closely related to elevated ventricular filling pressures, reduction of filling pressures in order to improve acute symptoms is a major goal of therapy. Recently, however, observational data from a variety of sources have led to questions about the appropriate use of diuretics in patients with ADHF. Studies of patients with both chronic HF and ADHF have shown that higher diuretic use is associated with a higher incidence of adverse events (especially worsening renal function) and mortality. Interpreting these types of data is highly problematic because of the issue of confounding by indication (i.e., patients who need higher diuretic doses are typically sicker, and thus it is impossible to determine if higher doses of diuretics are simply a marker of greater disease severity or whether they directly contribute to worsening outcomes).

Controversy also exists regarding whether continuous infusion (as opposed to intermittent bolus administration) may be a safer and more efficacious way of administering IV diuretics in ADHF. These questions have been recently addressed by a National Institutes of Health (NIH)-sponsored randomized clinical trial (the Diuretic Optimization Strategies Evaluation [DOSE]). Using a 2 × 2 factorial design, DOSE randomized 308 patients to either high (2.5 × chronic oral dose given IV) or low (1 × chronic oral dose given IV) and also to either continuous infusion or every-12-hour IV bolus. With regard to route of administration, there was no significant difference in either efficacy or safety when diuretics were given as intermittent boluses or as continuous infusion. With regard to dosing, there was a general trend toward greater decongestion and improved symptoms with higher dose diuretics (although the study did not meet its nominal primary efficacy endpoint of patient global assessment with a p value = .06). This suggestion of improved efficacy did appear to come at a cost of more episodes of renal dysfunction in the higher dose arm, but these changes were transient and did not appear to have any impact on post-discharge clinical outcome. Taken as a whole, the results from DOSE appear to generally support an aggressive approach to decongestion of volume-overloaded patients with ADHF, although renal function, electrolytes, and volume status need to be carefully monitored.

9. **What about vasodilators?**

Along with diuretic therapy, vasodilators are considered to be first-line agents in the treatment of ADHF. A combination of diuretic and vasodilator therapy has not only been shown to provide symptomatic relief but also to rapidly decrease neurohormonal activation. Nitrates such as nitroglycerin, isosorbide mononitrate, isosorbide dinitrate, and sodium nitroprusside have long been considered first-line agents for acute hypertensive HF, in patients with severe volume overload, or in acute pulmonary edema. As a class, these drugs work by offering an exogenous source of nitric oxide, which leads to relaxation of vascular smooth muscle. At low doses, nitrates mostly affect the venous circulation, reducing the preload via an increase in venous capacitance (mostly splanchnic). At higher doses nitrates result in additional arteriolar dilatation, leading to significant reduction in afterload. While the real-world experience with nitrates is extensive, there is a lack of robust data to show any significant benefit on mortality or hospital readmissions.

Beyond nitrates alone, there is proven benefit for the combination hydralazine and nitrate therapy in chronic HF, especially in African Americans with HFrEF. However, this combination is underused in clinical practice. The benefit of hydralazine includes additional afterload reduction and attenuation of nitrate tolerance. Other vasodilators such as nesiritide were not shown to be superior to placebo in the ASCEND-HF trial, despite initially promising data.

As a rule of thumb, vasodilators should be used in those who (1) present with ADHF and concomitant hypertension and/or (2) do not respond sufficiently to IV diuretic therapy.

Patients not responding to vasodilators may benefit from an inotrope. Inotropic therapies are discussed further in the next section.

10. What is the role of inotropes like dobutamine or milrinone in patients with acute decompensated heart failure?

Inotropic drugs, which increase cardiac contractility, are theoretically appealing as a therapy for ADHF. Despite this theoretical appeal, however, available data clearly demonstrate that such agents are not indicated for the vast majority of ADHF patients. In the OPTIME-CHF study, a large randomized trial of IV milrinone therapy in ADHF, randomization to milrinone did not shorten length of stay or improve other clinical outcomes and was associated with significantly higher rates of arrhythmias and hypotension than was placebo. These data suggest that the routine use of inotropes is not indicated in ADHF management. Importantly, OPTIME-CHF specifically excluded patients with shock or other apparent indications for inotropes. As noted earlier, the vast majority of ADHF patients do not have evidence of end-organ hypoperfusion or shock. In the subset of patients with cardiogenic shock or severe end-organ dysfunction, inotropic therapy may still be indicated as a method of achieving short-term stabilization until more definitive long-term therapy (such as revascularization, cardiac transplantation, or mechanical cardiac support) can be employed.

A comprehensive algorithm for the management of patients admitted with acute HF is given in Fig. 26.3.

11. What is cardiorenal syndrome in acute decompensated heart failure?

Worsening renal function during hospitalization for ADHF represents a major clinical challenge. Often termed *cardiorenal syndrome* (CRS), this clinical syndrome is characterized by persistent volume overload accompanied by worsening of renal function. Development of CRS, as defined by an increase in serum creatinine of 0.3 mg/dL or more from admission, occurs in as many as one-third of patients hospitalized with ADHF. CRS shows a strong correlation with central venous pressure and is independent of the cardiac index. Elevated intra-abdominal pressure is frequent in ADHF and related to renal dysfunction.

Development of CRS is associated with higher mortality and increased length of stay in patients with ADHF. Although the underlying mechanisms of CRS remain ill defined, data suggest that higher diuretic doses, preexisting renal disease, and diabetes mellitus are associated with an increased risk. The optimal therapeutic strategy for patients with ADHF and CRS remains unknown. A variety of clinical approaches (hemodynamically guided therapy, inotropes, temporarily holding diuretics, etc.) have all been used with varying results, and there are no large outcome studies to guide management of these challenging patients. Regardless of the therapy form, improvement in renal function is likely driven by cardiac and vascular decongestion.

Despite some promising initial studies, the supplementary decongestive therapies like ultrafiltration, used in addition to or instead of diuretic therapy, were ultimately not proven to be superior to usual therapy alone. In CARRESS-HF a stepped pharmacologic algorithm (primarily focused on diuretics) was shown to be superior and safer when compared to ultrafiltration.

12. How should we determine when to discharge patients?

The decision of when to discharge a patient with ADHF from the hospital is often based on clinical judgment rather than objective criteria. Criteria that should be met before consideration of hospital discharge have been published in various practice guidelines (Box 26.3). Most patients should have follow-up scheduled within 7 to 10 days of discharge, and high-risk patients should be considered for earlier follow-up (by phone or in person) or referral to a comprehensive disease management program. Early adjustment of diuretics may be required as patients transition from the hospital environment (with IV diuretics and controlled low-sodium diet) to home.

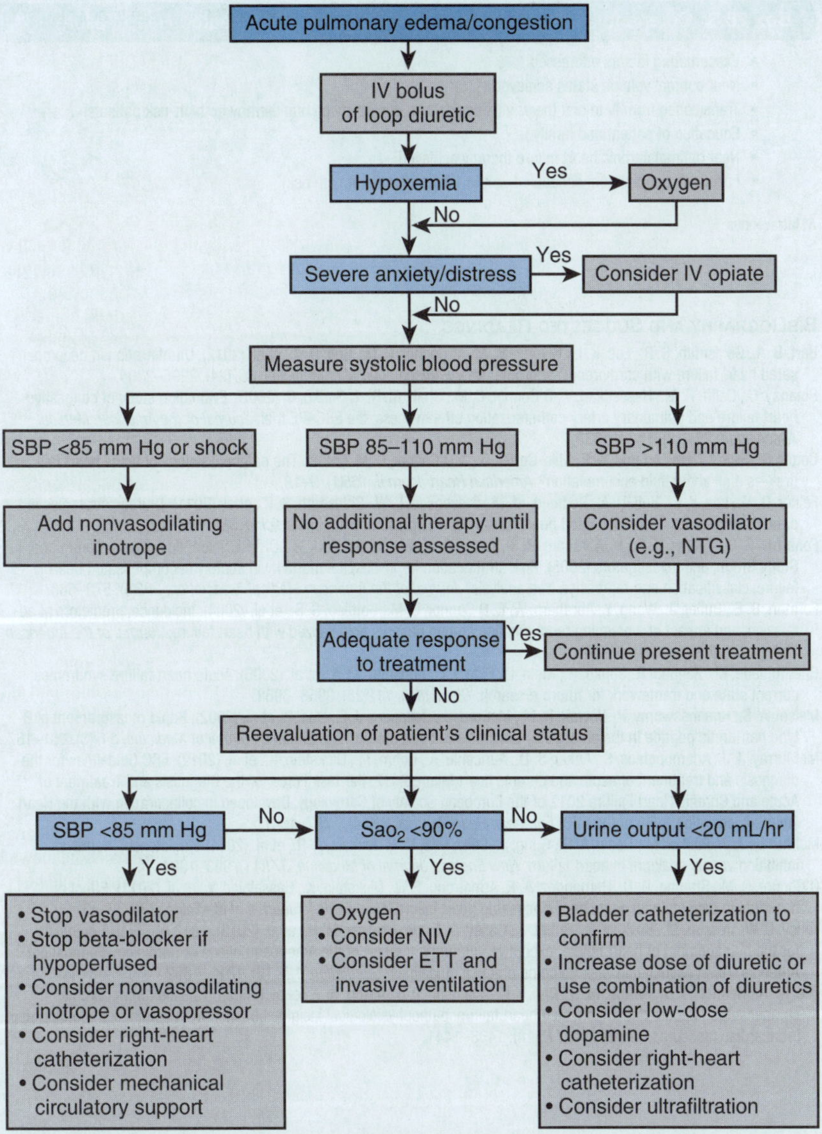

Fig. 26.3. Algorithm for management of patients admitted with AHF and pulmonary edema/congestion. *ETT*, Endotracheal tube; *IV*, intravenous; *NTG*, nitroglycerin. *(Image modified from McMurray, J. J., Adamopoulos, S., Anker, S. D., Auricchio, A., Böhm, M., Dickstein, K., et al. [2012]. ESC guidelines for the diagnosis and treatment of acute and chronic heart failure 2012: the Task Force for the Diagnosis and Treatment of Acute and Chronic Heart Failure 2012 of the European Society of Cardiology. Developed in collaboration with the Heart Failure Association [HFA] of the ESC.* European Heart Journal, 33*[14], 1787–1847.)*

Box 26.3. Criteria for Hospital Discharge in Acute Decompensated Heart Failure

- Exacerbating factors addressed
- Near optimal volume status achieved
- Transitioned from IV to oral therapy (consider 24 h of stability on oral therapy for high-risk patients)
- Education of patient and family
- Near optimal chronic heart failure therapy achieved
- Follow-up appointment scheduled in 7 to 10 days (earlier if high risk)

IV, Intravenous.

Bibliography and Suggested Readings

Bart, B. A., Goldsmith, S. R., Lee, K. L., Givertz, M. M., O'Connor, C. M., Bull, D. A., et al. (2012). Ultrafiltration in decompensated heart failure with cardiorenal syndrome. *New England Journal of Medicine, 367*(24), 2296–2304.

Binanay, C., Califf, R. M., Hasselblad, V., O'Connor, C. M., Shah, M. R., & Sopko, G. (2005). Evaluation study of congestive heart failure and pulmonary artery catheterization effectiveness: the ESCAPE trial. *Journal of the American Medical Association, 294*(13), 1625–1633.

Cotter, G., Felker, G. M., Adams, K. F., Milo-Cotter, O., & O'Connor, C. M. (2008). The pathophysiology of acute heart failure—is it all about fluid accumulation? *American Heart Journal, 155*(1), 9–18.

Felker, G. M., Lee, K. L., Bull, D. A., Redfield, M. M., Stevenson, L. W., Goldsmith, S. R., et al. (2011). Diuretic strategies in patients with acute decompensated heart failure. *New England Journal of Medicine, 364*, 797–805.

Fonarow, G. C., Adams, K. F., Jr., Abraham, W. T., Yancy, C. W., Boscardin, W. J., & ADHERE Scientific Advisory Committee, Study Group, and Investigators (2005). Risk stratification for in-hospital mortality in acutely decompensated heart failure: classification and regression tree analysis. *Journal of the American Medical Association, 293*(5), 572–580.

Forman, D. E., Butler, J., Wang, Y., Abraham, W. T., O'Connor, C. M., Gottlieb, S. S., et al. (2004). Incidence, predictors at admission, and impact of worsening renal function among patients hospitalized with heart failure. *Journal of the American College Cardiology, 43*(1), 61–67.

Gheorghiade, M., Zannad, F., Sopko, G., Klein, L., Piña, I. L., Konstam, M. A., et al. (2005). Acute heart failure syndromes: current state and framework for future research. *Circulation, 112*(25), 3958–3968.

Maisel, A. S., Krishnaswamy, P., Nowak, R. M., McCord, J., Hollander, J. E., Duc, P., et al. (2002). Rapid measurement of B-type natriuretic peptide in the emergency diagnosis of heart failure. *New England Journal of Medicine, 347*(3), 161–167.

McMurray, J. J., Adamopoulos, S., Anker, S. D., Auricchio, A., Böhm, M., Dickstein, K., et al. (2012). ESC Guidelines for the diagnosis and treatment of acute and chronic heart failure 2012: the Task Force for the Diagnosis and Treatment of Acute and Chronic Heart Failure 2012 of the European Society of Cardiology. Developed in collaboration with the Heart Failure Association (HFA) of the ESC. *European Heart Journal, 33*(14), 1787–1847.

McMurray, J. J., Packer, M., Desai, A. S., Gong, J., Lefkowitz, M. P., Rizkala, A. R., et al. (2014). Angiotensin–neprilysin inhibition versus enalapril in heart failure. *New England Journal of Medicine, 371*(11), 993–1004.

O'Connor, C. M., Starling, R. C., Hernandez, A. F., Armstrong, P. W., Dickstein, K., Hasselblad, V., et al. (2011). Effect of nesiritide in patients with acute decompensated heart failure. *New England Journal of Medicine, 365*, 32–43.

Yancy, C. W., Jessup, M., Bozkurt, B., Butler, J., Casey, D. E., Jr., Drazner, M. H., et al. (2013). 2013 ACCF/AHA guideline for the management of heart failure: executive summary: a report of the American College of Cardiology Foundation/American Heart Association Task Force on practice guidelines. *Circulation, 128*(16), 1810–1852.

Zile, M. R., Bennett, T. D., Sutton, M. S., Cho, Y. K., Adamson, P. B., Aaron, M. F., et al. (2008). Transition from chronic compensated to acute decompensated heart failure: pathophysiological insights obtained from continuous monitoring of intracardiac pressures. *Circulation, 118*(14), 1433–1441.

HEART FAILURE: LONG-TERM MANAGEMENT

CHAPTER 27

Luke Cunningham, Glenn Levine, Biykem Bozkurt

This chapter deals specifically with the long-term management of patients with heart failure with reduced (depressed) ejection fraction (HFrEF). The management of patients with heart failure with preserved ejection fraction (HFpEF, previously referred to as "diastolic dysfunction") is discussed in Chapter 23. The management of patients with acute decompensated heart failure is discussed in Chapter 26. Specific discussions of the evaluation and management of myocarditis, dilated cardiomyopathy, hypertrophic cardiomyopathy, and restrictive/infiltrative cardiomyopathy, as well as consideration with cardiac transplantation, are discussed in other dedicated chapters in this section of the book. The roles of pacemakers and implantable cardioverter defibrillators (ICDs) in patients with heart failure are discussed in this chapter, as well as in the chapters on pacemakers (Chapter 38) and ICDs (Chapter 39).

1. How are heart failure symptoms classified?

Symptoms are most commonly classified using the New York Heart Association (NYHA) classification system:

- **Class I:** No limitation; ordinary physical activity does not cause excess fatigue, shortness of breath, or palpitations.
- **Class II:** Slight limitation of physical activity; ordinary physical activity results in fatigue, shortness of breath, palpitations, or angina.
- **Class III:** Marked limitation of physical activity; ordinary activity will lead to symptoms.
- **Class IV:** Inability to carry on any physical activity without discomfort; symptoms of congestive heart failure are present even at rest; increased discomfort is experienced with any physical activity.

2. What is the stage system for classifying heart failure?

In 2001 the American College of Cardiology/American Heart Association (ACC/AHA) introduced a system to categorize the stages of heart failure. This system is somewhat different in focus than the previous NYHA classification system by highlighting the structural development and progression of heart failure. It was intended in part to emphasize the prevention of the development of symptomatic heart failure. In addition, the 2013 Heart Failure Guidelines suggest appropriate therapy for each stage, emphasizing the differences in HFrEF and HFpEF at Stage C (Fig. 27.1).

- **Stage A:** Patient at high risk for developing heart failure but without structural heart disease or symptoms of heart failure. Includes patients with hypertension, coronary artery disease (CAD), obesity, diabetes, history of drug or alcohol abuse, history of rheumatic fever, family history of cardiomyopathy, and treatment with cardiotoxins.
- **Stage B:** Patient with structural heart disease but without signs or symptoms of heart failure. Includes patients with previous myocardial infarction (MI), left ventricular (LV) remodeling including left ventricular hypertrophy (LVH) and low ejection fraction (EF), and asymptomatic valvular disease.
- **Stage C:** Patient with structural heart disease with prior or current symptoms of heart failure.
- **Stage D:** Patient with refractory heart failure requiring specialized interventions.

3. Which medical treatments have been shown to decrease mortality in patients with heart failure?

Pharmacotherapies that have been shown to decrease mortality in patients with HFrEF (Table 27.1) include the following.

- Angiotensin-converting enzyme (ACE) inhibitors are first-line agents in those with depressed EF because they have been convincingly shown to improve symptoms, decrease hospitalizations, and reduce mortality. Angiotensin II receptor blockers (ARBs) are used in those who are ACE-inhibitor intolerant because of persistent cough or in some cases after an episode of angioedema.

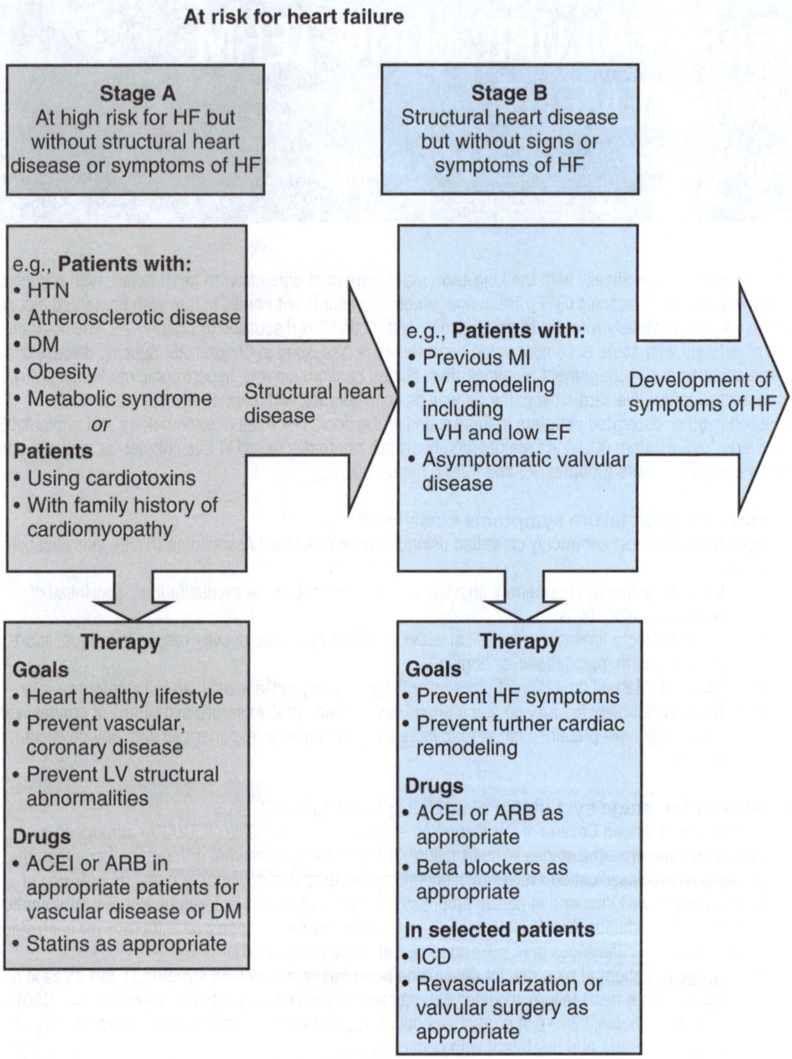

Fig. 27.1. The 2013 ACC/AHA Guidelines for the Diagnosis and Management of Heart Failure in Adults. The figure was created before approval of sacubitril/valsartan and ivabradine, which would now be included under Stage C, HFrEF therapies. *(Reproduced from Yancy, C. W., Jessup, M., Bozkurt, B., Butler, J., Casey, D. E., Jr., Drazner, M. H., et al. [2013]. 2013 ACCF/AHA guideline for the management of heart failure: a report of the American College of Cardiology Foundation/American Heart Association Task Force on Practice Guidelines.* Journal of the American College of Cardiology, 62*[16], e148–e239.)*

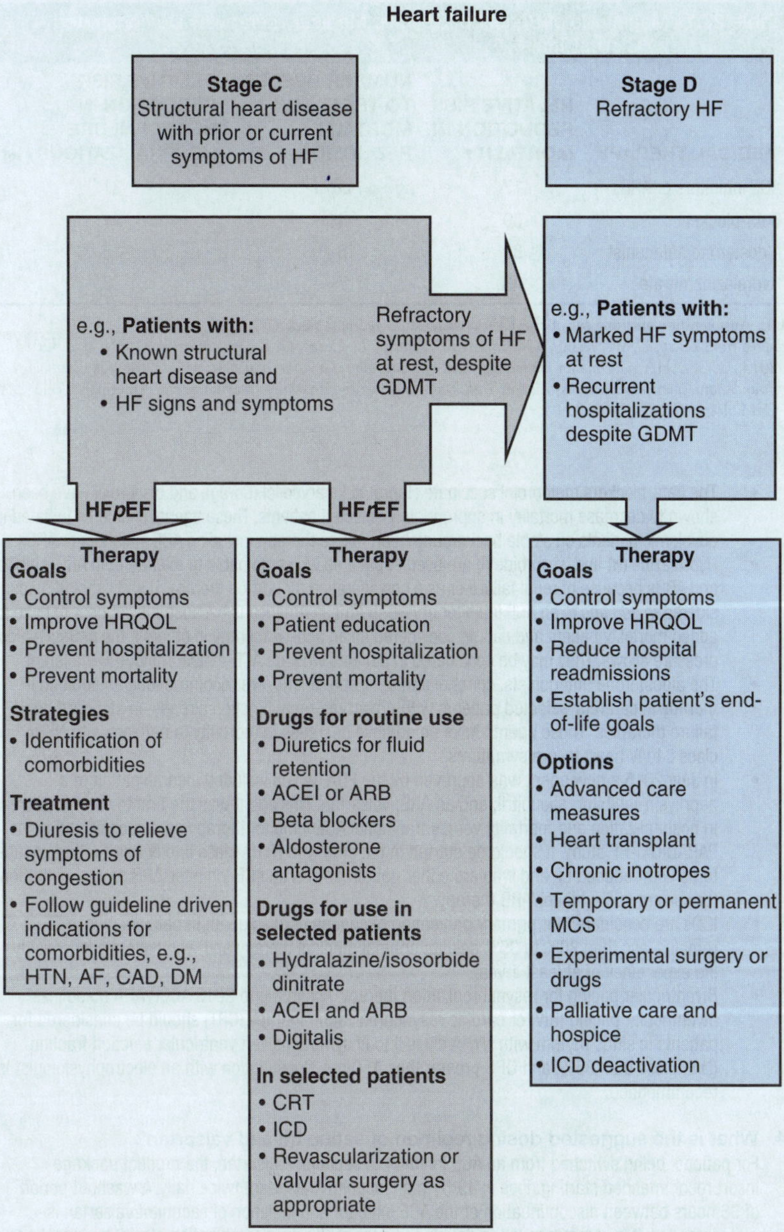

Fig. 27.1. cont'd

Table 27.1. Magnitude of Benefit of Specific Medical Therapy as Demonstrated by Clinical Trials

MEDICAL THERAPY	RELATIVE RISK REDUCTION IN MORTALITY	NUMBER NEEDED TO TREAT FOR MORTALITY REDUCTION	RELATIVE RISK REDUCTION IN HEART FAILURE HOSPITALIZATIONS (%)
ACE inhibitors or ARBs	17	26	31
Beta-blocker	39	4	41
Aldosterone antagonist	30	6	35
Hydralazine/nitrate	43	7	33

ACE, *Angiotensin-converting enzyme;* ARBs, *angiotensin II receptor blockers.*

Adapted from Yancy, C. W., Jessup, M., Bozkurt, B., Butler, J., Casey, D. E., Jr., Drazner, M. H., et al. [2013]. 2013 ACCF/AHA guideline for the management of heart failure: a report of the American College of Cardiology Foundation/American Heart Association Task Force on Practice Guidelines. Journal of the American College of Cardiology, 62[16], e148–e239.

- The beta-blockers metoprolol succinate (Toprol XL), carvedilol (Coreg), and bisoprolol have been shown to decrease mortality in appropriately selected patients. These agents should be initiated in euvolemic patients on stable background heart failure therapy, including ACE inhibitors or ARBs.
- Hydralazine (H) and isosorbide (I) are used in patients who are unable to tolerate both ACE inhibitors and ARBs because of renal failure or as a consideration for add-on therapy. H and I should be considered *in addition* to an ACE inhibitor or ARB in African Americans because they appear to have an added mortality benefit and can be considered as an add-on therapy in others if the patient's blood pressure allows. They may be considered in patients who are ACE-inhibitor and ARB intolerant.
- The aldosterone antagonists, spironolactone or eplerenone, are recommended as additional therapy in carefully selected patients with preserved renal function already on standard heart failure therapies. These agents have an additive decrease in mortality in patients with NYHA class II to IV heart failure symptoms.
- In July 2015 a new agent was approved by the FDA, which included a combination of a neprilysin-inhibitor; sacubitril; and an ARB, valsartan. This agent was the first to show a decrease in hospitalization and mortality versus traditional ACE inhibitor therapy as demonstrated in the PARADIGM-HF study. It should be started in patients with NYHA class II to IV heart failure symptoms with reduced EF and who are either not already on an ACE inhibitor/ARB or in substitution for current ACE inhibitor/ARB therapy.
- ICDs are considered for primary prevention of sudden cardiac death in patients whose EF remains less than 30% to 35% despite optimal medical therapy and who have a good-quality life expectancy of at least 1 year.
- Biventricular pacing for resynchronization therapy. According to 2013 ACCF/AHA guidelines biventricular pacing (BiV) or cardiac resynchronization therapy (CRT) should be considered for patients in sinus rhythm with NYHA class II to IV symptoms, left ventricular ejection fraction (LVEF) less than 35%, and QRS greater than 150 ms. Consultation with an electrophysiologist is recommended.

4. What is the suggested dosing regimen of sacubitril and valsartan?

For patients being switched from an ACE inhibitor to sacubitril/valsartan, the product package insert recommended starting dose is 49/51 mg (sacubitril/valsartan) twice daily. A washout period of 36 hours between discontinuation of the ACE inhibitor and initiation of sacubitril/valsartan is recommended. It is recommended to double the dose of the drug combination after 2 to 4 weeks to the target maintenance dose of 97/103 mg twice daily, as tolerated.

It is recommended that the starting dose be reduced to 24/26 mg twice daily for:

- Patients not currently taking an ACE inhibitor or ARB or previously taking a low dose of these agents
- Patients with severe chronic kidney disease (eGFR <30 mL/min/1.73 m^2)
- Patients with moderate hepatic impairment

Sacubitril/valsartan should not be used in patients with severe liver disease, pregnancy, concomitant use of ACE inhibitors (allow a washout period of 36 hours), and those with a history of angioedema related to previous ACE inhibitor or ARB therapy.

Important side effects of the drug combination include hyperkalemia, renal impairment, hypotension, and angioedema.

5. Which therapies in heart failure have been shown to reduce hospitalization?

All the previously mentioned medical therapies reduce heart failure symptoms and to a degree heart failure hospitalizations. There are also two other medications that appear to impact only heart failure hospitalization.

Digoxin has been shown to decrease heart failure symptoms and long-term risk of re-hospitalization in patients already on medical therapy. The Digitalis Investigation Group (DIG) trial was a multicenter, randomized, double-blinded, placebo-controlled study of 6801 symptomatic patients with heart failure and EF less than 45%. Digoxin did not improve total mortality or deaths from cardiovascular causes. However, hospitalizations as a result of worsening heart failure (a secondary endpoint) were significantly reduced by digoxin.

Ivabradine was a medication introduced in April 2015 as a new therapy for those with chronic systolic heart failure (LVEF less than 35%), already on maximally tolerated beta-blocker doses, but with persistent resting heart rates over 70 beats per minute. In the randomized SHIFT study it was found to decrease hospitalization from heart failure.

6. What is the suggested dosing regimen of ivabradine?

Per the package insert, ivabradine is indicated to reduce the risk of hospitalization for worsening heart failure in patients with stable, symptomatic chronic heart failure with LVEF ≤35% who are in sinus rhythm with a resting heart rate ≥70 beats/min and either are on maximally tolerated doses of beta-blockers or have a contraindication to beta-blocker use.

Contraindications to ivabradine include acute decompensated heart failure, hypotension, sick sinus syndrome, third-degree heart block (unless a pacemaker is present), resting heart rate less than 60 beats/min, severe liver disease, and pacemaker dependence (heart rate maintained exclusively by a pacemaker).

The recommended starting dose of ivabradine is 5 mg twice daily. After 2 weeks of treatment, the dose can be adjusted based on heart rate. The maximum drug dose is 7.5 mg twice daily.

In patients with conduction defects or in whom bradycardia could lead to hemodynamic compromise, the initial recommended dose is 2.5 mg twice daily.

Suggested dose adjustments are as follows:

- For HR greater than 60 beats/min, increase dose by 2.5 mg (given twice daily) up to a maximum dose of 7.5 mg twice daily.
- For HR 50 to 60 beats/min, maintain current dose.
- For HR less than 50 beats/min or signs/symptoms of bradycardia, decrease dose by 2.5 mg (given twice daily). If current dose is 2.5 mg twice daily, discontinue therapy.

7. How do angiotensin-converting enzyme inhibitors and angiotensin II receptor blockers work?

ACE inhibitors inhibit ACE, thus blocking the conversion of angiotensin I to angiotensin II. ACE is predominantly found in the pulmonary and to a lesser extent in the renal endothelium. By decreasing the production of angiotensin II, ACE inhibitors attenuate sympathetic tone, decrease arterial vasoconstriction, and attenuate myocardial hypertrophy. Because angiotensin II stimulates aldosterone production, circulating levels of aldosterone are reduced. This results in decreased sodium chloride absorption, decreased potassium excretion in the distal tubules, and decreased water retention. Through a decrease in antidiuretic hormone (ADH) production, ACE inhibitors also decrease water absorption in the collecting ducts.

ARBs selectively block the binding of angiotensin II to the AT_1 receptor, thereby blocking the effect of angiotensin II on end organs. This results in attenuation of sympathetic tone, decrease in arterial vasoconstriction, and attenuation of myocardial hypertrophy. Because angiotensin II stimulates aldosterone production, circulating levels of aldosterone are reduced. This results in a decrease in sodium chloride absorption, potassium excretion in the distal tubules, and water retention.

8. What approach should be taken if a patient treated with an angiotensin-converting enzyme inhibitor develops a cough?

Nonproductive cough related to ACE inhibitors occurs in 5% to 10% of white patients of European descent and in up to 50% of Chinese patients. The cough is believed related to kinin potentiation.

The cough usually develops within the first months of therapy and disappears within 1 to 2 weeks of discontinuation of therapy. ACC/AHA guidelines suggest one should first make sure the cough is related to treatment and not another condition. The guidelines state that the demonstration that the cough disappears after drug withdrawal and recurs after re-challenge with another ACE inhibitor strongly suggests that ACE inhibition is the cause of the cough. They emphasize that patients should be *re-challenged*, because many will not redevelop a cough, suggesting the initial development of cough was coincidental and may have been related to heart failure. Patients who do have ACE inhibitor--related cough and cannot tolerate symptoms should be treated with an ARB.

9. How do aldosterone antagonists work?

Aldosterone receptor blockers block the mineralocorticoid receptor in the distal renal tubules, thereby decreasing sodium chloride absorption, potassium excretion, and water retention. In addition, they block the direct deleterious effects of aldosterone on the myocardium and may thus decrease myocardial fibrosis and its consequences.

10. List the two primary indications of aldosterone antagonists in heart failure.

Current primary indications of aldosterone antagonists in heart failure include the following:

- Chronic NYHA class II to IV heart failure and LV EF 35% or less in patients who are already receiving standard therapy for heart failure, including ACE inhibitors, beta-blockers, and diuretics (based on the evaluation of spironolactone in the RALES trial and eplerenone in the EMPHASIS trial)
- Post-MI patients with LV dysfunction (EF less than 40%) and heart failure symptoms who are already receiving standard therapy, including ACE inhibitors and beta-blockers (EPHESUS study of eplerenone)

11. What is the recommended dosing of aldosterone antagonists in heart failure?

Dosing of aldosterone antagonists in heart failure is as follows:

- **Spironolactone:** 12.5 to 25 mg daily, increased to up to 25 mg twice daily
- **Eplerenone:** 25 mg daily, increased to 50 mg daily

12. Can all patients with heart failure safely be started on an aldosterone antagonist?

No. Aldosterone antagonists should not be started in

- Men with creatinine more than 2.5 mg/dL or women with creatinine more than 2 mg/dL
- Patients with potassium more than 5 mEq/L
- Those in whom monitoring for hyperkalemia and renal function is not anticipated to be feasible
- Those not already on other diuretics

13. Describe common adverse effects of angiotensin-converting enzyme inhibitors, angiotensin II receptor blockers, and aldosterone antagonists.

Common adverse effects of ACE inhibitors, ARBs, and aldosterone antagonists include the following:

- **ACE inhibitors:** Hypotension, worsening renal function, hyperkalemia, cough, and angioedema
- **ARBs:** Hypotension, worsening renal function, and hyperkalemia
- **Aldosterone antagonists:** Hyperkalemia, worsening renal dysfunction, hypotension, and hyponatremia

ARBs are as likely as ACE inhibitors to produce hypotension, worsening renal function, and hyperkalemia. Otherwise, ARBs are better tolerated than ACE inhibitors. The incidence of cough is much lower in ARBs (approximately 1%) compared with ACE inhibitors (approximately 10%). The incidence of angioedema with ACE inhibitors is rare (less than 1%; more common in African Americans) and even rarer with ARBs. However, because there have been case reports of patients developing angioedema on ARBs, the guidelines advise that ARBs may be considered in patients who have had angioedema while taking an ACE inhibitor, albeit with extreme caution. Practically, if a patient develops angioedema while taking an ACE inhibitor, an ARB is generally not initiated.

Gynecomastia and other antiandrogen effects can occur with spironolactone and are not generally seen with eplerenone.

14. What are the indications for combination therapy with nitrates plus hydralazine in patients with chronic heart failure?

The vasodilator combination of I/H has been shown to produce modest benefits in patients with heart failure compared with placebo. The combination has, however, been shown to be less effective than

ACE inhibitors. The A-Heft trial, which was limited to African American patients with class III and IV heart failure, showed that the addition of I/H to standard therapy with an ACE inhibitor or a beta-blocker conferred significant morbidity and mortality benefit. Taking all the study data together, the I/H combination is indicated in the following patients:

- Those who cannot take an ACE inhibitor or ARB because of renal insufficiency or hyperkalemia
- Those who are hypertensive/symptomatic despite taking ACE inhibitor, ARB, and beta-blockers
- The combination of hydralazine and nitrates is recommended to improve outcomes for patients self-described as African Americans with moderate to severe symptoms on optimal medical therapy with ACE inhibitors, beta-blockers, and diuretics.

15. What dosing is used in treating patients with nitrates and hydralazine?

A dosing regimen that is used in treating patients with I + H is

- **Hydralazine:** Start at 37.5 mg three times a day, and increase to a goal of 75 mg three times a day.
- **Isosorbide dinitrate:** Start at 20 mg three times a day, and increase to a goal of 40 mg three times a day.

16. How should patients be treated with beta-blockers?

Certain beta-blockers have been convincingly shown to decrease mortality in patients with depressed EF and symptoms of heart failure, and thus it is a class I indication to treat such patients with beta-blockers, with an attempt to reach target doses. The beta-blockers shown to decrease mortality, their starting doses, and their target doses are given in Table 27.2. Recommendations from the Heart Failure Society of America and other organizations include the following:

- Patients should not be initiated on beta-blocker therapy during decompensated or hemodynamically unstable heart failure.
- Beta-blocker therapy should only be initiated when patients are euvolemic and hemodynamically stable, are usually on a good maintenance dose of diuretics (if indicated), and receiving ACE inhibitors or ARBs.
- Beta-blockers should be initiated at low doses, uptitrated gradually (in at least 2-week intervals), and titrated to target doses shown to be effective in clinical trials. Practitioners should aim to achieve target doses in 8 to 12 weeks from initiation of therapy and to maintain patients at maximal tolerated doses.
- If patient symptoms worsen during initiation or dose titration, the dose of diuretics or other concomitant vasoactive medications should be adjusted, and titration to target dose should be continued after the patient's symptoms return to baseline.
- If uptitration continues to be difficult, the titration interval can be prolonged, the target dose may have to be reduced, or the patient should be referred to a heart failure specialist.
- If an acute exacerbation of chronic heart failure occurs, therapy should be maintained if possible; the dose can be reduced if necessary, but abrupt discontinuation should be avoided. If the dose is reduced (or discontinued), the beta-blocker (and prior dose) should be gradually reinstated before discharge if possible.

17. What diuretics should be used and at what doses should they be initiated in heart failure patients?

Diuretics are indicated for volume overload. Starting doses of furosemide are often 20 to 40 mg once or twice a day, but higher doses will be required in patients with significant renal dysfunction. The dose should be uptitrated to a maximum of up to 600 mg daily (see Table 27.1). Failure of therapy is often the result of inadequate diuretic dosing. Torsemide is more expensive than furosemide but has superior absorption and longer duration of action. Bumetanide is approximately 40 times more potent milligram-for-milligram than furosemide. It can also be used in patients who are unresponsive or poorly responsive to furosemide, as it is thought to have better absorption.

Synergistic diuretics that act on the distal portion of the tubule (thiazides, such as metolazone, or potassium-sparing agents) are often added in those who fail to respond to high-dose loop diuretics alone.

18. Should all heart failure patients be placed on statins?

While statins have been shown to have significant effects in reducing the rate of MI and progression of vascular disease in those with coronary or peripheral vascular disease, the benefits have not been

Table 27.2. Initial and Target Doses for Commonly Utilized Drugs for Patients with Depressed Systolic Ejection Fraction and/or Congestive Heart Failure

DRUG	INITIAL DAILY DOSES	TARGET/MAXIMUM DOSES
Angiotensin Converting Enzyme Inhibitors		
Captopril	6.25 mg TID	50 mg TID
Enalapril	2.5 mg BID	10-20 mg BID
Lisinopril	2.5-5 mg qD	20-40 mg qD
Perindopril	2 mg qD	8-16 mg qD
Ramipril	1.25-2.5 mg qD	10 mg qD
Trandolapril	1 mg qD	4 mg qD
Angiotensin Receptor Blockers		
Candesartan	4-8 mg qD	32 mg qD
Valsartan	20-40 mg BID	160 mg BID
Angiotensin Receptor Neprilysin Inhibitor		
Sacubitril/valsartan	24/26-49/51 mg BID	97/103 mg BID
Aldosterone Antagonists		
Spironolactone	12.5-25 mg qD	25 mg qD
Eplerenone	25 mg qD	50 mg qD
Beta-Blockers		
Bisoprolol	1.25 mg qD	10 mg qD
Carvedilol	3.125 mg BID	25 mg BID (50 mg BID if >85 kg)
Metoprolol succinate	12.5-25 mg qD	200 mg qD
Cyclic Nucleotide-Gated Channel Blocker		
Ivabradine	2.5-5 mg BID	2.5-7.5 mg BID (based on HR)
Loop Diuretics		
Bumetanide	0.5-1.0 mg qD-BID	Max daily dose 10 mg
Furosemide	20-40 mg qD-BID	Max daily dose 600 mg
Torsemide	10-20 mg qD	Max daily dose 200 mg
Thiazide Diuretics		
Chlorothiazide	250-500 mg qD-BID	Max daily dose 1000 mg
Chlorthalidone	12.5-25 mg qD	Max daily dose 100 mg
Hydrochlorothiazide	25 mg qD-BID	Max daily dose 200 mg
Metolazone	2.5 mg qD	Max daily dose 20 mg
Potassium-Sparing Diuretics		
Amiloride	5 mg qD	Max daily dose 20 mg
Eplerenone	25 mg qD	50 mg qD
Spironolactone	12.5-25 mg qD	Max daily dose 50 mg
Triamterene	50-75 mg BID	Max daily dose 200 mg

Adapted from Yancy, C. W., Jessup, M., Bozkurt, B., Butler, J., Casey, D. E., Jr., Drazner, M. H., et al. [2013]. 2013 ACCF/AHA guideline for the management of heart failure: a report of the American College of Cardiology Foundation/American Heart Association Task Force on Practice Guidelines. Journal of the American College of Cardiology, *62[16], e148–e239*.

translated to heart failure patients with such atherosclerotic disease. Two large clinical trials, the CORONA trial and the GISSI-HF trial, demonstrated no clinical benefit in the use of statin therapy in addition to recommended medical therapy. Of note, the CORONA trial excluded patients with a history of MI within 6 months and those with a prior percutaneous coronary intervention or stroke but still noted to significantly decrease cardiovascular and heart failure hospitalization in those on statin therapy. The 2013 ACC/AHA guidelines do not currently recommend statin therapy in heart failure patients unless there is another indication.

19. What is the mechanism of action of digoxin?

Digoxin is a cardiac glycoside and is an inhibitor of the Na^+-K^+ ATPase pump in the sarcolemmal membrane of the myocyte and other cells. This inhibition causes intracellular accumulation of Na^+, which makes the Na^+-Ca^{2+} pump extrude less Ca^{2+}, causing Ca^{2+} to accumulate inside the cell. This effect results in increased force of contraction. Cardiac glycosides also have effects in the central nervous system, enhancing parasympathetic and reducing sympathetic outputs to the heart, through carotid sinus baroreflex sensitization. This is the mechanism that underlies the reduction in sinus node activity and slowing in atrioventricular (AV) conduction, which makes digoxin the only agent with a positive inotropic-bradycardic effect and is the basis for its use in the control of some supraventricular arrhythmias.

20. What are some of the relevant drug interactions of digoxin?

Relevant drug interactions of digoxin include the following:

- Quinidine, verapamil, amiodarone, propafenone, and quinine (used for muscle cramps) may double digoxin levels, and the dose of digoxin should be halved when used in combination with any of these drugs.
- Tetracycline, erythromycin, and omeprazole can increase digoxin absorption, whereas cholestyramine and kaolin-pectin can decrease it.
- Thyroxine and albuterol increase the volume of distribution, resulting in decreased levels.
- Cyclosporine and paroxetine and other selective serotonin reuptake inhibitors (SSRIs) can increase serum digoxin levels.

21. What are the clinical manifestations of digoxin toxicity?

Digoxin has a narrow safety margin. (The difference in plasma drug concentrations between therapeutic and toxic levels is small.) Patients with digoxin toxicity may manifest nausea, vomiting, anorexia, diarrhea, fatigue, generalized malaise, visual disturbances (green or yellow halos around lights and objects), and arrhythmias. In the presence of hypokalemia, digoxin toxicity may occur within the therapeutic level. Digoxin dose should be reduced in elderly patients, in patients with renal insufficiency (glomerular filtration rate [GFR] less than 60 mL/min), and when combined with certain drugs. To guide dosing during chronic therapy, digoxin levels should be measured 6 to 8 hours after a dose.

22. What are the electrocardiographic findings of digoxin toxicity?

Digoxin toxicity can result in a variety of ventricular and supraventricular arrhythmias and AV conduction abnormalities. These arrhythmias result from the electrophysiologic effects of digoxin: Increased intracellular Ca^{2+} levels predispose to Ca^{2+}-induced delayed afterdepolarizations and hence increased automaticity (especially in the junction, Purkinje system, and ventricles); excessive vagal effects predispose to sinus bradycardia/arrest and AV block. Bradyarrhythmias and blocks are more common when the patient is also taking amiodarone. Specific ECG findings include the following:

- Sinus bradycardia
- Sinus arrest
- First- and second-degree AV block
- AV junctional escape
- Paroxysmal atrial tachycardia with AV block
- Bidirectional ventricular tachycardia (VT)
- Premature ventricular beats
- Bigeminy
- Regularized atrial fibrillation or atrial fibrillation with slow ventricular response (common)

23. How is digoxin toxicity treated?

It depends on the clinical severity. Digoxin withdrawal is sufficient with only suggestive symptoms. Activated charcoal may enhance the gastrointestinal (GI) clearance of digoxin if given within 6 hours of ingestion. Drugs that increase plasma digoxin levels (see Question 19) should be discontinued (except amiodarone because of its long half-life). Correction of hypokalemia is vital (intravenous [IV] replacement through a large vein is preferred with life-threatening arrhythmias), but judgment is needed in the presence of high degrees of AV block. Symptomatic AV block may respond to atropine or to phenytoin (100 mg IV every 5 minutes up to 1000 mg until response or side effects); if no response, use Digibind. The use of temporary transvenous pacing should be avoided. Patients with severe bradycardia should be given Digibind, even if they respond to atropine. Lidocaine and phenytoin may be used to treat ventricular arrhythmias, but for potentially life-threatening bradyarrhythmias or tachyarrhythmias, Digibind should be used. Dialysis has no role because of the high tissue binding of digoxin.

24. What are the indications for Digibind?

The indications for Digibind include life-threatening bradyarrhythmias and tachyarrhythmias; hemodynamic instability caused by digoxin; potassium level of more than 5 mEq/L in the setting of acute ingestion, regardless of symptoms or EKG findings; and digoxin level of more than 10 ng/mL or the ingestion of more than 10 mg of digoxin, regardless of symptoms or EKG findings. Digibind is an antibody that binds to digoxin in the plasma and interstitial space, creating a concentration gradient for the exit of intracellular digoxin. As poisoning of the Na^+-K^+ ATPase is relieved and K^+ is pumped intracellularly with the potential of causing hypokalemia, the potassium levels should be monitored when Digibind is used. The half-life of the digoxin-Digibind complex is 15 to 20 hours if renal function is normal. Serum digoxin concentration rises significantly after Digibind use (as tissue digoxin is released into the bloodstream bound to the antibody) and should not be measured.

25. What four classes of drugs exacerbate the syndrome of heart failure and should be avoided in most heart failure with reduced ejection fraction patients?

- Antiarrhythmic agents as a class are generally contraindicated in patients with HFrEF. Most can exert cardiodepressant and proarrhythmic effects. Only amiodarone and dofetilide appear to have a neutral effect on survival.
- Calcium channel blockers, more specifically the nondihydropyridine group, can lead to worsening heart failure and have been associated with an increased risk of cardiovascular events. Only the dihydropyridines or vasoselective calcium channel blockers have been shown not to adversely affect survival and can be used in select patients needing improved blood pressure control.
- Nonsteroidal anti-inflammatory drugs (NSAIDs) can cause sodium retention and peripheral vasoconstriction by directly inhibiting sodium resorption in the ascending loop of Henle and distal collecting ducts. This can attenuate the efficacy and enhance the toxicity of diuretics and ACE inhibitors.
- Thiazolidinediones were developed to increase insulin sensitivity by activating peroxisome proliferator-activated receptors (PPARs), which forces cells to increase reliance on oxidation of carbohydrates rather than fatty acids. However, these medications also have effects on the renal tubules, where PPARs act to direct sodium resorption in the collecting ducts. They can lead to sodium retention and onset of heart failure symptoms in those without a history of heart failure.

26. Is dietary restriction of sodium recommended in patients with symptomatic heart failure?

Yes. In general, patients should restrict themselves to 2 to 3 g sodium daily and less than 2 g daily in moderate to severe cases of heart failure.

27. Is fluid restriction recommended in all patients with heart failure?

Not necessarily. Fluid restriction is generally reserved for those patients with advanced or Stage D heart failure. Fluid restriction is recommended for patients with (1) hyponatremia (sodium less than 130 mEq/L) or (2) fluid retention difficult to control despite high doses of diuretics and sodium restriction. In such cases, patients are generally restricted to less than 2 L/day.

28. Should patients with heart failure be told to use salt substitutes instead of salt?

In some cases, the answer is no. Many salt substitutes contain potassium chloride in place of sodium chloride. This could lead to potential hyperkalemia in patients on potassium-sparing diuretics, ACE inhibitors or ARBs, aldosterone antagonists, and in those with chronic kidney disease (or those with the potential to develop acute renal failure). Patients who are permitted to use salt substitutes need to be cautioned about potassium issues.

29. What are the current criteria for consideration of cardiac resynchronization therapy with biventricular pacing?

The 2012 ACC/AHA/Heart Rhythm Society (HRS) guidelines on device-based therapy updated their recommendations for those who should receive CRT (with a class I indication) with or without ICD. The recommendation expanded to include those with NYHA class II heart failure symptoms. However, in the CRT for Mild to Moderate Heart Failure Study published in 2010 by the RAFT investigators, there was also a new finding that those who benefit from resynchronization predominantly have a QRS greater than 150 ms. Therefore current class I recommended criteria for CRT include

- Presence of sinus rhythm
- Class II, III, or ambulatory class IV symptoms despite good medical therapy
- LVEF less than or equal to 35%
- QRS more than 150 ms (especially if left bundle branch block morphology is present)

CRT may also be considered in those with less prolonged QRS duration (120 to 150 ms), although benefit is generally not as great and/or not as well established.

30. Which patients with heart failure should be considered for an implantable cardioverter defibrillator?

In the updated 2012 ACC/AHA/HRS guidelines on device-based therapy, the writing group stated that they believed guidelines for ICD implantation should reflect the ICD trials that were conducted. Thus, there are many very specific indications for ICD placement, based on symptom class, ischemic or nonischemic causes of heart failure, and EF. Because EF may improve significantly after MI (as a result of myocardial salvage and myocardial stunning) and with optimal medical therapy (including ACE inhibitors/ARBs and beta-blockers), patients being considered for ICD implantation for primary prevention should be optimally treated and have their EF reassessed on optimal medical therapy. ICD should only be considered in patients with a reasonable expectation of survival with an acceptable functional status for at least 1 year. Class I recommendations for ICD include the following:

- Secondary prevention (cardiac arrest survivors of VT/ventricular fibrillation [VF], hemodynamically unstable sustained VT)
- Structural heart disease and sustained VT, whether hemodynamically stable or unstable
- Syncope of undetermined origin with hemodynamically significant sustained VT or VF induced at electrophysiologic study
- LVEF less than or equal to 35% at least 40 days after MI and NYHA functional class II and III
- LVEF less than 30% at least 40 days after MI and NYHA functional class I
- LVEF less than or equal to 35% despite medical therapy in patient with nonischemic cardiomyopathy and NYHA functional class II and III
- Nonsustained VT caused by prior MI, LVEF less than 40%, and inducible VF or sustained VT at electrophysiologic study

31. How is advanced heart failure defined?

Advanced heart failure is recognized when heart failure patients follow the below clinical patterns:

- More than two hospitalizations or emergency room visits in the past 1 year for heart failure symptoms
- Progressive decline in renal function
- Progressive weight loss without other identifiable cause, known as cardiac cachexia
- Intolerance to beta-blockers due to worsening heart failure or hypotension
- Frequent systolic blood pressure less than 90 mm Hg
- Frequent dyspnea during dressing or bathing requiring rest
- Inability to walk one block on level ground due to dyspnea or fatigue
- Progressive decline in serum sodium, usually less than 133 mEq/L
- Frequent ICD shocks
- Need to escalate diuretic therapy to maintain volume status, usually reaching an equivalent daily dose of greater than 160 mg furosemide/day and/or need for daily supplemental metolazone therapy

Bibliography, Suggested Readings, and Websites

Cooper, L. T., Baughman, K. L., Feldman, A. M., Frustaci, A., Jessup, M., Kuhl, U., et al. (2007). The role of endomyocardial biopsy in the management of cardiovascular disease: a scientific statement from the American Heart Association, the American College of Cardiology, and the European Society of Cardiology. Endorsed by the Heart Failure Society of

America and the Heart Failure Association of the European Society of Cardiology. *Journal of the American College of Cardiology, 50*(19), 1914–1931.

Epstein, A. E., DiMarco, J. P., Ellenbogen, K. A., Estes, N. A., 3rd, Freedman, R. A., Gettes, L. S., et al. (2013). 2012 ACCF/AHA/HRS focused update incorporated into the ACCF/AHA/HRS 2008 guidelines for device-based therapy of cardiac rhythm abnormalities: a report of the American College of Cardiology/American Heart Association Task Force on Practice Guidelines and the Heart Rhythm Society. *Journal of the American College of Cardiology, 61*(3), e6–e75.

Heart Failure Society of America. <http://www.hfsa.org>.

Heart Failure Society of America, Lindenfeld, J., Albert, N. M., Boehmer, J. P., Collins, S. P., Ezekowitz, J. A., et al. (2010). HFSA 2010 comprehensive heart failure practice guideline. *Journal of Cardiac Failure, 16*, e1–e194.

Mann, D. L. (2008). Management of heart failure patients with reduced ejection fraction. In P. Libby, R. Bonow, & D. Mann (Eds.), *Braunwald's heart disease: a textbook of cardiovascular medicine* (8th ed.). Philadelphia, PA: Saunders.

Yancy, C. W., Jessup, M., Bozkurt, B., Butler, J., Casey, D. E., Jr., Drazner, M. H., et al. (2013). 2013 ACCF/AHA guideline for the management of heart failure: a report of the American College of Cardiology Foundation/American Heart Association Task Force on Practice Guidelines. *Journal of the American College of Cardiology, 62*(16), e148–e239.

HEART TRANSPLANTATION

Savitri Fedson

1. **How many heart transplants are performed in the United States each year? What are the most frequent causes of heart disease requiring cardiac transplantation?**
Dr. Christiaan Barnard performed the first human allograft transplant in 1967. Approximately 2200 to 2600 heart transplants occur each year, most commonly for nonischemic cardiomyopathy (53%) and coronary artery disease (CAD; 38%), and less commonly for congenital heart disease, valvular heart disease, and other indications, including retransplantation. There has been a slight increase in these numbers over the past 3 years after a decade of stable numbers.

2. **List common indications for heart transplantation.**
   - Severe heart failure (HF) (American College of Cardiology/American Heart Association [ACC/AHA] stage D, New York Heart Association [NYHA] class III or IV) with poor short-term prognosis despite maximal medical therapy, requiring continuous inotropic therapy, requiring mechanical support (balloon pump, left ventricular assist device [LVAD], extracorporeal membrane oxygenation [ECMO])
   - Restrictive or hypertrophic cardiomyopathy with NYHA III or IV symptoms
   - Refractory angina despite medical therapy, not amenable to revascularization, with poor short-term prognosis
   - Recurrent or refractory ventricular arrhythmias, despite medical and/or device therapy
   - Complex congenital heart disease with progressive ventricular failure not amenable to surgical or percutaneous repair
   - Retransplantation as a result of cardiac allograft vasculopathy (CAV)
   - Unresectable low-grade tumors confined to the myocardium, without evidence of metastasis

3. **What baseline evaluations are obtained in the pretransplant workup?**
Pretransplant evaluation assesses a patient's HF severity, mortality benefit from transplant, comorbidities that might shorten life expectancy or affect post-transplant survival, and potential contraindications to surgery. Factors important in transplant evaluation are given in Table 28.1.

4. **What are contraindications to heart transplantation?**
Contraindications include any noncardiac conditions that may decrease a patient's survival and increase risk of rejection or infection; contraindications are listed in Table 28.2.

5. **What do the terms *allotransplantation, xenotransplantation, orthotopic transplantation,* and *heterotopic transplantation* mean?**
   a) **Allotransplantation** involves transplantation of cells, tissue, or organs between the *same* species.
   b) **Xenotransplantation** involves transplantation of cells, tissue, or organs between *different* species.
   c) **Orthotopic heart transplantation:** The donor heart is transplanted *in the same position as* the recipient's heart. There are three anastomotic approaches used (Fig. 28.1).
      i. **Biatrial approach:** The donor atrial cuff is anastomosed to the recipient left atrium and right atrium, followed by aortic and pulmonary artery anastomosis.
      ii. **Bicaval approach:** The donor left atrial cuff is anastomosed to the recipient left atrium, followed by inferior vena cava, superior vena cava, aortic, and pulmonary artery anastomosis. This approach may be associated with improved atrial function, lower incidence of atrial arrhythmias, sinus node dysfunction, and tricuspid insufficiency.
      iii. **Total heart approach:** Similar to the bicaval approach, with only the cuffs of the recipient left atrium surrounding the pulmonary veins used for anastomosis.
   d) **Heterotopic heart transplantation:** The recipient's heart *remains in the mediastinum*, and the donor heart is attached "parallel" to the recipient heart (see Fig. 28.1).

Table 28.1. Factors Important in the Evaluation of the Patients for Cardiac Transplantation

History and Physical Examination
Immunocompatibility • ABO and HLA typing • PRA/flow
Infection • Screen for: hepatitis B and C, HIV, syphilis, TB (IGRA, such as QuantiFERON–Gold) > PPD). • Check titers for: IgG for HSV, CMV, *Toxoplasma,* EBV, and varicella.
Organ function • Basic metabolic panel • Complete blood count • Liver function tests • PT/INR • Urinalysis • Glomerular filtration rate, 24-h urine protein • Pulmonary function test with arterial blood gas • PA/lateral CXR • Abdominal imaging (ultrasound or other technique if needed) • Carotid Doppler • ABI • DEXA • Dental exam • Ophthalmologic exam if patient has DM
HF severity • Cardiopulmonary exercise test with respiratory exchange ratio • Echocardiogram (echo) • Right heart catheter with vasodilator challenge (if indicated) • ECG assessment for reversible ischemia/viability (if indicated)
Vaccination history • Influenza • Pneumococcal • Hepatitis B • Zoster • MMR
Preventive and age-appropriate screening • Colonoscopy • Mammography • Gynecologic/pap examination • Prostate evaluation • High-resolution CT if significant smoking history
Psychosocial evaluation

ABI, Ankle-brachial index; *CMV*, cytomegalovirus; *CT*, computed tomography; *CXR*, chest x-ray; *DEXA*, dual energy x-ray absorptiometry; *DM*, diabetes mellitus; *ECG*, electrocardiogram; *EBV*, Epstein-Barr virus; *HF*, heart failure; *HIV*, human immunodeficiency virus; *HLA*, human leukocyte antigen; *HSV*, herpes simplex virus; *Ig*, immunoglobulin; *IGRA*, interferon gamma release assay; *INR*, international normalized ratio; *MMR*, measles, mumps, and rubella; *PA*, posteroanterior; *PPD*, purified protein derivative; *PRA*, panel-reactive antibody; *PT*, prothrombin time; *TB*, tuberculosis.

6. **Define ischemic time of the donor heart. Why is it important?**
   The "cold ischemic time" is the time between cross-clamping of the donor heart and reperfusion of the heart in the recipient. During this interval, ischemic injury can occur to the heart because of lack of perfusion. Myocardial preservation is achieved with hypothermia and placement of the heart

Table 28.2. Absolute and Relative Contraindications to Heart Transplantation

Absolute Contraindications (for Solitary Heart Transplant):

- Systemic illness limiting survival despite heart transplant (e.g., active malignancy, HIV/AIDS with CD4 count <200 cells/mm^3, systemic lupus erythematosus)
- Systemic illness with high probability of recurrence in the transplanted heart (e.g., amyloidosis)
- Fixed pulmonary HTN (pulmonary vascular resistance >5 Wood units, transpulmonary gradient >15 mm Hg) unresponsive to pulmonary vasodilators
- Presence of any noncardiac conditions that would limit life expectancy
  - Irreversible hepatic disease
  - Irreversible renal failure
  - Severe symptomatic cerebrovascular disease
  - Severe symptomatic peripheral vascular disease irremediable by surgical/percutaneous intervention
  - Severe pulmonary dysfunction (FVC and FEV1 <40% of predicted)

Relative Contraindications

- Age >65 years (program dependent)
- DM with end-organ damage
- Morbid obesity (body mass index cut-off is program dependent, typically >35 kg/m^2)
- Psychosocial impairment (tobacco/alcohol/polysubstance abuse, psychiatric instability, noncompliance, poor social support)

AIDS, Acquired immunodeficiency syndrome; *CD4*, cluster of differentiation 4; *DM*, diabetes mellitus; *FEV1*, first forced expiratory volume; *FVC*, forced vital capacity; *HIV*, human immunodeficiency virus; *HTN*, hypertension.

in a solution mimicking the intracellular milieu to prevent cellular edema/acidosis (cardioplegia) and to maintain adenosine triphosphate (ATP) supply for membrane function. A prolonged ischemic time can lead to irreversible damage to the harvested organ. A cold ischemic time of greater than 5 hours is associated with a higher incidence of cardiac allograft dysfunction and decreased transplant recipient survival. There are ongoing studies of techniques for beating heart procurement, or "warm perfusion."

7. What is the estimated graft survival at 1 year, 3 years, 5 years, and 10 years posttransplant? What are the common causes of death?

Based on the 2014 US Organ Procurement and Transplantation Network (OPTN) and International Society for Heart and Lung Transplantation (ISHLT) report, graft survival is approximately 87% at 1 year, 73% at 5 years, and 50% 11.3 years post transplantation.

The major causes of posttransplant death are as follows:

- **Less than 30 days:** Graft failure, multiorgan failure, infection
- **Less than 1 year:** Infection, graft failure, acute allograft rejection
- **Greater than 5 years:** Allograft vasculopathy, late graft failure, malignancies, infection

8. What is cardiac allograft vasculopathy? Describe its pathophysiology, incidence, risk factors, and outcome.

Also known as transplant vasculopathy or transplant CAD, CAV is the progressive narrowing of the coronary arteries of the transplanted heart. Angiographic incidence of CAV is approximately 30% at 5 years and 50% at 10 years. CAV is associated with a significantly increased risk of death. After the first year post transplant, CAV is the second most common cause of death (after malignancy).

In CAV, there is diffuse, concentric proliferation of the intimal smooth muscle cells that typically involves the entire length of the coronary artery. In contrast, conventional atherosclerosis results from fibrofatty plaque resulting in concentric or eccentric focal lesions.

The etiology of CAV remains unclear, but immunologic (cellular/humoral rejection, human leukocyte antigen [HLA] mismatch) and nonimmunologic (cytomegalovirus [CMV] infection, hypercholesterolemia, older age/male donors, younger recipients, history of CAD, diabetes mellitus [DM], and insulin resistance) factors have been implicated.

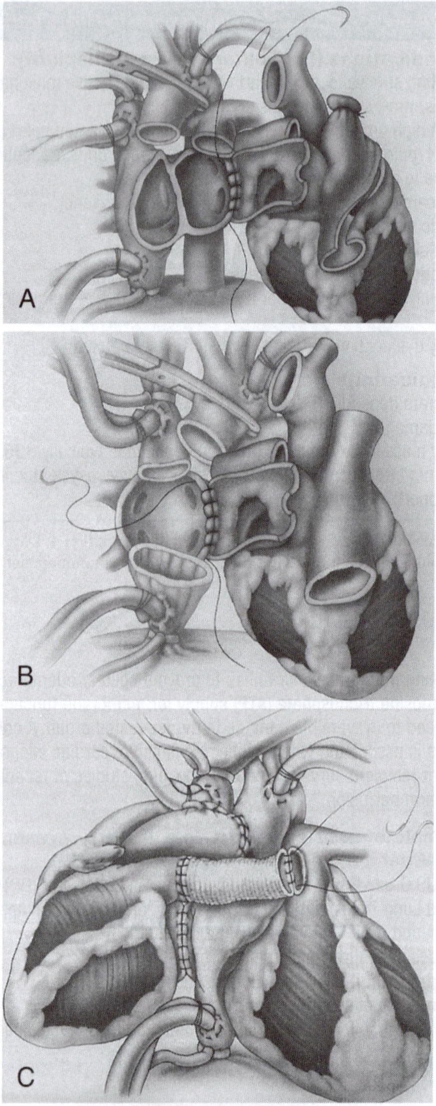

Fig. 28.1. Anastomotic approaches used in cardiac transplantation. **A,** Biatrial approach. The donor atrial cuff is anastomosed to the recipient left atrium, right atrium, followed by aortic and pulmonary artery anastomosis. **B,** Bicaval approach. The donor left atrial cuff is anastomosed to the recipient left atrium, followed by inferior vena cava, superior vena cava, aortic, and pulmonary artery anastomosis. This approach may be associated with improved atrial function, lower incidence of atrial arrhythmias, sinus node dysfunction, and tricuspid insufficiency. **C,** Heterotopic transplantation. The donor-recipient left atrial cuff is anastomosed, followed by superior vena cava, aortic, and pulmonary artery anastomosis via Dacron graft. This procedure is considered in donor-recipient body-size mismatch, when the recipient pulmonary artery systolic pressure is greater than 60 mm Hg, or when there is suboptimal donor heart systolic function. *(From Kirklin, J. K., Young, J. B., & McGiffin, D. C. [2002].* Heart transplantation. *Philadelphia, PA: Churchill Livingstone.)*

Cardiac transplant recipients can also develop conventional atherosclerosis through two main mechanisms:

- *Progression* of preexisting donor CAD
- *De novo* development as a result of transplant-related hypertension (HTN), DM, and dyslipidemia. Mammalian target of rapamycin (mTOR) inhibitors, also known as proliferation signal inhibitors, such as sirolimus and everolimus, may have a use in delaying progression of CAV when initiated early post transplant.

9. List infections that are encountered early and late after cardiac transplantation.

- **Early (less than 1 month):**
  - Donor-transmitted pathogens
  - Nosocomial infections related to surgery or invasive procedures (mediastinitis, wound/line/urinary tract infections, ventilator-associated pneumonia)
  - Early virus reactivation (typically herpes simplex virus, human herpesvirus-6)
- **Intermediate (1 to 6 months):**
  - Opportunistic infections
    - Bacterial (*Mycobacterium, Listeria, Nocardia*)
    - Viral (Cytomegalovirus (CMV), Epstein-Barr virus [EBV], varicella zoster virus [VZV], adenovirus, papovavirus)
    - Fungal (*Aspergillus*, pneumocystis, *Cryptococcus*)
    - Protozoal (*Strongyloides, Toxoplasma*)
- **Late (more than 6 months):** Most patients have stable graft function by this time, therefore the immunosuppressive regimen is reduced and the risk for opportunistic infection decreases. Typically, encountered infections include common viral and bacterial respiratory pathogens. However, some patients may develop chronic or recurrent opportunistic infections (i.e., CMV-related superinfection, EBV-associated lymphoproliferative disease). Reactivation of latent tuberculosis (TB) can occur within the first year of transplant.

10. What types of malignancies are encountered post transplant?

Malignancy risk in cardiac transplant recipients approaches 1% to 4% per year and is 10 to 100 times higher compared to age-matched controls. Malignancy is the major cause of late death in heart transplant recipients and is thought to be a result of chronic immunosuppression.

The most common malignancy encountered is skin cancer (29% at 15 years). Squamous cell carcinoma is more prevalent in transplant patients compared to basal celi cancer, which is more prevalent in the general population. Nonskin malignancies are seen in 18% of cardiac transplant recipients at 15 years and include prostate, lung, bladder, renal, breast, and colon cancer.

Posttransplant lymphoproliferative disorder (PTLD) is diagnosed in 6% of cardiac transplant recipients at 15 years. PTLD can be associated with primary or reactivated EBV infection, which leads to abnormal proliferation of lymphoid cells and can involve the gastrointestinal, pulmonary, and central nervous systems. PTLD usually presents as non-Hodgkin's lymphoma (predominately B-cell type). The risk of PTLD varies with allograft type, immunosuppression, EBV immunity prior to transplant, and previous CMV infection.

Because of the increased risk of malignancies, surveillance screening is recommended, including annual dermatologic skin checks.

11. Describe potential arrhythmias encountered post transplantation.

The donor heart is disconnected from sympathetic and parasympathetic innervation. Therefore, the resting heart rate is higher than normal (90 to 110 bpm) and atropine has no effect on the denervated heart. Early posttransplant arrhythmias can be a result of surgical trauma to the sinoatrial (SA) or atrioventricular (AV) nodes, prolonged ischemic time, surgical suture lines, and rejection. Late-occurring arrhythmias may suggest rejection or the presence of posttransplant vasculopathy.

- Sinus node dysfunction. Sinus node dysfunction occurs in up to 50% of cardiac transplant recipients. Sinus node dysfunction early after transplant does not appear to affect mortality but has been associated with increased morbidity. Treatment of sinus bradycardia includes temporary pacing, intravenous (isoproterenol or dobutamine) or oral (theophylline or terbutaline) therapy in the immediate postoperative period. However, severe persistent bradycardia may require permanent pacemaker placement, which is necessary in up to 15% of patients.
- AV nodal block. AV nodal block is rarely encountered; its occurrence may indicate the presence of transplant vasculopathy and has been associated with increased mortality.
- Atrial arrhythmias. Transient atrial arrhythmias, especially *premature atrial contractions (PACs)*, are common in the early postoperative period; their clinical significance remains unclear, but

frequent occurrences should prompt evaluation for rejection. *Atrial fibrillation or flutter* can occur in up to 25% of cardiac transplant recipients; late occurrence warrants evaluation for rejection. When atrial fibrillation or flutter occurs, treatment includes rate control with beta-blockers, cardioversion, overdrive pacing, and treatment for rejection. The non-dihydropyridine calcium-channel blockers can be used, but they inhibit the metabolism of calcineurin and mTOR inhibitors. Atrial flutter and other supraventricular tachycardias can be treated with radiofrequency ablation and may be intrinsic to the donor heart.

- Ventricular arrhythmias. Premature ventricular contractions (PVCs) are not uncommon early after cardiac transplantation, and their clinical significance is unknown. However, nonsustained ventricular tachycardia (greater than three consecutive PVCs) has been associated with rejection and transplant vasculopathy. Sustained ventricular tachycardia or ventricular fibrillation is associated with poor prognosis and indicates severe transplant vasculopathy or high-grade rejection. Treatment includes correcting electrolyte abnormalities, intravenous amiodarone or lidocaine, defibrillation, and prompt evaluation for rejection and transplant vasculopathy.

12. What are the clinical signs and symptoms associated with acute cardiac transplant rejection (allograft rejection)?

Between 40% and 70% of cardiac transplant recipients experience rejection within the first year posttransplant. Most episodes occur in the first 6 months, with a decrease in frequency after 12 months. Acute allograft rejection is the leading cause of death in the first year after transplant; this emphasizes the importance of early diagnosis and treatment. Most patients are asymptomatic early in the course of rejection; therefore, routine biopsies are necessary to assist in the diagnosis of rejection. In an appropriate low-risk group, gene expression profiling (GEP) may be used to identify those who warrant endomyocardial biopsy (EMB) for surveillance.

The clinical presentation of rejection can be variable. Patients may present with nonspecific constitutional symptoms such as fever, malaise, fatigue, myalgias, joint pain, and flu-like symptoms. Signs and symptoms of left ventricular (LV) and right ventricular (RV) dysfunction include severe fatigue, loss of energy, listlessness, weight gain, sudden onset of dyspnea, syncope/presyncope, orthopnea/paroxysmal nocturnal dyspnea, and abdominal bloating/nausea/vomiting. Physical exam can reveal elevated jugular venous pulse, peripheral edema, hepatomegaly, S3 or S4 gallop, and lower than usual blood pressure. Signs of cardiac irritation may include sinus tachycardia, bradycardia, arrhythmias, pericardial friction rub, or new pericardial effusion by echo. Acute rejection can occur at any time, including years after transplant.

13. List the different types of acute allograft rejections.

Allograft rejection occurs as a result of recipient immune response to donor heart antigens.

a) Hyperacute rejection occurs within minutes to hours of transplantation as a result of preformed recipient antibodies against donor ABO blood group, HLA, and endothelial cell antigens. Hyperacute rejection often results in loss of the graft.
b) Cellular rejection is a T-lymphocyte predominant, mononuclear inflammatory response directed against the allograft.
c) Noncellular or humoral/antibody-mediated rejection (AMR) is the result of de novo antibodies formed by the donor against recipient HLA antigens expressed on the vascular endothelium of the graft. Complement-mediated cytokine release leads to microvascular damage to the donor heart.

14. Describe the grading and immunohistologic findings of acute cellular rejection and acute antibody-mediated rejection.

The Standardized Biopsy Grading system for acute cellular rejection (ACR) and AMR was established in 1990 (later revised in 2004) by the ISHLT:

- The rejection grades and corresponding histologic findings for ACR are presented in Table 28.3A.
- The rejection grades and corresponding histologic findings for AMR are presented in Table 28.3B.

15. How is allograft rejection diagnosed?

- **Echocardiogram** may reveal increased ventricular wall thickness as a result of edema, alterations in diastolic function (decreased Ea, pseudonormal/restrictive filling pattern, shortened isovolumic relaxation time), decreased systolic function, and pericardial effusion.
- **Endomyocardial biopsy** remains the gold standard for the diagnosis of allograft rejection. *ACR* is characterized by lymphocytic infiltration and myocyte damage. *AMR* is supported by findings

Table 28.3A. Acute Cellular Rejection

REJECTION GRADE	HISTOLOGIC FINDINGS
Grade 0R	No rejection
Grade 1R, mild	Interstitial and/or perivascular infiltrate with ≤1 focus of myocyte damage
Grade 2R, moderate	≥2 foci of infiltrate with associated myocyte damage
Grade 3R, severe	Diffuse infiltrate with multifocal myocyte damage, ± edema, hemorrhage, or vasculitis

Table 28.3B. Acute Antibody-Mediated Rejection

REJECTION GRADE	HISTOLOGIC FINDINGS
AMR 0	Negative for acute AMR No histologic or immunopathologic features of AMR
AMR 1	Positive for AMR Histologic* features of AMR Positive immunofluorescence/immunoperoxidase** staining (+CD68, C4d)

AMR, Antibody-mediated rejection.

*Histologic features of AMR: myocardial capillary injury with endothelial swelling and accumulation of perivascular macrophage.

**Immunohistochemistry shows deposition of immunoglobulin (IgG, M, A), complement (C3d, C4d, C1q), and CD68 staining for macrophage in capillaries (using CD31 or CD34 vascular markers).

of myocardial capillary injury with intravascular macrophages; immunologic staining will identify antibody and complement deposits within capillaries.

- ECG can show a relative decrease in precordial lead amplitude, representing effusion or myocardial edema.
- **Rejection is a clinical event.** Even if biopsies do not support rejection, treatment can still be initiated on the basis of symptoms.

16. What is gene expression profiling, and how is it used in the diagnosis of rejection?

GEP evaluates the transcription of genes involved in acute rejection and myocardial injury. GEP is performed on peripheral blood analysis. The AlloMap score uses GEP to grade the risk of presence of rejection. The AlloMap score has been shown to have a high negative predictive value for lower scores, but the positive predictive value for high scores is low. Thus, the use of AlloMap is recommended only in select patients: to rule out the presence of ACR of grade 2R or greater in low-risk patients, between 6 months and 5 years after cardiac transplantation, who are on less than 20 mg of prednisone daily.

17. How is an endomyocardial biopsy performed, and what are potential complications?

EMB is the gold standard for the diagnosis of cardiac allograft rejection. During the first year post transplant, scheduled surveillance is performed with biopsies or with GEP. After the first year, these evaluations are performed at greater intervals or as dictated by clinical suspicion for rejection.

A sheath is placed into a central vein, typically the right internal jugular vein or femoral vein, and a flexible bioptome is introduced via the sheath and advanced into the right ventricle under fluoroscopic or echocardiographic guidance. Three to four samples are obtained from the interventricular septum.

Potential complications of biopsies include the following:

- Tricuspid valve, subvalvular damage, and chordal rupture can occur, resulting in flail leaflets and severe regurgitation.
- Right ventricular wall perforation resulting in cardiac tamponade
- Transient heart block and ventricular arrhythmia

- Complications associated with venous access include hematomas, nerve paresis, pneumothorax, thrombosis, and thromboembolism.

18. What is induction therapy? Describe its role in cardiac transplantation,

Induction therapy involves use of agents such as cytolytic antilymphocyte antibodies or T-cell signal inhibitors to suppress donor immune response, which is most vigorous shortly after transplantation. Induction agents have not consistently been shown to decrease rates of rejection and have been associated with increased risk of infection and malignancy (see Table 28.4).

However, induction therapy is beneficial in certain situations:

- Steroid-refractory, recurrent rejection
- Inability to use calcineurin inhibitors in the setting of profound renal insufficiency in the immediate postoperative period. Antilymphocyte antibodies can provide immunosuppression for at least 10 to 14 days until recovery of renal function.
- Higher immediate risk for rejection, such as with sensitized recipients

19. What is the incidence of acute cellular rejection? Describe predisposing factors and treatment.

Approximately 40% of cardiac transplant recipients have ACR (grade above 1R) in the first year after transplantation. Rejection frequency declines after the first year post transplant. Risk factors for ACR include early posttransplant period, female donor, young/African American/female recipients, and HLA mismatches.

ACR can present with or without hemodynamic compromise. Presentation determines the aggressiveness of treatment, which can include optimization of calcineurin inhibitors, increasing antimetabolites (mycophenolate mofetil [MMF]), and pulse dose steroids, intravenous immunoglobulins (IVIGs), and antithymocyte globulin (ATG).

Treatment generally consists of high-dose corticosteroids, or ATG.

20. Describe predisposing risk factors and treatment for acute antibody-mediated rejection.

AMR has a worse prognosis than ACR, with higher rates of mortality, graft loss, and incidence of transplant vasculopathy. Predisposing factors for AMR include prior cardiac transplant, transfusion, pregnancy (exposure to husband's HLA through the fetus), ventricular assist device placement (which can result in prominent B-cell activation and production of anti-HLA antibodies), CMV infection, and prior OKT3 therapy.

AMR treatment has not been standardized. Therapies currently include high-dose corticosteroids, plasmapheresis, IVIGs, rituximab, bortezomib, antilymphocyte antibodies (ATG), intravenous heparin, target of rapamycin (TOR) inhibitors, cyclophosphamide, and photopheresis.

Active CMV infection has been associated with AMR. Thus, patients with AMR should be evaluated for de novo or reactivation of CMV infection and treated if infection is present.

Table 28.4. Induction Agents

AGENT	MECHANISM OF ACTION	ADVERSE EFFECTS	THERAPEUTIC TARGET	INDICATIONS FOR USE
Polyclonal Antibodies (Derived from Animals Immunized with Human Thymocytes, Cultured B-Cells)				
ATG	Inhibits T-cell activation and B-cell proliferation Depletes T-cells and B-cells	Serum sickness, infection (especially CMV), rash, thrombocytopenia, leukopenia, anaphylaxis	T-cell to <10% of pretreatment level	• Induction therapy • Rejection grade >2R + symptoms/hemodynamic compromise • Steroid-refractory or recurrent rejection
Basiliximab (IL-2 receptor blocker)	Inhibits T- and B-cell proliferation	Severe, acute hypersensitivity reaction		• Induction therapy (shorter half-life of 7 days)

ATG, Antithymocyte globulin; *CMV*, cytomegalovirus.

21. Describe typical maintenance immunosuppression therapy.

The goal of maintenance immunosuppression is to suppress the recipient immune system from rejecting the transplanted heart. This "triple therapy" regimen consists of:

- *Calcineurin inhibitors*: cyclosporine or tacrolimus
- *Antimetabolites* or *cell cycle modulators*: MMF or azathioprine
- *Corticosteroids*

Approximately 60% of cardiac transplant recipients will not require long-term steroid use (see Table 28.5). Steroid withdrawal may be attempted post transplant in patients without episodes of rejection.

Table 28.5. Agents Used for Maintenance Immunosuppression

AGENT	MECHANISM OF ACTION	ADVERSE EFFECTS	THERAPEUTIC TARGET (ng/mL)	INDICATIONS FOR USE
1 Calcineurin Inhibitors				
Cyclosporine	Inhibits IL-2 production, B-cell proliferation	Nephrotoxicity, HTN, dyslipidemia, hepatotoxicity, hirsutism, gingival hyperplasia, hyperuricemia, neurotoxicity, hyperkalemia, acidosis. Potential nephrotoxicity with aminoglycoside, amphotericin, NSAID, trimethoprim-sulfamethoxazole, sirolimus use. Metabolized by hepatic cytochrome P450, 3A4, therefore monitor for potential drug interactions.	0-6 months: 250-350 6-12 months: 200-250 >12 months: 100-200	Maintenance immunosuppression
Tacrolimus	Inhibits IL-2 production, B-cell proliferation	Nephrotoxicity, headache, tremor, glucose intolerance, hyperkalemia. Rarely TTP. Metabolized by hepatic cytochrome P450, 3A4, therefore monitor for potential drug interactions.	0-6 months: 12-15 6-12 months: 8-12 >12 months: 5-10	• Alternative to cyclosporine as maintenance immunosuppression • "Rescue" agent with recurrent rejection on cyclosporine
2 Antimetabolites				
MMF	Inhibits purine synthesis, B-cell, and smooth muscle proliferation	Gastrointestinal complaints (nausea, vomiting, diarrhea), and leukopenia. Should be administered on an empty stomach (antacids decrease enteric absorption).	Blood levels not routinely monitored (2-5)	Maintenance immunosuppression
Azathioprine	Inhibits purine synthesis, B-cell proliferation	Bone marrow suppression, hepatotoxicity, pancreatitis, alopecia, cutaneous malignancies with chronic use. Allopurinol interferes with azathioprine metabolism, thus potentiates myelosuppression.	Blood levels not monitored	Maintenance immunosuppression

Continued on following page

Table 28.5. Agents Used for Maintenance Immunosuppression *(Continued)*

AGENT	MECHANISM OF ACTION	ADVERSE EFFECTS	THERAPEUTIC TARGET (ng/mL)	INDICATIONS FOR USE
3 Other				
Corticosteroids	Inhibits T-cell activation, B/T-cell proliferation	DM, impaired wound healing, HTN, peptic ulcer, obesity, avascular necrosis, osteoporosis, cataract, and psychosis.	Blood levels not monitored	Maintenance therapy and pulse therapy for acute rejection
Inhibitors of Target of Rapamycin*				
Sirolimus (rapamycin) and everolimus	Inhibits G1-S cell cycle progression, B/T-cell, smooth muscle proliferation	Thrombocytopenia, dyslipidemia, anemia, lower extremity edema, renal insufficiency, oral ulcers, lung nodules, and impaired wound healing.	5-20	• Can be used with lower dose of calcineurin inhibitor in calcineurin-related RI • Alternative to antimetabolites in accelerated transplant vasculopathy • Everolimus has been approved for use in Europe, but not in the United States.

DM, Diabetes mellitus; *HTN*, hypertension; *MMF*, mycophenolate mofetil; *NSAID*, nonsteroidal anti-inflammatory drug; *RI*, renal insufficiency; *TTP*, thrombotic thrombocytopenic purpura.
*Not part of routine maintenance therapy. TOR inhibitors are added in certain situations (see the text).

Newer agents include the mTOR inhibitors (sirolimus, everolimus). Currently, the mTOR inhibitors are not used as part of the standard maintenance therapy but are added in patients with accelerated transplant vasculopathy, worsening renal function on calcineurin inhibitors, and frequent rejections on standard triple maintenance therapy. Note that MMF or azathioprine is often stopped when sirolimus or everolimus is added to avoid excessive immunosuppression and side effects.

22. What are common medical conditions encountered in posttransplant patients?

- HTN: Attributed to sympathetic stimulation, neurohormonal activation, renal vasoconstriction by calcineurin inhibitors, and mineralocorticoid effect of steroids
- Renal impairment: As a result of low cardiac output pretransplant, ischemic injury during transplantation, and calcineurin-related renal arteriolar vasoconstriction and tubulointerstitial fibrosis
- Dyslipidemia: As a result of weight gain, corticosteroid and cyclosporine use
- Diabetes: As a result of corticosteroid use, weight gain
- Osteoporosis: Resulting from corticosteroid use
- Gout: Hyperuricemia from decreased uric acid clearance with cyclosporine use

23. Describe adverse effects encountered with calcineurin inhibitor use and potential drug interactions that may lead to calcineurin toxicity.

- **HTN:** Greater than 70% by 1 year and 95% by 5 years
- **Renal dysfunction:** Greater than 25% by 1 year and 5% progress to end-stage renal disease within 7 years
- **Rhabdomyolysis** when used concurrently with 3-hydroxy-3-methylglutaryl-coenzyme (HMG-CoA) reductase inhibitors (statins), because calcineurin inhibitors inhibit metabolism of certain statins (lovastatin, simvastatin, cerivastatin, and atorvastatin). Fluvastatin, pravastatin, and rosuvastatin are less likely to be involved in this type of interaction.

- **Calcineurin toxicity** is characterized by neurologic symptoms (headaches, tremor, confusion, agitation, delirium, expressive aphasia, and seizures), nephrotoxicity, and HTN. The enzyme cytochrome P450 3A4 (CYP3A4) metabolizes calcineurin inhibitors, and inhibitors of CYP3A4 can lead to increased drug levels and adverse effects.
  CYP3A4 inhibitors include:
  - Azole antifungal agents (ketoconazole, itraconazole)
  - Macrolide antibiotics (erythromycin, clarithromycin)
  - Grapefruit juice
  - Non-dihydropyridine calcium antagonists (diltiazem, verapamil)
  - Dihydropyridine calcium-channel blockers (nicardipine, nifedipine); amlodipine has minimal effect on CYP3A4.
  - Some highly active antiretroviral therapies (HAARTs)
  - Isoniazid (INH)

  CYP3A4 inducers include:
  - Antiepileptics (phenytoin, valproic acid)
  - Rifampin
  - Some HAARTs

24. How do patients with transplant vasculopathy clinically present? What invasive and noninvasive tests are used to assist in the diagnosis of transplant vasculopathy?

Because transplanted hearts are denervated, cardiac transplant recipients typically do not present with angina when they develop transplant vasculopathy. Clinical manifestations include silent myocardial infarctions, symptoms of HF, syncope, sudden cardiac death, and arrhythmias.

Most centers have adopted surveillance angiographies for early diagnosis of transplant vasculopathy. However, transplant vasculopathy is often diffuse and concentric in its distribution and may be underestimated by angiography. To improve detection and sensitivity, intravascular ultrasound and/or quantitative coronary angiography are used as adjunctive modalities.

Dobutamine stress echo or myocardial perfusion imaging can be used to diagnose transplant vasculopathy, but each has a lower sensitivity when compared to angiography. To avoid contrast-induced nephropathy, noninvasive stress testing is used in patients with renal insufficiency.

25. Describe strategies to prevent and treat cardiac allograft vasculopathy.

Although no effective preventive strategy for transplant vasculopathy has been identified, several factors have been associated with a lower incidence of transplant vasculopathy:

- **Lipid lowering therapy** (pravastatin has fewer drug interactions and is better tolerated)
- **mTOR inhibitors** (may decrease transplant vasculopathy incidence)
- **Blood pressure control** (diltiazem may also limit intimal thickening but needs careful drug-drug monitoring)

Treatment options for transplant vasculopathy are limited. Percutaneous and surgical revascularizations have limited roles in the setting of diffuse vasculopathy. Retransplantation is the only definitive therapy. In some cases, immunosuppression regimen adjustment and trial of TOR inhibitor may be attempted (Fig. 28.2).

26. When should mechanical circulatory support device implantation be considered?

A limited number of donor hearts and an increasing number of patients with NYHA class IV symptoms have created a demand for alternative treatments for end-stage HF. One strategy is the implantation of a mechanical circulatory support device (MCSD) or LVAD.

Indications for LVAD implantation include:

- An attempt to extend life in a deteriorating transplant candidate who is listed for a donor heart (bridge-to-transplant)
- In patients with multiorgan failure, an LVAD may help determine transplant eligibility. If pulmonary HTN or renal insufficiency improves after LVAD, a heart transplant would be more likely of benefit (bridge-to-decision).
- Support for patients whose surgery is complicated by cardiogenic shock
- Permanent support for nontransplant candidates (destination therapy)

27. What is the Interagency Registry for Mechanically Assisted Circulatory Support profile?

The Interagency Registry for Mechanically Assisted Circulatory Support (INTERMACS) patient profiles describe the clinical status of advanced HF patients who are being considered for mechanical circulatory support. INTERMACS profile levels are summarized in Table 28.6.

28. How are the Interagency Registry for Mechanically Assisted Circulatory Support profiles helpful?

The INTERMACS profiles are used to help with risk estimates for survival and to compare clinical outcomes from trial data.

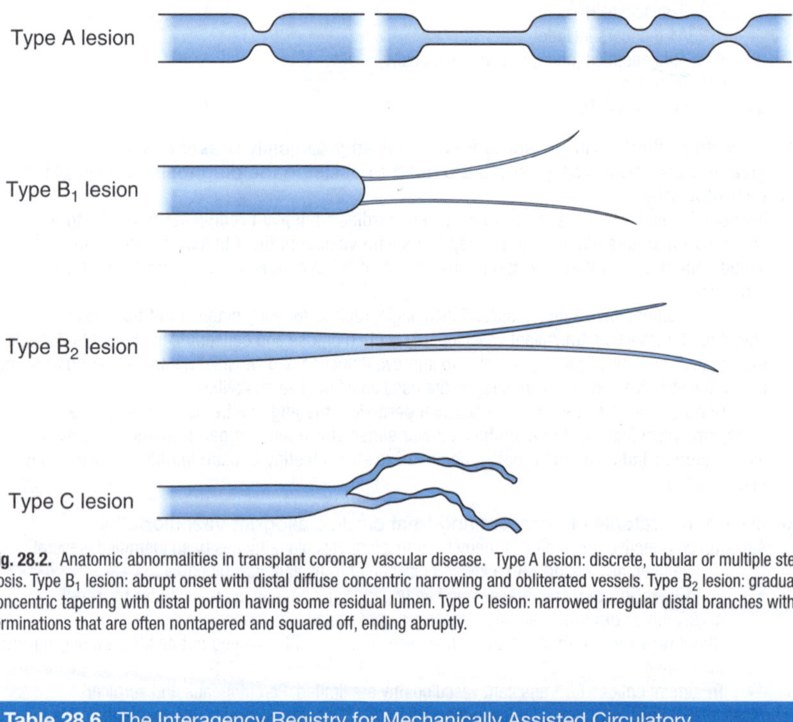

Fig. 28.2. Anatomic abnormalities in transplant coronary vascular disease. Type A lesion: discrete, tubular or multiple stenosis. Type B_1 lesion: abrupt onset with distal diffuse concentric narrowing and obliterated vessels. Type B_2 lesion: gradual, concentric tapering with distal portion having some residual lumen. Type C lesion: narrowed irregular distal branches with terminations that are often nontapered and squared off, ending abruptly.

Table 28.6. The Interagency Registry for Mechanically Assisted Circulatory Support Patient Profile Classification System

PROFILE LEVEL	CLINICAL STATUS	COLLOQUIALLY	EXPECTED SURVIVAL
1	Critical cardiogenic shock	Crashing and burning	Hours
2	Progressive decline on inotropes	Sliding on inotropes	1-7 days
3	Stable, inotrope dependent	Dependent stability	Weeks
4	Resting symptoms on oral therapy (NYHA IV)	Frequent flyer	Weeks to a few months
5	Exertion intolerant	Housebound	Weeks to months
6	Exertion limited	Walking wounded	Months
7	Advanced NYHA III (b)		

NYHA, New York Heart Association.

Bibliography and Suggested Readings

Aliabadi, A., Grömmer, M., & Zuckermann, A. (2011). Is induction therapy still needed in heart transplantation? *Current Opinion in Organ Transplantation, 16*(5), 536–542.

Alraies, M. C., & Eckman, P. (2014). Adult heart transplant: indications and outcomes. *Journal of Thoracic Disease, 6*(8), 1120–1128.

Cooper, L. T., Baughman, K., Feldman, A. M., Frustaci, A., Jessup, M., Kuhl, U., et al. (2007). The role of endomyocardial biopsy in the management of cardiovascular disease: a scientific statement from the American Heart Association, the American College of Cardiology, and the European Society of Cardiology. *Journal of the American College of Cardiology, 50*, 1914–1931.

Hunt, S. A., & Haddad, F. (2008). The changing face of heart transplantation. *Journal of the American College of Cardiology, 52*(8), 587–598.

Jessup, M., Banner, N., Brozena, S., Campana, C., Costard-Jäckle, A., Dengler, T., et al. (2006). Optimal pharmacologic and non-pharmacologic management of cardiac transplant candidates: approaches to be considered prior to transplant evaluation: International Society for Heart and Lung Transplantation guidelines for the care of cardiac transplant candidates—2006. *The Journal of Heart and Lung Transplantation, 25*(9), 1003–1023.

Kobashigawa, J. A. (2007). Contemporary concepts in noncellular rejection. *Heart Failure Clinics, 3*(1), 11–15.

Stewart, S., Winters, G. L., Fishbein, M. C., Tazelaar, H. D., Kobashigawa, J., Abrams, J., et al. (2005). Revision of the 1990 working formulation for the standardization of nomenclature in the diagnosis of heart rejection. *The Journal of Heart and Lung Transplantation, 24*(11), 1710–1720.

Yancy, C. W., Jessup, M., Bozkurt, B., Butler, J., Casey, D. E., Jr., Drazner, M. H., et al. (2013). 2013 ACCF/AHA guideline for the management of heart failure: a report of the American College of Cardiology Foundation/American Heart Association Task Force on Practice Guidelines. *Journal of the American College of Cardiology, 62*, e147–e239.

BIBLIOGRAPHY AND SUGGESTED READINGS

IV
Valvular Heart Disease

AORTIC STENOSIS

Douglas R. Johnston, Ahmad Zeeshan, Blaise A. Caraballo

1. What is the prevalence of aortic stenosis? What are the trends in aortic stenosis with age?

Aortic stenosis (AS) is a very common form of valvular heart disease that has been estimated to occur in 0.3% to 0.5% of the general population and 2% to 7% of individuals older than 65 years of age. The prevalence of severe AS, for which intervention should be considered, may be as high as 3% to 4% in older adult (>75 years of age) populations.

2. What are the risk factors for, and common causes of, aortic stenosis?

In the developing world, rheumatic fever remains the most common cause of AS. In developed countries, progressive calcification of tricuspid or bicuspid aortic valves represents the primary pathophysiology. Though AS is sometimes called "degenerative," evidence would suggest the underlying pathology is inflammatory and that it shares similarities with atherosclerosis including deranged lipid metabolism. Less common causes include prosthetic AS related to degeneration of biological prostheses, mechanical prostheses limited by pannus or thrombus, and failed aortic valve repair. Subaortic obstruction to left ventricular outflow may mimic many of the features of AS.

A normal aortic valve, a bicuspid aortic valve, a rheumatic aortic valve with stenosis, and a valve with calcific AS are shown in Fig. 29.1A-D, respectively.

3. What is the pathophysiology of aortic stenosis, and what effect does it have on the left ventricle?

AS exerts a pressure overload on the left ventricle (LV). Normally, pressure in the LV and aorta are similar during systole, as the normal aortic valve permits free flow of blood from LV to aorta.

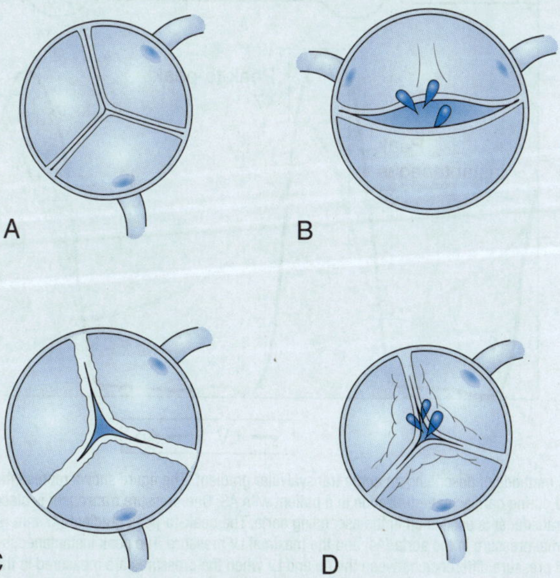

Fig. 29.1. A, Normal aortic valve. **B,** Congenital bicuspid aortic valve. **C,** Rheumatic AS. **D,** Calcific degenerative AS. *(Cleveland Clinic ImageBank, used by permission.)*

However, in AS the stenotic valve forces the LV to generate higher pressure to drive blood through the stenosis, causing a pressure difference (gradient) from the LV to the aorta. The LV compensates for this pressure overload by increasing its mass (left ventricular hypertrophy [LVH]). The transvalvular gradient is measured and quantified as shown in Fig. 29.2.

4. **What are the symptoms of aortic stenosis? How are they related to outcome?**
   The classic symptoms of AS are angina, syncope, and dyspnea. It is generally thought that manifestations of heart failure (dyspnea, orthopnea, lower extremity edema, etc.) represent a more severe form of the pathology and a worse prognosis. The commonly accepted paradigm for survival and symptoms is represented in Fig. 29.3. Risk of sudden death in the asymptomatic phase is relatively low at 1% per year, and risk of mortality increases dramatically with symptom onset, with three-quarters of patients dead within 3 years. Onset of symptoms may be subtle in active patients, however. In many patients, fatigue, or even an unconscious decrease in previous activity levels that is noticed by family members, may precede the onset of overt symptoms.

5. **What are the signs of aortic stenosis?**
   AS is usually recognized by the presence of a harsh systolic ejection murmur that radiates to the neck. In mild disease, the murmur peaks in intensity early in systole, peaking progressively later as severity of disease increases (Fig. 29.4). The carotid upstrokes become delayed in timing and reduced in volume because the stenotic valve steals energy from the flow of blood as it passes the valve. The apical beat is forceful. Palpation of this strong apical beat with one examining hand while the other hand palpates the weakened delayed carotid upstroke is dynamic proof of the obstruction that exists between the LV and the systemic circulation. Because the severely stenotic aortic valve barely opens, there is little valve movement upon closing. Thus, the A2 component of S2 is lost, rendering a soft single second sound. An S4 is usually present in patients in sinus rhythm, reflecting impaired filling of the thickened, noncompliant LV.

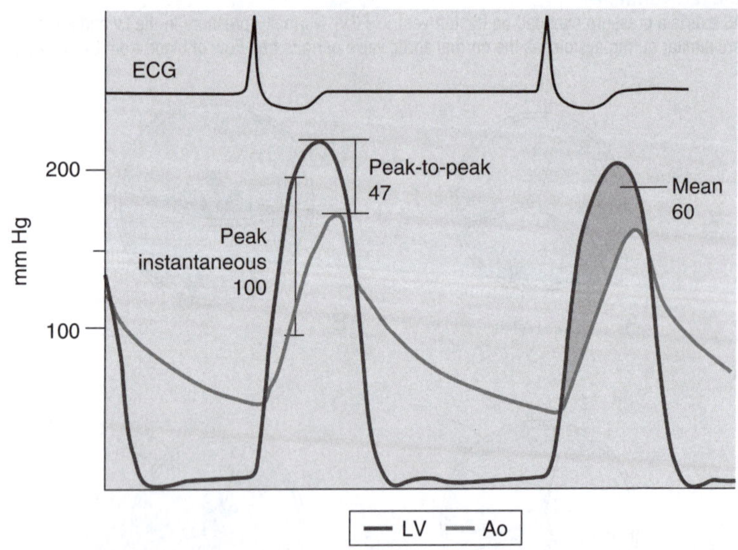

Fig. 29.2. Various methods of describing an aortic transvalvular gradient. The figure shows representative pressure tracings measured during cardiac catheterization in a patient with AS. One pressure transducer is placed in the LV, and a second pressure transducer is positioned in the ascending aorta. The peak-to-peak gradient (47 mm Hg) is the difference between the maximal pressure in the aorta (Ao) and the maximal LV pressure. The peak instantaneous gradient (100 mm Hg) is the maximal pressure difference between the Ao and LV when the pressures are measured in the same moment (usually during early systole). The mean gradient *(shaded area)* is the integral of the pressure difference between the LV and Ao during systole (60 mm Hg). *ECG,* Electrocardiogram. *(From Bashore, T. M. [1990].* Invasive cardiology: principles and techniques *[p. 258]. Philadelphia, PA: BC Decker.)*

6. What are the preferred modalities for diagnosis of aortic stenosis?

Two-dimensional (2D) echocardiography is the primary diagnostic tool in valvular heart disease. AS is characterized by decreased mobility of the aortic valve leaflets, the presence of calcification, and flow acceleration across the valve (Fig. 29.5).

Three-dimensional (3D) echocardiography may provide additional information on valve morphology (bicuspid or tricuspid) and location of calcification, which is helpful for procedure planning if the patient is referred for surgical or transcatheter aortic valve replacement (TAVR).

Four-dimensional (4D) computed tomography (CT) is increasingly used for determination of specific valve anatomy, particularly in planning transcatheter valve interventions. 4D CT and magnetic resonance imaging (MRI) can provide aortic valve area data that correlate well with echocardiography and may be valuable in patients with poor echo windows, in particular when additional anatomic data are desirable, for example, ascending aortic diameter or arch calcification.

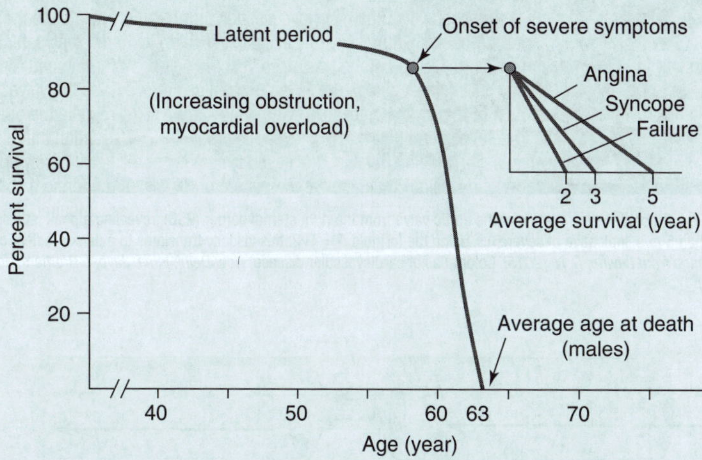

Fig. 29.3. The natural history of medically treated AS. Once symptoms develop in a patient with AS, the average survival with medical treatment (e.g., no curative surgery) is only 2 to 5 years. *(From Townsend, C. M. Jr., Beauchamp, R. D., Evers, B. M., & Mattox, K. L. [2008].* Sabiston textbook of surgery: the biological basis of modern surgical practice *[18th ed.]. Philadelphia, PA: Saunders.)*

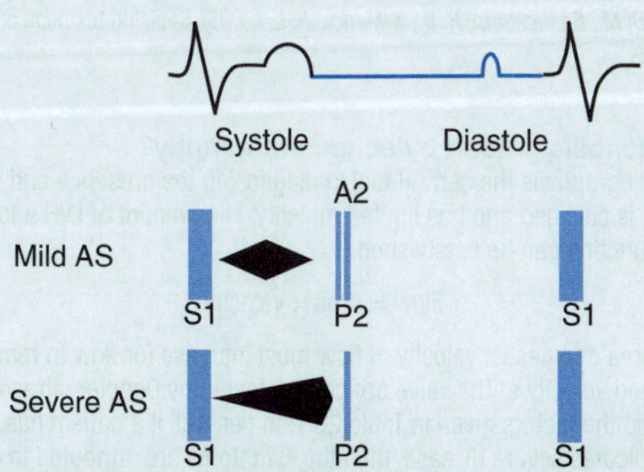

Fig. 29.4. The auscultatory findings for a patient with mild *(upper panel)* and severe *(lower panel)* AS are shown. As the disease severity worsens, the systolic ejection murmur peaks progressively later in systole and the A_2 component of the second heart sound is often lost. *(Image adopted from Ursula, P., & Wolfgang, D. [2011]. Asymptomatic aortic stenosis—prognosis, risk stratification and follow-up. In M. Hirota [Ed.].* Aortic stenosis—etiology, pathophysiology and treatment. *Croatia: Intechweb.org.)*

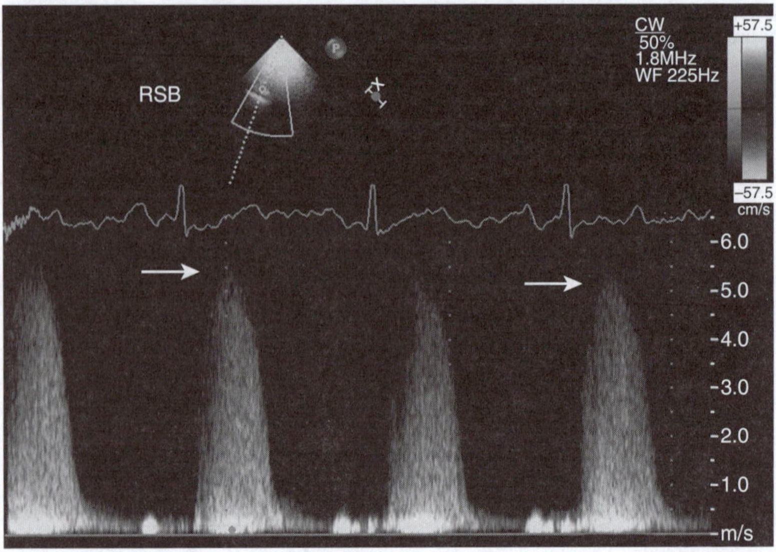

Fig. 29.5. Pedoff Doppler interrogation of the aortic valve from the right sternal border (RSB), revealing a peak jet velocity of greater than 5 m/s, indicative of severe AS. Using the formula $G = 4V2$, this velocity translates to a peak gradient of 100 mm Hg. *(Image from Levine, G. N. [2015].* Color atlas of cardiovascular disease. *New Delhi, India: Jaypee Brothers Medical Publishers.)*

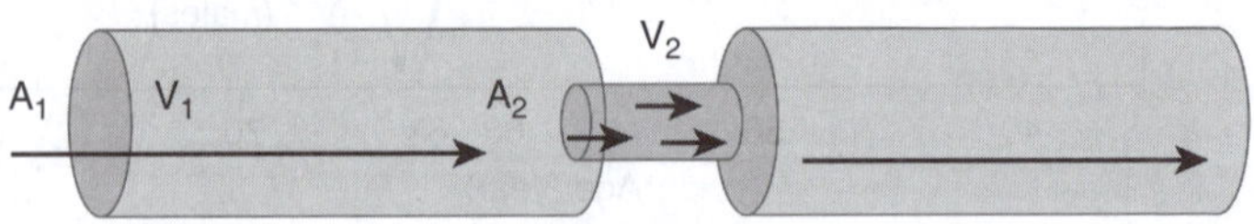

$$A_1 \times V_1 = A_2 \times V_2$$

Fig. 29.6. Determination of aortic valve area using the continuity equation. For blood flow ($A_1 \times V_1$) to remain constant when it reaches a stenosis (A_2), velocity must increase to V_2. Determination of the increased velocity V_2 by Doppler ultrasound permits calculation of the aortic valve gradient and solution of the equation for A_2. *A*, Area; *V*, velocity. *(From Townsend, C. M. Jr., Evers, B. M., Beauchamp, R. D., & Mattox, K. L. [2008].* Sabiston textbook of surgery *[18th ed.]. Philadelphia, PA: Saunders.)*

7. How is aortic stenosis graded by echocardiography?

Currently, echocardiography is the central tool in diagnosing the presence and severity of AS. In severe AS, the aortic valve is calcified and has limited mobility. The amount of LVH and the presence or absence of LV dysfunction can be established.

$$\text{Flow} = \text{Area} \times \text{Velocity}$$

As the valve area decreases, velocity of flow must increase for flow to remain constant (Fig. 29.6). This increase in blood velocity at the valve orifice is detected by Doppler ultrasound. The severity of AS is assessed using the factors given in Table 29.1. In general, if a patient has the symptoms of AS and assessment indicates severe disease, then the symptoms are attributed to AS. However, it must be emphasized that the benchmarks listed here are only guidelines to severity and some patients are exceptions to them.

Severity of AS can also be assessed by direct measurement of valve area using planimetry; however, jet velocity measurements more consistently reflect the physiology of AS in relation to the ventricle and are, in general, a better means of assessing severity.

Table 29.1. Echocardiographic Criteria for the Degree of Aortic Stenosis

	MILD	MODERATE	SEVERE
Peak jet velocity (m/s)	<3.0	3.0-4.0	>4.0
Mean gradient (mm Hg)	<25	25-40	>40
Aortic valve area (cm^2)	>1.5	1.0-1.5	<1.0
Valve area index (cm^2/m^2)			<0.6
Outflow track velocity-to-aortic valve velocity			<0.25

Modified from Bonow, R. O., Carabello, B. A., Chatterjee, K., de Leon, A. C. Jr., Faxon, D. P., Freed, M. D. et al. (2006). ACC/AHA 2006 *guidelines for the management of patients with valvular heart disease*. Journal of the American College of Cardiology, 48, *e1–e148*.

8. What is the role of exercise stress testing in aortic stenosis?

Exercise stress testing in AS is a matter of some controversy. Because of the risk of sudden death, there is no role for stress testing in symptomatic patients. The usefulness of exercise stress testing falls into two categories. The first are patients with severe AS and no or equivocal symptoms. Surprisingly, one-third of patients who are asymptomatic will develop symptoms with stress. A positive stress test portends a significantly worse prognosis and should prompt a discussion of surgical intervention.

The second category of patients are those with symptoms potentially attributable to AS but with lower gradients at rest. In these patients, stress echocardiography may be helpful to demonstrate ventricular reserve and also to document an increase in gradient with exercise, which may be more reflective of the patient's actual physiology.

9. What medical therapies are effective in the treatment of aortic stenosis? What is the risk of mortality in severe symptomatic aortic stenosis managed medically?

Although lipid metabolism is thought to be involved in the pathogenesis and progression of AS, several trials have failed to document an effect of lipid-lowering therapy on AS progression. Medically managed severe AS is believed to carry a risk of mortality of 50% at 2 years, comparable to many malignancies.

10. When is surgery indicated in aortic stenosis?

According to the most recent American College of Cardiology/American Heart Association (ACC/AHA) guidelines for AS, class I indications for aortic valve replacement (AVR) are as follows:

- Symptomatic patients with severe AS
- Severe AS with left ventricular systolic dysfunction (left ventricular ejection fraction [LVEF] less than 50%)
- Severe AS in patients undergoing coronary artery bypass grafting, other heart valve surgery, or thoracic aortic surgery (if AS is instead moderate, then AVR in these situations is considered a class IIa indication, *reasonable*)

In addition, surgery may be considered in asymptomatic patients with left ventricular dysfunction, very severe stenosis (a mean transaortic gradient >60 mm Hg), or with a positive exercise test as a class IIa indication.

Asymptomatic patients with at least moderate stenosis may be considered for surgery *if* surgical risk is low, a class IIb indication.

Fig. 29.7 and Table 29.2 summarize indications for aortic valve intervention.

11. What are the indications for surgical aortic valve replacement versus transcatheter aortic valve replacement?

Surgical aortic valve replacement (SAVR) is indicated in patients at low or moderate risk for surgery.

Based on initial studies of TAVR, guidelines state that TAVR could be considered in patients at high risk for surgery provided that patients are evaluated and treated using a heart team approach. More recent studies demonstrate comparable outcomes of patients with severe AS treated with SAVR or TAVR.

12. What are the outcomes with aortic valve replacement?

Mortality for surgical AVR has fallen dramatically over the past two decades. Mortality at experienced aortic valve centers has been consistently less than 1% as compared with 2% to 3% across the spectrum of aortic valve implantation in the United States.

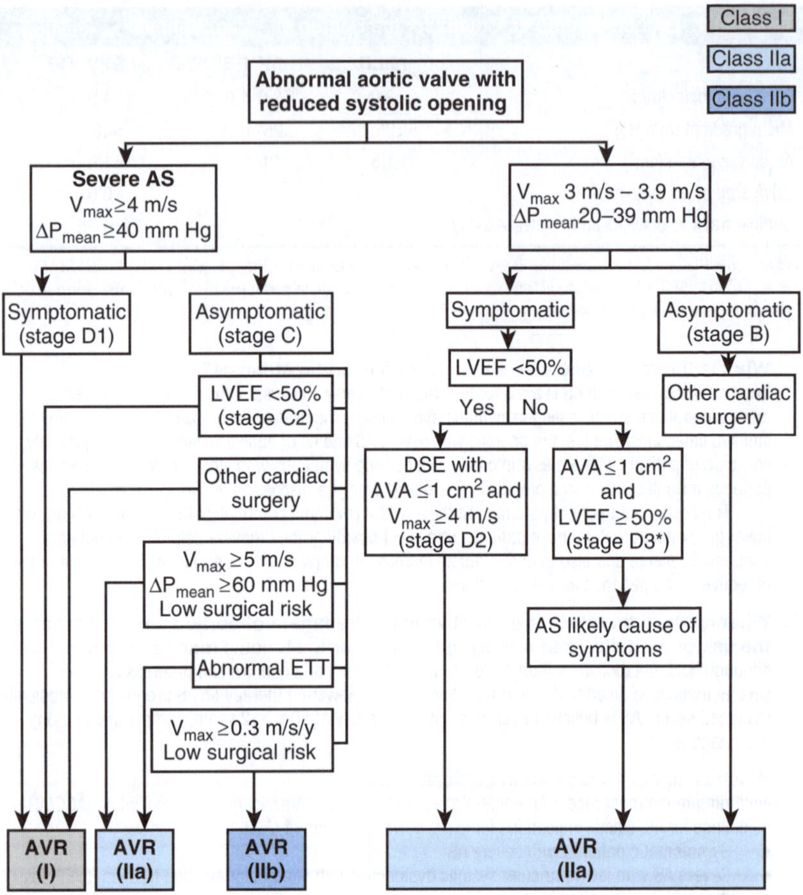

Fig. 29.7. *Arrows* show the decision pathways that result in a recommendation for AVR. Periodic monitoring is indicated for all patients in whom AVR is not yet indicated, including those with asymptomatic AS (stage D or C) and those with low-gradient AS (stage D2 or D3) who do not meet the criteria for intervention. *AVR should be considered with stage D3 AS only if valve obstruction is the most likely cause of symptoms, stroke volume index is less than 35 mL/m^2, indexed AVA is ≤0.6 cm^2/m^2, and data are recorded when the patient is normotensive (systolic BP <140 mm Hg). *AS,* Aortic stenosis; *AVA,* aortic valve area; *AVR,* aortic valve replacement by surgical or transcatheter approach; *BP,* blood pressure; *DSE,* dobutamine stress echocardiography; *ETT,* exercise treadmill test; *LVEF,* left ventricular ejection fraction; ΔP_{mean}, mean pressure gradient; and V_{max}, maximum velocity. *(Reprinted from Nishimura, R. A., Otto, C. M., Bonow, R. O., Carabello, B. A., Erwin, J. P. 3rd, Guyton, R. A., et al. [2014]. 2014 AHA/ACC guideline for the management of patients with valvular heart disease: a report of the American College of Cardiology/American Heart Association Task Force on Practice Guidelines.* Journal of the American College of Cardiology, 63*[22], e57–e185.)*

Minimally invasive aortic valve surgery has been shown to improve early recovery and reduce hospital stay, without an impact on long-term survival.

TAVR has been shown to be effective in moderate- and high-risk populations, albeit with increased risk of paravalvular leak. Major in-hospital complications and long-term survival rates are similar to SAVR in select patients, with shorter recovery times.

Balloon aortic valvuloplasty (BAV) was previously a treatment option for high-risk patients with AS. However, rates of iatrogenic aortic insufficiency are high, and recurrence of AS within several months is the norm. The availability of TAVR has largely supplanted BAV in most cases.

Table 29.2. Summary of Recommendations for Aortic Valve Intervention

RECOMMENDATIONS	CLASS OF RECOMMENDATION	LEVEL OF EVIDENCE
AVR is recommended for symptomatic patients with severe high-gradient AS who have symptoms by history or on exercise testing (stage D1).	I	B
AVR is recommended for asymptomatic patients with severe AS (stage C2) and LVEF <50%.	I	B
AVR is indicated for patients with severe AS (stage C or D) when undergoing other cardiac surgery.	I	B
AVR is reasonable for asymptomatic patients with very severe AS (stage C1, aortic velocity >5.0 m/s) and low surgical risk.	IIa	B
AVR is reasonable in asymptomatic patients (stage C1) with severe AS and decreased exercise tolerance or an exercise fall in BP.	IIa	B
AVR is reasonable in symptomatic patients with low-flow/low-gradient severe AS with reduced LVEF (stage D2) with a low-dose dobutamine stress study that shows an aortic velocity >4.0 m/s (or mean pressure gradient >440 mm Hg) with a valve area <1.0 cm^2 at any dobutamine dose.	IIa	B
AVR is reasonable in symptomatic patients who have low-flow/low-gradient severe AS (stage D3) who are normotensive and have an LVEF >50% if clinical hemodynamic and anatomic data support valve obstruction as the most likely cause of symptoms.	IIa	C
AVR is reasonable for patients with moderate AS (stage B) (aortic velocity 3.0-3.9 m/s) who are undergoing other cardiac surgery.	IIa	C
AVR may be considered for asymptomatic patients with severe AS (stage C1) and rapid disease progression and low surgical risk.	IIb	C

AS, Aortic stenosis; *AVR*, aortic valve replacement by surgical or transcatheter approach; *BP*, blood pressure; *LVEF*, left ventricular ejection fraction; *N/A*, not applicable.

Reproduced from Nishimura, R. A., Otto, C. M., Bonow, R. O., Carabello, B. A., Erwin, J. P. 3rd, Guyton, R. A., et al. (2014). 2014 AHA/ACC guideline for the management of patients with valvular heart disease: a report of the American College of Cardiology/American Heart Association Task Force on Practice Guidelines. Journal of the American College of Cardiology, *63(22), e57–e185.*

Long-term survival after AVR is excellent. For elderly patients, survival is similar to age- and census-matched controls. In all age groups with severe AS, surgery confers far superior survival to medical therapy. Survival after AVR is independent of the type of prosthesis implanted (tissue vs. mechanical).

Bibliography and Suggested Readings

Johnston, D. R., Atik, F. A., Rajeswaran, J., Blackstone, E. H., Nowicki, E. R., Sabik, J. F., 3rd, et al. (2012). Outcomes of less invasive *J*-incision approach to aortic valve surgery. *Journal of Thoracic and Cardiovascular Surgery, 144*(4), 852–858.

Leon, M. B., Smith, C. R., Mack, M., Miller, D. C., Moses, J. W., Svensson, L. G., et al. (2010). Transcatheter aortic-valve implantation for aortic stenosis in patients who cannot undergo surgery. *New England Journal of Medicine, 363*(17), 1597–1607.

Nishimura, R. A., Otto, C. M., Bonow, R. O., Carabello, B. A., Erwin, J. P., 3rd, Guyton, R. A., et al. (2014). 2014 AHA/ACC guideline for the management of patients with valvular heart disease: a report of the American College of Cardiology/

American Heart Association Task Force on Practice Guidelines. *Journal of the American College of Cardiology*, *63*(22), e57–e185.

Tommaso, C. L., Bolman, R. M., 3rd, Feldman, T., Bavaria, J., Acker, M. A., Aldea, G., et al. (2012). Multisociety (AATS, ACCF, SCAI, and STS) expert consensus statement: Operator and institutional requirements for transcatheter valve repair and replacement, Part 1: transcatheter aortic valve replacement. *Journal of Thoracic and Cardiovascular Surgery*, *143*(6), 1254–1263.

Vahanian, A., Baumgartner, H., Bax, J., Butchart, E., Dion, R., Filippatos, G., et al. (2007). Guidelines on the management of valvular heart disease: the Task Force on the Management of Valvular Heart Disease of the European Society of Cardiology. *European Heart Journal*, *28*(2), 230–268.

AORTIC REGURGITATION

Edward Soltesz, Blase Carabello

CHAPTER 30

1. **What are the causes of aortic regurgitation?**
   Abnormalities of the aortic root or the aortic valve leaflets can cause aortic regurgitation (AR). Aortic root dilatation leads to AR in the absence of leaflet abnormalities in conditions such as Marfan's syndrome, annuloaortic ectasia, and ascending aortic dissections. Leaflet causes of AR include infective endocarditis, rheumatic heart disease, collagen vascular disease, and a congenitally bicuspid aortic valve.

2. **What are the most common causes of acute aortic regurgitation?**
   The most common causes of acute aortic regurgitation are infective endocarditis, aortic dissection, or iatrogenic causes such as complication after percutaneous aortic balloon dilation or transcatheter aortic valve replacement (TAVR). Blunt chest trauma can rarely cause acute aortic regurgitation (AR).

3. **What are the most common causes of chronic aortic regurgitation?**
   In the United States and other developed countries, the most common causes of chronic AR are bicuspid aortic valve, calcific valve disease, and dilation of the ascending aorta of sinuses of Valsalva. In developing countries, the leading cause of chronic AR is rheumatic heart disease.

4. **What is the pathophysiology of aortic regurgitation?**
   The incompetent aortic valve allows ejected blood to return to the left ventricle during diastole. This regurgitant volume is lost from the effective cardiac output. In turn, the left ventricle must pump extra blood to make up for this loss; thus, AR constitutes an LV volume overload. Compensation comes from an increase in LV volume (eccentric hypertrophy) in cases of chronic aortic regurgitation. The larger left ventricle can pump more blood to compensate for the blood lost to AR. Because all the stroke volume is pumped into the aorta during systole (while some leaks back into the left ventricle during diastole), pulse pressure, which is dependent on stoke volume, widens as systolic pressure increases and diastolic pressure decreases. Thus, AR imparts not only a volume overload on the left ventricle but also a pressure overload. Because of this second load, left ventricle thickness in chronic AR patients is slightly greater than normal. Increased wall thickness and the increased diastolic LV volume lead to increased LV diastolic filling pressure. In acute AR, there is no time for adaptation to additional blood volume. The left ventricle is not able to adequately compensate for the regurgitant volume, and excessive backward blood flow impairs forward stroke volume. Compensatory tachycardia may preserve cardiac output initially, but eventually hypotension, organ failure, and other evidence of cardiogenic shock will develop.

5. **What are the symptoms of aortic regurgitation?**
   Dyspnea and fatigue are the main symptoms of AR. Occasionally patients experience angina because reduced diastolic aortic pressure reduces coronary filling pressure, impairing coronary blood flow. Reduced diastolic systemic pressure may also cause syncope or presyncope. In acute aortic regurgitation, patients usually present with symptoms of low cardiac output and cardiogenic shock.

6. **Is the presentation of acute aortic regurgitation different from that of chronic aortic regurgitation?**
   Yes, dramatically. In chronic AR there has been no time for progressive LV dilation so that the increased forward stroke volume and widened pulse pressure that drive the dynamic examination of a patient with chronic AR are absent. Thus the examination of a patient with severe acute AR may be misleadingly bland, belying a potentially fatal condition. Acute AR occurs most commonly in the patient with infective endocarditis. When such patients develop evidence of heart failure, AR should be suspected even if there is only a faint murmur or no murmur at all.

7. **What are the findings of aortic regurgitation on physical examination?**
   Chronic AR produces myriad physical findings because of the large stroke volume pumped by the left ventricle. The pulse pressure is wide. The dynamic LV apical beat is displaced downward and to

the left and is often visible several feet away from the patient. A diastolic blowing murmur is present and is heard best along the left sternal border with the patient sitting upward and leaning forward. A second murmur (Austin Flint), believed to be due to vibration of the mitral valve caused by the impinging AR, is a low-pitched diastolic rumble heard toward the LV apex.

The widened pulse pressure and high total stroke volume cause several physical signs of AR:

- The head may bob with each heartbeat (de Musset's sign).
- Auscultation of the femoral artery may produce a sound similar to a pistol shot (pistol shot pulse).
- If the bell of the stethoscope is compressed over the femoral artery, a to-and-fro bruit (Duroziez sign) may be heard.
- Compression of the nailbed may demonstrate systolic plethora and diastolic blanching of the nail bed (Quincke pulse).

8. How is the diagnosis of aortic regurgitation confirmed?

Echocardiography remains the mainstay of diagnosis and can fully characterize cardiac size and function as well as the degree of regurgitation. Often the anatomic abnormality responsible for the patient's AR can be established as well. As shown in Fig. 30.1, Doppler interrogation of the valve reveals the jet of blood leaking across the valve in diastole. Table 30.1 displays current criteria for establishing the severity of AR.

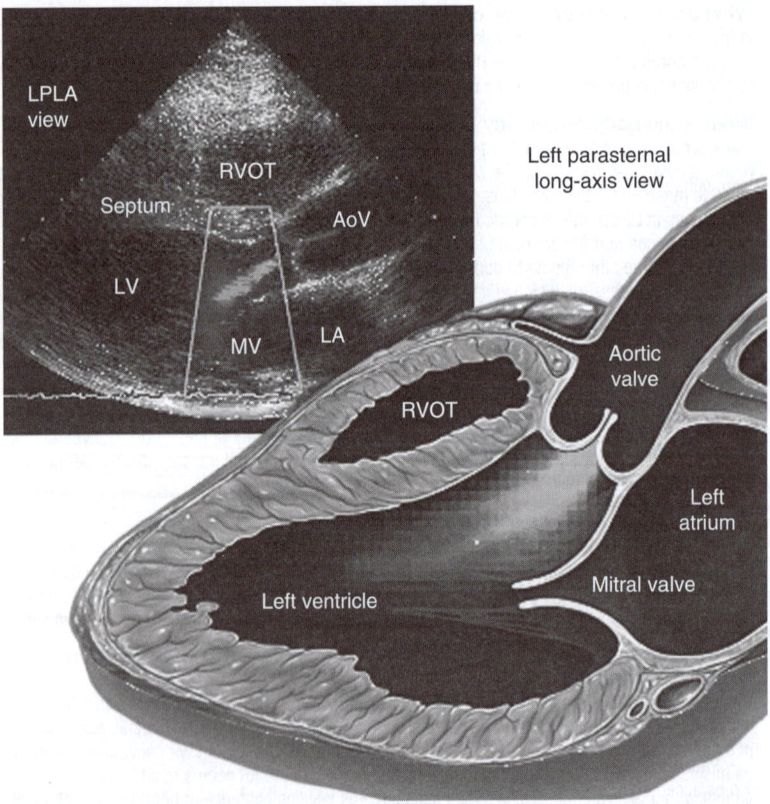

Fig. 30.1. Aortic regurgitation (AR). Left parasternal long-axis (LPLA) view of the heart, demonstrating AR seen on Doppler echocardiogram, along with the corresponding anatomic illustration. In actuality, the regurgitant jet is displayed in color, reflecting the direction of blood flow. *LV,* Left ventricle; *MV,* mitral valve; *LA,* left atrium; *AoV,* aortic valve; *RVOT,* right ventricular outflow track. *(From Yale Atlas of Echocardiography.)* http://www.med.yale.edu/intmed/cardio/echo_atlas/entities/aortic_regurgitation.html. Accessed 30.08.08.

Table 30.1. Cardiac Catheterization and Echocardiographic Criteria for the Degree of Aortic Regurgitation

	MILD	MODERATE	SEVERE
Angiographic grade	1+	2+	3-4+
Color Doppler central jet width	<25% LVOT		>65% LVOT
Doppler vena contracta width	<0.3 cm	0.3-0.6 cm	>0.6 cm
Regurgitant volume (mL/beat)	<30 mL	30-59 mL	≥60 mL
Regurgitant fraction	<30%	30%-49%	≥50%
Regurgitant orifice area	<0.10 cm^2	0.10-0.29 cm^2	≥0.30 cm^2
LV size			Increased
Pressure half-time			<250 ms

LV, Left ventricle; *LVOT*, left ventricular outflow tract.

Modified from Bonow, R. O., Carabello, B. A., Chatterjee, K., de Leon, A. C. Jr., Faxon, D. P., Freed, M. D., et al. (2006). ACC/AHA 2006 *guidelines for the management of patients with valvular heart disease*. Journal of the American College of Cardiology, 48, e1–e148.

9. What imaging test should be obtained when echocardiography is indeterminate?

Cardiac magnetic resonance (CMR) imaging is indicated (class I recommendation) in patients with moderate to severe AR (stages B, C, or D) and suboptimal echocardiographic images. CMR can provide accurate measurements of regurgitant volume, regurgitant fraction, LV volume, and LV function. Importantly, CMR can also provide a morphologic assessment of the aorta.

10. What other testing may be useful in select patients?

When noninvasive and clinical findings remain uncertain or discordant (or CMR cannot be performed), cardiac catheterization can be used to assess hemodynamics, severity of AR, and coronary artery anatomy.

In patients with unclear functional capacity or symptoms, exercise stress testing can be used to assess functional capacity and symptomatic status.

11. How is aortic regurgitation classified?

In addition to the traditional severity of AR (mild, moderate, severe), AR is now also classified by stage. The stages are A-D, and include at risk of AR, progressive AR, asymptomatic severe AR, and symptomatic severe AR. These stages are summarized in Table 30.2.

12. How is aortic regurgitation managed?

Patients with severe AR should be seen at least once a year or more often to evaluate symptomatic status and to perform repeat echocardiograms to assess LV size and function.

Aortic valve replacement (AVR) is indicated (ACC/AHA and European Society of Cardiology [ESC] class I recommendations) for the following patients:

- Symptomatic patients with severe AR, irrespective of LV systolic function
- Asymptomatic patients with chronic severe AR and LV systolic dysfunction (left ventricular ejection fraction [LVEF] 50% or less)
- Patients with chronic severe AR who are undergoing coronary artery bypass grafting (CABG), other heart valve surgery, or thoracic aortic surgery

Class IIa and class IIb indications for AVR in asymptomatic patients include those with severe AR with normal LV systolic function (LVEF more than 50%) but with LV dilation (end-systolic dimension greater than 50 mm [class IIa] or end-diastolic dimension greater than 65 mm and low surgical risk [class IIb]).

Patients with mild or moderate AR who are undergoing other cardiac surgical operations may also be acceptable candidates for AVR (ACC/AHA and ESC class IIa recommendation).

At present, transcatheter AVR (TAVR) is not indicated in the United States for patients with native isolated AR, though it is used in Europe. Transcatheter valve-in-valve may be an option for selected patients with prosthetic AR.

Recommendations for intervention in patients with AR are summarized in Table 30.3. The suggested algorithm for management of patients with AR is given in Fig. 30.2.

Table 30.2. The Stages of Chronic Aortic Regurgitation

STAGE	DEFINITION	VALVE ANATOMY	VALVE HEMODYNAMICS	HEMODYNAMIC CONSEQUENCES	SYMPTOMS
A	At risk of AR	Bicuspid aortic valve (or other congenital valve anatomy) Aortic valve sclerosis Diseases of the aortic sinuses or ascending aorta History of rheumatic fever or known rheumatic heart disease IE	AR severity: none or trace	None	None
B	Progressive AR	Mild-to-moderate calcification or a trileaflet valve bicuspid aortic valve (or other congenital valve anomaly) Dilated aortic sinuses Rheumatic valve changes Pervious IE	Mild AR: Jet width <25% of LVOT; Vena contracta <0.3 cm; RVol <30 mL/beat; RF <30%; ERO <0.10 cm^2; Angiography grade 1+ Moderate AR: Jet width 25%-64% of LVOT; Vena contracta 0.3-0.6 cm; RVol 30-59 mL/beat; RF 30%-49%: ERO 0.10-0.29 cm^2; Angiography grade 2+	Normal LV systolic function Normal LV volume or mild LV dilation	None

C	Asymptomatic severe AR	Calcific aortic valve disease Bicuspid valve (or other congenital abnormality) Dilated aortic sinuses or ascending aorta Rheumatic valve changes Previous IE with abnormal leaflet closure or perforation	Severe AR: Jet width >65% of LVOT; Vena contracta >0.6 cm; Holodiastolic flow reversal in the proximal abdominal aorta RVol >60 mL/beat; RF >50%; ERO >0.3 cm^2; Angiography grade 3+ to 4+; In addition, diagnosis of chronic severe AR requires evidence of LV dilation	C1: Normal LVEF (>50%) and mild-to-moderate LV dilation (LVESD <50 mm) C2: Abnormal LV systolic function with depressed LVEF (<50%) or severe LV dilatation (LVESD >50 mm or indexed LVESD >25 mm/m^2)	None: exercise testing is reasonable to confirm symptom status
D	Symptomatic severe AR	Calcific aortic valve disease Bicuspid valve (or other congenital abnormality) Dilated aortic sinuses or ascending aorta Rheumatic valve changes Previous IE with abnormal leaflet closure or perforation	Doppler jet width >65% of LVOT; Vena contracta >0.6 cm; Holodiastolic flow reversal in the proximal abdominal aorta; RVol >60 mL/beat; RF >50%; ERO >0.3 cm^2; Angiography grade 3+ to 4+; In addition, diagnosis of chronic severe AR requires evidence of LV dilation	Symptomatic severe AR may occur with normal systolic function (LVEF >50%), mild-to-moderate LV dysfunction (LVEF 40%-50%), or severe LV dysfunction (LVEF <40%); Moderate-to-severe LV dilation is present	Exertional dyspnea or angina or more severe HF symptoms

AR, Aortic regurgitation; *ERO*, effective regurgitant orifice; *HF*, heart failure; *IE*, infective endocarditis; *LV*, left ventricular; *LVEF*, left ventricular ejection fraction; *LVESD*, left ventricular end-systolic dimension; *LVOT*, left ventricular outflow tract; *RF*, regurgitant fraction; *RVol*, regurgitant volume.

Reproduced from Nishimura, R. A., Otto, C. M., Bonow, R. O., Carabello, B. A., Erwin, J. P. III, Guyton, R. A., et al. (2014). 2014 AHA/ACC guideline for the management of patients with valvular heart disease: a report of the American College of Cardiology/American Heart Association Task Force on Practice Guidelines. Journal of the American College of Cardiology, 63, e57–e185.

Table 30.3. Summary of Recommendations for Aortic Regurgitation Intervention

RECOMMENDATIONS	CLASS OF RECOMMENDATION	LEVEL OF EVIDENCE
AVR is indicated for symptomatic patients with severe AR regardless of LV systolic function (stage D).	I	B
AVR is indicated for asymptomatic patients with chronic severe AR and LV systolic dysfunction (LVEF <50%) (stage C2).	I	B
AVR is indicated for patients with severe AR (stage C or D) while undergoing cardiac surgery for other indications.	I	C
AVR is reasonable for asymptomatic patients with severe AR with normal LV systolic function (LVEF >50%) but with severe LV dilation (LVESD >50 mm, stage C2).	IIa	B
AVR is reasonable in patients with moderate AR (stage B) who are undergoing other cardiac surgery.	IIa	C
AVR may be considered for asymptomatic patients with severe AR and normal LV systolic function (LVEF >50%, stage C1) but with progressive severe LV dilation (LVEDD >65 mm) if surgical risk is low.*	IIb	C

AR, Aortic regurgitation; *AVR*, aortic valve replacement; *LV*, left ventricular; *LVEDD*, left ventricular end-diastolic dimension; *LVEF*, left ventricular ejection fraction; *LVESD*, left ventricular end-systolic dimension.

*Practically, in the setting of progressive LV enlargement.

Reproduced from Nishimura, R. A., Otto, C. M., Bonow, R. O., Carabello, B. A., Erwin, J. P. III, Guyton, R. A., et al. (2014). 2014 AHA/ACC guideline for the management of patients with valvular heart disease: a report of the American College of Cardiology/American Heart Association Task Force on Practice Guidelines. Journal of the American College of Cardiology, 63, e57–e185.

13. Is there any medical therapy for aortic regurgitation?

As with aortic stenosis (AS), there is no proven medical therapy for AR. Treatment of hypertension is recommended in patients with chronic AR, preferably with a dihydropyridine calcium channel blocker, angiotensin-converting enzyme (ACE) inhibitor, or angiotensin II receptor blocker (ARB). Medical therapy with ACE inhibitors, ARBs, and beta-blockers is considered reasonable (class IIa) in patients with severe AR who have symptoms and/or LV dysfunction (stages C2 and D) when surgery is not performed because of comorbidities.

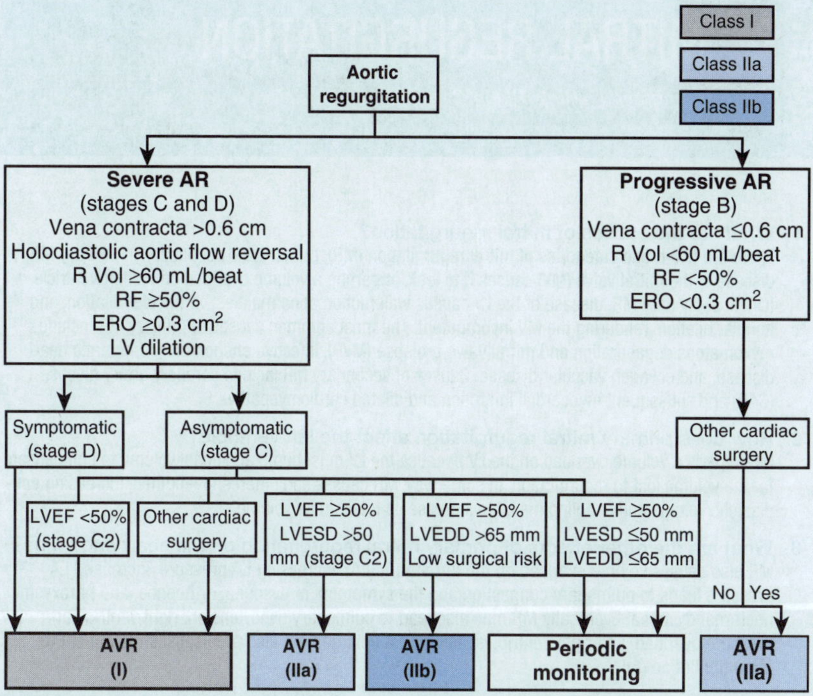

Fig. 30.2. Flow diagram of the indications for AVR in chronic AR. *AR,* Aortic regurgitation; *AVR,* aortic valve replacement; *LV,* left ventricle; *ERO,* effective orifice area; *RF,* regurgitant fraction; *LVEF,* left ventricular ejection fraction; *LVESD,* left ventricular end-systolic dimension; *LVEDD,* left ventricular end-diastolic dimension. *(Image from Nishimura, R. A., Otto, C. M., Bonow, R. O., Carabello, B. A., Erwin, J. P. III, Guyton, R. A., et al. [2014]. 2014 AHA/ACC guideline for the management of patients with valvular heart disease: a report of the American College of Cardiology/American Heart Association Task Force on Practice Guidelines.* Journal of the American College of Cardiology, 63, *e57–e185).*

Bibliography and Suggested Readings

Goldbarg, S. H., & Halperin, J. L. (2008). Aortic regurgitation: disease progression and management. *Nature Reviews Cardiology*, *5*, 269–279. http://dx.doi.org/10.1038/ncpcardio1179.

Hamirani, Y. S., Dietl, C. A., Voyles, W., Peralta, M., Begay, D., & Raizada, V. (2012). Acute aortic regurgitation. *Circulation*, *126*, 1121–1126.

Maganti, K., Rigolin, V. H., Sarano, M. E., & Bonow, R. O. (2010). Valvular heart disease: diagnosis and management. *Mayo Clinic Proceedings*, *85*(5), 483–500. http://dx.doi.org/10.4065/mcp.2009.0706.

Nishimura, R. A., Otto, C. M., Bonow, R. O., Carabello, B. A., Erwin, J. P., III, Guyton, R. A., et al. (2014). 2014 AHA/ACC guideline for the management of patients with valvular heart disease: a report of the American College of Cardiology/American Heart Association Task Force on Practice Guidelines. *Journal of the American College of Cardiology*, *63*, e57–e185.

Vahanian, A., Alfieri, O., Andreotti, F., Antunes, M. J., Barón-Esquivias, G., Baumgartner, H., et al. (2012). Guidelines on the management of valvular heart disease (version 2012). *European Heart Journal*, *33*(19), 2451–2496. http://dx.doi.org/10.1093/eurheartj/ehs109.

CHAPTER 31

MITRAL REGURGITATION

Stephanie L. Mick, Blase Carabello

1. **What are the causes of mitral regurgitation?**
   There are two broad categories of mitral regurgitation (MR), primary and secondary. In primary MR, disease of the mitral valve (MV) causes it to leak, imparting a volume overload on the left ventricle (LV). In secondary MR, disease of the LV causes wall motion abnormalities, ventricular dilation, and annular dilation, rendering the MV incompetent. The most common causes of primary MR include myxomatous degeneration and mitral valve prolapse (MVP), infective endocarditis, rheumatic heart disease, and collagen vascular disease. Causes of secondary MR include coronary artery disease (CAD) and subsequent myocardial infarction and dilated cardiomyopathy.

2. **How does primary mitral regurgitation affect the left ventricle?**
   MR imparts a volume overload on the LV because the LV must pump additional volume to compensate for the volume lost to regurgitation. In some way, MR causes sarcomeres to lengthen, increasing end-diastolic volume and enabling the LV to increase its total stroke volume.

3. **What are the other effects of primary mitral regurgitation on the heart and lungs?**
   MR also causes volume overload on the left atrium (LA), increasing LA pressure. Increased LA pressure leads to pulmonary congestion and the symptoms of dyspnea, orthopnea, and paroxysmal nocturnal dyspnea. Eventually MR may also lead to pulmonary hypertension, right ventricular pressure overload, and right ventricular failure. LA enlargement also predisposes the patient to atrial fibrillation (AF).

4. **What are the clues to mitral regurgitation on physical examination?**
   The typical murmur of MR is holosystolic, radiating to the axilla. It may be accompanied by a systolic apical thrill; the apical beat is displaced downward and to the left, indicating LV enlargement. In severe MR, an S3 is usually heard. Here, the S3 may not indicate heart failure (HF) but rather is caused by the increased LA volume emptying into the LV at higher than normal pressure.

5. **How is the diagnosis of mitral regurgitation confirmed?**
   Although the chest radiograph and the electrocardiogram (ECG) may indicate LV enlargement, as with other valvular heart diseases, echocardiography is the diagnostic modality of choice. It demonstrates LA and LV size and volume, allows assessment of LV function and pulmonary artery pressure, and can reliably quantify the amount of MR present.

6. **How is the severity of mitral regurgitation classified?**
   The degree (severity) of MR is traditionally classified as mild, moderate, or severe. Ventriculography (Fig. 31.1) during cardiac catheterization was used in the past to assess the degree of MR. In current practice, this has been supplanted by the use of echocardiography (Fig. 31.2), which can qualitatively and quantitatively assess the severity of MR. Echocardiographic findings suggestive of severe MR include enlarged LA or LV, the color Doppler MR jet occupying a large proportion (more than 40%) of the LA, a regurgitant volume (RVol) of 60 mL or more, a regurgitant fraction (RF) of 50% or greater, a regurgitant orifice of 0.40 cm^2 or greater, and a Doppler vena contracta width of 0.7 cm or larger.

   Angiographic and echocardiographic criteria for the assessment of the severity of MR are given in Table 31.1.

7. **How are the stages of mitral regurgitation classified?**
   In addition to the traditional severity classification of MR (mild, moderate, severe), MR is now also classified by stage. The stages are A-D and include at risk of MR, progressive MR, asymptomatic severe MR, and symptomatic severe MR. These stages are summarized in Tables 31.2 and 31.3.

8. **Are there effective medical therapies for chronic primary mitral regurgitation?**
   No. The asymptomatic patient will not benefit from medical therapy, and once symptoms develop, MR should be treated surgically. It should be noted that some patients with MR also have systemic

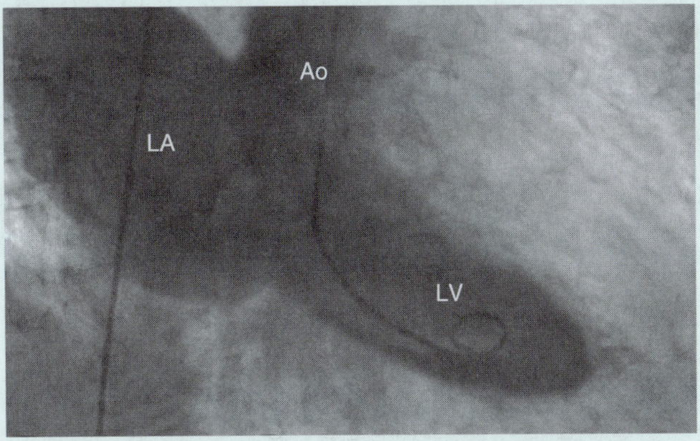

Fig. 31.1. Left ventriculography demonstrating severe mitral regurgitation (MR). *Ao,* Aorta; *LA,* left atrium; *LV,* left ventricle.

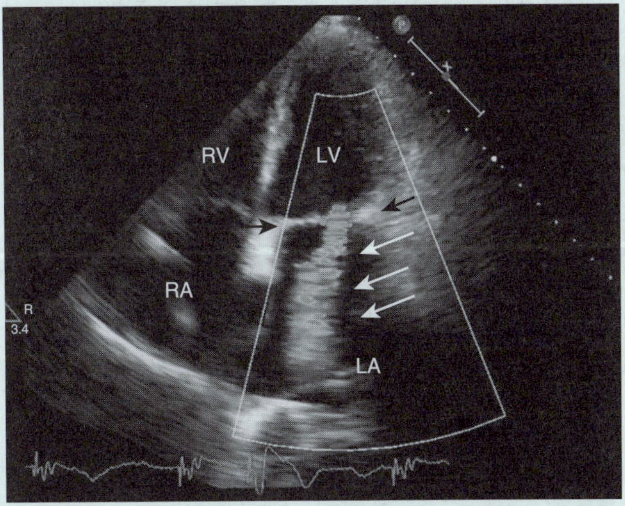

Fig. 31.2. Mitral regurgitation. Apical four-chamber view with color Doppler revealing severe mitral regurgitation (MR) *(white arrows). Black arrows* point to the mitral valve (MV). Note that in actuality, the regurgitant jet is displayed in color, corresponding to the flow of blood. *LA,* Left atrium; *LV,* left ventricle; *RA,* right atrium; *RV,* right ventricle.

Table 31.1. Angiographic and Echocardiographic Criteria for the Assessment of the Severity of Mitral Regurgitation

	MILD	MODERATE	SEVERE
Angiographic grade	1+	2+	3-4+
Color Doppler jet area	Small central jet (<4 cm^2 or <20% LA area)	—	Vena contracta width >0.7 cm with large central MR jet (area >40% LA), any wall-impinging jet, or any swirling in LA
Doppler vena contracta width	<0.3 cm	0.3-0.69 cm	≥0.7 cm
RVol	<30 mL	30-59 mL	≥60 mL
RF	<30%	30%-49%	≥50%
Regurgitant orifice	<0.20 cm^2	0.20-0.39 cm^2	≥0.40 cm^2
Chamber size	—	—	Enlarged LA or LV

LA, Left atrium; *LV,* left ventricle; *MR,* mitral regurgitation; *RF,* regurgitant fraction; *RVol,* regurgitant volume.
Modified from Bonow, R. O., Carabello, B. A., Chatterjee, K., de Leon A. C., Faxon, D. P., Freed M. D., et al. (2006). *ACC/AHA 2006 guidelines for the management of patients with valvular heart disease.* Journal of the American College of Cardiology, 48, *e1–e148.*

Table 31.2. Stages of Primary Mitral Regurgitation

GRADE	DEFINITION	VALVE ANATOMY	VALVE HEMODYNAMICS*	HEMODYNAMIC CONSEQUENCES	SYMPTOMS
A	At risk of MR	Mild MVP with normal coaptation Mild valve thickening and leaflet restriction	No MR jet or small central jet area <20% LA on Doppler Small vena contracta <0.3 cm	None	None
B	Progressive MR	Severe MVP with normal coaptation Rheumatic valve changes with leaflet restriction and loss of central coaptation Prior IE	Central jet MR 20%-40% LA or late systolic eccentric jet MR Vena contracta <0.7 cm RVol <60 mL RF <50% ERO <0.40 cm^2 Angiographic grade 3-4+	Mild LA enlargement No LV enlargement Normal pulmonary pressure	None
C	Asymptomatic severe MR	Severe MVP with loss of coaptation or flail leaflet Rheumatic valve changes with leaflet restriction and loss of central coaptation Prior IE Thickening of leaflets with radiation heart disease	Central jet MR >40% LA or holosystolic eccentric jet MR Vena contracta >0.7 cm RVol >60 mL RF >50% ERO >0.40 cm^2 Angiographic grade 3-4+	Moderate or severe LA enlargement LV enlargement Pulmonary hypertension may be present at rest or with exercise C1: LVEF >60% and LVESD <40 mm C2 : LVEF <60% and LVESD >40 mm	None
D	Symptomatic severe MR	Severe MVP with loss of coaptation or flail leaflet Rheumatic valve changes with leaflet restriction and loss of central coaptation Prior IE Thickening of leaflets with radiation heart disease	Central jet MR >40% LA or holosystolic eccentric jet MR Vena contracta >0.7 cm RVol >60 mL RF >50% ERO >0.40 cm^2 Angiographic grade 3-4+	Moderate or severe LA enlargement LV enlargement Pulmonary hypertension present	Decreased exercise tolerance Exertional dyspnea

ERO, Effective regurgitant orifice: *IE*, infective endocarditis; *LA*, left atrium/atrial; *LV*, left ventricular; *LVEF*, left ventricular ejection fraction; *LVESD*, left ventricular end-systolic dimension; *MR*, mitral regurgitation; MVP, mitral valve prolapse; *RF*, regurgitant fraction; *RVol*, regurgitant volume.

*Several valve hemodynamic criteria are provided for assessment of MR severity, but not all criteria for each category will be present in each patient. Categorization of MR severity as mild, moderate, or severe depends on data quality and interrogation of these parameters in conjunction with other clinical evidence.

Adapted from Nishimura, R. A., Otto, C. M., Bonow, R. O., Carabello, B. A., Erwin, J. P. III, Guyton, R. A., et al. (2014). 2014 AHA/ACC guideline for the management of patients with valvular heart disease: a report of the American College of Cardiology/American Heart Association Task Force on Practice Guidelines. Journal of the American College of Cardiology, 63, e57–e185.

Table 31.3. Stages of Secondary Mitral Regurgitation

GRADE	DEFINITION	VALVE ANATOMY	VALVE HEMODYNAMIC	ASSOCIATED CARDIAC FINDINGS	SYMPTOMS
A	At risk of MR	Normal valve leaflets, chords, and annulus in a patient with coronary disease or cardiomyopathy	No MR jet or small central jet area <20% LA on Doppler Small vena contracta <0.20 cm	Normal or mildly dilated LV size with fixed (infraction) or inducible (ischemia) regional wall motion abnormalities Primary myocardial disease with LV dilation and systolic dysfunction	Symptoms due to coronary ischemia or HF may be present that respond to revascularization and appropriate medical therapy.
B	Progressive MR	Regional wall motion abnormalities with mild tethering of mitral leaflet Annular dilation with mild loss of central coaptation of the mitral leaflets	ERO <2.0 mL RVol <30 mL RF <50%	Regional wall motion abnormalities with reduced LV systolic function LV dilation and systolic dysfunction due to primary myocardial disease	Symptoms due to coronary ischemia or HF may be present that respond to revascularization and appropriate medical therapy.
C	Asymptomatic severe MR	Regional wall motion abnormalities and/or LV dilation with severe tethering of mitral leaflets Annular dilation with severe loss of central coaptation of the mitral leaflets	ERO >0.20 cm^2 RVol >30 mL RF >50%	Regional wall motion abnormalities with reduced LV systolic function LV dilation and systolic dysfunction due to primary myocardial disease	Symptoms due to coronary ischemia or HF may be present that respond to revascularization and appropriate medical therapy.
D	Symptomatic severe MR	Region wall motion abnormalities and/or LV dilation with severe tethering of mitral leaflet Annular dilation with severe loss of central coaptation of the mitral leaflets	ERO >0.20 cm^2 RVol >30 mL RF >50%	Regional wall motion abnormalities with reduced LV systolic function LV dilation and systolic dysfunction due to primary myocardial disease	HF symptoms due to MR persist even after revascularization and optimization of medical therapy. Decreased exercise tolerance Exertional dyspnea

2D, Two-dimensional; *ERO*, efficiency regurgitant orifice; *HF*, heart failure; *LA*, left atrium; *LV*, left ventricle; *MR*, mitral regurgitation; *RF*, regurgitant fraction; *RVol*, regurgitant volume; *TTE*, transthoracic echocardiogram.

Several valve hemodynamic criteria are provided for assessment of MR severity, but not all criteria for each category will be present in each patient. Categorization of MR severity as mild, moderate, or severe depends on data quality and integration of these parameters in conjunction with other clinical evidence.

The measurement of the proximal isovelocity surface area by 2D TTE in patients with secondary MR underestimates the true ERO due to crescentic shape of the proximal convergence.

Adapted from Nishimura, R. A., Otto, C. M., Bonow, R. O., Carabello, B. A., Erwin, J. P. III, Guyton, R. A., et al. (2014). 2014 AHA/ACC guideline for the management of patients with valvular heart disease: a report of the American College of Cardiology/American Heart Association Task Force on Practice Guidelines. Journal of the American College of Cardiology, 63, e57–e185.

hypertension, which should be treated in the same manner in which hypertension is routinely treated.

9. What is the definitive therapy for primary mitral regurgitation, and when should it be employed?

As with all primary valve disease, MR is a mechanical problem requiring a mechanical solution. Here, however, the therapy for MR departs from that of other valve lesions. Unlike the aortic valve, the MV serves to do more than just direct forward cardiac flow. The MV is also an integral part of the LV, coordinating LV contraction and maintaining LV shape. When the valve is destroyed at the time of surgery, there is a precipitous fall in LV function postoperatively, which does not occur when the valve apparatus is conserved. Further, operative mortality is lower with valve repair than with valve replacement. Thus, every attempt should be made to repair rather than replace the valve at the time of surgery.

Because the onset of symptoms worsens prognosis for patients with MR, MV repair should be performed when symptoms begin. However, some patients fail to develop symptoms even though LV dysfunction has ensued. To guard against permanent LV dysfunction, mitral surgery should be performed before ejection fraction falls to 60% or less or before the LV can no longer contract to an end-systolic dimension of 40 mm. The onset of AF or pulmonary hypertension is also an indication for

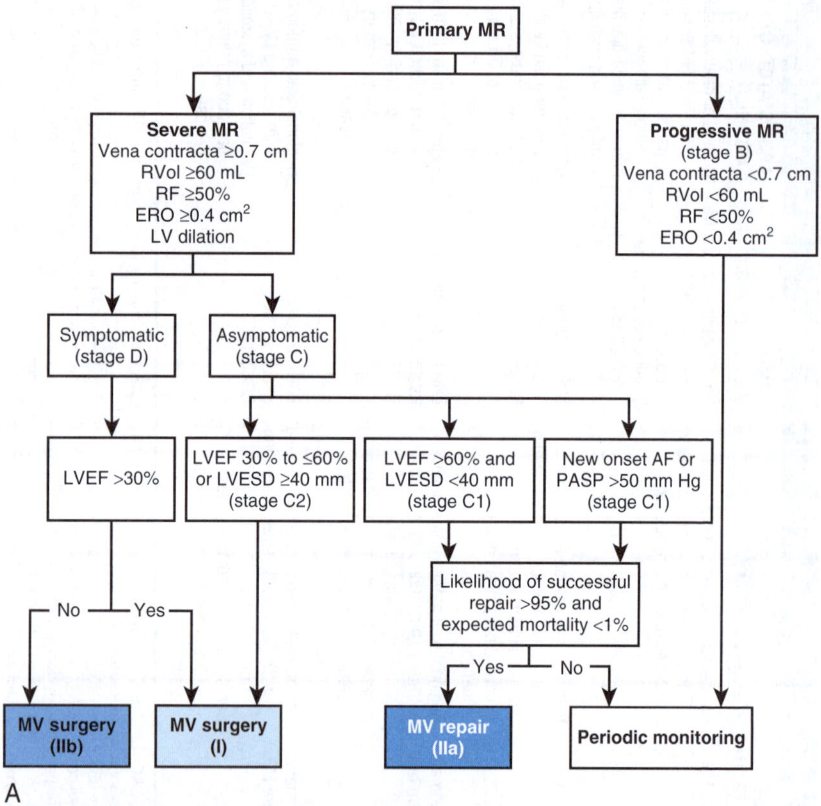

Fig. 31.3. A and B, Indications for surgery for primary MR. *AF,* Atrial fibrillation; *CAD,* coronary artery disease; *CRT,* cardiac resynchronization therapy; *ERO,* effective regurgitant orifice; *HF,* heart failure; *LV,* left ventricle; *LVEF,* left ventricular ejection fraction; *LVESD,* left ventricular end-systolic dimension; *MR,* mitral regurgitation, *MV,* mitral valve; *MVR,* mitral valve replacement; *NYHA,* New York Heart Association; *PASP,* pulmonary artery systolic pressure; *RF,* regurgitant fraction; *RVol,* regurgitant volume; *Rx,* therapy. *(Adapted from Nishimura, R. A., Otto, C. M., Bonow, R. O., Carabello, B. A., Erwin, J. P. III, Guyton, R. A., et al. [2014]. 2014 AHA/ACC guideline for the management of patients with valvular heart disease: a report of the American College of Cardiology/American Heart Association Task Force on Practice Guidelines.* Journal of the American College of Cardiology, *63, e57–e185.)*

surgery. Repair is recommended over replacement. However, it should be noted that not all MVs can be repaired. In such cases, MV replacement is performed.

Recommendations for MV repair and replacement in patients with chronic primary MR are given in Table 31.4.

10. What percutaneous options are available to patients with primary mitral regurgitation?

Although a number of technologies for mitral repair or replacement are in clinical development, an edge-to-edge leaflet repair device (the MitraClip) is currently the only US Food and Drug Administration (FDA)-approved device for transcatheter mitral valve repair (TMVR). The MitraClip and the CARILLON mitral annuloplasty device are approved for use in Europe.

The MitraClip is a transcatheter technology based on the surgical Alfieri edge-to-edge repair, which involves suturing the regurgitant orifice of the MV leaflets together and creates a "double orifice" MV. The clip is cobalt chromium covered with a polypropylene fabric that grasps both the MV leaflets, thereby reducing MR by increasing the coaptation between the leaflets. In some cases, multiple (two or more) may be used to adequately reduce the MR toward a goal of final regurgitant severity less than 2+. Although the MitraClip has been used to treat both primary and secondary MR, it is FDA-approved for commercial use only in patients with 3 to 4+ primary MR.

Anatomic characteristics should be assessed with transthoracic echocardiogram (TEE) to determine candidacy for TMVR. These include an MV area greater than 4 cm^2 (measured in the parasternal short-axis view at tips of the MV), gradient less than 5 mm Hg, and a graspable leaflet (e.g., minimal calcification, adequate length for grasping, etc.).

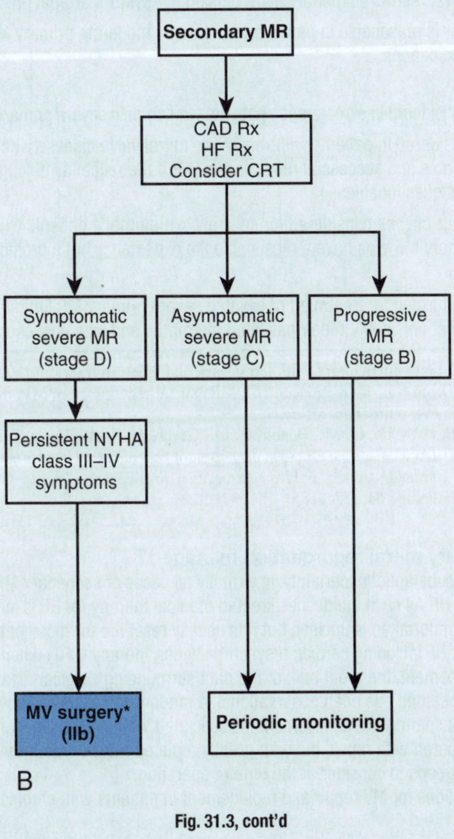

Fig. 31.3, cont'd

Table 31.4. Summary of American Heart Association/American College of Cardiology Recommendations in Chronic Primary Mitral Regurgitation

Class I
MV surgery is recommended for symptomatic patients with chronic severe primary MR and LVEF >30%.
Mitral valve surgery is recommended for asymptomatic patients with chronic severe primary MR and LV dysfunction (LVEF 30%-60% and/or LVESD ≥40 mm).
MV repair is recommended in preference to MVR when surgical treatment is indicated for patients with chronic severe primary MR limited to the posterior leaflet.
MV repair is recommended in preference to MVR when surgical treatment is indicated for patients with chronic severe primary MR involving the anterior leaflet or both leaflets when a successful and durable repair can be accomplished.
Concomitant MV repair or replacement is indicated in patients with chronic severe primary MR undergoing cardiac surgery for other indications.
Class IIa
MV repair is reasonable in asymptomatic patients with chronic severe primary MR with preserved LV function (LVEF >60% and LVESD <40 mm) in whom the likelihood of a successful and durable repair without residual MR is >95% with an expected mortality rate of <1% when performed at a Heart Valve Center of Excellence.
MV repair is reasonable for asymptomatic patients with chronic severe nonrheumatic primary MR and preserved LV function in whom there is a high likelihood of a successful and durable repair with (1) new onset of AF or (2) resting pulmonary hypertension (PA systolic arterial pressure >50 mm Hg).
Concomitant MV repair is reasonable in patients with chronic moderate primary MR undergoing cardiac surgery for other indications.
Class IIb
MV surgery may be considered in symptomatic patients with chronic severe primary MR and LVEF <30%.
MV repair may be considered in patients with rheumatic mitral valve disease when surgical treatment is indicated if a durable and successful repair is likely or if the reliability of long-term anticoagulation management is questionable.
Transcatheter MV repair may be considered for severely symptomatic patients (NYHA class III/IV) with chronic severe primary MR who have a reasonable life expectancy but a prohibitive surgical risk.
Class III
MVR should not be performed for treatment of isolated severe primary MR limited to less than one-half of the posterior leaflet unless MV repair has been attempted and was unsuccessful.

AF, Atrial fibrillation; *LV*, Left ventricular; *LVEF*, left ventricular ejection fraction; *LVESD*, left ventricular end-systolic dimension; *MVR*, mitral valve replacement; *MR*, mitral regurgitation; *MV*, mitral valve; *NYHA*, New York Heart Association; *PA*, pulmonary artery.

Adapted from Nishimura, R. A., Otto, C. M., Bonow, R. O., Carabello, B. A., Erwin, J. P. III, Guyton, R. A., et al. (2014). 2014 AHA/ACC guideline for the management of patients with valvular heart disease: a report of the American College of Cardiology/American Heart Association Task Force on Practice Guidelines. Journal of the American College of Cardiology, *63, e57–e185.*

11. How is secondary mitral regurgitation managed?

This area is one of substantial uncertainty. In virtually all cases of secondary MR, there is also severe LV dysfunction and HF. As such, guideline-directed medical therapy for HF is indicated. When mitral surgery should be undertaken is unclear, but it is usually reserved for those patients who have failed medical therapy for HF including cardiac resynchronization therapy (CRT) when appropriate. Regarding repair versus replacement, the great bulk of the data surrounding surgical repair (annuloplasty) versus replacement in this setting has been observational. A randomized trial has shown that when surgery is undertaken, chordal sparing MV replacement is associated with similar rates of surgical mortality and survival when compared with repair, but with greatly reduced rates of recurrent MR. This information is important for surgeons to consider at the time of operation.

Recommendations for MV repair and replacement in patients with chronic secondary MR are given in Table 31.5.

Table 31.5. Summary of American Heart Association/American College of Cardiology Recommendations in Chronic Severe Secondary Mitral Regurgitation

Class IIa
MV surgery is reasonable for patients with chronic severe secondary MR who are undergoing CABG or AVR.
Class IIb
MV surgery may be considered for severely symptomatic patients (NYHA class III/IV) with chronic severe secondary MR.
MV repair may be considered for patients with chronic moderate secondary MR (stage B) who are undergoing other cardiac surgery.

AVR, Aortic valve replacement; *CABG*, coronary artery bypass grafting; *MR*, mitral regurgitation; *MV*, mitral valve; *NYHA*, New York Heart Association.

Adapted from Nishimura, R. A., Otto, C. M., Bonow, R. O., Carabello, B. A., Erwin, J. P. III, Guyton, R. A., et al. (2014). 2014 AHA/ACC guideline for the management of patients with valvular heart disease: a report of the American College of Cardiology/American Heart Association Task Force on Practice Guidelines. Journal of the American College of Cardiology, 63, e57–e185.

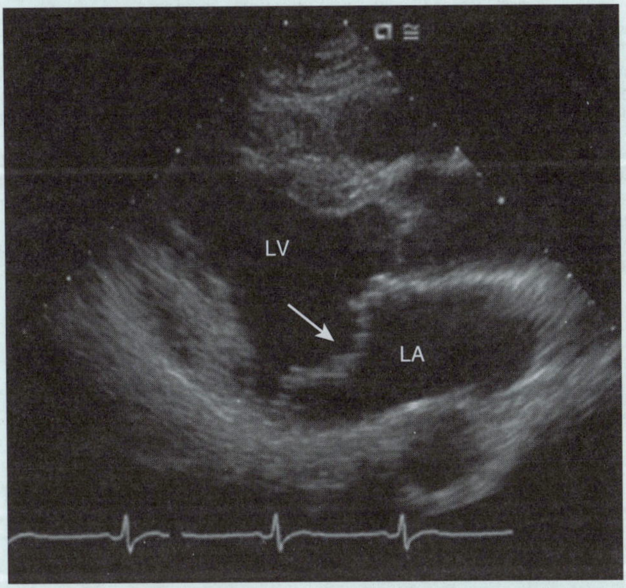

Fig. 31.4. Mitral valve prolapse. The mitral leaflets *prolapse* across the plain of the mitral valve (MV), into the LA *(arrow). LA,* Left atrium; *LV,* left ventricle. *(Modified from Libby, P., Bonow, R. O., Mann, D. L., & Zipes, D. P. [2008].* Braunwald's heart disease: a textbook of cardiovascular medicine *[8th ed.]. Philadelphia, PA: Saunders.)*

12. What percutaneous options are available to patients with secondary mitral regurgitation?

Although the MitraClip is only approved for use in patients with moderate to severe or severe primary MR, observational data suggest that selected patients with secondary MR may benefit from TMVR. Ongoing randomized trials are evaluating the potential benefit of MitraClip therapy in patients with HF and secondary MR. A number of technologies for mitral repair or replacement are in clinical development, and the field is evolving rapidly. It is reasonable to expect that additional percutaneous options will be available to patients with secondary MR in the next decade.

13. What is mitral valve prolapse?

MVP is the condition in which there is systolic billowing of one or both mitral leaflets into the LA (Fig. 31.4), with or without resulting MR. It is usually diagnosed by echocardiography according to established criteria (valve prolapse of 2 mm or more beyond the mitral annulus, as seen in the parasternal long-axis view). Its prevalence is 1% to 2.5%.

14. **What is the classic auscultatory finding in mitral valve prolapse?**
The classic finding is a mid-systolic click and late systolic murmur, although the click may actually vary somewhat within systole, depending on changes in left ventricular dimension. There may actually be multiple clicks. The clicks are believed to result from the sudden tensing of the MV apparatus as the leaflets prolapse into the LA during systole.

15. **What is the natural history of asymptomatic mitral valve prolapse?**
The course of patients with MVP can range from benign, with a normal life expectancy, to worsening MR and progressive left atrial dilation and left ventricular dysfunction and congestive HF.

Bibliography and Suggested Readings

Carabello, B. A. (2008). The current therapy for mitral regurgitation. *Journal of the American College of Cardiology*, *52*(5), 319–326.

Carabello, B. A. (2000). The pathophysiology of mitral regurgitation. *The Journal of Heart Valve Disease*, *9*(5), 600–608.

Feldman, T., Foster, E., Glower, D. D., Kar, S., Rinaldi, M. J., Fail, P. S., et al. (2011). Percutaneous repair or surgery for mitral regurgitation. *The New England Journal of Medicine*, *364*(15), 1395–1406. http://dx.doi.org/10.1056/NEJMoa1009355.

Maganti, K., Rigolin, V. H., Sarano, M. E., & Bonow, R. O. (2010). Valvular heart disease: diagnosis and management. *Mayo Clinic Proceedings*, *85*(5), 483–500. http://dx.doi.org/10.4065/mcp.2009.0706.

Mick, S. L., Keshavamurthy, S., & Gillinov, A. M. (2015). Mitral repair versus replacement. *Annals of Cardiothoracic Surgery*, *4*(3), 230–237.

Nishimura, R. A., Otto, C. M., Bonow, R. O., Carabello, B. A., Erwin, J. P., III, Guyton, R. A., et al. (2014). 2014 AHA/ACC guideline for the management of patients with valvular heart disease: a report of the American College of Cardiology/American Heart Association Task Force on Practice Guidelines. *Journal of the American College of Cardiology*, *63*, e57–e185.

O'Gara, P. T., Calhoon, J. H., Moon, M. R., & Tommaso, C. L. (2014). Transcatheter therapies for mitral regurgitation: a professional society overview from the American College of Cardiology, the American Association for Thoracic Surgery, Society for Cardiovascular Angiography and Interventions Foundation, and the Society of Thoracic Surgeons. *Journal of the American College of Cardiology*, *63*(8), 840–852.

Vahanian, A., Alfieri, O., Andreotti, F., Antunes, M. J., Barón-Esquivias, G., Baumgartner, H., et al. (2012). Guidelines on the management of valvular heart disease (version 2012). *European Heart Journal*, *33*, 2451–2496.

CHAPTER 32

MITRAL STENOSIS

Edward Soltesz, Blase Carabello

1. What is the usual cause of mitral stenosis?

Almost all cases of mitral stenosis (MS) stem from previous episodes of rheumatic fever. Most cases of rheumatic heart disease are seen in patients who emigrate from areas of the world where rheumatic fever is still common, including the Middle East, Asia, and South Africa. Although the rate of rheumatic fever is similar in men and women, MS is 3 times more common in women than in men.

2. What is the pathophysiology of mitral stenosis?

MS inhibits the normal free flow of blood from left atrium (LA) to left ventricle (LV) in diastole. Normally, diastolic left atrial and left ventricular pressures equalize shortly after mitral valve opening. In MS, the stenotic valve impedes left atrial emptying, inducing a diastolic gradient between the LA and LV (Fig. 32.1). Elevated LA pressure is referred to the lungs, where it causes

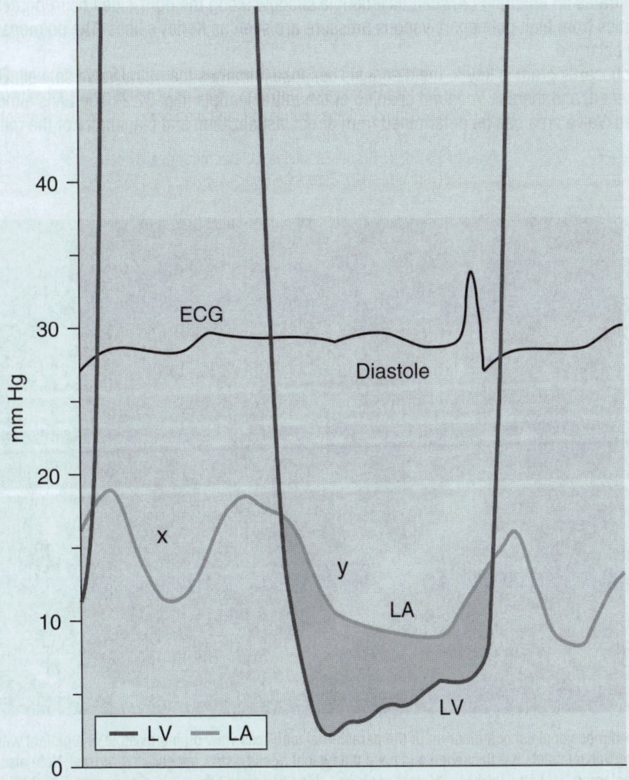

Fig. 32.1. Pressure gradient in a patient with mitral stenosis. The pressure in the left atrium (LA) exceeds the pressure in the left ventricle (LV) during diastole, producing a diastolic pressure gradient *(shaded area). ECG,* Electrocardiogram. *(Modified from Bashore, T. M. [1990].* Invasive cardiology: principles and techniques *[p. 264]. Philadelphia, PA: BC Decker.)*

pulmonary congestion. Simultaneously, impaired emptying of the LA reduces filling of the LV filling and limits cardiac output. Thus, the combination of increased LA pressure and decreased cardiac output produce the syndrome of heart failure. Because increased LA pressure increases pulmonary pressure, the right ventricle becomes pressure overloaded, eventually leading to right ventricular (RV) failure.

3. What are the typical symptoms of mitral stenosis?

Patients with mild disease are likely to be asymptomatic. As MS worsens, dyspnea appears, as does orthopnea and paroxysmal nocturnal dyspnea. If RV failure ensues, it may be accompanied by edema and ascites. During exercise, sudden increases in LA pressure and pulmonary venous pressure may cause rupture of anastomoses between pulmonary and systemic veins, leading to hemoptysis.

4. What are the signs of mitral stenosis at physical examination?

The gradient across the mitral valve holds the valve open throughout diastole, so that when it closes, S1 may be quite loud. The murmur of MS is a soft diastolic rumble heard near the apex. The murmur is often preceded by an opening snap, caused by sudden opening of the stiffened mitral valve from higher than normal atrial pressure. If pulmonary hypertension has developed, P2 is increased in intensity. If RV failure has occurred, elevated neck veins, ascites, and edema are likely to be present.

5. How is the diagnosis made?

The chest radiograph used to be at the forefront of diagnosis and still can be helpful today. It demonstrates an enlarged LA, seen as a double shadow along the right-sided heart border. Thickened lymphatics from high pulmonary venous pressure are seen as Kerley's lines. The pulmonary artery is usually enlarged.

Echocardiogram is key to the diagnosis because it images the mitral valve so well. The valve is thickened, and there is impaired opening of the mitral leaflets (Fig. 32.2). The LA is almost always enlarged. Valve area can be determined from direct visualization and planimetry of the mitral orifice,

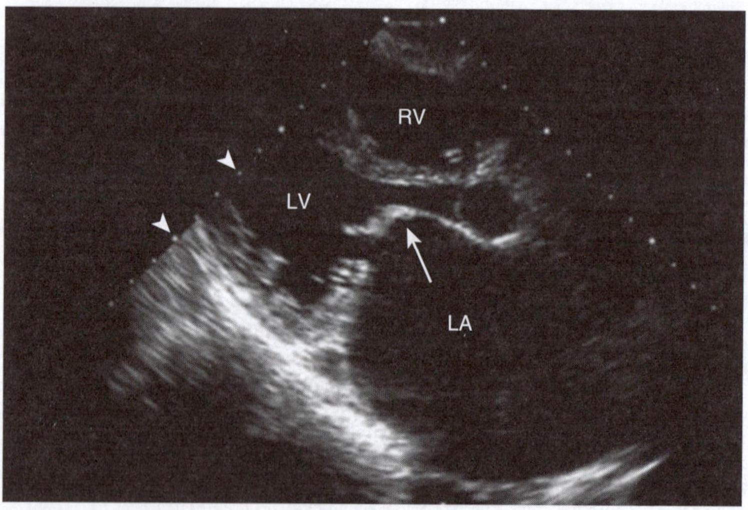

Fig. 32.2. Two-dimensional echocardiogram of the parasternal long-axis view during diastole of a patient with mitral stenosis. The mitral valve leaflets are thickened and have the typical *hockey-stick* appearance *(arrow).* Note also that the left atrium (LA) is enlarged. *LV,* Left ventricle; *RV,* right ventricle. *(Modified from Libby, P., & Braunwald, E. [2008].* Braunwald's heart disease: a textbook of cardiovascular medicine *[8th ed.]. Philadelphia, PA: Saunders.)*

from Doppler assessment of the transvalvular gradient, and from measuring the delay in LA emptying. Pulmonary pressure, left ventricular function, and RV function are also evaluated. In general, the main criteria for severe MS are as follows:

- Mean gradient more than 10 mm Hg
- Valve area less than 1.0 cm^2
- Pulmonary arterial (PA) systolic pressure greater than 50 mm Hg

The severity of MS is estimated using the criteria given in Table 32.1.

6. What are the four states of mitral stenosis?

Similar to other valvular lesions, MS is now classified not only by severity but more generally by stage. The four states are (A) at risk of MS, (B) progressive MS, (C) asymptomatic severe MS, and (D) symptomatic severe MS. These four stages are described in detail in Table 32.2.

7. Is there effective medical management for mitral stenosis?

Yes. Patients with mild symptoms and normal pulmonary artery pressure can be treated with diuretics to lower left atrial pressure and relieve pulmonary congestion. The combination of LA enlargement and continued inflammation from a smoldering rheumatic process predisposes patients with MS to develop atrial fibrillation (AF). AF with rapid heart rate affects the MS patient gravely because it diminishes transit time for blood flow from the LA to LV, further increasing LA pressure and diminishing cardiac output. Rate control with beta-blockers, calcium-channel blockers, or digoxin is imperative. If these agents fail to control the heart, cardioversion is indicated. Once AF has developed in the MS patient, the risk of stroke approaches 10% per year. Thus, anticoagulation to an international normalized ratio (INR) of 2.5 to 3.5 is mandatory unless a contraindication exists.

8. What is the definitive management for severe mitral stenosis?

If symptoms cannot be easily controlled medically or if asymptomatic pulmonary hypertension develops, this mechanical lesion must be treated by mechanical relief of the stenosis, because both conditions worsen MS prognosis. In most cases, mitral balloon valvotomy is the preferred therapy. In this procedure, a balloon is passed percutaneously from the femoral vein across the atrial septum (by needle puncture) through the mitral valve, where it is inflated (Fig. 32.3). Balloon inflation ruptures the adhesions at the commissures caused by the rheumatic process, allowing as much as doubling of the mitral valve area (MVA) and normalizing cardiac output, left atrial pressure, and pulmonary artery pressure, in turn relieving symptoms.

Criteria have been established to determine whether balloon valvotomy should be performed or the patient referred for surgery. These four criteria are valve mobility, subvalvular thickening, leaflet thickening, and degree of valvular calcification. In addition to these characteristics, the degree of mitral regurgitation is assessed, because balloon valvotomy can worsen the degree of mitral regurgitation.

Fig. 32.4 summarizes the indications for intervention for rheumatic MS. Recommendations for MS intervention are given in Table 32.3.

Table 32.1. Echocardiographic Criteria for the Assessment of the Severity of Mitral Stenosis

MILD	MODERATE	SEVERE
Mean gradient	<5 mm Hg	5-10 mm Hg > 10 mm Hg
PA systolic	>30 mm Hg	30-50 mm Hg > 50 mm Hg
Valve area	<1.5 cm^2	1.0-1.5 cm^2 < 1.0 cm^2

Modified from Bonow, R. O., Carabello, B. A., Chatterjee, K., de Leon, A. C. Jr., Faxon, D. P., Freed, M. D., et al. (2006). ACC/AHA 2006 *guidelines for the management of patients with valvular heart disease*. Journal of the American College of Cardiology, 48, *e1–e148*.

Table 32.2. The Four Stages of Mitral Stenosis

STAGE	DEFINITION	VALVE ANATOMY	VALVE HEMODYNAMICS	HEMODYNAMIC CONSEQUENCE	SYMPTOMS
A	At risk of MS	Mild valve doming during diastole	Normal transmitral flow velocity	None	None
B	Progressive MS	Rheumatic valve changes with commissural fusion and diastolic doming of the mitral valve leaflets Planimetered MVA >1.5 cm^2	Increased transmitral flow velocities MVA >1.5 cm^2 Diastolic pressure half-time <150 ms	Mild to moderate LA enlargement Normal pulmonary pressure at rest	None
C	Asymptomatic severe MS	Rheumatic valve changes with commissural fusion and diastolic doming of the mitral valve leaflets Planimetered MVA <1.5 cm^2 (MVA <1.0 cm^2 with very severe MS)	MVA <1.5 cm^2 (MVA <1.0 cm^2 with very severe MS) Diastolic pressure half-time >150 ms (Diastolic pressure half-time >220 ms with very severe MS)	Severe LA enlargement Elevated PASP >30 mm Hg	None
D	Symptomatic severe MS	Rheumatic valve changes with commissural fusion and diastolic doming of the mitral valve leaflets Planimetered MVA <1.5 cm^2	MVA <1.5 cm^2 (MVA <1.0 cm^2 with severe MS) Diastolic pressure half-time >150 ms (Diastolic pressure half-time >220 ms with very severe MS)	Severe LA enlargement Elevated PASP >30 mm Hg	Decreased exercise tolerance Exertional dyspnea

LA, Left atrial; *LV*, left ventricular; *MS*, mitral stenosis; *MVA*, mitral valve area; *PASP*, pulmonary artery systolic pressure.

The transmitral mean pressure gradient should be obtained to further determine the hemodynamic effect on the MS and is usually ≥5 mmHg, 10 mmHg in severe MS; however, because of the variability of the mean pressure gradient with heart rate and forward flow, it has not yet been included in the criteria for severity.

Table from Nishimura, R. A, Otto, C. M., Bonow, R. O., Carabello, B. A., Erwin, J. P. III, Guyton, R. A., et al. (2014). 2014 AHA/ACC guideline for the management of patients with valvular heart disease: a report of the American College of Cardiology/American Heart Association Task Force on Practice Guidelines. Journal of the American College of Cardiology, 63, e57–e185.

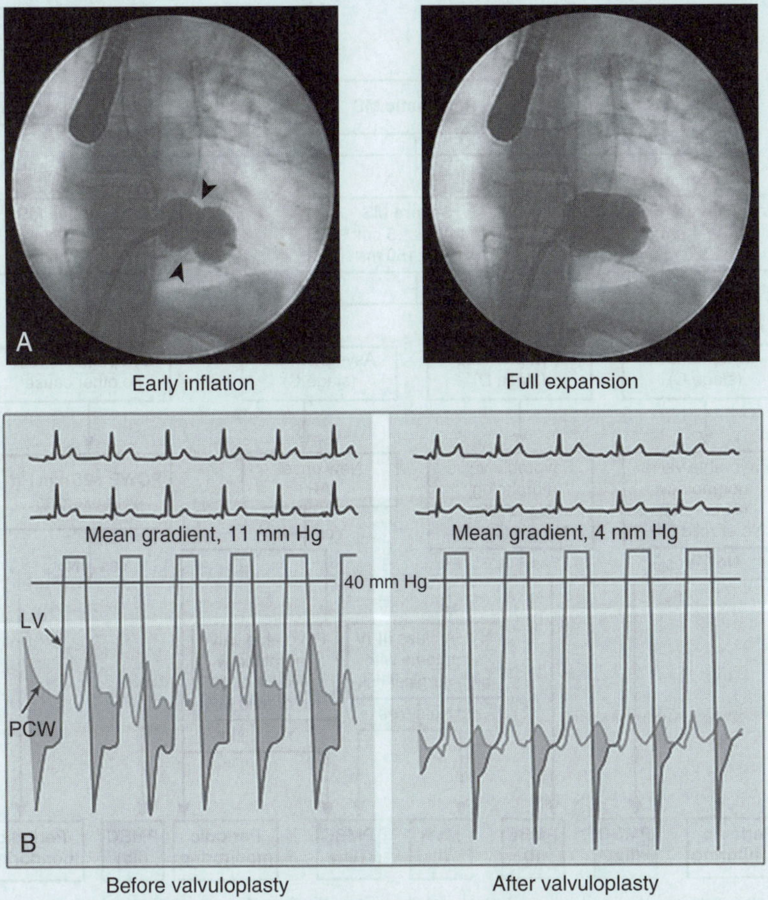

Fig. 32.3. Percutaneous balloon mitral valvotomy (BMV) for mitral stenosis using the Inoue technique. **A**, The catheter is advanced into the left atrium via the transseptal technique and guided antegrade across the mitral orifice. As the balloon is inflated, its distal portion expands first and is pulled back so that it fits snugly against the orifice. With further inflation, the proximal portion of the balloon expands to center the balloon within the stenotic orifice *(left).* Further inflation expands the central *waist* portion of the balloon *(right),* resulting in commissural splitting and enlargement of the orifice. **B**, Successful BMV results in significant increase in mitral valve area, as reflected by reduction in the diastolic pressure gradient between left ventricle (LV) and pulmonary capillary wedge (PCW) pressure, as indicated by the *shaded area. (From Delabays, A., & Goy, J. J. [2001]. Images in clinical medicine: percutaneous mitral valvuloplasty.* New England Journal of Medicine, *345, e4.)*

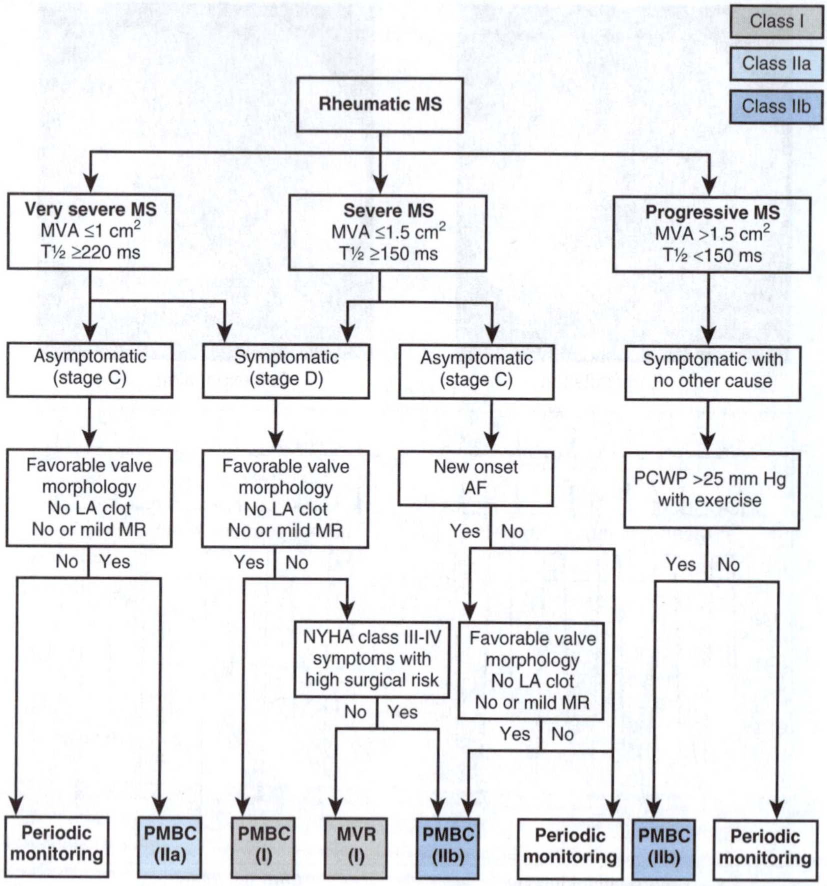

Fig. 32.4. Indications for intervention for rheumatic MS. *(Image from Nishimura, R. A., Otto, C. M., Bonow, R. O., Carabello, B. A., Erwin, J. P. III, Guyton, R. A., et al. [2014]. 2014 AHA/ACC guideline for the management of patients with valvular heart disease: a report of the American College of Cardiology/American Heart Association Task Force on Practice Guidelines.* Journal of the American College of Cardiology, *63, e57–e185.)*

Table 32.3. Summary of Recommendations for Mitral Stenosis Intervention

RECOMMENDATIONS	COR	LOE	REFERENCES
PMBC is recommended for symptomatic patients with severe MS (MVA <1.5 cm^2, stage D) and favorable valve morphology in the absence of contraindications.	I	A	(280-248, 286)
Mitral valve surgery is indicated in severely symptomatic patients (NYHA class III/IV) with severe MS (MVA <1.5 cm^2, stage D) who are not at high risk for surgery and who are not candidates for or failed previous PMBC.	I	B	(319-324)
Concomitant mitral valve surgery is indicated for patients with severe MS (MVA <1.5 cm^2, stage C or D) undergoing other cardiac surgery.	I	C	N/A
PMBC is reasonable for asymptomatic patients with very severe MS (MVA <1.0 cm^2, stage C) and favorable valve morphology in the absence of contraindications.	IIa	C	(239, 325, 327)
Mitral valve surgery is reasonable for severely symptomatic patients (NYHA class III/IV) with severe MS (MVA <1.5 cm^2, stage D), provided there are other operative indications.	IIa	C	N/A
PMBC may be considered for asymptomatic patients with severe MS (MVA <1.5 cm^2, stage C) and favorable valve morphology who have new onset of AF in the absence of contraindications.	IIb	C	N/A
PMBC may be considered for asymptomatic patients with MVA >1.5 cm^2. If there is evidence of hemodynamically significant MS during exercise,	IIb	C	N\A
PMBC may be considered for severely symptomatic patients (NHYA class III/IV) with severe MS (MVA <1.5 cm^2, stage D) who have suboptimal valve anatomy and are not candidates for surgery or are at high risk for surgery.	IIb	C	N/A
Concomitant mitral valve surgery may be considered for patients with moderate MS (MVA 1.6-2.0 cm^2) undergoing other cardiac surgery.	IIb	C	N/A
Mitral valve surgery and excision of the left atrial appendage may be considered for patients with severe MS (MVA <1.5 cm^2, stages C and D) who have had recurrent embolic events while receiving adequate anticoagulation.	IIb	C	N/A

AF, Atrial fibrillation; *COR*, Class of Recommendation; *LOE*, Level of Evidence; *MS*, mitral stenosis; *MVA*, mitral valve area; *NYHA*, New York Heart Association; *PMBC*, percutaneous mitral balloon commissurotomy.

Table from Nishimura, R. A., Otto, C. M., Bonow, R. O., Carabello, B. A., Erwin, J. P. III, Guyton, R. A., et al. (2014). 2014 AHA/ACC guideline for the management of patients with valvular heart disease: a report of the American College of Cardiology/American Heart Association Task Force on Practice Guidelines. Journal of the American College of Cardiology, 63, e57–e185.

Bibliography and Suggested Readings

Bonow, R. O., Carabello, B. A., Chatterjee, K., de Leon, A. C., Jr., Faxon, D. P., Freed, M. D., et al. (2006). ACC/AHA 2006 guidelines for the management of patients with valvular heart disease. *Journal of the American College of Cardiology, 48*, e1–e148.

Carabello, B. A. (2005). Modern management of mitral stenosis. *Circulation, 112*(3), 432–437.

Nishimura, R. A., Otto, C. M., Bonow, R. O., Carabello, B. A., Erwin, J. P., III, Guyton, R. A., et al. (2014). 2014 AHA/ACC guideline for the management of patients with valvular heart disease: a report of the American College of Cardiology/American Heart Association Task Force on practice guidelines. *Journal of the American College of Cardiology, 63*, e57–e185.

Vahanian, A., Alfieri, O., Andreotti, F., Antunes, M. J., Barón-Esquivias, G., Baumgartner, H., et al. (2012). Guidelines on the management of valvular heart disease (version 2012). *European Heart Journal, 33*, 2451–2496.

TRANSCATHETER AORTIC VALVE REPLACEMENT

CHAPTER 33

Jimmy Kerrigan, Amar Krishnaswamy, Faisal Bakaeen, Stephanie Mick

1. **What is transcatheter aortic valve replacement?**

Transcatheter aortic valve replacement (TAVR, alternately known as transcatheter aortic valve implantation [TAVI]) is a procedure in which a diseased aortic valve is replaced via an endovascular or transapical approach, using an expandable valve delivered with a catheter (Figs. 33.1 and 33.2). Traditionally, TAVR has been used to ameliorate severe aortic stenosis (AS). The alternative, surgical aortic valve replacement (SAVR), is the gold standard; however, 30% to 40% of patients evaluated for SAVR are considered to present with high or prohibitive risks to proceed with surgery. In appropriately selected patients, randomized clinical trials have demonstrated that TAVR reduces mortality compared to medical therapy alone in inoperable patients and is noninferior (or in some cases superior) to SAVR in intermediate- and high-risk patients.

2. **How is risk assessed for patients in whom aortic valve replacement is being considered?**

For patients who would be deemed potentially high risk for SAVR, evaluation by a heart valve team, consisting of healthcare professionals with experience in valvular heart disease, cardiac imaging, interventional cardiology, and cardiac surgery, is recommended.

The decision on SAVR versus TAVR should be based upon an individual risk-benefit analysis, performed for each patient by the heart valve team. An estimate of operative mortality can be derived from multiple different scoring systems, most commonly the Society of Thoracic Surgeons Predicted Risk of Mortality (STS-PROM) Calculator (riskcalc.sts.org/stswebriskcalc/#/), which considers typical factors including age, renal function, lung disease, cardiac function, and prior cardiac surgeries. However,

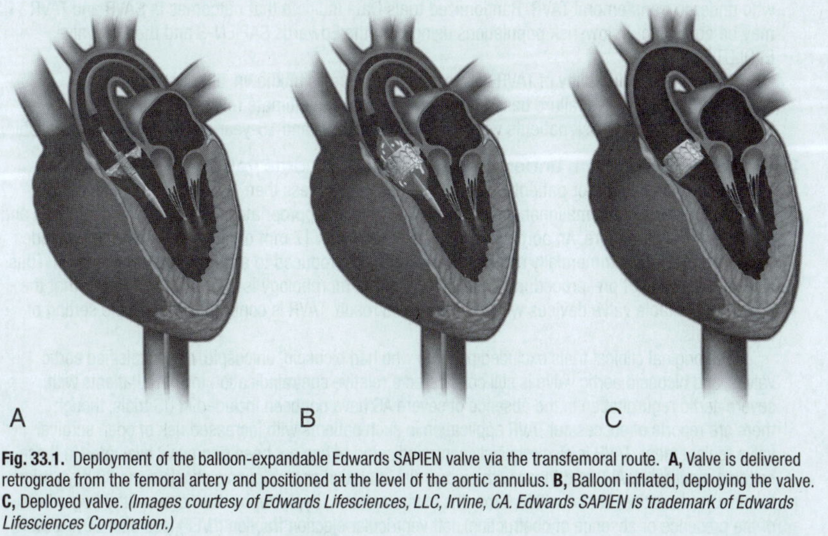

Fig. 33.1. Deployment of the balloon-expandable Edwards SAPIEN valve via the transfemoral route. **A,** Valve is delivered retrograde from the femoral artery and positioned at the level of the aortic annulus. **B,** Balloon inflated, deploying the valve. **C,** Deployed valve. *(Images courtesy of Edwards Lifesciences, LLC, Irvine, CA. Edwards SAPIEN is trademark of Edwards Lifesciences Corporation.)*

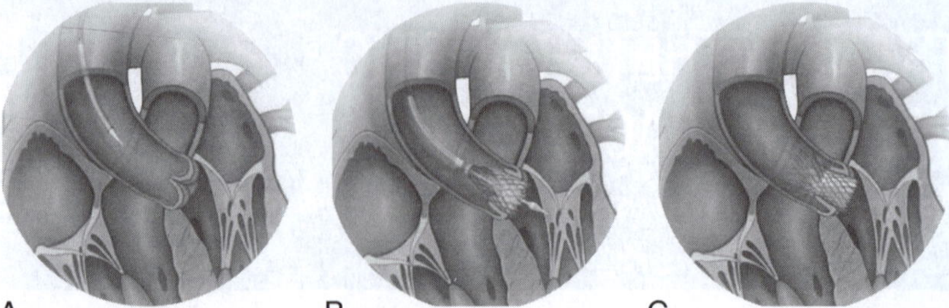

A B C

Fig. 33.2. Deployment of the self-expanding Medtronic Core-Valve via the transapical route. **A,** Valve is delivered retrograde from the femoral artery. **B,** Valve is positioned at the level of the aortic annulus. The sheath is retracted, allowing expansion of the valve. **C,** Deployed valve. *(Images courtesy of Medtronics.)*

often- encountered comorbidities, including cirrhosis, heavily calcified ("porcelain") ascending aorta, and frailty, are not considered in the current STS-PROM. Therefore, a comprehensive approach that factors the STS score and patient-specific factors must be considered. Table 33.1 gives one suggested approach to categorizing SAVR risk that incorporates both STS-PROM score and other factors.

3. What options are there for low- and intermediate-risk patients?

At this time, TAVR is only approved by the US Food and Drug Administration (FDA) for patients at high or prohibitive surgical risk. In these patients, based upon results from various observational studies, multicenter registries, and randomized controlled trials, in whom the alternative was medical treatment alone for inoperable patients and SAVR for high-risk patients, survival and rates of repeat hospitalization were significantly decreased in patients who underwent TAVR as opposed to those undergoing medical therapy and noninferior or better than SAVR in the high-risk group. Current American College of Cardiology/American Heart Association (ACC/AHA) guidelines give TAVR a class I recommendation for patients at prohibitive risk for SAVR and a class IIa recommendation for those at high risk for SAVR.

Trials performed in Europe indicate that TAVR and SAVR may be equivalent in low- and intermediate-risk patients. Recently data indicate that SAVR and TAVR, when using the Edwards SAPIEN XT valve, are equivalent in intermediate-risk patients (as at 2 years' time, with a potential trend towards superiority (improved survival and lower rate of stroke) in intermediate-risk patients who undergo transfemoral TAVR. Randomized trials Data indicate that outcomes in SAVR and TAVR may be equivalent in low-risk populations using both the Edwards SAPIEN-3 and the CoreValve EVOLUT R.

Currently, the durability of TAVR valves beyond 5 years is unknown, although there is no suggestion of early valve failure based on *ex vivo* testing. The ultimate role of TAVR in young intermediate- and low-risk patients will not be clear until 10- and 15-year durability data are available.

4. Who is excluded from undergoing transcatheter aortic valve replacement?

TAVR is contraindicated for patients with a life expectancy of less than 1 year based on noncardiac factors (e.g., metastatic malignancies), in order to strike an appropriate balance between the risks and benefits of the procedure. An aortic annulus size of less than 17 mm or larger than 29 mm precludes TAVR, as currently commercially available valves are not produced to accommodate these sizes. Thus, a careful analysis of pre-procedural/baseline aortic root morphology is imperative to ensure that the currently available valve devices will provide a good result. TAVR is contraindicated in the setting of endocarditis.

The original clinical trials excluded patients who had bicuspid, unicuspid, or noncalcified aortic valves, and bicuspid aortic valve is still considered a relative contraindication to TAVR. Patients with severe aortic regurgitation in the absence of severe AS have not been included in US trials, though there are reports of successful TAVR application in such patients with increased risk of open surgical valve replacement. TAVR is also relatively contraindicated or has not been rigorously evaluated in those needing emergency AVR and those with myocardial infarction or cardiogenic shock in the 30 days prior to valve implantation, stroke within 6 months of implantation, hypertrophic cardiomyopathy (regardless of the presence or absence of obstruction), left ventricular ejection fraction (LVEF) less than 20%, severe

Table 33.1. Risk Assessment Combining STS Risk Estimate, Frailty, Major Organ System Dysfunction, and Procedure-Specific Impediments

	LOW RISK (MUST MEET ALL CRITERIA IN THIS COLUMN)	INTERMEDIATE RISK (ANY 1 CRITERION IN THIS COLUMN)	HIGH RISK (ANY 1 CRITERION IN THIS COLUMN)	PROHIBITIVE RISK (ANY 1 CRITERION IN THIS COLUMN)
STS-PROM*	<4% AND	4%-8% OR	>8% OR	Predicted risk with surgery of death or major morbidity (all-cause) >50% at 1 y OR
Frailty†	None AND	1 Index (mild) OR	≥2 Indices (moderate to severe) OR	
Major organ system compromise not to be improved postoperatively‡	None AND	1 Organ system OR	No more than 2 organ systems OR	≥3 Organ systems OR
Procedure-specific impediment§	None	Possible procedure-specific impediment	Possible procedure-specific impediment	Severe procedure-specific impediment

*Use of the STS PROM to predict risk in a given institution with reasonable reliability is appropriate only if institutional outcomes are within 1 standard deviation of STS average observed/expected ratio for the procedure in question.

†Seven frailty indices: Katz Activities of Daily Living (independence in feeding, bathing, dressing, transferring, toileting, and urinary continence) and independence in ambulation (no walking aid or assist required or 5-meter walk in <6 s). Other scoring systems can be applied to calculate no, mild, or moderate to severe frailty.

‡Examples of major organ system compromise: Cardiac—severe LV systolic or diastolic dysfunction or RV dysfunction, fixed pulmonary hypertension; CKD stage 3 or worse; pulmonary dysfunction with *FEV1* <50% or $DLCO_2$ <50% of predicted; CNS dysfunction (dementia, Alzheimer's disease, Parkinson's disease, CVA with persistent physical limitation); GI dysfunction—Crohn's disease, ulcerative colitis, nutritional impairment, or serum albumin <3.0; cancer—active malignancy; and liver—any history of cirrhosis, variceal bleeding, or elevated INR in the absence of VKA therapy.

§Examples: tracheostomy present, heavily calcified ascending aorta, chest malformation, arterial coronary graft adherent to posterior chest wall, or radiation damage.

CKD, chronic kidney disease; *CNS*, central nervous system; *CVA*, stroke; *DLCO₂*, diffusion capacity for carbon dioxide; *FEV1*, forced expiratory volume in 1 s; *GI*, gastrointestinal; *INR*, international normalized ratio; *LV*, left ventricular; *PROM*, predicted risk of mortality; *RV*, right ventricular; *STS*, Society of Thoracic Surgeons; and *VKA*, vitamin *K* antagonist.

From Nishimura, R. A., Otto, C. M., Bonow, R. O., Carabello, B. A., Erwin, J. P. III, Guyton, R. A., O'Gara, P. T., Ruiz, C. E., Skubas, N. J., Sorajja, P., Sundt, T. M. III, Thomas, J. D. 2014 AHA/ACC guideline for the management of patients with valvular heart disease: a report of the American College of Cardiology/American Heart Association Task Force on Practice Guidelines. J Am Coll Cardiol 2014:63:e57–185.

Table 33.2. Summary of ACC/AHA Guidelines for Choice of Surgical Aortic Valve Replacement or Transcatheter Aortic Valve Replacement in Patients with Aortic Stenosis

Class I (Recommended)
• Surgical AVR is recommended in patients who meet an indication for AVR with low or intermediate surgical risk.
• For patients in whom TAVR or high-risk surgical AVR is being considered, members of a heart valve team should collaborate to provide optimal patient care.
• TAVR is recommended in patients who meet an indication for AVR for AS who have a prohibitive surgical risk and a predicted post-TAVR survival >12 mo.
Class IIa (Reasonable)
• TAVR is a reasonable alternative to surgical AVR in patients who meet an indication for AVR and who have high surgical risk.
Class III (No benefit)
• TAVR is not recommended in patients in whom existing comorbidities would preclude the expected benefit from correction of AS.

AS, Aortic stenosis; *AVR*, aortic valve replacement; *TAVR*, transcatheter aortic valve replacement.

Adapted from Nishimura, R. A., Otto, C. M., Bonow, R. O., Carabello, B. A., Erwin, J. P. III, Guyton, R. A., et al. (2014). 2014 AHA/ACC guideline for the management of patients with valvular heart disease: a report of the American College of Cardiology/American Heart Association Task Force on Practice Guidelines. Journal of the American College of Cardiology, *63, e57–e185.*

right ventricular dysfunction due to pulmonary hypertension (whether primary or secondary), inability to be anticoagulated (with agents described later in the chapter), severe dementia, and severe mitral regurgitation. As these are all relative contraindications, decision making by the heart team is imperative in weighing the relative risks and benefits of the procedure for each individual patient.

Access-specific contraindications include aortic atheroma, intracardiac masses or thrombi, aortic aneurysm, iliac/femoral aneurysm, iliac/femoral stenosis, or severe tortuosity of the aorta.

5. What are the indications for aortic valve replacement?

At this time, AVR (whether SAVR or TAVR) is indicated in

- Symptomatic patients with severe AS (aortic velocity of >4 m/s or mean pressure gradient of >40 mm Hg)
- Severe AS if LVEF is less than 50%
- Severe AS with decreased exercise tolerance or fall in systolic blood pressure on exercise testing
- Symptomatic patients with low-flow/low-gradient AS and an LVEF greater than 50% if clinical, hemodynamic, and anatomic data support valve obstruction as the most likely cause of symptoms. (Low flow is defined as a stroke volume index <35 mL/m^2.)
- Symptomatic patients with low-flow/low-gradient severe AS with LVEF less than 50% where with low-dose dobutamine stress testing these parameters increase (aortic velocity becomes >4 m/s, mean pressure gradient becomes greater than 40 mm Hg, and valve area remains ≤1.0 cm^2).

6. What are the current recommendations regarding when to choose transcatheter aortic valve replacement over surgical aortic valve replacement?

Both American and European guidelines emphasize that decisions regarding TAVR or SAVR should be made by a heart valve team approach. Specific recommendations regarding TAVR are summarized in Tables 33.2 and 33.3.

7. What testing is needed prior to transcatheter aortic valve replacement?

Multiple pre-procedural tests are required in order to evaluate the aortic valve (number of leaflets, degree of calcification, and annular dimensions) and root (sinus and ST junction dimensions and coronary ostial clearance) anatomy. In addition, the severity of AS is evaluated and incidence of concomitant coronary or other valvular disease is investigated. The adequacy of the peripheral vasculature for the catheters required to perform the procedure and to determine the severity of any existing comorbidities is also an important part of patient workup and planning for TAVR.

- Transthoracic echocardiography (TTE), is the procedure of choice for is the assessing for severity of AS. In cases of low flow low-gradient AS, dobutamine echocardiography should be performed.

Table 33.3. Summary of the European Society of Cardiology and European Association for Cardio-Thoracic Surgery Guidelines for Transcatheter Aortic Valve Implantation.*

Class I (Recommended and indicated)
• TAVR should only be undertaken with a multidisciplinary heart team. • TAVR should only be performed in hospitals with on-site cardiac surgery capability. • TAVR should be performed in patients with severe AS who are not suitable for AVR, as assessed by a heart team, and who are likely gain improvement in their quality of life and to have a life expectancy of >1 y after consideration of their comorbidities.
Class IIa (Should be considered)
• TAVR should be considered in high-risk patients with severe symptomatic AS who may still be suitable for surgery but in whom TAVI is favored by a heart team based on individual risk profile and anatomic suitability.

AS, Aortic stenosis; *AVR*, aortic valve replacement; *TAVI*, transcatheter aortic valve implantation; *TAVR*, transcatheter aortic valve replacement.

Adapted from Vahanian, A., Alfieri, O., Andreotti, F., Antunes, M. J., Barón-Esquivias, G., Baumgartner, H., et al. (2012). The joint task force on the management of valvular heart disease of the European Society of Cardiology (ESC) and the European Association for Cardio-Thoracic Surgery (EACTS). European Heart Journal, 33, 2451–2496.

*These Recommendations Were Formulated Before the Results of Several Pivotal Trials of Transcatheter Aortic Valve Replacement in Patients at Intermediate Surgical Risk Were Known.

- Computed tomography (CT) of the aortic root, aorta, and peripheral vasculature. This provides information on the size of the aortic annulus, the spatial relationship between the coronary arteries and the aortic valve annulus, and adequacy of the peripheral vasculature to accept the cannulas necessary to perform the procedure. With patients for whom administration of intravenous contrast is relatively or absolutely contraindicated (i.e., renal insufficiency), CT may either be performed with intravenous administration of contrast via a pigtail catheter placed in the abdominal aorta or, in some cases, without contrast administration. These techniques, however, allow only for assessment of the iliofemoral system, and annulus assessment for valve sizing requires either cardiac magnetic resonance imaging (cMRI) or three-dimensional transesophageal echocardiography (TEE).
- Cardiac catheterization is required in order to evaluate for coronary disease. On left heart catheterization, angiography of the coronary arteries is performed, and clinically significant lesions may be stented prior to TAVR if the patient is not a candidate for combined SAVR and CABG. If the degree of AS remains uncertain after echocardiography, the aortic valve may be crossed so that pressure gradients may be accurately measured. At the time of left heart catheterization, right heart catheterization is performed in order to obtain information on pulmonary hypertension and cardiac output (which allows calculation of the aortic valve area, if the valve is crossed).
- Pulmonary function testing is performed in order to assess for obstructive or restrictive lung disease; information gained from this is combined with radiographic data (CT or chest roentgenograms) and used to evaluate the presence and severity of pulmonary problems.
- Rarely, ultrasound of the peripheral vasculature is used for access planning, most commonly in patients with chronic kidney dysfunction (CKD) in whom it is desirable to minimize exposure to iodinated contrast.

8. What vascular approaches are commonly used in transcatheter aortic valve replacement?

TAVR is most commonly performed via a transfemoral approach (TF-TAVR) using a delivery sheath placed in the common femoral artery. An alternate approach is the transapical approach (TA-TAVR), in which the delivery cannula is placed into the apex of the left ventricle via a small left thoracotomy (Fig. 33.3). With both approaches, the femoral vessels are still used for placement of the remainder of the required accessory catheters.

Additional delivery approaches include transsubclavian artery via axillary artery cutdown, transcarotid artery, transseptal (puncturing the interatrial septum via a venous approach), transaortic (TAo-TAVR, performed via partial sternotomy or right anterior thoracotomy) (Fig. 33.4), and transcaval (where a connection is made between the inferior vena cava and the abdominal aorta,

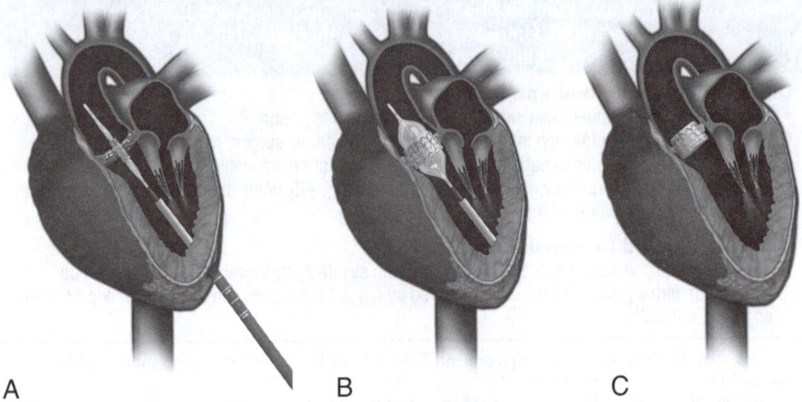

Fig. 33.3. Deployment of the balloon-expandable Edwards SAPIEN valve via the transapical route. **A,** Valve delivered antegrade to the aortic annulus via a small incision in the left ventricular apex. **B,** Balloon inflated, deploying the valve. **C,** Deployed valve. *(Images courtesy of Edwards Lifesciences, LLC, Irvine, CA. Edwards SAPIEN is trademark of Edwards Lifesciences Corporation.)*

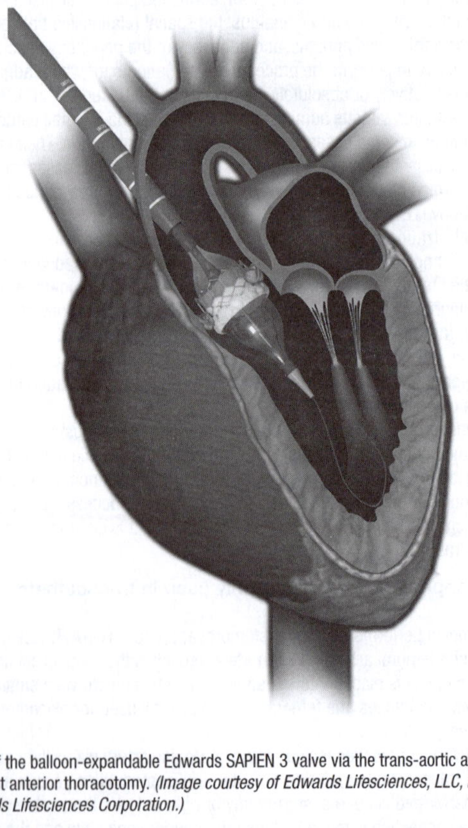

Fig. 33.4. Deployment of the balloon-expandable Edwards SAPIEN 3 valve via the trans-aortic approach, performed via partial sternotomy or right anterior thoracotomy. *(Image courtesy of Edwards Lifesciences, LLC, Irvine, CA. Edwards SAPIEN 3 is trademark of Edwards Lifesciences Corporation.)*

which is subsequently closed with an occluder device). Decisions on which alternate approach to use in patients with prohibitive peripheral vascular disease are made based upon comorbidities, anatomy, and the type of valve to be used.

9. What valves are currently being used for transcatheter aortic valve replacement in the United States?

At present, two valves are approved for commercial (i.e., not in clinical trials) use in the United States. The Edwards SAPIEN valve is a balloon-expandable valve. The SAPIEN valve, like a coronary stent, is provided compressed over a balloon. Once the device is in position, this balloon is inflated, expanding the stent into the patient's aortic annulus and securing the valve in place. Once placed, it is irretrievable.

Medtronic's self-expanding CoreValve ReValving system is delivered to the level of the aortic annulus surrounded by a sheath, which is subsequently slowly retracted to allow the valve frame to expand into place. Unlike the balloon-expandable valve, this system may be recaptured if malpositioning is observed early in its deployment.

Historically, the CoreValve has been associated with higher rates of aortic insufficiency and heart block, requiring placement of a permanent pacemaker when compared with the SAPIEN valve. The SAPIEN valve, in contrast, carries a very small but higher risk of aortic annular rupture (especially in patients with calcified, small aortic annuli). Despite these differences, multiple registries have indicated that overall long-term outcomes between the two valves are similar concerning procedural success and mortality. A decision on which prosthesis is used is based upon several factors, including annular size, annular geometry, calcification, and distance between the aortic annulus and the coronary ostia.

10. What antiplatelet regimen is used after transcatheter aortic valve replacement?

Patients are typically placed on dual antiplatelet therapy (aspirin 81 mg and clopidogrel 75 mg daily) for some period of time (usually 3 to 6 months). Following this, clopidogrel is discontinued and patients remain on lifelong aspirin. Patient-specific factors, particularly bleeding risk, will often dictate the specific regimen and duration of antiplatelet therapy.

11. What are the possible complications of transcatheter aortic valve replacement?

The most common post-TAVR complication is paravalvular aortic regurgitation. While initial studies of the first-generation valve systems demonstrated moderate or severe paravalvular aortic regurgitation in almost 16% of patients, with improvements in valve design and a better understanding of valve sizing and implantation techniques, the newest trials demonstrate significant paravalvular aortic regurgitation in a much smaller percentage of patients (generally <3%).

A second important complication is complete heart block. The rates of heart block vary depending on the valve type (balloon-expandable vs. self-expanding) and generation of prosthetic valve used. In some cases, the conduction system recovers and heart block abates, but not infrequently, implantation of a permanent pacemaker may be required.

Other complications include bleeding, embolic stroke, obstruction of a coronary ostium, annular rupture, ventricular perforation, aortic dissection, Acute kidney injury (AKI), cardiogenic shock, and embolization of the valve prosthesis.

Longer term complications include development of aortic regurgitation (both paravalvular and transvalvular, AS, and valve thrombosis).

12. Can transcatheter aortic valve replacement be performed in patients with aortic insufficiency?

In Europe, TAVR is used commercially for the treatment of pure aortic insufficiency. In the United States, TAVR has not been approved for the treatment of aortic regurgitation, although it has been used off-label in some patients. The main concern in patients with aortic regurgitation is the lack of valvular and annular calcification that may prevent secure anchoring of currently available valves.

13. Can patients with prior aortic valve replacement undergo transcatheter aortic valve replacement?

In patients with mechanical AVRs, TAVR is not feasible. In patients with bioprosthetic valves that have failed (either placed surgically or via TAVR), TAVR can be used to treat either AS or aortic regurgitation. Use of TAVR in patients with prior bioprosthetic valves is referred to as "valve-in-valve" TAVR.

Bibliography and Suggested Readings

Achenbach, S., Delgado, V., Hausleiter, J., Schoenhagen, P., Min, J. K., & Leipsic, J. A. (2012). SCCT expert consensus document on computed tomography imaging before transcatheter aortic valve implantation (TAVI)/transcatheter aortic valve replacement (TAVR). *Journal of Cardiovascular Computed Tomography, 6*(6), 366–380.

Holmes, D. R., Jr., & Mack, M. J. (2011). Transcatheter valve therapy a professional society overview from the American College of Cardiology Foundation and the Society of Thoracic Surgeons. *Journal of the American College of Cardiology, 58*(4), 445–455.

Holmes, D. R., Jr., Rich, J. B., Zoghbi, W. A., & Mack, M. J. (2013). The heart team of cardiovascular care. *Journal of the American College of Cardiology, 61*(9), 903–907.

Mack, M. J. (2012). Transcatheter aortic valve implantation: changing patient populations and novel indications. *Heart, 98*(Suppl. 4), iv73–iv79.

Nishimura, R. A., Otto, C. M., Bonow, R. O., Carabello, B. A., Erwin, J. P., III, Guyton, R. A., et al. (2014). 2014 AHA/ACC guideline for the management of patients with valvular heart disease: a report of the American College of Cardiology/American Heart Association Task Force on Practice Guidelines. *Journal of the American College of Cardiology, 63*, e57–e185.

Vahanian, A., Alfieri, O., Andreotti, F., Antunes, M. J., Barón-Esquivias, G., Baumgartner, H., et al. (2012). Guidelines on the management of valvular heart disease (version 2012). *European Heart Journal, 33*, 2451–2496.

CHAPTER 34

ENDOCARDITIS AND ENDOCARDITIS PROPHYLAXIS

Nadeen Faza, Tina Shah

1. What are believed to be the first steps in the development of infective endocarditis?

Infective endocarditis (IE) is believed to occur only after one first develops what is termed *nonbacterial thrombotic endocarditis* (NBTE). According to the American Heart Association (AHA) statement on endocarditis, it is believed that turbulent blood flow produced by certain types of congenital or acquired heart diseases traumatizes the endothelium. This turbulent blood flow may be the result of flow from a high- to a low-pressure chamber or across a narrowed orifice. This trauma of the endothelium then creates a predisposition for deposition of platelets and fibrin on the surface of the endothelium, resulting in NBTE. If bacteremia (or fungemia) occurs, the organisms may then colonize this site, resulting in IE.

2. What are risk factors for developing infective endocarditis?

Important risk factors for the development of IE include the following:

- Age greater than 60 years
- Poor dentition or dental infection
- Rheumatic heart disease (in underdeveloped countries)
- Prosthetic valves
- History of congenital heart disease
- Previous history of endocarditis
- Intracardiac devices
- Intravenous drug abuse
- Immunocompromised state
- Diabetes mellitus
- Chronic hemodialysis

3. Has the incidence or mortality from endocarditis decreased over the past 3 decades?

IE has an annual incidence of 3 to 7 per 100,000 person in the most recent surveys. Although the overall IE incidence has remained stable, the incidence of IE caused by *Staphylococcus aureus* has increased.

4. How often does routine tooth brushing and flossing cause transient bacteremia?

Transient bacteremia occurs 20% to 68% of the time with routine tooth brushing and flossing. It occurs 20% to 40% of the time with use of wooden toothpicks, and 7% to 71% of the time with chewing food. This is part of the rationale of the latest AHA guidelines deemphasizing antibiotic prophylaxis during certain dental and other procedures—namely, that the vast majority of the time bacteremia is due to daily activities and not to the occasional or rare dental or other procedure. The emphasis now is more on maintaining good oral hygiene and access to routine dental care.

5. True or false: Prospective randomized placebo-controlled trials have demonstrated that antibiotic prophylaxis before dental or other procedures reduces the risk of infective endocarditis

False. Despite the fact that for 50 years antibiotic prophylaxis has been recommended, there has never been a prospective randomized placebo-controlled trial to support this recommendation. In fact, the data on whether antibiotic prophylaxis even significantly affects bacteremia are contradictory, with some studies showing some reduction and others showing no reduction.

6. What are the four conditions identified as having the highest risk of adverse outcome from endocarditis, for which prophylaxis with dental procedures is still recommended?

- Prosthetic cardiac valve or prosthetic material used in valve repair
- Previous endocarditis
- Congenital heart disease only in the following categories:
  - Unrepaired cyanotic congenital heart disease, including those with palliative shunts and conduits
  - Completely repaired congenital heart disease with prosthetic material or device, whether placed by surgery or catheter intervention, during the first 6 months after the procedure
  - Repaired congenital heart disease with residual defects at the site or adjacent to the site of a prosthetic patch or prosthetic device (which inhibit endothelialization)
- Cardiac transplantation recipients with cardiac valvular disease

7. In the American Heart Association guidelines, for those patients with conditions listed in Question 6, which dental procedures carry a recommendation of endocarditis prophylaxis?

The guidelines emphasize that *all dental procedures* that involve the manipulation of gingival tissue or the periapical region of teeth or perforation of the oral mucosa should receive endocarditis prophylaxis. Antibiotic prophylaxis is *not recommended* for local anesthetic injections in non-infected tissues, treatment of superficial caries, removal of sutures, dental X-rays, placement or adjustment of removable prosthodontic or orthodontic appliances or braces, or following the shedding of deciduous teeth or trauma to the lips and oral mucosa.

8. For what other procedures may prophylaxis be considered in patients with high-risk lesions?

The AHA guidelines deemphasize prophylaxis for most other procedures. Antibiotic prophylaxis solely to prevent IE is not recommended for genitourinary (GU) or gastrointestinal (GI) tract procedures. Antibiotic therapy is mainly needed only when invasive procedures are performed in the context of infection. Procedures where prophylaxis may be considered (class IIb, level of evidence C) are

- Invasive procedures of the respiratory tract that involve incision or biopsy of the respiratory mucosa (e.g., tonsillectomy, adenoidectomy)
- Bronchoscopy with incision of the respiratory tract mucosa (but not otherwise for bronchoscopy)
- Invasive respiratory tract procedures to treat an established infection (e.g., drainage or an abscess or empyema)
- Surgical procedures that involve infected skin, skin structures, or musculoskeletal tissue
- Non-elective cystoscopy or other urinary tract manipulation in patients with enterococcal urinary tract infection or colonization

9. In patients who need antibiotic prophylaxis, what is the recommended regimen prior to dental procedures?

Antibiotic treatment should be administered as a single dose before the procedure, with antimicrobial therapy directed against viridans group streptococci. Amoxicillin (2 g orally [PO]), administered 30 to 60 minutes before the procedure, is the first-line recommendation. Those unable to take oral medication can be treated with ampicillin (2 g intramuscularly [IM] or intravenously [IV]) or cefazolin or ceftriaxone (1 g IM or IV). For those allergic to penicillins or ampicillin, potential agents to use include cephalexin, clindamycin, azithromycin, clarithromycin, cefazolin, and ceftriaxone. Table 34.1 summarizes the antibiotic regimens used for prophylaxis.

10. Is endocarditis prophylaxis recommended in patients treated with coronary stents, pacemakers, or defibrillators; those undergoing transesophageal echocardiography; or those who have undergone coronary artery bypass grafting (without valve replacement)?

No. However, some electrophysiologists will pretreat or posttreat patients undergoing pacemaker/defibrillator with antibiotics to prevent local infection (but not endocarditis).

11. What factors should raise the suspicion for endocarditis?

Factors that should raise the suspicion for endocarditis include

- Bacteremia/sepsis of unknown cause
- Fever
- Constitutional symptoms, such as unexplained malaise, weakness, arthralgias, and weight loss

Table 34.1. Antibiotic Prophylaxis Regimens for Infective Endocarditis

SITUATION	AGENT	REGIMEN—SINGLE DOSE 30-60 MIN BEFORE PROCEDURE	
		Adults	Children
Oral	Amoxicillin	2 g	50 mg/kg
Unable to take oral medication	Ampicillin OR Cefazolin or ceftriaxone	2 g IM or IV 1 g IM or IV	50 mg/kg IM or IV 50 mg/kg IM or IV
Allergic to penicillins or ampicillin—oral regimen	Cephalexin OR Clindamycin OR Azithromycin or clarithromycin	2 g 600 mg 500 mg	50 mg/kg 20 mg/kg 15 mg/kg
Allergic to penicillins or ampicillin and unable to take oral medication	Cefazolin or ceftriaxone OR Clindamycin	1 g IM or IV 600 mg IM or IV	50 mg/kg IM or IV 20 mg/kg IM or IV

IM, Intramuscularly; *IV*, intravenously.

Adapted from Nishimura, R. A., Otto, C. M., Bonow, R. O., Carabello, B. A., Erwin, J. P. 3rd., Guyton, R. A., et al. (2014). 2014 AHA/ACC guideline for the management of patients with valvular heart disease: a report of the American College of Cardiology/American Heart Association task force on practice guidelines. Journal of the American College of Cardiology, *63(22), e57–e185.*

- Hematuria, glomerulonephritis, and suspected renal infarction
- Embolic event of unknown origin (to the brain, lungs, spleen, kidney)
- New heart murmur (primarily regurgitant murmurs)
- Unexplained new atrioventricular (AV) nodal conduction abnormality (prolonged PR interval, heart block)
- Multifocal or rapid changing pulmonic infiltrates
- Peripheral abscesses
- Cutaneous lesions (Osler nodes, Janeway lesions)
- Ophthalmic manifestations (Roth's spots)

12. Which patients can present with endocarditis in an atypical manner?

A classic history and oslerian manifestations of endocarditis (bacteremia, active valvulitis, peripheral emboli, and immunologic phenomena) are present in a minority of patients. In most patients, these "textbook" findings may be absent. Hence, a high index of suspicion and low threshold for investigation are essential in these high-risk groups. Some specific patients who can present with endocarditis in an atypical manner include

- Those with right-sided endocarditis
- Elderly and immunocompromised patients

13. In which patients is right-sided endocarditis frequently seen?

- Patients with pacemakers, implantable cardioverter defibrillators, or central venous catheters
- Intravenous drug users, especially if with concomitant immunosuppression

14. When should echocardiography be ordered in cases of suspected endocarditis?

This should be done as quickly as possible. Echocardiographic evidence of an oscillating intracardiac mass or vegetation, an annular abscess, prosthetic valve dehiscence, and new valvular regurgitation are major criteria in the diagnosis of IE. Transthoracic echocardiography (TTE) has a sensitivity of 60% to 75% in the detection of native valve endocarditis (NVE). It can detect 70% of vegetations larger than 6 mm but only 25% of vegetations less than 5 mm. In cases where the clinical suspicion of endocarditis is low, a good-quality TTE is usually adequate. In cases where the suspicion of endocarditis is higher, a negative or non-diagnostic TTE should be followed by transesophageal echocardiography (TEE), which has a sensitivity of 88% to 100% and a specificity of 91% to 100% for native valves. TTE is not considered a sensitive test when a prosthetic valve or intracardiac device is present, and a TEE is recommended in such cases. Figs. 34.1 and 34.2 demonstrate a mitral valve vegetation visualized by TEE.

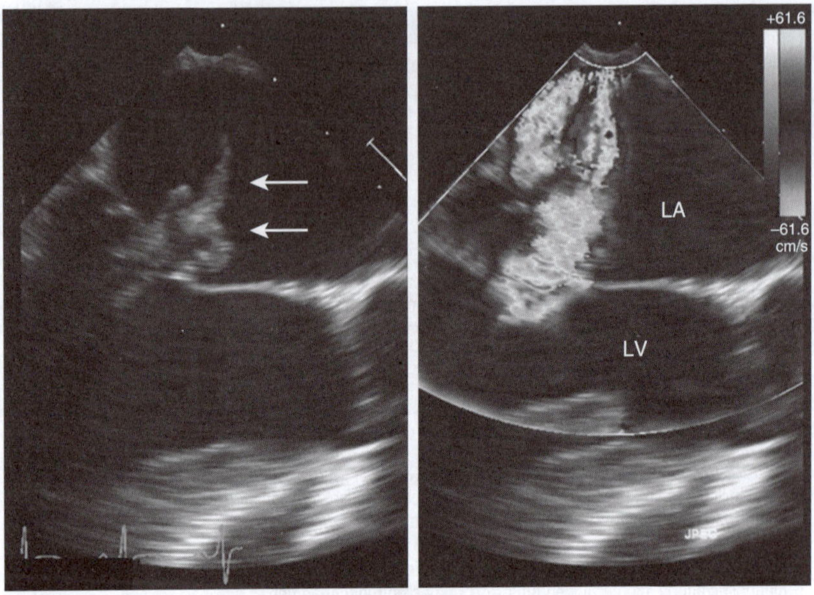

Fig. 34.1. Transesophageal echocardiography (TEE) imaging showing endocarditis on the mitral valve. The left panel shows a large vegetation *(arrow)* on the mitral valve. The right panel shows the resultant severe mitral regurgitation. A large turbulent jet of blood is demonstrated going from the LV, across the damaged mitral valve, into the LA. *LA,* Left atrium; *LV,* left ventricle.

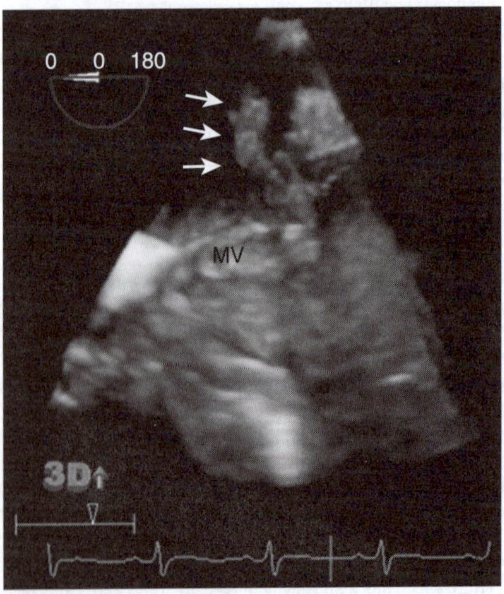

Fig. 34.2. 3D transesophageal echo showing large vegetation *(arrow)* on the MV. *MV,* Mitral valve.

15. When is repeat imaging indicated in patients with infective endocarditis?
Repeat imaging is indicated with acute changes in the patient's signs and symptoms. Examples include development of a new murmur, embolic phenomena, or AV conduction blocks. Persistence of fever despite adequate antibiotic therapy is also an indication for repeat echocardiography. Repeat echocardiography can also be considered during follow-up of uncomplicated IE, to detect new occult complications and monitor size of large vegetations. In these cases, timing of repeat imaging depends on the initial findings and response to therapy.

16. What is the procedure for obtaining blood cultures in cases of suspected endocarditis?
Three separate sets of blood cultures should be obtained from different venipuncture sites, with the first and last sample drawn at least 1 hour apart. For what is called *subacute* IE, some experts recommend the cultures be drawn over a period of 24 hours. These blood cultures should not be obtained from intravenous lines (although some may recommend additional blood cultures should be obtained from indwelling lines). At least 5 mL, and ideally 10 mL, of blood should be added to each culture bottle. In patients treated for a short period with antibiotics, one should wait, if possible, for at least 3 days after antibiotic discontinuation before obtaining new blood cultures.

17. What is the role of other imaging modalities (besides echocardiography) in the diagnosis of infective endocarditis?
A multislice CT scan (MSCT) can be used to detect abscesses/pseudoaneurysms and is probably superior to echocardiography in providing information on the extent of perivalvular extension. It is also helpful to diagnose embolic complications to the spleen, kidney, and brain. MRI is more sensitive than a CT scan to diagnose neurologic complications of IE. ^{18}F-FDG PET/CT significantly improves diagnostic accuracy in patients with prosthetic valve IE or cardiac device-related IE.

18. What is the most common overall organism reported to cause endocarditis?
The most common organism is *Staphylococcus aureus,* followed by viridans group streptococci and then enterococci and coagulase-native staphylococci.

19. What is the most common organism causing subacute native valve endocarditis?
Streptococcus viridans is the most common.

20. What is the most common organism causing endocarditis in intravenous drug abusers?
Staphylococcus aureus is the most common.

21. What is the most common organism causing early prosthetic valve endocarditis?
Staphylococcus infection is the most common, particularly *S. epidermidis* and *S. aureus.*

22. What is *Enterococcus faecalis* endocarditis often associated with?
It is associated with malignancy or manipulation of the GI or GU tract.

23. What is the most common cause of *culture-negative* endocarditis?
The most common cause of culture-negative endocarditis is prior use of antibiotics. Other causes include fastidious organisms (HACEK group, *Legionella, Chlamydia, Brucella*, certain fungal infections, etc.) and noninfectious causes. The HACEK group of organisms may cause large vegetations and large-vessel embolism.

24. How does one diagnose endocarditis caused by fastidious and non-culturable agents?
Diagnosis can be achieved through serologic testing and polymerase chain reaction (PCR)-based testing. However, there are limitations to these methods, and hence they are not included as major criteria in the Duke ischemia. Cross-reaction is a limitation of serologic testing, and low sensitivity (unless cardiac valvular tissue is available for testing) is a limitation of PCR.

25. What are the Duke criteria for the diagnosis of endocarditis?
The Duke criteria are a set of criteria proposed for the *definite* and *possible* diagnosis of IE, published in 1994 (see Bibliography), based on both pathologic and clinical criteria. These criteria were a

Table 34.2. The Modified Duke Criteria Definitions of Definite, Possible, and Rejected Endocarditis

Definite IE
• Pathologic criteria 1. Microorganisms demonstrated by culture or histologic examination of a vegetation, a vegetation that has embolized, or an intracardiac abscess specimen; or 2. Pathologic lesions; vegetation or intracardiac abscess confirmed by histologic examination showing active endocarditis
• Clinical criteria (see Table 34.3) 1. Two major criteria 2. One major criterion and three minor criteria 3. Five minor criteria
Possible IE (see Table 34.3) 1. One major criterion and one minor criterion 2. Three minor criteria
Rejected 1. Firm alternate diagnosis explaining evidence of IE 2. Resolution of infection endocarditis syndrome with antibiotic therapy for ≤4 days 3. No pathologic evidence of IE at surgery or autopsy, with antibiotic therapy for ≤4 days 4. Does not meet criteria for possible IE, as described previously

IE, Infective endocarditis.

Modified from Li, J. S., Sexton, D. J., Mick, N., Nettles, R., Fowler, V. G., Ryan, T., et al. (2000). Proposed modifications to the Duke criteria for the diagnosis of infective endocarditis. Clinical Infectious Diseases, 30(4), 633–638.

modification of previously proposed criteria (the *Von Reyn criteria*). They were slightly modified in 2000, with the criteria incorporating the value of transesophageal echo, special recognition of *Coxiella burnetti,* and several other issues (see Bibliography). These revisions became known as the "modified Duke criteria" and are presented in Tables 34.2 and 34.3.

26. What are among the complications of endocarditis?

IE may present the following complications:

- Cardiac complications
  - Heart failure (HF)
  - Myocarditis/pericarditis
  - Perivalvular extension including abscess formation, fistulae, and pseudoaneurysms
  - Conduction disturbances (e.g., AV blocks)
- Extracardiac complications
  - Uncontrolled and persistent infection
  - Embolic phenomena to spleen, kidneys
  - Neurologic complications (e.g., stroke, transient ischemic attack (TIA), brain abscess, meningitis, toxic encephalopathy, and silent cerebral emboli)
  - Mycotic aneurysms

27. What are poor prognostic factors in patients presenting with infective endocarditis?

Prognosis in IE is influenced by patient characteristics, the presence of complications (cardiac or extracardiac) of IE, the type of infecting organism, and the echocardiographic findings. They are summarized in the recent European Society of Cardiology (ESC) guidelines as follows:

- Older age
- Prosthetic valve IE
- Comorbidities (e.g., immunosuppression, renal disease)
- HF
- Renal failure
- Large area of ischemic stroke

Table 34.3. The Modified Duke Criteria for the Diagnosis of Endocarditis

Major Criteria

- Blood culture positive for IE
  - Typical microorganisms consistent with IE from two separate blood cultures
    - Viridans streptococci; *Streptococcus bovis*, HACEK group, *Staphylococcus aureus*; or
    - Community-acquired enterococci, in the absence of a primary focus
  - Microorganisms consistent with IE from persistently positive blood cultures, defined as follows:
    - At least two positive blood cultures of blood samples drawn >12 h apart; or
    - All of three or a majority of ≥4 separate cultures of blood (with first and last sample drawn at least 1 h apart)
  - Single positive blood culture for *Coxiella burnetii* or antiphase I IgG antibody titer >1:800
- Evidence of endocardial involvement
- Echocardiogram positive for IE (TEE recommended in patients with prosthetic valves, rated at least "possible IE" by clinical criteria, or complicated IE [paravalvular abscess]; TTE as first test in other patients), defined as follows:
  - Oscillating intracardiac mass on valve or supporting structures, in the path of regurgitant jets, or on implanted material in the absence of an alternative anatomic explanation; or
  - Abscess; or
  - New partial dehiscence of prosthetic valve
- New valvular regurgitation (worsening or changing or preexisting murmur not sufficient)

Minor Criteria

- Predisposition, predisposing heart condition or injection drug use
- Fever, temperature >38°C
- Vascular phenomena, major arterial emboli, septic pulmonary infarcts, mycotic aneurysm, intracranial hemorrhage, conjunctival hemorrhages, and Janeway lesions
- Immunologic phenomena: Glomerulonephritis, Osler nodes, Roth's spots, and rheumatoid factor
- Microbiological evidence: Positive blood culture but does not meet a major criterion as noted previously (excluding single positive cultures for coagulase-negative staphylococci and organisms that do not cause endocarditis) or serologic evidence of active infection with organisms consistent with IE
- Echocardiographic minor criteria eliminated

IE, Infective endocarditis; *TEE*, transesophageal echocardiography, *TTE*, transthoracic echocardiography.
Modified from Li, J. S., Sexton, D. J., Mick, N., Nettles, R., Fowler, V. G., Ryan, T., et al. (2000). Proposed modifications to the Duke criteria for the diagnosis of infective endocarditis. Clinical Infectious Diseases, 30(4), 633–638.

- Brain hemorrhage
- Septic shock
- IE caused by *S. aureus,* fungi, or non-HACEK gram-negative bacilli
- High-risk features on echocardiography
  - Large vegetation
  - Severe prosthetic or left-sided valve dysfunction
  - Low ejection fraction (EF)
  - Periannular complications

28. What are generally accepted indications for surgery in patients with left-sided infective endocarditis?

Decisions regarding surgery will depend on both the indications for surgery and the patient's overall status and risks of surgery. Recommendations vary among the American College of Cardiology Foundation (ACCF)/AHA guidelines on valvular disease, the ESC guidelines on IE, and other experts who have weighed in on the topic. In general, accepted indications include acute valvular regurgitation (or valvular stenosis) leading to HF, infection caused by fungi or other organisms not likely to be successfully treated with antibiotics, complications such as abscess formation, or recurrent embolism. Other potential indications for surgery include pseudoaneurysm, perforation, fistula, valve aneurysm, and dehiscence of a prosthetic valve. ACCF/AHA guidelines for surgery in cases of IE are summarized in Tables 34.4 to 34.7; ESC guidelines for surgery are summarized in Table 34.8.

Table 34.4. Summary of the American College of Cardiology Foundation/American Heart Association Recommendations for Surgery for Left-Sided Native Valve Infective Endocarditis

Class I (Recommended)
- IE with valve dysfunction resulting in symptoms or signs of heart failure
- IE complicated by heart block, annular or aortic abscess, or destructive penetrating lesions
- Evidence of persistent infection (manifested by persistent bacteremia or fever lasting >5-7 days and provided that other sites of infection and fever have been excluded) after the start of appropriate antimicrobial therapy

Class IIa (Reasonable)
- IE with recurrent emboli and persistent vegetations despite appropriate antibiotic therapy
- IE with severe valve regurgitation and mobile vegetations >10 mm

Class IIb (May be reasonable)
- IE with mobile vegetations >10 mm, particularly when involving the anterior leaflet of the mitral valve and associated with other relative indications for surgery

IE, Infective endocarditis.
From Bonow, R. O., Carabello, B. A., Chatterjee, K., de Leon, A. C. Jr., Faxon, D. P., Freed, M. D., et al. (2008). *2008 Focused update incorporated into the ACC/AHA 2006 guidelines for the management of patients with valvular heart disease*. Journal of the American College of Cardiology, 52(13), e1–e142.

Table 34.5. Summary of the American College of Cardiology Foundation/American Heart Association Recommendations for Surgery for Prosthetic Valve and Device Infective Endocarditis

Class I (Recommended)
- IE in patients with symptoms or signs of heart failure resulting from valve dehiscence, intracardiac fistula, or severe prosthetic valve dysfunction
- IE in patients with PVE caused by fungi or highly resistant organisms
- IE complicated by heart block, annular or aortic abscess, or destructive penetrating lesions
- Persistent bacteremia despite appropriate antibiotic therapy for 5-7 days in whom other sites of infection have been excluded
- Complete removal of pacemaker or defibrillator systems, including all leads and the generator, is indicated as part of the early management plan in patients with IE with documented infection of the device or leads.

Class IIa (Reasonable)
- IE with persistent bacteremia or recurrent emboli despite appropriate antibiotic treatment
- Complete removal of pacemaker or defibrillator systems, including all leads and the generator, is reasonable in patients with valvular IE caused by *S. aureus* or fungi, even without evidence of device or lead infection.
- Complete removal of pacemaker or defibrillator systems, including all leads and the generator, is reasonable in patients undergoing valve surgery for valvular IE.

Class IIb (May be reasonable)
- IE with mobile vegetations >10 mm

IE, Infective endocarditis; *PVE*, prosthetic valve endocarditis.
From Bonow, R. O., Carabello, B. A., Chatterjee, K., de Leon, A. C. Jr., Faxon, D. P., Freed, M. D., et al. (2008). *2008 Focused update incorporated into the ACC/AHA 2006 guidelines for the management of patients with valvular heart disease*. Journal of the American College of Cardiology, 52(13), e1–e142.

Table 34.6. Summary of the American College of Cardiology Foundation/American Heart Association Recommendations for Surgery for Right-Sided Native Valve Infective Endocarditis

Class IIa (Reasonable)

- IE with certain complications such as
  - Right heart failure secondary to severe tricuspid regurgitation with poor response to medical therapy
  - Sustained infection caused by difficult-to-treat organisms
  - Tricuspid valve vegetations that are ≥20 mm in diameter and recurrent pulmonary embolism despite antimicrobial therapy
- It is reasonable to avoid surgery when possible in patients who are IDUs.

IDU, Injecting drug users; *IE*, infective endocarditis.

From Bonow, R. O., Carabello, B. A., Chatterjee, K., de Leon, A. C. Jr., Faxon, D. P., Freed, M. D., et al. (2008). *2008 Focused update incorporated into the ACC/AHA 2006 guidelines for the management of patients with valvular heart disease*. Journal of the American College of Cardiology, 52(13), e1–e142.

Table 34.7. Indications and Timing of Surgery in Left-Sided Valve Infective Endocarditis (Native Valve Endocarditis and Prosthetic Valve Endocarditis)

INDICATIONS FOR SURGERY	TIMING*	CLASS†	LEVEL‡	REF.§
Heart Failure				
Aortic or mitral NVE or PVE with severe acute regurgitation, obstruction, or fistula causing refractory pulmonary edema or cardiogenic shock	Emergency	I	B	111,115, 213,216
Aortic or mitral NVE or PVE with severe regurgitation or obstruction causing symptoms of HF or echocardiographic signs of poor hemodynamic tolerance	Urgent	I	B	37,115, 209,216, 220,221
Uncontrolled Infection				
Locally uncontrolled infection (abscess, false aneurysm, fistula, enlarging vegetation)	Urgent	I	B	37,209, 216
Infection caused by fungi or multiresistant organisms	Urgent/ elective	I	C	
Persisting positive blood cultures despite appropriate antibiotic therapy and adequate control of septic metastatic foci	Urgent	I la	B	123
PVE caused by staphylococci or non-HACEK gram-negative bacteria	Urgent/ elective	I la	C	—
Prevention of Embolism				
Aortic or mitral NVE or PVE with persistent vegetations >10 mm after one or more embolic episode despite appropriate antibiotic therapy	Urgent	I	B	9,58,72, 113,222
Aortic or NVE with vegetations >10 mm, associated with severe valve stenosis or regurgitation and low operative risk	Urgent	I la	B	9
Aortic or mitral NVE or PVE with isolated very large vegetations (>30 mm)	Urgent	I la	B	113
Aortic or mitral NVE or PVE with isolated large vegetations (>15 mm) and no other indication for surgery**	Urgent	I lb	C	—

HF, Heart failure; *NVE*, native valve endocarditis; *PVE*, prosthetic valve endocarditis.

*Emergency surgery: Surgery performed within 24 h; urgent surgery: within a few days; elective surgery: after at least 1-2 weeks of antibiotic therapy.

†Class of recommendation.

‡Level of evidence.

§Reference(s) supporting recommendations.

**Surgery may be preferred if a procedure preserving the native valve is feasible.

Table 34.8. Recommendations from the European Society of Cardiology Guidelines on the Prevention, Diagnosis, and Treatment of Infective Endocarditis: Indications and Timing of Surgery in Left-Sided Native Valve Infective Endocarditis

RECOMMENDATIONS: INDICATIONS FOR SURGERY	TIMING	CLASS OF RECOMMENDATION
Heart Failure		
Aortic or mitral IE with severe acute regurgitation, valve obstruction, or fistula causing refractory pulmonary edema or cardiogenic shock	Emergency	I
Aortic or mitral IE with severe acute regurgitation or valve obstruction and persisting HF or echocardiographic signs of poor hemodynamic tolerance (early mitral closure or pulmonary hypertension)	Urgent	I
Uncontrolled Infection		
Locally uncontrolled infection (abscess, false aneurysm, fistula, enlarging vegetation)	Urgent	I
Infection caused by fungi or multiresistant organisms	Urgent	I
Persisting positive blood cultures despite appropriate antibiotic therapy and adequate control of septic metastatic foci	Urgent	IIa
PVE caused by staphylococci or non-HACEK gram-negative bacteria	Urgent/elective	IIa
Prevention of Embolism		
Aortic or mitral IE with large vegetations (>10 mm) following one or more embolic episodes despite appropriate antibiotic therapy	Urgent	I
Aortic or mitral IE with large vegetations (>10 mm), associated with severe valve stenosis or regurgitation and low operative risk	Urgent	IIa
Aortic or mitral NVE or PVE with isolated very large vegetations (0.30 mm)	Urgent	IIa
Isolated very large vegetations (>15 mm) and no other indications for surgery	Urgent	IIb

HF, Heart failure; *IE*, infective endocarditis; *NVE*, native valve endocarditis; *PVE*, prosthetic valve endocarditis.
Adapted from Habib, G., Lancellotti, P., Antunes, M. J., Bongiorni, M. G., Casalta, J. P., Del Zotti, F., et al. (2015). 2015 ESC Guidelines for the management of infective endocarditis: the task force for the management of infective endocarditis of the European Society of Cardiology (ESC). Endorsed by European Association for Cardio-Thoracic Surgery (EACTS), the European Association of Nuclear Medicine (EANM). European Heart Journal, *36(44), 3075–3128.*

29. What are the indications for surgery in patients with right-sided endocarditis?

There is a high recurrence rate of IE in Intravenous Drug Use (IVDU), and thus surgery is generally avoided in patients with right-sided endocarditis unless they have one of the following indications as delineated in the ESC 2015 guidelines:

- Right HF due to severe tricuspid regurgitation (TR) not responding to diuretics
- Tricuspid valve vegetations greater than 20 mm that persist after recurrent pulmonary emboli with or without concomitant right HF
- IE caused by organisms that are difficult to eradicate or bacteremia for at least 7 days despite adequate antimicrobial therapy

30. How is infective endocarditis of cardiac implantable electronic devices managed?

Infections of cardiac implantable electronic devices are associated with a very high morbidity and mortality. Staphylococci, and especially coagulase-negative *Staphylococcus* species, account for a majority of the cases. TTE and TEE play a complementary and vital role in the diagnosis of vegetations

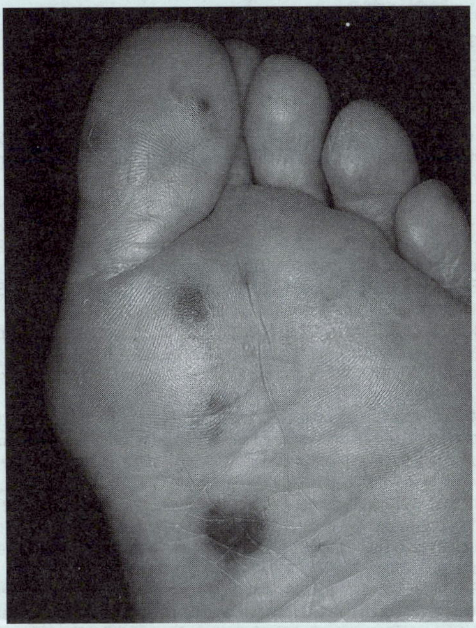

Fig. 34.3. Janeway lesions in a patient with *Staphylococcus aureus* endocarditis. *(From Sande, M. A., & Strausbaugh, L. J. [1977]. Infective endocarditis. In E. W. Hook, G. L. Mandell, J. M. Gwaltney Jr., & M. A. Sande [Eds.],* Current concepts of infectious diseases. *New York, NY: Wiley Press, Fig. 77.3.)*

on the leads and associated involvement of the tricuspid valve. A recent study showed that ^{18}F-FDG PET/CT significantly improved diagnostic accuracy in these patients. Treatment includes prolonged antibiotic therapy with complete hardware removal.

31. Are patients with mechanical prosthetic heart valves more likely to develop endocarditis than those with bioprosthetic heart valves?

No. The incidence for patients with both types of prosthetic heart valves is approximately 1% per year of follow-up.

32. What are Osler nodes?

Osler nodes are small, tender red-purple nodules. They most commonly occur on the fingers, hands, toes, and feet. They may be caused by circulating immunocomplexes.

33. What are Janeway lesions?

Janeway lesions are irregular macules located on the hands and feet. As opposed to Osler nodes, they are painless (Fig. 34.3).

34. What is marantic endocarditis?

Marantic endocarditis is the term previously used for what is now referred to as NBTE. The term reportedly derived from the Greek *marantikos,* meaning "wasting away." The vegetations in NBTE are sterile and believed to be composed of platelets and fibrin. The finding of such sterile vegetations occurs in the setting of chronic wasting diseases, chronic infections (e.g., tuberculosis [TB], osteomyelitis), certain cancers, and disseminated intravascular coagulation. These often large vegetations may embolize to the brain, the coronary arteries, and the periphery.

35. What is Libman-Sacks endocarditis?

Libman-Sacks endocarditis is a form of NBTE seen in patients with systemic lupus erythematosus (SLE). Described in 1924, the vegetations most commonly occur on the mitral valve, although they can affect all four cardiac valves. The lesions are due to accumulations of immune complexes, fibrin, and mononuclear cells. Most lesions do not cause symptoms, although valvular regurgitation or stenosis can occasionally occur because of the lesions. Embolization of the lesions is rare.

Bibliography and Suggested Readings

Baddour, L. M., Wilson, W. R., Bayer, A. S., Fowler, V. G., Jr., Tleyjeh, I. M., Rybak, M. J., et al. (2015). Infective endocarditis in adults: diagnosis, antimicrobial therapy, and management of complications: a scientific statement for healthcare professionals from the American Heart Association. *Circulation, 132*, 1435–1486.

Durack, D. T., Lukes, A. S., & Bright, D. K. (1994). New criteria for diagnosis of infective endocarditis: utilization of specific echocardiographic findings. Duke Endocarditis Service. *American Journal of Medicine, 96*(3), 200–209.

Habib, G., Lancellotti, P., Antunes, M. J., Bongiorni, M. G., Casalta, J. P., Del Zotti, F., et al. (2015). 2015 ESC Guidelines for the management of infective endocarditis: the task force for the management of infective endocarditis of the European Society of Cardiology (ESC). Endorsed by: European Association for Cardio-Thoracic Surgery (EACTS), the European Association of Nuclear Medicine (EANM). *European Heart Journal, 36*(44), 3075–3128.

Li, J. S., Sexton, D. J., Mick, N., Nettles, R., Fowler, V. G., Ryan, T., et al. (2000). Proposed modifications to the Duke criteria for the diagnosis of infective endocarditis. *Clinical Infectious Diseases, 30*(4), 633–638.

Mylonakis, E., & Calderwood, S. B. (2001). Infective endocarditis in adults. *New England Journal of Medicine, 345*(18), 1318–1330.

Nishimura, R. A., Otto, C. M., Bonow, R. O., Carabello, B. A., Erwin, J. P., 3rd, Guyton, R. A., et al. (2014). 2014 AHA/ACC Guideline for the management of patients with valvular heart disease: a report of the American College of Cardiology/American Heart Association task force on practice guidelines. *Journal of the American College of Cardiology, 63*(22), e57–e185.

Pizzi, M. N., Roque, A., Fernández-Hidalgo, N., Cuéllar-Calabria, H., Ferreira-González, I., Gonzàlez-Alujas, M. T., et al. (2015). Improving the diagnosis of infective endocarditis in prosthetic valves and intracardiac devices with 18F-fluordeoxyglucose positron emission tomography/computed tomography angiography: initial results at an infective endocarditis referral center. *Circulation, 132*(12), 1113–1126.

Wilson, W., Taubert, K. A., Gewitz, M., Lockhart, P. B., Baddour, L. M., Levison, M., et al. (2007). Prevention of infective endocarditis: guidelines from the American Heart Association: a guideline from the American Heart Association Rheumatic Fever, Endocarditis, and Kawasaki Disease Committee, Council on Cardiovascular Disease in the Young, and the Council on Clinical Cardiology, Council on Cardiovascular Surgery and Anesthesia, and the Quality of Care and Outcomes Research Interdisciplinary Working Group. *Circulation, 116*(15), 1736–1754.

V
ARRHYTHMIAS

CHAPTER 35

ATRIAL FIBRILLATION

Michael E. Field

1. What is the difference between atrial fibrillation and atrial flutter?

Atrial fibrillation (AF) is a supraventricular tachyarrhythmia with uncoordinated atrial activation and consequently ineffective atrial contraction with ECG characteristics of (1) irregular R-R intervals (when atrioventricular conduction is present), (2) absence of distinct repeating P waves, and (3) irregular atrial activity (Fig. 35.1). In contrast, atrial flutter is characterized by the presence of discrete P waves and atrial activation sequences. An important characteristic of atrial flutter is that the atrial activation is the same from beat to beat. Often times, patients with coarse AF with large-amplitude fibrillatory waves are mistaken for atrial flutter.

2. How common is atrial fibrillation?

The prevalence is 1% in the general population and increases with age (>10% in octogenarians). The number of patients with AF is likely to increase due to the aging population, improved survival for conditions predisposing to AF (such as myocardial infarction and heart failure), and improved detection strategies.

3. What are the primary goals of atrial fibrillation management?

The primary goals of AF management consist of

- Prevention of thromboembolism, including stroke
- Control of ventricular rate in AF and prevention of tachycardia-mediated cardiomyopathy *(rate control)*
- Alleviation of symptoms by restoring and/or maintaining sinus rhythm *(rhythm control)*

4. What is the current classification of atrial fibrillation?

- *Paroxysmal AF*—AF that terminates spontaneously or with intervention within 7 days of onset
- *Persistent AF*—Continuous AF that is sustained more than 7 days
- *Long-standing persistent AF*—Continuous AF more than 12 months in duration
- *Permanent AF*—This term is used when the patient and clinician make a joint decision to stop further attempts to restore or maintain sinus rhythm

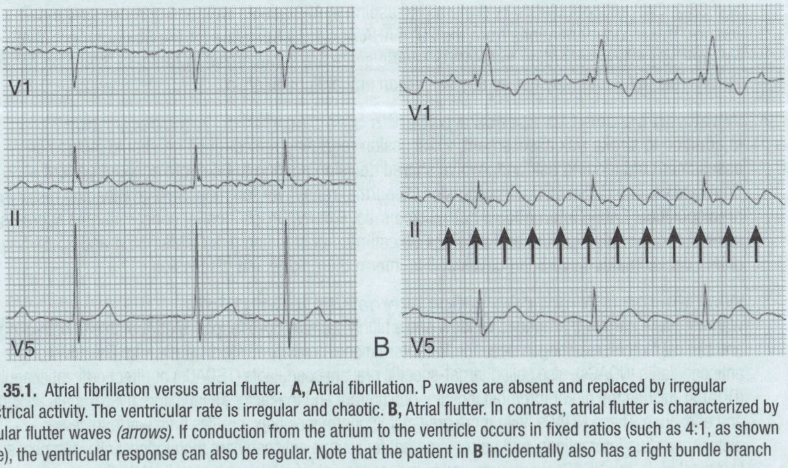

Fig. 35.1. Atrial fibrillation versus atrial flutter. **A,** Atrial fibrillation. P waves are absent and replaced by irregular electrical activity. The ventricular rate is irregular and chaotic. **B,** Atrial flutter. In contrast, atrial flutter is characterized by regular flutter waves *(arrows)*. If conduction from the atrium to the ventricle occurs in fixed ratios (such as 4:1, as shown here), the ventricular response can also be regular. Note that the patient in **B** incidentally also has a right bundle branch block.

Table 35.1. The CHA2DS2-VASc Scoring System

CHA2DS2-VASc RISK	SCORE
CHF or LVEF <40%	1
Hypertension	1
Age >75	2
Diabetes	1
Stroke/TIA/thromboembolism	2
Vascular disease	1
Age 65-74	1
Female	1
Maximum score	9

Each clinical risk factor shown is assigned either 1 or 2 points, and the sum of all risks factors is the patient's score (maximum 9 points). Shown on the right is the event rate per 100 person-years at 1 year, including hospitalization or death due to TIA, ischemic stroke, peripheral artery embolism, and pulmonary embolism. With increasing score, there is a gradient of increased risk of stroke. Abbreviations: *CHF*, congestive heart failure; LVEF, left ventricular ejection fraction; TIA, transient ischemic attack.

Modified from Olesen, J. B., Lip, G. Y., Hansen, M. L., Hansen, P. R., Tolstrup, J. S., Lindhardsen, J., et al. (2011). Validation of risk stratification schemes for predicting stroke and thromboembolism in patients with atrial fibrillation: nationwide cohort study. British Medical Journal, 342, *d124*.

5. What are the most common etiologic factors contributing to atrial fibrillation?

Although AF can present in the absence of any risk factors, the most common associated risk factors are hypertension and advanced age. AF is also associated with ischemic heart disease, heart failure, and valvular heart disease. It is also important to consider sleep apnea and obesity, which are important modifiable risk factors for AF that may be underrecognized. There is also an association with high-intensity endurance exercise and hereditary components.

In the inpatient setting the majority of cases of new-onset AF occur after noncardiac surgery or in patients with infections and, to a much lesser extent, associated with pulmonary embolism, thyrotoxicosis, or pericarditis.

6. What is the CHA2DS2-VASc score, and how is it used?

Several scoring systems have been developed for stratification of stroke risk with AF to identify who is likely to benefit from anticoagulation. The most commonly used tool is the CHA2DS2-VASc score, which takes into account several clinical risk factors and is summarized in Tables 35.1 and 35.2. Oral anticoagulation is preferred to aspirin in AF patients with one or more stroke risk factors. The recommendations from the 2014 AHA/ACC/HRS Guideline for the Management of AF for anticoagulation according to CHA2DS2-VASc score are summarized in Table 35.3. Aspirin has a limited role in AF and may not be any safer than oral anticoagulation.

7. What can be used to assess a patient's bleeding risk on anticoagulation?

In addition to stroke risk assessment, a discussion regarding anticoagulation should include an assessment of bleeding risk and involve shared decision making to take into account patient preferences. The HAS-BLED (Hypertension, Abnormal renal/liver function, Stroke, Bleeding history or predisposition, Labile international normalized ratio, Elderly, Drugs/alcohol concomitantly) score uses several common risk factors and provides an estimate of bleeding risk (Tables 35.4 and 35.5). Several online decision aids have been developed to inform the risk/benefit discussion.

8. What are the different medication alternatives to warfarin?

Warfarin has a narrow therapeutic window and a highly variable dose response attributable to both genetic and clinical factors, resulting in need for INR (international normalized ratio) monitoring. The novel oral anticoagulants (NOACs), also called target-specific oral anticoagulants (TSOACs) or direct oral anticoagulants (DOACs), include the direct thrombin inhibitor dabigatran) and the factor Xa inhibitors rivaroxaban, apixaban, and edoxaban. These NOACs have more predictable pharmacokinetic profiles than warfarin, fewer dietary and drug interactions, and no requirement for routine anticoagulant monitoring. Following phase III clinical trials, the NOACs were approved to reduce the risk of stroke or systemic embolism in patients with nonvalvular AF after showing either similar or increased efficacy for reduction of the risk of stroke or systemic embolism compared with warfarin and a decreased risk of intracranial hemorrhage.

Table 35.2. The CHA2DS2-VASc Scoring System

CHA2DS2-VASc	EVENT RATE AT 1 YEAR
0	0.78
1	2.01
2	3.71
3	5.92
4	9.27
5	15.26
6	19.74
7	21.50
8	22.38
9	23.64

The event rate per 100 person-years at 1 year, including hospitalization or death due to transient ischemic attack, ischemic stroke, peripheral artery embolism, and pulmonary embolism. With increasing score, there is a gradient of increased risk of stroke.

Modified from Olesen, J. B., Lip, G. Y., Hansen, M. L., Hansen, P. R., Tolstrup, J. S., Lindhardsen, J., et al. (2011). Validation of risk stratification schemes for predicting stroke and thromboembolism in patients with atrial fibrillation: nationwide cohort study. British Medical Journal, 342, *d124.*

Table 35.3. Anticoagulation Recommendation for Atrial Fibrillation Based on Patients' CHA2DS2-VASc Score

CHA2DS2-VASc SCORE	RECOMMENDATION
≥2	Oral anticoagulants are recommended
1	Either anticoagulation, no therapy, aspirin
0	No antithrombotic therapy

Modified from January, C. T., Wann, L. S., Alpert, J. S., Calkins, H., Cleveland, J. C. Jr., Cigarroa, J. E., et al. (2014). 2014 AHA/ACC/HRS guideline for the management of patients with atrial fibrillation: a report of the American College of Cardiology/American Heart Association Task Force on Practice Guidelines and the Heart Rhythm Society. Journal of the American College of Cardiology, 64*(21), e1–e76.*

Table 35.4. HAS-BLED Score Risk Factors

RISK FACTOR
Hypertension (systolic BP >160 mm Hg)
Abnormal liver or renal function (1 point each)
Stroke history
Bleeding history (or anemia)
Labile INR (<60% of the time therapeutic)
Elderly (age >65)
Drugs (antiplatelet, NSAIDs) or alcohol (1 point each)

BP, Blood pressure. INR, international normalized ratio; NSAIDs, nonsteroidal antiinflammatory drugs.

Modified from Pisters, R., Lane, D. A., Nieuwlaat, R., de Vos, C. B., Crijns, H. J., & Lip, G. Y. (2010). A novel user-friendly score (HAS-BLED) to assess 1-year risk of major bleeding in patients with atrial fibrillation: the Euro Heart Survey. Chest, 138, *1093–1100.*

Table 35.5. HAS-BLED Score

SCORE	BLEEDING RISK (%)
0	1
1	2
2	3
3	4
4	9
>5	13

Modified from Pisters, R., Lane, D. A., Nieuwlaat, R., de Vos, C. B., Crijns, H. J., & Lip, G. Y. (2010). A novel user-friendly score (HAS-BLED) to assess 1-year risk of major bleeding in patients with atrial fibrillation: the Euro Heart Survey. Chest, 138, *1093–1100.*

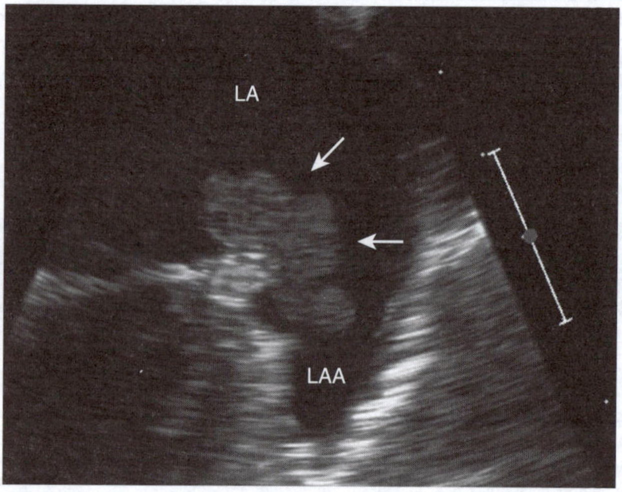

Fig. 35.2. Left atrial appendage thrombus. Transesophageal echocardiographic image of thrombus in the left atrial appendage *(arrows). LA,* Left atrium; *LAA,* left atrial appendage.

9. What are the alternatives to anticoagulation for the prevention of stroke and systemic embolism with atrial fibrillation?

The left atrial appendage (LAA) is thought to be the primary source of stroke in patients with nonvalvular AF (Fig. 35.2). Several nonpharmacologic approaches to LAA occlusion exist and represent potential alternatives to anticoagulation. The WATCHMAN device (Boston Scientific , Marlborough, MA) is a self-expanding nitinol frame covered with a membrane that can be placed percutaneously in the LAA and appears to be an effective therapy for stroke prevention. Surgical occlusion of the LAA can also be performed at the time of concomitant cardiac surgery or as a stand-alone procedure using a minimally invasive approach with a specialized device, such as the AtriClip (AtriCure, Inc., Mason, OH).

10. What options exist for rate control of atrial fibrillation?

Multiple agents have been used for rate control in AF and are summarized in the AHA/ACC/HRS 2014 AF guidelines. The most commonly used agents are beta-blockers, followed by nondihydropyridine calcium channel blockers (which include diltiazem and verapamil). Digoxin is less commonly used but has a role in more sedentary patients and in those with reduced left ventricular function. Amiodarone may rarely be used as a rate control agent in patients when other agents have failed or are contraindicated, such as in critically ill patients.

11. What is the optimal target heart rate for rate control in atrial fibrillation?

Most patients with AF will require some degree of ventricular rate control, which can be used to reduce symptoms and prevent tachycardia-mediated cardiomyopathy. The RACE ((Rate Control Efficacy in Permanent Atrial Fibrillation: a Comparison between Lenient versus Strict Rate Control)) II trial formally assessed the optimal target by randomizing patients to a "lenient" (resting heart rate <110 bpm) versus "strict" (resting heart rate <80 bpm) strategy. At 3 years the primary composite endpoint of cardiovascular death, hospitalization for heart failure, stroke, embolism, bleeding, or life-threatening arrhythmic events was similar between the two groups (12.9% lenient rate control vs. 14.9% strict rate control), suggesting that a strict rate control strategy did not improve outcomes. Although there are a number of caveats to this trial, it is reasonable in clinical practice to use a more permissive ventricular target rate as long as symptoms are controlled and the left ventricular function is preserved.

12. What are the reasons to pursue maintenance of sinus rhythm in patients with atrial fibrillation?

The main goal of strategies to maintain sinus rhythm (termed *rhythm control strategies*) is to reduce symptoms by decreasing the frequency and duration of AF episodes. However, data from rate versus rhythm control trials, such as AFFIRM (Atrial Fibrillation Follow-up Investigation of Rhythm Management) and RACE, do not support any mortality benefit of a rhythm control strategy. An important reason to consider a rhythm control approach is inability to achieve adequate rate control, especially when associated with a tachycardia-mediated cardiomyopathy. Other factors that might favor trying to maintain sinus rhythm include patient preference and young patient age. In theory, leaving a patient in AF may eliminate for them new rhythm control options that might arise in the future.

13. Are anticoagulation recommendations different for patients with paroxysmal versus persistent atrial fibrillation?

No, the assessment of stroke risk is based on the individual patient's stroke risk based on other clinical risk factors using scoring systems, such as the CHA2DS2-VASc score. It is not based on whether the AF is paroxysmal or persistent, whether the patient has short duration or longer duration AF episodes, or whether the AF is apparently well controlled on antiarrhythmics or after AF ablation.

14. When is anticoagulation indicated around the time of cardioversion?

For AF that is less than 48 hours in duration, cardioversion may be performed without prior anticoagulation. If the duration is more than 48 hours or unknown (regardless of the baseline CHA2DS2-VASc score), the patient should be treated with anticoagulation therapy for 3 weeks before and at least 4 weeks after cardioversion. Alternatively, for AF of more than a 48-hour duration or unknown duration, a transesophageal echocardiogram (TEE) may be performed in patients recently initiated on anticoagulation to assess for thrombus prior to cardioversion. If no thrombus is seen, it is reasonable to proceed with cardioversion and then continue anticoagulation for at least 4 weeks afterward. In each of these scenarios, longer term anticoagulation may be indicated based on the patient's stroke risk assessment (CHA2DS2-VASc score).

15. What can be done if cardioversion for atrial fibrillation is unsuccessful?

It is important to differentiate between a cardioversion in which no sinus rhythm occurred from one in which sinus rhythm was transiently seen but then AF recurred. In the former scenario, in which no beats of sinus rhythm are seen, the issue is energy delivery. Things that can improve energy delivery include increasing shock strength (joules), using a biphasic rather than monophasic waveform, changing the shock vector by altering the electrode pad position, pressing on the anterior electrode pad during shock delivery with a gloved hand, or using a drug such as ibutilide prior to energy delivery. Patients in whom sinus rhythm is transiently seen but then AF recurs can be pretreated with an antiarrhythmic drug prior to cardioversion. A baseline eye exam is also recommended.

16. What are some common side effects with amiodarone?

Side effects due to amiodarone treatment are common and include organ toxicity to the lung, thyroid, and liver. Amiodarone can also cause or exacerbate sinus bradycardia. It also can cause bluish discoloration of the skin, photosensitivity, tremor, peripheral neuropathy, ocular deposits, and optic neuropathy. Monitoring of patients while on amiodarone varies by clinician but includes periodic laboratory testing for liver and thyroid dysfunction, as well as chest radiography and pulmonary function testing. A baseline eye exam is also recommended.

17. Why do some patients taking propafenone have a pronounced beta-blocking effect?

The cytochrome P450 enzyme activity CYP2D6 metabolizes propafenone to 5-hydroxypropafenone, a metabolite that has less beta-blocking activity than the parent compound. Approximately 6% of white people in the US population are naturally deficient in CYP2D6 activity. In patients lacking the CYP2D6 enzyme, propafenone levels are markedly higher (and levels of 5-hydroxy propafenone are lower), resulting in an exaggerated beta-blocking effect.

18. What are some risk factors for torsades de pointes associated with antiarrhythmic drug therapy?

The common pathway for drug-induced torsades de pointes is inhibition of the IKr (rapidly activating potassium current.) Sotalol and dofetilide (and rarely amiodarone or dronedarone) can be associated with torsades de pointes. Risk factors include hypokalemia, hypomagnesemia, female gender, concomitant use of other QT-prolonging drugs, baseline QT prolongation, or ventricular hypertrophy.

19. What is the target of atrial fibrillation catheter ablation?

The electrical triggers associated with AF originate from the region where the pulmonary veins join the left atrium and represent the common targets for AF catheter ablation. Ablation, using energy, such as radiofrequency or cryoablation, results in isolation of the electrically active sleeves of myocardium at the pulmonary vein junctions in what is termed *pulmonary vein isolation.*

20. What are the indications for atrial fibrillation catheter ablation?

Ablation is reserved primarily for symptomatic patients refractory to antiarrhythmic medication, although in select patients it may be appropriate as first-line treatment.

21. When is it appropriate to stop anticoagulation after atrial fibrillation catheter ablation?

The decision to discontinue anticoagulation more than 2 to 3 months after AF catheter ablation should be based on the patient's CHA2DS2-VASc score rather than the apparent success of the procedure. This conservative approach reflects that recurrences of AF following ablation are not uncommon, can be asymptomatic, and escape detection with intermittent monitoring.

22. What are some complications of atrial fibrillation catheter ablation?

A worldwide survey on AF catheter ablation showed an overall incidence of major complications around 5% to 6%. Potential complications include access site complications, cardiac tamponade, stroke, pericarditis, phrenic nerve paralysis, pulmonary vein stenosis, and esophageal fistula. Reentrant and focal left atrial tachycardias, which in some cases can be more symptomatic than the initial AF due to difficult-to-control heart rate, may be seen after the procedure and may be transient or require repeat ablation.

23. What is "pre-excited" atrial fibrillation?

Pre-excited AF occurs in a patient with Wolff-Parkinson-White (WPW) syndrome who develops AF. There is anterograde conduction to varying degrees over the AV node and the accessory pathway. This results in a wide complex tachycardia characterized by irregular ventricular response and varying QRS complexes. (See fig. 35.3) If the accessory pathway is capable of rapid conduction, the ventricular response can be very rapid and potentially degenerate to ventricular fibrillation and subsequent sudden death. Treatment of these patients includes synchronized cardioversion if the patient is unstable or intravenous (IV) procainamide infusion.

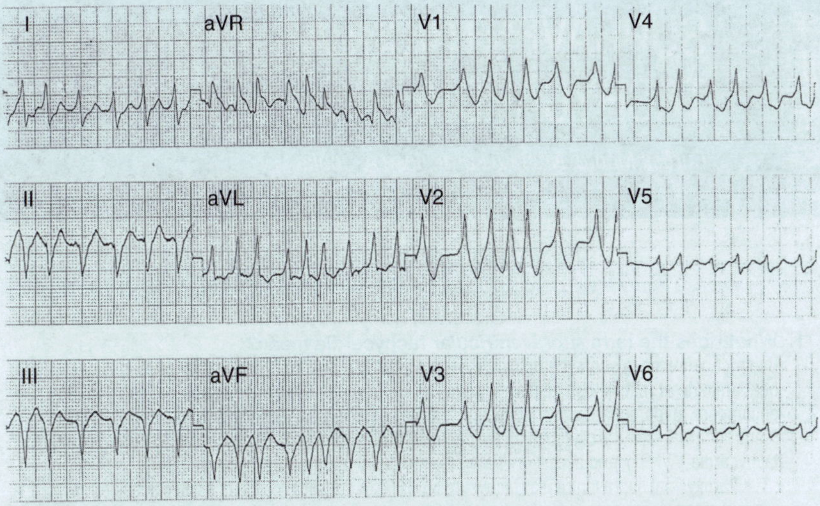

Fig. 35.3. Atrial fibrillation in a patient with Wolff-Parkinson-White syndrome ("pre-excited" atrial fibrillation). Twelve-lead ECG with wide complex tachycardia characterized by irregular ventricular response and varying QRS complexes. This pattern is characteristic of atrial fibrillation in a patient with Wolff-Parkinson-White syndrome in which anterograde conduction occurs to varying degrees over the atrioventricular node and the accessory pathway. If the accessory pathway is capable of rapid conduction, the ventricular response can be very rapid and potentially degenerate to ventricular fibrillation and subsequent sudden death.

Bibliography, Suggested Readings, and Websites

January, C. T., Wann, L. S., Alpert, J. S., Calkins, H., Cleveland, J. C., Jr., Cigarroa, J. E., et al. (2014). 2014 AHA/ACC/HRS guideline for the management of patients with atrial fibrillation: a report of the American College of Cardiology/American Heart Association Task Force on Practice Guidelines and the Heart Rhythm Society. *Journal of the American College of Cardiology*, *64*(21), e1–e76.

Lip, G. Y., Nieuwlaat, R., Pisters, R., Lane, D. A., & Crijns, H. J. (2010). Refining clinical risk stratification for predicting stroke and thromboembolism in atrial fibrillation using a novel risk factor-based approach: the Euro Heart Survey on Atrial Fibrillation. *Chest*, *137*, 263–272.

Pisters, R., Lane, D. A., Nieuwlaat, R., de Vos, C. B., Crijns, H. J., & Lip, G. Y. (2010). A novel user-friendly score (HAS-BLED) to assess 1-year risk of major bleeding in patients with atrial fibrillation: the Euro Heart Survey. *Chest*, *138*, 1093–1100.

Van Gelder, I. C., Hagens, V. E., Bosker, H. A., Kingma, J. H., Kamp, O., Kingma, T., et al. (2002). A comparison of rate control and rhythm control in patients with recurrent persistent atrial fibrillation. *New England Journal of Medicine*, *347*, 1834.

Van Gelder, I. C., Groenveld, H. F., Crijns, H. J., Tuininga, Y. S., Tijssen, J. G., Alings, A. M., et al. (2010). Lenient versus strict rate control in patients with atrial fibrillation. *New England Journal of Medicine*, *362*, 1363.

Walkey, A. J., Benjamin, E. J., & Lubitz, S. A. (2014). New-onset atrial fibrillation during hospitalization. *Journal of the American College of Cardiology*, *64*(22), 2432–2433.

Wyse, D. G., Waldo, A. L., DiMarco, J. P., Domanski, M. J., Rosenberg, Y., Schron, E. B., et al. (2002). A comparison of rate control and rhythm control in patients with atrial fibrillation. *New England Journal of Medicine*, *347*, 1825.

Zimetbaum, P. (2012). Antiarrhythmic drug therapy for atrial fibrillation. *Circulation*, *125*, 381–389.

HealthDecision™,<www.HealthDecision.org> Accessed Nov 2016.

AFib Toolkit, American College of Cardiology,<www.acc.org/tools-and-practice-support/clinical-toolkits/atrial-fibrillation-afib> Accessed June 2016.

CHAPTER 36

SUPRAVENTRICULAR TACHYCARDIA

Curtiss Moore, Nitin Kulkarni, Jose A. Joglar

1. **What does the term *supraventricular* tachycardia mean?**
   By strict definition, a supraventricular tachycardia (SVT) is any tachycardia with rates in excess of 100 beats/minute at rest, whose genesis involves tissue from the His bundle or above. Thus, the term can encompass inappropriate sinus tachycardia, atrial tachycardia (AT) (focal and multifocal), macro-reentrant atrial tachycardia (such as typical atrial flutter), junctional tachycardia, AV nodal reentrant tachycardia (AVNRT), and accessory pathway–mediated reentrant tachycardia (AVRT).

   Paroxysmal supraventricular tachycardia (PSVT), a subset of SVTs, is a clinical syndrome characterized by the presence of a regular and rapid tachycardia of abrupt onset and termination, frequently seen with AVNRT and AVRT and less frequently seen with AT.

   Of note, we will not discuss in detail the management of atrial fibrillation (AF) in this chapter (which is also technically an SVT), since we aim to highlight the treatment of SVT as a general category and AF will be discussed elsewhere.

2. **How common is supraventricular tachycardia in the general population?**
   In the United States, the prevalence of SVT in the general population has been estimated at 2.25 per 1000 persons, with approximately 89,000 newly diagnosed cases per year. Compared to men, women have twice the risk of developing SVT, while individuals older than 65 years of age have five times the risk, compared to the younger population.

3. **What is the most common cause of paroxysmal supraventricular tachycardia?**
   AVNRT accounts for 60% to 70% of paroxysmal SVTs in adult patients, followed by AVRT.

4. **What factors are part of the *generic* workup for supraventricular tachycardia?**
   - History, including type and duration of symptoms (palpitations, lightheadedness, chest pains, dyspnea, presyncope, syncope, precipitating factors)
   - Questions regarding the intake of alcohol, caffeine, and illicit drugs
   - Cardiac history (myocardial infarction, valvular disease, cardiac surgery, prior ablation)
   - Physical examination (although often unrevealing)
   - 12-lead electrocardiogram (ECG) (looking for chamber enlargement, preexcitation, etc.)
   - Echocardiogram (often unrevealing because paroxysmal SVT often occurs in the normal heart; nevertheless structural heart disease must to be ruled out)
   - Laboratory tests (electrolyte abnormalities, hyperthyroidism)

5. **What are the causes of narrow complex regular tachycardias (regular referring to fixed R-R intervals—the time or *distance* between QRS complexes)?**
   - Sinus tachycardia (not an abnormal rhythm but still in the differential)
   - Atrial tachycardia
   - Atrial flutter with "fixed atrioventricular conduction"
   - AVNRT
   - AVRT
   - Inappropriate sinus tachycardia (IST), defined as sinus heart rate greater than 100 beats per minute (bpm) at rest with a mean 24-hour heart rate greater than 90 bpm not due to appropriate physiologic response
   - Sinoatrial nodal reentrant tachycardia and junctional tachycardia, rare causes of narrow complex tachycardia that are difficult to diagnose and usually more suited for discussion at the cardiology fellow or attending level (Fig. 36.1)

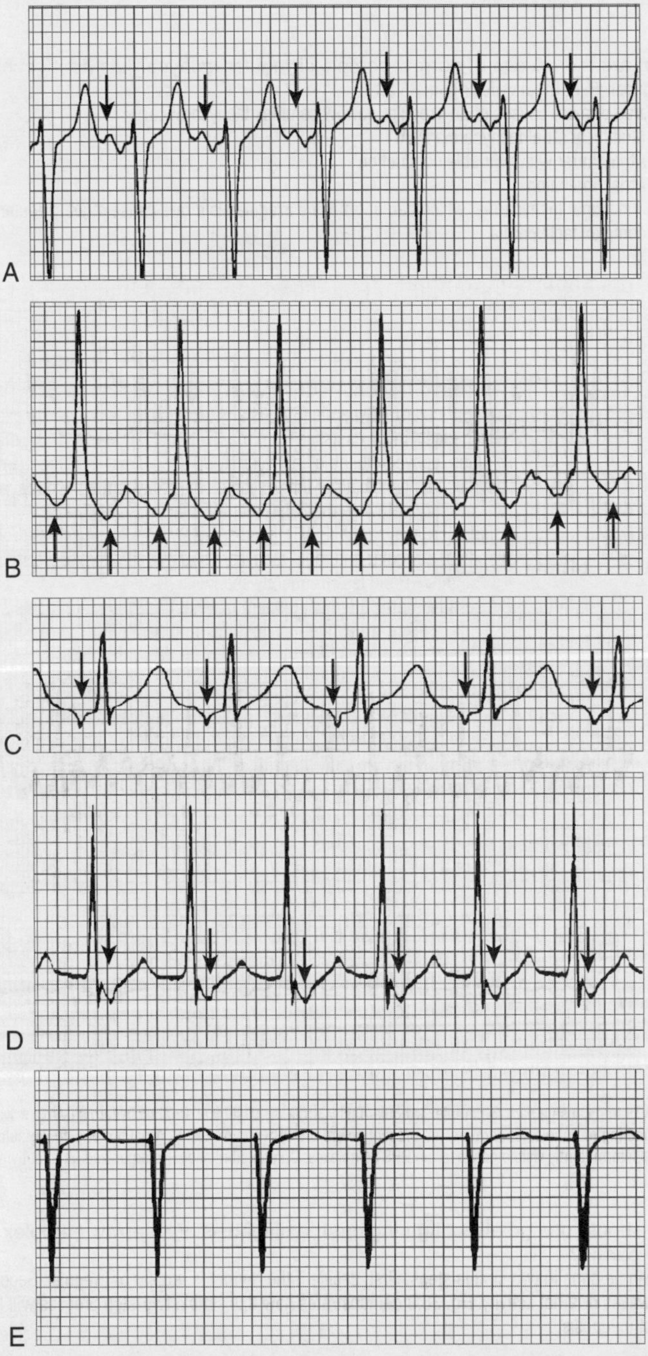

Fig. 36.1. SVTs that cause a narrow complex regular tachycardia. **A,** Sinus tachycardia—Normal appearing P waves *(arrows)* are present before each QRS complex. **B,** Atrial flutter—Flutter waves *(arrows)* are present. There is 2:1 conduction. **C,** Atrial tachycardia—Abnormal, inverted P waves *(arrows)* are present before each QRS complex. **D,** AVNRT—No P waves are present before the QRS complexes. Retrograde, inverted P waves *(arrows)* are visible immediately after the QRS complexes. **E,** No R-P tachycardia—No P waves are present before the QRS complexes. This is often seen in AVNRT, although junctional tachycardia and atrial tachycardia cannot be excluded.

6. What are the causes of narrow complex irregular tachycardias (tachycardias with irregular R-R intervals)? (Fig. 36.2.)

The three primary causes of an irregular narrow complex tachycardia are

- Multifocal atrial tachycardia (MAT)
- Atrial flutter with "variable conduction"
- Atrial fibrillation
- Junctional tachycardia, which can at times be irregular, is a rare cause of an irregular narrow complex tachycardia

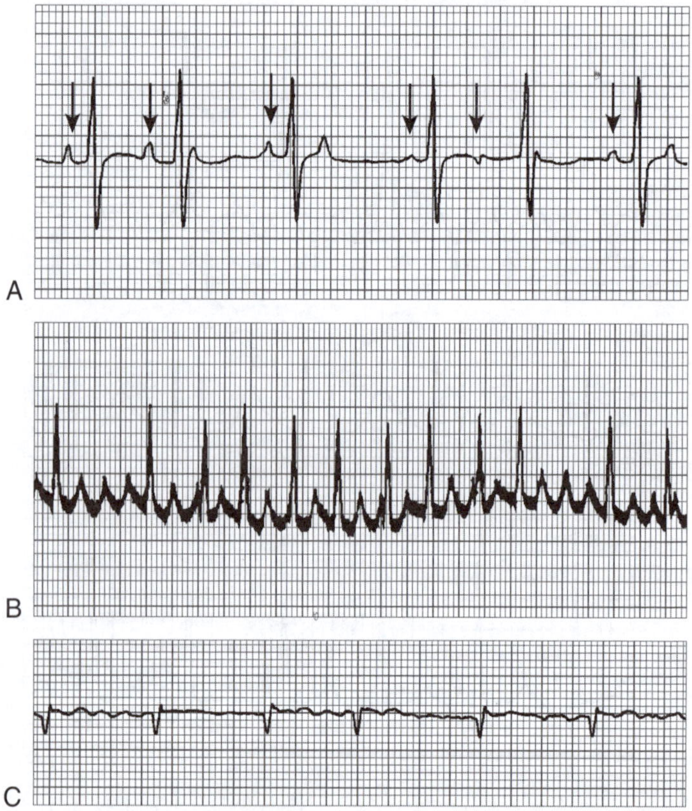

Fig. 36.2. SVTs that cause a narrow complex irregular tachycardia. **A,** Multifocal atrial tachycardia (MAT). P waves of at least three differing morphologies *(arrows)* are present before the QRS complexes. **B,** Atrial flutter with variable block. Flutter waves are intermittently visible between the QRS complexes. **C,** Atrial fibrillation. No organized atrial activity is present.

7. How should one go about figuring out the diagnosis of a narrow complex tachycardia?

This can be done in two simple steps. First, decide if the rhythm is regular or irregular. Second, look for P waves or atrial activity. Fig. 36.3 demonstrates how this simple two-step process will lead to the correct diagnosis.

8. What is the initial treatment for acute conversion of supraventricular tachycardia?

Vagal maneuvers, including Valsalva and carotid sinus massage, should be first-line interventions for acute conversion of SVT. These maneuvers should be performed with the patient in the supine position. The Valsalva maneuver requires the patient to bear down against a closed glottis for 10 to 30 seconds to increase intrathoracic pressure. Carotid massage should be performed after carotid bruit is ruled out by applying steady pressure over the carotid sinus for 5 to 10 seconds. Vagal maneuvers are effective just over 20% of the time, but a recently described "modified Valsalva" appears to be more effective, where immediately after bearing down a member of the medical team would raise the patient's legs to 45 degrees for 15 seconds.

9. What pharmacologic therapies are used for acute conversion of supraventricular tachycardia?

Adenosine is effective in terminating SVT due to AVNRT, AVRT, and some atrial tachycardias (78% to 96% in nonrandomized emergency department studies). In some instances, adenosine may be useful in diagnosing other SVTs such as atrial flutter and atrial tachycardia, since the slow ventricular response induced by adenosine often allows for examination of the underlying atrial rate and rhythm. Adenosine should be administered quickly through a large-bore intravenous (IV) line inserted in a proximal vein, starting with a dose of 6 mg followed by a subsequent dose of 12 mg if necessary. Adenosine should be used with caution, if at all, in patients after heart transplant (discuss with attending). Adenosine has a short half-life, so recurrent SVT is often seen, necessitating alternative longer acting therapies. Intravenous nondihydropyridine calcium channel blockers (diltiazem and verapamil) have been shown to terminate SVT in 64% to 98% of patients. This therapy is contraindicated in patients with depressed LVEF and pre-excited AF. In fact, all AV nodal blocking agents are contraindicated in pre-excited AF because blocking the AV node leads to faster conduction over the accessory pathway, which can at times lead to ventricular fibrillation. Beta-blockers are less effective in terminating SVT when compared to nondihydropyridine calcium channel blockers, but they are not contraindicated in patients with history of heart failure and have a long record of safety, making them a reasonable choice when attempting to terminate SVT in hemodynamically stable patients without pre-excited AF.

10. What therapies are used for patients who are hemodynamically unstable from supraventricular tachycardia?

Synchronized cardioversion and adenosine are commonly used. Per the 2010 adult ACLS guidelines, patients suffering from SVT who present with hypotension, acutely altered mental status, signs of shock, and chest pain should undergo synchronized cardioversion immediately, but adenosine should be considered initially if readily available and the SVT is deemed regular with a narrow QRS complex.

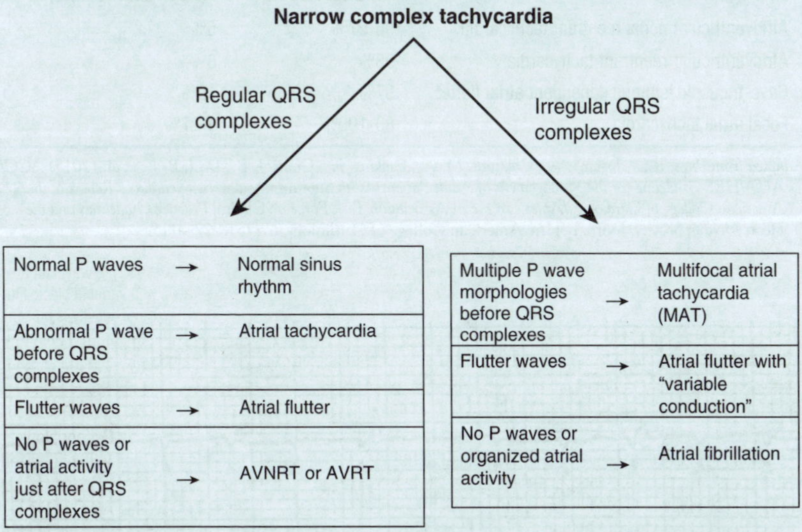

Fig. 36.3. Simple algorithm for the diagnosis of narrow complex tachycardias. Step one is to decide if the rhythm is regular or irregular. (Are the QRS complexes occurring at regular or irregular intervals?) Step two is to search for the presence of P waves or organized atrial activity.

11. **What are the success and complication rates for ablation of supraventricular tachycardia?**
Ablation for SVT has a high success rate (>90% for most SVTs) and low recurrence rate (≤10% for most SVTs). These rates are given in Table 36.1.

12. **Which drugs should be considered for treatment of idiopathic sinus tachycardia?**
Beta-blockers can be effective, although often IST patients cannot tolerate them. Ivabradine, a new drug recently FDA approved for patients with systolic heart failure, has been shown to lower heart rate and improve symptoms and exercise tolerance in patients with IST.

13. **Which drug is most commonly implicated in cases of drug-induced atrial tachycardia?**
Digoxin is most commonly implicated in drug-induced atrial tachycardia. Digoxin toxicity can cause many arrhythmias; a "classic one" is *paroxysmal atrial tachycardia with block.* In paroxysmal atrial tachycardia (PAT) with block, there is atrial tachycardia but also AV nodal blocks, leading to a slow ventricular response rate (Fig. 36.4). Therefore, in cases of PAT with block, digoxin toxicity should be suspected and the drug discontinued.

14. **What is the most common ventricular response rate in patients who develop atrial flutter?**
Atrial activity in atrial flutter most commonly occurs at a rate around 300 bpm, although the rate can be somewhat slower in patients on antiarrhythmic agents that slow conduction (such as amiodarone) or in diseased and dilated atria. Most commonly, there is 2:1 AV block, meaning that only every other atrial impulse is conducted down to the ventricles through the AV node. Thus, the most common ventricular response rate is approximately 150 bpm (see Fig. 36.1B). Therefore, finding a regular narrow complex tachycardia at exactly 150 bpm should raise suspicion of atrial flutter as the causative arrhythmia.

Table 36.1. Success and Recurrence Rates for Ablation Therapy for Supraventricular Tachycardia

ARRHYTHMIA	SUCCESS RATE	RECURRENCE RATE
Atrioventricular nodal reentrant tachycardia	96-97%	5%
Atrioventricular reentrant tachycardia	93%	8%
Cavo-tricuspid isthmus dependent atrial flutter	97%	10%
Focal atrial tachycardia	80-100%	4-27%

Adapted from Page, R.L., Joglar J. A., Caldwell, M. A., Calkins, H., Conti, J. B., Deal, B. J., et al. (2015) ACC/AHA/HRS Guideline for the Management of Adult Patients With Supraventricular Tachycardia: a Report of the American College of Cardiology/American Heart Association Task Force on Clinical Practice Guidelines and the Heart Rhythm Society. Journal of the American College of Cardiology, *67(13), e27–e115.*

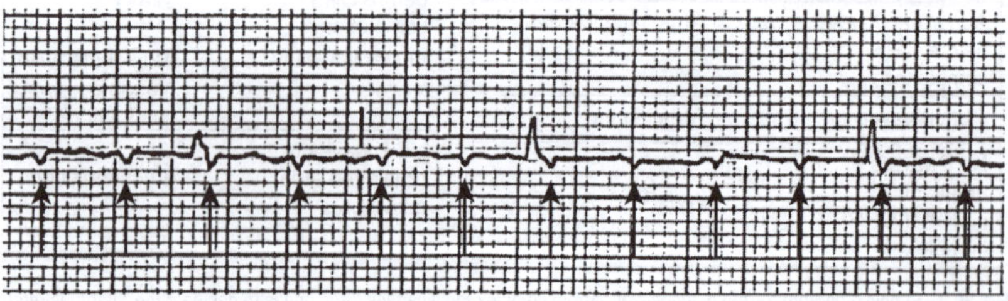

Fig. 36.4. Atrial tachycardia with block. The finding of atrial tachycardia with significant AV node block is highly suggestive of digoxin toxicity.

15. Which is more common, AV nodal reentrant tachycardia or accessory pathway–mediated reentrant tachycardia?

AVNRT is more common in the general adult population. In patients with known preexcitation syndrome (Wolff-Parkinson-White syndrome [WPW]), AVRT, which requires an accessory pathway, is more common. Thus, statistically, the cause of a narrow complex regular tachycardia is more likely to be AVNRT than AVRT, unless the patient has known WPW (or evidence of it on a baseline ECG).

16. What is the most common cause of focal atrial tachycardia?

Focal atrial tachycardia (see Fig. 36.1C) is most commonly caused by a discrete autonomic focus, although a micro-reentrant circuit can cause a small percentage of atrial tachycardias. Precipitating factors and causes of atrial tachycardia include

- Diseased atrial tissue (fibrosis, inflammation, etc.)
- Increased sympathetic stimulation (hyperthyroidism, caffeine, etc.)
- Excessive alcohol consumption
- Digoxin toxicity
- Electrolyte abnormalities
- Hypoxemia

Although textbooks describe the rate of atrial tachycardia as anywhere between 100 and 220 bpm, a rate of approximately 160 to 180 bpm is most common. AV conduction is usually 1:1 unless the tachycardia is very rapid, in which 2:1 conduction may occur. Because most cases of atrial tachycardia are due to an autonomic focus and not a reentry, the arrhythmia most commonly does not terminate with cardioversion. Adenosine only terminates the arrhythmia in a small portion of patients, yet still may be useful in cases in which the mechanism of regular SVT is unclear.

17. What is concealed conduction?

In many patients with preexcitation syndrome (WPW), conduction from the atrium to the ventricle will result in the appearance of a *delta wave* on the 12-lead ECG. However, in some patients with WPW, the accessory bypass tract does not conduct in an antegrade direction but only in a retrograde direction (*up* from the ventricle to the atrium). No delta wave appears on the baseline ECG because there is no antegrade conduction, but the accessory pathway is capable of retrograde conduction and participating in the genesis of orthodromic AVRT (impulse travels down the His-Purkinje system, into the ventricle, and then up the accessory pathway into the atrium).

18. For what arrhythmia should AV nodal blocking agents *not* be administered?

In rare cases of atrial fibrillation in the setting of an accessory bypass tract (WPW syndrome), some conduction of impulses will occur down the AV node and His-Purkinje system into the ventricle and some conduction down the bypass tract. In such cases, administration of AV nodal blocking agents (adenosine, digoxin, beta-blockers, and calcium channel blockers) may lead to increased conduction down the accessory bypass tract, producing an increased ventricular response rate and possibly precipitating ventricular fibrillation.

19. Do patients with atrial flutter require anticoagulation before cardioversion?

Previously it was believed that the risk of embolization during cardioversion for atrial flutter was negligible. However, observational studies have reported rates of embolization with cardioversion of atrial flutter ranging between 1.7% and 7%. Although a collective review showed that the rate of embolization with cardioversion for atrial flutter was lower than the rate with atrial fibrillation (2.2% vs. 5% to 7%), expert consensus is that the risk of thromboembolism is sufficient to warrant anticoagulation (and/or transesophageal echocardiogram) similar to that used in patients with atrial fibrillation undergoing cardioversion.

20. Can supraventricular tachycardia cause a wide QRS complex tachycardia?

Yes. SVT occurring in the setting of preexisting bundle branch block will produce a wide complex (QRS ≥120 ms) tachycardia. At faster heart rates, patients who may have a narrow QRS complex at baseline can also develop what is called *rate-related* bundle branch block. In the setting of preexcitation, a wide complex SVT rarely can also be caused by AVRT with antidromic conduction or any SVT occurring in setting of an accessory pathway that results in pre-excitation, which can appear as a wide complex tachycardia.

21. What is accessory pathway–mediated reentrant tachycardia with antidromic conduction?

In 95% of cases of AVRT, the reentrant circuit is composed of conduction *down* the AV node and His-Purkinje system, into the ventricle, and then *up* the bypass tract (which is called orthodromic conduction). However, in less than 5% of cases of AVRT, the reentrant circuit is reversed, with conduction from the atrium *down* the bypass tract, into the ventricle, and then *up* the His-Purkinje system and AV node and into the atrium. This is termed *antidromic conduction.* Because ventricular depolarization occurs without the use of the His-Purkinje system (the ventricle being activated first), the QRS complexes appear wide and resemble ventricular tachycardia (VT).

22. Which factors make the diagnosis of a wide QRS complex more likely to be ventricular tachycardia than supraventricular tachycardia?

- **P-wave dissociation** (also called AV dissociation): In P-wave dissociation, the QRS complexes occur at a greater rate than the P waves, and there is no fixed relationship between the QRS complexes and the P waves. This finding is highly suggestive of VT. Unfortunately, P-wave dissociation can only be clearly discerned in 21% of cases of VT.
- **QRS complexes in leads V_1–V_6:** R-S interval greater than 100 ms in any precordial lead is consistent with VT.
- **QRS complex in a VR:** The presence of an initial R wave. Initial Q wave greater than 40 ms and/or the presence of a notch on the descending limb at the onset of a predominantly negative QRS are consistent with VT, as they both signify prolonged conduction (cell-to-cell conduction as opposed to use of the His-Purkinje system).
- **Concordance:** Concordance is the finding of all negative or positive precordial QRS complexes (also referred to as lack of RS complex). This finding is essentially diagnostic for VT.
- **Ventricular fusion beats:** Fusion beats are QRS complexes that may be formed from the *fusion* of an impulse originating in the ventricle with an impulse originating in the atria and traveling down the AV node and His-Purkinje system. The finding of fusion beats indicates VT.
- **R-wave peak time in lead II:** R-wave peak time ≥50 ms suggests VT.
- Importantly, the presence of stable hemodynamics and no cardiac symptoms does not distinguish between SVT and VT.

Bibliography and Suggested Readings

Page, R. L., Joglar, J. A., Caldwell, M. A., Calkins, H., Conti, J. B., Deal, B. J., et al. (2015). ACC/AHA/HRS Guideline for the Management of Adult Patients With Supraventricular Tachycardia: a Report of the American College of Cardiology/American Heart Association Task Force on Clinical Practice Guidelines and the Heart Rhythm Society. *Journal of the American College of Cardiology*, *67*(13), e27–e115.

Appelboam, A., Reuben, A., Mann, C., Gagg, J., Ewings, P., Barton, A., et al. (2015). Postural modification to the standard Valsalva manoeuvre for emergency treatment of supraventricular tachycardias (REVERT): a randomised controlled trial. *Lancet*, *386*(10005), 1747–1753.

Link, M. S., Atkins, D. L., Passman, R. S., Halperin, H. R., Samson, R. A., White, R. D., et al. (2010). Part 6: electrical therapies: automated external defibrillators, defibrillation, cardioversion, and pacing: 2010 American Heart Association Guidelines for Cardiopulmonary Resuscitation and Emergency Cardiovascular Care. *Circulation*, *122*(18 Suppl 3), S706–S719.

CHAPTER 37

VENTRICULAR ARRHYTHMIAS

Jose L. Baez-Escudero

1. **What is the differential diagnosis of a wide complex tachycardia?**
The differential includes the following:
   - Ventricular tachycardia (VT) (monomorphic or polymorphic)
   - Supraventricular tachycardia (SVT) with aberrant conduction or underlying bundle branch block
   - Antidromic SVT using an accessory pathway for antegrade conduction (Wolff-Parkinson-White syndrome)
   - Toxicity related (hyperkalemia, digoxin, other drugs) (Fig. 37.1)
   - Pacemaker-mediated tachycardia
   - Telemetry artifacts

   Of note, a wide-QRS tachycardia should always be presumed to be VT if the diagnosis is unclear.

2. **What is the definition of ventricular tachycardia?**
VT is defined as three or more consecutive QRS complexes arising from the ventricles. *Sustained VT* is that which causes symptoms or lasts more than 30 seconds. *Nonsustained VT (NSVT)* is VT that does not meet criteria for sustained VT.

3. **What is the pathophysiologic substrate of ventricular tachycardia?**
It depends on the clinical scenario, but the most common mechanism is reentry, followed by automaticity.

4. **What is the most common underlying heart disease predisposing to ventricular tachycardia?**
The most common conditions predisposing to VT are coronary artery disease and coronary ischemia. VT in the setting of acute ischemia and immediately after myocardial infarction (MI) is related to excess ventricular ectopy as a result of increased automaticity (Na^+, K^+ ATPase pump malfunction, increase in intracellular calcium, tissue acidosis, and locally released catecholamines). After completion of a transmural MI, patients with resultant ischemic cardiomyopathy can suffer from recurrent sustained monomorphic VT. In this case, VT originates in scarred myocardium, where islands of infarcted tissue surrounded by strands of functional myocytes provide the substrate for the creation of a reentrant circuit.

5. **Can ventricular tachycardia occur in other nonischemic heart diseases?**
Scar-related VT can occur in other nonischemic conditions whenever an inflammatory or infiltrative disorder damages the myocardium with resultant disruption of healthy myocardial cell architecture. Sarcoidosis and Chagas disease are typical examples in which VT can occur as a result of such nonischemic scars. The myocardial disarray seen in hypertrophic cardiomyopathy (HCM) patients often creates a substrate for reentry and VT. Fatty infiltration of the right ventricle leads to areas

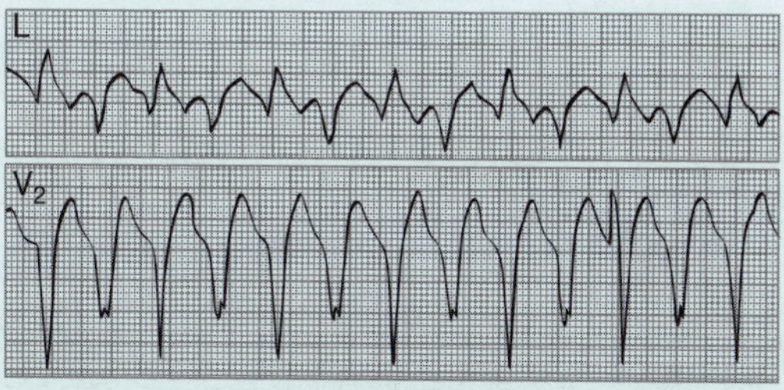

Fig. 37.1. Bidirectional ventricular tachycardia in a patient with digitalis toxicity. *(Modified from Marriott, H. J. L., & Conover, M. B. [1989].* Advanced concepts in arrhythmias *[2nd ed.]. St. Louis, MO: Mosby.)*

of unexcitable myocardium that can facilitate the formation of reentrant circuits in patients with arrhythmogenic right ventricular dysplasia (ARVD). Myocardial scars leading to reentry also occur after surgical correction of congenital heart diseases. Dilated cardiomyopathies (DCMs) often have scar sites located near the base of the LV, facilitating VT. DCM can also lead to reentry within a diseased conduction system, the so-called bundle branch reentry, where impulses use the right and left bundles as antegrade and retrograde pathways (less commonly in the opposite direction). Conceivably, any structural heart disease can lead to reentry.

6. Can ventricular tachycardia occur in the absence of structural heart disease?

VT can occur in the structurally normal heart. Monomorphic VT occurs in two distinct clinical entities in the absence of heart disease, *outflow tract VT* and *idiopathic fascicular VT*.

Outflow tract VT: This condition often presents not as sustained VT but rather as isolated premature ventricular complexes (PVCs), which can be very frequent (e.g., bigeminy) (Fig. 37.2) and can cause a variety of symptoms, such as effective bradycardia and frequent palpitation or the sensation of skipped beats. If the PVC burden is high, it can cause deterioration of the left ventricular function, or so-called PVC-induced cardiomyopathy. Sustained outflow tract VT (Fig. 37.3) typically occurs during or after exercise or with enhanced catecholamine states. It is thought to be generated by triggered activity in the form of delayed afterdepolarizations, typically created in situations of calcium overload. In outflow tract VT the PVCs and VT originate most commonly from the right ventricular outflow tract, under the pulmonic valve, but occasionally can arise from the left ventricular outflow tract, aortomitral continuity, and even the aortic cusps. Although it is a wide complex tachycardia (WCT), when sustained, it may respond to intravenous (IV) adenosine therapy.

Idiopathic fascicular VT (also known as verapamil-sensitive or Belhassen VT): Idiopathic fascicular VT typically occurs in young, healthy individuals with normal hearts and most commonly involves a right bundle branch block (RBBB) and left anterior fascicular block pattern because it arises from the left posterior fascicle.

Both these forms of VT are curable with mapping and catheter ablation. PVC-induced cardiomyopathy can be reversed, and normalization of LV function is often achievable with successful catheter ablation.

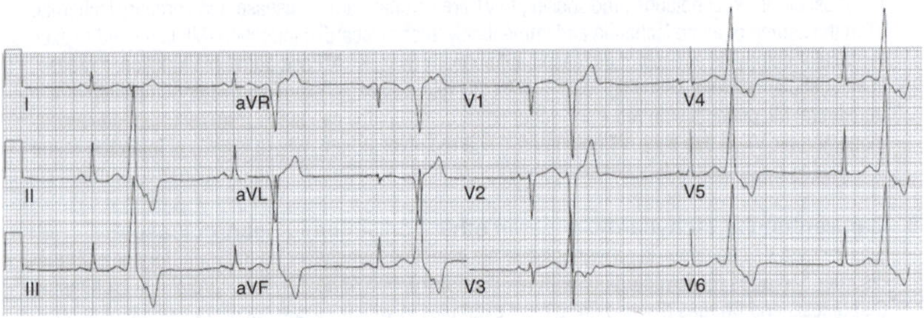

Fig. 37.2. Right ventricular outflow tract bigeminal premature ventricular complex originating under the pulmonic valve.

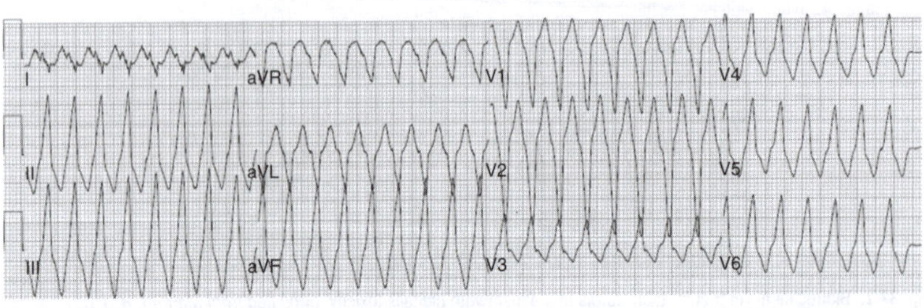

Fig. 37.3. Left ventricular outflow tract sustained ventricular tachycardia originating under the aortic cusp.

7. What are channelopathies, and how do they relate to ventricular arrhythmias?

Primary electrical disorders or congenital **channelopathies** are a group of clinical syndromes that specifically affect the myocardial ion channels (including Na^+, K^+, and Ca^{2+} channels). Channelopathies occur because of disturbed functioning of ion channel subunits or the proteins that regulate them and are either congenital (mutations in encoding genes) or acquired (often acquired from an autoimmune attack on an ion channel). As a result, normal myocardial depolarization and repolarization is altered, changing the surface electrocardiogram (ECG) and predisposing the carrier to potentially fatal ventricular arrhythmia. *Familial long QT syndromes* typically lead to torsades de pointes (TdP), as does *short QT syndrome*. *Brugada syndrome* causes a typical right bundle branch pattern with ST-segment elevation in the early precordial leads at baseline (Fig. 37.4). It often causes sudden death due to ventricular fibrillation (VF) (Fig. 37.5). *Catecholaminergic polymorphic ventricular tachycardia (CPVT)* is a mutation of the ryanodine receptor that typically causes exercise-induced bidirectional and polymorphic VT.

8. What is idiopathic ventricular fibrillation?

Idiopathic VF, or primary VF, is a disease of unknown etiology that occurs in young adults in the absence of structural heart disease or identifiable channelopathies. In this rare syndrome, spontaneous VF is invariably triggered by a very short coupled ventricular extrasystole or PVC arising from the Purkinje fibers. Most survivors of sudden cardiac death will need a secondary prevention implantable cardiac defibrillator (ICD). In some patients, recurrent ICD shocks for primary VF can be prevented by successful targeted ablation of the triggering PVC.

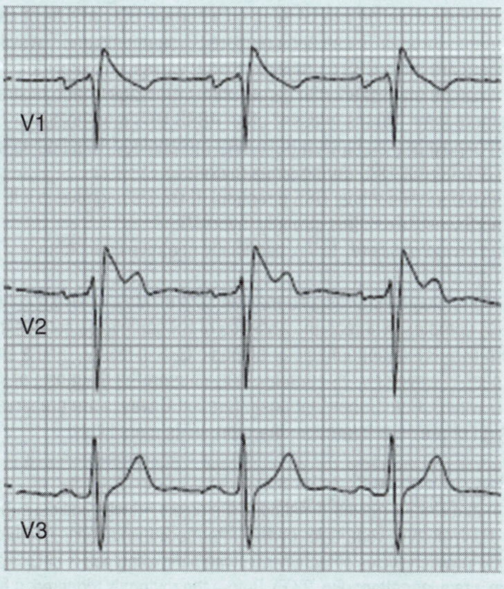

Fig. 37.4. Type I Brugada electrocardiogram pattern with right bundle branch block and ST elevation in V_1 to V_3.

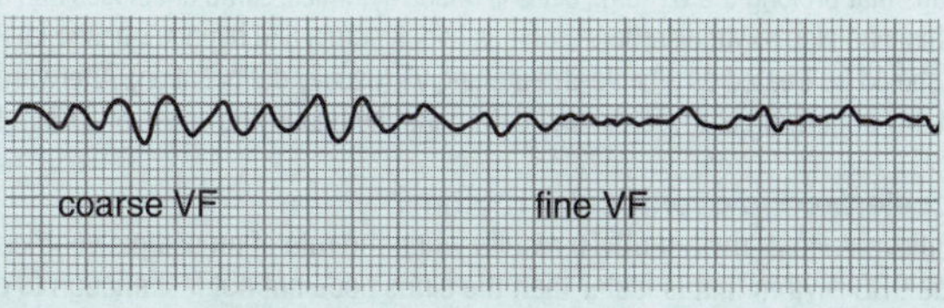

Fig. 37.5. Coarse VF, which then degenerates further into fine VF. *VF*, Ventricular fibrillation. *(From Goldberger, E. [1990]. Treatment of cardiac emergencies [5th ed.]. St. Louis, MO: Mosby.)*

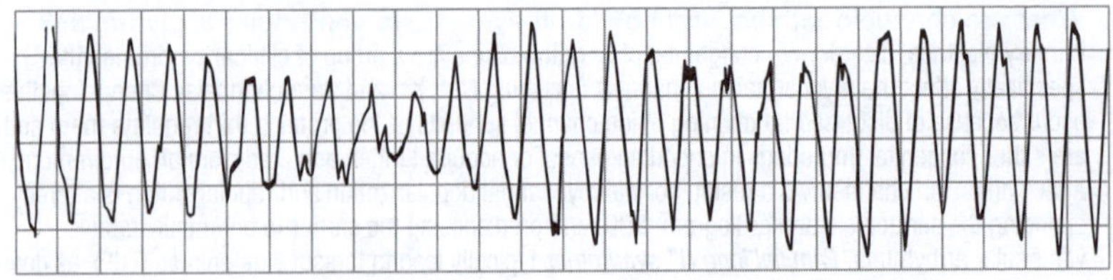

Fig. 37.6. Torsades de pointes, in which the QRS axis seems to rotate about the isoelectric point. *(Modified from Olgin, J. E., & Zipes, D. P. [2008]. Specific arrhythmias: diagnosis and treatment. In R. O. Bonow, D. L. Mann, D. P. Zipes, and P. Libby,* Braunwald's heart disease: a textbook of cardiovascular medicine *[8th ed.]. Philadelphia, PA: Saunders.)*

9. What electrocardiogram features favor ventricular tachycardia (over supraventricular tachycardia with bundle branch block) as the cause of a wide complex tachycardia?

VT rhythms have rates between 100 and 280 beats/minute and can be monomorphic or polymorphic. Typical ECG clues that favor VT include the following:

- Presence of *fusion beats,* which identify simultaneous depolarization of the ventricle by both the normal conduction system and an ectopic impulse originating in the ventricle.
- *Capture beats,* which are normally conducted sinus beats with a narrow QRS complex that generally occur at a shorter interval than the tachycardia.
- *Atrioventricular (AV) dissociation,* the finding of independent atrial and ventricular activity at differing rates. AV dissociation can be seen on a surface ECG in 30% of cases. Look for visible P waves that "march through" (scan and compare ST segments and T waves, look for subtle QRS changes). If there are more QRS complexes than P waves, it is likely to be VT. If AV dissociation is not obvious, it can be unmasked with carotid sinus massage or administration of adenosine.
- A *QRS width* more than 140 ms in cases of an RBBB QRS morphology or more than 160 ms in cases of a left bundle branch block (LBBB) QRS morphology. This finding suggests VT, especially in the setting of a normal QRS during sinus rhythm.
- *Limb lead concordance* (identical QRS direction). If QRS is negative in I, II, and III (an extreme leftward or "northwest" axis), this strongly favors VT.
- *Precordial lead concordance* (V_1 to V_6), especially negative concordance. This is highly specific for the diagnosis of VT.
- Certain QRS morphologic features also may be helpful. Most aberrant conduction patterns have a precordial RS complex, whereas the absence of RS complexes suggests VT. An atypical right bundle pattern (R > R′), a monophasic or biphasic QRS in lead V_1, and a small R wave coupled with a large deep S wave or a QS complex in V_6 support the diagnosis of VT.
- Presence of Q waves. Remember that postinfarction Q waves are preserved in VT. Their presence in WCT is a sign of previous infarction; therefore VT is more likely.

10. What is torsades de pointes?

TdP is a French term that literally means "twisting of the points." It was first described by Dessertenne in 1966 and refers to a polymorphic ventricular rhythm intermediate in appearance between VT and VF. It has a distinct morphology in which cycles of tachycardia with alternating peaks of QRS amplitude turn about the isoelectric line in a regular pattern (Fig. 37.6). Before the rhythm is triggered, a baseline prolonged QT interval and pathologic U waves are present, reflecting abnormal ventricular repolarization. A short-long-short sequence between the R-R interval (marked bradycardia or preceding pause) occurs before the trigger response. Drugs that prolong the QT (e.g., class III antiarrhythmics, some antibiotics and antifungals, tricyclic antidepressants) and electrolyte disorders (such as hypokalemia and hypomagnesemia) are common triggers. TdP should be treated as any life-threatening VT (usually defibrillation). Afterward, efforts must be made to treat any underlying bradycardia and determine the underlying cause of QT lengthening.

11. What is accelerated idioventricular rhythm?

Accelerated idioventricular rhythm (AIVR) results when the rate of an ectopic ventricular pacemaker causes a wide QRS rhythm that is faster than the sinus node but not fast enough to cause tachycardia (<100 bpm) (Fig. 37.7). AIVR is often associated with increased vagal tone and decreased sympathetic tone. A proposed mechanism is enhanced automaticity of a ventricular natural pacemaker, although

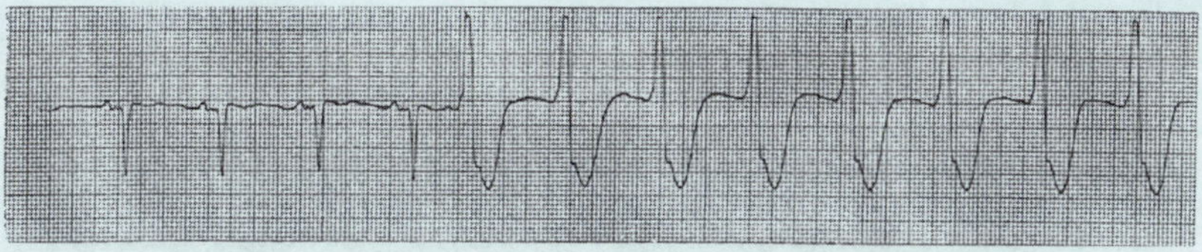

Fig. 37.7. Accelerated idioventricular rhythm. Note the wide QRS that appears spontaneously during sinus rhythm. The rhythm is slower than 100 bpm and is thus not fast enough to be called ventricular tachycardia.

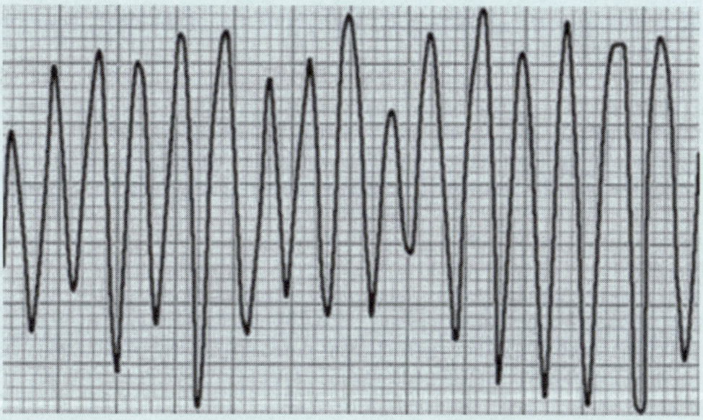

Fig. 37.8. Ventricular flutter. The electrocardiogram recording shows a continuous sine wave that looks identical when viewed upside down, without identifiable P waves, QRS complexes, or T waves.

triggered activity may play a role, especially in ischemia and digoxin toxicity. AIVR is classically seen in the reperfusion phase of an acute ST-segment-elevation myocardial infarction (STEMI; post thrombolytic therapy or primary percutaneous coronary intervention). It can also occur in normal athletic hearts and during return of spontaneous circulation (ROSC) following cardiac arrest. It is usually a well-tolerated, benign, self-limiting arrhythmia and does not usually require treatment.

12. What is ventricular flutter?

Ventricular flutter is an extreme form of VT with loss of organized electrical activity. It is associated with rapid and profound hemodynamic compromise. It is usually short lived due to rapid progression to VF. As with VF, rapid initiation of resuscitative efforts is required. The ECG shows often a continuous sine wave that looks identical when viewed upside down, without identifiable P waves, QRS complexes, or T waves (Fig. 37.8). The rate is usually greater than 200 bpm.

13. What critical decisions must be made in the management of sustained ventricular tachycardia?

The critical decision in the management of a patient with sustained VT is the urgency with which to treat the rhythm. In a hemodynamically stable and minimally symptomatic patient, treatment should be delayed until a 12-lead ECG can be obtained. The axis and morphology help to make the diagnosis of VT, as well as shed light on the potential mechanism and origin of the rhythm. During the delay, a brief medical history and baseline laboratory values can be obtained (especially serum levels of potassium and magnesium, as well as cardiac biomarkers). Specific attention should be paid to a history of MI, systolic heart failure, history of structural heart disease, family history of sudden cardiac death, and potentially proarrhythmic drugs.

14. What methods are used to terminate sustained ventricular tachycardia?

With any question of hemodynamic instability, termination should be done immediately with synchronized direct current electrical cardioversion. Hemodynamic instability is defined as symptomatic hypotension, congestive heart failure, myocardial ischemia (infarction or angina), or signs or symptoms of inadequate cerebral perfusion. It is important to ensure that the energy is delivered in a synchronized fashion before cardioversion. Failure to do so may accelerate the rhythm or induce VF. If the patient is conscious, adequate IV sedation should always be provided. Termination of hemodynamically stable VT may be attempted medically. Reasonable drugs of choice are IV procainamide (or ajmaline in some European countries), lidocaine, and IV amiodarone. For ischemic monomorphic VT, IV lidocaine is also a reasonable option. Pace termination (either through transvenous insertion of a temporary pacer or by reprogramming an ICD) can be useful to treat patients with sustained monomorphic VT that is refractory to cardioversion or is recurrent despite the use of the previously mentioned drugs. If VT is associated with acute ischemia, urgent angiography and revascularization are paramount.

In those overtly hemodynamically compromised, frankly unresponsive, or pulseless, prompt defibrillation should be used.

15. After the acute episode of ventricular tachycardia is terminated, what are the next management strategies?

This depends on the clinical situation and on the individual patient. Any potentially reversible cause should be sought and treated aggressively—specifically, ischemia, heart failure, or electrolyte abnormalities. In general, beta-blockers are usually safe and effective and should be administered in most patients in whom concomitant antiarrhythmic drugs are indicated. Amiodarone (and in expert hands, sotalol) has been the mainstay of preventive therapy, especially in patients with left ventricle (LV) dysfunction. However, the long-term clinical success of medical regimens is low, and amiodarone carries a risk of serious side effects.

All patients should be risk stratified for the likelihood of recurrence and subsequent risk of sudden cardiac death. Appropriate consultation with an electrophysiologist should be obtained to assess the need for ICD implantation (indications for ICDs are discussed in Chapter 39). Although cardiac device therapy has revolutionized treatment, providing excellent protection from sudden cardiac death, it does not prevent recurrences. Patients with defibrillators may remain symptomatic with palpitations, syncope, and recurrent shocks for VT. Ablation of the reentrant circuits that cause VT also provides a nonpharmacologic option for the reduction of symptoms.

16. How is catheter ablation of ventricular tachycardia performed?

VT ablation remains challenging and is offered primarily at experienced centers. Endocardial mapping of VT to identify an optimal region for ablation can be time consuming because of the complexity of the reentry circuits and the existence of certain circuit portions deep into the endocardium, although modern, three-dimensional, voltage-mapping technologies that reconstruct and relate electrophysiologic characteristics to specific anatomy have greatly facilitated the ablation procedure. Ablation can be achieved using traditional radiofrequency or with other technologies, such as cryoablation or laser.

When endocardial circuits are resistant to ablation, the technique of transthoracic pericardial access with epicardial mapping of VT is used. This approach facilitates localization and ablation of deep and epicardial circuits and requires the insertion of a sheath into the pericardial space, using a needle and guidewire under fluoroscopic guidance.

If a separate indication for heart surgery is present (e.g., need for surgical revascularization, LV aneurysmectomy, mitral valve repair or replacement), surgical ablation may be considered.

17. When is catheter ablation used to treat ventricular tachycardia?

Ablation has traditionally been used for secondary prevention after an ICD-terminated VT and as an alternative to chronic antiarrhythmic therapy. It may also be considered as an option for reducing ICD therapies in patients with recurrent appropriate shocks and as an alternative to drug therapy for outflow tract or fascicular VT. The success rates vary depending on an individual's substrate for the arrhythmia. A patient with a VT arising from the right ventricular outflow tract in a structurally normal heart will likely have a much higher success rate when compared with a patient with a severely reduced ejection fraction from a large anterior wall MI with multiple VT morphologies.

18. How can autonomic modulation treat ventricular tachycardia?

In the hyperadrenergic state of VT storm in which ICD shocks are psychologically and physiologically traumatizing, and for incessant VTs that are refractory to conventional therapy, suppression of sympathetic outflow from the organ level of the heart up to higher brain centers plays a significant role in reducing the propensity for VT recurrence. The autonomic nervous system continuously receives input from the heart (afferent signaling), integrates the signals, and sends efferent signals to modify or maintain arrhythmogenesis. Spinal anesthesia with thoracic epidural infusion of bupivacaine and surgical vagal denervation with removal of the sympathetic chain including the stellate ganglion has been shown to decrease recurrences of VT. Excess sympathetic outflow with catecholamine release can be also modified with catheter-based renal denervation.

Bibliography and Suggested Readings

Brugada, P., Brugada, J., Mont, L., Smeets, J., & Andries, E. W. (1991). A new approach to the differential diagnosis of a regular tachycardia with a wide QRS complex. *Circulation, 83*, 1649–1659.

Jacobson, J. T., & Weiner, J. B. (2010). Management of ventricular tachycardia in patients with structural heart disease. *Cardiovascular Therapeutics, 28*(5), 255–263.

Pellegrini, C. N., & Scheinman, M. M. (2010). Clinical management of ventricular tachycardia. *Current Problems in Cardiology, 35*(9), 453–504. http://dx.doi.org/10.1016/j.cpcardiol.2010.08.001.

Priori, S. G., Blomström-Lundqvist, C., Mazzanti, A., Blom, N., Borggrefe, M., Camm, J., et al. (2015). 2015 ESC Guidelines for the management of patients with ventricular arrhythmias and the prevention of sudden cardiac death. *European Heart Journal, 36*, 2793–2867.

Reddy, V. Y., Reynolds, M. R., Neuzil, P., Richardson, A. W., Taborsky, M., Jongnarangsin, K., et al. (2007). Prophylactic catheter ablation for the prevention of defibrillator therapy. *New England Journal of Medicine, 357*, 2657–2665.

Roberts-Thomson, K. C., Lau, D. H., & Sanders, P. (2011). The diagnosis and management of ventricular arrhythmias. *Nature Reviews Cardiology, 8*, 311–321. http://dx.doi.org/10.1038/nrcardio.2011.15.

Tung, R., & Shivkumar, K. (2015). Neuraxial modulation for treatment of VT storm. *Journal of Biomedical Research, 29*(1), 56–60.

Zipes, D. P., Camm, A. J., Borggrefe, M., Buxton, A. E., Chaitman, B., Fromer, M., et al. (2006). ACC/AHA/ESC 2006 guidelines for management of patients with ventricular arrhythmias and the prevention of sudden cardiac death: a report of the American College of Cardiology/American Heart Association Task Force and the European Society of Cardiology Committee for Practice Guidelines (writing committee to develop guidelines for management of patients with ventricular arrhythmias and the prevention of sudden cardiac death). *Circulation, 114*, e385–e484.

CHAPTER 38

CARDIAC PACING FOR BRADYCARDIA, HEART BLOCK, AND HEART FAILURE

Paul Schurmann, Miguel Valderrábano

1. **What is sick sinus syndrome?**

   Sinus node dysfunction, commonly referred to as *sick sinus syndrome,* refers to a broad array of abnormalities of the sinus node, ranging from atrial impulse formation through propagation of the depolarization impulse. Sick sinus syndrome can manifest as sinus bradycardia, paroxysmal sinus arrest, sinus node exit block, or chronotropic insufficiency. Tachycardia-bradycardia ("tachy-brady") syndrome is a common appearance of sick sinus syndrome in patients with paroxysmal atrial fibrillation or atrial flutter.

   Sick sinus syndrome is primarily a disease of older adults and a common cause of bradyarrhythmias. The prevalence of sick sinus syndrome can range from 0% to 4.5%, and the syndrome accounts for approximately 40% to 60% of pacemaker implantations in the United States. Patients with sick sinus syndrome can be asymptomatic or have mild nonspecific symptoms, depending on the severity of the bradycardia or the duration of the pauses. If symptoms are present, usually they present for months or even years. Most commonly they include dizziness, near-syncope, recurrent falls, and/or syncope, and exercise intolerance due to chronotropic incompetence may also be present.

   Sick sinus syndrome may be due to intrinsic causes, such as replacement of nodal tissue with fibrous tissue at the sinus node itself, or it may be due to extrinsic causes, such as offending drugs, electrolyte imbalance, hypothermia, hypothyroidism, hypoxemia, increased intracranial pressure, sleep apnea, and excessive vagal tone. The use of a permanent pacemaker is usually the therapy of choice for symptomatic sick sinus syndrome, but first it is important to identify transient or reversible causes that could correct sick sinus syndrome. Pharmacologic therapies with isoproterenol or atropine are effective only as short-term solutions or in the case of an emergency.

2. **What are the three types of atrial ventricular blocks?**

   Bradyarrhythmia can be caused by atrioventricular (AV) block. There are three degrees of AV block: first, second, and third (complete). This classification is based on the electrocardiogram (ECG).

   First-degree block refers to a stable prolongation of the PR interval to more than 200 ms and represents delays in conduction at the level of the AV node. There are no indications for pacing in isolated asymptomatic first-degree block.

   Second-degree block is divided into two types. Mobitz type I ("Wenckebach") exhibits progressive prolongation of the PR interval before an atrial impulse fails to stimulate the ventricle. Anatomically this form of block occurs above the bundle of His. Type II exhibits no prolongation of the PR interval before a dropped beat and anatomically occurs at the level of the bundle of His or below. This rhythm may be associated with a prolonged QRS complex.

   Third-degree or *complete heart block* defines the absence of AV conduction and refers to complete dissociation of the atrial and ventricular rhythms, with a ventricular rate less than the atrial rate. The width and rate of the ventricular escape rhythm helps to identify an anatomic location for the block: narrow QRS is associated with minimal slowing of the rate, generally at the AV node, and wide QRS is associated with considerable slowing of the rate at or below the bundle of His.

   High-grade or *advanced AV block* refers to instances in which more than one consecutive P wave fails to conduct through the AV node, regardless of the anatomic location. Permanent pacemaker implantation is indicated for third-degree and type II second-degree AV block at any anatomic level associated with bradycardia with symptoms.

   Examples of first-, second-, and third-degree heart block are shown in Fig. 38.1.

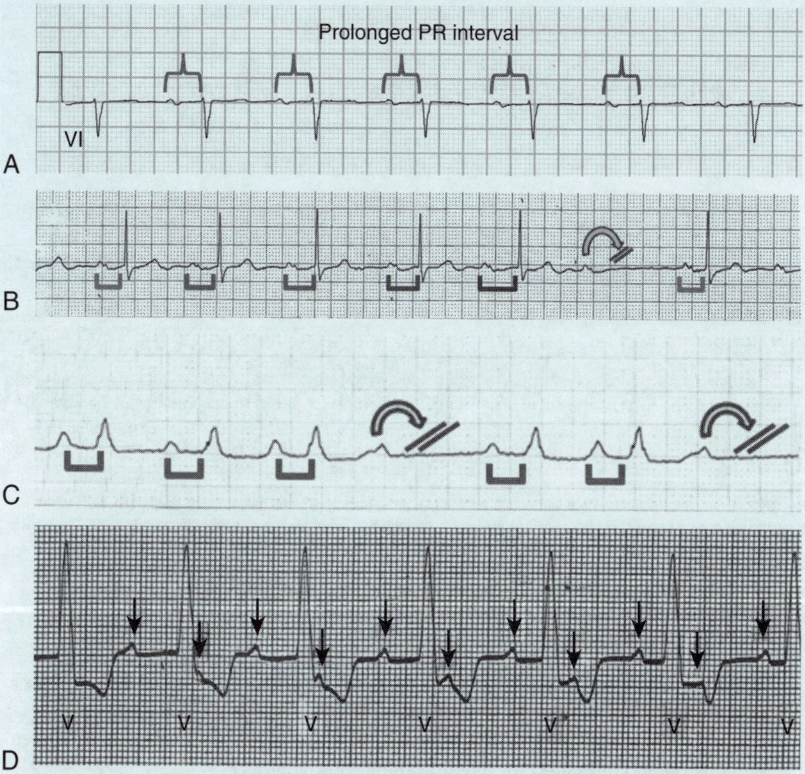

Fig. 38.1. Examples of heart block. In first-degree heart block **(A)**, the PR interval is prolonged but all atrial impulses ("p waves") are conducted. In second-degree type I heart block **(B)**, the PR interval is progressively prolonged until an atrial impulse is no longer conducted. In second-degree heart block type II **(C)**, the PR interval is constant in the setting of a non-conducted atrial impulse. In complete heart block **(D)**, no atrial impulses are conducted. *(Images reproduced from Levine, G. N. [2014].* Color atlas of cardiovascular disease. *New Delhi, India: Jaypee Brothers Medical Publishers.)*

3. What is bifascicular or trifascicular block?

Bifascicular block is located below the AV node and involves a combination of blocks at the level of the right bundle with blocks within one of the fascicles of the left bundle (left anterior or left posterior fascicle).

Trifascicular block refers to the presence of a prolonged PR interval, in addition to a bifascicular block. Based on the surface ECG, it is impossible to tell whether the prolonged PR interval is due to delay at the AV node *(suprahisian)* or in the remaining conducting fascicle (*infrahisian*, hence the term *trifascicular block*).

Pacing is indicated when bifascicular or trifascicular block is associated with the following:

- Complete heart block and symptomatic bradycardia
- Alternating bundle branch block
- Intermittent type II second-degree block with or without related symptoms
- Symptoms suggestive of bradycardia and an HV interval greater than 100 ms on invasive electrophysiology study or evidence of infra-His block
- Neuromuscular disease such as muscular dystrophy or Erb dystrophy

4. When is permanent cardiac pacing indicated?

The most important clinical criterion for permanent pacemaker implantation is the presence of symptoms that are clearly associated with the bradyarrthymia, tachy-brady syndrome refractory

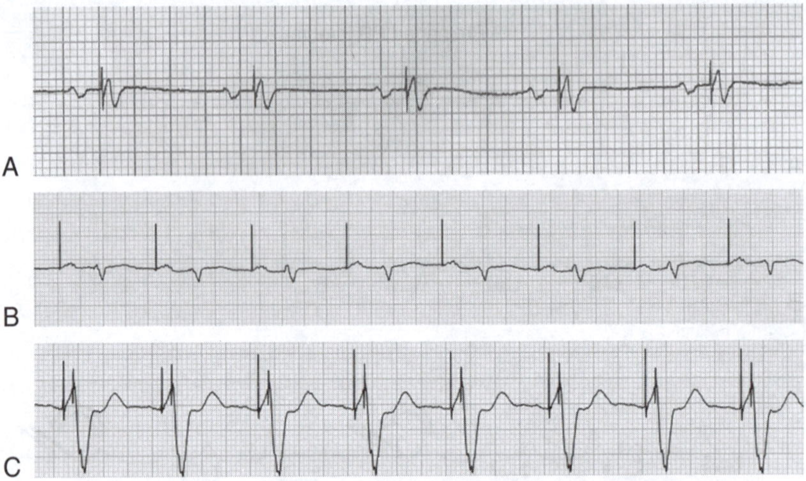

Fig. 38.2. Example of standard right ventricular pacing (A), atrial pacing (B), and biventricular pacing (C). Note with biventricular pacing two distinct pacer spikes are visible (though this is not always so easily visualized).

to medical therapy, and/or chronotropic insufficiency. The clinical manifestations of symptomatic bradycardia include fatigue, dyspnea on exertion, decreased exercise tolerance, lightheadedness, dizziness, presyncope, and syncope.

Biventricular pacing is indicated when symptoms of congestive heart failure are associated with severe left ventricular dysfunction (ejection fraction [EF] <35%) and prolonged QRS (>120 ms in cases of left bundle branch block [LBBB] and >150 ms in cases of non-LBBB).

Examples of right ventricular and biventricular pacing are shown in Fig. 38.2.

5. When is pacing indicated for asymptomatic bradycardia?

There are a few clear indications for pacing in patients with bradycardia who are asymptomatic. These include the following:

- Third-degree AV block with documented asystole lasting 3 or more seconds (in sinus rhythm) or junctional or ventricular escape rates below 40 beats per minute (bpm) in patients while awake
- Third-degree AV block or second-degree AV Mobitz type II block in patients with chronic bifascicular and trifascicular block
- Congenital third-degree AV block with a wide QRS escape rhythm, ventricular dysfunction, or bradycardia markedly inappropriate for age

Potential (class II) other indications for pacing in asymptomatic patients include the following:

- Third-degree AV block with faster escape rates in patients who are awake
- Second-degree AV Mobitz type II block in patients without bifascicular or trifascicular block
- The finding in an electrophysiologic study of a block below or within the bundle of His or an HV interval of 100 ms or longer

Importantly, when bradycardia is present only during sleep, even if extreme, pacing is not indicated.

6. Is pacing indicated for neurocardiogenic syncope?

Neurocardiogenic syncope occurs when triggering of a neural reflex results in a usually self-limited episode of systemic hypotension characterized by both bradycardia and peripheral vasodilation. If bradycardia occurs only in specific situations, patient education, pharmacologic trials, and prevention strategies are indicated before pacing in most patients. Permanent pacemaker implantation is considered in cases of syncope without a provocative event or with ventricular pauses greater than or equal to 3 seconds. Permanent pacemaker implantation can be considered in syncope with documented bradycardia on tilt table testing. Unfortunately, many patients with neurocardiogenic syncope have a prominent vasodepressor (peripheral vasodilation) component to their syndrome, and implantation of a pacemaker may not completely relieve symptoms.

7. What are the indications for pacing after myocardial infarction?

Unlike many other indications for pacemaker implantation, indications for pacemaker implantation after myocardial infarction (MI) do not require the presence of symptoms. Pacing is indicated in the setting of acute MI for the following:

- Persistent complete third-degree block or advanced second-degree block that is associated with block in the His-Purkinje system (wide complex ventricular rhythm) after ST-segment elevation MI or if the patients are symptomatic.
- Transient advanced second-degree or complete heart block with a new bundle branch block.

Importantly, the temporary implantation of a transvenous pacemaker in the immediate MI period by itself does not constitute an indication for permanent pacemaker implantation.

8. What other medical condition could require permanent pacing?

Permanent pacing may be considered in medically refractory symptomatic patients with significant resting or provoked LV outflow tract obstruction, such as in patients with hypertrophic cardiomyopathy (HCM). Although pacemaker implantation at one point was believed to have substantial benefit in such patients, its benefits in general appear to be quite modest, and first-line treatment in patients with HCM and continued symptoms despite medical therapy are surgical myomyectomy (or percutaneous alcohol septal ablation).

Permanent pacing can also be used to prevent pause-dependent VT and VT in high-risk patients with congenital long QT syndrome. Heart transplant patients with persistent inappropriate bradycardia should also be considered for permanent pacing.

9. What are the components of a pacing system?

Standard pacing systems consist of a pulse generator and pacing leads (Fig. 38.3). The pulse generator is usually implanted in the left upper chest area. The pacing leads are implanted into the atria, the ventricles, or both, depending on the indication for pacemaker implantation.

Pacemakers function by providing an electrical stimulus resulting in cardiac depolarization during periods when intrinsic cardiac electrical activity is inappropriately slow or absent. The battery most commonly used in permanent pacers has a life span of 6 to 10 years.

10. What is a leadless pacemaker system?

Unlike standard pacemaker systems, a leadless pacemaker is placed directly in the heart without the need for pacing leads (Fig. 38.4). The device is much smaller than a conventional pacemaker and is comprised of a pulse generator that includes a battery and an electrode that is all intracardiac. The device can be implanted in various locations in the right ventricle (Fig. 38.5). This new technology eliminates long-term lead and subcutaneous pocket complications that can occur with standard pacemakers.

11. What is the accepted pacing nomenclature for the different pacing modalities?

The North American Society of Pacing and Electrophysiology and the British Pacing and Electrophysiology Group (NBG) have modified the code to describe various pacing modes matching the new advances in technologies. It assumes that all pacemakers are communicative and programmable and consists of five letters:

- Letter 1: Chamber that is paced (*A* = atria, *V* = ventricles, *D* = dual chamber)
- Letter 2: Chamber that is sensed (*A* = atria, *V* = ventricles, *D* = dual chamber, *0* = none)
- Letter 3: Response to a sensed event (*I* = pacing inhibited, *T* = pacing triggered, *D* = dual, *0* = none)
- Letter 4: Rate-responsive features, is an activity sensor in the pulse generator that detects bodily movement and increases the pacing rate according to a programmable algorithm (*R* = rate-responsive pacemaker, *0* = none)
- Letter 5: Chamber that is paced in multisite pacing (*A* = atria, *V* = ventricles, *D* = dual chamber).

A pacemaker in VVI mode denotes that it paces and senses the ventricle and is inhibited by a sensed ventricular event. The DDD mode denotes that both chambers are capable of being sensed and paced.

12. What are potential complications associated with pacemaker implantation?

Complications in the hands of experienced operators are rare (approximately 1% to 2%) and include the following: bleeding, infection, pneumothorax, hemothorax, cardiac arrhythmias, cardiac perforation causing tamponade, diaphragmatic/phrenic nerve pacing, pocket hematoma, coronary sinus trauma, and prolonged radiation exposure.

Late complications of pacemaker implantation include erosion of the pacer through the skin (requires pacer replacement, lead extraction, and systemic antibiotics), and lead malfunction (lead fracture, break in lead insulation, or dislodgment).

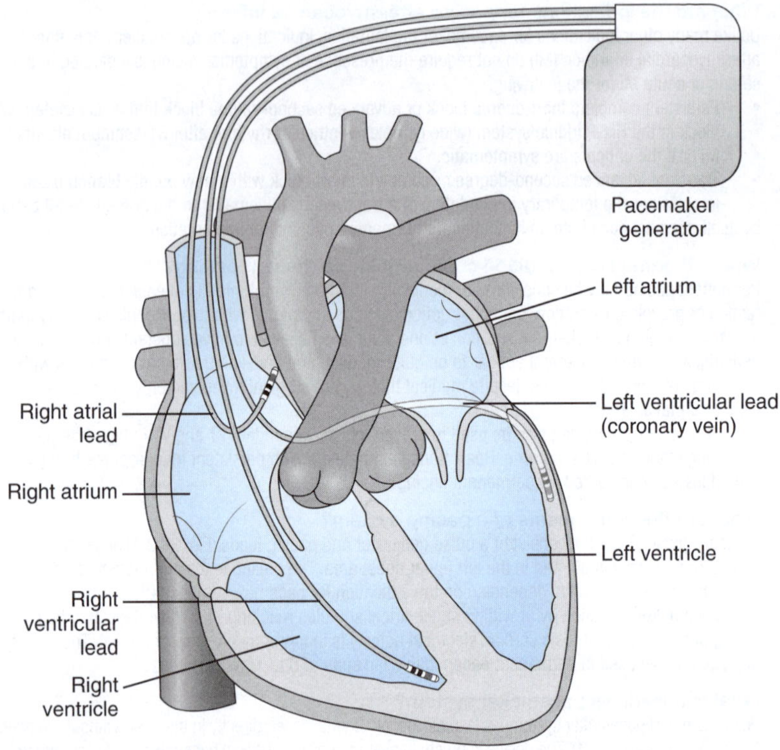

Fig. 38.3. Example of the components of a biventricular pacing system, with pacemaker generator a right atrial lead, a right ventricular lead, and a left ventricular lead. *(Image adopted from Goldberger, A. L. [2006].* Clinical electrocardiography: a simplified approach, *[7th ed.]. Philadelphia, PA: Mosby).*

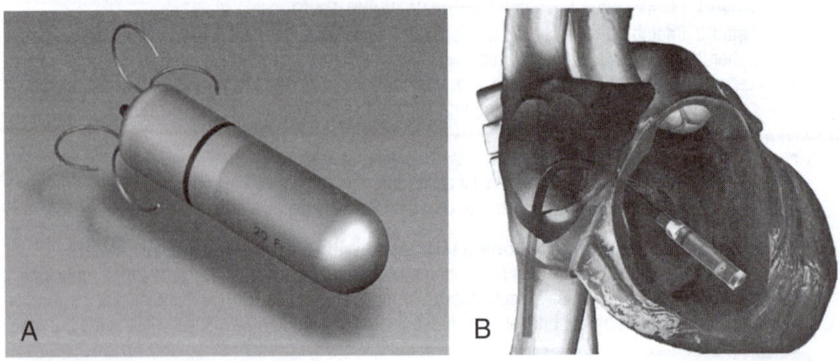

Fig. 38.4. Leadless pacemaker. **A,** Example of a leadless pacemaker. The pacemaker is only approximately 1 inch in length. **B,** Illustration of implantation of the leadless pacemaker. The pacemaker is percutaneously inserted into the right ventricular apex via a femoral venous approach.

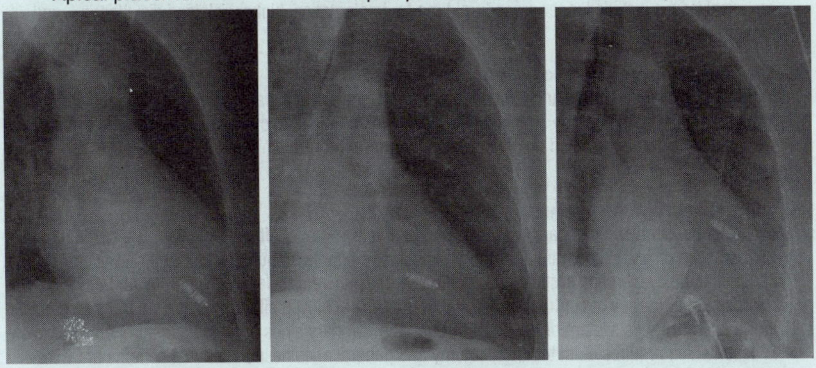

Fig. 38.5. Chest x-rays showing the various positions in the right ventricle that the leadless pacemaker can be implanted. The device can be implanted in the right ventricular apex *(left panel)*, mid septum *(middle panel)*, or right ventricular outflow tract *(right panel)*. *(Image from Ritter, P., Duray G. Z., Steinwender, C., Soejima, K., Omar, R., Mont L., et al. [2015]. Early performance of a miniaturized leadless cardiac pacemaker: the Micra Transcatheter Pacing Study.* European Heart Journal, *36, 2510–2519).*

13. What is pacemaker syndrome?

Historically, *pacemaker syndrome* refers to progressive worsening of symptoms, particularly congestive heart failure, after single-chamber ventricular pacing. This was due to asynchronous ventricular pacing, leading to inappropriately timed atrial contractions, including those occurring during ventricular systole. Dual-chamber pacing and appropriate pacing mode selection prevent the occurrence of pacemaker syndrome.

Pseudopacemaker syndrome occurs when a patient without a pacemaker has PR prolongation so severe that the P waves are closer to the preceding R waves than to the following ones, leading to atrial contractions during the preceding ventricular systole.

14. What is twiddler syndrome?

Twiddler syndrome is a rare complication of pacemaker implantation caused by repetitive and often unintentional twisting of the generator in the pacemaker pocket, producing lead dislodgment or fracture and subsequent pacemaker failure. It is most commonly observed in patients with behavioral disorders.

15. What is pacemaker-mediated tachycardia?

Pacemaker-mediated tachycardia (PMT) is a form of reentrant tachycardia that can occur in patients who have a dual-chamber pacemaker. If the AV node retrogradely conducts a ventricular-paced beat or a premature ventricular contraction (PVC) back to the atrium and depolarizes the atrium before the next atrial-paced beat, this atrial activation will be sensed by the pacemaker atrial lead and interpreted as an intrinsic atrial depolarization. Consecutively, the pacemaker will then pace the ventricle after the programmed AV delay and perpetuate the cycle of ventricular pacing–retrograde ventriculoatrial (VA) conduction–atrial sensing–ventricular pacing (the pacemaker forms the antegrade limb of the circuit, and the AV node is the retrograde limb). Consider PMT in patients with a dual-chamber pacemaker who experience palpitations, rapid heart rates, lightheadedness, syncope, or chest discomfort. It is corrected by programming the pacemaker with a postventricular atrial refractory period (PVARP) so that the pacemaker ignores atrial events occurring shortly after ventricular events.

16. What is permanent para-Hisian pacing?

Permanent para-Hisian pacing is direct His bundle activation by the pacemaker system with subsequent ventricular activation. It is known to prevent desynchronization and negative inotropic effects that can be seen with right ventricular apical pacing. When activated, the His bundle creates a more efficient ventricular activation than conventional pacing (apical pacing). However, this method of pacing requires a normal His and infra-Hisian conduction system.

The presence of a healthy intrinsic conduction system is necessary for para-Hisian pacing. Other technical issues include longer procedural time for implantation, higher risk lead dislodgment, and higher thresholds.

17. Can right ventricular pacing be deleterious?

In patients with left ventricular dysfunction, right ventricular pacing alone can lead to significant intraventricular dyssynchrony, precipitate heart failure, and lead to overall worse outcomes. In such patients, consideration should be given to cardiac resynchronization therapy (CRT). CRT is discussed below.

18. What is cardiac resynchronization therapy?

CRT refers to simultaneous pacing of both the right ventricle and left ventricle (LV). The rationale for CRT is based on the observation that the presence of a bundle branch block or other intraventricular conduction delay worsens systolic heart failure by causing ventricular dyssynchrony and thereby reduces the efficiency of contraction. Pacing of the LV is achieved either by placing a transvenous lead in the lateral venous system of the heart through the coronary sinus or by placement of an epicardial LV lead (which requires a limited thoracotomy and general anesthesia). Potential benefits of CRT include improved contractile function (increase in ejection fraction, increase in cardiac index, and decrease in pulmonary capillary wedge pressure) and reverse ventricular remodeling (reductions in LV end-systolic and end-diastolic dimensions, severity of mitral regurgitation, and LV mass).

19. When is cardiac resynchronization therapy indicated?

CRT is indicated in patients with sinus rhythm being treated with guideline-directed medical therapy who present with symptoms of heart failure (New York Heart Association [NYHA] class II, III, and ambulatory IV), severe left ventricular systolic dysfunction (left ventricular ejection fraction 35% or less), and intraventricular conduction delay (QRS more than 120 ms for LBBB or greater than 150 ms for non-LBBB). CRT is also indicated in patients with an expected high percentage of ventricular pacing (>40%).

CRT can be considered in other patients with wide QRS complex, including those with NYHA class I and those with atrial fibrillation (including those who require AV node ablation of inadequately controlled ventricle response rates).

CRT can be achieved with a device designed only for pacing or can be combined with a defibrillator, because many patients who are candidates for an implantable cardioverter defibrillator [ICD] are also candidates for CRT. CRT has been shown not only to improve quality of life and decrease heart failure symptoms (improvement in NYHA class by one class or increased 6-minute walk distance) but also to reduce mortality.

Indications for CRT are summarized in Table 38.1.

20. Do all patients with dyssynchrony respond to cardiac resynchronization therapy?

Not all patients who undergo CRT have a clinical response to it. The magnitude of response is also different. Those who do derive benefit have a lower mortality, fewer heart failure events, and fewer symptoms than nonresponses. Factors that favor a good response to CRT are female gender, nonischemic cardiomyopathy, LBBB, and wider QRS.

The incidence of nonresponders is approximately 25%. Interestingly though, some who initially do not have a positive response to CRT may manifest symptomatic improvement a year or more after implantation.

21. What is multipoint pacing in cardiac resynchronization therapy?

Despite the improvements seen with standard CRT technology, nonresponders to this therapy remain a significant issue. The addition of *multipoint pacing* to conventional CRT allows more capture of left ventricular tissue by delivering two pacing pulses. Multipoint left ventricular pacing from a quadripolar LV lead has been shown to improve CRT response and decrease the nonresponder rate. Multipoint pacing has been shown to improve LV electrical activation. Reducing LV dyssynchrony, decreasing end-systolic volume, and improving LV function at 3 and 12 months when compared with conventional CRT.

22. What is anodal stimulation?

Anodal stimulation is a phenomenon of activation of the myocardium in proximity to the anode. At the anode the hyperpolarization tissue can trigger depolarization in the surrounding tissue. This phenomenon can be seen as pectoral stimulation with unipolar pacing or right ventricular stimulation when CRT is programed from LV tip electrode (cathode) to right ventricular lead coil ring (anode). Right ventricular anodal stimulation has been associated with decreased CRT response.

Table 38.1. Indications for Cardiac Resynchronization Therapy in Patients with Stage C Heart Failure

Class I (is indicated)
- LVEF <35%, sinus rhythm, LBBB with a QRS ≥150 ms, and NYHA class II, III, or ambulatory IV symptoms on GDMT

Class IIa (is reasonable, can be useful)
- LVEF of 35% or less, sinus rhythm, a non-LBBB pattern with a QRS duration of 150 ms or greater, and NYHA class III/ambulatory class IV symptoms on GDMT
- LVEF ≤35%, sinus rhythm, LBBB with a QRS 120-149 ms, and NYHA class II, III, or ambulatory IV symptoms on GDMT LVEF ≤35%, sinus rhythm, LBBB with a QRS 120-149 ms, and NYHA class II, III, or ambulatory IV symptoms on GDMT
- CRT can be useful in patients with AF and LVEF ≤35% on GDMT if (a) the patient requires ventricular pacing or otherwise meets CRT criteria and (b) AV nodal ablation
- LVEF ≤35% and undergoing new or replacement device implantation with anticipated ventricular pacing (>40%)

Class IIb (may be considered)
- LVEF ≤35%, sinus rhythm, a non-LBBB pattern with a QRS duration of 120-149 ms, and NYHA class III/ambulatory class IV on GDMT
- LVEF ≤35%, sinus rhythm, a non-LBBB pattern with QRS ≥150 ms, and NYHA class II symptoms on GDMT
- LVEF ≤30%, ischemic etiology of HF, sinus rhythm, LBBB with QRS ≥150 ms, and NYHA class I symptoms on GDMT

Class III—no benefit (is not recommended)
- NYHA class I or II symptoms and non-LBBB pattern with QRS <150 ms
- Patients whose comorbidities and/or frailty limit survival to <1 year

AF, Atrial fibrillation; *CRT*, cardiac resynchronization therapy; *GDMT*, guideline-directed medical therapy; *HF*, heart failure; *IV*, intravenous; *LBBB*, left bundle branch block; *LVEF*, left ventricular ejection fraction; *NYHA*, New York Heart Association.

Adapted from Yancy, C. W., Jessup, M., Bozkurt, B., Butler, J., Casey, D. E. Jr., Drazner, M. H., et al. [2013]. ACCF/AHA *guideline for the management of heart failure: a report of the American College of Cardiology Foundation/American Heart Association Task Force on Practice Guidelines.* Journal of the American College of Cardiology, 62, *e147–e239.*

BIBLIOGRAPHY AND SUGGESTED READINGS

Bristow, M. R., Saxon, L. A., Boehmer, J., Krueger, S., Kass, D. A., De Marco, T., et al. (2004). Cardiac-resynchronization therapy with or without an implantable defibrillator in advanced chronic heart failure. *New England Journal of Medicine, 350,* 2140.

Epstein, A. E., Dimarco, J. P., Ellenbogen, K. A., Estes, N. A., 3rd, Freedman, R. A., Gettes, L. S., et al. (2008). ACC/AHA/HRS 2008 guidelines for device-based therapy of cardiac rhythm abnormalities. *Heart Rhythm, 5,* e1–e62.

Epstein, A. E., DiMarco, J. P., Ellenbogen, K. A., Estes, N. A., 3rd, Freedman, R. A., Gettes, L. S., et al. (2013). 2012 ACCF/AHA/HRS focused update incorporated into the ACCF/AHA/HRS 2008 guidelines for device-based therapy of cardiac rhythm abnormalities: a report of the American College of Cardiology Foundation/American Heart Association Task Force on Practice Guidelines and the heart rhythm society. *Journal of the American College of Cardiology, 61,* e6–e75.

Jarcho, J. A. (2005). Resynchronizing ventricular contraction in heart failure. *New England Journal of Medicine, 352,* 1594.

Miller, M. A., Neuzil, P., Dukkipati, S. R., & Reddy, V. Y. (2015). Leadless cardiac pacemakers. *Journal of the American College of Cardiology, 66*(10), 1179–1189. http://dx.doi.org/10.1016/j.jacc.2015.06.1081.

Pappone, C., Calovic, Z., Vicedomini, G., Cuko, A., McSpadden, L. C., Ryu, K., et al. (2015). Improving cardiac resynchronization therapy response with multipoint left ventricular pacing: twelve-month follow up study. *Hearth Rhythm, 12,* 1250–1258.

Yancy, C. W., Jessup, M., Bozkurt, B., Butler, J., Casey, D. E., Jr., Drazner, M. H., et al. (2013). 2013 ACCF/AHA guideline for the management of heart failure: a report of the American College of Cardiology Foundation/American Heart Association Task Force on Practice Guidelines. *Journal of the American College of Cardiology, 62,* e147–e239.

CHAPTER 39

IMPLANTABLE CARDIAC DEFIBRILLATOR

Paul Schurmann, Moises Rodriguez-Manero

1. What are the components of an implantable cardioverter defibrillator?

An implantable cardioverter defibrillator (ICD) is composed of a pulse generator (typically implanted in the left upper chest) and one or more leads. The generator uses lithium-vanadium batteries, which are reliable energy sources with predictable discharge curves. An ICD is able to deliver a charge larger than its battery voltage because of a system of internal capacitors.

Since many patients in whom an ICD is indicated are also candidates for cardiac resynchronization therapy, many current ICDs also have biventricular pacing capabilities (Fig. 39.1).

2. What are the types of implantable cardioverter defibrillators?

There are two types of ICDs:

- Transvenous ICDs (having one or multiple leads, with a transvenous lead attached directly to the heart)
- Subcutaneous ICDs (S-ICDs) (with only one subcutaneous lead)

Transvenous ICDs are commonly used and can work as pacemakers. The transvenous lead contains two distal electrodes (tip and ring) that sense local electrical signals or are paced. The right ventricular lead is essential for defibrillators, but additional leads may be used for atrial and biventricular pacing.

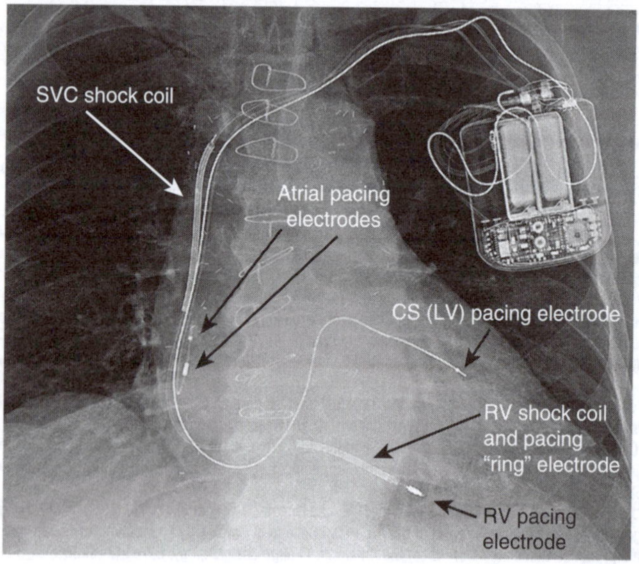

Fig. 39.1. A radiograph of a patient with an implantable cardioverter defibrillator (ICD). With this ICD, shock coils are present in both the right ventricle (RV) and the superior vena cava (SVC). There is also a coronary sinus (CS) lead present for biventricular pacing. *LV,* left ventricle. *(From Miller, R., Eriksson, L., Fleisher, L., Wiener-Kronish, J. P., Cohen, N. H., & Young, W. L. [2009].* Miller's anesthesia *[7th ed.].* Philadelphia, PA: Churchill Livingstone.)

The right ventricular lead differs from a pacemaker owing to its ability to deliver high-energy shocks. ICDs may contain one or two coils (located in the right ventricle and the superior vena cava) specifically designed to create a circuit to capture most of the myocardium with a high-energy shock.

3. How does the implantable cardioverter defibrillator work?

The ICD is always sensing the electrical signals of the heart and processes them to classify the rhythm. The arrhythmia criteria are met by counting intervals between successive electrograms. If the detected arrhythmia meets the criteria for ventricular tachycardia (VT), the ICD often first tries to restore a normal rhythm by pacing the ventricle faster than the intrinsic rhythm, which is known as antitachycardia pacing (ATP). If the VT is not terminated with ATP, the ICD sends a high-energy shock to the heart to restore a normal rhythm. The device then goes back to its watchful mode.

The criteria to detect arrhythmia and therapies can be reprogrammed based on the patient's clinical needs. The criteria for arrhythmia are based on beat-to-beat intervals and usually consist of three zones: a monitor zone, a VT zone, and a ventricular fibrillation (VF) zone. The monitor zone usually captures the slowest arrhythmia of all three zones. Tachycardia is only recorded and no therapies are delivered. Shorter RR intervals in the arrhythmia would fall in the VT zone and even shorter RR intervals (corresponding to faster heart rates) in the VF zone.

Once the arrhythmia is classified into a zone, algorithms can often distinguish whether the rhythm is more likely to be VT, atrial fibrillation with rapid ventricular response, or another supraventricular rhythm (or sinus tachycardia). Criteria used by the algorithms to distinguish VT from supraventricular tachycardia (SVT, or sinus tachycardia) include abrupt versus gradual tachycardia onset, regularity or irregularity of the rhythm, QRS morphology, and QRS vector (Fig. 39.2). If the ICD algorithms determine that the rhythm is ventricular in origin, the programmed therapy for the selected zone will be delivered. Once therapy is delivered, the ICD monitors the following intervals to redetect sinus rate (which means the therapy was successful) or redetect the arrhythmia (which results in additional therapy).

4. How does implantable cardioverter defibrillator therapy improve survival?

ICD therapy, compared with conventional or traditional antiarrhythmic drug therapy, has been associated with reductions in mortality of 23% to 55%, with the improvement in survival due almost exclusively to a reduction in sudden cardiac death (SCD). ICD defibrillation can terminate VT, torsades de pointes, and VF (Figs. 39.3 and 39.4).

Trials of ICDs are categorized into two types:

- *Primary prevention trials*, in which the subjects have not experienced life-threatening sustained VT, VF, or resuscitated cardiac arrest but are at risk Table 39.1
- *Secondary prevention trials*, involving subjects who have had an abortive cardiac arrest, a life-threatening VT, or VT as the cause of syncope

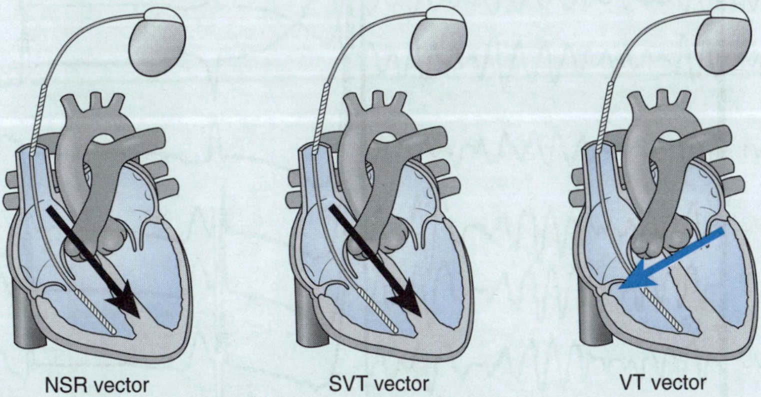

Fig. 39.2. Demonstration of an ICD rhythm-discrimination algorithm based on the vector of the QRS complex. Black arrow are the QRS vector of Normal sinus rhythm and SVT. Blue arrow shows the difference vector from *VT. NSR*, normal sinus rhythm; *SVT*, supraventricular; *VT*, ventricular. *(Image from Seifert M. Tachycardia discrimination algorithms in ICDs. In D. Erkapic & T. Bauernfeind [Eds.],* Cardiac defibrillation. Heart. *2007 Nov; 93(11): 1478–1483. doi: 10.1136/hrt.2006.095190intechweb.org.)*

5. What are the current class I indications for implantable cardioverter defibrillator implantation for primary prevention of sudden cardiac death?

Assuming that patients are receiving guideline-directed medical therapy and have a reasonable expectation of survival with good functional status for more than 1 year, class I indications are as follows:

- Patients with left ventricular (LV) ejection fraction (LVEF) less than 35% as a result of prior myocardial infarction (MI) who are at least 40 days post MI and are in New York Heart Association (NYHA) functional class II or III

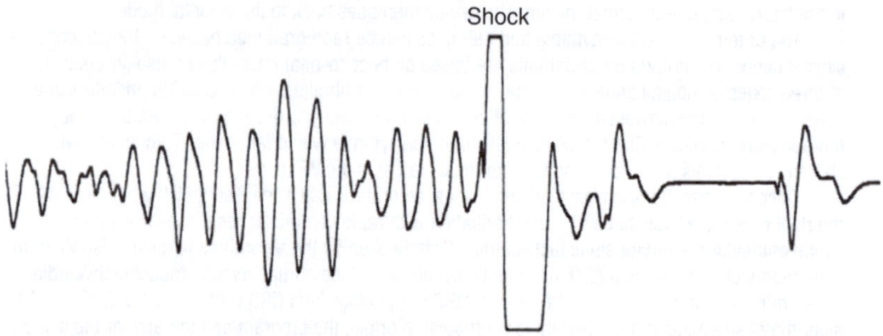

Fig. 39.3. Example of successful ICD shock in a patient with torsades de pointes. *(Image from Rosenheck, S. Defibrillation shock amplitude, location and timing. In J. J. Harris [Ed.],* Cardiac defibrillation—prediction, prevention and management of cardiovascular arrhythmic events. *intechweb.org.)*

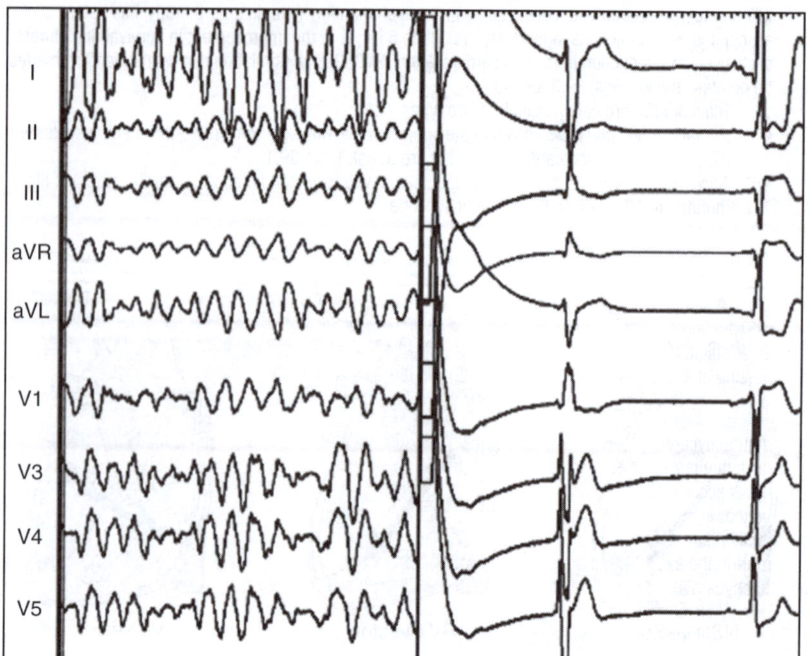

Fig. 39.4. An example of ICD termination of ventricular fibrillation with an appropriately delivered shock. *(Image from Rosenheck, S. Defibrillation shock amplitude, location and timing. In J. J. Harris [Ed.],* Cardiac defibrillation—prediction, prevention and management of cardiovascular arrhythmic events. *intechweb.org.)*

- Patients with LV dysfunction as a result of prior MI who are at least 40 days post MI, have an LVEF less than 30%, and are in NYHA functional class I
- Patients with nonischemic dilated cardiomyopathy (DCM) who have an LVEF of 35% or less and are in NYHA functional class II or III
- Patients with nonsustained VT as a result of prior MI, LVEF less than 40%, and inducible VF or sustained VT at electrophysiologic study

6. What are the current class I indications for implantable cardioverter defibrillator implantation for secondary prevention of sudden cardiac death?

ICDs are indicated for secondary prevention of SCD in patients who

- Survive sudden cardiac arrest without completely reversible causes
- Have structural heart disease with spontaneous sustained VT
- Have syncope of unexplained etiology with clinically relevant inducible sustained VT or VF on electrophysiologic study

7. What other special populations may benefit from implantable cardioverter defibrillator therapy?

ICD implantation is performed in other patient populations and those at high risk for SCD including patients with

- Hypertrophic cardiomyopathy (HCM) with one or more risk factors for SCD (VF, VT, family history of SCD, unexplained syncope, LV thickness 30 mm or more, abnormal blood pressure response to exercise)
- Brugada syndrome with a history of previous cardiac arrest, documented sustained VT, or unexplained syncope
- Nonhospitalized patients awaiting transplantation
- Noncompaction of the left ventricle
- Long and short QT syndromes with previous cardiac arrest or unexplained syncope
- Catecholaminergic polymorphic VT who have syncope and/or VT while receiving beta-blockers
- Arrhythmogenic right ventricular dysplasia/cardiomyopathy who have one or more risk factors for SCD
- Infiltrative cardiomyopathies such as sarcoidosis, amyloidosis, Fabry disease, hemochromatosis, giant cell myocarditis, or Chagas disease
- Certain muscular dystrophies

8. What is defibrillator threshold testing?

The defibrillation threshold (DFT) is defined as the amount of energy required to reliably defibrillate the heart during an arrhythmia. During implant, the electrophysiologist may elect to perform DFT testing, in which VF is induced, detected, and then terminated by the device with a high-energy shock to find the reliable level of energy needed to achieve defibrillation. Defibrillation efficacy has traditionally been initiated with successive DFT attempts using approximately 20 J in a device that delivered 25 to 30 J. A safety margin of 10 J was required for the implantation of the earliest defibrillators. Because DFT testing involves inducing potentially fatal VF several times, it requires deep conscious sedation. In addition, lack of evidence for routine use has led some electrophysiologists to stop performing DFT testing at implantation and instead to program the device to the highest output settings.

9. What is antitachycardia pacing?

Antitachycardia pacing (ATP) has long been recognized as a way to pace-terminate certain types of arrhythmias, particularly slow monomorphic VT involving a reentry circuit. The idea is to deliver a few seconds of pacing stimuli to the heart at a rate faster than the tachycardia. The basic principle is that in most reentrant circuits there is an excitable gap—that is, a time between successive activations when the myocardium is available to respond to excitations. Pacing in a reentrant circuit during the excitable gap introduces new activation wavefronts that collide with one of the preexisting tachycardias and can terminate it. Advantages offered by ATP include the following:

- ATP is not painful (sometimes barely noticed by some patients).
- ATP may reduce battery drainage by terminating the arrhythmia without the need for shocks.
- ATP is an easily programmable feature on most ICDs.

On the other hand, ATP has potential disadvantages. If ineffective, it can delay defibrillation therapies and prolong the time during which the patient is in tachycardia, which may lead to syncope. ATP can also accelerate VT into faster rhythms and even VF.

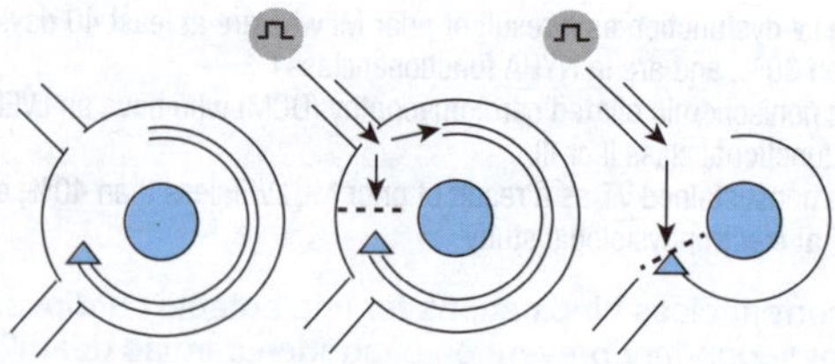

Fig. 39.5. Schematic example of how antitachycardia pacing (overdrive pacing) disrupts the reentrant circuit in the ventricle, terminating the arrhythmia.

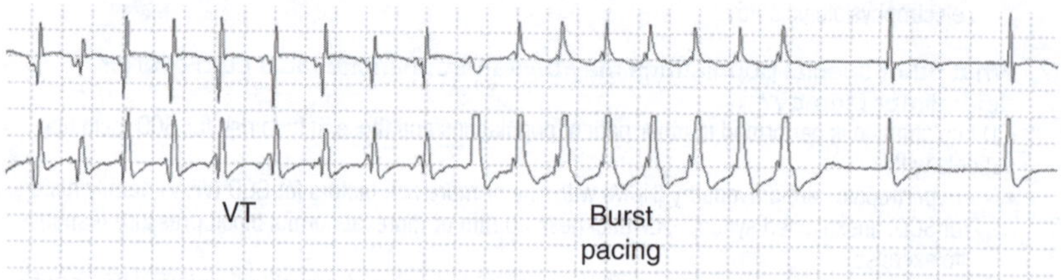

Fig. 39.6. Intracardiac tracing showing burst pacing (overdrive pacing or antitachycardia pacing) terminating an episode of ventricular tachycardia. *(Image from Raatikainen, M. J. P., & Koivisto, U. M. Remote monitoring of implantable cardioverter-defibrillator therapy. In N. Trayanova [Ed.],* Cardiac defibrillation—mechanisms, challenges and implications. *intechweb.org.)*

For this reason ATP is mostly used in patients who remain stable and asymptomatic during episodes of slow VT, generally below 200 beats per minute. However, more aggressive ATP programming has been shown to decrease ICD shocks, and newer ICDs incorporate ATP while charging for a shock. A schematic example of ATP is shown in Fig. 39.5. An actual intracardiac tracing showing burst pacing terminating VT is shown in Fig. 39.6.

10. How common are inappropriate shocks in patients with implantable cardioverter defibrillators?

Inappropriate shocks occur when a device delivers therapy for a fast supraventricular rhythm or for abnormal sensing in the ventricle. They occur in up to 11% of patients with ICDs and can constitute up to a third of all shock episodes a patient experiences. The most common rhythm triggering an inappropriate shock is atrial fibrillation with rapid ventricular response. Other inappropriate shocks can result from other SVTs, including sinus tachycardia. Smoking, atrial fibrillation, diastolic hypertension, young age, nonischemic cardiomyopathy, and prior appropriate shocks increase the chance of receiving an inappropriate shock.

Inappropriate shock can also result from what is called ventricular oversensing by the ICD. One example of this is when the ICD mistakes the T waves for QRS complexes, so that the ICD mistakenly calculates the ventricular rate at twice the actual rate. T-wave oversensing remains the most frequent cause of ventricular oversensing and has been reported in up to 14% of patients with ICDs. Ventricular oversensing is associated with increased mortality in patients with ICDs and has important psychological effects in this population. ICD programming options can be used to reduce oversensing.

11. What is a subcutaneous defibrillator?

A totally subcutaneous defibrillator (S-ICD) is a recently developed device that is capable of providing the same proven defibrillation protection as a transvenous ICD but without the complications associated with the presence of transvenous endocardial leads. The S-ICD electrode is implanted in the parasternal area in the subcutaneous space and then connected to an active high voltage can (Fig. 39.7). Defibrillation is delivered between the coil on the electrode and the active can. Sensing is accomplished using both or either of the proximal and distal ring electrodes and the electrically conductive pulse generator enclosure. An S-ICD eliminates problems such as failure to achieve vascular access, intravascular injury, or intracardiac injury and makes it possible to avoid radiation

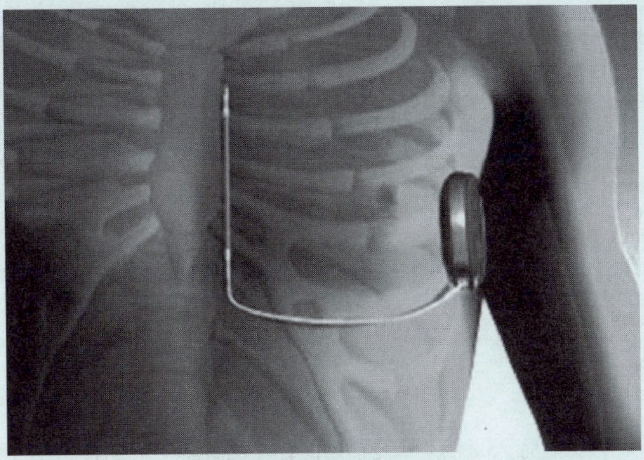

Fig. 39.7. A subcutaneous ICD.

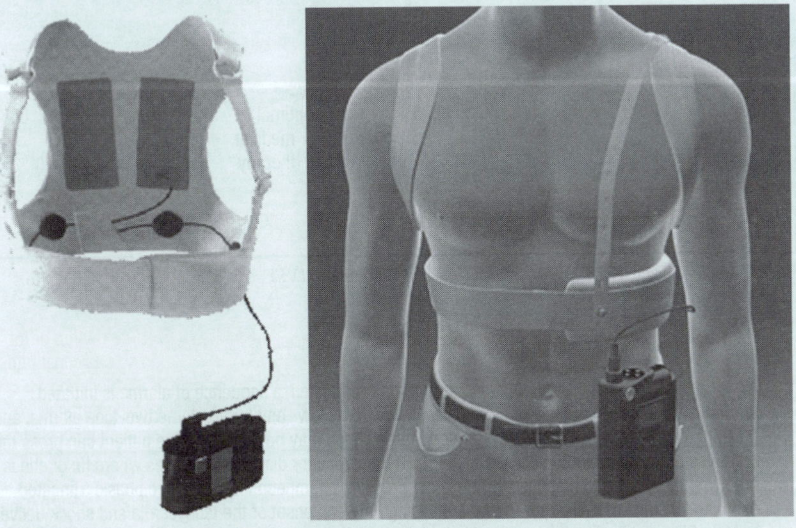

Fig. 39.8. A wearable ICD.

exposure. The disadvantage of the S-ICD is the limited pacing capability up to 30 seconds after a shock at a rate of 50 beats per minute and the lack of ATP.

12. What is a wearable implantable cardioverter defibrillator?

A wearable ICD system (also referred to as a LifeVest) is a vest-like system worn by the patient that can deliver defibrillation (Fig. 39.8). The wearable ICD has three defibrillation and four electrocardiographic (ECG) sensing electrodes fitted within a garment worn by the patient. The defibrillation electrodes are self-gelling, and the ECG electrodes are nonadhesive dry tantalum oxide capacitive electrodes. The defibrillator unit is carried on a waist belt. Two ECG channels can be monitored with the two pairs of ECG electrodes from front-to-back and right-to-left lead sets. Microampere alternating current is used to check electrode contacts, as in conventional monitoring systems.

Table 39.1. Primary prevention for sudden cardiac death with implantable cardiac defibrillator

TRIAL	# OF PTS	AGE (YEARS)	LVEF (%)	FOLLOW-UP (MONTHS)	CONTROL THERAPY	Mortality (%) CONTROL	ICD	P
MUSTT (Multicentre unstable tachycardia trial)	704	67 + 12	30	39	No EP-guided therapy	48	24	.06
MADIT (Multicentre automatic defibrillator implantation Trial)	196	63 + 9	26	27	Conventional	38.6	15.7	.009
DEFINITE (Defibrillators in non-ischemic cardiomyopathy treatment evaluation)	458	58	21	29.0 + 14.4	Optimal medical therapy	14.1	7.9	.08
ACD-HeFT (Sudden cardiac death in heart failure)	2521	60.1	25	45.5	Optimal medical therapy	36.1	28.9	.007

EP, Electrophysiologic; *ICD*, implantable cardioverter defibrillator; *LVEF*, left ventricular ejection fraction.

Once the programmed detection parameters are fulfilled, a sequence of alarms is initiated, starting with vibration in the belt electronics, followed by low- and high-volume two-tone alarms, and finishing with a voice warning to bystanders that a shock may be delivered. The patient can press the response buttons within 20 seconds to withhold the capacitor discharge in cases where he or she is not symptomatic. If the response button is not pressed, an impedance-adapted biphasic truncated exponential shock is delivered. The time elapsing between onset of the tachycardia and shock delivery is 45 to 55 seconds. The LifeVest is able to deliver up to five successive shocks in case the arrhythmia continues after the first shock.

At present no study has convincingly demonstrated that utilization of a wearable ICD reduces mortality. Nevertheless there are certain situations in which some practitioners consider the use of prophylaxis with this device. An American Heart Association (AHA) scientific advisory concluded that the use of a wearable ICD is reasonable when there is a clear indication for an implanted permanent device but a transient contraindication to implantation and that use of these devices might be reasonable in patients at risk for SCD but in whom ventricular function may improve after medical therapy or revascularization.

Bibliography and Suggested Readings

Bardy, G. H., Lee, K. L., Mark, D. B., Poole, J. E., Packer, D. L., Boineau, R., et al. (2005). Amiodarone or an implantable cardioverter-defibrillator for congestive heart failure. *New England Journal of Medicine, 352*, 225–237.

Bardy, G. H., Smith, W. M., Hood, M. A., Crozier, I. G., Melton, I. C., Jordaens, L., et al. (2010). An entirely subcutaneous implantable cardioverter-defibrillator. *New England Journal of Medicine, 363*, 36–44.

Daubert, J. P., Zareba, W., Cannom, D. S., McNitt, S., Rosero, S. Z., Wang, P., et al. (2008). Inappropriate implantable cardioverter-defibrillators shocks in the MADIT II study: frequency, mechanisms, predictors, and survival impact. *Journal of the American College of Cardiology*, *51*, 1357–1365.

DiMarco, J. P. (2003). Implantable cardioverter-defibrillators. *New England Journal of Medicine*, *349*, 1836–1847.

Epstein, A. E., DiMarco, J. P., Ellenbogen, K. A., Mark Estes, N. A., Freedman, R. A., Gettes, L. S., et al. (2008). ACC/AHA/HRS 2008 guidelines for device-based therapy of cardiac rhythm abnormalities: executive summary: a report of the American College of Cardiology/American Heart Association Task Force on Practice Guidelines (Writing Committee to Revise the ACC/AHA/NASPE 2002 Guideline Update for Implantation of Cardiac Pacemakers and Antiarrhythmia Devices). *Journal of the American College of Cardiology*, *51*, 2085–2105.

Hohnloser, S. H., Kuck, K. H., Dorian, P., Roberts, R. S., Hampton, J. R., Hatala, R., et al. (2004). Prophylactic use of an implantable cardioverter-defibrillator after acute myocardial infarction. *New England Journal of Medicine*, *351*, 2481–2488.

Kadish, A., Dyer, A., Daubert, J. P., Quigg, R., Estes, N. A., Anderson, K. P., et al. (2004). Prophylactic defibrillator implantation in patients with nonischemic dilated cardiomyopathy. *New England Journal of Medicine*, *350*, 2151–2158.

Moss, A. J., Zareba, W., Hall, W. J., Klein, H., Wilber, D. J., Cannom, D. S., et al. (2002). Prophylactic implantation of a defibrillator in patients with myocardial infarction and reduced ejection fraction. *New England Journal of Medicine*, *346*, 877–883.

Piccini, J. P., Sr., Allen, L. A., Kudenchuk, P. J., Page, R. L., Patel, M. R., & Turakhia, M. P. (2016). Wearable cardioverter-defibrillator therapy for the prevention of sudden cardiac death: a science advisory from the American Heart Association. *Circulation*, *133*, 1715–1727. http://dx.doi.org/10.1161/CIR.0000000000000394.

CHAPTER 40

CARDIAC ARREST AND RESUSCITATION

Vu Hoang, Glenn N. Levine

1. **Why was the airway, breathing, compression ("ABC") sequence of cardiopulmonary resuscitation changed to compression, airway, breathing?**
According to American Heart Association (AHA) guidelines for cardiopulmonary resuscitation (CPR) and emergency cardiovascular care (ECC), chest compressions were often delayed while the rescuer opened the airway to give mouth-to-mouth breaths, retrieved a barrier device, or gathered and assembled ventilation equipment. Starting the resuscitation sequence with chest compressions will reduce delay to first chest compression.

2. **What factors constitute "high-quality cardiopulmonary resuscitation"?**
Components of high-quality CPR are given below and summarized in Table 40.1.
    - Chest compressions should be at a rate between 100 and 120 times per minute.
    - Depth of chest compressions for adults is at least 2 inches but not more than 2.4 inches (6 cm); for children compressions of 2 inches (5 cm); and for infants compressions of 1.5 inches (4 cm).
    - Allowing for complete chest recoil after each compression
    - Minimizing interruptions in chest compressions
    - Avoiding excessive ventilation

3. **What is the first step to do if you are alone and come across an unresponsive adult victim with no signs of breathing?**
Activate an emergency response system, get an automated external defibrillator (AED) if available in the area, and then return to the victim. If you return with an AED, turn it on and follow the prompt. If no AED is available, check for a pulse and begin CPR until emergency medical services (EMS) arrives to take over. These steps are summarized in Fig. 40.1.

4. **In patients with respiratory arrest (with a perfusing rhythm), how often are breaths delivered?**
For respiratory arrest with a perfusion cardiac rhythm, breaths should be delivered every 6 seconds, for a total of 10 breaths per minute.

5. **What is the most common cause of airway obstruction in the unconscious adult patient?**
In adults the most common cause of airway obstruction in an unconscious patient is loss of tone in the throat muscles, leading to airway occlusion by the tongue. This may be treated by head tilt–chin lift, jaw thrust, or insertion of an oropharyngeal airway.

6. **How many joules (J) are indicated for the treatment of ventricular fibrillation or pulseless ventricular tachycardia when using a biphasic defibrillator?**
Biphasic defibrillators are now used at most institutions, replacing the older monophasic defibrillators. The number of joules will often be device specific, ranging from 120 to 200 J. If the appropriate setting is unknown, use 200 J. Additional shocks should be equivalent or higher. This is in contrast to the older monophasic defibrillators, in which 360 J is recommended.

7. **In order, what are the preferred routes of drug administration?**
    - Intravenous (IV) is the preferred route of drug administration. The guidelines emphasize that resuscitation attempts should not be delayed by trying to achieve central IV access when peripheral IV access can be easily achieved.
    - When IV access is not possible, intraosseous (IO) is preferred over endotracheal (ET). IO can be used in both children and adults.

Table 40.1. Summary of High-Quality Cardiopulmonary Resuscitation Components for BLS Providers

COMPONENT	ADULTS AND ADOLESCENTS	CHILDREN (AGE 1 YEAR TO PUBERTY)	INFANTS (AGE LESS THAN 1 YEAR, EXCLUDING NEWBORNS)
Scene safety	Make sure the environment is safe for rescuers and victims		
Recognition of cardiac arrest	Check for responsiveness No breathing only gasping (i.e., no normal breathing) No definite pulse felt within 10 s Breathing and pulse checks can be performed simultaneously in less than 10 s		
Activation of emergency response system	If you are alone with no mobile phone, leave the victim to activate the emergency response system and get the AED before beginning CPR Otherwise, send someone and begin CPR immediately; use the AED as soon as it is available	**Witnessed collapse** Follow steps for adults and adolescents on the left **Unwitnessed collapse** Give 2 min of CPR Leave the victim to activate the emergency response system and get the AED Return to the child or infant and resume CPR; use the AED as soon as it is available	
Compression ventilation ratio without advanced airway	**1 or 2 rescuers** 30:2	**1 rescuer** 30:2 **2 or more rescuers** 15:2	
Compression ventilation ratio with advanced airway	Continuous compressions at a rate of 100-120 min Give 1 breath every 6 s (10 breaths/min)		
Compression rate	100-120/min		
Compression depth	At least 2 inches (5 cm)	At least one-third AP diameter of chest Approximately 2 inches (5 cm)	At least one-third AP diameter of chest Approximately 1.5 inches (2 cm)
Hand placement	2 hands on the lower half of the breastbone (sternum)	2 hands or 1 hand (optional for very small child) on the lower half of the breastbone (sternum)	**1 rescuer** 2 fingers in the center of the chest, just below the nipple line **2 or more rescuers** 2 thumb-encircling hands in the center of the chest, just below the nipple line

Continued on following page

Table 40.1. Summary of High-Quality Cardiopulmonary Resuscitation Components for BLS Providers *(Continued)*

COMPONENT	ADULTS AND ADOLESCENTS	CHILDREN (AGE 1 YEAR TO PUBERTY)	INFANTS (AGE LESS THAN 1 YEAR, EXCLUDING NEWBORNS)
Chest recoil	Allow full recoil of the chest after each compression; do not lean on the chest after each compression		
Minimizing interruptions	Limit interruptions in chest compressions to less than 10 s		

AED, Automated external defibrillator; *AP*, anteroposterior; *BLS*, Basic Life Support; *CPR*, cardiopulmonary resuscitation.

*Compression depth should be no more than 2.4 inches (6 cm).

Adapted with permission from AHA Guidelines Update for CPR and ECC. <https://eccguidelines.heart.org/wp-content/uploads/2015/10/2015-AHA-Guidelines-Highlights-English.pdf>.

- Absorption of drugs given via the ET route is considered to be less reliable and predictable. In addition, the optimal dose of most drugs given via the ET route is unknown; the typical dose of drugs administered via the ET route is reported to be 2 to 2.5 times the IV route. Drugs delivered via the ET route should be diluted in 5 to 10 mL of water or normal saline. Advanced cardiac life support (ACLS) drugs that can be given via the ET route are naloxone, atropine, epinephrine, and lidocaine (NAVEL).

8. What are the two most important components of resuscitation for cardiac arrest?

High-quality CPR and rapid defibrillation. Guidelines emphasize that high-quality CPR is critical for cerebral perfusion and to increase the chances of successful defibrillation and resuscitation. Defibrillation should be performed as soon as possible. Defibrillation is followed by 2-minute rounds of CPR and then reassessment of the rhythm and pulse (not immediate assessment after defibrillation of the rhythm and pulse). The ACLS Adult Cardiac Arrest Algorithm is given in Fig. 40.2.

9. In a patient with ventricular fibrillation or pulseless ventricular tachycardia, after the first unsuccessful shock, which two drugs should be considered?

- Epinephrine 1 mg IV/IO is the traditional medication to be considered. Additional similar doses of epinephrine can be administered every 3 to 5 minutes. If ET administration is necessary, the suggested dose is epinephrine 1:1000, 2 to 2.5 mg diluted in 5 to 10 mL or water or normal saline, injected directly into the ET tube. Although a mainstay of the American Heart Association's ACLS VT/VF algorithm, it is acknowledged that there are actually very few data to support the use of epinephrine in this situation.
- The 2015 resuscitation guidelines concluded that the treatment strategy of vasopressin and/or epinephrine offered no advantage over epinephrine alone. For the purpose of simplicity, the 2015 guideline update eliminated vasopressin from the adult cardiac arrest algorithm.

10. After several unsuccessful shocks, and treatment with epinephrine, what other drugs (and their doses) should be considered?

Amiodarone (or lidocaine if amiodarone is not available) should be considered. No antiarrhythmic has ever actually been shown to improve survival to hospital discharge, although amiodarone has been shown to increase rates of survival to hospital admission.

- The dose of amiodarone is 300 mg IV/IO once, with consideration of a subsequent 150 mg IV/IO if indicated, 3 to 5 minutes after the first 300-mg dose.
- The dose of lidocaine is 1 to 1.5 mg/kg IV/IO, with subsequent doses of 0.5 to 0.75 mg/kg IV/IO given over 5- to 10-minute intervals, to a maximum total lidocaine dose of 3 mg/kg. The suggested ET dose of lidocaine is 2 to 4 mg/kg.

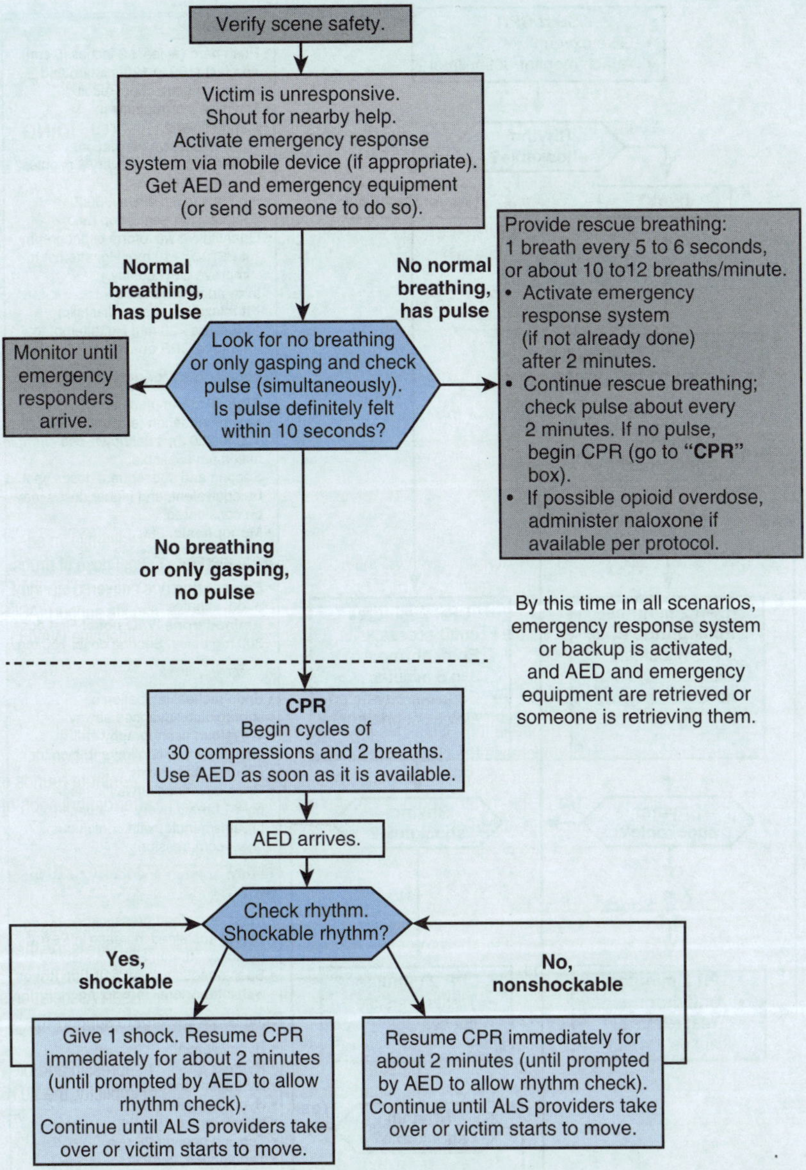

Fig. 40.1. The BLS Healthcare Provider Adult Cardiac Arrest Algorithm. *AED,* Automated external defibrillator; *ALS,* advances life support; *CPR,* cardiopulmonary resuscitation. *(Reprinted with permission from* 2015 Highlights of the AHA Guidelines Update for CPR and ECC. <https://eccguidelines.heart.org/wp-content/uploads/2015/10/2015-AHA-Guidelines-Highlights-English.pdf>.*)*

11. If the patient is in torsades de pointes, in addition to defibrillation, what medication can be considered?

Magnesium, administered as a dose of 1 to 2 g IV/IO, can be given. It is recommended that it be diluted in 10 mL of 5% dextrose in water (D_5W) and administered over 5 to 20 minutes.

The readers should be aware that, although it is commonly taught and present in algorithms that the treatment of this arrhythmia is magnesium, such infusion usually takes many minutes. Thus,

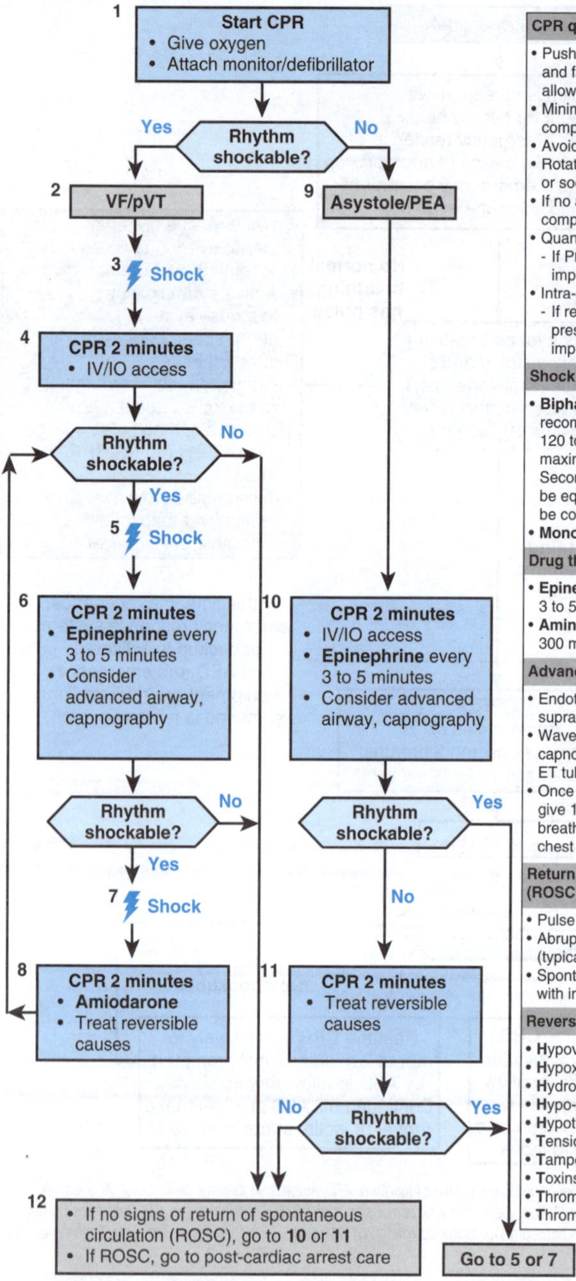

CPR quality

- Push hard (at least 2 inches [5 cm]) and fast (100 to 120/minute) and allow complete chest recoil.
- Minimize interruptions in compressions.
- Avoid excessive ventilation.
- Rotate compressor every 2 minutes, or sooner if fatigued.
- If no advanced airway, 30:2 compression-ventilation ratio.
- Quantitative waveform capnography
  - If P_{ETCO_2} <10 mm Hg, attempt to improve CPR quality.
- Intra-arterial pressure
  - If relaxation phase (diastolic) pressure <20 mm Hg, attempt to improve CPR quality.

Shock energy for defibrillation

- **Biphasic:** Manufacturer recommendation (e.g. initial dose of 120 to 200 J); if unknown, use maximum available.
  Second and subsequent doses should be equivalent, and higher doses may be considered.
- **Monophasic:** 360 J

Drug therapy

- **Epinephrine IV/IO dose:** 1 mg every 3 to 5 minutes
- **Aminodarone IV/IO dose:** First dose: 300 mg bolus. Second dose: 150 mg.

Advanced airway

- Endotracheal intubation or supraglottic advanced airway
- Waveform capnography or capnometry to confirm and monitor ET tube placement
- Once advanced airway in place, give 1 breath every 6 seconds (10 breaths/minute) with continuous chest compressions

Return of spontaneous circulation (ROSC)

- Pulse and blood pressure
- Abrupt sustained increase in P_{ETCO_2} (typically 40 mm Hg)
- Spontaneous arterial pressure waves with intra-arterial monitoring

Reversible causes

- Hypovolemia
- Hypoxia
- Hydrogen ion (acidosis)
- Hypo-/hyperkalemia
- Hypothermia
- Tension pneumothorax
- Tamponade, cardiac
- Toxins
- Thrombosis, pulmonary
- Thrombosis, coronary

Fig. 40.2. Algorithm for the treatment of patients with cardiac arrest. *ROSC*, Returns of spontaneous circulation. *CPR*, Cardiopulmonary resuscitation; *ET*, endotracheal; *IO*, intraosseous; *IV*, intravenous; *PEA*, pulseless electrical activity; *pVT*, pulseless ventricular tachycardia; *ROSC*, return of spontaneous circulation; *VF*, ventricular fibrillation. *(Reprinted with permission from Link, M. S., Berkow, L. C., Kudenchuk, P. J., Halperin, H. R., Hess, E. P., Moitra, V. K., et al. [2015]. Part 7: adult advanced cardiovascular life support: 2015 American Heart Association Guidelines Update for Cardiopulmonary Resuscitation and Emergency Cardiovascular Care.* Circulation, *132[Suppl 2]:S444–S464).*

Table 40.2. Potentially Treatable Causes of Pulseless Electrical Activity

H's	T's
Hypovolemia	Toxins
Hypoxia	Tamponade (cardiac)
Hydrogen ion (acidosis)	Tension pneumothorax
Hyperkalemia/hypokalemia	Thrombosis (coronary and pulmonary)
Hypoglycemia	Trauma
Hypothermia	

Adapted from Advanced Cardiovascular Life Support Provider Manual. Modified from Sinz, E., Navarro, K., Soderberg, E. S., Callaway, C. W.; American Heart Association. (2011). Advanced cardiovascular life support provider manual. *Dallas, TX: American Heart Association.*

given that patients are almost always hemodynamically unstable or pulseless, prompt defibrillation is usually indicated.

12. After administering a drug via a peripheral intravenous line, what steps should be taken to promote delivery of the drug to the central circulation?

After administering a drug via a peripheral IV line, a 20-mL bolus of IV fluid should be administered, and the extremity should be elevated for 10 to 20 seconds.

13. Can one shock a hypothermic patient who is in ventricular fibrillation/ventricular tachycardia?

Yes, with caveats. For the hypothermic patient (temperature less than 30°C [86°F]) in VF/VT, a single defibrillation is deemed appropriate.

14. If a person who was in ventricular fibrillation/ventricular tachycardia is successfully defibrillated, assuming he or she has not already received any amiodarone, what is the dosing of amiodarone if this is to be started to prevent further ventricular fibrillation/ventricular tachycardia?

The following regimen is what is given in the ACLS booklet and is the "classic" loading of amiodarone. An initial "bolus" of 150 mg IV is given over 10 minutes. This is followed by an infusion of 1 mg/minute for 6 hours (total 360 mg) and then an infusion of 0.5 mg/minute over the next 18 hours (540 mg).

15. What are the treatable causes of pulseless electrical activity?

Because pulseless electrical activity (PEA) has such a poor prognosis unless a reversible cause of the rhythm is quickly identified and addressed, it is important to commit to memory the treatable causes of PEA. The *Hs* and *Ts* of PEA are given in Table 40.2. Hypovolemia and hypoxemia are reported to be the two most common and easily reversible causes of PEA.

16. What drugs can be considered in a patient with pulseless electrical activity?

Epinephrine can be used, as described earlier for the treatment of VF/VT, although known vasopressor has been shown to increase survival in PEA. Atropine is no longer recommended for asystole or PEA.

17. In bradycardic patients, such as those with heart block, what are the primary treatments if they are symptomatic and suffering from poor perfusion?

The immediate use of transcutaneous pacing is now emphasized for patients with symptomatic bradycardia. Although preparations are being made for transcutaneous pacing, the following pharmaceutical interventions should be considered:

- Atropine 0.5 mg IV: This may be repeated every 3 to 5 minutes to a total dose of 3 mg. The use of atropine should not be relied on in patients with Mobitz II second-degree atrioventricular (AV) block or third-degree (complete) AV block. Some have considered the use of atropine in Mobitz II or third-degree heart block ("infra-Hisian" heart block) contraindicated, although this is not explicitly stated in the latest ACLS guidelines.
- Epinephrine 2 to 10 μg/minute
- Dopamine 2 to 10 μg/kg per minute

18. Is transcutaneous pacing recommended for the treatment of a patient in asystole?

As noted in the ACLS algorithm, several randomized controlled trials have failed to show benefit from attempted transcutaneous pacing in patients in asystole. Thus it is not currently recommended in this situation.

19. In a *symptomatic yet stable* patient with a regular narrow complex tachyarrhythmia, what drug is recommended as a first-line agent?

Adenosine has become the drug of choice for a *symptomatic yet stable* patient with a narrow complex tachyarrhythmia. The distinction between *stable* and *unstable* is subjective, but the symptomatic yet stable patient might be described as one who is slightly lightheaded (systolic blood pressure [SBP] of approximately 80 mm Hg) or having mild shortness of breath or chest discomfort. Patients experiencing more severe symptoms would be those with altered mentation because of low blood pressure or moderate to severe shortness of breath or chest discomfort. Note that although adenosine, which blocks AV conduction, may terminate some narrow complex tachycardias, such as AV nodal reentrant tachycardia (AVNRT) or AV reentrant tachycardia (AVRT), it will not terminate rhythms, such as atrial flutter or atrial tachycardia (although it may lead to a transient decrease in conduction through the AV node and slower ventricular response rate, allowing identification of the rhythm). Adenosine would not be expected to terminate an irregular narrow complex tachycardia, because the genesis of these rhythms does not involve the AV node.

20. What is the dosing regimen for adenosine, and what are its primary side effects?

The adenosine dosing regimen is 6 mg rapid IV push, followed, if no rhythm conversion, by 12 mg rapid IV push. The half-life of adenosine is only several seconds, so every effort must be made to administer this quickly and ensure its quick delivery to the central circulation. The effects of adenosine may be potentiated by dipyridamole or carbamazepine (consider starting dose of 3 mg) and blocked by theophylline and caffeine. Adenosine may cause the patient to experience flushing, shortness of breath, or chest discomfort. Because it can cause bronchospasm, it should be avoided in patients with significant reactive airway disease. The practitioner should also be aware that because of its profound effects on AV nodal conduction, it may result in asystole for several seconds or more, an often disconcerting occurrence to the practitioner watching the telemetry monitor. Prolonged asystole has been reported in patients with transplanted hearts and following central venous administration; a lower dose of 3 mg should be considered in such situations.

21. After return of spontaneous circulation, what intervention has been shown to improve neurologic recovery in comatose patients?

Therapeutic hypothermia improves neurologic recovery in comatose patients. Patients are cooled to 32°C to 36°C for at least 24 hours via surface cooling devices (ice bags and/or cooling blankets) and cold, non–dextrose-containing, isotonic fluids (30 mL/kg). Decisions on percutaneous coronary intervention (PCI) are not affected by therapeutic hypothermia.

Coronary angiogram should be performed in all post–cardiac arrest patients with returns of spontaneous circulation (ROSC) with suspected cardiac etiology regardless if the patient is comatose or awake.

Bibliography and Suggested Readings

American Heart Association. (2015). *Highlights of the AHA Guidelines Update for CPR and ECC.* < https://eccguidelines.heart.org/wp-content/uploads/2015/10/2015-AHA-Guidelines-Highlights-English.pdf. > Accessed Nov 2016.

Link, M. S., Berkow, L. C., Kudenchuk, P. J., Halperin, H. R., Hess, E. P., Moitra, V. K., et al. (2015). Part 7: adult advanced cardiovascular life support 2015 American Heart Association Guidelines Update for Cardiopulmonary Resuscitation and Emergency Cardiovascular Care. *Circulation, 132*(Suppl. 2), S444–S464. http://dx.doi.org/10.1161/CIR.0000000000000261.

Lundin, A., Djärv, T., Engdahl, J., Hollenberg, J., Nordberg, P., Ravn-Fischer, A., et al. (2015). Drug therapy in cardiac arrest: a review of the literature. *European Heart Journal—Cardiovascular Pharmacotherapy, 2*, 54–75. http://dx.doi.org/10.1093/ehjcvp/pvv047.

Pearson, D. A. (2015). Review of clinical guidelines for cardiopulmonary resuscitation. *North Carolina Medical Journal, 76*(4), 257–259.

Scirica, B. M. (2013). Therapeutic hypothermia after cardiac arrest. *Circulation, 127*, 244–250.

VI
Primary and Secondary Prevention

HYPERTENSION

Gabriel B. Habib

CHAPTER 41

1. **What is the prevalence of hypertension in men and women across various age groups?**

Hypertension affects more than 70 million persons in the United States and more than a billion adults worldwide. Hypertension is the leading cause of death and disability worldwide and is the most important global risk factor for cardiovascular risk (coronary artery disease and stroke).

The prevalence of hypertension varies markedly worldwide, from as low as 3% of men in rural India to 72% of men in Poland. Hypertension prevalence is higher among younger (<60 years) men than younger women. However, starting at 60 years of age, the prevalence of hypertension in women catches up with and eventually exceeds that in men. Approximately 78% of women and only 67% of men older than 75 years are hypertensive. Overall, hypertension is directly related to mortality in a greater number of women than men.

2. **What are the "stages of hypertension"?**

Hypertension has been classified as follows:

- Normal: blood pressure (BP) less than 120/80 mm Hg
- Prehypertension: BP 120 to 139/80 to 89 mm Hg
- Hypertension stage 1: BP 140 to 159/90 to 99 mm Hg
- Hypertension stage 2: BP ≥160/100 mm Hg

3. **What are the four primary complications of hypertension?**

The four most important complications of hypertension are

- Coronary artery disease and myocardial infarction (MI)
- Heart failure (systolic and "diastolic")
- Chronic kidney disease and renal failure
- Stroke

4. **What are the goals of hypertension treatment?**

Reducing elevated blood pressure levels is an important strategy to prevent various complications of systemic hypertension, including stroke, heart attacks, heart failure, and renal disease. The best predictor of the efficacy in preventing various cardiorenal complications is the degree of reduction of blood pressure. The risk of death from ischemic heart disease or stroke in longitudinal cohort studies is lowest at a blood pressure of approximately 115/75 mm Hg and doubles with each 20 mm Hg increment in systolic blood pressure greater than 115/75 mm Hg (Fig. 41.1).

Although blood pressure less than 120/80 mm Hg is associated in observational cohort studies with the lowest risk of death from ischemic heart disease and stroke, the goal of blood pressure treatment has traditionally been a blood pressure less than 140/90 mm Hg, with some organizations recommending a goal of less than 130/80 in diabetic patients and those with chronic kidney disease. Although one group has recommended that in patients older than 60 years the goal be 150/90 mm Hg, this recommendation is controversial and has not been adopted by most health organizations.

Two major studies have examined the potential benefit of lowering blood pressure below a target of 140/90. The Action to Control Cardiovascular Risk in Diabetes (ACCORD) trial found that targeting a systolic BP of less than 120 mm Hg as compared with less than 140 mm Hg in patients with type 2 diabetes mellitus did not reduce the rate of a composite outcome of fatal and nonfatal major cardiovascular events, although stroke risk (a secondary study endpoint) was significantly reduced. The Systolic Blood Pressure Intervention Trial (SPRINT) found that targeting a systolic BP less than 120 mm Hg compared with less than 140 mm Hg in patients at high risk for cardiovascular events but without diabetes resulted in lower rates of fatal and nonfatal major cardiovascular events and death from any cause, although significantly higher rates of some adverse events were observed in the intensive treatment group. These study results will likely impact future hypertension guidelines.

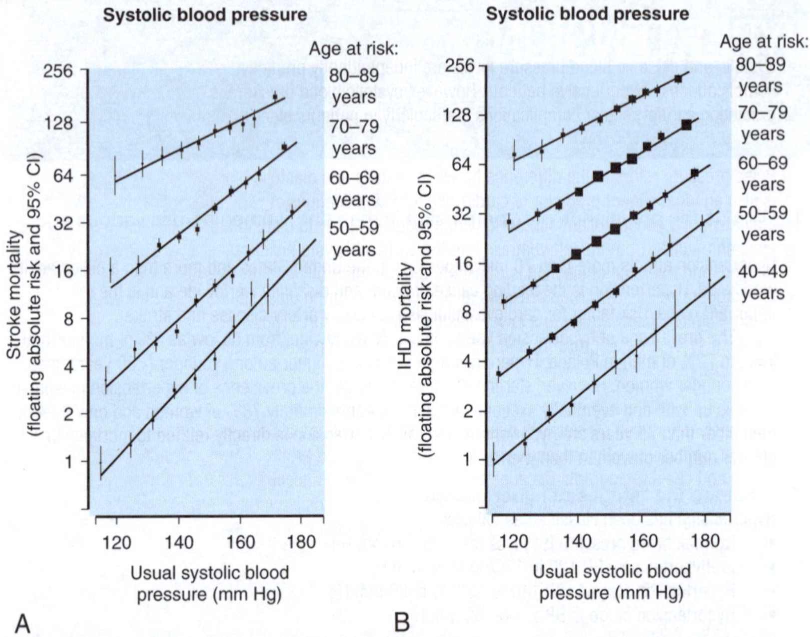

Fig. 41.1. The relationship between blood pressure, age, and risk of stroke and ischemic heart disease (IHD) death. **A,** Stroke Mortality and **B,** Ischemic Heart Disease Mortality. The risk of stroke and IHD death are lowest at a blood pressure (BP) of 115/75 mm Hg and double every 20-mm Hg increment. *(Image from Lewington, S., Clarke, R., Qizilbash, N., Peto, R., Collins, R., & Prospective Studies Collaboration. [2002]. Age-specific relevance of usual blood pressure to vascular mortality: a meta-analysis of individual data for one million adults in 61 prospective studies.* Lancet, *360, 1903–1913.)*

5. What are the steps in managing a patient with newly diagnosed hypertension?

The first step in a newly diagnosed hypertensive patient is to advise optimal lifestyle interventions, including low-salt diet, regular exercise, weight control, and avoidance of smoking. This is followed by initiation of single- or two-drug antihypertensive therapy (separately or as a fixed dose combination). Initial medications include a thiazide diuretic, a calcium channel blocker, and an angiotensin-converting enzyme inhibitor (ACEI) or angiotensin receptor blocker (ARB).

If blood pressure remains greater than 140/90 mm Hg on one or two drugs, additional drugs are added. After all three initially recommended antihypertensive drugs—diuretic, calcium channel blocker, and ACEI or ARB—are prescribed in maximally tolerated doses without achieving a goal BP less than 140/90 mm Hg, additional antihypertensive drugs are added, such as beta-blockers, aldosterone antagonists, or others. Beta-blockers are NOT recommended as a first-, second-, or third-line antihypertensive drug in the treatment of hypertensive patients but can be added as a fourth-line drug.

These recommendations apply to the “generic” hypertensive patient. There may be compelling reasons to use certain antihypertensive agents as first- or second-line therapies.

6. What are the recommended antihypertensive drugs in African American hypertensive patients?

In the general African American population, including those with diabetes, initial antihypertensive treatment usually includes a thiazide-type diuretic or calcium channel blocker.

7. What are the recommended antihypertensive drugs in hypertensive patients with chronic kidney disease?

In patients with chronic kidney disease, initial or add-on antihypertensive treatment should include an ACEI or ARB. These medications have been shown to have some “renoprotective” effects, delaying the progression of renal disease.

8. Is systolic or diastolic blood pressure more powerful as a predictor of cardiovascular complications of hypertension?

Systolic and diastolic blood pressure levels are independently predictive of the risk of cardiovascular complications in hypertensive patients. However, systolic blood pressure is more powerful in predicting cardiovascular complications, particularly in patients older than 50 years.

9. What does the term *pulse pressure* refer to?

Pulse pressure refers to the difference between systolic and diastolic blood pressure. Pulse pressure is also an independent predictor of cardiovascular complications. A wide pulse pressure is usually indicative of a noncompliant stiff aorta with a reduced ability to distend and recoil. During systolic ejection of blood from the left ventricle into the aorta and systemic circulation, the aorta does *not* distend, and the force of ejection is transmitted more forcefully into the peripheral vessels, causing an exaggerated systolic blood pressure level recording. During diastole, the elastic recoil of the aorta is more limited, contributing to a lower diastolic blood pressure. Thus a noncompliant aorta would increase systolic blood pressure and reduce diastolic blood pressure, resulting in a widened pulse pressure.

10. What is the recommended initial diagnostic workup for a hypertensive patient?

Any newly diagnosed patient with hypertension should have measurements of serum creatinine, sodium, potassium, calcium, and hematocrit, full fasting lipid profile, 12-lead electrocardiogram (ECG), and chest radiograph. Because essential hypertension accounts for the large majority—more than 95%—of all hypertension, a thorough and costly diagnostic workup for secondary causes of hypertension (discussed later) is not routinely recommended unless there are clinical or laboratory clues suggesting secondary hypertension.

11. What findings in a patient with newly diagnosed hypertension suggest kidney involvement?

Signs of kidney involvement range from minimal proteinuria or slight increase of serum creatinine to end-stage renal disease. Kidney function is calculated using blood tests and patient demographic data. Kidney size is evaluated by a variety of imaging methods and has prognostic significance. Hypertension is the second leading cause of renal failure in the United States, particularly in African Americans.

12. What findings in a patient with newly diagnosed hypertension suggest neurologic involvement?

The eye fundus appearance is the *mirror* of the brain circulation. Findings range from minor atherosclerotic changes to papilledema and hemorrhages, which are consistent with malignant hypertension. A careful neurologic examination may reveal signs of previously undiagnosed strokes, and history may reveal previous transient ischemic attacks. Carotid ultrasound or cerebral angiography may demonstrate cerebrovascular disease. Computed tomography (CT) and magnetic resonance imaging (MRI) may demonstrate old strokes.

13. What findings in a patient with newly diagnosed hypertension suggest cardiac involvement?

A direct consequence of hypertension is left ventricle hypertrophy (LVH) with increased left ventricular mass. The finding of high QRS voltage or "left ventricular hypertrophy" on the ECG is suggestive of, although not diagnostic for, true left ventricular hypertrophy. LVH is definitively diagnosed by echocardiography, cardiac CT, or cardiac MRI. The finding of LVH is strongly associated with an increased risk of sudden death and MI. LVH is a frequent cause of decreased LV compliance and "diastolic dysfunction" (more properly termed *heart failure with preserved ejection fraction*).

Hypertension can lead to coronary artery disease, which may be reflected in the patient's history and symptomatology (angina, history of MI), ECG (Q waves), and imaging studies (focal hypokinesis or akinesis, scarred and thinned walls).

Untreated or poorly treated hypertension can lead to left ventricular dilation, depressed left ventricular systolic function, and heart failure.

14. What is resistant hypertension, and how prevalent is it?

Resistant hypertension is defined as blood pressure that remains above goal despite the concurrent use of three antihypertensive agents of different classes. Ideally, one of the three agents should be a diuretic, and all agents should be prescribed at optimal dose amounts.

Resistant hypertension identifies patients who are at risk of having reversible causes of hypertension or patients who by virtue of persistently elevated blood pressure levels may benefit from special diagnostic and therapeutic considerations. In an analysis of the National Health and Nutrition Examination Survey (NHANES), only 53% of hypertensive patients were controlled to less than 140/90; the majority of the remaining 47% of these patients probably have resistant hypertension. Although the exact prevalence of resistant hypertension is unknown, it is estimated from published hypertension clinical trials, including the Antihypertensive and Lipid-Lowering Treatment to Prevent Heart Attack trial (ALLHAT), that approximately 20% to 30% of hypertensives have resistant hypertension.

Factors recognized to be associated with resistant hypertension include older age, high baseline blood pressure, obesity, excessive dietary salt ingestion, chronic kidney disease, diabetes mellitus, LVH, African American race, female gender, and residence in southeastern United States regions. Medications that interfere with blood pressure control should be specifically inquired about in poorly controlled hypertensive patients that may interfere with blood pressure control (see Tables 41.1 and 41.2).

15. **What is secondary hypertension?**

Up to 5% of all hypertension cases are *secondary*, meaning that a specific cause can be identified. Some of these cases are curable if the source of hypertension can be treated, such as surgery for an adrenal tumor, stenting of a renal artery stenosis, and correction of an aortic coarctation. Given the low prevalence of secondary hypertension, routine screening for secondary hypertension is not routinely recommended. A targeted approach is much more cost effective, and clinical and laboratory clues are critically important in evaluating patients for specific causes of secondary hypertension. Signs, symptoms, and findings suggestive of secondary hypertension are given in Table 41.3.

Table 41.1. Patient Characteristics Associated with Resistant Hypertension

- Older age
- High baseline blood pressure
- Obesity
- Excessive dietary salt ingestion
- Chronic kidney disease
- Diabetes
- Left ventricular hypertrophy
- African American race
- Female gender
- Residence in southeastern United States

Table 41.2. Medications That Can Interfere with Blood Pressure Control

- Nonnarcotic analgesics
- Nonsteroidal anti-inflammatory agents, including aspirin
- Selective COX-2 inhibitors
- Sympathomimetic agents (decongestants, diet pills, cocaine)
- Stimulants (methylphenidate, dexmethylphenidate, dextroamphetamine, amphetamine, methamphetamine, modafinil)
- Alcohol
- Oral contraceptives
- Cyclosporine
- Erythropoietin
- Natural licorice
- Herbal compounds (ephedra or ma huang)

COX-2, Cyclooxygenase-2.

16. **What are the most common causes of secondary hypertension among patients with treatment-resistant or uncontrolled hypertension, when do you suspect them, and how do you confirm them?**

Secondary hypertension is common among patients with resistant hypertension. The most common causes of secondary hypertension among patients with resistant hypertension are obstructive sleep apnea (see Chapter 53), renal parenchymal and vascular disease, and, possibly, primary aldosteronism. Rare causes of secondary hypertension include pheochromocytoma, Cushing syndrome, hyperparathyroidism, aortic coarctation, and intracranial tumors. The following are important clinical or laboratory clues to these secondary hypertension causes:

- **Obstructive sleep apnea:** Untreated obstructive sleep apnea is an increasingly recognized cause of secondary hypertension. Clues include loud snoring, witnessed apnea, and excessive daytime somnolence. Diagnosis is confirmed with a sleep study.
- **Renal artery stenosis:** This is suspected in patients with atherosclerotic peripheral or coronary vascular disease, early age (younger than 35 years) or late age (older than 55 years) at onset of hypertension, abnormal renal function or worsening renal function with the use of an ACEI or in patients with a unilateral small kidney. Renal ultrasonography is not recommended, and magnetic resistance angiography is the most specific and reliable noninvasive diagnostic imaging modality. Contrast angiography is also useful for the diagnosis and for possible renal angioplasty. It is important to recognize that the anatomic diagnosis of a renal artery stenosis, independent of its cause, does not imply that the stenosis is the cause of hypertension. Causation can be confirmed by documenting the *functionality* of the lesion by measuring renal vein renin activity and documenting a renin activity ratio greater than 1.5 between the two sides.
- **Primary hyperaldosteronism:** This is suspected in hypertensive patients with unexplained hypokalemia. Diagnosis is suspected by a suppressed renin activity and a high 24-hour urinary aldosterone excretion in the course of a high dietary sodium intake and is confirmed radiographically with a localizing imaging procedure, such as CT or MRI, with specific adrenal protocol.
- **Renal parenchymal disease:** This is suspected by impaired renal function, but causation is difficult to confirm because longstanding untreated hypertension may also cause renal parenchymal disease. Imaging techniques that evaluate kidney size, presence of hydronephrosis and obstructive nephropathy, calculi, polycystic kidney disease, or congenital malformations are useful to detect specific causes of renal parenchymal disease.

Table 41.3. Clinical Signs, Symptoms, and Findings Suggestive of Secondary Causes of Hypertension

SIGNS, SYMPTOMS, AND FINDINGS	SUGGESTED SECONDARY CAUSE
Onset at a young age (<35 years) in female patient	Renal artery medial fibromuscular dysplasia
Onset at a late age (>55 years), especially in a patient with atherosclerosis-exaggerated drop in blood pressure and/or kidney function with initiation of ACEI abdominal bruit	Renal artery stenosis
Unexplained hypokalemia	Primary hyperaldosteronism
Paroxysmal episodes of palpitations, sweating, and headaches	Pheochromocytoma
Use of birth control pills, laxatives, or licorice	Drug-induced due to mineralocorticoid effects
Renal calculi, elevated calcium level	Hyperparathyroidism
Reduced femoral pulses with high blood pressure values only in the upper extremities	Aortic coarctation
Abdominal striae, truncal obesity	Cushing disease
Loud snoring, witnessed apnea	Obstructive sleep apnea
Worsening renal function, polycystic kidneys or small kidneys on ultrasound	Renal parenchymal disease

ACEI, Angiotensin-converting enzyme inhibitor.

- **Pheochromocytoma:** A rare secondary cause of hypertension that often presents with paroxysmal and postural hypotension, usually in a younger adult, with intermittent episodes of headache, palpitation, and sweating. The best screening test is plasma free metanephrines (normetanephrine and metanephrine).

17. What is the secondary cause of hypertension suggested by these findings and scenarios?

- Onset at a young age (younger than 35 years) in female patients → renal artery medial fibromuscular dysplasia
- Onset at a late age (older than 55 years) → renal vascular disease (renal artery stenosis)
- Unexplained hypokalemia—sometimes manifested by generalized weakness—either in the absence of diuretic use or an exaggerated hypokalemia following low doses of diuretics → primary hyperaldosteronism
- Paroxysmal episodes of palpitations, sweating, and headaches → pheochromocytoma
- A transient episode of periorbital swelling and dark-colored urine that went untreated → chronic glomerulonephritis
- Multiple episodes of cystitis or urinary infection left untreated or with incomplete treatment → chronic pyelonephritis
- Use of birth control pills by young women and laxative use by older adults or licorice use, which has a mineralocorticoid effect → mineralocorticoid-induced hypertension
- A history of chronic pain → analgesic nephropathy
- Renal calculi (possibly due to hyperparathyroidism) → obstructive nephropathy
- Reduced femoral pulses with high BP values only in the upper extremities → aortic coarctation
- Abdominal bruits → renal artery stenosis
- Exaggerated drop in BP following initiation of treatment with ACEIs or ARBs → renal artery stenosis
- Bilateral abdominal palpable masses renal artery stenosis → polycystic kidney disease
- Abdominal striae and truncal obesity → Cushing disease

18. A 32-year-old man complains of intermittent episodes of headaches, palpitations, and profuse sweating. Over the past year, he has been treated three times in the emergency department for hypertensive crisis. In your office, he always has a blood pressure below 120/70 mm Hg.

This is a typical presentation for a pheochromocytoma. The clues given by the patient's history are invaluable for diagnosis: many patients with pheochromocytoma have a normal baseline BP, with high BP values only on occasion. *Postural hypotension* is a classic feature. High serum catecholamine levels explain the sweating and palpitations and the low fever, elevation of serum glucose, and leukocytosis. Gentle palpation of the abdomen during physical examination may sometimes trigger a crisis. Because of the general and metabolic manifestations of the disease, it may mimic a large variety of conditions (e.g., vasculitis, diabetes), and a high level of suspicion is always necessary.

Some patients present with a high BP that is constant rather than paroxysmal. A *rule of 10* may be applied: 10% of all cases are familial, 10% are bilateral, 10% are due to a malignant adrenal tumor, 10% recur, 10% are extraadrenal, 10% occur in children, 10% are associated with a multiple endocrine neoplasia (MEN) syndrome, and 10% present with a stroke as the inaugural symptom.

Diagnosing the presence of pheochromocytoma is important because this very sick patient, who is prone to life-threatening complications, can be virtually cured. The current recommendation for biochemical diagnosis of pheochromocytoma is urine testing for metanephrines and fractionated catecholamines. These tests only certify the presence of a catecholamine-secreting tumor; therefore the next step is to localize the tumor. In 90% of cases the location of the pheochromocytoma is the adrenal medulla. In the other 10% of cases of pheochromocytoma, the tumor is scattered where chromaffin tissue is found. The preferred treatment is laparoscopic adrenalectomy.

19. How important are nonpharmacologic strategies in hypertension treatment?

Hypertension treatment is a lifelong commitment regardless of the recommended treatment modality. Thus compliance to treatment is critically important in achieving the expected clinical benefits of treatments. Hypertensive patients should be appropriately educated about the natural history and complications of hypertension and the critical importance of compliance with any treatment recommendation. Goal blood pressure attainment is much more likely to be achieved with earlier initiation of combination antihypertensive drug therapies—particularly in stage 2 hypertension, characterized by blood pressure levels greater than 160/100 mm Hg—and by frequent monitoring of blood pressure at home and in the physician's office and appropriate uptitration of antihypertensive medications to reach accepted goals of blood pressure treatments.

Patients and some physicians tend to be skeptical about the importance of lifestyle changes. Often the skepticism of the physician may be communicated to the patient even without the physician's conscious effort. It is critically important that patients and their physicians believe in the benefit of lifestyle changes. Current hypertension guidelines describe lifestyle changes as *therapeutic* to emphasize their proven benefit. Therapeutic lifestyle changes—weight loss; reduced intake of saturated fat and salt; reduced dietary calorie intake; regular exercise and moderation of alcohol intake; consumption of adequate amounts of calcium, potassium, magnesium, and fiber; and smoking cessation—are emphasized in treatment algorithms. Therapeutic lifestyle changes have been demonstrated to be effective in reducing blood pressure levels by 10 to 20 mm Hg, changes that are at times similar to the efficacy of one additional antihypertensive drug. In patients with prehypertension, therapeutic lifestyle changes, but not pharmacologic treatment, are generally recommended to prevent hypertension development. Pharmacologic treatment is generally recommended in addition to, not as sole therapy, in hypertensive patients.

20. True or false: beta-blockers are preferred initial antihypertensive agents in hypertensive patients with no known hypertensive complications.

False. Based on study results, guidelines generally recommend initial antihypertensive therapy with thiazide diuretics, calcium channel blockers, ACEIs, or ARBs. However, in patients with exertional angina, prior MI, or reduced ejection fraction, there may be a compelling reason to initiate beta-blocker therapy.

21. Are alpha-blockers effective in preventing cardiovascular complications of hypertension, and when is it appropriate to use them in hypertensive patients?

Alpha-blockers are effective antihypertensive agents but have not been shown in either placebo-controlled or active-controlled clinical prospective trials to be effective in preventing cardiovascular complications of hypertension. In the ALLHAT, the largest hypertensive clinical trial that randomized hypertensive patients to an ACEI, a calcium channel blocker, or an alpha-blocker versus a thiazide diuretic, the alpha-blocker arm of the trial was prematurely terminated because of an almost doubling of the risk of heart failure and a 25% excess cardiovascular death among patients treated with an alpha-blocker compared with a thiazide diuretic. Thus alpha-blockers are *not* recommended as initial antihypertensive therapy. However, alpha-blockers may be considered after a thiazide-type diuretic, a calcium channel blocker, an ACEI, or an ARB have already been used and blood pressure remains uncontrolled.

22. When are angiotensin-converting enzyme inhibitors or angiotensin receptor blockers specifically recommended in hypertensive patients?

Compelling indications for selection of an ACEI as initial antihypertensive drug include heart failure, previous MI, diabetes mellitus, chronic kidney disease, high coronary artery disease (CAD) risk, and recurrent stroke prevention. These recommendations are based on several randomized, prospective, controlled clinical trials confirming the benefits of ACEIs in preventing cardiovascular or renal complications in these patients. ACEIs prevent myocardial remodeling, heart failure progression, progressive ventricular enlargement after a recent MI, and stroke in patients with cardiovascular disease (CVD) and have also been demonstrated to prevent progression of renal disease among diabetic patients with established diabetic renal disease.

23. What is the prevalence of hypertension among African Americans and Hispanic Americans compared with non-Hispanic whites?

Overall, hypertension affects approximately 33% of adults 20 years or older in the United States. In African Americans the prevalence is 44%. In Hispanics the prevalence is 25%. From 1988 to 2008, the prevalence of hypertension has risen more in African Americans than in whites or Hispanics.

24. What are the goals for hypertension treatment in African Americans recommended by the International Society of Hypertension in Blacks?

African Americans have a significantly higher prevalence of hypertension than any other racial ethnic group in the United States and suffer a much higher risk of hypertensive complications. Unlike the seventh report of the Joint National Committee (JNC), the International Society of Hypertension in Blacks consensus report recommends lower BP goals in African Americans: specifically a BP goal of less than 135/85 for primary prevention of CVD in African Americans without target organ damage and a BP goal of less than 130/80 in African Americans with target organ damage or preclinical or clinical CVD.

Bibliography and Suggested Readings

ACCORD Study Group, Cushman, W. C., Evans, G. W., Byington, R. P., Goff, D. C., Jr., Grimm, R. H., Jr., et al. (2010). Effects of intensive blood-pressure control in type 2 diabetes mellitus. *New England Journal of Medicine, 362*, 1575–1585.

ALLHAT Officers and Coordinators for the ALLHAT Collaborative Research Group, & the Antihypertensive and Lipid-Lowering Treatment to Prevent Heart Attack Trial. (2002). Major outcomes in high-risk hypertensive patients randomized to angiotensin-converting enzyme inhibitor or calcium channel blocker vs diuretic: the Antihypertensive and Lipid-Lowering Treatment to Prevent Heart Attack Trial (ALLHAT). *Journal of the American Medical Association, 288*, 2981–2997.

Calhoun, D. A., Jones, D., Textor, S., Goff, D. C., Murphy, T. P., Toto, R. D., et al. (2008). Resistant hypertension: diagnosis, evaluation, and treatment: a scientific statement from the American Heart Association Professional Education Committee of the Council for High Blood Pressure Research. *Hypertension, 51*(6), 1403–1419.

Flack, J. M., Sica, D. A., Bakris, G., Brown, A. L., Ferdinand, K. C., Grimm, R. H., Jr., et al. (2010). Management of high blood pressure in Blacks: an update of the International Society on Hypertension in Blacks consensus statement. *Hypertension, 56*, 780–800.

Go, A. S., Mozaffarian, D., Roger, V. L., Benjamin, E. J., Berry, J. D., Blaha, M. J., et al. (2014). Heart disease and stroke statistics—2014 update: a report from the American Heart Association. *Circulation, 129*(3), e28–e292.

James, P. A., Oparil, S., Carter, B. L., Cushman, W. C., Dennison-Himmelfarb, C., Handler, J., et al. (2014). 2014 evidence-based guideline for the management of high blood pressure in adults: report from the panel members appointed to the Eighth Joint National Committee (JNC 8). *Journal of the American Medical Association, 311*(5), 507–520.

Kearney, P. M., Whelton, M., Reynolds, K., Whelton, P. K., & He, J. (2004). Worldwide prevalence of hypertension: a systematic review. *Journal of Hypertension, 22*(1), 11–19.

Lewington, S., Clarke, R., Qizilbash, N., Peto, R., Collins, R., & Prospective Studies Collaboration. (2002). Age-specific relevance of usual blood pressure to vascular mortality: a meta-analysis of individual data for one million adults in 61 prospective studies. *Lancet, 360*, 1903–1913.

Lim, S. S., Vos, T., Flaxman, A. D., Danaei, G., Shibuya, K., Adair-Rohani, H., et al. (2012). A comparative risk assessment of burden of disease and injury attributable to 67 risk factor clusters in 21 regions, 1990-2010: a systematic analysis for the Global Burden of Disease Study 2010. *Lancet, 380*, 2224–2260.

National Heart, Lung, and Blood Institute. (2003). *Seventh Report of the Joint National Committee on Prevention, Detection, Evaluation, and Treatment of High Blood Pressure.* < http://www.nhlbi.nih.gov/guidelines/hypertension/express.pdf. >

Roger, V. L., Go, A. S., Lloyd-Jones, D. M., Benjamin, E. J., Berry, J. D., Borden, W. B., et al. (2012). Heart disease and stroke statistics—2012 update: a report from the American Heart Association. *Circulation, 125*(1), e2–e220.

Rosendorff, C., Black, H. R., Cannon, C. P., Gersh, B. J., Core, J., Izzo, J. L., Jr., et al. (2007). Treatment of hypertension in the prevention and management of ischemic heart disease: a scientific statement from the American Heart Association Council for High Blood Pressure Research and the Councils on Clinical Cardiology and Epidemiology and Prevention. *Circulation, 115*, 2761–2788.

SPRINT Research Group, Wright, J. T., Jr., Williamson, J. D., Whelton, P. K., Snyder, J. K., Sink, K. M., et al. (2015). A randomized trial of intensive versus standard blood-pressure control. *New England Journal of Medicine, 373*(22), 2103–2116.

Yusuf, S., Sleight, P., Pogue, J., Bosch, J., Davies, R., & Dagenais, G. (2000). Effects of an angiotensin-converting-enzyme inhibitor, ramipril, on cardiovascular events in high-risk patients. The Heart Outcomes Prevention Evaluation Study Investigators. *New England Journal of Medicine, 342*, 145–153.

CHAPTER 42

HYPERLIPIDEMIA

Ozlem Bilen, Salim Virani, Vijay Nambi

1. What is dyslipidemia?

Dyslipidemia can be thought of as abnormal lipid values. The following are considered generally to be values above the "desirable" range:

- Total cholesterol greater than 200 mg/dL
- Low-density lipoprotein cholesterol (LDL-C) greater than 130 mg/dL
- High-density lipoprotein cholesterol (HDL-C) less than 40 mg/dL (men) and less than 50 mg/dL (women)
- Triglycerides greater than 150 mg/dL

2. Who should be screened for dyslipidemias?

As per the 2013 American College of Cardiology/American Heart Association (ACC/AHA) guidelines, all adults aged 20 years or older should undergo fasting lipoprotein profile testing every 4 to 6 years. Testing should include fasting total cholesterol, LDL-C, HDL-C, and triglycerides. If an individual is not fasting, then only the total cholesterol and HDL-C can be adequately interpreted.

3. What are important *secondary* causes of dyslipidemias?

Table 42.1 summarizes secondary causes of hyperlipidemia most likely encountered in clinical practice. It is noted that in a lipid specialty clinic the most frequently encountered secondary conditions were excessive alcohol intake, uncontrolled diabetes mellitus, and overt albuminuria.

4. What are the suggested low-density lipoprotein cholesterol goals based on the 2013 American College of Cardiology/American Heart Association Cholesterol Treatment Guidelines?

The 2013 ACC/AHA guidelines removed LDL-C goals and instead recommended use of moderate- to high-intensity statin therapy for atherosclerotic cardiovascular disease (ASCVD) risk reduction. The new guidelines include data from individual randomized trials, as well as comprehensive meta-analyses and, on the basis of this large and consistent body of evidence, identified four major statin benefit groups in which ASCVD risk reduction using statin therapy outweighs the risk of adverse events.

5. What are the outcomes ascertained by the 2013 American College of Cardiology/American Heart Association atherosclerotic cardiovascular disease risk estimator, and how does it differ from the Framingham coronary artery heart risk estimator used in the Adult Treatment Panel III guideline?

ASCVD risk as defined by the 2013 ACC/AHA guideline includes nonfatal myocardial infarction (MI), Coronary Heart disease (CHD) death, and nonfatal and fatal stroke. In contrast, the traditional Framingham risk score (as recommended by the National Cholesterol Education Program [NCEP] Adult Treatment Panel [ATP] III cholesterol guidelines) includes nonfatal MI and coronary heart disease death (note that there is also a Framingham cardiovascular disease [CVD] risk estimator). Unlike the Framingham CHD risk estimator, the new Pooled Cohort Equations were developed in cohorts that included African Americans and hence thought to improve accuracy in ASCVD prediction in African American individuals.

6. Should a lipid panel be checked after starting a patient on statin therapy?

Although there are no lipid goals, the new guidelines still support and recommend the use of a lipid panel 4 to 12 weeks after initiation of statin therapy to determine a patient's response to treatment and to monitor adherence. It is important to note that this is a class I recommendation.

7. What are the four groups in whom statin therapy should be considered based on the 2013 American College of Cardiology/American Heart Association cholesterol guideline?

The new guidelines focus on statins because they are demonstrated to be effective, safe when taken as directed, and inexpensive. The guidelines endorse clinician-patient discussions to ensure that

Table 42.1. Common Secondary Causes of Dyslipidemia

- Hypothyroidism
- Diabetes mellitus
- Obstructive liver disease
- Chronic renal failure/nephrotic syndrome
- Drugs (e.g., progestins, anabolic steroids, corticosteroids)
- Weight gain, obesity, pregnancy

issues, such as adherence to a healthy lifestyle, treatment of reversible risk factors, and appropriate use of statin therapy, are addressed along with patient's understanding of risks and benefits and making a decision based on the same. The four groups in which statin therapy should be considered are

- Individuals with clinical ASCVD (i.e., acute coronary syndromes, or a history of MI, stable or unstable angina, coronary or other arterial revascularization, stroke, transient ischemic attack, or peripheral artery disease presumed to be of atherosclerotic origin)
- Individuals with primary elevations of LDL-C (defined as LDL-C ≥190 mg/dL; i.e., familial hypercholesterolemia)
- Individuals 40 to 75 years of age with diabetes and LDL-C 70 to 189 mg/dL
- Individuals without clinical ASCVD or diabetes who are 40 to 75 years of age with LDL-C 70 to 189 mg/dL and an estimated 10-year ASCVD risk of 7.5% or higher

The suggested treatment algorithm for statin therapy for primary and secondary prevention is given in Fig. 42.1.

8. In addition to the four statin benefit groups defined previously, when could statin initiation be considered?

In patients who do not fall into the four major statin benefit groups discussed previously, certain other factors can be considered to inform clinical judgment about statin treatment. These other factors include:

- Primary LDL-C greater than or equal to 160 mg/dL or other evidence of genetic hyperlipidemias
- Family history of premature ASCVD with onset less than 55 years of age in a first-degree male relative or less than 65 years of age in a first-degree female relative
- High-sensitivity C-reactive protein greater than 2 mg/L
- Coronary calcium score greater than or equal to 300 Agatston units or greater than or equal to 75 percentile for age, gender, and ethnicity
- Ankle-brachial index less than 0.9
- Elevated lifetime risk of ASCVD

Of note, there is a weak recommendation to consider treatment with a moderate-intensity statin to adults 40 to 75 years of age, with LDL-C 70 to 189 mg/dL, without clinical ASCVD or diabetes and an estimated 10-year ASCVD risk of 5% to less than 7.5%.

9. What are high-, moderate-, and low-intensity statins?

The intensity of a statin relates to its ability to lower LDL-C. High-intensity statins are those that can lower LDL-C by 50% or greater, whereas moderate-intensity statins lower LDL-C by 30 to less than 50% and low-intensity statins lower LDL-C less than 30%. Drugs and doses of high-, moderate-, and low-intensity statins are summarized in Table 42.2.

10. How often do statins cause elevations of liver function tests?

Clinical studies of statins have demonstrated a 0.5% to 3.0% occurrence of transient elevations in aminotransferases in patients receiving statins. This is primarily noticed during the first 3 months of therapy and is dose dependent. In 2012 the US Food and Drug Administration (FDA) revised its labeling information on statins to recommend only liver function testing prior to initiation of statin therapy and to repeat such testing for clinical reasons only but not on a routine basis.

11. How often do statins cause musculoskeletal side effects?

Information about the frequency of statin-associated musculoskeletal side effects varies between randomized clinical trials and observational studies. In placebo-controlled trials of statin therapy, the incidence of nonspecific muscle aches (myalgia) or joint pains in patients treated with statins is

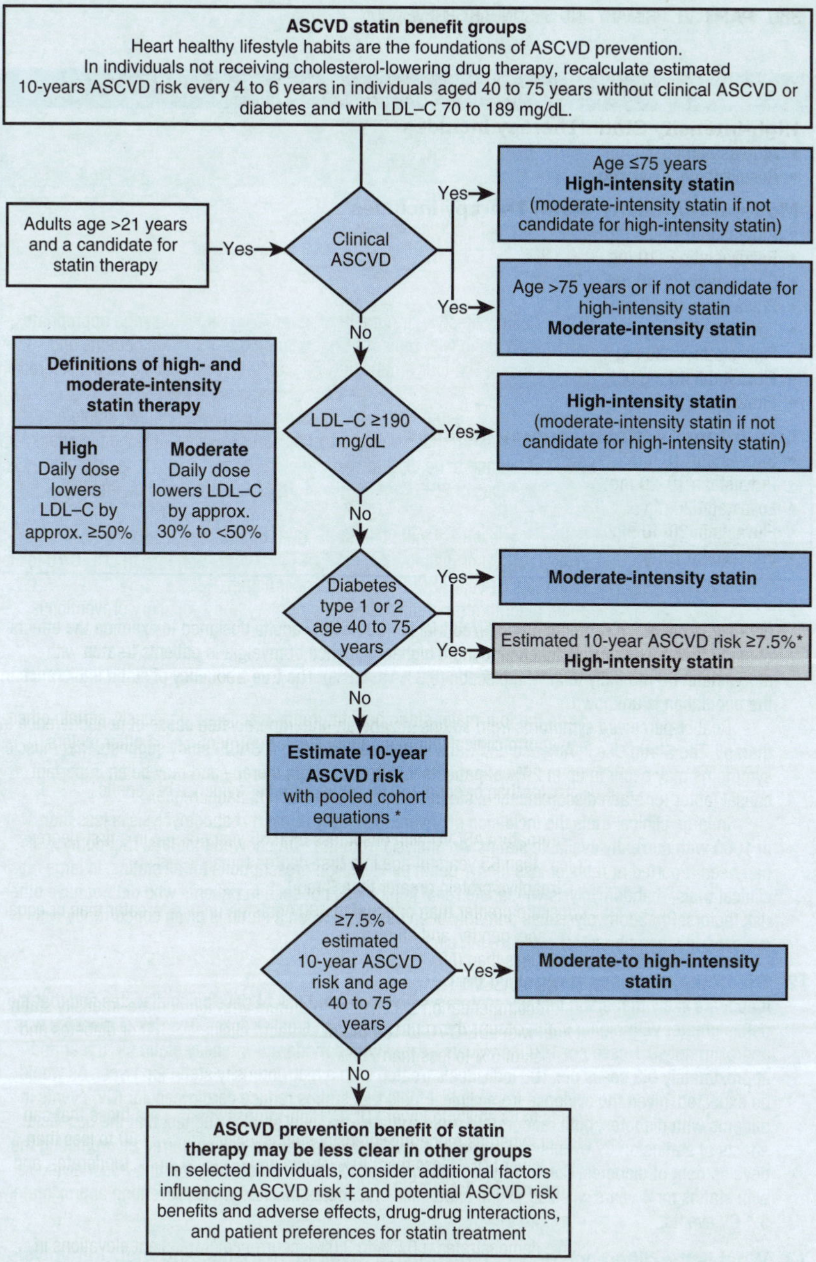

Fig. 42.1. Major recommendations for statin therapy for atherosclerotic cardiovascular disease prevention.
‡yThe Pooled Cohort Equations can be used to estimate 10-year ASCVD risk in individuals with and without diabetes. The estimator within this application should be used to inform decision making in primary prevention patients not on a statin.
*xFor those in whom a risk assessment is uncertain, consider factors such as primary LDL-C 160 mg/dL or other evidence of genetic hyperlipidemias, family history of premature ASCVD with onset <55 years of age in a first-degree male relative or <65 years of age in a first-degree female relative, hs-CRP 2 mg/L, CAC score 300 Agatston units, or 75th percentile for age, sex, and ethnicity (for additional information, see http://www.mesa-nhlbi.org/CACReference.aspx), ABI <0.9, or lifetime risk of ASCVD. Additional factors that may aid in individual risk assessment may be identified in the future. *(From Stone, N. J., Robinson, J., Lichtenstein, A. H., Bairey Merz, C. N., Lloyd-Jones, D. M., Blum, C. B., et al. [2013]. 2013 ACC/AHA guideline on the treatment of blood cholesterol to reduce atherosclerotic cardiovascular risk in adults.* Journal of the American College of Cardiology. *63, 2889–2934. doi:10.1016/j.jacc.2013.11.002.)*

Table 42.2. High-, Moderate-, and Low-Intensity Statin Therapy

High-Intensity Statin Therapy Includes
- Atorvastatin 40-80 mg
- Rosuvastatin 20-40 mg

Moderate-Intensity Statin Therapy Includes
- Atorvastatin 10-20 mg
- Rosuvastatin 5-10 mg
- Simvastatin 20-40 mg
- Pravastatin 40-80 mg
- Lovastatin 40 mg
- Fluvastatin XL 80 mg
- Fluvastatin 40 mg bid
- Pitavastatin 2-4 mg

Low-Intensity Statin Therapy Includes
- Simvastatin 10 mg
- Pravastatin 10-20 mg
- Lovastatin 20 mg
- Fluvastatin 20-40 mg
- Pitavastatin 1 mg

approximately 5%. A 6-month randomized trial in 420 healthy adults designed to examine the effects of statin therapy on muscle function found a higher incidence of myalgia in patients treated with atorvastatin 80 mg daily than with placebo (9.3% vs. 4.6%). The true frequency of statin intolerance in the population is unknown.

Real or perceived symptoms from statins may be an underappreciated cause of nonadherence to therapy. The Statin Use in America and Gaps in Patient Education (USAGE) study suggests that muscle symptoms may occur in up to 29% of patients initiated on statin therapy and may be an important causal factor for statin discontinuation, statin switching, and statin nonadherence.

In large clinical trials the incidence of severe myopathy or overt rhabdomyolysis is less than 1 in 1000 with currently available statins. An analysis from the FDA showed that fatal rhabdomyolysis had been reported at rates of less than 1 death per 1 million prescriptions for all statins. In large clinical trials, rhabdomyolysis with acute renal failure was not seen in patients who did not have other risk factors. Rhabdomyolysis has primarily been observed when a statin is given concurrently with cyclosporine, gemfibrozil, or protease inhibitors.

12. Do statins increase the risk of diabetes?

It appears likely that statin therapy confers a small increased risk of developing diabetes and that the risk is greater with higher statin doses when compared with smaller doses. The risk of diabetes was approximately 0.1 case per 100 individuals treated with a moderate-intensity statin for 1 year and approximately 0.3 cases per 100 individuals treated with a high-intensity statin for 1 year. As would be expected, given the evidence from clinical trials that statins reduce cardiovascular (CV) events in patients with diabetes, both randomized trials and observational studies suggest that the beneficial effects of statins on CV events and mortality outweigh any increased risk conferred by promoting the development of diabetes. Combining information from 13 individual studies, treating 255 individuals with statins for 4 years will lead to one extra case of diabetes mellitus while preventing approximately 5.4 CV events.

13. What is the difference between myopathy, myalgia, myositis, and rhabdomyolysis?

- Myopathy: General term referring to any disease of muscles
- Myalgia: Muscle ache or weakness without creatine kinase (CK) elevation
- Myositis: Muscle symptoms with increased CK levels
- Myonecrosis: Elevation in muscle enzymes compared with either baseline CK levels or the Upper limit of Normal (ULN) (mild: 3-fold to 10-fold elevation in CK; moderate: 10- to 50-fold elevation in CK; severe: 50-fold or greater elevation in CK)
- Clinical rhabdolyolysis: Myonecrosis associated with myoglobinuria or acute renal failure (an increase in serum creatinine of least 0.5 mg/dL)

14. What are other strategies and non-statin agents considered for management of low-density lipoprotein cholesterol–related atherosclerotic cardiovascular disease risk?

Clinicians treating high-risk patients who have a less-than-anticipated response to statins, who need further LDL-C reduction beyond that conferred by high-intensity statin therapy, who are unable to tolerate the recommended intensity of a statin, or who are completely statin intolerant may consider the addition of a non-statin cholesterol-lowering therapy. The 2016 American College of Cardiology Expert Consensus Decision Pathway on the Role of Non-Statin Therapies for LDL-Cholesterol Lowering in the Management of Atherosclerotic Cardiovascular Disease Risk gives suggested treatment algorithms for non-statin therapy based on the presence or absence of comorbidities and whether treatment is for primary or secondary prevention. Two such treatment algorithms for secondary prevention are given in Figs. 42.2 and 42.3. Table 42.3 summarizes non-statin agents that can be used for management of LDL-C–related ASCVD risk reduction.

15. When used in combination with a statin in treatment after an acute coronary syndrome, which agent can provide additional reduction in cardiovascular events?

IMProved Reduction of Outcomes: Vytorin Efficacy International Trial (IMPROVE-IT) was the first large trial to directly assess clinical outcomes with ezetimibe plus a moderate-dose statin therapy compared with a moderate-dose statin alone. Over a period of 7 years the addition of ezetimibe to simvastatin 40 mg led to a relative reduction in the primary endpoint—a composite of CV death, MI, unstable angina requiring rehospitalization, coronary revascularization, or stroke—by 6.4% when compared with patients who received simvastatin alone ($p = .016$). The absolute reduction in risk over 7 years was 2.0%, with 32.7% in the ezetimibe/simvastatin arm experiencing a primary endpoint compared with 34.7% in the simvastatin arm. It is important to note that in IMPROVE-IT, moderate-intensity statins were used (either alone or in combination with ezetimibe), and therefore, it is not known whether ezetimibe therapy would improve outcomes when used in combination with a high-intensity statin therapy.

16. What are proprotein convertase subtilisin kexin 9 inhibitors?

Proprotein convertase subtilisin kexin 9 (PCSK9) is a serine protease produced predominantly in the liver that leads to the degradation of hepatocyte LDL receptors and increased plasma LDL-C levels. Genetic studies have shown that gain of function mutations in the PCSK9 gene are responsible for some cases of familial hypercholesterolemia and loss of function mutations are associated with very low LDL-C levels and markedly reduced incidence of CV disease. Monoclonal antibodies that inhibit PCSK9 have been shown to reduce LDL-C levels in a dose-dependent manner (as much as 70% with monotherapy and by an additional 60% in patients on statin therapy). These monoclonal antibodies have become available for clinical use. At the time of this writing, two agents, evolocumab and alirocumab, have been approved by the FDA for clinical use, with others under study. In a post hoc analysis of the Long-term Safety and Tolerability of Alirocumab in High Cardiovascular Risk Patients with Hypercholesterolemia Not Adequately Controlled with Their Lipid Modifying Therapy (ODYSSEY), a long-term trial of alirocumab, the rate of major adverse CV events (death from coronary heart disease, nonfatal MI, fatal or nonfatal ischemic stroke, or unstable angina requiring hospitalization) was lower with alirocumab than with placebo (1.7% vs. 3.3%; hazard ratio: 0.52; 95% confidence interval: 0.31 to 0.90; nominal $p = .02$). In addition, extension studies of Open-Label Study of Long-Term Evaluation Against LDL-C (OSLER)-1 and OSLER-2 trials were performed, and the rate of CV events at 1 year was reduced from 2.18% in the standard therapy group to 0.95% in the evolocumab group (hazard ratio in the evolocumab group: 0.47; 95% confidence interval: 0.28 to 0.78; $p = .003$). Large-scale, phase III studies will better define the benefit and role of these agents.

17. When does triglyceride reduction become the initial goal of therapy and why?

An elevated triglyceride level is not a target of therapy per se, except when very high (≥500 mg/dL), due to the risk of developing acute pancreatitis with severe hypertriglyceridemia.

18. What are the components of therapy for elevated triglyceride levels?

Patients with very elevated triglyceride levels (≥500 mg/dL) are at increased risk for pancreatitis. Therapy should always include nonpharmacologic interventions, such as weight loss in obese patients, aerobic exercise, and dietary changes to avoid concentrated sugars and fats, because triglycerides are very sensitive to lifestyle changes. In addition, attention should be paid to medications that raise serum triglyceride levels and to strict glycemic control in diabetics. Pharmacologic options typically include the use of fibrates, niacin, and fish oil (omega fatty acids).

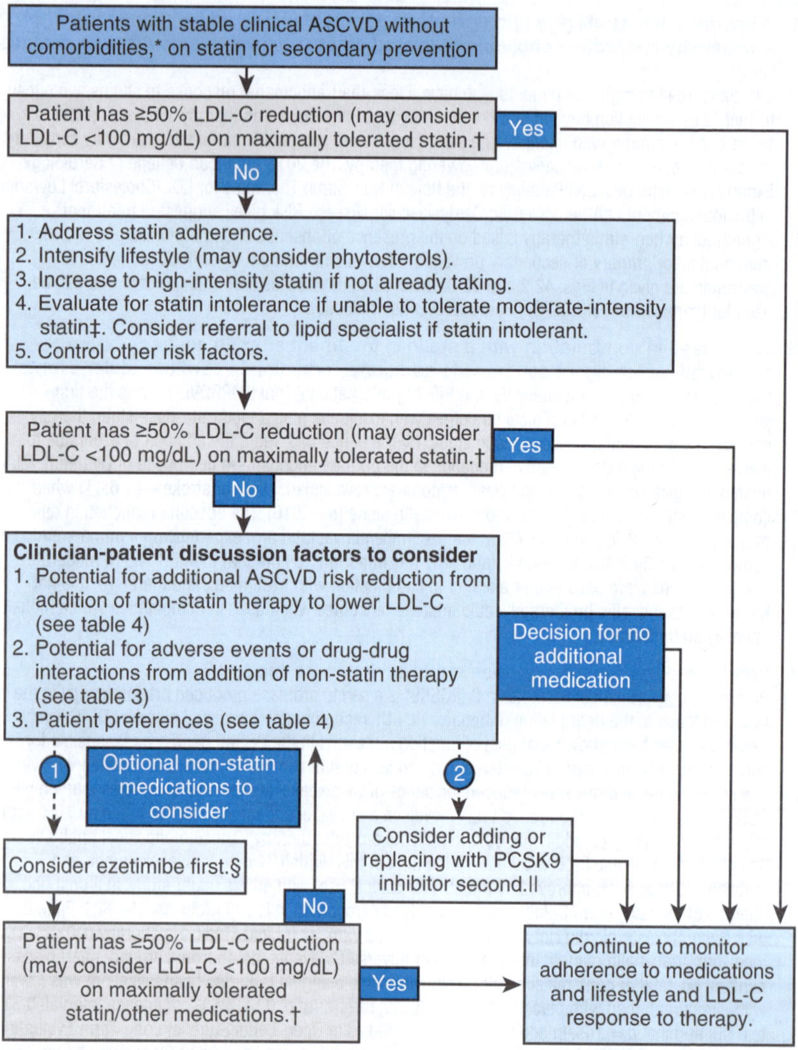

Fig. 42.2. Summary of Statin Initiation Recommendations for the Treatment of Blood Cholesterol to Reduce ASCVD Risk in Adults without Comorbidities. *ASCVD*, Atherosclerotic cardiovascular disease; *BAS*, bile acid sequestrant; *LDL-C*, low-density lipoprotein cholesterol; *PDSK9*, proprotein convertase subtilisin/kexin 9; *RDN*, registered dietitian nutritionist.

*Comorbidities are defined as diabetes, recent (<3 months) acute ASCVD event, ASCVD event while already taking a statin, baseline LDL-C ≥190 mg/dL not due to secondary causes, poorly controlled major ASCVD risk factors, elevated lipoprotein(a), and chronic kidney disease. Patients with ASCVD and baseline LDL-C ≥190 mg/dL are addressed in a separate algorithm. Patients with symptomatic heart failure, those on maintenance hemodialysis, and those with planned or current pregnancy require individualized care.

†The Expert Panel emphasizes that these are not firm triggers for adding medication, but they are factors that may be considered within the broader context of an individual patient's clinical situation.

‡See section on strategy for assessment and management of statin intolerance.

§May consider BAS if ezetimibe intolerant and triglycerides <300 mg/dL.

||Consider only if on maximally tolerated statin and either ezetimibe or BAS, with persistent <50% LDL-C reduction or LDL-C ≥100 mg/dL. Strongly consider if fully statin intolerant and attempts to lower LDL-C with ezetimibe and/or BAS result in persistent <50% LDL-C reduction or LDL-C ≥100 mg/dL. (*From Lloyd-Jones, D. M., Morris, P. B., Ballantyne, C. M., Birtcher, K. K., Daly, D. D. Jr., DePalma, S. M., et al. [2016]. 2016 ACC expert consensus decision pathway on the role of non-statin therapies for LDL-cholesterol lowering in the management of atherosclerotic cardiovascular disease risk.* Journal of the American College of Cardiology, 68, *92–125).*

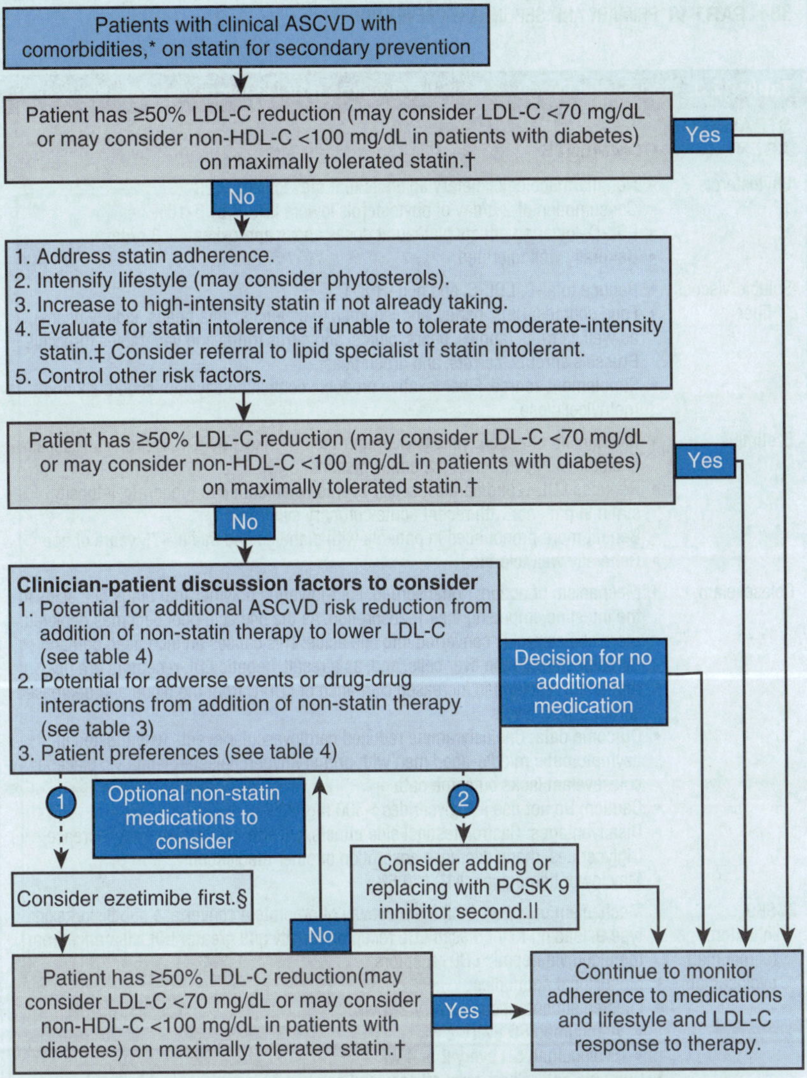

Fig. 42.3. Summary of Statin Initiation Recommendations for the Treatment of Blood Cholesterol to Reduce ASCVD Risk in Adults with Comorbidities. *ASCVD*, Atherosclerotic cardiovascular disease; *BAS*, bile acid sequestrant; *LDL-C*, low-density lipoprotein cholesterol; *PDSK9*, proprotein convertase subtilisin/kexin 9; *RDN*, registered dietitian nutritionist.

*Comorbidities are defined as diabetes, recent (<3 months) acute ASCVD event, ASCVD event while already taking a statin, baseline LDL-C ≤190 mg/dL not due to secondary causes, poorly controlled major ASCVD risk factors, elevated lipoprotein(a), and chronic kidney disease. Patients with ASCVD and baseline LDL-C 190 mg/dL are addressed in a separate algorithm. Patients with symptomatic heart failure, those on maintenance hemodialysis, and those with planned or current pregnancy require individualized care.

†The Expert Panel emphasizes that these are not firm triggers for adding medication, but they are factors that may be considered within the broader context of an individual patient's clinical situation. Due to increase in triglycerides often present in diabetes, may also consider combination therapy if non–HDL-C ≥100 mg/dL.

‡See section on strategy for assessment and management of statin intolerance.

§Consider BAS if ezetimibe intolerant and triglycerides <300 mg/dL. Colesevelam may have modest salutary effects on HbA1c and may worsen hypertriglyceridemia.

‖Consider only if on maximally tolerated statin and either ezetimibe or BAS, with persistent <50% LDL-C reduction or LDL-C ≥70 mg/dL. Strongly consider if fully statin intolerant and attempts to lower LDL-C with ezetimibe and/or BAS result in persistent <50% LDL-C reduction or LDL-C ≥70 mg/dL. *(From Lloyd-Jones, D. M., Morris, P. B., Ballantyne, C. M., Birtcher, K. K., Daly, D. D. Jr., DePalma, S. M., et al. [2016]. 2016 ACC expert consensus decision pathway on the role of non-statin therapies for LDL-cholesterol lowering in the management of atherosclerotic cardiovascular disease risk.* Journal of the American College of Cardiology, 68,*92–125).*

Table 42.3. Non-Statin Drugs Used in the Treatment of Hypercholesterolemia

STRATEGY/ AGENT	COMMENTS
Phytosterols	• Nonpharmacologic, dietary adjuncts that may lower LDL-C • Consumption of 2 g/day of phytosterols lowers LDL-C by 5-10% • LDL-C–lowering effects plateau at doses above approximately 3 g/day • Generally well tolerated
Soluble/viscous fiber	• Reduce total-C, LDL-C, and non–HDL-C • Food sources: Oats, barley, and legumes (e.g., lentils, lima beans, kidney beans), as well as fruits (apples, pears, plums, and citrus fruits) and vegetables (broccoli, Brussels sprouts, carrots, and green peas) • Supplement source: Fiber laxative products containing psyllium seed husk and methylcellulose
Ezetimibe	• Mechanism of action: Inhibits Niemann-Pick C1-like 1 (NPC1L1) protein; reduces cholesterol absorption in the small intestine • Reduced LDL-C and cardiovascular events when added to moderate-intensity statin in patients with recent acute coronary syndrome • Benefit more pronounced in patients with diabetes and those >75 years of age • Generally well tolerated
Colesevelam	• Mechanism of action: Nonabsorbed, lipid-lowering polymer that binds bile acids in the intestine, impeding their reabsorption. As the bile acid pool becomes depleted, more cholesterol is converted into bile acids. This causes an increased demand for cholesterol in the liver cells, and, as a result, hepatic LDL receptors are up-regulated, resulting in increased clearance of LDL-C from the blood and decreased serum LDL-C levels • Outcome data: Cholestyramine reduced cardiovascular events when tested in asymptomatic middle-aged men with primary hypercholesterolemia vs. placebo; colesevelam lacks outcome data • Caution: Do not use if triglycerides >300 mg/dL • Disadvantages: Gastrointestinal side effects, pill size, pill burden, may increase triglycerides, many decrease absorption of other medications • May lower hemoglobin A1C (–0.5%)

PCSK9 inhibitors (alirocumab, evolocumab)	• Mechanism of action: Inhibit the activity of proprotein convertase subtilisin/kexin type 9, leading to increased LDL receptor density and greater LDL clearance from the blood via hepatic LDL receptors
	• Monoclonal antibodies
	• Injected subcutaneously every 2-4 wk
	  • Alirocumab SQ every 2 wk
	  • Evolocumab SQ every 2 or 4 wk
	• Outcome data: Short-term efficacy and safety data have been published. Longer term, large-scale, randomized clinical trials are ongoing
	• Expensive
	• Adverse reactions: Injection site reactions, nasopharyngitis, flulike symptoms

Niacin	• Reduces LDL-C and non–HDL-C; increases HDL-C • Outcome data: Immediate-release niacin reduced in coronary events in middle-aged men with coronary heart disease and marked hypercholesterolemia • Long-acting niacin preparation in combination with moderate-intensity statin in secondary prevention populations reduced LDL-C but did not reduce cardiovascular events • Niacin therapy was also associated with an increased incidence of adverse effects

HDL-C, high-density lipoprotein cholesterol; *LDL*, low-density lipoprotein; *LDL-C*, low-density lipoprotein cholesterol.

From Stone, N. J., Robinson, J., Lichtenstein, A. H., Bairey Merz, C. N., Lloyd-Jones, D. M., Blum, C. B., et al. (2013). *2013 ACC/AHA guideline on the treatment of blood cholesterol to reduce atherosclerotic cardiovascular risk in adults*. Journal of the American College of Cardiology. 63, 2889–2934. doi:10.1016/j.jacc.2013.11.002.

19. What are recommended treatment goals for low high-density lipoprotein cholesterol?

There are no recommended goals for the treatment of low HDL-C. In individuals with low HDL-C, LDL-C remains the primary target for therapy.

20. What factors make up metabolic syndrome?

The factors that make up metabolic syndrome are

- Abdominal obesity (waist circumference in men more than 40 inches [102 cm] or in women more than 35 inches [88 cm])
- Triglycerides of 150 mg/dL or more
- Low HDL-C (less than 40 mg/dL in men or less than 50 mg/dL in women)
- Blood pressure of 135/85 mm Hg or higher
- Fasting glucose 100 mg/dL or more

21. What is a lipoprotein?

A lipoprotein is the particle that transports cholesterol and triglycerides. Lipoproteins are composed of proteins (called apolipoproteins), phospholipids, triglycerides, and cholesterol (Fig. 42.4).

22. What is lipoprotein (a)?

Lipoprotein (a) (Lp(a)) is a circulating lipoprotein composed of liver-derived apolipoprotein (a) (apo(a)) covalently bound to apoB, which is similar in lipid composition to apoB of LDL particle (LDL-P). Apo(a) has potent lysine-binding domains, similar to those on plasminogen, and binds to damaged endothelial cells and exposed or injured subendothelial matrix proteins. As a result, it delivers cholesterol for cell membrane growth, which unfortunately contributes to increased atherogenicity. Elevated Lp(a) levels have shown to be associated with an increased risk of CV event in certain patient populations. Lp(a) is one of the factors that the 2013 ACC/AHA guideline suggests to consider and discuss with patients when patient are not in the four main statin-treatment groups.

23. What is non–high-density lipoprotein cholesterol?

Non–HDL-C is the cholesterol carried by all potentially atherogenic particles, including LDL, Intermediate density lipoprotein (IDL), very low density lipoprotein (VLDL), and VLDL remnants, chylomicron remnants and Lp(a). The level of non-HDL-C is calculated by subtracting HDL-C from total cholesterol. Epidemiologic studies have shown that non–HDL-C levels are more strongly associated with ASCVD events compared with LDL-C.

24. What is apolipoprotein B?

ApoB is a primary protein that is carried by each potentially atherogenic lipoprotein particle (i.e., chylomicrons, VLDL, IDL, LDL, Lp(a)). The apoB concentration is therefore a direct indicator of the number of circulating atherogenic particles.

25. What is the importance of low-density lipoprotein particle number and particle size?

LDL-C is a measure of the cholesterol mass, which is carried within LDL-Ps. The amount of cholesterol carried by each LDL-P varies among individuals, in response to therapy and by triglycerides (TG) and VLDL remnant concentration. Two individuals with same LDL-C may have different LDL-P size and number. Individuals with elevated TGs tend to have a higher concentration of LDL-Ps compared with those with normal TG levels.

Most of the atherogenic lipoproteins in patients with metabolic syndrome, diabetes, and insulin resistance are small, dense LDL-Ps. Thus there is usually "discordance" between measurements of LDL-C and LDL-P in these individuals. When there is discordance between these measurements, studies have shown that ASCVD risk tracks better with LDL-P compared with LDL-C. However, it is not entirely clear whether LDL-P provides substantial benefit in ASCVD risk prediction beyond regular lipid parameters (e.g., non–HDL-C), and recently released ACC/AHA guidelines on cholesterol management have not endorsed the use of this lipid parameter in routine clinical practice.

26. What is vertical auto profile and nuclear magnetic resonance?

A regular lipid profile testing includes such measurements as total cholesterol, LDL-C, HDL-C, triglycerides, and non–HDL-C. Vertical auto profile (VAP) and nuclear magnetic resonance (NMR) spectroscopy profile are specialized panels, in addition to standard lipid testing. They include additional lipid measurements, such as LDL and HDL subgroups, LDL-P concentration, Lp(a), apoB levels, and other CV risk assessment markers, such as insulin resistance score, hs-CRP (C-reactive protein), homocysteine, and Brain natriuretic peptide or B-type natriuretic peptide (BNP). VAP measures the relative distribution of cholesterol within various lipoprotein subfractions, quantifying the cholesterol content of lipoprotein subclasses. The VAP

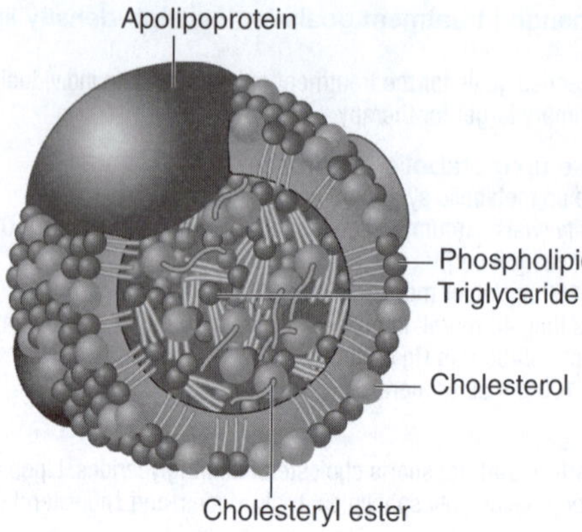

Fig. 42.4. A lipoprotein particle. The polar surface coat is composed of apoproteins, phospholipids, and free cholesterol. The nonpolar lipid core is composed of cholesterol esters and triglycerides. *(Reproduced with permission from Genest, J., & Libby, P. [2007]. Lipoprotein disorders and cardiovascular disease. In D. L. Mann, D. P. Zipes, P. Libby, & R. O. Bonow [Eds.].* Braunwald's heart disease: a textbook of cardiovascular medicine *[8th ed.]. Philadelphia, PA: Saunders.)*

also determines the predominant LDL size distribution (e.g., A "buoyant LDL"; AB "mixed phenotype"; or B "small, dense LDL" phenotypes) but does not provide concentrations of the lipoprotein particles themselves.

In contrast, NMR is based on the concept that each lipoprotein particle in plasma of a given size has its own characteristic lipid methyl group NMR signal. Particle concentrations of lipoprotein subfractions of different size are obtained from the measured amplitudes of their lipid methyl group NMR signals. Lipoprotein particle sizes are then derived from the sum of the diameter of each subclass multiplied by its relative mass percentage based on the amplitude of its methyl NMR signal. NMR simultaneously quantifies lipoprotein concentrations of VLDL, IDL, LDL, and HDL particles and their subfractions, each expressed as a lipoprotein particle concentration (number of particles per liter) or as an average particle size for each of VLDL, LDL, and HDL.

These specialized tests may have roles in certain individuals who would benefit from additional risk assessment. These tests should be interpreted by physicians who have expertise and understanding of them.

Bibliography and Suggested Readings

Ganda, O. P. (2015). Deciphering cholesterol treatment guidelines: a clinician's perspective. *Journal of the American Medical Association, 313*(10), 1009–1010.

Lloyd-Jones, D. M., Morris, P. B., Ballantyne, C. M., Birtcher, K. K., Daly, D. D., Jr., DePalma, S. M., et al. (2016). 2016 ACC expert consensus decision pathway on the role of non-statin therapies for LDL-cholesterol lowering in the management of atherosclerotic cardiovascular disease risk. *Journal of the American College of Cardiology, 68*, 92–125.

Perk, J., Backer, G. D., Gohlke, H., Graham, I., Reiner, Z., Verschuren, W. M., et al. (2012). European guidelines on cardiovascular disease prevention in clinical practice (version 2012). *European Heart Journal, 33*, 1635–1701.

Stone, N. J., Robinson, J., Lichtenstein, A. H., Bairey Merz, C. N., Lloyd-Jones, D. M., Blum, C. B., et al. (2013). 2013 ACC/AHA guideline on the treatment of blood cholesterol to reduce atherosclerotic cardiovascular risk in adults. *Journal of the American College of Cardiology, 63*, 2889–2934. http://dx.doi.org/10.1016/j.jacc.2013.11.002.

DIABETES AND CARDIOVASCULAR DISEASE

Mandeep S. Sidhu, Michael E. Farkouh

1. **What is the current global burden of diabetes, and what is its impact on the epidemiology of cardiovascular disease?**

The World Health Organization report of 2016 estimated the global burden of diabetes mellitus (DM) to be 422 million adults older than 18 years. It was estimated there were approximately 108 million individuals with DM in 1980, and this has nearly quadrupled by 2014. Furthermore, the global prevalence has nearly doubled from 4.7% in 1980 to approximately 8.5% by 2014. It is projected that by 2035 the increasing prevalence of DM will lead to approximately 592 million individuals inflicted with the disease. However, due to the rapid urbanization and adoption of Western lifestyle choices with sedentary living and dietary habits, the developing world is having a rapid progression in the proportion of diabetics—particularly in low-income populations.

Knowledge of the epidemiology of DM is important to place the expected contribution of DM to the global cardiovascular (CV) disease burden into perspective. The relationship between type 1 and type 2 DM and CV disease is well established. In particular, DM is a very strong risk factor for the development of coronary artery disease (CAD) and stroke. The hazard ratio for CAD death in diabetic patients is considered as high as 2.03 (95% confidence interval [CI]: 1.60 to 2.59) for men and 2.54 (95% CI: 1.84 to 3.49) for women.

Atherosclerosis accounts for 80% of all deaths in diabetic persons, compared with approximately 30% among nondiabetic persons. Atherosclerotic disease also accounts for greater than 75% of hospitalizations for diabetes-related complications.

Patients with diabetes but without previous myocardial infarction (MI) carry the same level of risk for subsequent acute coronary events as nondiabetic patients with previous MI. These results had prompted the Adult Treatment Panel III of the National Cholesterol Education Program to establish diabetes as a CAD risk equivalent, mandating aggressive antiatherosclerotic therapy. More recently, the 2013 American College of Cardiology/American Heart Association (ACC/AHA) Guideline on the Treatment of Blood Cholesterol to Reduce Atherosclerotic Cardiovascular Risk in Adults has further delineated diabetic patients as a specific high-risk subgroup warranting more aggressive lipid management.

2. **What is the impact of diabetes on cardiovascular disease outcomes?**

In addition to its salutary effects on stable atherosclerotic disease, diabetic patients experience an increased rate of early and late complications following acute coronary syndrome. Diabetic patients with non–ST-elevation acute coronary syndromes also experience more in-hospital MIs and associated complications and higher death rates. Diabetic patients also respond less optimally to fibrinolytic therapy, an effect that is sex-dependent—diabetic women fare worse than men. In patients with acute coronary syndromes complicated by hypotension and cardiogenic shock, diabetes is an independent risk variable for adverse outcomes, including death. In the short and long term, diabetic patients with acute coronary syndromes experience higher rates of heart failure, death, and repeat infarction and require more frequent coronary revascularization.

3. **What effect, if any, does diabetes have on the clinical manifestations and prognosis of peripheral arterial disease and cerebrovascular disease?**

Diabetes increases the risk of peripheral arterial disease (PAD) approximately twofold to fourfold. It is more commonly associated with femoral bruits and absent pedal pulses and with a high rate of abnormal ankle-brachial indices, ranging from 11% to 16% in different studies. The duration and severity of diabetes correlate with incidence and extent of PAD. The pattern of PAD in diabetic patients is characterized by a preponderance of infrapopliteal occlusive disease and vascular calcification. Clinically, PAD in diabetic patients manifests more commonly with claudication and also a higher rate of amputation—the most common cause of nontraumatic amputations.

Diabetic patients also have a higher rate of intracranial and extracranial cerebrovascular atherosclerosis and calcifications. Patients with a history of stroke have a threefold higher likelihood of being diabetic than controls, with a risk of stroke that may be up to threefold to fourfold higher than nondiabetic patients. Compared with nondiabetic subjects, the mortality from stroke in diabetic patients is almost threefold higher. Diabetes also results in a disproportionately higher stroke rate in younger patients and increases the risk of severe carotid disease. In patients younger than 55 years, diabetes increases the risk of stroke approximately 10 times, according to one study. Diabetic patients also suffer worse post-stroke outcomes, including a higher mortality rate and recurrence risk and a greater probability of vascular dementia.

4. What is the overall impact of diabetes on the vascular tree?

CV complications in diabetic patients can be the result of macrovascular disease, including CAD, PAD, and cerebrovascular disease, or they can be due to microvascular disease that can result in nephropathy, retinopathy, and neuropathy. Often diabetic cardiomyopathy is considered to be a distinct entity that is thought to result primarily from hyperglycemia-induced myocardial adverse effects.

5. What is the burden of additional cardiovascular risk factors in diabetic patients, and what is their cumulative impact on the atherosclerosis morphology and burden?

Diabetic patients are known to have a higher burden of CV risk factors, including nearly twice the prevalence of hypertension, and a higher prevalence of dyslipidemia, including lower high-density lipoprotein cholesterol (HDL-C), higher triglycerides, and low-density lipoprotein cholesterol (LDL-C) levels. The clustering of CV risk factors appears to have a multiplicative effect in diabetic patients, who experience a threefold higher CV mortality than nondiabetic persons for each risk factor present. In addition, CAD in diabetic patients involves a greater number of coronary vessels and more diffuse atherosclerotic lesions, including significantly more severe proximal and distal CAD.

Atherosclerotic plaque ulceration and thrombosis also occur more often in diabetic patients. Atherosclerotic plaques in diabetic patients are also considered high-risk plaques because of a greater propensity for erosion or rupture, which account for a higher incidence of acute coronary syndromes in this population. Diabetic plaques are characterized by high levels of inflammatory cell infiltration, large lipid cores, thin fibrous caps, and the presence of new vessel formation (neovascularization) and hemorrhage within the plaque.

6. What characteristics of the atherosclerotic plaque in diabetic patients make it unstable compared with plaque in nondiabetic patients?

Diabetic patients harbor proinflammatory and prothrombotic milieu with higher C-reactive protein (CRP), matrix metalloproteinase 3 and 9 (MMP-3 and MMP-9), intercellular adhesion molecule (ICAM), NFκ-beta, monocyte chemotactic protein-1 (MCP-1), plasminogen activator inhibitor-1 (PAI-1), and superoxide concentrations. In addition to its adverse effects on the endothelium, diabetes promotes processes that lead to monocyte transmigration across the endothelium into the vessel wall and uptake of oxidized LDLs into these cells, resulting in foam cell and fatty streak formation. In addition to plaque initiation, diabetes renders the atherosclerotic plaque unstable. Endothelial cells in diabetic patients release cytokines and enzymes (MMPs) that impair collagen synthesis by vascular smooth muscle cells and also accelerate its breakdown. Because collagen is an essential component of the plaque fibrous cap, weakening it renders the plaque unstable.

Plaque rupture or erosion triggers an intense local prothrombotic milieu, resulting in thrombus formation. In addition, following plaque rupture, diabetic platelets aggregate more aggressively and are more likely to deaggregate with more efficacious antiplatelet agents, especially prasugrel and ticagrelor, when compared with clopidogrel, as demonstrated in the diabetic cohorts of the Trial to Assess Improvement in Therapeutic Outcomes by Optimizing Platelet Inhibition with Prasugrel-Thrombolysis in Myocardial Infarction (TRITON-TIMI 38) and Platelet Inhibition and Patient Outcomes (PLATO) trials. Diabetes also results in elevated factor VII levels (procoagulant) and reduced protein C and antithrombin III levels (naturally occurring anticoagulants). Finally, diabetic endothelial cells produce more tissue factor, the major procoagulant found in atherosclerotic plaques.

7. What broad management strategy is advocated for diabetic patients with cardiovascular disease?

A multidisciplinary approach is the cornerstone in the successful management of diabetes and CV disease. Because the presence of diabetes is considered equivalent to having CAD, aggressive management of all potential risk factors, including hypertension, dyslipidemia, and the hypercoagulable state, are recommended. In addition to measures to promote weight loss by dietary modification and exercise, diabetic patients benefit from aggressively managing conventional risk factors. The strongest evidence supporting a multifaceted and comprehensive approach in the management of diabetic patients comes from the STENO-2 trial. It demonstrated that a strategy including lifestyle and pharmacologic interventions intended to reduce CV risk in type 2 diabetic patients with microalbuminuria was significantly more effective in reducing CV events and mortality than usual care in the long term.

Fig. 43.1 summarizes therapies to stem the onset and progression of atherosclerosis in patients with diabetes.

8. How does the treatment of hyperglycemia and insulin resistance impact outcomes in diabetic patients with cardiovascular disease?

Tight glycemic control has been shown to improve microvascular complications, including diabetic nephropathy. The 2016 American Diabetes Association target for HbA_{1C} is less than 7% and for the 2015 American College of Clinical Endocrinology target is less than 6.5%. Diabetic nephropathy occurs in 40% of patients with type 1 and type 2 diabetes, and the main risk factors for its development include poor glycemic control, hypertension, and ethnicity. The Diabetes Control and Complications Trial (DCCT) and the United Kingdom Prospective Diabetes Study group trial (UKPDS) demonstrated that the development and progression of microalbuminuria can be prevented through strict glycemic control. This was also demonstrated for type 2 patients in the Action in Diabetes and Vascular Disease: Preterax and Diamicron Modified Release Controlled Evaluation (ADVANCE) trial.

Despite epidemiologic evidence linking poor glycemic control with CV disease, the role of aggressive glucose control in reduction of CV risk is controversial and potentially harmful in susceptible populations. This has been an area of considérable debate because of the results of two recent large randomized controlled trials: ACCORD and ADVANCE. The means used to attain glycemic

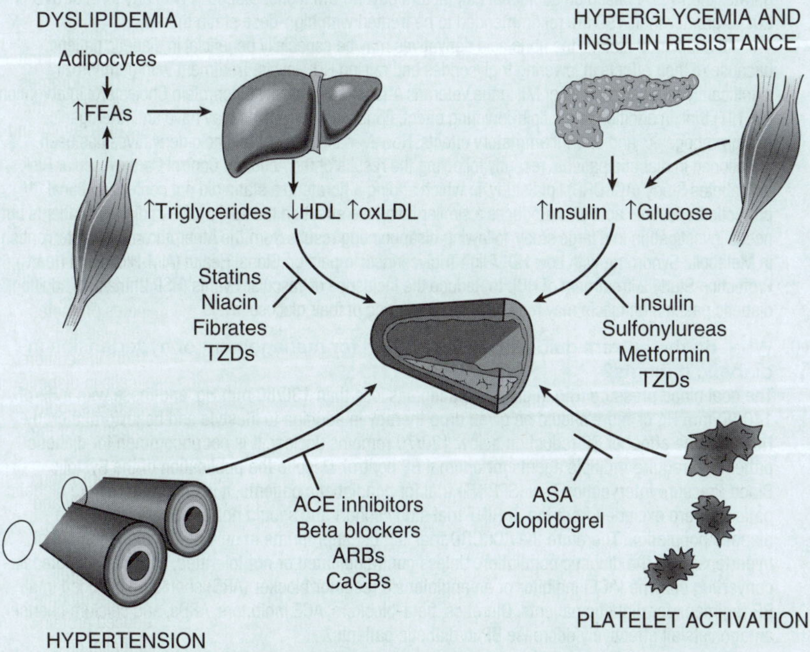

Fig. 43.1. Diabetes requires therapy for each metabolic abnormality to stem the onset and progression of atherosclerosis. Statins improve the lipid profile and decrease the risk of MI and death. Treatment of hypertension decreases the rate of myocardial infarction (MI) and stroke in patients with diabetes. Therapy should include ACE inhibitors or angiotensin receptor blockers (ARBs) for their microvascular and possible atherosclerosis benefits. The heightened thrombotic potential of the diabetic state supports the use of platelet antagonists, such as aspirin or clopidogrel. Although strict treatment of hyperglycemia does not significantly reduce the incidence of MI or death, the improvement in microvascular outcomes itself warrants vigorous pursuit of rigorous glycemic control in diabetes. *ACE*, Angiotensin-converting enzyme; *ASA*, aspirin; *CaCBs*, calcium channel blockers; *FFAs*, free fatty acids; *HDL*, high-density lipoprotein; *oxLDL*, oxidized low-density lipoprotein; *TZDs*, thiazolidinediones. *(Modified from Libby, P., & Plutzky, J. [2002]. Diabetic macrovascular disease: the glucose paradox?* Circulation, *106, 2760–2763.)*

control have received much scrutiny because of reports suggesting increased risk of CV disease, including mortality, MI, and fluid retention/heart failure with thiazolidinediones (TZD), and in particular rosiglitazone. Another TZD, pioglitazone, which is believed to have a relatively benign CV profile, has recently been associated with a higher incidence of bladder carcinoma and bone fractures.

For these reasons, metformin remains the first-line treatment option in most type 2 diabetes patients and seems to have a beneficial effect on insulin resistance without an adverse effect on CV disease. The Bypass Angioplasty Revascularization Investigation 2 Diabetes (BARI 2D) trial has demonstrated that an insulin-sensitizing strategy led by metformin was superior to an insulin provision strategy in reducing CV events in diabetic patients with established coronary disease. This landmark study also demonstrated the efficacy of medical management in diabetic patients with less extensive coronary disease.

9. What are the currently recommended strategies for the management of diabetic dyslipidemia?

The lipid abnormalities in diabetes improve with lifestyle modifications, including weight loss, exercise, smoking cessation, and dietary changes, which are the first line of treatment. The most effective intervention in the management of diabetic patients with CAD is the use of statin medications, which have proven especially useful in this population. In the Scandinavian Simvastatin Survival Study (4S) and Cholesterol and Recurrent Events (CARE) trials and the Heart Protection Study, simvastatin demonstrated a significantly greater benefit in mortality and MI compared with nondiabetic subjects. The 2013 ACC/AHA Guidelines on the Treatment of Blood Cholesterol to Reduce Atherosclerotic Cardiovascular Risk in Adults recommended all patients between the ages of 40 to 75 with diabetes and LDL-C 70 to 189 mg/dL without evidence of cardiovascular disease (CVD) should receive statin therapy with moderate-dose statin; however, high-dose statin should be considered if the 10-year risk by new risk calculator is greater than 7.5% based on additional risk factors beyond DM alone. Diabetics with any form of CVD or LDL-C greater than 190 are recommended to be treated with high-dose statin therapy.

In addition to statins, the fibric acid derivatives may be especially beneficial in diabetic patients because of their effects in lowering triglycerides and raising HDL levels. Treatment with gemfibrozil significantly reduced the risk of MI, in the Veterans Affairs High-Density Lipoprotein Cholesterol Intervention (VA-HIT) trial. In addition to the lipid-lowering effect, fibric acid derivatives may have antiatherogenic, antithrombogenic, and anti-inflammatory effects. However, the role of fibric acid derivatives has been questioned in diabetic patients recently following the results of the Action to Control Cardiovascular Risk in Diabetes Study (ACCORD) lipid study, in which adding a fibrate to a statin did not confer additional CV protection. Nicotinic acid also produces a similar favorable effect on the lipid profile in diabetic patients but needs investigation in a large study, following disappointing results from the Atherothrombosis Intervention in Metabolic Syndrome with Low HDL/High Triglycerides: Impact on Global Health (AIM-HIGH) and Heart Protection Study 2 Treatment of HDL to Reduce the Incidence of Vascular Events (HSP 2) trials. In addition, diabetic patients on niacin may require close monitoring of their glucose levels.

10. What do the current guidelines recommend for management of hypertension in diabetic patients?

The goal blood pressure (BP) in diabetic patients is less than 130/80 mm Hg, and those with a BP of 140/90 mm Hg or more should be given drug therapy in addition to lifestyle and behavioral therapy. However, the effect of BP reduction below 120/70 remains unclear. It is not uncommon for diabetic patients to require multiple agents for optimal BP control. Despite the publication of the Systolic Blood Pressure Intervention Trial (SPRINT) trial for nondiabetic patients, it is important to note diabetic patients were excluded from the SPRINT trial study cohort and should not be generalized to the diabetic population. Therefore the ACCORD trial is most appropriate in guiding the management of hypertension in the diabetic population. Unless contraindicated or not tolerated, either an angiotensin-converting enzyme (ACE) inhibitor or an angiotensin receptor blocker (ARB) should be included in all BP regimens for diabetic patients. Diuretics, beta-blockers, ACE inhibitors, ARBs, and calcium channel antagonists all effectively decrease BP in diabetic patients.

Regardless of the agent chosen, evidence from prior randomized clinical trials overwhelmingly favors good BP control. The recommendations given here are based on the results of trials of hypertension or CV prevention. In the Heart Outcomes and Prevention Evaluation (HOPE) study, ramipril significantly decreased the rates of MI, stroke, and death in patients with diabetes and one additional CV risk factor. The Losartan Intervention for Endpoint Reduction in Hypertension (LIFE) study demonstrated that losartan was more effective than atenolol for reducing CV mortality in diabetic patients with hypertension and left ventricle hypertrophy (LVH).

A summary of recommendations as of 2015 for CVD risk factor management in type 2 DM is given in Table 43.1.

Table 43.1. Summary of Current Recommendations as of 2015 for Cardiovascular Disease Risk Factor Management in Type 2 Diabetes Mellitus

RISK FACTOR	SPECIFIC RECOMMENDATIONS
Nutrition	• Reduction of energy intake for overweight or obese patients • Individualized medical nutrition therapy for all patients with diabetes mellitus • Carbohydrate monitoring as an important strategy for glycemic control • Consumption of fruits, legumes, vegetables, whole grains, and dairy products in place of other carbohydrate sources • Pattern may improve glycemic control and CVD risk factors • Limit of sodium to less than 1500-2300 mg/day, similar to recommendations for the general population • ADA Level of Evidence B; note that the AHA differs and recommends sodium less than 1500 mg/day
Obesity	• Overweight and obese patients should be counseled that lifestyle changes can produce a 3% to 5% rate of weight loss that can be sustained over time and that this can be associated with clinically meaningful health benefits • For patients with BMI ≥40 kg/m^2 or BMI ≥35 kg/m^2 with an obesity-related comorbidity who want to lose weight but have not responded to behavioral treatment with or without pharmacologic treatment, bariatric surgery may improve health
Blood glucose	• Lower A1c to ≤7.0% in most patients to reduce the incidence of microvascular disease; this can be achieved with a mean plasma glucose of ≈8.3 to 8.9 mmol/L (≈150-160 mg/dL); ideally, fasting and premeal glucose should be maintained at less than 7.2 mmol/L (<130 mg/dL) and postprandial glucose at less than 10 mmol/L (<180 mg/dL) • More stringent A1c targets (e.g., <6.5%) might be considered in selected patients (with short disease duration, long life expectancy, no significant CVD) if this can be achieved without significant hypoglycemia or other adverse effects of treatment • Less stringent A1c goals (e.g., <8.0% or even slightly higher) are appropriate for patients with a history of severe hypoglycemia, limited life expectancy, advanced complications, cognitive impairment, and extensive comorbid conditions and those in whom the target is difficult to attain despite intensive self-management education, repeated counseling, and effective doses of multiple glucose-lowering agents, including insulin
Blood pressure	• For most individuals with diabetes mellitus, achieve a goal of less than 140/90 mm Hg; lower targets may be appropriate for some individuals, although the guidelines have not yet been formally updated to incorporate this new information • Pharmacologic therapy should include a regimen with either an ACEI or an ARB (ADA Level of Evidence B); if one class is not tolerated, the other should be substituted • For patients with CKD, antihypertension treatment should include an ACEI or ARB • Hypertension/blood pressure control has been revised to suggest that the systolic blood pressure goal for many people with diabetes mellitus and hypertension should be less than 140 mm Hg but that lower systolic targets (e.g., <130 mm Hg) may be appropriate for certain individuals, such as younger patients, if it can be achieved without undue treatment burden
Cholesterol	• Patients with diabetes mellitus between 40 and 75 years of age with LDL-C between 70 and 189 mg/dL should be treated with a moderate-intensity statin • Statin therapy of high intensity should be given to individuals with diabetes mellitus between 40 and 75 years of age with a ≥7.5% estimated risk of ASCVD • Among individuals with diabetes mellitus who are 75 years of age, practitioners should evaluate the benefit of statin treatment. Evaluate and treat patients with fasting triglycerides greater than 500 mg/dL

ADA, American Diabetes Association; *ARB*, Angiotensin receptor blocker; *ASCVD*, atherosclerotic cardiovascular disease; *A1c*, glycated hemoglobin; *BMI*, body mass index; *CKD*, chronic kidney disease; *CVD*, cardiovascular disease; *LDL-C*, low-density lipoprotein cholesterol.

Adapted from Fox, C. S., Golden, S. H., Anderson, C., Bray, G. A., Burke, L. E., de Boer, I. H., et al. (2015). Update on prevention of cardiovascular disease in adults with type 2 diabetes mellitus in light of recent evidence: a scientific statement from the American Heart Association and the American Diabetes Association. Circulation, 132, 691–718.

11. **What are the principles of management of chronic coronary artery disease in diabetic patients?**
Diabetic patients are more likely to experience painless cardiac ischemia and suffer more silent MIs and sudden cardiac death. Evidence from observational studies and randomized trials has shown significant mortality benefit with beta-blockers in diabetic patients. Beta-blockers are well tolerated in diabetic patients; masking or prolongation of hypoglycemic symptoms is infrequent, particularly with cardioselective agents. Recommendations include continuing antiplatelet therapy; ACE inhibitors and ARBs should be used as appropriate for BP control, and beta-blockers are recommended in diabetic patients after an MI. However, routine screening for CAD in diabetic patients is not recommended, as demonstrated in the Detection Of Ischemia In Asymptomatic Diabetics (DIAD) trial. The multifaceted approach to the diabetic patient is illustrated in Fig. 43.1.

12. **What strategies for coronary revascularization are currently recommended for the management of multivessel coronary artery disease in diabetic patients?**
The optimal revascularization strategy in stable diabetic patients with multivessel coronary disease has been debated extensively in recent years. The BARI trial substudy of diabetic patients indicated that coronary artery bypass grafting (CABG) offered a clinically meaningful and statistically significant survival advantage in diabetic patients when compared with balloon angioplasty. Even in nondiabetic patients, the need for future revascularization has been traditionally higher in the angioplasty group compared with CABG, and these differences are even more pronounced in diabetic patients. However, BARI was conducted in an era when stents were not available. The BARI-2D trial suggested that diabetic patients with three vessel and severe coronary disease should preferably be managed with open revascularization. Because BARI-2D did not compare percutaneous coronary intervention (PCI) and CABG in patients with multivessel disease, the landmark Future Revascularization Evaluation in Patients with Diabetes Mellitus: Optimal Management of Multivessel Disease (FREEDOM) trial results suggest that in patients with DM and multivessel CAD, the superiority of CABG to PCI was mainly driven by differences in rates of MI and all-cause mortality.

13. **What alternative pharmacologic therapies should be considered in the diabetic population?**
Sodium-glucose co-transporter 2 (SGLT2)-inhibitors are a class of oral antidiabetic agents with a distinctive mechanism of action. In the renal glomeruli, approximately 180 g of glucose is filtered daily and reabsorbed thereafter in the proximal convoluted tubule via passive facilitated glucose transporters (GLUTs) and active cotransporters, SGLTs. There are six identified SGLTs, two of which (SGLT1 and SGLT2) are considered to be the most promising targets. SGLT2-inhibitors work by inhibiting SGLT2 in the PCT. This in turn prevents the reabsorption of glucose, facilitating its urinary excretion. Ultimately, excretion of glucose decreases its plasma levels, leading to an improvement in all glycemic parameters.

The Empagliflozin, Cardiovascular Outcomes, and Mortality in Type 2 Diabetes (EMPA-REG OUTCOME) trial studied the effects of empagliflozin, an SGLT2-inhibitor, in addition to standard care, on CV morbidity and mortality in patients with type 2 DM at high CV risk and showed that in the empagliflozin group there were significantly lower rates of death from CV causes (3.7% vs. 5.9% in the placebo group; 38% relative risk reduction; $p = <.001$), hospitalization for heart failure (2.7% and 4.1%, respectively; 35% relative risk reduction; $p = .02$), and death from any cause (5.7% and 8.3%, respectively; 32% relative risk reduction, $p = <.001$). In the future, this new class of pharmacologic agents may have a larger role in managing diabetic patients with an elevated CV risk, and further investigation is warranted to better understand these agents and their effects.

Bibliography and Suggested Readings

Action to Control Cardiovascular Risk in Diabetes Study Group, Gerstein, H. C., Miller, M. E., Byington, R. P., Goff, D. C., Jr., Bigger, J. T., et al. (2008). Effects of intensive glucose lowering in type 2 diabetes. *New England Journal of Medicine, 358*(24), 2545–2559.

ADVANCE Collaborative Group, Patel, A., MacMahon, S., Chalmers, J., Neal, B., & Billot, L. (2008). Intensive blood glucose control and vascular outcomes in patients with type 2 diabetes. *New England Journal of Medicine, 358*(24), 2560–2572.

American Diabetes Association. (2006). Standards of medical care in diabetes—2006. *Diabetes Care, 29*(Suppl. 1), S4–S42.

American Diabetes Association. (2016). Standards of medical care in diabetes—2016. *Diabetes Care, 39*(Suppl. 1), S1–S2.

Beckman, J. A., Creager, M. A., & Libby, P. (2002). Diabetes and atherosclerosis: epidemiology, pathophysiology, and management. *Journal of the American Medical Association, 287*(19), 2570–2581.

Berry, C., Tardif, J. C., & Bourassa, M. G. (2007). Coronary heart disease in patients with diabetes: part I: recent advances in prevention and noninvasive management. *Journal of the American College of Cardiology, 49*(6), 631–642.

Farkouh, M. E., Domanski, M., Sleeper, L. A., Siami, F. S., Dangas, G., Mack, M., et al. (2012). Strategies for multivessel revascularization in patients with diabetes. *New England Journal of Medicine, 367*, 2375–2384.

Fox, C. S., Golden, S. H., Anderson, C., Bray, G. A., Burke, L. E., de Boer, I. H., et al. (2015). Update on prevention of cardiovascular disease in adults with type 2 diabetes mellitus in light of recent evidence: a scientific statement from the American Heart Association and the American Diabetes Association. *Circulation, 132*, 691–718.

Gaede, P., Lund-Andersen, H., Parving, H. H., & Pedersen, O. (2008). Effect of a multifactorial intervention on mortality in type 2 diabetes. *New England Journal of Medicine, 358*(6), 580–591.

Goldberg, R. B., Mellies, M. J., Sacks, F. M., Moyé, L. A., Howard, B. V., Howard, W. J., et al. (1998). Cardiovascular events and their reduction with pravastatin in diabetic and glucose-intolerant myocardial infarction survivors with average cholesterol levels: subgroup analyses in the cholesterol and recurrent events (CARE) trial: the CARE investigators. *Circulation, 98*, 2513–2519.

Grundy, S. M., Cleeman, J. I., Merz, C. N., Brewer, H. B., Jr., Clark, L. T., Hunninghake, D. B., et al. (2004). Implications of recent clinical trials for the National Cholesterol Education Program Adult Treatment Panel III Guidelines. *Journal of the American College of Cardiology, 44*(3), 720–732.

Gu, K., Cowie, C. C., & Harris, M. I. (1999). Diabetes and decline in heart disease mortality in US adults. *Journal of the American Medical Association, 281*, 1291–1297.

Guariguata, L., Whiting, D. R., Hambleton, I., Beagley, J., Linnenkamp, U., & Shaw, J. E. (2014). Global estimates of diabetes prevalence for 2013 and projections for 2035. *Diabetes Research and Clinical Practice, 103*, 137–149.

Handelsman, Y., Bloomgarden, Z. T., Grunberger, G., Umpierrez, G., Zimmerman, R. S., Bailey, T. S., et al. (2015). American Association of Clinical Endocrinologists and American College of Endocrinology—Clinical Practice Guidelines for developing a diabetes mellitus comprehensive care plan—2015. *Endocrine Practice, 21*(Suppl. 1), 1–87.

Heart Outcomes Prevention Evaluation Study Investigators. Effects of ramipril on cardiovascular and microvascular outcomes in people with diabetes mellitus: results of the HOPE study and MICRO-HOPE substudy.*Lancet, 355*, (2000), 253–259.

Malmberg, K., Yusuf, S., Gerstein, H. C., Brown, J., Zhao, F., Hunt, D., et al. (2000). Impact of diabetes on long-term prognosis in patients with unstable angina and non-Q-wave myocardial infarction: results of the OASIS (Organization to Assess Strategies for Ischemic Syndromes) registry. *Circulation, 102*, 1014–1019.

McCullock, D. K. Overview of Medical Care in Adults with Diabetes Mellitus. < http://www.utdol.com >.

NCD Risk Factor Collaboration (NCD-RisC). (2016). Worldwide trends in diabetes since 1980: a pooled analysis of 751 population-based studies with 4.4 million participants. *Lancet, 387*(10027), 1513–1530. http://dx.doi.org/10.1016/S0140-6736(16)00618-8.

Pyörälä, K., Pedersen, T. R., Kjekshus, J., Faergeman, O., Olsson, A. G., Thorgeirsson, G., et al. (1997). Cholesterol lowering with simvastatin improves prognosis of diabetic patients with coronary heart disease. A subgroup analysis of the Scandinavian Simvastatin Survival Study (4S). *Diabetes Care, 20*, 614–620.

Skyler, J. S., Bergenstal, R., Bonow, R. O., Buse, J., Deedwania, P., Gale, E. A., et al. (2009). Intensive glycemic control and the prevention of cardiovascular events: implications of the ACCORD, ADVANCE, and VA Diabetes Trials: a position statement of the American Diabetes Association and a Scientific Statement of the American College of Cardiology Foundation and the American Heart Association. *Journal of the American College of Cardiology, 53*(3), 298–304.

Smith, S. C., Jr., Allen, J., Blair, S. N., Bonow, R. O., Brass, L. M., Fonarow, G. C., et al. (2006). ACC/AHA guidelines for secondary prevention for patients with coronary and other atherosclerotic vascular disease: 2006 update: endorsed by the National Heart, Lung, and Blood Institute. *Circulation, 113*(19), 2363–2372.

Stone, N. J., Robinson, J. G., Lichtenstein, A. H., Bairey Merz, C. N., Blum, C. B., Eckel, R. H., et al. (2013). 2013 ACC/AHA guideline on the treatment of blood cholesterol to reduce atherosclerotic cardiovascular risk in adults: a report of the American College of Cardiology/American Heart Association Task Force on Practice Guidelines. *Journal of the American College of Cardiology, 63*(25 Pt B), 2889–2934.

Tuomilehto, J. (2013). The emerging global epidemic of type 1 diabetes. *Current Diabetes Reports, 13*(6), 795–804.

WHO. (2016). *WHO Mortality Database* [online database]. Geneva: World Health Organization. <http://apps.who.int/healthinfo/statistics/mortality/causeofdeath_query/>.

Zinman, B., Wanner, C., Lachin, J. M., Fitchett, D., Bluhmki, E., Hantel, S., et al. (2015). Empagliflozin, cardiovascular outcomes, and mortality in type 2 diabetes. *New England Journal of Medicine, 373*(22), 2117–2128.

CHAPTER 44

SMOKING CESSATION

Andrew Pipe

1. **Why is smoking cessation of fundamental importance in managing the cardiac patient?**
   Smoking cessation is the most important of the modifiable risk factors for cardiovascular disease. The products of tobacco smoke contribute directly and distinctly to the development of atherosclerosis and its adverse consequences (Table 44.1). The benefits of smoking cessation cannot be exaggerated. A rapid and sustained reduction in the likelihood of cardiac disease or a cardiac event occurs in those who successfully stop smoking; following cessation, those with established cardiac disease experience a dramatic reduction in the likelihood of recurrence, complication, or death. In both instances the benefits of smoking cessation accrue rapidly and reflect the elimination rather than the ongoing management of a major risk factor (Table 44.2). The benefits of hypertension control and the management of dyslipidemia are attenuated by the persistence of smoking; continued smoking following coronary artery revascularization is associated with higher rates of adverse clinical outcomes. Smoking cessation should be accorded a priority in those with cardiac disease in every professional setting; to do otherwise should be seen as reflecting substandard care.

2. **Why have cardiologists neglected the treatment of tobacco addiction in the past?**
   For too long dogmas and misconceptions have surrounded the management of the patient who smokes; prominent among these were the perceptions that smoking was a "habit" or a "lifestyle choice" and that successful smoking cessation required little more than "grit and determination."

Table 44.1. Smoking and the Genesis of Cardiovascular Disease and Cardiac Events

The Products of Tobacco Smoke
1. Contribute to a proinflammatory state
2. Damage endothelial surfaces
3. Induce endothelial dysfunction
4. Distort the lipid profile and oxidize lipoproteins
5. Facilitate platelet aggregation and activation
6. Elevate fibrinogen levels
7. Potentiate the development of atheromas
8. Contribute to plaque "instability"
9. Produce elevated levels of carboxyhemoglobin and impair oxygen transport

Table 44.2. Mortality Risk Reduction in Those with Coronary Heart Disease

Smoking cessation	36%
Statin therapy	29%
Beta-blocker therapy	23%
ACE-I therapy	23%
ASA therapy	15%

ACE-I, Angiotensin-converting enzyme I; ASA, acetylsalicylic acid.

Critchley, J. A., & Capewell, S. (2003). Mortality risk reduction associated with smoking cessation in patients with coronary heart disease. A systematic review. Journal of the American Medical Association, 290, 86–97.

Such outdated beliefs have impeded our ability to address this fundamental, major cardiovascular risk factor. Assumptions and misconceptions have also clouded clinicians' understanding of the role that pharmacotherapy can play in aiding cessation. Misplaced concerns regarding the safety of nicotine-replacement therapy in the cardiac setting, for example, have precluded the use of this effective cessation pharmacotherapy.

3. What should every healthcare professional know about smoking?

Nicotine is the most addictive substance encountered in the community. Nicotine addiction is established in only a few days once inhalation has been "mastered." Thereafter brain function, structure, and neurochemistry are transformed. Smokers smoke to maintain levels of nicotine—and the elevated levels of dopamine and other neurotransmitters—whose release follows the stimulation of nicotine receptors. The cigarette is a perversely engineered drug delivery device designed to deliver a precise aliquot of nicotine as rapidly as possible. Smokers are "intra-arterial" drug users: following the inhalation of tobacco smoke, nicotine is delivered rapidly via the arterial system to the brainstem, where it initiates a cascade of neurologic activity and dopamine release.

Components of cigarette smoke stimulate the metabolism of caffeine (and several medications) via the cytochrome P450 system. Caffeine levels rise substantially when smoking stops, producing restlessness and discomfort. Advice to reduce caffeine levels by 50% or to switch to decaffeinated beverages should be provided to all coffee drinkers who are trying to stop smoking.

Most smokers know why they should not smoke; most smokers do not want to be smokers; and many smokers will make one or two unassisted quit attempts each year—most of which will fail. Smokers typically do not need more education or lectures. They want help. Optimal cessation strategies involve the following:

- The delivery of personally relevant, unambiguous, nonjudgmental advice regarding the fundamental importance of smoking cessation in the management of cardiac disease and the offer of specific assistance with cessation
- The use of pharmacotherapy to eliminate or curb the symptoms of withdrawal and craving that lead to the use of cigarettes
- The provision of strategic, tactical advice regarding the management or avoidance of those circumstances, settings, and situations that typically accompany and stimulate smoking

4. How might smokers with cardiac disease be better helped with cessation?

A systematic approach to the identification and documentation of the smoking status of all patients in every clinical setting permits the provision of advice regarding the fundamental importance of cessation in the management of any cardiac condition and, more importantly, prompts the delivery of specific cessation assistance and appropriate follow-up. Serendipitous considerations of smoking status, offhand advice regarding the need for cessation, or the assumption that this is the responsibility of others (typically the family physician) have contributed in the past to substandard care of the cardiac patient who smokes.

The management of tobacco addiction can be addressed in exactly the same way as other cardiovascular risk factors: once a risk factor is identified, a strategy for its management is outlined; medication is provided, monitored, and titrated appropriately until a desired endpoint is reached. Contemporary approaches to smoking cessation are no different. They involve the provision of strategic, tactical advice and counseling in association with the use of appropriately prescribed (titrated as necessary) cessation pharmacotherapy until a patient—free of the discomfort of cravings and withdrawal symptoms—acquires a repertoire of nonsmoking behaviors and is able to comfortably navigate all the daily circumstances and situations previously associated with smoking.

In hospitals and many other settings, clinical protocols, care maps, and other systematized approaches to the identification and treatment of smokers are becoming the norm; they facilitate and enhance the care of patients addicted to tobacco (Table 44.3).

5. What is a good starting point for smoking cessation?

In the past, approaches to smoking cessation have placed an emphasis on the patient's "preparation and planning" prior to reaching a quit date. There is increasing evidence that asking about willingness to embark on a quit attempt at every patient encounter can be helpful, capitalizing on recent clinical events and a patient's interest in cessation. Even among those expressing disinterest in cessation, the provision of smoking cessation pharmacotherapy can result in a decline in cigarette consumption and has been demonstrated to be effective in stimulating a quit attempt and cessation. This reduce-to-quit (RTQ) paradigm may be particularly appropriate in the cardiac setting, where further follow-up is likely

Table 44.3. A Systematic Approach to Smoking Cessation in Every Cardiac Setting

IDENTIFY	Identify the smoking status of all patients: "Have you used any form of tobacco in the past 6 months?" "Have you used any form of tobacco in the past 7 days?"
DOCUMENT	Make sure that smoking status and history are documented in the medical record and prompt an appropriate cessation intervention.
ADVISE	Make sure that the patient is advised of the importance of cessation in an unambiguous, nonjudgmental, personally relevant manner.
ACT	Provide cessation pharmacotherapy and strategic cessation advice as appropriate.
FOLLOW-UP	Arrange appropriate follow-up (smoking cessation clinic, primary-care practitioner, community services, quit-lines, etc.)

Reid, R. D., Mullen, K. A., Pipe, A. L. (2011). *Systematic approaches to smoking cessation in the cardiac setting.* Current Opinion in Cardiology, *26*(5), 443–438.

to occur. Both patient and clinician will be pleasantly surprised to note that cigarette consumption has fallen appreciably, serving as an appropriate entrée to a more carefully planned cessation attempt with ongoing follow-up (perhaps in association with the family physician).

6. How can one best use pharmacotherapy to optimize the likelihood of cessation?

The appropriate use of pharmacotherapy, titration if necessary, and follow-up will substantially increase the likelihood of successful cessation. Three first-line pharmacotherapies are currently available: Nicotine replacement therapy (NRT), bupropion, and varenicline. Patient experience or preference may be the fundamental determinant of choice of therapy. Combination NRT (patch plus short-acting NRT) and varenicline have demonstrated the greatest overall effectiveness, tripling the likelihood of successful cessation. In all cases the titration and/or prolongation of therapy may be necessary to ensure effectiveness or to mitigate certain side effects. We have been comfortable and confident in asking patients to take medications to address hypertension and dyslipidemia—for decades! Ironically, however, we have been reluctant to offer smoking cessation treatment beyond a few short weeks despite evidence that prolonged treatment can be beneficial.

7. Can nicotine replacement therapy be initiated in the inpatient setting for patients with cardiac disease?

Yes. NRT may be offered to smokers within hours of patient admission. In many smokers nicotine withdrawal occurs rapidly, producing discomfort for them and a variety of behavioral challenges for clinical staff. These factors complicate compliance with treatment of such patients' cardiac conditions. For years, evidence has been accumulating attesting to the safety of NRT in cardiac patients. Nicotine in this setting is delivered slowly via the venous system (not the arterial system, as is the case with smoking); it achieves steady-state levels that will always be far less than those to which a smoker has been accustomed. Such treatment is not accompanied by the inhalation of carbon monoxide and countless other toxins, and it is provided to patients who have developed a marked tolerance to the cardiovascular effects of nicotine. A standardized order template may be helpful in guiding the use of NRT (Table 44.4).

8. What if a smoker reports that nicotine replacement therapy has not decreased his or her desire to smoke?

Smokers may report that the use of NRT was not associated with any decrease in the desire to smoke; this is a classic indication of underdosing. It has been calculated that the standard doses of NRT will not meet the nicotine "needs" of a majority of today's smokers. Smokers are able to titrate nicotine intake with considerable precision; thus the use of a nicotine "inhaler" in association with a

Table 44.4.

University of Ottawa Heart Institute	
Standard Orders for Nicotine Replacement Therapy	
20 Cigarettes per day	21-mg NRT patch +/– short-acting NRT
30 Cigarettes per day	21 + 7-mg NRT patches +/– short-acting NRT
40 Cigarettes per day	2 × 21-mg NRT patches +/– short-acting NRT
Short-acting NRT = NRT "inhaler," NRT lozenge, NRT spray, NRT gum	
Standard Orders for Bupropion	
Days 1-3	150 mg daily
Day 4-Week 12	150 mg twice daily
Standard Orders for Varenicline	
Days 1-3	0.5 mg daily
Days 4-7	0.5 mg twice daily
Weeks 2-12	1 mg twice daily

NRT, Nicotine replacement therapy.
In each case be prepared to titrate therapy to ensure control of withdrawal and craving or to address dose-related side effects. Therapy may be prolonged as necessary in order to prevent relapse to smoking. Consideration may be given to combining therapies in those who find single-agent treatments insufficient to address symptoms of withdrawal and craving and/or for whom total cessation has not been achieved.

nicotine patch will allow the emerging nonsmoker to titrate nicotine to meet particular needs, usually at times of more intense craving or withdrawal. Use of NRT, as with every cessation pharmacotherapy, can be continued until its discontinuation is not accompanied by an urge to smoke or a lapse to smoking in response to certain stimuli or surroundings. It is exceptionally rare for patients to become NRT-dependent.

9. Can bupropion be useful for smoking cessation?

As an antidepressant, bupropion was found also to be efficacious in smoking cessation; it stimulates noradrenergic and dopaminergic centers in the brain associated with withdrawal and craving, respectively. It is contraindicated in those with a history of or propensity for seizures. Like all smoking cessation medications, it may cause transient insomnia or sleep disturbance and can be associated with dose-related side effects (e.g., dry mouth, skin rash, tremor), which will typically respond to titration of therapy—in this case a reduction in dose. Over an initial 7-day period doses are gradually increased to achieve therapeutic levels, at which point a quit date is reached.

10. Can varenicline be useful for smoking cessation?

Varenicline acts as a nicotinic acetylcholine receptor (nAChR) partial agonist and antagonist; as such it stimulates this receptor, triggering a degree of dopamine release in the forebrain while occupying and blocking the receptor site, thus preventing nicotine from exerting its effects when and if smoking occurs. Most patients receiving varenicline experience little or no craving for nicotine and, if they do smoke, derive no sensation or "benefit" typically associated with smoking. Varenicline has been shown to be the most effective single agent for inducing cessation and has demonstrated effectiveness in those with stable cardiovascular disease (CVD). Concerns have been raised about an increase in cardiovascular events among those using this medication; however, no clear evidence of a causal relationship has been identified, nor has a biologically plausible reason for any such effects been suggested. The publication of a recent meta-analysis has dispelled those concerns. There is now clear evidence that varenicline does not induce neuropsychiatric side effects—a concern that persisted despite accumulating evidence to the contrary. The risks of any smoking cessation pharmacotherapy must always be considered against the risks of continued smoking. The principal side effects of varenicline are nausea, which can typically be managed by taking the medication with meals and a full glass of water or by reducing the dose, and sleep disturbances, usually short-lived. Both side effects are produced by varenicline's stimulation of nicotine receptors in the gut and brain.

Bibliography and Suggested Readings

Aboyans, V., Thomas, D., & Lacroix, P. (2010). The cardiologist and smoking cessation. *Current Opinion in Cardiology, 25*(5), 469–477.

Ambrose, J., & Barua, R. (2004). The pathophysiology of cigarette smoking and cardiovascular disease: an update. *Journal of the American College of Cardiology, 43*(10), 1731–1737.

Anthenelli, R. M., Benowitz, N. L., West, R., St Aubin, L., McRae, T., Lawrence, D., et al. (2016). Neuropsychiatric safety and efficacy of varenicline, bupropion, and nicotine patch in smokers with and without psychiatric disorders (EAGLES): a double-blind, randomised, placebo-controlled trial. *Lancet.* Published online April 22, 2016. http://dx.doi.org/10.1016/S0140-6736(16)30294-X.

Baker, T. B., Piper, M. E., Stein, J. H., Smith, S. S., Bolt, D. M., Fraser, D. L., et al. (2016). Effects of nicotine patch vs. varenicline vs. combination nicotine replacement therapy on smoking cessation at 26 weeks: a randomized clinical trial. *Journal of the American Medical Association, 315*, 371–379.

Benowitz, N. L. (2003). Cigarette smoking and cardiovascular disease: pathophysiology and implications for treatment. *Progress in Cardiovascular Diseases, 46*(1), 91–111.

Benowitz, N. L. (2008). Neurobiology of nicotine addiction: implications for smoking cessation treatment. *American Journal of Medicine, 121*(4A), S3–S10.

Benowitz, N., & Gourlay, S. (1997). Cardiovascular toxicity of nicotine: implications for nicotine replacement therapy. *Journal of the American College of Cardiology, 29*(7), 1422–1431.

Critchley, J. A., & Capewell, S. (2003). Mortality risk reduction associated with smoking cessation in patients with coronary heart disease: a systematic review. *Journal of American Medical Association, 290*(1), 86–97.

Ebbert, J. O., Burke, M. V., Hays, J. T., & Hurt, R. D. (2009). Combination treatment with varenicline and nicotine replacement therapy. *Nicotine & Tobacco Research, 11*(5), 572–576.

Erhardt, L. (2009). Cigarette smoking: an undertreated risk factor for cardiovascular disease. *Atherosclerosis, 205*(1), 23–32.

Fiore, M. C., Jaen, C. R., Baker, T. B., et al. (2008). *Treating tobacco use and dependence: 2008 update. Clinical practice guideline.* Rockville, MD: US Dept of Health and Human Services, Public Health Service.

Frey, P., Waters, D. D., De Micco, D. A., Breazna, A., Samuels, L., Pipe, A., et al. (2011). Impact of smoking on cardiovascular events in patients with coronary disease receiving contemporary medical therapy (from the Treating to New Targets [TNT] and the Incremental Decrease in End Points Through Aggressive Lipid Lowering [IDEAL] Trials). *American Journal of Cardiology, 107*, 145–150.

Hubbard, R., Lewis, S., Smith, C., Godfrey, C., Smeeth, L., Farrington, P., et al. (2005). Use of nicotine replacement therapy and the risk of acute myocardial infarction, stroke, and death. *Tobacco Control, 14*(6), 416–421.

Hurt, R. D., Dale, L. C., Offord, K. P., Lauger, G. G., Baskin, L. B., Lawson, G. M., et al. (1993). Serum nicotine and cotinine levels during nicotine-patch therapy. *Clinical Pharmacology and Therapeutics, 54*(1), 98–106.

Hurt, R. D., Sachs, D. P., Glover, E. D., Offord, K. P., Johnston, J. A., Dale, L. C., et al. (1997). A comparison of sustained-release bupropion and placebo for smoking cessation. *New England Journal of Medicine, 337*(17), 1195–1202.

Jorenby, D. E., Hays, J. T., Rigotti, N. A., Azoulay, S., Watsky, E. J., Williams, K. E., et al. (2006). Efficacy of varenicline, an alpha4beta2 nicotinic acetylcholine receptor partial agonist, vs placebo or sustained-release bupropion for smoking cessation: a randomized controlled trial. *Journal of the American Medical Association, 296*(1), 56–63.

Pipe, A. (2010). Tobacco and cardiovascular disease: achieving smoking cessation in cardiac patients. In S. Yusuf (Ed.), *Evidence based cardiology* (3rd ed.). Oxford: Blackwell Publishing.

Pipe, A. L., Eisenberg, M. J., Gupta, A., Reid, R. D., Suskin, N. G., & Stone, J. A. (2011). Smoking cessation and the cardiovascular specialist: Canadian Cardiovascular Society position paper. *Canadian Journal of Cardiology, 27*(2), 132–137.

Prochaska, J. J., & Hilton, J. F. (2012). Risk of cardiovascular serious adverse events associated with varenicline use for tobacco cessation: systematic review and meta-analysis. *British Medical Journal, 344*, e2856.

Rigotti, N. A., Pipe, A. L., Benowitz, N. L., Arteaga, C., Garza, D., & Tonstad, S. (2010). Efficacy and safety of varenicline for smoking cessation in patients with cardiovascular disease: a randomized trial. *Circulation, 121*(2), 221–229.

Zhang, Y. J., Iqbal, J., van Klaveren, D., Campos, C. M., Holmes, D. R., Kappetein, A. P., et al. (2015). Smoking is associated with adverse clinical outcomes in patients undergoing revascularization with PCI or CABG: the SYNTAX trial at 5-year follow-up. *Journal of the American College of Cardiology, 65*(11), 1107–1115.

PHYSICAL ACTIVITY, EXERCISE, AND THE HEART

CHAPTER 45

Megan Titas, Eric Awtry, Gary J. Balady

1. What is the difference between physical activity and exercise?

Physical activity is skeletal muscle contraction causing body movement that requires energy use. *Exercise* is a type of planned physical activity that is performed to attain or maintain physical fitness. Physical activity can be classified metabolically as *anaerobic* (energy derived in the absence of oxygen) or *aerobic* (energy derived in the presence of oxygen). Physical activity is defined mechanically as activities that produce limb movement without a change in muscle tension (*isotonic* exercise, more commonly known as aerobic, endurance, or dynamic exercise, includes activities such as walking, running, swimming, cycling), versus activities that cause muscle tension without limb movement (*isometric* exercise, more commonly known as resistance exercise, such as weight lifting). Most physical activity and exercise include a combination of isometric and isotonic activities.

2. How is physical activity intensity defined?

Intensity is the rate of energy expenditure during physical activity per unit of time. It can be measured directly using respiratory gas analysis during exercise to quantify oxygen uptake. Intensity is usually expressed in relation to resting energy expenditure, where 1 metabolic equivalent (MET) equals a resting energy expenditure of approximately 3.5 mL O_2/kg per minute. Light activities are less than 4 METs, moderate activities 4 to 6 METs, and vigorous activities greater than 6 METs.

Relative intensity is related to individual cardiorespiratory fitness. It is expressed as percentage of maximal exercise capacity performed during exercise and can be reported as a percentage of maximal heart rate (HR) or maximal oxygen uptake (VO_{2max}).

Relative intensity can further delineate the intensity of activity interpretation. For example, walking is considered a moderate-intensity (4 to 6 METs) activity. Walking briskly at 3 mph has an intensity of about 4 METs; however, the relative intensity is considered light for a healthy 20-year-old, as opposed to vigorous for an 80-year-old. Activities with moderate relative intensity usually occur at 40% to 60% of VO_{2max}.

3. How is physical activity measured?

Traditionally, physical activity measurements have been obtained through self-report, which is limited by over- and underestimation of true physical activity. New mobile health technologies, such as pedometers, accelerometers, and HR monitors via smartphone applications and wearable devices that are commercially available are able to directly and accurately measure physical activity. Most simple devices can measure activity such as steps/day or distance walked. Advanced models can provide reliable information on frequency, intensity, and duration of physical activity.

4. What are the acute cardiovascular changes that occur with physical activity and exercise?

Aerobic activities cause HR and stroke volume (SV) to increase, producing a four- to six-fold increase in cardiac output among healthy individuals. This occurs through several mechanisms. With aerobic activities, there is decreased vagal tone and increased sympathetic tone, resulting in increased HR. HR can gradually increase to a maximum, predicted from the following formula:

$$\text{Maximum predicted HR} = 220 - \text{age (in years)}$$

Increased venous return from exercising muscle coupled with increased left ventricular emptying from decreased systemic vascular resistance due to vasodilation in exercising muscle and improved myocardial contractility yield a 20% to 50% increase in SV. Vascular beds outside the heart, brain, and exercising muscle vasoconstrict, and with increased cardiac output, systolic blood pressure (SBP) increases and diastolic blood pressure (DBP) remains the same to slightly lower.

Resistance activities cause increased HR and thereby increased cardiac output. Contraction in exercising muscle increases peripheral vascular resistance, resulting in increased SBP and DBP (Fig. 45.1).

5. **What are the chronic cardiovascular changes that occur with exercise?**
Over time, isotonic activities associated with increased venous return and cardiac output result in left ventricular dilation with minimal increase in wall thickness. Chronic isometric activities result in increased left ventricular wall thickness with normal left ventricular dimensions.

6. **What is the training effect?**
Regular participation in aerobic exercise improves exercise capacity, whereas regular participation in resistance exercise increases strength. The *training effect* refers to these physiologic changes, which allow individuals to exercise at a higher intensity for longer duration and achieve lower HRs at submaximal levels of exercise.

7. **Do endurance training and resistance training have similar benefits?**
Both types of activities improve insulin resistance, bone mineral density, and body composition. Both types of training can have beneficial effects on reducing fat mass. Endurance activities improve peak exercise capacity and increase caloric expenditure while performing these activities. Resistance training increases strength and resting energy expenditure through increased muscle mass.

8. **What is an exercise prescription?**
A recommended exercise regimen that is individualized for each patient and takes into account the patient's physical abilities, cardiac status, and medical comorbidities is an *exercise prescription.* It includes the four components of *intensity, duration, frequency,* and *modality*. The exercise prescription for healthy adults is detailed in the following question, "How much exercise is necessary to improve or maintain cardiovascular fitness?" More specific exercise prescriptions can be provided for several

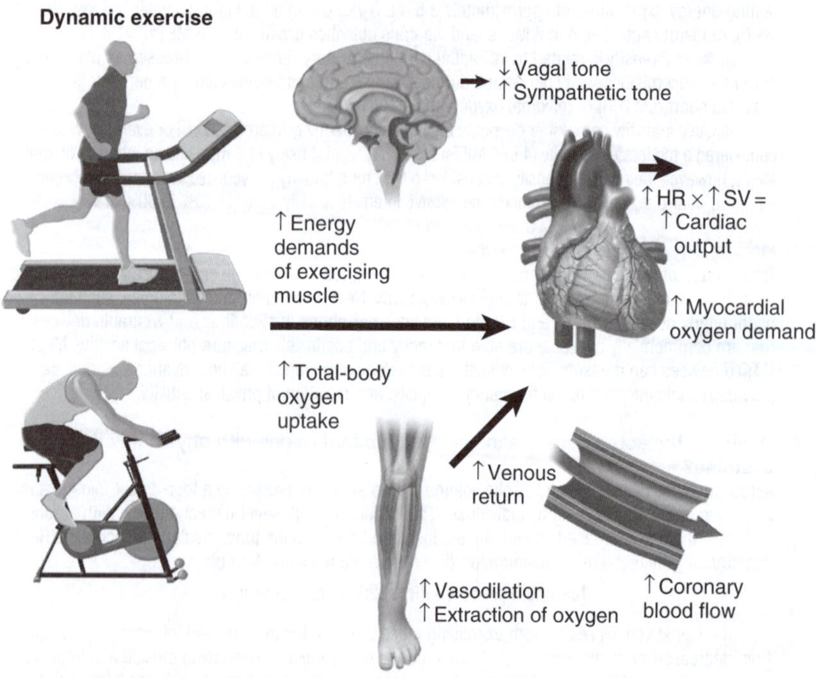

Fig. 45.1. Physiologic responses to acute exercise. See the text for details. *HR*, Heart rate; *SV*, stroke volume. *(From Mann, D. L., Zipes, D. P., Libby, P., & Bonow, R. O. [Eds.]. [2015].* Braunwald's heart disease: a textbook of cardiology *[10th ed., pp. 155–178]. Philadelphia, PA: Elsevier Saunders.)*

cardiovascular conditions including coronary artery disease (CAD), heart failure, and peripheral arterial disease (PAD). These are further addressed in the following questions.

9. **How much exercise is necessary to maintain or improve cardiovascular fitness?**
Guidelines from the American Heart Association (AHA) and American College of Sports Medicine (ACSM) recommend that healthy adults perform at least 30 minutes of moderate-intensity activities (e.g., brisk walking) for at least 5 days per week or 20 minutes of vigorous-intensity activities (e.g., jogging) at least 3 times per week, plus resistance training at least 2 days per week. This daily activity goal does not need to be attained in one sitting, but smaller quantities throughout the day can be accrued for the daily goal. Individuals who would like to achieve weight loss or increased physical fitness may need to exceed these baseline recommendations of weekly activity. The Physical Activity Guidelines for Americans also recommend avoidance of inactivity or prolonged sedentary behavior.

10. **What is the effect of exercise on cardiac risk factors?**
Exercise has numerous beneficial effects on hypertension, diabetes, and obesity as well as thrombosis, endothelial function, autonomic tone, and inflammation (Table 45.1).

11. **What is the effect of physical activity on mortality?**
Observational studies show that there is an inverse relationship between all-cause mortality and the amount of physical activity for healthy individuals and those with chronic diseases such as diabetes and cardiovascular disease, including heart failure. Individuals who participate in regular physical activity may be able to decrease cardiovascular risk 30% to 50% as compared with inactive individuals. An individual's maximal physical exertion, or *exercise capacity* (as measured in METs), is a strong predictor of risk of death in those with and without cardiovascular disease. Higher exercise capacity is associated with longer survival.

12. **Is there an age limit on the benefits of physical activity/exercise?**
In every age group and ethnic group, including older individuals, those who are physically active appear to have a mortality benefit. Those who become more active also gain a mortality benefit compared with those individuals who remain sedentary. Conversely, individuals who were physically active when younger but do not remain physically active do not appear to gain any long-term mortality benefit.

13. **Is it safe for patients with known coronary artery disease to exercise?**
Yes! Exercise is not only safe but confers many benefits: reduced risk of death, improved cardiac risk factor profiles, less angina and ischemia at any level of exertion, and increased exercise capacity. Patients with known CAD enrolled in cardiac rehabilitation programs have a 20% decreased risk of death and 25% decreased risk of cardiac death when compared to those with CAD not enrolled in an exercise program. Furthermore, individuals who have undergone percutaneous coronary intervention (PCI) who participate in cardiac rehabilitation have a 40% reduction in all-cause mortality.

Table 45.1. Beneficial Effects of Endurance Exercise on Atherosclerotic Risk Factors

FACTOR	EFFECT OF EXERCISE
Hypertension	Modest ↓ in SBP (approximately 4 mm Hg) and DBP (approximately 3 mm Hg)
Diabetes	↑ Insulin sensitivity, ↓ hepatic glucose production, preferential use of glucose over fatty acids by exercising muscle
Hyperlipidemia	Significant ↓ in TG, modest ↑ in HDL, minimal change in LDL
Obesity	Modest weight loss (2-3 kg), ↓ in body fat necessary to maintain weight loss
Thrombosis	↓ Fibrinogen, ↓ platelet activation
Endothelial function	Improved vasodilation, possibly through ↑ NO synthesis
Autonomic tone	↑ Vagal tone, ↓ sympathetic tone
Inflammation	↓ Inflammatory markers (CRP, TNF-α, IL-6)

CRP, C-reactive protein; *DBP*, diastolic blood pressure; *HDL*, high-density lipoprotein; *IL*, interleukin; *LDL*, low-density lipoprotein; *NO*, nitric oxide; *SBP*, systolic blood pressure; *TG*, triglycerides; *TNF*, tumor necrosis factor.

There is an important incremental benefit between the number of cardiac rehabilitation sessions attended and the magnitude of the benefit obtained. Analysis of 30,161 persons in the Medicare database who had suffered a recent myocardial infarction (MI), had acute coronary syndrome, or had undergone recent coronary artery bypass surgery who attended all 36 cardiac rehabilitation sessions had an incrementally lower risk of death and MI than patients who attended 24 sessions (14% and 12% reduction, respectively), 12 sessions (22% and 23% reduction, respectively), or only 1 session (47% and 31% reduction, respectively). Unfortunately, only a minority of patients attend the full cardiac rehabilitation course; addressing barriers to participation in these programs is crucial to ensure success.

14. How soon after a myocardial infarction can a patient begin an exercise program?

As long as patients are clinically stable, physical activity can begin 1 to 2 days post MI, as part of inpatient cardiac rehabilitation programs. Activities may start with range of motion and rapidly progress to assisted walking and finally independent activities of daily living upon hospitalization discharge. Current guidelines from the AHA and American College of Cardiology (ACC) recommend that all clinically stable post-infarction patients be referred to formal cardiac rehabilitation programs at time of discharge. This is especially important in patients with multiple risk factors and those of higher risk (residual CAD and/or reduced left ventricular systolic function) where supervised exercise is warranted. Most patients can start cardiac rehabilitation programs in 2 to 3 weeks.

15. Is exercise safe for patients with heart failure?

Yes! As long as they are clinically stable and not decompensated. The physiologic changes that occur with isotonic physical activity (increased SV and decreased systemic vascular resistance) are favorable changes for those with decreased left ventricular systolic function. Studies have shown that supervised exercise training in patients with stable heart failure increases functional capacity, decreases heart failure symptoms, increases quality of life scores, and decreases all-cause mortality and all-cause hospitalization. Conversely, participation in cardiac rehabilitation exercise training is generally safe in patients with stable well-controlled heart failure, including those patients with implanted cardioverter-defibrillators (ICD). Light- to moderate-resistance training is also safe and beneficial for patients with heart failure.

16. Does exercise benefit patients who are limited by claudication?

Yes! Walking exercise programs are currently recommended as first-line therapy for treatment of intermittent claudication. Exercise training in patients with claudication improves exercise capacity, decreases symptoms of claudication, and improves quality of life scores, which is similar to outcomes attained by invasive techniques (surgery or percutaneous peripheral intervention). Exercise training in those with PAD improves exercise capacity and leg strength. Patients who suffer from claudication should be encouraged to exercise until mild to moderate claudication symptoms occur, rest until symptoms resolve, and then resume activity. PAD is a strong predictor of CAD; thus, aggressive risk factor modification should also be pursued.

17. How is an exercise prescription developed for patients with known coronary artery disease?

Ideally, patients with known CAD should undergo formal exercise testing to quantify their exercise capacity, assess for inducible ischemia, and thereby derive an exercise intensity that is safe and effective. To prescribe exercise *intensity*, an HR range is recommended by determining 50% to 85% of the *HR reserve*, which is the difference between resting HR and peak HR on the exercise test. This is then added to resting HR to provide a target training HR range. If ischemia occurs during exercise testing (by symptoms or ECG changes), then the peak training HR is prescribed 10 beats below the HR at which the ischemia occurred. If a patient has an ICD, the peak training HR is prescribed at least 20 beats below ICD therapy HR. Exercise *duration* should be at least 20 to 30 minutes and at an exercise *frequency* of 3 to 5 days/week. Exercise *modalities* for aerobic training include walking/jogging (treadmill), elliptical trainer, rowing, cycling, and stair climbing.

18. Should patients with heart disease perform resistance training?

Yes! Resistance training is an important part of the exercise program for patients with and without heart disease and is particularly beneficial in those with diabetes, stable heart failure, and older adults. Improvements in muscle strength and endurance with resistance training help with activities of daily living and returning to the workplace. Resistance training is prescribed at the following levels:

- *Intensity:* 10 to 15 repetitions per set, using a load that is based on the maximum load (ML) that the patient can lift a single time (upper body: 30% to 40% ML; lower body: 50% to 60% ML).

- *Duration:* Patients should perform 1 to 3 sets of 8 to 10 different upper- and lower-body exercises at a *frequency* of 2 to 3 times per week.
- *Modality:* Common *modalities* for resistance training include free weights, weight machines, wall pulleys, elastic bands, and calisthenics.

19. What about interval training?

Standard training programs involve constant moderate-intensity exercise. *Aerobic interval training* refers to regimens where periods (several minutes) of high-intensity activities (90% to 95% peak exercise HR) alternate with moderate-intensity activities (60% to 70% peak exercise HR). Aerobic interval training appears to improve cardiovascular fitness in patients with heart failure and after coronary artery bypass as compared to standard exercise programs; however, limited safety and efficacy data preclude the routine inclusion of aerobic interval training in physical activity recommendations for individuals with cardiovascular disease at this time.

20. How can we encourage our patients to engage in regular physical activity or exercise?

Healthcare providers should promote physical activity by assessing activity levels in routine office visits and then prescribing it when warranted. Wearable devices that can measure physical activity are now commercially available and are reasonably accurate. Use of these devices to encourage and monitor physical activity offers promise in this effort, and they are currently being investigated in many ongoing studies.

Referral to cardiac rehabilitation programs is recommended by AHA/ACC guidelines for patients with recent MI, acute coronary syndrome, chronic stable angina, heart failure, and patients who have undergone recent coronary bypass surgery, PCI, valve surgery, or heart transplant. The use of cardiac rehabilitation programs by eligible patients is unfortunately very low (14% to 35% of post-MI patients and approximately 31% of patients after coronary bypass surgery). Lower referral and enrollment/completion of cardiac rehabilitation programs are found more commonly in patients who are female, older, and minorities and have lower socioeconomic status and lower education levels, speak languages other than English, lack insurance coverage and social support, and have work constraints. Efforts to address these barriers and improve participation rates are being explored: new home- and Internet-based cardiac rehabilitation programs for lower risk patients and offering individualized programs (woman-specific, lower cost, less intensive options, with counseling and coaching help by nonphysician medical professionals by all means of communication—in person, phone, apps, and Internet).

21. Are there cardiovascular risks of exercise?

The risk of adverse cardiac events in healthy individuals is extremely low and varies depending on age, gender, level of fitness, and medical conditions. Adverse cardiac events are mostly related to underlying structural or congenital abnormalities (hypertrophic cardiomyopathy, coronary anomalies, arrhythmogenic right ventricular cardiomyopathy) in young individuals, or underlying CAD in older individuals. Vigorous exercise is associated with a transient increase in MI and sudden cardiac death, especially in sedentary individuals with underlying CAD.

22. Should patients be screened before enrolling in an exercise program?

Per AHA/ACC guidelines, athletes in high school and college should have personal and family history evaluated as well as a cardiovascular exam prior to participation in competitive athletics. Abnormal findings should guide further testing. Routine screening electrocardiography for all athletes is not presently recommended. Healthy individuals without cardiovascular disease or symptoms can start mild- to moderate-intensity exercise programs without pre-participation medical evaluation. Pre-participation exercise stress testing should be performed in those individuals with known CAD or symptoms suggestive of CAD and should be considered in asymptomatic men older than 45 and women older than 55 with risk factors of cardiovascular disease and/or diabetes.

23. What are the contraindications to participation in an exercise program?

Unstable coronary heart disease, decompensated heart failure, symptomatic valvular stenosis, severe systemic hypertension, and uncontrolled arrhythmias are absolute contraindications to exercise. Further guidance regarding exercise participation can be found in the 2015 AHA/ACC Guidelines of Eligibility and Disqualification Recommendations for Competitive Athletes with Cardiovascular Abnormalities, the ACSM Guidelines for Testing and Prescription, and the AHA Exercise Standards for Testing and Training.

Bibliography and Suggested Readings

Ades, P. A., Keteyian, S. J., Balady, G. J., Houston-Miller, N., Kitzman, D. W., Mancini, D. M., et al. (2013). Cardiac rehabilitation exercise and selfcare for chronic heart failure. *JACC: Heart Failure*, *1*, 540–547.

American Association of Cardiovascular and Pulmonary Rehabilitation. <http://www.aacvpr.org/>. Accessed 11.02.16.

American College of Sports Medicine. <http://www.acsm.org/>. Accessed 11.02.16.

American Heart Association (search *Exercise*) Heartorg Home Page. <http://www.americanheart.org/>. Accessed 18.03.16.

Balady, G. J., Ades, P. A., Bittner, V. A., Franklin, B. A., Gordon, N. F., Thomas, R. J., et al. (2011). Referral, enrollment, and delivery of cardiac rehabilitation/secondary prevention programs at clinical centers and beyond: a presidential advisory from the American Heart Association. *Circulation*, *124*, 2951–2960.

Balady, G. J., Williams, M. A., Ades, P. A., Bittner, V., Comoss, P., Foody, J. M., et al. (2007). Core components of cardiac rehabilitation/secondary prevention programs: 2007 update: a scientific statement from the American Heart Association Exercise, Cardiac Rehabilitation, and Prevention Committee, the Council on Clinical Cardiology; the Councils on Cardiovascular Nursing, Epidemiology and Prevention, and Nutrition, Physical Activity, and Metabolism; and the American Association of Cardiovascular and Pulmonary Rehabilitation. *Circulation*, *115*, 2675–2682.

Colberg, S. R., Sigal, R. J., Fernhall, B., Regensteiner, J. G., Blissmer, B. J., Rubin, R. R., et al. (2010). Exercise and type 2 diabetes: the American College of Sports Medicine and the American Diabetes Association: joint position statement executive summary. *Diabetes Care*, *33*, 2692–2696.

Downing, J., & Balady, G. J. (2011). The role of exercise training in heart failure. *Journal of the American College of Cardiology*, *58*, 561–569.

Fletcher, G. F., Ades, P. A., Kligfield, P., Arena, R., Balady, G. J., Bittner, V. A., et al. (2013). Exercise standards for testing and training: a scientific statement from the American Heart Association. *Circulation*, *128*, 873–934.

Hamburg, N. M., & Balady, G. J. (2011). Exercise rehabilitation in peripheral artery disease: functional impact and mechanisms of benefits. *Circulation*, *123*, 87–97.

Hammill, B. G., Curtis, L. H., Schulman, K. A., & Whellan, D. J. (2009). Relationship between cardiac rehabilitation and long-term risks of death and myocardial infarction among elderly Medicare beneficiaries. *Circulation*, *121*, 63–70.

Haskell, W. L., Lee, I.-M., Pate, R. R., Powell, K. E., Blair, S. N., Franklin, B. A., et al. (2007). Physical activity and public health: updated recommendation for adults from the American College of Sports Medicine and the American Heart Association. *Circulation*, *116*, 1081–1093.

Maron, B. J., Zipes, D. P., Kovacs, R. J., & on behalf of the American Heart Association Electrocardiography and Arrhythmias Committee of the Council on Clinical Cardiology, Council on Cardiovascular Disease in the Young, Council on Cardiovascular and Stroke Nursing, Council on Functional Genomics and Translational Biology, and the American College of Cardiology. (2015). Eligibility and disqualification recommendations for competitive athletes with cardiovascular abnormalities: preamble, principles, and general considerations: a scientific statement from the American Heart Association and American College of Cardiology. *Circulation*, *132*, e256–e261. The Task Force reports for these proceedings are available online at http://circ.ahajournals.org (*Circulation*. 2015;132:e262-e349).

Murphy, T. P., Cutlip, D. E., Regensteiner, J. G., Mohler, E. R., Cohen, D. J., Reynolds, M. R., et al. (2011). Supervised exercise versus primary stenting for claudication resulting from aortoiliac peripheral artery disease: six-month outcomes from the claudication: exercise versus endoluminal revascularization (CLEVER) study. *Circulation*, *125*, 130–139.

O'Connor, C. M., Whellan, D. J., Lee, K. L., Keteyian, S. J., Cooper, L. S., Ellis, S. J., et al. (2009). Efficacy and safety of exercise training in patients with chronic heart failure: HF-ACTION randomized controlled trial. *Journal of the American Medical Association*, *301*, 1439.

Piscetello, J. (Ed.). (2014). *American College of Sports Medicine guidelines for exercise testing and prescription* (9th ed.). Philadelphia, PA: Lippincott Williams and Wilkins.

US Department of Health and Human Services. (2008). *Physical activity guidelines for Americans*. <http://www.health.gov/paguidelines>. Accessed 10.02.16.

Williams, M. A., Haskell, W. L., Ades, P. A., Amsterdam, E. A., Bittner, V., Franklin, B. A., et al. (2007). Resistance exercise in individuals with and without cardiovascular disease: 2007 update: a scientific statement from the American Heart Association Council on Clinical Cardiology and Council on Nutrition, Physical Activity, and Metabolism. *Circulation*, *116*, 572–584.

VII
The Heart In Specific Populations and Conditions

CARDIAC MANIFESTATIONS OF HIV/AIDS

Amy French, Sheilah Bernard

CHAPTER 46

1. **How have the cardiac manifestations of human immunodeficiency virus/acquired immunodeficiency syndrome changed over the years?**

Cardiac manifestations of acquired immunodeficiency syndrome (AIDS) until the early 1990s frequently included pericardial disease, myocarditis, dilated and infiltrative cardiomyopathies, pulmonary hypertension, arrhythmias, and marantic or infectious endocarditis. Because patients tended to be younger, very little coronary atherosclerosis was noted. Since highly active antiretroviral therapy (ART) has emerged as an effective treatment for human immunodeficiency virus (HIV), HIV has transformed from a fatal infection to a chronically managed disease, and HIV-infected patients are now facing the challenges of chronic diseases, including cardiovascular disease. When compared to the general population, patients with HIV are at increased risk of cardiovascular disease, which may occur earlier and progress more rapidly.

HIV patients have a higher incidence of traditional cardiovascular risk factors, including male gender, smoking, advanced age, glucose intolerance, insulin resistance, and dyslipidemia. They also have a higher incidence of nontraditional cardiac risk factors, including polysubstance abuse, lifestyle choices, immune dysregulation, chronic inflammation associated with HIV, and effects of ART. Furthermore, children born with vertically transmitted HIV are now surviving to adulthood, with attendant cardiac complications associated with chronic inflammation, drug therapy, and immunosuppression.

2. **What are HIV-related cardiac complications?**

Since the advent of ART in the 1990s, the incidence of HIV-related complications has significantly decreased but include the following:

- Pericardial effusion/tamponade
- Dilated cardiomyopathy
- Left ventricular systolic or diastolic dysfunction
- Myocarditis
- Marantic (thrombotic) or infectious endocarditis
- Cardiac tumors (Kaposi sarcoma, lymphoma)
- Pulmonary arterial hypertension (PAH)
- Accelerated coronary artery disease
- Peripheral vascular disease
- Sudden cardiac death

A summary of HIV-associated cardiovascular complications is given in Table 46.1.

3. **How common is a pericardial effusion in an HIV-infected patient?**

Pericardial effusion is an incidental finding in about 11% of HIV-infected patients and up to 30% of AIDS patients with CD4 counts less than 400 who have echocardiograms. The effusions are typically small, and patients are usually asymptomatic. It only rarely progresses to tamponade, which is more common in end-stage, cachectic patients who develop elevated intrapericardial pressures caused by low right-sided filling pressures *(low-pressure tamponade).* The presence of an effusion, however, is an independent predictor of mortality in these patients. Effusions are most often transudative. *T. mycobacterium* and *T. aviarum* are the principal causes of infectious pericarditis. Rarely, Kaposi sarcoma can bleed into the pericardium, resulting in tamponade physiology.

4. **What are the incidence and pathophysiology of HIV-associated myocarditis and cardiomyopathy?**

In different series, one-third to one-half of patients in the pre-ART era (or where ART therapy was not available) dying of AIDS had lymphocytic infiltration at autopsy. Eighty percent of these patients had no other pathogens identified. Additionally, up to 10% of endomyocardial specimens in HIV patients have

Table 46.1. Summary of HIV-Associated Cardiovascular Diseases

DISEASE	POSSIBLE CAUSES	TREATMENT
Accelerated atherosclerosis	PIs, atherogenesis with virus-infected macrophages, chronic inflammation, glucose intolerance, dyslipidemia, endothelial dysfunction	Smoking cessation, low-fat diet, aerobic exercise, blood pressure control, guideline-based statin use, percutaneous coronary intervention, coronary artery bypass surgery
Left ventricular systolic dysfunction	CAD, drug related (AZT, IL-2, doxorubicin, interferon), infectious, cytokines, autoimmune	Standard heart failure therapies, treatment of infection, nutritional replacement, IVIG, intensify ART
Left ventricular diastolic dysfunction	TNF, IL-6, hypertension, chronic viral infection	Treat hypertension, intensify ART
Right ventricular dysfunction	Recurrent pulmonary infections, pulmonary arteritis/arterial hypertension, microvascular pulmonary emboli, COPD	Diuretics, treat underlying lung infection or disease, anticoagulation as clinically indicated
Arrhythmias	Drug therapy, pentamidine, autonomic dysfunction, acidosis, electrolyte abnormalities	Discontinue drug, electrolyte replacement
Pericardial	Bacterial, viral, other pathogens, malignancy, uremia	Treat underlying cause, intensify ART, serial echocardiograms, pericardiocentesis or window
Endocarditis	Nonbacterial thrombotic, autoimmune, bacterial, fungal	Intravenous antibiotics, valve replacement

ART, Antiretroviral therapy; *AZT*, azidothymidine; *CAD*, coronary artery disease; *COPD*, chronic obstructive pulmonary disease; *IL*, interleukin; *IVIG*, intravenous immunoglobulin; *PIs*, protease inhibitors; *TNF*, tumor necrosis factor.

Adapted from Fisher, S. D., & Lipshultz S. E. Cardiovascular abnormalities in HIV-infected individuals. In Braunwald's heart disease: a textbook of cardiovascular medicine *(10th ed., chapter 70, pages 1624–1635); Philadelphia, PA: Saunders.*

evidence of other infections (coxsackie B, Epstein-Barr virus, adenovirus, cytomegalovirus). Studies have demonstrated the role of computed tomography (CT) and magnetic resonance imaging (MRI) to noninvasively identify myocarditis of all etiologies, which can be applied to the HIV population.

The initiation of ART therapy has significantly reduced the incidence of cardiomyopathy, likely as a result of reduction in HIV itself and reduction in the presence of opportunistic infections.

HIV is thought to cause myocarditis from direct action of HIV on myocytes or indirectly through toxins. Patients with HIV and cardiomyopathy have a worse prognosis than those with cardiomyopathy due to other causes of cardiomyopathy. Heart failure caused by HIV-associated left ventricular dysfunction is most commonly found in patients with the lowest CD4 counts and is a marker of poor prognosis. Despite the association of HIV and myocarditis/cardiomyopathy, other causes of heart failure (e.g., ischemic, valvular, toxin-related) should be excluded in these patients.

5. How is HIV cardiomyopathy treated?

Standard heart failure regimens should be used as tolerated, including angiotensin-converting enzyme (ACE) inhibitors or angiotensin-receptor blockers (ARBs), beta-blockers, aldosterone antagonists, diuretics for volume overload, and digoxin for advanced disease. Additionally, nutritional and electrolyte deficiencies should be repleted. Treatment of HIV and any co-infections is also key.

6. How is infective endocarditis managed in patients with HIV and AIDS?

The valvular devastation often seen with bacterial infections may not occur in HIV and AIDS patients due to an impaired autoimmune response. However, fulminant infective endocarditis can occur in late AIDS and can be associated with a high mortality. Management of infective endocarditis in HIV-infected patients is the same as in patients without HIV, and patients with hemodynamically significant valvular disease warrant valve replacement.

7. What malignancies can affect the heart in AIDS and HIV?

Kaposi sarcoma is associated with herpesvirus-8 in homosexual AIDS patients. This tumor is often found in the subepicardial fat around surface coronary arteries. About 25% of AIDS patients with systemic Kaposi sarcoma had incidental cardiac involvement, with death as a result of underlying opportunistic infections. Non-Hodgkin's lymphoma is more common in HIV-positive patients, with a poor prognosis. Leiomyosarcoma is rarely associated with Epstein-Barr virus in AIDS patients.

8. Can nutritional deficiencies be responsible for HIV myopathy?

HIV leads to immune impairment and malnutrition, which can contribute to rapid progression to AIDS. Malnutrition can be secondary to poor appetite, poor absorption in the GI tract, or functional limitations, such as odynophagia or dysphagia associated with thrush or esophagitis (seen commonly in AIDS patients). Nutritional deficiencies are seen in late-stage, untreated AIDS and may ultimately lead to electrolyte losses. Selenium deficiency increases the virulence of coxsackievirus to cardiac tissue and is reversed by repleting selenium. Low levels of B_{12}, carnitine, growth hormone, and T4 can cause a reversible myopathy.

9. How common is HIV-associated pulmonary arterial hypertension?

The prevalence of PAH was estimated to be 0.5% of HIV-infected patients in 1997, before the advent of ART. Since that time, despite the increase of ART, the prevalence of PAH remains similar. PAH can be diagnosed in any stage and is not thought to be related to CD4 count; up to 84% of patients survive to 1 year, with a median survival of 3.6 years. On histology, HIV-infected PAH patients do not differ from uninfected patients and exhibit concentric laminar fibrosis, medial hypertrophy, and plexiform lesions. It is not known whether HIV infects the pulmonary vascular system, but HIV proteins can lead to abnormal endothelial function. Therapy includes those used for primary pulmonary hypertension, including intravenous epoprostenol and endothelin antagonists. The benefit of ART on stemming the progression of PAH is controversial.

10. How should HIV patients be screened for coronary artery disease?

The Framingham Risk Score (age, gender, blood pressure, total cholesterol, high-density lipoprotein [HDL], diabetes, and smoking) has been applied to HIV patients on therapy and reasonably predicts coronary artery disease (CAD) events. It has been shown to underestimate the risk of cardiovascular disease in HIV patients who are also smokers. The Data Collection on Adverse Events of Anti-HIV Drugs (DAD) group has tried to incorporate HIV-specific risks (such as exposure to protease inhibitors [PIs]) in addition to traditional risk factors, but these risk models are not yet validated. The Infectious Disease Society of America (IDSA) recommends fasting lipid panels and fasting glucose levels prior to and 1 to 3 months after initiation of highly active ART. Use of diagnostic stress testing is performed in these patients according the current guidelines for the general population. Carotid intimal medial thickening, coronary artery calcium scores, highly sensitive C-reactive protein (CRP), adiponectin, and other markers of cardiovascular disease are also being investigated in the HIV population to predict early disease (Table 46.2).

11. What is the pathophysiology of accelerated atherosclerosis in HIV patients?

Histopathologically, atherosclerosis in HIV patients is distinct from that in noninfected patients. Based on autopsy studies, these lesions have features of both atherosclerosis and transplant vasculopathy. These lesions reveal diffuse circumferential involvement with smooth muscle cell proliferation and elastic fibers, leading to endoluminal projections.

The relative risk of MI in HIV compared to non-HIV patients is increased 1.7- to 1.8-fold, and may increase further with increasing age. There is a complex relationship between HIV-related, ART-related side effects and traditional risk factors that result in a higher prevalence of atherosclerotic disease in HIV patients (Fig. 46.1). ART is associated with increased visceral adiposity, insulin resistance, and abnormal glucose tolerance and therefore increases the risk of cardiovascular disease. Traditional risk factors, such as hypertension (which may be associated with ART use) and tobacco use, are highly prevalent in this population. HIV is known to lead to a state of increased inflammation, which has been identified as a factor for early atherosclerosis. HIV directly leads to endothelial dysfunction, and HIV envelope proteins have been linked to higher levels of endothelin-1 concentrations. Viral levels and CD4 counts are predictive of cardiovascular disease.

12. What are the effects of antiretroviral therapy on cardiovascular risk?

Many ARTs have been associated with dyslipidemia. PIs are associated with a small to moderate increase in total cholesterol and low-density lipoprotein (LDL) and a significant rise in triglyceride

Table 46.2. Antiretroviral Therapies and Specific Drugs, and Their Effects on Lipid Profiles

	PROTEASE INHIBITORS (PIs)	NONNUCLEOSIDE REVERSE TRANSCRIPTASE INHIBITORS (NNRTIs)	NUCLEOSIDE REVERSE TRANSCRIPTASE INHIBITORS (NRTIs)
Specific drugs	Atazanavir Ritonavir Tipranavir Darunavir Lopinavir Saquinavir Fosamprenavir Nelfinavir	Efavirenz Nevirapine Etravirine	Stavudine Tenofovir Abacavir
Total cholesterol	↑	Slight ↑	Slight ↑
LDL	↑	Slight ↑	Slight ↑
HDL		Slight ↑	
Triglycerides	↑↑		
Insulin resistance			Slight ↑

HDL, High-density lipoprotein; *LDL*, low-density lipoprotein.

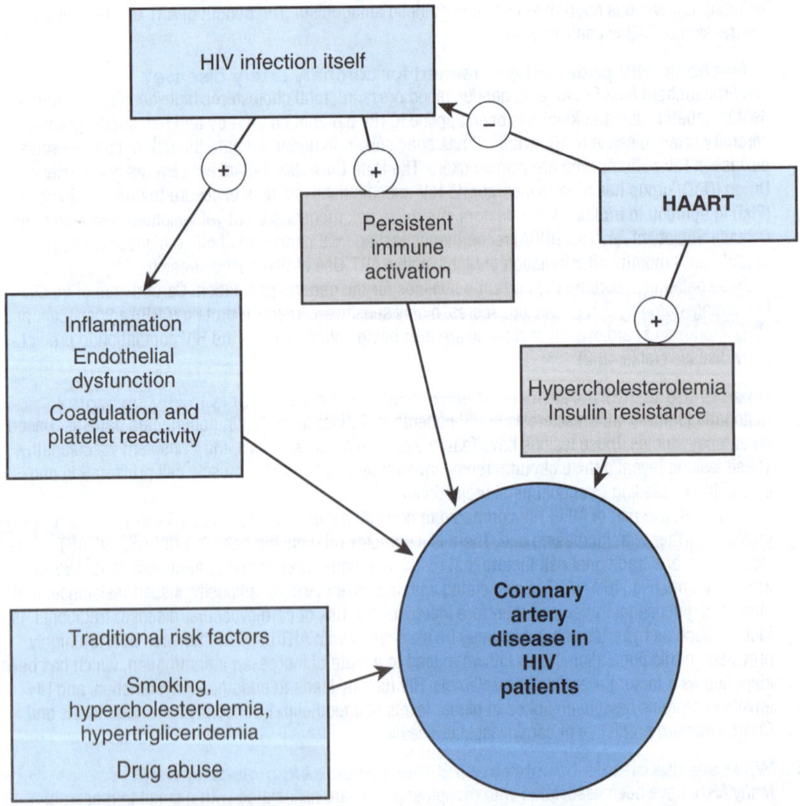

Fig. 46.1. Pathogenesis of coronary artery disease in HIV infection. *(Adapted from Cerrato, E., Calcagno, A., D'Ascenzo, F., Biondi-Zoccai, G., Quadri, G., Omede, P., et al. [2013]. Acute coronary syndrome in human immunodeficiency virus patients: exploiting physiopathology to inform the clinical practice.* OA Evidence-Based Medicine, 1[1], *5.* http://www.oapublishinglondon.com/article/542.*)*

levels. Nonnucleoside reverse transcriptase inhibitors (NNRTIs) are associated with dyslipidemia, but less so than PIs. They typically result in a small increase in total cholesterol, LDL, as well as HDL (which is potentially beneficial). In general, the nucleoside reverse transcriptase inhibitors (NRTIs) have been associated with insulin resistance, and the lipid profile changes are less severe than with PIs and NNRTIs. While PIs and NNRTIs have well-established effects on lipid profiles, the new agents such as fusion inhibitors, chemokine inhibitors, or integrase inhibitors have not shown these changes.

13. What is acquired lipodystrophy?

This is a disorder characterized by selective loss of adipose tissue from subcutaneous areas of the face, arms, and legs, with redistribution to the posterior neck *(buffalo hump)* and visceral abdomen. Visceral adiposity is associated with increased inflammatory markers. Lipodystrophy is also associated with attendant development of diabetes mellitus (DM), dyslipidemia, hepatic steatosis, hypertension, and acanthosis nigricans. It can occur in 20% to 40% of HIV patients taking PIs for more than 1 to 2 years. Exercise with or without treatment with metformin has been reported to improve body composition in patients with lipodystrophy.

14. What dyslipidemias occur with HIV infection, and how are they treated?

In early HIV infection, prior to initiation of therapy, triglycerides increase and HDL and LDL levels decline. After ART is initiated, LDL and total cholesterol levels appear to increase. This may be due to general improvement in health or due to medication effects. The prevalence of hyperlipidemia in HIV patients is variable, ranging from 28% to 80% in various studies.

Treatment of dyslipidemia should include attempts to manage common comorbid conditions, including obesity, hypertension, and diabetes. Patients should be counseled with regard to the importance of dietary modification, regular exercise, weight loss, tobacco cessation, and adherence to prescribed medical therapy for other comorbid conditions. Physicians can consider transitioning to a different class of antiretrovirals, such as replacing PIs with NNRTIs and/or NRTIs if the new regimen has the same ability to suppress viral replication. Several statins are degraded by cytochrome P450 isoform 3A4, which is inhibited by PIs. Therefore, simvastatin is contraindicated with PI use, but other statins, including atorvastatin and rosuvastatin, are less affected and are still used to treat HIV-associated dyslipidemia. Pravastatin and ezetimibe, which are not metabolized by the cytochrome P450 pathway, are also safe to use in this setting. Niacin has been shown to reduce triglyceride levels, but it does increase insulin resistance; its benefit is therefore unclear. Fish oil (omega-3 fatty acids) is well tolerated and has been shown to decrease triglyceride levels. Unfortunately, some studies have also noted an increase in LDL with fish oil, so its overall clinical benefit is unclear.

15. Can cardiothoracic surgery be performed safely in HIV patients?

HIV patients can undergo cardiothoracic surgery (valve replacement, coronary artery bypass grafting [CABG]) with similar mortality to non-HIV patients but slightly higher morbidity (as a result of sepsis, sternal infection, bleeding, prolonged intubation, and readmission). There have not been large surgical series, but smaller studies have shown 81% event-free survival at 3 years for HIV patients undergoing CABG. CD4 counts do not drop postoperatively. Needle sticks remain a healthcare issue in all patients.

16. What other drugs used in AIDS/HIV treatment can have cardiac complications?

The nucleoside analogue abacavir can cause hypotension and lactic acidosis. Zidovudine (also known as azidothymidine [AZT]) can cause a reversible, dose-dependent skeletal and cardiac myopathy, which has been attributed to mitochondrial injury, and has also been linked to systolic and diastolic dysfunction. The antiparasitic pentamidine, antiviral ganciclovir, and antibiotic erythromycin have been associated with acquired QT prolongation and torsades de pointes (polymorphic ventricular tachycardia).

Bibliography and Suggested Readings

Barbaro, G. (2010). Heart and HAART: two sides of the coin for HIV-associated cardiology issues. *World Journal of Cardiology, 2*(3), 53–57.

Barbaro, G., & Lipshultz, S. E. (2001). Pathogenesis of HIV-associated cardiomyopathy. *Annals of the New York Academy of Sciences, 946*, 57–81.

Bloomfield, G. S., Alenezi, F., Barasa, F. A., Lumsden, R., Mayosi, B. M., & Velazquez, E. J. (2015). Human immunodeficiency virus and heart failure in low- and middle-income countries. *JACC: Heart Failure, 3*(8), 579–590.

Cicalini, S., Almodovar, S., Grilli, E., & Flores, S. (2011). Pulmonary hypertension and human immunodeficiency virus infection: epidemiology, pathogenesis, and clinical approach. *Clinical Microbiology and Infection, 17*, 25–33.

Cotter, B. R. (2003). Epidemiology of HIV cardiac disease. *Progress in Cardiovascular Diseases, 45*, 319–326.

Duggal, S., Chugh, T. D., & Duggal, A. S. (2012). HIV and malnutrition: effects on immune system. *Clinical and Developmental Immunology, 2012*, 1–8.

Feeney, E., & Mallon, P. W. G. (2011). HIV and HAART-associated dyslipidemia. *Open Cardiovascular Medicine Journal, 5*, 49–63.

Feinstein, M. J., Bahiru, E., Achenbach, C., Longenecker, C. T., Hsue, P., So-Armah, K., et al. (2016). Patterns of cardiovascular mortality for HIV-infected adults in the United States: 1999 to 2013. *American Journal of Cardiology, 117*, 214–220.

Friis-Moller, N., Reiss, P., Sabin, C. A., Sabin, C. A., Weber, R., Monforte, Ad, et al. (2007). Class of antiretroviral drugs and the risk of myocardial infarction. *New England Journal of Medicine, 356*, 1723–1735.

Green, M. I. (2002). Evaluation and management of dyslipidemia in patients with HIV infection. *Journal of General Internal Medicine, 17*, 797–810.

Grinspoon, S. K., Grunfeld, C., Kotler, D. P., Currier, J. S., Lundgren, J. D., Dubé, M. P., et al. (2008). State of the science conference: initiative to decrease cardiovascular risk and increase quality of care for patients living with HIV/AIDS: executive summary. *Circulation, 118*, 198–210.

Hakeem, A., Bhatti, S., & Cilingiroglu, M. (2010). The spectrum of atherosclerotic coronary artery disease in HIV patients. *Current Atherosclerosis Reports*, *12*, 119–124.

Ho, E., & Hsue, P. Y. (2009). Cardiovascular manifestations of HIV infection. *Heart, 95*, 1193–1202.

Hsue, Y., & Waters, D. D. (2005). What a cardiologist needs to know about patients with human immunodeficiency virus infection. *Circulation, 112*, 3947–3957.

Janda, S., Quon, B. S., & Swiston, K. (2010). HIV and pulmonary arterial hypertension: a systematic review. *HIV Medicine, 11*, 620–634.

Kaplan, R. C., Hanna, D. B., & Kizer, J. R. (2016). Recent insights into cardiovascular disease (CVD) risk among HIV-infected adults. *Current HIV/AIDS Reports, 13*, 44–52.

Katz, A. S., & Sadaniantz, A. (2003). Echocardiography in HIV cardiac disease. *Progress in Cardiovascular Diseases, 45*, 285–292.

Malvestuttom, C., & Aberg, J. (2010). Coronary heart disease in people infected with HIV. *Cleveland Clinic Journal of Medicine, 77*(8), 547–556.

Nakazono, R., Jeudy, J., & White, C. (2012). HIV-related cardiac complications: CT and MRI findings. *American Journal of Roentgenology, 198*, 364–369.

Shah, M., Cook, N., Wong, R., Hsue, P., Ridker, P., Currier, J., et al. (2015). Stimulating high impact HIV-related cardiovascular research: recommendations from a multidisciplinary NHLBI Working Group on HIV-related heart, lung, and blood disease. *Journal of the American College of Cardiology, 65*(7), 738–744.

Thienemann, F., Sliwa, K., & Rockstroh, J. K. (2013). HIV and the heart: the impact of antiretroviral therapy: a global perspective. *European Heart Journal, 34*(46), 3538–3546.

CARDIOVASCULAR COMPLICATIONS OF RHEUMATIC DISEASES

CHAPTER 47

Stephen A. Gannon, Nishant R. Shah

1. **What is the leading cause of mortality in patients with rheumatoid arthritis, and what are the most common cardiac manifestations of rheumatoid arthritis?**
Ischemic heart disease is the leading cause of mortality in patients with rheumatoid arthritis (RA), accounting for nearly 25% of all deaths. Even in the absence of traditional risk factors, RA is associated with increased risk of fatal myocardial infarction (MI). Other cardiac manifestations of RA include pericarditis, valvular heart disease (most commonly mitral regurgitation), heart failure, and arrhythmias.

2. **What pathophysiologic mechanisms contribute to accelerated atherosclerosis in patients with rheumatoid arthritis?**
As depicted in Fig. 47.1, chronic release of proinflammatory cytokines in patients with RA is associated with dyslipidemia (e.g., decreased high-density lipoprotein [HDL], increased low-density lipoprotein [LDL]), endothelial dysfunction and activation (e.g., expression of monocyte-chemotactic protein-1, upregulation of vascular cell adhesion protein-1), subendothelial macrophage activation, T-cell activation, insulin resistance, and expression of matrix metalloproteinases associated with fibrous cap thinning and increased plaque vulnerability.

3. **What are the most common cardiac manifestations of systemic lupus erythematosus?**
Similar to RA, systemic lupus erythematosus (SLE) is an independent risk factor for premature atherosclerosis and coronary artery disease. Antinuclear antibodies may play a role in the development of coronary artery disease (CAD). Pericarditis, with or without pericardial effusion, is common with SLE, occurring in up to 60% of patients, although severe manifestations including constrictive pericarditis and cardiac tamponade are rare. Nonbacterial valvular vegetations (Libman-Sacks vegetations; Fig. 47.2) have also been reported in up to 60% of patients and are generally univalvular, small, left-sided, and associated with antiphospholipid and/or anticardiolipin antibodies. These vegetations carry a high risk of thromboembolism, necessitating lifelong anticoagulation. Infants born to mothers with anti-Ro/SSA and anti-La/SSB antibodies are at increased risk of congenital complete heart block, and the most common arrhythmias in adult patients with SLE are sinus tachycardia, atrial fibrillation, and ectopic atrial beats.

4. **What cardiovascular medications are associated with drug-induced lupus erythematosus?**
Cardiovascular medications associated with drug-induced lupus erythematosus (DILE) are separated into three categories as shown in Table 47.1, based on whether they are definitely, probably, or possibly causative.

5. **Who is at risk for antiphospholipid syndrome, what are its most common cardiovascular manifestations, and how is it typically treated?**
Antiphospholipid syndrome (APS) affects women more commonly than men. Nearly half of APS cases are not associated with another rheumatic disease (and are thus labeled as primary APS). Antiphospholipid antibodies are present in up to 40% of patients with SLE, the most common cause of secondary APS, but less than half of these patients develop clinical manifestations. The most common clinical manifestations of APS are spontaneous venous and arterial thrombosis (e.g., deep vein thrombosis, stroke, MI, digital ischemia), recurrent spontaneous abortions, thrombocytopenia, and livedo reticularis. In addition, as with RA and SLE, APS is independently associated with

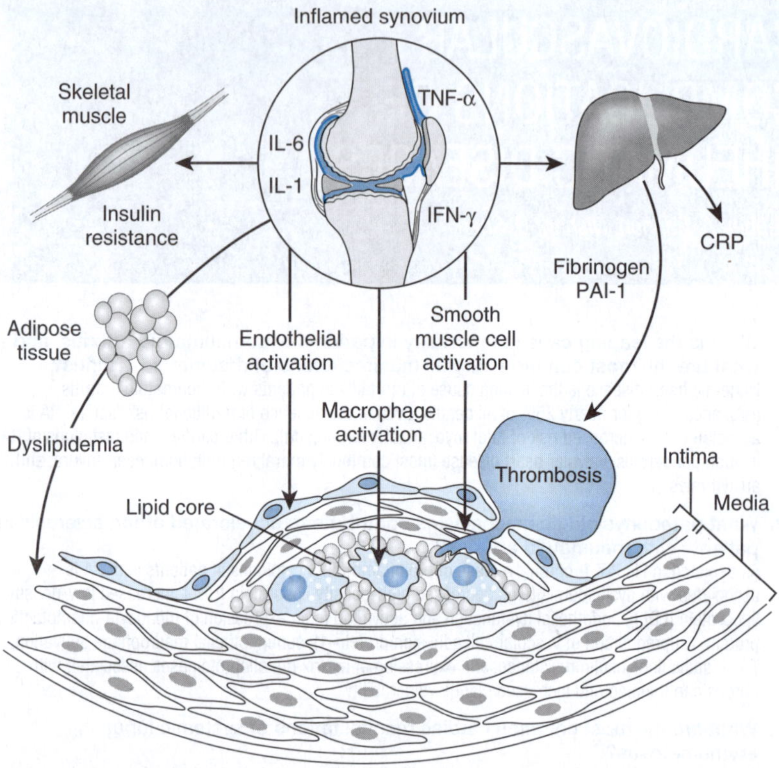

Fig. 47.1. Pathophysiologic mechanisms associated with accelerated atherosclerosis in patients with rheumatoid arthritis. *CRP*, C-reactive protein; *IFN*, interferon; *IL*, interleukin; *PAI*, plasminogen activator inhibitor; *TNF*, tumor necrosis factor. *(Libby P. [2008]. Role of inflammation in atherosclerosis associated with rheumatoid arthritis.* American Journal of Medicine, *121[10 Suppl. 1], S21–S31.)*

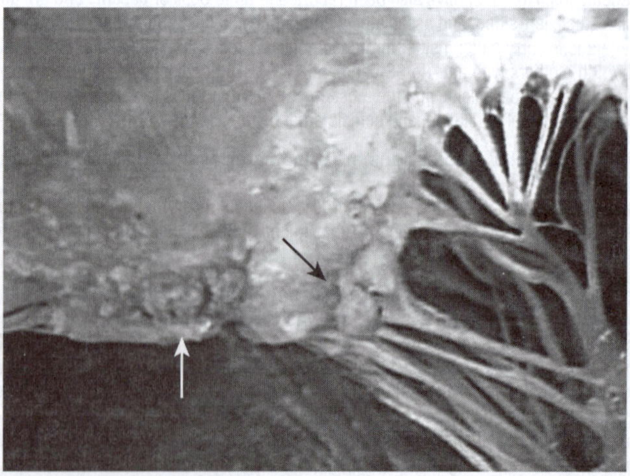

Fig. 47.2. Nonbacterial valvular vegetations (Libman-Sacks vegetations) *(arrows)* on the mitral valve. Libman-Sacks endocarditis can be observed in patients with systemic lupus erythematosus and is a form of non-bacterial endocarditis. *(Image from Armed Forces Institute of Pathology.)*

Table 47.1. Cardiovascular Medications Associated with Drug-Induced Lupus Erythematosus

DEFINITELY CAUSATIVE	PROBABLY CAUSATIVE	POSSIBLY CAUSATIVE
Procainamide	Beta-blockers	Statins
Hydralazine	Captopril	Lisinopril
Diltiazem	Hydrochlorothiazide	Enalapril
Quinidine	Amiodarone	Spironolactone
Methyldopa	Ticlopidine	Clonidine Minoxidil Reserpine

accelerated atherosclerosis. Primary prophylaxis with low-dose aspirin has unproven benefit but may be reasonable in patients with increased cardiovascular risk. Acute thrombotic events are generally treated with heparin followed by long-term anticoagulation with warfarin (target international normalized ratio of 2.0 to 3.0).

6. **What are the most common cardiac manifestations of systemic sclerosis?**
The hallmark of cardiac involvement in systemic sclerosis is patchy biventricular myocardial fibrosis. Fibrosis can directly cause systolic and/or diastolic heart failure or can do so indirectly via impaired coronary artery flow reserve (e.g., accelerated epicardial coronary atherosclerosis, microvascular ischemia). Fibrosis can also lead to recurrent coronary artery vasospasm (also known as myocardial Raynaud phenomenon), supraventricular and ventricular tachyarrhythmias, and/or heart block. Concurrent pulmonary involvement, associated with pulmonary fibrosis and pulmonary hypertension, increases the risk of right ventricular dysfunction in patients with systemic sclerosis.

7. **What are the most common cardiovascular manifestations of ankylosing spondylitis?**
Ankylosing spondylitis typically affects young men with human leukocyte antigen B27 (HLA-B27), and the most common cardiovascular complication is aortic root dilation with or without aortic regurgitation. The underlying pathophysiology is driven by inflammation-mediated fibroblast hyperactivity, resulting in tissue thickening and shortening of the aortic root, aortic annulus and cusps, and subaortic tissue. Extension into the aortomitral continuity and the anterior mitral leaflet can cause mitral regurgitation, and extension into the muscular septum can cause complete atrioventricular nodal or bundle branch block.

8. **What are the most common cardiovascular complications of polyarteritis nodosa?**
Polyarteritis nodosa (PAN) is necrotizing vasculitis not associated with antineutrophil cytoplasmic antibodies (ANCA) that predominantly affects medium-sized muscular arteries. Involvement of the renal arteries can cause renal ischemia, activation of the renin-angiotensin system, and hypertension. Involvement of the coronary arteries can result in serial small aneurysms with intervening irregular constrictions (Fig. 47.3) and myocardial ischemia that clinically manifests most commonly as angina and/or heart failure. Overt MI is uncommon.

9. **What are the most common cardiovascular manifestations of Takayasu arteritis, and how is it typically treated?**
Takayasu arteritis is a granulomatous vasculitis of the aorta and its branches that typically affects women younger than 50 years old. Lesions produced by the inflammatory process can be stenotic (Fig. 47.4) or aneurysmal. Arterial stenoses can cause claudication (particularly of the upper extremities) and hypertension. Aneurysms of the aortic root can cause significant aortic regurgitation. Evaluation of the entire aorta and its primary branches with invasive, computed tomography (CT) or magnetic resonance (MR) angiography is recommended to determine the distribution and severity of vascular lesions. Addition of 18F-fluorodeoxyglucose positron emission tomography can provide adjunctive information about current disease activity. High-dose corticosteroids, strict management of traditional cardiovascular risk factors, and anatomic correction of clinically significant lesions comprise the preferred initial treatment strategy.

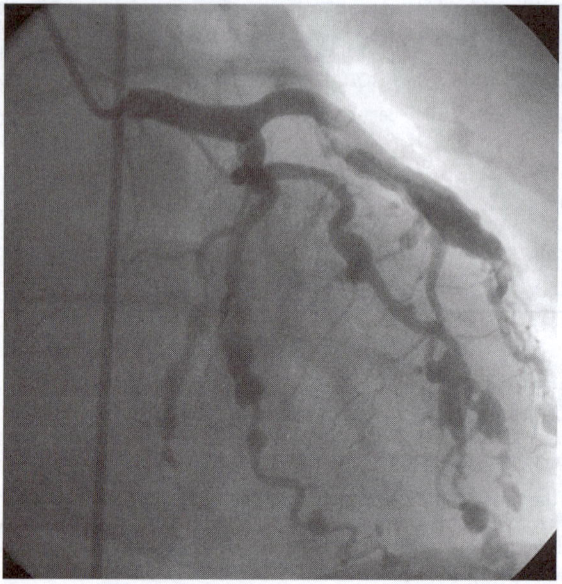

Fig. 47.3. Numerous coronary artery aneurysms are present in this patient with polyarteritis nodosa (PAN). *(Image from Bonow, R. O., Mann, D. L., Zipes, D. P., & Libby, P. [Eds.], [2012].* Braunwald's heart disease: a textbook of cardiovascular medicine *(9th ed.). Philadelphia, PA: Saunders.)*

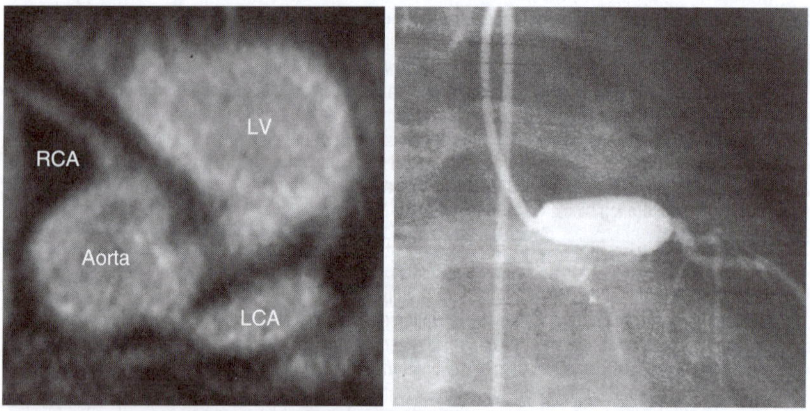

Fig. 47.4. Left coronary artery aneurysm visualized by MRA *(left panel)* and coronary angiography *(right panel). MRA,* Magnetic resonance angiography. *(Image from Mavrogeni, S., Papadopoulos, G., Douskou, M., Kaklis, S., Seimenis, I., Baras, P., et al. [2004]. Magnetic resonance angiography is equivalent to X-ray coronary angiography for the evaluation of coronary arteries in Kawasaki disease.* Journal of the American College of Cardiology*, 43[4], 649–652.)*

10. What is the leading cause of mortality in patients with Kawasaki disease (mucocutaneous lymph node syndrome)?

Kawasaki disease is most common in young children and is characterized by polyarteritis accompanied by high fever, cervical adenopathy, desquamative skin rash, nonexudative conjunctivitis, and mucous membrane lesions (e.g., strawberry tongue). Although rare, MI is the leading cause of mortality in patients with Kawasaki disease and typically results from thrombosis of a coronary artery aneurysm (Fig. 47.5). These aneurysms occur most commonly in the proximal left anterior descending

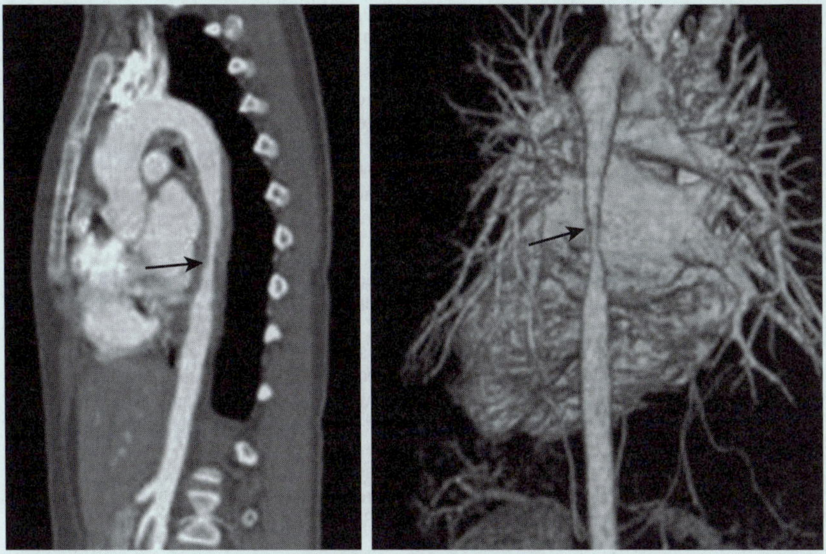

Fig. 47.5. Takayasu arteritis. CT scan images demonstrating stenosis *(arrow)* of the descending thoracic aorta in a patient with Takayasu arteritis. *(Image from Bao, N. [2011]. Aortic isthmus arteritis: report of one case.* Cardiology Research, *2[6], 301–303.)*

and right coronary arteries and can first be detected by echocardiography 7 days after the onset of fever. Treatment consists of high-dose aspirin and intravenous immune globulin.

11. What are the most common cardiovascular manifestations of Marfan syndrome?

Marfan syndrome (MFS) is caused by an autosomal dominant fibrillin-1 gene defect. The most common cardiovascular complication is asymptomatic progressive aortic root enlargement beginning at the sinuses of Valsalva. The development of an ascending aortic aneurysm places patients at high risk for type A aortic dissection, aortic rupture, and aortic regurgitation. Mitral valve prolapse is present in 50% of patients with MFS and can be associated with significant mitral regurgitation.

12. How should Marfan syndrome be managed?

Patients with MFS should have an echocardiogram, CT, or magnetic resonance imaging (MRI) at diagnosis to measure baseline aortic root and ascending aorta diameter and again with the same noninvasive imaging modality 6 months later to assess the rate of enlargement. In adults, if the baseline aortic diameter is less than 45 mm and remains stable, then annual noninvasive imaging surveillance is reasonable. More frequent surveillance should be considered if the baseline aortic diameter is greater than 45 mm, if there is rapid expansion (≥0.5 cm/year), or if there is new-onset or worsening aortic regurgitation.

Criteria for earlier consideration of surgery include aortic diameter greater than 50 mm, aortic diameter growth greater than 1 cm/year, family history of dissection less than 5 cm, or moderate to severe aortic regurgitation. Adults with MFS should be on beta-blocker therapy to maintain a heart rate less than 100 beats/minute after submaximal exercise; losartan is an alternative in patients intolerant to beta-blocker therapy. High-intensity exercise and other activities associated with marked increases in blood pressure should be avoided.

13. How is vascular (type IV) Ehlers-Danlos syndrome different from the other types?

Patients with vascular (type IV) Ehlers-Danlos syndrome (EDS) have an autosomal dominant defect in type III procollagen and typically lack the large joint hyperextensibility seen in the other forms of EDS. Instead, they are at markedly higher risk for spontaneous vascular or visceral rupture prior to age 40. The most common vascular sites of rupture are the iliac, splenic, and renal arteries, as well as the aorta. Aneurysms are typically pseudoaneurysms and are therefore rarely detected prior to rupture. Patients with type IV EDS should be followed by a cardiovascular disease expert and undergo intermittent surveillance echocardiography. Celiprolol and/or losartan may reduce the risk of arterial rupture. Arterial punctures and arteriography should be avoided unless necessary, and bleeding should be managed with endovascular procedures rather than open surgery, because collagen-deficient tissues do not hold sutures well.

14. What are the most common cardiovascular complications of Behçet syndrome?

Vasculitis associated with Behçet syndrome is more prevalent in males and involves arterial and venous vessels of all sizes (small, medium, and large). Superficial and deep vein thromboses are the most common venous manifestations. Although small-vessel vasculitis is the most common arterial manifestation, proximal pulmonary artery aneurysms are nearly pathognomonic for Behçet syndrome. Cardiac manifestations are very uncommon, and unlike RA and SLE, atherosclerosis does not appear to be accelerated in these patients.

15. Why are non-aspirin nonselective and cyclooxygenase-2 selective nonsteroidal anti-inflammatory drugs associated with increased risk of adverse cardiovascular events?

Non-aspirin nonselective and cyclooxygenase (COX)-2 selective nonsteroidal anti-inflammatory drugs (NSAIDs) promote platelet activation and thrombotic events primarily due to inhibition of anti-thrombotic endothelial prostacyclin production with relative sparing of pro-thrombotic platelet thromboxane A_2 production. In addition, all non-aspirin NSAIDs increase sodium retention, predisposing patients to hypertension and heart failure exacerbations. Of all non-aspirin NSAIDs, naproxen is associated with the lowest risk of cardiovascular events and can be combined with a proton pump inhibitor to reduce the risk of gastrointestinal bleeding. Given the increased cardiovascular risk associated with COX-2 selective NSAIDs, they should be avoided in patients with known coronary artery disease and if used, concurrent low-dose aspirin should be considered.

16. What treatments for rheumatic diseases are associated with cardiotoxicity?

Tumor necrosis factor (TNF)-α inhibitors have a possible association with heart failure and are therefore generally contraindicated in patients with moderate to severe heart failure (New York Heart Association [NYHA] class III–IV symptoms). For patients with RA, NYHA class I–II symptoms, and arthritis refractory to other disease-modifying antirheumatic drugs, TNF-α inhibitors may be reasonable, but cardiology consultation before initiation of therapy is advised. Antimalarial medications, particularly hydroxychloroquine, are often used to treat rheumatic diseases and rarely cause a restrictive or dilated cardiomyopathy with or without conduction system abnormalities (e.g., atrioventricular block, bundle branch block).

Bibliography and Suggested Readings

Danelich, I. M., Wright, S. S., Lose, J. M., Tefft, B. J., Cicci, J. D., & Reed, B. N. (2015). Safety of nonsteroidal anti-inflammatory drugs in patients with cardiovascular disease. *Pharmacotherapy: the Journal of Human Pharmacology and Drug Therapy, 35*(5), 520–535.

De Virgilio, A., Greco, A., Magliulo, G., Gallo, A., Ruoppolo, G., Conte, M., et al. (2016). Polyarteritis nodosa: a contemporary overview. *Autoimmunity Reviews, 15*(6), 564–570.

Hollan, I., Meroni, P. L., Ahearn, J. M., Cohen Tervaert, J. W., Curran, S., Goodyear, C. S., et al. (2013). Cardiovascular disease in autoimmune rheumatic diseases. *Autoimmunity Reviews, 12*(10), 1004–1015.

Keser, G., Direskeneli, H., & Aksu, K. (2014). Management of Takayasu arteritis: a systematic review. *Rheumatology (Oxford), 53*(5), 793–801.

Lum, Y. W., Brooke, B. S., & Black, J. H., 3rd. (2011). Contemporary management of vascular Ehlers–Danlos syndrome. *Current Opinion in Cardiology, 26*(6), 494–501.

Nurmohamed, M. T., Heslinga, M., & Kitas, G. D. (2015). Cardiovascular comorbidity in rheumatic diseases. *Nature Reviews Rheumatology, 11*(12), 693–704.

Prasad, M., Hermann, J., Gabriel, S. E., Weyand, C. M., Mulvagh, S., Mankad, R., et al. (2015). Cardiorheumatology: cardiac involvement in systemic rheumatic disease. *Nature Reviews Cardiology, 12*(3), 168–176.

Radke, R. M., & Baumgartner, H. (2014). Diagnosis and treatment of Marfan syndrome: an update. *Heart, 100*(17), 1382–1391.

Villa-Forte, A., & Mandell, B. F. (2012). Rheumatic diseases and the cardiovascular system. In R. O. Bonow, D. L. Mann, D. P. Zipes, & P. Libby (Eds.), *Braunwald's heart disease: a textbook of cardiovascular medicine* (9th ed.) (pp. 1876–1892). Philadelphia, PA: W.B. Saunders.

CARDIO-ONCOLOGY

Kara A. Thompson

CHAPTER 48

1. **What is type I versus type II cardiotoxicity?**

Type I drugs cause irreversible cell loss and cumulative dose-related cardiotoxicity. Anthracyclines are type I drugs. Clinical manifestations of irreversible damage may not present for years owing to compensatory mechanisms. Stress factors such as hypertension and coronary artery disease (CAD) might later lead to cardiac decompensation. Other type I drugs include mitoxantrone and cyclophosphamide.

Type II drugs can cause cellular dysfunction by altering mitochondrial and protein function and can thereby induce reversible cardiotoxicity. Trastuzumab, a monoclonal antibody against the HER2/erbB2 receptor, is a type II drug, although irreversible damage can occur with trastuzumab in the setting of preexisting cardiac disease or with concomitant use of anthracyclines. Concomitant use of trastuzumab with an anthracycline greatly increases the risk of cardiotoxicity (16% vs. 0%–3.9% New York Health Association [NYHA] class III–IV heart failure). A time interval of 3 months is recommended before starting trastuzumab after anthracycline. Other type II drugs include angiogenesis inhibitors such as bevacizumab, sunitinib, and sorafenib.

2. **What is the mechanism of anthracycline-induced cardiotoxicity?**

The cellular target for doxorubicin is topoisomerase II (Top 2). There are two Top 2 enzymes, Top 2 alpha and Top 2 beta. Top 2 alpha is overexpressed in tumors and is the molecular basis of anticancer activity. Cardiomyocytes express Top 2 beta but not Top 2 alpha. Doxorubicin also targets Top 2 beta and forms a complex that induces DNA double-stranded breaks and leads to cell death as well as an increase in reactive oxygen species.

3. **What is a safe dose of anthracycline?**

There is no safe dose of anthracycline. The risk of cardiac dysfunction increases with increasing cumulative dose. The risk is less than 5% for doses of less than 250 mg/m^2, 10% for doses between 250 mg/m^2 and 600 mg/m^2, and greater than 30% for doses greater than 600 mg/m^2.

4. **What are primary prevention strategies for anthracycline-induced cardiotoxicity?**

- *Continuous infusion.* Bolus administration of anthracycline leads to a higher cardiac concentration and higher cardiac toxicity. Continuous infusion does not compromise antitumor efficacy but does reduce cardiac toxicity. This finding does not apply to children. In children cardiac toxicity is the same with a bolus or a continuous infusion.
- *Liposomal doxorubicin.* Liposomal encapsulation does not penetrate healthy vasculature as readily as tumor vasculature and thus provides an equivalent antitumor effect with less cardiac toxicity. Use is limited owing to cost and is approved by the US Food and Drug Administration (FDA) only for ovarian cancer, HIV-related Kaposi sarcoma, and multiple myeloma after failure of another therapy.
- *Dexrazoxane.* Dexrazoxane prevents anthracyclines from binding to the Top 2 complex and thereby provides cardioprotection. Dexrazoxane is FDA-approved only for breast cancer patients who have already received 300 mg/m^2 of anthracyclines. There is concern that dexrazoxane might interfere with the antitumor effect of anthracyclines. In children there is concern that there may be an increased risk for the development of a secondary malignancy.
- It is uncertain whether beta-blockers or angiotensin-converting enzyme (ACE) inhibitors are useful in primary prevention. There are short-term studies suggesting benefit, but further study is needed.

5. **How should cardiac function be monitored in patients receiving anthracyclines?**

Prior to treatment patients should have a history and physical, electrocardiogram (ECG), and measurement of left ventricular ejection fraction (LVEF), preferably by echocardiogram. Patients under age 65 with normal EF are considered to be at low risk. Those with prior cardiac disease are at intermediate or high risk, and the oncologist and cardiologist must weigh the risk and benefit of treatment with anthracyclines versus using a less cardiotoxic regimen. If the LVEF is less than 40%, anthracyclines should not be used.

Cardiac function should be reassessed at 3, 6, and 9 months during treatment and at 12 and 18 months after initiation of treatment. If the EF decreases to less than 40%, the anthracycline should be discontinued. If the EF decreases to 40% to 50%, recommendations are slightly variable. At MD Anderson, if the EF is less than 45%, chemotherapy is held, treatment with an angiotensin-converting enzyme (ACE) inhibitor and beta-blocker is initiated, and the LVEF is reassessed after 1 month. If the LVEF is 45% to 49%, treatment with an ACE inhibitor and beta-blocker is initiated. Chemotherapy is held if the LVEF decrease is greater than 10% from baseline and continued if the LVEF decrease is less than 10% from baseline. LVEF is reassessed after 1 month.

6. How long is cardiac monitoring recommended after treatment with anthracyclines?

Lifelong cardiac monitoring is recommended because the incidence of cardiac toxicity increases with length of time since treatment. There is no time limit on the development of cardiac toxicity. Assessment by echocardiography of LVEF is as follows:

- Anthracycline dose less than 200 mg/m^2: every 5 years
- Anthracycline dose between 200 and 300 mg/m^2: every 2 years
- Anthracycline dose greater than 300 mg/m^2: every year

More frequent monitoring is recommended in patients who received radiation therapy in addition to anthracyclines. More frequent monitoring is also recommended in patients who received anthracyclines at age less than 5 years.

7. How should cardiac function be monitored in patients receiving trastuzumab?

Baseline evaluation and discontinuation for EF less than 40% is the same as for anthracyclines. If the EF decreases to 40% to 50%, management is different and slightly variable. At MD Anderson, if the EF decrease is less than 15% compared with baseline, trastuzumab is continued with initiation of an ACE inhibitor and a beta-blocker. If the EF decrease is greater than 15% compared with baseline, trastuzumab is held, an ACE inhibitor and beta-blocker are started, and the EF is reassessed after 1 month.

8. What tyrosine kinase inhibitor was featured on the cover of *TIME* magazine as "the magic bullet" against cancer?

Imatinib (Gleevec). Chronic myelogenous leukemia (CML) was the first cancer treated with a tyrosine kinase inhibitor (TKI). CML is caused by the Philadelphia chromosome, which creates the BCR-ABL protein. Imatinib is a "break point cluster region" - Abelson (BCR-ABL) inhibitor. Treatment with imatinib improved 5-year survival in CML patients from 40% to 50% initially to 90%, essentially converting a fatal cancer into a manageable chronic condition. Imatinib has been associated with a low incidence of cardiomyopathy and asymptomatic cardiac dysfunction. However, patients can develop resistance to imatinib. Thus newer generation BCR-ABL kinase inhibitors have been developed.

9. What are tyrosine kinase inhibitors?

TKIs are the most common targeted cancer drugs. Kinases are enzymes that control diverse cellular functions by transferring a phosphate group from adenosine triphosphate (ATP). Most cancers are associated with an overactivation of kinases. Drugs that target kinases have less toxic side effects than older chemotherapies. There are 20 lipid kinases and 518 protein kinases. Tyrosine kinases are protein kinases and can be categorized into receptor tyrosine kinases (RTKs) and nonreceptor tyrosine kinases.

10. What are the mechanisms of tyrosine kinase inhibitors?

The mechanisms of action of TKIs are shown in Fig. 48.1. These include

- Monoclonal Ab directed against circulating vascular endothelial growth factor (VEGF)
- Monoclonal Ab directed against the VEGF RTK. One such TKI is trastuzumab.
- Small-molecule TKI that blocks the intracellular pathway. These are attractive because they can be administered orally.
- Soluble decoy receptor

11. Is there a "class effect" for cardiovascular side effects of tyrosine kinase inhibitors?

No. The side-effect profiles of TKIs are different owing to different targets and variable selectivity and potency against targets. TKIs can be broadly categorized as those that are VEGF inhibitors and those that are not VEGF inhibitors, but there is overlap of activity and side effects.

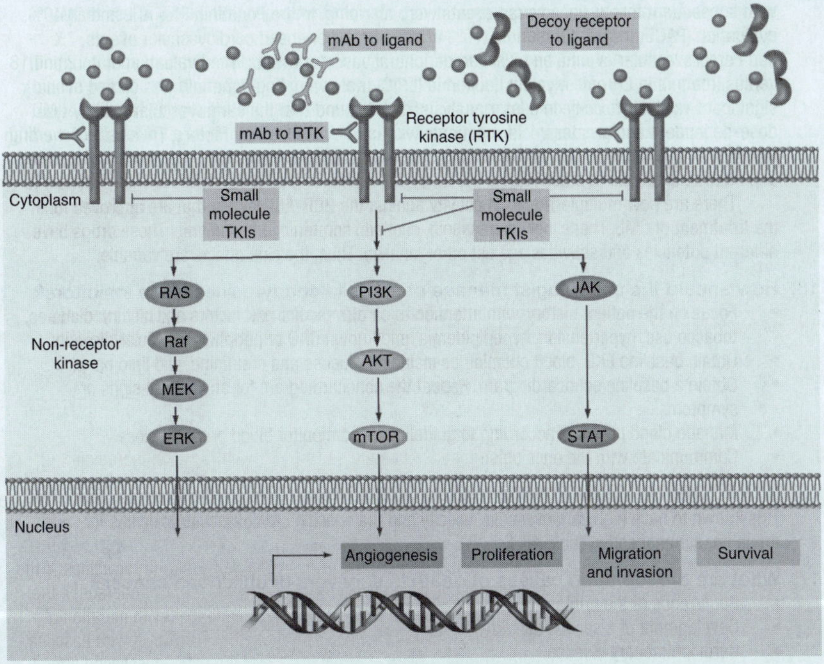

Fig. 48.1. The mechanisms of action of a tyrosine kinase inhibitor. *(Image from Li, W., Croce, K., Steensma, D. P., McDermott, D. F., Ben-Yehuda, O., & Moslehi, J. [2015]. Vascular and metabolic implications of novel targeted cancer therapies: focus on kinase inhibitors.* Journal of the American College of Cardiology, 66, *1160–1178.)*

12. What are the important effects of vascular endothelial growth factor and blocking vascular endothelial growth factor?

VEGF maintains vascular tone by (1) producing nitric oxide, which relaxes arteries, and (2) by producing prostacyclin, which decreases the vasoconstrictor endothelin-1. VEGF also promotes angiogenesis and cell growth. Tumors depend on vascularization for growth and metastasis. Inhibition of angiogenesis can inhibit tumor growth.

13. What is the main side effect of drugs that inhibit vascular endothelial growth factor?

Hypertension is the most common cardiotoxicity of targeted drugs that inhibit VEGF and is described as an "on-target" side effect. With VEGF inhibitors, 100% of patients develop an increase in blood pressure, and 25% develop frank hypertension. Hypertension is considered a marker of response to therapy. Treatment of hypertension has not been shown to impair the oncologic efficiency of VEGF inhibitors. The hypertension is reversible when the VEGF inhibitor is stopped.

The goal of the healthcare provider is to manage the hypertension in order to avoid more sequelae of hypertension, such as heart failure and stroke, and to enable the oncologist to continue therapy. ACE inhibitors, beta-blockers, and dihydropyridine calcium channel blockers are commonly used. Nondihydropyridine calcium channel blockers (verapamil and diltiazem) are generally avoided as they are inhibitors of cytochrome P450 34A and can interact with the metabolism of several cancer drugs. Diuretics are often not a first-choice therapy because some TKIs can cause diarrhea and dehydration.

VEGF inhibitors can cause other cardiovascular side effects including arterial thromboembolism and cardiomyopathy.

14. What drug was suspended from marketing in October, 2013, owing to serious arterial thrombotic events?

Ponatinib. Ponatinib is a newer generation BCR-ABL kinase inhibitor that is highly effective in CML patients resistant to other TKIs. At 1 year, cardiovascular toxicity was found to be acceptable. But, with subsequent follow-up, adverse events were alarming. In the Ponatinib Ph+ ALL and CML evaluation (PACE) trial, at 28 months, 10% of patients experienced cardiovascular events, 7% had cerebrovascular events, and 7% had peripheral vascular events. The Evaluation of Ponatinib versus Imatinib in Chronic Myeloid Leukemia (EPIC) trial evaluating ponatinib was closed owing to significant vascular toxicity. In a later analysis, it was found that the cardiovascular toxicity was dose-dependent and greater in older patients with cardiovascular risk factors. Thus sale of the drug resumed in 2014 with a black-box warning; it is restricted to patients with a BCR-ABL-1 mutation and contraindications to other TKIs.

There are now multiple TKIs with activity against the BCR-ABL kinase that are approved for the treatment of CML. These include dasatinib, nilotinib, sorafenib, and sunitinib. These drugs have different potencies and activities against other kinases. Thus, the side effects are variable.

15. How should the cardiologist manage patients taking tyrosine kinase inhibitors?

- Focus on the patient history, with attention to cardiovascular risk factors and history: diabetes, tobacco use, hypertension, hyperlipidemia, and known CAD or peripheral vascular disease.
- Obtain baseline EKG, blood chemistries including glucose and creatinine, and lipid panel.
- Obtain a baseline echocardiogram. Repeat the echocardiogram for any clinical signs or symptoms.
- Manage blood pressure according to guidelines, and monitor blood pressure closely.
- Communicate with the oncologist.

16. Which tyrosine kinase inhibitors are known to have high cardiovascular toxicity?

TKIs known to have high cardiovascular toxicity and the specific cardiovascular toxicities for such drugs are summarized in Table 48.1.

17. What are the top three causes of death in survivors of childhood cancer?

- Recurrence of the primary cancer
- Development of a second cancer
- Cardiopulmonary disease

18. What chemotherapy drugs have Food and Drug Administration–mandated specific guidelines for monitoring the QT interval?

- Vandetanib
- Vemurafenib
- Nilotinib
- Arsenic

Many cancer drugs cause prolongation of the QT interval. This can be exacerbated by the concomitant administration of other drugs commonly used in cancer patients (e.g., antiemetics, antipsychotics, methadone, antibiotics, antifungal agents, antiviral agents, antiarrhythmic agents). In addition, cancer patients often develop electrolyte depletion. It is important to monitor the QT interval and maintain potassium and magnesium homeostasis. Arsenic is the most prominent chemotherapy that causes QT prolongation. It is used for relapsed acute promyelocytic leukemia. It causes QT prolongation in up to 40% of treated patients and is associated with a significant risk of torsades de pointes.

Table 48.1. TKIs Known to Pose a High Risk of Cardiovascular Toxicity

TKI	CV toxicity
Trastuzumab (Herceptin)	Left ventricular (LV) dysfunction
Dasatinib (Sprycel)	Edema, pulmonary hypertension
Nilotinib (Tasigna)	Peripheral arterial disease, edema, hypertension (HTN)
Sunitinib (Suntent)	HTN, heart failure
Sorafenib (Nexavar)	HTN
Bevacizumab (Avastin)	HTN, edema, thromboembolism
Ponatinib	Arterial thrombotic events, HTN, edema, heart failure

HTN, Hypertension; *LV*, left ventricular; *TKI*, tyrosine kinase inhibitor.

19. True or false: Thrombocytopenia protects cancer patients from ischemic coronary events.

False. Thrombocytopenia in cancer patients is associated with an increased risk of thrombus formation due to increased platelet function.

20. What is the minimum platelet count required for performing a coronary angiogram?

There is no minimum platelet count below which a coronary angiogram is contraindicated. In the absence of coagulation abnormalities, interventional procedures can generally be performed safely with a platelet count of greater than 40,000/mL. For coronary artery bypass surgery, a platelet count greater than 50,000/mL is recommended.

21. Are antiplatelet agents administered in cancer patients with thrombocytopenia and coronary artery disease?

Yes. Aspirin is often administered when platelet counts are greater than 10,000/mL. Dual antiplatelet therapy with aspirin and clopidogrel is often administered when the platelet count is greater than 30,000/mL. Prasugrel and ticagrelor should not be given to patients with platelet counts less than 50,000/mL. Glycoprotein IIb/IIIa inhibitors are not administered to patients with platelet counts less than 50,000 to 100,000.

For patients with a platelet count less than 30,000/mL who need revascularization, a multidisciplinary evaluation is recommended to assess the relative risks and benefits of revascularization and potential use of dual antiplatelet therapy (in those treated with coronary stent implantation). Techniques such as thromboelastography (TEG) to evaluate platelet and coagulation function may be useful in the decision process.

22. How does radiation-induced coronary artery disease differ from age-related atherosclerosis?

Radiation-induced CAD is pathologically indistinguishable from age-related atherosclerosis. CAD due to radiation generally develops approximately 10 years after treatment and can occur in young patients with no other coronary risk factors. At the 10-year follow-up visit, screening with a stress test or coronary computed tomography (CT) angiogram is recommended, as radiation-induced coronary ischemia can be silent due to radiation damage to the innervation of the heart.

The anatomic distribution can differ from that in age-related CAD. Isolated ostial disease has been reported after radiation treatment of Hodgkin lymphoma. Left anterior descending disease occurs with greater frequency after irradiation for breast cancer. Treatment of radiation-induced CAD is not different from standard treatment. Aggressive treatment of risk factors is warranted as conventional risk factors increase the risk of radiation-induced disease. Coronary artery bypass surgery is associated with increased perioperative complications due to mediastinal scarring and fibrosis after radiation therapy.

23. What is the most reproducible technique for measurement of ejection fraction in patients undergoing cancer chemotherapy?

3D echocardiography.

24. What causes pericardial effusions in cancer patients, and what is the prognosis for cancer patients with pericardial effusions?

Pericardial effusions occur in up to 21% of patients with cancer. Malignancies commonly associated with pericardial effusions include lung cancer, leukemia, lymphoma, and breast cancer. In a recent study from MD Anderson of patients with pericardial effusions who underwent pericardiocentesis, 41% had malignant cells in the pericardial fluid, 2% had infectious etiologies, and 57% had an undetermined etiology. Possible causes of effusion in those with undetermined etiologies include lymphatic obstruction by tumor, radiation-induced fibrosis, or inflammation related to chemotherapies such as anthracyclines or dasatinib.

Overall 1-year survival for patients with malignant cells in the pericardial fluid was 12%, compared with 50% for those with no malignant cells. However, when cancer type was considered, lung cancer patients with malignant cells had significantly shorter median survival times compared with patients with other cancer types (95 days vs. 166 days); the presence of malignant cells did not affect survival in patients with breast cancer.

25. **What should the cardiologist know about renal cell cancer?**

Most cardiac tumors that metastasize to the heart are managed by systemic treatment of the underlying cancer. Renal cell cancer with cardiac metastasis is an exception to this general rule. Surgical resection improves survival. Ten percent of cases involve the inferior vena cava, and 40% of those that involve the inferior vena cava also involve the right atrium. Pulmonary embolism occurs in less than 6%, but mortality is 60% to 65% if it occurs. It is important to look for tumor thrombus in the inferior vena cava in reading the echocardiogram of a patient with renal cell cancer.

Bibliography and Suggested Readings

Children's Oncology Group. (2013). *Long-term follow-up guidelines for survivors of childhood, adolescent, and young adult cancer.* www.survivorshipguidelines.org.

Curigliano, G., Cardinale, D., Suter, T., Plataniotis, G., de Azambuja, E., Sandri, M. T., et al. (2012). Cardiovascular toxicity induced by chemotherapy, targeted agents and radiotherapy: ESMO Clinical Practice Guidelines. *Annals of Oncology, 23*(Suppl. 7), vii155–vii166.

Cutter, D., Taylor, C., Rahimi, K., McGale, P., Ferreira, V., & Darby, S. C. (2013). Effects of radiation therapy on the cardiovascular system. In M. Ewer & E. Yeh (Eds.), *Cancer and the heart* (2nd ed.). Shelton, CT: People's Medical Publishing House.

Dispenzieri, A., Gertz, M. A., Kyle, R. A., Lacy, M. Q., Burritt, M. F., Therneau, T. M., et al. (2004). Serum cardiac troponins and N-terminal pro-brain natriuretic peptide: a staging system for primary systemic amyloidosis. *Journal of Clinical Oncology, 22,* 3751–3757.

El Haddad, D., Iliescu, C., Yusuf, S. W., William, W. N., Khair, T. H., Song, J., et al. (2015). Outcomes of cancer patients undergoing percutaneous pericardiocentesis for pericardial effusion. *Journal of the American College of Cardiology, 66,* 1119–1128.

Force, T., Krause, D. S., & Van Etten, R. A. (2007). Molecular mechanisms of cardiotoxicity of tyrosine kinase inhibition. *Nature Reviews Cancer, 7,* 332–344.

Hall, P. S., Harshman, L. C., Srinivas, S., & Witteles, R. M. (2013). The frequency and severity of cardiovascular toxicity from targeted therapy in advanced renal cell carcinoma patients. *JACC: Heart Failure, 1,* 72–78.

Iliescu, C. A., Grines, C. L., Herrmann, J., Yang, E. H., Cilingiroglu, M., Charitakis, K., et al. (2016). SCAI expert consensus statement: evaluation, management, and special considerations of cardio-oncology patients in the cardiac catheterization laboratory (Endorsed by the Cardiological Society of India, and Sociedad Latino Americana de Cardiologia Intervencionista). *Catheterization and Cardiovascular Interventions, 87,* 895–899.

Li, W., Croce, K., Steensma, D. P., McDermott, D. F., Ben-Yehuda, O., & Moslehi, J. (2015). Vascular and metabolic implications of novel targeted cancer therapies: focus on kinase inhibitors. *Journal of the American College of Cardiology, 66,* 1160–1178.

Lipshultz, S. E., Adams, M. J., Colan, S. D., Constine, L. S., Herman, E. H., Hsu, D. T., et al. (2013). Long-term cardiovascular toxicity in children, adolescents, and young adults who receive cancer therapy: pathophysiology, course, monitoring, management, prevention, and research directions: a scientific statement from the American Heart Association. *Circulation, 128,* 1927–1995.

Lipshultz, S. E., Alvarez, J. A., & Scully, R. E. (2008). Anthracycline associated cardiotoxicity in survivors of childhood cancer. *Heart, 94,* 525–533.

Moslehi, J. J., & Deininger, M. (2015). Tyrosine kinase inhibitor-associated cardiovascular toxicity in chronic myeloid leukemia. *Journal of Clinical Oncology, 33,* 4210–4218.

Neragi-Miandoab, S., Kim, J., & Vlahakes, G. J. (2007). Malignant tumours of the heart: a review of tumour type, diagnosis and therapy. *Clinical Oncology (Royal College of Radiologists [Great Britain]), 19,* 748–756.

Nesbitt, J. C., Soltero, E. R., Dinney, C. P., Walsh, G. L., Schrump, D. S., Swanson, D. A., et al. (1997). Surgical management of renal cell carcinoma with inferior vena cava tumor thrombus. *Annals of Thoracic Surgery, 63,* 1592–1600.

Selvanayagam, J. B., Hawkins, P. N., Paul, B., Myerson, S. G., & Neubauer, S. (2007). Evaluation and management of the cardiac amyloidosis. *Journal of the American College of Cardiology, 50,* 2101–2110.

Suter, T. M., & Ewer, M. S. (2013). Cancer drugs and the heart: importance and management. *European Heart Journal, 34,* 1102–1111.

Vejpongsa, P., & Yeh, E. T. (2014). Prevention of anthracycline-induced cardiotoxicity: challenges and opportunities. *Journal of the American College of Cardiology, 64,* 938–945.

Woodruff, D. Y., Van Veldhuizen, P., Muehlebach, G., Johnson, P., Williamson, T., & Holzbeierlein, J. M. (2013). The perioperative management of an inferior vena caval tumor thrombus in patients with renal cell carcinoma. *Urologic Oncology, 31,* 517–521.

Yeh, E. (2016). *MD Anderson practices in onco-cardiology.* Dallas, TX: Primedia E-launch LLC.

Yusuf, S. W., Solhpour, A., Banchs, J., Lopez-Mattei, J. C., Durand, J. B., Iliescu, C., et al. (2014). Cardiac amyloidosis. *Expert Review of Cardiovascular Therapy, 12,* 265–277.

Zhang, S., Liu, X., Bawa-Khalfe, T., Lu, L. S., Lyu, Y. L., Liu, L. F., et al. (2012). Identification of the molecular basis of doxorubicin-induced cardiotoxicity. *Nature Medicine, 18,* 1639–1642.

CHAPTER 49

COCAINE AND THE HEART

Fawad Virk, James McCord

1. **How common is cocaine use in the United States?**
Cocaine is the second most commonly used illicit drug in the United States, with only marijuana being used more often. Between 1994 and 1998, the number of new cocaine users per year increased by 82%. In 2005, there were approximately 450,000 cocaine-related emergency department visits in the United States. In 2007, there were 2.1 million cocaine users age 12 or older, comprising 0.8% of the population. Users are more likely to be young, between 18 and 20 years of age. Males are more likely to be users than females by a 2:1 ratio. Cocaine-associated chest pain accounts for approximately 16% of all cocaine-related admissions, leading to the evaluation of approximately 64,000 patients annually. Of these, approximately 57% are admitted to the hospital for further evaluation. The annual cost incurred by premature deaths related to regular cocaine use was $1.1 billion.

2. **What are the pharmacologic effects of cocaine?**
Cocaine is a powerful sympathomimetic that acts by directly stimulating central sympathetic outflow and blocking presynaptic uptake of norepinephrine and dopamine. This augmentation in postsynaptic catecholamine increases heart rate, mean arterial pressure, and left ventricular (LV) contractility by stimulating of both alpha- and beta-adrenergic receptors. Through enhanced alpha-adrenergic receptor activation, increased endothelin production, and diminished nitric oxide generation, cocaine leads to coronary artery vasoconstriction.

    Cocaine may also enhance platelet aggregation and thrombus formation through heightened production of adenosine diphosphate, thromboxane A_2, and tissue plasminogen activator inhibitors as well as reductions in protein C and antithrombin III. A study has demonstrated that intravenous cocaine administration can activate circulating platelets via increased expression of P-selectin found on surfaces of the activated platelets.

    Cocaine has toxic effects on cardiac muscle that arise primarily from Ca^{2+} overload during excessive beta-adrenergic stimulation. Adventitial mast cells may potentiate atherosclerosis, vasospasm, thrombosis, and premature sudden death in long-term cocaine abusers.

    Cocaine is well absorbed through all body mucous membranes and can be administered by nasal, sublingual, intramuscular, intravenous, and respiratory routes. The onset of action varies from 3 seconds to 5 minutes, depending on the route of administration. The proposed potential mechanism of the cardiovascular effects of cocaine when beta-blockers are administered in cocaine-induced acute coronary syndrome (ACS) are summarized in Fig. 49.1.

3. **What are the typical symptoms after cocaine ingestion?**
Cardiopulmonary complaints are the most commonly reported symptoms after cocaine use, occurring in 56% of cases. Chest pain is the most common symptom and is typically described as a pressure sensation. Other common symptoms include dyspnea, anxiety, palpitations, syncope, dizziness, and nausea. The onset of symptoms usually occurs soon after ingestion, with two-thirds of patients presenting within 3 hours.

4. **What are the consequences of cocaine use?**
The cardiac and systemic effects of cocaine are complex. Most complications occur in the first 24 hours, but a case report suggests late effects even after 2 weeks, resulting in LV thrombus due to LV dysfunction. A cocaine-induced increase in sympathomimetic activity results in increased myocardial contractility, heart rate, blood pressure, and myocardial oxygen demand while simultaneously decreasing myocardial oxygen supply owing to vasoconstriction.

    The clinical cardiovascular consequences of cocaine use include hypertensive crises, acute myocardial infarction (AMI), aortic dissection, and stroke. Premature coronary atherosclerosis has been seen in young cocaine abusers, with obstructive coronary artery disease (CAD) seen in 35% to 40% of patients who undergo angiography for cocaine-associated chest pain. Cocaine may depress LV function in the absence of acute coronary ischemia because of its direct effect on cardiac muscle,

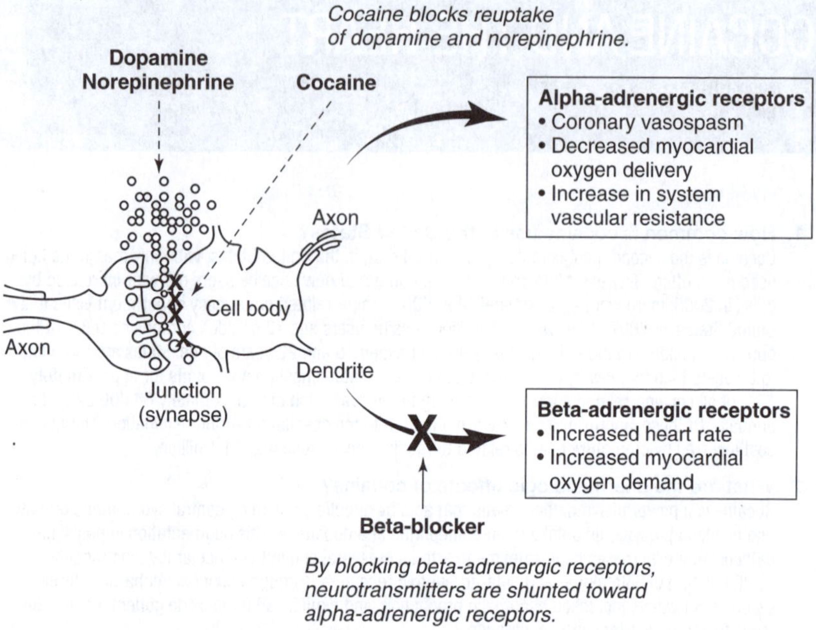

Fig. 49.1. Proposed potential mechanism of the cardiovascular effects of cocaine when beta-blockers are administered in cocaine-induced acute coronary syndrome.

Table 49.1. Summary of the Clinical Cardiovascular Complications of Cocaine
• Tachycardia and hypertension • Premature coronary artery disease • Chest pain, myocardial ischemia, and angina pectoris • Acute myocardial infarction (demand ischemia, NSTE–ACS and STEMI) • Arrhythmias (supraventricular and ventricular) • Sudden cardiac death • Pulmonary edema and crack lung • Myocarditis and cardiomyopathy • Aortic dissection • Stroke

ACS, Acute coronary syndrome; *NSTE*, non–ST-segment elevation; *STEMI*, ST-segment elevation myocardial infarction.

therefore leading to myocarditis and cardiomyopathy. Oxidative stress is major mechanism of cocaine-induced cardiomyopathy.

Cocaine exhibits properties of a class I antiarrhythmic agent by Na-channel blockade. It also prolongs the duration of the QT interval by inhibiting myocyte repolarization, which occurs by the efflux of potassium. Cocaine also increases intracellular calcium with resultant afterdepolarizations, reduces vagal activity, and increases myocyte irritability by inducing ischemia. Ischemia due to vasospasm and fatal ventricular arrhythmias due to ischemia are presumed to be important mechanisms of sudden death in these patients.

The clinical cardiovascular complications of cocaine are summarized in Table 49.1.

5. How often does acute myocardial infarction occur after cocaine ingestion?

Reported rates of AMI vary widely (1% to 31%); the variance in the incidence of AMI in studies likely relates to the difference in patient populations, AMI diagnostic criteria, and the use of newer, more sensitive troponin assays that can detect smaller levels of myocardial necrosis in patients who were previously classified as having unstable angina. AMI occurs within minutes to days after cocaine exposure independent of dose, length of use, or route of administration. However, the time during which individuals are at higher risk for developing AMI is within the first hour of cocaine use.

6. What else should be considered in the differential diagnosis of chest pain or shortness of breath after cocaine use?

Because patients who present to the emergency department with chest pain after cocaine use are commonly hypertensive and tachycardic, aortic dissection must be considered in the differential diagnosis. Information concerning cocaine-induced aortic dissection is limited, but one study of 38 consecutive cases of aortic dissection demonstrated that a surprisingly high percentage (37%) of cases were associated with cocaine use. However, among 921 patients in the International Registry of Aortic Dissection (IRAD), only 0.5% of the cases of aortic dissection were associated with cocaine use.

In addition, an acute pulmonary syndrome, "crack lung," has been described after inhalation of freebase cocaine. The syndrome presents with hypoxemia, hemoptysis, respiratory failure, and diffuse pulmonary infiltrates.

Chronic cocaine use can lead to decreased LV systolic function and congestive heart failure. This may relate to accelerated atherosclerosis or myocarditis, both of which are associated with cocaine use. Cocaine-induced takatsubo cardiomyopathy has been described in a patient with typical echocardiographic findings of apical ballooning 2 days after cocaine use.

7. How does cocaine ingestion lead to acute myocardial infarction?

Cocaine can lead to AMI in a multifactorial fashion, including the following:

- Increasing myocardial oxygen demand by increasing heart rate, blood pressure, and contractility
- Decreasing oxygen supply as a result of vasoconstriction
- Inducing a prothrombotic state by altering the balance between procoagulant and anticoagulant factors
- Accelerating the atherosclerotic process

Coronary vasospasm, rather than plaque rupture, likely constitutes the primary pathogenesis. In patients with preexisting high-grade coronary arterial narrowing, acute ischemia may be the result of increased myocardial oxygen demand associated with hypertension and tachycardia. In those presenting with no underlying atherosclerotic obstruction, coronary occlusion may be due to vasospasm, thrombus formation, or both. For many years the conventional assumption was that AMI after cocaine exposure was due solely to coronary vasospasm. Current knowledge suggests that vasospasm may only be the initiating pathophysiologic event leading to thrombus formation rather than plaque rupture.

8. Should younger patients with chest pain have a cocaine screening test?

The American Heart Association (AHA) recommends that the establishment of cocaine use should depend primarily on self-reporting. Because the use of cocaine influences treatment strategies, patients being evaluated for possible AMI should be queried about cocaine use; this applies especially to younger patients. Even if a young patient with chest pain denies cocaine use, its use should be considered. Young patients with nontraumatic chest pain should be questioned regarding cocaine use.

9. Are there any specific electrocardiographic findings in patients who use cocaine?

Abnormal electrocardiograms (ECGs) have been reported in 56% to 84% of patients with cocaine-associated chest pain. Many of these patients are young and have the normal variant findings of early repolarization—namely, elevation of the J point as well as concave ST-segment elevation and prominent T waves. In a study of 101 patients who had used cocaine, 42% manifested ST-segment elevation on the ECG, but all AMI was ultimately excluded by serial testing of cardiac markers. LV hypertrophy can also be noted on the ECG. In a study comparing the ECGs of cocaine users versus a normal population, bradycardia was found more commonly in chronic cocaine users, which could be due to beta-receptor downregulation resulting from chronic exposure. In a series of 238 individuals who used cocaine, 33% had a normal ECG, 23% had nonspecific findings, 13% had LV hypertrophy, 6% had LV hypertrophy and early repolarization, and 13% had early repolarization alone.

10. Should all patients with cocaine-associated chest pain be admitted to the hospital?

No. Most patients with cocaine-associated chest pain do not have ACS and can safely and efficiently be evaluated in a chest pain observation unit. In a prospective study of 344 patients with cocaine-associated chest pain, 42 (12%) high-risk patients with ST-segment elevation or depression, elevated cardiac markers, or hemodynamic instability were directly admitted. The other 302 were evaluated in an observation unit over 9 to 12 hours with telemetry monitoring, serial troponin I measurement, and selective stress testing. Among the patients in the observation unit there were no cardiac deaths, 4 (2%) nonfatal AMIs, and 158 (52%) patients who underwent stress testing.

11. Should all patients with cocaine-associated chest pain have a stress test?

No. The AHA states that stress testing is optional in patients who have an uneventful 9 to 12 hours of observation. Patients should be counseled about the cessation of cocaine use. Patients can be followed in the outpatient setting, and stress testing may be considered later, depending on cardiac risk factors and ongoing symptoms.

12. How should patients with ST-segment elevation or non–ST-segment elevation myocardial infarction be treated in the setting of cocaine use?

Rapid reperfusion by percutaneous coronary intervention (PCI) in a high-volume center by experienced operators is preferred over fibrinolytic therapy in the setting of ST-segment elevation myocardial infarction (STEMI), and this is even more desirable after cocaine use. Many young patients will have early repolarization, and only a small percentage of these will actually be experiencing an AMI. Furthermore, after cocaine use, hypertensive patients are at higher risk for significant bleeding complications. There have been case reports of intracranial hemorrhage after fibrinolytic therapy in the setting of STEMI associated with cocaine use. Fibrinolytic therapy should be considered only for patients who are clearly having a STEMI and cannot receive timely PCI. Patients with non–ST-elevation myocardial infarction (NSTEMI) should be treated in the same way as other patients, with a notable exception regarding beta-blockers (see Question 14).

13. How should patients with cocaine-associated chest pain be treated?

Patients who ingest cocaine are commonly hypertensive, tachycardic, and anxious. In patients who use cocaine, the AHA recommends the early use of intravenous benzodiazepines, which decrease the central stimulating characteristics of cocaine and thus lessen anxiety. Their use has been shown to relieve chest pain and have beneficial hemodynamic effects. Many times the hypertension and tachycardia will not require direct treatment after treatment with benzodiazepines. Aspirin should also be given. In patients who remain hypertensive, nitroglycerin or nitroprusside can be administered. Phentolamine is also an alternative. Calcium channel blockers have not been well studied in this population but can be considered in patients who do not respond to benzodiazepines and nitroglycerin. However, short-acting nifedipine should not be used, and verapamil and diltiazem should be avoided in the setting of heart failure or decreased LV systolic function. Atorvastatin could be beneficial as it has been shown *in vitro,* to reduce pro-adhesive and pro-thrombotic properties of endothelial cells induced by cocaine. Therapeutic hypothermia can be applied to cocaine-induced cardiac arrest; one study reported full neurologic recovery. Novel therapy with dexmedetomidine (an anxiolytic and sedative) has been shown to reduce sympathetic drive as well as heart rate and blood pressure as compared with placebo in patients who have used cocaine. An algorithm for the management of patients with cocaine-associated chest pain is given in Fig. 49.2.

14. Should beta-blockers be given to patients with cocaine-associated chest pain?

No. The AHA recommends that beta-blockers not be administered acutely in patients with ACS or undifferentiated chest pain in the setting of cocaine use. After cocaine use the administration of propranolol leads to worsening coronary vasoconstriction and increased systemic blood pressure because of the unopposed alpha-adrenergic effect. Multiple experimental animal models have shown that beta-blockers in this setting elevate coronary vascular resistance and decrease coronary blood flow, increase seizure activity, and increase mortality. There have been case reports of sudden cardiac death in humans shortly after the administration of beta-blockers in the setting of cocaine use.

Despite these concerns, however, one retrospective study of 376 cocaine users who presented with chest pain found no difference in outcome between beta-blocker use and nonuse. Another study of 331 cocaine users who presented to an emergency room with chest pain found no meaningful difference in ECG changes, cardiac troponin levels, length of stay, ventricular tachycardia, ventricular

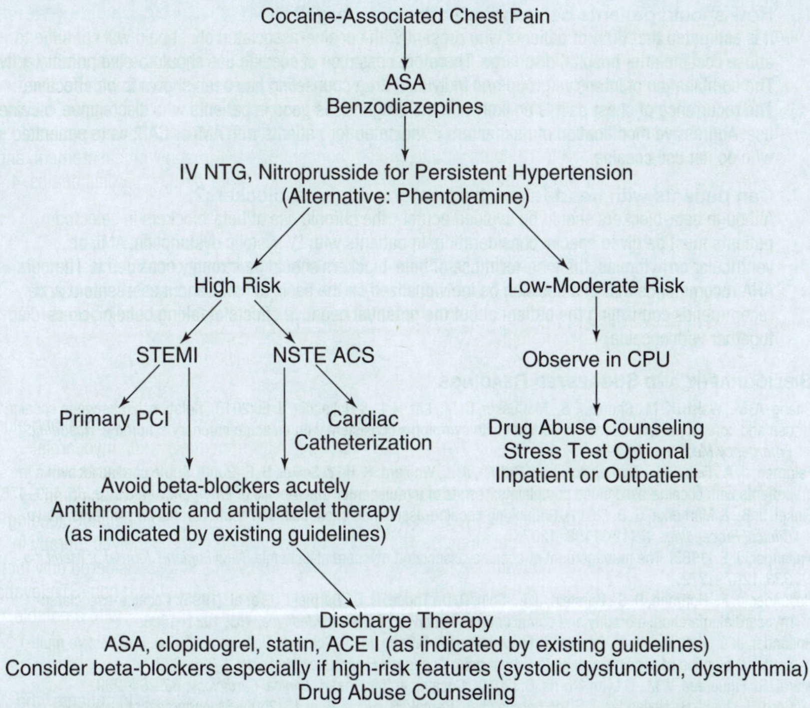

Fig. 49.2. Therapeutic and diagnostic recommendations in cocaine-associated chest pain. *ACE,* Angiotensin-converting enzyme; *ACS,* acute coronary syndrome; *ASA,* aspirin; *beta-blockers,* beta-adrenergic receptor blocking agents; *CPU,* chest pain unit; *IV,* intravenous; *NSTE,* non–ST-segment elevation; *NTG,* nitroglycerin; *PCI,* percutaneous coronary intervention; *STEMI,* ST-segment elevation myocardial infarction. *(Adapted from McCord, J., Jneid, H., Hollander, J. E., de Lemos, J. A., Cercek, B., Hsue, P., et al. [2008]. Management of cocaine-associated chest pain and myocardial infarction: a scientific statement from the American Heart Association acute cardiac care committee of the Council on Clinical Cardiology.* Circulation, *117[14], 1897–1907.)*

fibrillation, or death among those who received beta-blockers versus those who did not. These findings notwithstanding, experts still recommend against the acute administration of a beta-blocker.

Although theoretically more attractive, the administration of labetalol in the setting of cocaine use is not recommended. Labetalol has substantially more beta-blocking than alpha-blocking effects. In animal models, labetalol leads to increased seizure activity and death after cocaine administration and does not reverse coronary vasoconstriction in humans. The β_1-selective agent metoprolol has not been evaluated in the setting of cocaine, but the β_1-selective agent esmolol has been associated with an increase in systemic blood pressure after cocaine use. Compared with labetalol, carvedilol, an alpha-receptor blocker, may be 4 times more potent and, unlike labetalol, carvedilol at recommended doses may attenuate the physiologic and behavioral response to smoked cocaine. However, strong clinical evidence to change current recommendations is still lacking.

15. How should tachyarrhythmias be treated after cocaine use?

Sinus tachycardia and atrial tachyarrhythmias may respond to benzodiazepines. In cases of atrial tachyarrhythmias that do not respond to benzodiazepines, verapamil or diltiazem can be considered. Ventricular arrhythmias that occur immediately after cocaine use are thought to result from the Na-channel blocking effect of cocaine and may respond to the administration of sodium bicarbonate, similar to arrhythmias associated with type IA agents. Ventricular arrhythmias that occur several hours after cocaine use are usually due to ischemia, which should be treated as directed earlier. In case of persistent ventricular arrhythmias, lidocaine can be used. Radiofrequency ablation is safe and effective in patients who have drug-refractory ventricular tachycardia due to chronic cocaine use.

16. How should patients be managed after discharge?

It is estimated that 60% of patients who present with cocaine-associated chest pain will continue to abuse cocaine after hospital discharge. Therefore cessation of cocaine use should be the primary goal. The combination of intensive group and individual drug counseling has been shown to be effective. The recurrence of chest pain is unlikely and the prognosis is good in patients who discontinue cocaine use. Aggressive modification of risk factors is indicated for patients with AMI or CAD, as in patients who do not use cocaine.

17. Can patients with heart failure be treated with beta-blockers?

Although beta-blockers should be avoided acutely, the chronic use of beta-blockers in selected patients must be given special consideration. In patients with LV systolic dysfunction, AMI, or ventricular arrhythmias, the long-term use of beta-blockers should be strongly considered. The AHA recommends that this decision be individualized on the basis of risk-benefit assessment and recommends counseling the patient about the potential negative effects of taking beta-blockers together with cocaine.

Bibliography and Suggested Readings

Chang, A. M., Walsh, K. M., Shofer, F. S., McCusker, C. M., Litt, H. I., & Hollander, J. E. (2010). Relationship between cocaine use and coronary artery disease in patients with symptoms consistent with an acute coronary syndrome. *Academic Emergency Medicine*, *18*, 1–9.

Feldman, J. A., Fish, S. S., Beshansky, J. R., Griffith, J. L., Woolard, R. H., & Selker, H. P. (2000). Acute cardiac ischemia in patients with cocaine-associated complaints: results of a multicenter trial. *Annals of Emergency Medicine*, *36*, 469–476.

Finkel, J. B., & Marhefka, G. D. (2011). Rethinking cocaine-associated chest pain and acute coronary syndromes. *Mayo Clinical Proceedings*, *86*(12), 1198–1207.

Hollander, J. E. (1995). The management of cocaine-associated myocardial ischemia. *New England Journal of Medicine*, *333*, 1267–1272.

Hollander, J. E., Hoffman, R. S., Burstein, J. L., Shih, R. D., Thode, H. C., Bartfield, J., et al. (1995). Cocaine-associated myocardial infarction: mortality and complications. *Archives of Internal Medicine*, *155*, 1081–1086.

Hollander, J. E., Hoffman, R. S., Gennis, P., Fairweather, P., DiSano, M. J., Schumb, D. A., et al. (1994). Prospective multicenter evaluation of cocaine-associated chest pain. *Academic Emergency Medicine*, *1*, 330–339.

Maraj, S., Figueredo, V. M., & Lynn Morris, D. (2010). Cocaine and the heart. *Clinical Cardiology*, *33*, 264–269.

McCord, J., Jneid, H., Hollander, J. E., de Lemos, J. A., Cercek, B., Hsue, P., et al. (2008). Management of cocaine-associated chest pain and myocardial infarction a scientific statement from the American Heart Association acute cardiac care committee of the Council on Clinical Cardiology. *Circulation*, *117*(14), 1897–1907.

Weber, J. E., Shofer, F. S., Larkin, G. L., Kalaria, A. S., & Hollander, J. E. (2003). Validation of a brief observation period for patients with cocaine-associated chest pain. *New England Journal of Medicine*, *348*, 510–517.

HEART DISEASE IN THE ELDERLY

Tomoya T. Hinohara, E. Magnus Ohman

CHAPTER 50

1. **Who are the elderly?**
   Although there is no universal definition for the elderly, guidelines and clinical studies typically designate individuals over the age of 75 years as elderly.

2. **What are important considerations when treating the elderly?**
   Guidelines are less clear when treating the elderly population due to underrepresentation of this population in clinical trials. A study examining the representation of the elderly in cardiovascular randomized controlled trials found that despite efforts to make trials more inclusive (trial enrollment of the elderly increased from 2% during 1966–1990 to 9% during 1991–2000), the elderly remained underrepresented relative to their disease prevalence. Additionally, the elderly represent a heterogeneous population with a wide variety of life expectancies and comorbidities that are not encapsulated by chronologic age alone. Therefore, management should focus on shared decision making and individualized care based on factors including frailty, life expectancy, comorbidities, functional and cognitive capacities, and goals of care.

3. **What is frailty, and how does it affect decision making?**
   Frailty is a syndrome characterized by functional decline and vulnerability to stressors due to the loss of physiologic reserve. Frailty is an important prognosticator associated with increased morbidity and mortality in patients with cardiovascular diseases, including congestive heart failure and myocardial infarction, and in those requiring cardiac surgery. An analysis of frailty in the Targeted Platelet Inhibition to Clarify the Optimal Strategy to Medically Manage Acute Coronary Syndromes (TRILOGY ACS) study demonstrated that frailty in patients with acute coronary syndromes was associated with a higher incidence of all-cause mortality (frail vs. non-frail: 30.2% vs. 15.0%, hazard ratio 1.98, 95% confidence interval 1.47 to 2.68) as well as a higher incidence of a composite of cardiovascular death, myocardial infarction, and stroke (hazard ratio 1.52, 95% confidence interval 1.18 to 1.98). Identification of frailty is an important step to tailor individualized care. The most commonly cited frailty evaluation tool is the Fried Frailty Criteria (Table 50.1).

4. **What are unique challenges in prescribing medications for the elderly?**
   Prescribing medications for the elderly presents special challenges that can result in avoidable but serious adverse drug events if not done cautiously. The elderly are at greater risk of harm due to age-related changes in pharmacokinetics, comorbidities, and polypharmacy. In addition, many medications were not studied in the elderly. It is important to dose medications appropriately with attention to dose adjustments based on age, weight, and renal function. Renal function should be estimated by

Table 50.1. The Fried Frailty Criteria: The Presence of ≥3 Criteria Indicates Frailty

FRAILTY CRITERIA	INDICATORS
Weight loss	Greater than 10 pounds of unintentional weight loss in the prior year
Exhaustion	Affirmation of either of the following criteria: 1. I felt everything I did was an effort in the past week. 2. I could not get going in the past week.
Weakness	Maximal grip strength is lowest quintile (by age, body mass index) using Jamar hand dynamometer.
Slowness	Time to walk 15 feet is the slowest quintile (by gender, height).
Low physical activity level	Kilocalories expended per week is the lowest quintile (by gender).

calculating a creatinine clearance using the Cockroft-Gault equation or Modification of Diet in Renal Disease (MDRD) equation rather than utilizing creatinine alone, as elderly patients may have a near normal serum creatinine but still have significant renal impairment. One study showed that in patients with acute coronary syndromes, older age is a predictor of receiving excess doses of antithrombotic therapy with an estimated 15% of major bleeding attributable to excess dosing. When starting a new medication, it is important to consider the proper dose, potential drug-drug interactions, drug adherence that may be limited by poor cognitive function, adverse drug events, and patient goals.

5. **What is the approach to treating hypertension in the elderly?**
Both initiation and continuation of anti-hypertensive therapy is recommended in the elderly, as it is shown to reduce all-cause mortality. The SPRINT trial demonstrated a mortality benefit, including among the elderly, when systolic blood pressure is targeted to a goal of less than 120 mm Hg, suggesting that more intensive blood pressure is beneficial. It is recommended to start with lower initial drug dosages and slower medication titration, with close monitoring for side effects, including hypotension, syncope, electrolyte abnormalities, and acute kidney injury.

6. **What are the current guidelines for initiating statin therapy for primary prevention in the elderly?**
Statin therapy reduces the risk of major vascular events by 25% in those without clinical atherosclerotic cardiovascular disease (ASCVD), as demonstrated in the Cholesterol Treatment Trialists' Collaboration. However, the magnitude of benefit in the elderly is less known because the elderly population was not well represented in the clinical trials. Therefore, the 2013 American College of Cardiology/American Heart Association (ACC/AHA) blood cholesterol guideline recommends individualized care including a discussion of benefits, risk of adverse events, drug-drug interactions, and patient preferences. The Pooled Cohort Equations is recommended to calculate a 10-year ASCVD risk for those 76 to 79 years of age.

7. **What are the current guidelines for initiating statin therapy for secondary prevention in the elderly?**
The 2013 ACC/AHA blood cholesterol guideline recommends the use of moderate-intensity statin therapy but not high-intensity statin for secondary prevention in individuals greater than 75 years of age with clinical ASCVD. This is based on the Cholesterol Treatment Trialists' Collaboration, which demonstrated a reduction in major vascular events in patients greater than 75 years of age with ASCVD when comparing statin versus control (rate ratio 0.85, 95% confidence interval 0.73 to 0.99) but no significant difference when comparing more versus less intensive statin therapy (rate ratio 0.78, 95% confidence interval 0.52 to 1.18). Continuation of statin therapy is recommended in those who are already taking and tolerating these medications.

8. **How is stable ischemic heart disease managed in the elderly?**
Management by goal-directed medical therapy is the preferred initial approach in the elderly. The goals of medical therapy include symptom relief, risk factor modification, and prevention of myocardial infarction and death. Several studies including the COURAGE trial have demonstrated that initial medical therapy is not significantly less effective than revascularization in relieving angina in the elderly, and the latter is associated with higher mortality rates in the elderly. Despite this recommendation, the elderly are less frequently treated with evidence-based medical therapies.

9. **Do elderly patients with acute coronary syndrome present differently from younger patients?**
Younger patients are much more likely to present with typical chest pain characterized by substernal chest pressure with radiation to the arm or jaw. Symptoms concerning acute coronary syndrome among the elderly include dyspnea, altered mental status, confusion, fatigue, and syncope. ECG changes are also more likely to be nondiagnostic.

10. **How should non–ST-segment elevation acute coronary syndrome be managed in the elderly?**
Elderly patients have high incidence and prevalence of non–ST-segment elevation acute coronary syndrome (NSTE-ACS). The 2014 ACC/AHA NSTE-ACS guideline recommends treating all elderly patients with antiplatelet and anticoagulant agents as well as early invasive revascularization (less than 48 hours). However, in clinical practice, elderly patients are less likely to receive evidence-based pharmacotherapy and early invasive revascularization despite reduced morbidity and mortality as well

as greater absolute benefit than younger patients treated with the same therapy. This is in part due to atypical presentation delaying care as well as concern for increased risk of complications including bleeding. Earlier and increased implementation of evidence-based care should be the focus of treating elderly patients with NSTE-ACS. Table 50.2 summarizes dosing recommendations in elderly patients for pharmacologic agents used in the treatment of acute coronary syndromes.

Table 50.2. Pharmacologic Agents and Dosing Recommendations in Elderly Patients for Acute Coronary Syndromes

DRUG	DRUG CLASS	STANDARD DOSE	ADJUSTED DOSE
Aspirin	Antiplatelet, COX inhibitor	325-mg loading dose, 81-mg daily maintenance dose	None
Cangrelor	Antiplatelet, thienopyridine P2Y12 inhibitor	30-mcg/kg loading dose, 4-mcg/kg per minute maintenance infusion	None
Clopidogrel	Antiplatelet, thienopyridine P2Y12 inhibitor	300-600-mg loading dose, 75-mg daily maintenance dose	None
Prasugrel	Antiplatelet, thienopyridine P2Y12 inhibitor	60-mg loading dose, 10-mg daily maintenance dose	Avoid use if ≥75 years old
Ticagrelor	Antiplatelet, non-thienopyridine P2Y12 inhibitor	180-mg loading dose, 80-mg twice daily maintenance dose	None
Abciximab	Antiplatelet, glycoprotein IIb/IIIa inhibitor	UA/NSTEMI: 0.25-mg/kg bolus and 10-mcg/minute infusion STEMI: 0.25-mg/kg bolus and 0.125-mcg/kg per minute infusion	None
Eptifibatide	Antiplatelet, glycoprotein IIb/IIIa inhibitor	180-mcg/kg bolus and 2-mcg/kg per minute infusion	If CrCl <50 mL/minute, 180-mcg/kg bolus and 1-mcg/kg per minute infusion Contraindicated in end-stage renal disease
Tirofiban	Antiplatelet, glycoprotein IIb/IIIa inhibitor	25-mcg/kg loading dose and 0.15-mcg/kg per minute infusion	If CrCl ≤60 mL/min, 25-mcg/kg loading dose, 0.075-mcg/kg maintenance infusion
Bivalirudin	Anticoagulant, direct thrombin inhibitor	UA/NSTEMI: Prior to PCI: 0.1-mg/kg bolus and 0.25-mg/kg per hour infusion During PCI: Additional 0.5-mg/kg bolus and increase infusion to 1.75 mg/kg per hour or 0.75-mg/kg bolus and 1.75 mg/kg per hour infusion if patient did not receive initial medical management STEMI: 0.75-mg/kg bolus and 1.75-mg/kg per hour infusion	During PCI or for STEMI, if CrCl is 10-29 mL/min, bolus is unchanged and infusion rate is decreased to 1 mg/kg per hour. If dialysis dependent, bolus is unchanged and infusion rate is decreased to 0.25 mg/kg per hour.

Continued on following page

Table 50.2. Pharmacologic Agents and Dosing Recommendations in Elderly Patients for Acute Coronary Syndromes *(Continued)*

DRUG	DRUG CLASS	STANDARD DOSE	ADJUSTED DOSE
Enoxaparin	Anticoagulant, low-molecular-weight heparin	UA/NSTEMI: 1 mg/kg subcutaneously every 12 hours STEMI: 30-mg IV bolus and 1 mg/kg subcutaneously every 12 hours	UA/NSTEMI: If CrCl less than 30: 1 mg/kg subcutaneously daily STEMI: If ≥75 years old: 0.75 mg/kg subcutaneously every 12 hours without IV bolus If less than 75 years old and CrCl less than 30 mL/min: 30-mg IV bolus and 1 mg/kg once daily If ≥75 years old and CrCl less than 30 mL/min: 1 mg/kg subcutaneously once daily without IV bolus
Fondaparinux	Anticoagulant, factor Xa inhibitor	UA/NSTEMI: 2.5 mg subcutaneously daily STEMI: 2.5 mg intravenously and 2.5 mg subcutaneously daily	Contraindicated if CrCl less than 30 mL/min
Unfractionated heparin	Anticoagulant	60-unit/kg bolus (maximum 4000 units) and 12-unit/kg per hour infusion (maximum 1000 units per hour) for goal aPTT of 50-70 s	None

aPTT, Activated partial thromboplastin time; *COX*, cyclooxygenase; *CrCl*, creatinine clearance; *IV*, intravenous; *NSTEMI*, non–ST-segment elevation myocardial infarction; *STEMI*, ST-segment elevation myocardial infarction; *UA*, unstable angina.

11. What is the preferred treatment for ST-segment elevation myocardial infarction in the elderly?

The gold standard is prompt coronary artery reperfusion by primary percutaneous coronary intervention (PCI) in individuals with ischemic symptoms of less than 12 hours' duration. Current guidelines give preference to primary PCI over fibrinolytic therapy in the elderly. Unfortunately, the elderly are less likely to receive primary PCI or fibrinolytic therapy due to delayed diagnosis attributable to atypical symptoms or nondiagnostic ECGs and relative or absolute contraindications to fibrinolytic therapy.

12. What is the most common arrhythmia in the elderly, and how should it be treated?

Atrial fibrillation is the most common arrhythmia among the elderly, occurring in up to 9% of individuals older than 80 years of age. Symptoms are typically subtle (e.g., fatigue or generalized lack of energy) or even absent. A rate control strategy is the preferred initial therapy rather than rhythm control due to diminished clearance of antiarrhythmic medications resulting in a higher likelihood of adverse effects including bradyarrhythmias. Rate control is typically achieved with beta-blockers or non-dihydropyridine calcium channel blockers. Caution must be taken when initiating therapy, as the elderly are more susceptible to bradycardia and orthostatic hypotension.

13. What is the preferred method of stroke prevention in the elderly with atrial fibrillation?

Yearly stroke risk increases with age and is reduced by the use of aspirin or chronic anticoagulation. The decision for pharmacologic therapy can be guided by CHA2DS2-VASc and HAS-BLED scores. Current guidelines recommend that all individuals age 75 years or older be treated with anticoagulants. According to a meta-analysis of randomized controlled trials, novel oral anticoagulants (apixiban,

Table 50.3. Pharmacologic Agents and Dosing Recommendations for Prevention of Stroke and Systemic Embolism in Nonvalvular Atrial Fibrillation in Elderly Patients

DRUG	MECHANISM OF ACTION	STANDARD DOSE	ADJUSTED DOSE
Dabigatran	Direct thrombin inhibitor	150 mg twice daily	Avoid use if CrCl ≤30 mL/min
Apixiban	Direct factor Xa inhibitor	5 mg twice daily	2.5 mg twice daily if ≥80 years old *and* either weight ≤60 kg *or* serum creatinine ≥1.5 mg/dL
Edoxaban	Direct factor Xa inhibitor	60 mg daily	Avoid use if CrCl less than 15 mL/min
Rivaroxaban	Direct factor Xa inhibitor	20 mg daily	Avoid use if CrCl ≤30 mL/min

CrCl, Creatinine clearance.

dabigatran, and rivaroxaban) are preferred over warfarin in the elderly because they significantly lower the risk of stroke and systemic embolism (OR 0.65, 95% CI 0.48 to 0.87) without increasing the risk of bleeding (OR 1.02, 95% CI 0.73 to 1.43). For patients with absolute or relative contraindications to anticoagulation, including a previous life-threatening bleeding episode, aspirin is the preferred alternative. Warfarin is the drug of choice for patients with chronic renal failure (creatinine clearance [CrCl] <30 mL/min). Table 50.3 summarizes the commonly prescribed anticoagulants and dosing recommendations in the elderly.

14. **What is the most common valvular disease in the elderly?**
Aortic stenosis is the most common valvular disease, affecting approximately 15% of individuals age 65 years and older. Symptom monitoring is important, as the 2-year mortality rate increases to around 50% after symptom onset.

15. **What is the preferred treatment strategy for symptomatic aortic stenosis?**
Treatment strategy is similar to the younger population and relies on surgical aortic valve replacement as the first-line option. The Society of Thoracic Surgery (STS) risk score is a useful tool to calculate an individual's risk of mortality and various morbidities with surgery. Individuals who are nonsurgical or high-risk surgical candidates may be considered for transcatheter aortic valve replacement (TAVR). This is a minimally invasive treatment option that was demonstrated in the PARTNER A and B trials to be superior to medical therapy in nonsurgical candidates and to have similar outcomes compared to surgery in high-risk surgical candidates.

16. **How does management of heart failure differ in the elderly?**
Landmark trials in heart failure management primarily enrolled middle-aged individuals, although more recent studies have also included the elderly population. Studies that include the elderly suggest a benefit of beta-blockers, ACE inhibitors or ARBs, and aldosterone antagonists in individuals with heart failure with reduced ejection fraction. Direct vasodilators including hydralazine and nitrates have a limited role due to orthostatic hypotension. The elderly are also less likely to tolerate doses studied in the trials due to adverse effects, and individualized dose titration to tolerability is important.

Bibliography and Suggested Readings

Amsterdam, E. A., Wenger, N. K., Brindis, R. G., Casey, D. E., Ganiats, T. G., Holmes, D. R., et al. (2014). 2014 AHA/ACC guideline for the management of patients with non-ST-elevation acute coronary syndromes: a report of the American College of Cardiology/American Heart Association Task Force on Practice Guidelines. *Journal of the American College of Cardiology*, *64*(24), e139–e228.

Baigent, C., Blackwell, L., Emberson, J., Holland, L. E., Reith, C., Bhala, N., et al. (2010). Efficacy and safety of more intensive lowering of LDL cholesterol: a meta-analysis of data from 170,000 participants in 26 randomised trials. *Lancet*, *376*(9753), 1670–1681.

Boden, W. E., O'Rourke, R. A., Teo, K. K., Hartigan, P. M., Maron, D. J., Kostuk, W. J., et al. (2007). Optimal medical therapy with or without PCI for stable coronary disease. *New England Journal of Medicine*, *356*(15), 1503–1516.

James, P. A., Oparil, S., Carter, B. L., Cushman, W. C., Dennison-Himmelfarb, C., Handler, J., et al. (2014). 2014 evidence-based guideline for the management of high blood pressure in adults: report from the panel members appointed to the Eighth Joint National Committee (JNC 8). *Journal of the American Medical Association*, *311*(5), 507–520.

Lee, P. Y., Alexander, K. P., Hammill, B. G., Pasquali, S. K., & Peterson, E. D. (2001). Representation of elderly persons and women in published randomized trials of acute coronary syndromes. *Journal of the American Medical Association, 286*(6), 708–713.

Leon, M. B., Smith, C. R., Mack, M., Miller, D. C., Moses, J. W., Svensson, L. G., et al. (2010). Transcatheter aortic-valve implantation for aortic stenosis in patients who cannot undergo surgery. *New England Journal of Medicine, 363*(17), 1597–1607.

Lip, G. Y., & Lane, D. A. (2015). Stroke prevention in atrial fibrillation: a systematic review. *Journal of the American Medical Association, 313*(19), 1950–1962.

Nishimura, R. A., Otto, C. M., Bonow, R. O., Carabello, B. A., Erwin, J. P., Guyton, R. A., et al. (2014). 2014 AHA/ACC guideline for the management of patients with valvular heart disease: executive summary: a report of the American College of Cardiology/American Heart Association Task Force on Practice Guidelines. *Journal of the American College of Cardiology, 63*(22), 2438–2488.

O'Gara, P. T., Kushner, F. G., Ascheim, D. D., Casey, D. E., Chung, M. K., De Lemos, J. A., et al. (2013). 2013 ACCF/AHA guideline for the management of ST-elevation myocardial infarction: a report of the American College of Cardiology Foundation/American Heart Association Task Force on Practice Guidelines. *Journal of the American College of Cardiology, 61*(4), e78–e140.

Prystowsky, E. N., Padanilam, B. J., & Fogel, R. I. (2015). Treatment of atrial fibrillation. *Journal of the American Medical Association, 314*(3), 278–288.

Sardar, P., Chatterjee, S., Chaudhari, S., & Lip, G. Y. (2014). New oral anticoagulants in elderly adults: evidence from a meta-analysis of randomized trials. *Journal of the American Geriatrics Society, 62*(5), 857–864.

Singh, M., Stewart, R., & White, H. (2014). Importance of frailty in patients with cardiovascular disease. *European Heart Journal, 35*(26), 1726–1731.

Smith, C. R., Leon, M. B., Mack, M. J., Miller, D. C., Moses, J. W., Svensson, L. G., et al. (2011). Transcatheter versus surgical aortic-valve replacement in high-risk patients. *New England Journal of Medicine, 364*(23), 2187–2198.

Stone, N. J., Robinson, J. G., Lichtenstein, A. H., Merz, C. N., Blum, C. B., Eckel, R. H., et al. (2014). 2013 ACC/AHA guideline on the treatment of blood cholesterol to reduce atherosclerotic cardiovascular risk in adults: a report of the American College of Cardiology/American Heart Association Task Force on Practice Guidelines. *Journal of the American College of Cardiology, 63*(25 Pt B), 2889–2934.

White, H. D., Westerhout, C. M., Alexander, K. P., Roe, M. T., Winters, K. J., Cyr, D. D., et al. (2015). Frailty is associated with worse outcomes in non-ST-segment elevation acute coronary syndromes: insights from the TaRgeted platelet Inhibition to cLarify the Optimal strateGy to medicallY manage Acute Coronary Syndromes (TRILOGY ACS) trial. *European Heart Journal: Acute Cardiovascular Care, 5*, 231–242.

Wright, J. T., Jr., Whelton, P. K., & Reboussin, D. M. (2015). A randomized trial of intensive versus standard blood-pressure control. *New England Journal of Medicine, 373*(22), 2103–2116.

HEART DISEASE IN PREGNANCY

Heidi Nicewarner, Sheilah Bernard

CHAPTER 51

1. What cardiac physiologic changes occur during pregnancy?

Hormonal changes cause an increase in both plasma volume (from water and sodium retention) and red blood cell volume (from erythrocytosis) during a normal pregnancy (Fig. 51.1). A disproportionate increase in plasma volume explains the physiologic anemia of pregnancy. Maternal heart rate (HR) increases throughout the 40 weeks, mediated partially by increased sympathetic tone and heat production. Stroke volume subsequently continues to increase until the third trimester, when inferior vena cava (IVC) return may be compromised by the gravid uterus. Maternal cardiac output (CO) increases by 30% to 50% during a normal pregnancy. Systolic blood pressure drops during the first half of pregnancy and returns to normal levels by delivery. The physiologic changes that occur during pregnancy are shown in Fig. 51.2 and summarized in Table 51.1.

2. Are there independent vascular changes that occur during a normal pregnancy?

The vascular wall weakens during pregnancy as a result of estrogen and prostaglandin, leading to increased risk for vascular dissection. As the placenta develops, it creates a low-resistance circulation. These factors, in addition to heat production, contribute to the reduced systemic vascular resistance (SVR) that is a normal part of pregnancy.

3. What are normal cardiac signs and symptoms of pregnancy?

Normal cardiac signs and symptoms of pregnancy include the following:

- *Hyperventilation* (as a result of increased minute ventilation)
- *Peripheral edema* (from volume retention and vena caval compression by the gravid uterus)
- *Dizziness/lightheadedness* (from reduced SVR and vena caval compression)
- *Palpitations* (where normal HR increases by 10 to 15 beats/minute)

4. What are pathologic cardiac signs and symptoms of pregnancy?

Pathologic cardiac signs and symptoms of pregnancy include the following:

- *Anasarca*, or generalized edema, and *paroxysmal nocturnal dyspnea* are not components of normal pregnancy and warrant workup.
- *Syncope* warrants evaluation for pulmonary embolism, tachy/bradyarrhythmias, pulmonary hypertension, obstructive valvular pathology (aortic, mitral, or pulmonic stenosis), or hypotension.
- *Chest pain* may be due to aortic dissection, pulmonary embolism, angina, or even myocardial infarction. As more women delay childbearing, there is a higher incidence of preexisting cardiac disease and risk factors in pregnant women.
- *Hemoptysis* may be a harbinger of occult mitral stenosis, although rheumatic heart disease is becoming less common in developed countries.

5. What are normal cardiac examination findings during pregnancy?

Normal cardiac examination findings during pregnancy include the following:

- Blood pressure (BP) will decline and HR will increase.
- The point of maximum impulse will be displaced laterally as the uterus enlarges.
- S3 is common because of increased rapid filling of the left ventricle (LV) in early diastole.
- A physiologic pulmonic flow murmur is common because of elevated stroke volume passing through a normal valve.
- *A mammary soufflé* (due to increased blood flow into the breasts) and *venous hum* (due to increased blood flow through jugular veins) are two continuous, superficial murmurs that can be obliterated by compressing the site with the diaphragm of the stethoscope. If the murmur does not change, consider patent ductus arteriosus or coronary arteriovenous (AV) fistula.

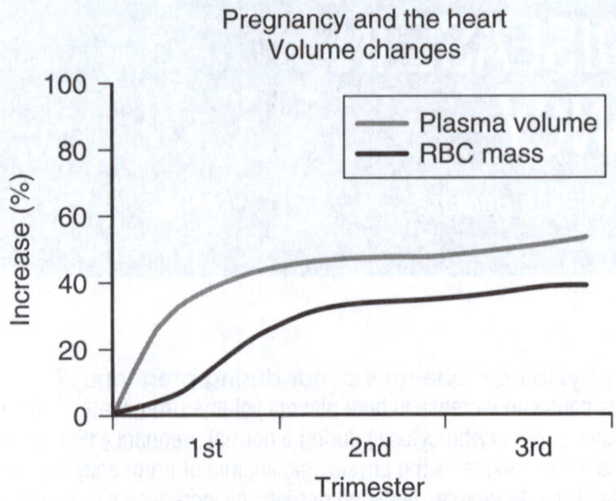

Fig. 51.1. Blood volume changes in pregnancy. Plasma volume and red blood cell (RBC) mass increase during the trimesters of pregnancy. The plasma volume approaches 50% above baseline by the second trimester and then virtually plateaus until delivery. *(Image from Warnes, C. Pregnancy and heart disease. In* J. R. Teerlink, & E. Foster (Eds.), Valvular heart disease in pregnancy. A contemporary perspective. Cardiol Clin, Philadelphia: WB Saunders Company. 16(3), 574, 1998 Aug.

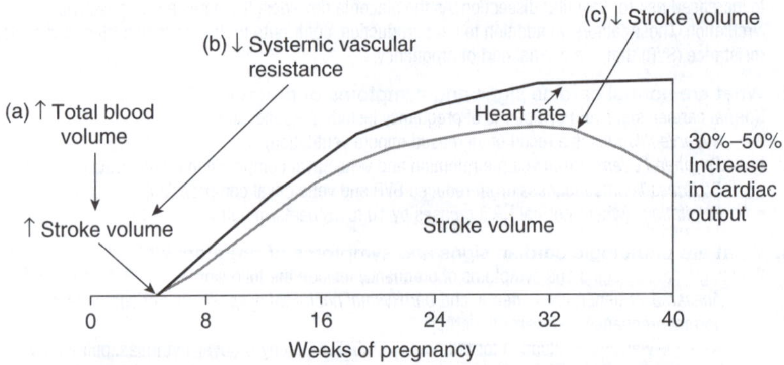

Fig. 51.2. Time course and mechanisms for increased cardiac output during pregnancy.

Table 51.1. Hemodynamic Changes in Pregnancy

PARAMETER	CHANGE
Peripheral resistance	↓
Blood volume	↑40-50%
Heart rate	↑10-20%
Cardiac output	↑30%
Blood pressure	↔ or ↓
Pulmonary vascular resistance	↓
Venous pressure in lower extremities	↑

Table adapted from figure in Warnes, C. Pregnancy and heart disease. In Braunwald's heart disease: a textbook of cardiovascular medicine *(10th ed., chapter 78, pp. 1755–1770). Philadelphia, PA: Saunders.*

Table 51.2. Normal and Pathologic Cardiovascular Findings, Signs, and Symptoms with Pregnancy

NORMAL	PATHOLOGIC
Cardiac Examination	
Decrease in blood pressure	Elevated jugular venous pressure (JVP)
Increase in heart rate	Systolic murmur 3/6 or louder
Displaced point of maximum impulse (PMI)	Any diastolic murmur
Physiologic pulmonary flow murmur	S4
Mammary souffle or venous hum	Right ventricular heave, loud P2
Peripheral edema	Anasarca
Hyperventilation	Clubbing Cyanosis Hypoxia
Symptoms	
Dizziness/lightheadedness	Syncope
Palpitations	Hemoptysis Paroxysmal nocturnal dyspnea Chest pain

6. What are pathologic cardiac exam findings during pregnancy?

Pathologic cardiac exam findings during pregnancy include the following:

- *Clubbing* and *cyanosis* are not a part of normal pregnancy; desaturation for any reason is abnormal and warrants investigation.
- *Elevated jugular venous pressure (JVP)* is abnormal, reflecting elevated right atrial pressure. Although edema is common in this population, it is important to evaluate neck veins in any pregnant woman with peripheral edema.
- *Pulmonary hypertension* (right ventricular heave, loud P2, JVP elevation) findings should be investigated early. Women with preexisting pulmonary hypertension (pulmonary pressure greater than 75% of systemic pressure) should be counseled prior to pregnancy as to the risks.
- *Systolic murmur 3/6 or louder* and any *diastolic murmur* audible in pregnancy are considered abnormal and warrant evaluation.
- *S4* is unusual during pregnancy and may reflect underlying hypertension.

The normal and pathologic cardiovascular findings, signs, and symptoms with pregnancy are summarized in Table 51.2.

7. What are the cardiac changes that occur during labor and delivery?

With each contraction, 300 to 500 mL of blood are autotransfused from the uterus into the maternal circulatory system. CO drops less with vaginal delivery than cesarean, so this form of delivery is recommended more commonly in patients with cardiac disease. Vacuum-assisted delivery is used to shorten stage II of labor for women who may not tolerate pushing. After delivery, intravascular volume increases from release of the IVC compression, and HR slows. BP, CO, and HR generally normalize post-partum; however, CO remains elevated in lactating women while they continue to breastfeed.

8. Which women should undergo infective endocarditis prophylaxis at the time of delivery?

Infective endocarditis (IE) prophylaxis is currently not recommended by the European Society of Cardiology (ESC) at the time of vaginal or cesarean delivery for patients with prior IE, prosthetic valves, or congenital heart disease (CHD).

9. What maternal cardiac tests can be performed safely?

All tests utilizing radiation should be performed only after a thorough review and justification of the risks and benefits to the mother and fetus.

- Electrocardiograms and echocardiograms are safe with no known risk to the fetus.
- Chest radiographs can be performed with proper pelvic shielding.
- MRI is considered safe (although there are few data during the first trimester).
- Low-level exercise tolerance testing to 70% of maternal maximal heart rate is safe with low risk of fetal distress/bradycardia.
- Transesophageal echocardiography (TEE) can be performed with appropriate sedation and monitoring.
- Cardiac catheterization, balloon valvuloplasty, angioplasty, and percutaneous intervention are invasive diagnostic and therapeutic tests that may be lifesaving to the mother with appropriate pelvic shielding for the fetus.
- Computerized tomography is relatively contraindicated due to radiation risk to the fetus.
- Nuclear imaging is contraindicated due to radiation risk to the fetus.

10. What are the highest risk maternal cardiac conditions during pregnancy?

Moderate to severe mitral, aortic, and pulmonic stenosis are tolerated poorly during pregnancy. Patients should be counseled, with consideration of valvuloplasty or valve replacement before conception. These procedures can be performed during high-risk pregnancies if the patient decompensates. Pulmonary hypertension (pHTN) is also a high-risk condition, with historic maternal mortality rates between 30% and 56%. While mortality remains prohibitively high, improvements in both the treatment of pHTN as well as the management of high-risk pregnancy have led to significant mortality reductions. Women with pHTN should be counseled regarding these risks.

11. How are the common congenital lesions tolerated during pregnancy?

In developed countries, CHD has superseded rheumatic heart disease as the most common preexisting heart disease in pregnancy. Repaired atrial septal defects (ASDs) and ventricular septal defects (VSDs) confer no increased cardiac risk. Unrepaired left-to-right intracardiac shunts (ASD and VSD) are well tolerated because of the reduction in SVR, which decreases left-to-right shunting during pregnancy. Patients are at an increased risk for paradoxic embolization if they develop deep venous thrombosis.

Right-to-left (cyanotic) shunting is poorly tolerated in pregnancy. Women with tetralogy of Fallot should undergo repair before contemplating pregnancy. Right-to-left shunting worsens during pregnancy because of reduction of SVR. Women with Eisenmenger's syndrome risk a 30% to 50% maternal mortality with pregnancy. Such high-risk women are counseled to avoid pregnancy or undergo therapeutic termination.

12. Are regurgitant valvular lesions equally risky?

Both mild to moderate aortic insufficiency and mitral regurgitation are tolerated well during pregnancy. The reduction in SVR can lessen the degree of regurgitation. Only patients with severe symptomatic regurgitation (New York Heart Association [NYHA] class III–IV) should be considered for valve replacement before pregnancy. The only indication for valve replacement for regurgitant lesions during pregnancy is infective endocarditis (Table 51.3).

Table 51.3. Cardiovascular Conditions Associated with High-Risk Pregnancies
• Dilated cardiomyopathy, ejection fraction <40%
• Aortic stenosis, moderate to severe
• Mitral stenosis, moderate to severe
• Mechanical prosthetic valves
• Congenital cyanotic lesions
• Pulmonary hypertension
• Pulmonary stenosis
• Coarctation of the aorta
• Marfan syndrome with aortic root >40 mm

Adapted from Warnes, C. Pregnancy and heart disease. In Braunwald's heart disease: a textbook of cardiovascular medicine *(10th ed., chapter 78, pp. 1755–1770). Philadelphia, PA: Saunders.*

13. What are maternal complications seen in pregnant women with cardiac disease? What are some predictors of fetal complications?

Pulmonary edema, stroke, arrhythmia, and cardiac death are complications noted in a study of 599 such pregnancies. Fetal complications were seen more often in pregnancies with maternal cyanosis, left heart obstruction, anticoagulation, concomitant smoking, multiple gestations, and heart failure symptoms greater than NYHA class II.

14. How is maternal hypertension treated during pregnancy?

Identification of maternal hypertension is essential during pregnancy, as hypertensive disorders are a major cause of maternal and perinatal morbidity and mortality as reviewed by the American College of Obstetricians and Gynecologists (ACOG) in 2013.

- *Preeclampsia* is defined as new-onset hypertension (SBP ≥140 and/or DBP ≥90 measured on two occasions at least 4 hours apart after 20 weeks' gestation) and new-onset proteinuria (≥300 mg per 24-hour urine collection or a protein/creatinine ratio ≥0.3). However, some women may not have proteinuria, and its presence is not required to make the diagnosis. In its absence, the definition includes hypertension (as defined previously) in association with thrombocytopenia (a platelet count <100,000/μL), impaired liver function (elevated blood levels of liver transaminases to twice the normal concentration), the development of new renal insufficiency (elevated serum creatinine >1.1 mg/dL or a doubling of serum creatinine in the absence of other renal disease), pulmonary edema, or new-onset cerebral or visual disturbances.
- *Eclampsia* occurs in women with preeclampsia who develop new-onset grand mal seizures.
- *Gestational hypertension* is a BP elevation after 20 weeks of gestation in the absence of proteinuria or the systemic findings associated with preeclampsia.
- *Chronic hypertension* is hypertension that has been diagnosed prior to pregnancy.
- *Superimposed preeclampsia* is chronic hypertension in association with preeclampsia.

In general, labetalol, nifedipine, methyldopa, and hydralazine are safe antihypertensives to use during pregnancy, with goal BPs being 120 to 160/80 to 110. ACE inhibitors, angiotensin receptor blockers, renin inhibitors, and mineralocorticoid receptor antagonists are contraindicated during pregnancy.

15. How are pregnant women anticoagulated during pregnancy?

Per AHA/ACC valvular heart disease guidelines, it is reasonable for patients who maintain a therapeutic INR on warfarin doses ≤5 mg daily to continue this low dose throughout pregnancy until delivery. Because daily doses >5 mg warfarin are contraindicated during the first trimester and at term, 2012 American College for Chest Physicians (ACCP) guidelines recommend one of the following grade 1A strategies:

- Aggressive adjusted-dose twice-daily low-molecular-weight heparin (LMWH) throughout pregnancy with doses adjusted to achieve target peak anti-Xa level 4 hours post injection
- Aggressive adjusted-dose twice-daily unfractionated heparin (UFH) throughout pregnancy administered subcutaneously to a therapeutic partial thromboplastin time (PTT)
- UFH or LMWH until the 13th week of pregnancy with substitution by vitamin K antagonists (warfarin) until close to delivery. At that point, UFH or LMWH is resumed.

Long-term anticoagulants should be resumed postpartum with all regimens, as early as the same evening. Low-dose aspirin can be optionally added for high-risk patients with mechanical heart valves. Mothers taking warfarin may nurse after delivery.

Pregnant women have been excluded from participation in clinical trials of the new oral direct thrombin inhibitors and anti-Xa inhibitors, and the ACCP recommends avoiding their use.

16. Which cardiac arrhythmias can complicate pregnancy?

Patients may develop atrial and ventricular ectopy because of myocardial stretch. Reentrant pathways may emerge, leading to atrial arrhythmias. These can be treated acutely with vagal maneuvers or adenosine if the mother is unstable. Recurrent supraventricular arrhythmias can be prevented with digitalis or beta-blockers. Symptomatic ventricular arrhythmias are treated medically or with implantable cardioverter/defibrillators.

17. How do you treat a pregnant woman with an acute myocardial infarction?

Pregnant women with ST-segment elevation myocardial infarction (STEMI) should be taken to the catheterization laboratory for primary Percutaneous Coronary Intervention (PCI). Heparin can be used safely; however, there are few data on the use of stents, as clopidogrel has not been extensively studied in pregnancy. It is currently categorized by the US Food and Drug Administration (FDA) as class B. Beta-blockers and low-dose aspirin can be used in pregnancy, but ACE inhibitors, angiotensin receptor blockers (ARBs), and statins should be avoided. Risk factors should be treated.

18. How do you treat a pregnant woman with cardiac arrest?

In the pregnant patient, supine positioning causes aortocaval compression, which impairs CO during cardiopulmonary resuscitation (CPR). Relief of aortocaval compression is recommended using manual left uterine displacement (LUD) in all pregnant women who are in cardiac arrest, in which the uterus is palpated at or above the umbilicus. Manual LUD can be performed from the left side of the patient where the uterus is cupped and lifted up and leftward off the maternal vessels, or from the right of the patient, where the uterus is pushed upward and leftward off the maternal vessels.

Hypoxemia develops more rapidly in pregnancy; therefore, rapid, high-quality, and effective airway and breathing interventions are an important part of resuscitation. The current recommendations are to implement the use of early bag-mask ventilation with 100% oxygen.

If no return of spontaneous maternal circulation has occurred, perimortem cesarean delivery (PMCD) should be strongly considered after approximately 4 minutes of resuscitative efforts.

19. How do women with hypertrophic cardiomyopathy tolerate pregnancy?

The management of pregnancy in women with hypertrophic cardiomyopathy is similar to that for the nongravid state. Women with HCM will experience left ventricular end-diastolic pressure (LVEDP) elevations because of increased volume of pregnancy. If the LV is able to dilate, outflow obstruction may improve. At the time of delivery, anesthesia is critical to reduce sympathetic stimulation from pain; most anesthetic agents reduce myocardial contractility. Preload and afterload changes during delivery must be minimized to avoid increased outflow obstruction. Short-acting vasoconstrictors, diuretics, or volume adjustments may be necessary.

20. What are the recommendations for patients with Marfan syndrome?

Women with Marfan syndrome are at risk for aortic dissection because of the additional vascular changes of pregnancy. Genetic counseling should be performed before conception because of autosomal dominant transmission. Those with an aortic root diameter of more than 40 mm are at highest risk and are advised to avoid pregnancy. Management includes beta-blockers, serial echocardiograms, and bed rest to avoid further root dilation. Type A dissection (involving the ascending aorta) should be managed surgically, with delivery of the viable fetus before repair. Type B dissection (descending aortic involvement) can be managed medically with labetalol or nitroprusside.

Thoracic endovascular aortic repair (TEVAR) is an emerging alternative to open surgery in patients with Marfan syndrome but is not currently recommended as a first-line treatment per a recent position statement of the European Association for Cardio-Thoracic Surgery (EACTS) and the ESC. TEVAR has not been studied in pregnant women with Marfan syndrome.

21. Which commonly used cardiac medications should be avoided during pregnancy?

- Women should be counseled that warfarin and statins are currently FDA class X. Investigations on the use of statins in pregnancy are under way, with a recent meta-analysis suggesting that statin use may be safer than previously thought.
- ACE inhibitors, ARBs, atenolol, and amiodarone are class D.
- LMWH or UFHs should replace warfarin at certain periods of pregnancy.
- The oral factor Xa inhibitors have not been well studied in pregnancy and are class B (apixaban) or class C (rivaroxaban).
- Hydralazine with nitrates should replace ACE inhibitors/ARBs in patients with heart failure.
- ACE inhibitors can be used in nursing mothers.
- Metoprolol, propranolol, or labetalol should be used instead of atenolol.

Table 51.4 summarizes the safety of cardiac medications in pregnancy.

22. What is peripartum cardiomyopathy?

This is a syndrome of congestive heart failure diagnosed from the last month of pregnancy up to 5 months postpartum, with demonstration of reduced systolic function by echocardiogram, without identifiable or reversible cause. This is distinct from preexisting cardiac disease, which usually presents before the final month due to physiologic changes of pregnancy. Women are treated

Table 51.4. Safety of Cardiac Medications in Pregnancy

- Women should be counseled that warfarin is a class X drug per the US Food and Drug Administration. LMWH or UFHs should replace warfarin in the first trimester and after 36 weeks of pregnancy.
- Statins are also class X, although investigations on the use of statins in pregnancy are under way, with a recent meta-analysis suggesting that statin use may be safer than previously thought.
- ACE inhibitors, ARBs, atenolol, and amiodarone are class D.
- Hydralazine with nitrates should replace ACE inhibitors and ARBs in patients with heart failure.
- ACE inhibitors can be used in nursing mothers.
- Metoprolol, propranolol, or labetalol should be used instead of atenolol.
- The oral factor Xa inhibitors have not been well studied in pregnancy and are class B (apixaban) or class C (rivaroxaban).

ACE, Angiotensin-converting enzyme; *ARB*, angiotensin II receptor blocker; *LMWH*, low-molecular-weight heparin; *UFH*, unfractionated heparin.

with standard heart failure medications (hydralazine/nitrates while pregnant and ACE inhibitors after delivery). Prognosis is determined by degree of systolic function recovery. Maternal risk is higher during subsequent pregnancies if LVEF dysfunction (EF <40%) persists. B-type natriuretic peptide (BNP) levels do not rise in a normal pregnancy; increased levels suggest cardiomyopathy, preeclampsia, eclampsia, and/or diabetes.

Bibliography and Suggested Readings

Baddour, L. M., Wilson, W. R., Bayer, A. S., Fowler, V. G., Jr., Tleyjeh, I. M., & Rybak, M. J. (2015). Infective endocarditis in adults: diagnosis, antimicrobial therapy and management of complications: a scientific statement for healthcare professionals from the American Heart Association. *Circulation, 132*, 1435–1486.

Bates, S. M., Greer, I. A., Middeldorp, S., Veenstra, D. L., Prabulos, A. M., Vandvik, P. O., et al. (2012). VTE, thrombophilia, antithrombotic therapy, and pregnancy: antithrombotic therapy and prevention of thrombosis, 9th ed: American College of Chest Physicians Evidence-Based Clinical Practice Guidelines. *Chest, 141*, e691S–e736.

Bédard, E., Dimopoulos, K., & Gatzoulis, M. A. (2009). Has there been any progress made on pregnancy outcomes among women with pulmonary arterial hypertension? *European Heart Journal, 30*, 256–265.

Drenthen, W., Pieper, P., Roos-Hesselink, J., van Lottum, W. A., Voors, A. A., Mulder, B. J., et al. (2007). Outcome of pregnancy in women with congenital heart disease: a literature review. *Journal of the American College of Cardiology, 49*, 2303–2311.

Grabenwöger, M., Alfonso, F., Bachet, J., Bonser, R., Czerny, M., Eggebrecht, H., et al. (2012). Thoracic Endovascular Aortic Repair (TEVAR) for the treatment of aortic diseases: a position statement from the European Association for Cardio-Thoracic Surgery (EACTS) and the European Society of Cardiology (ESC), in collaboration with the European Association of Percutaneous Cardiovascular Interventions (EAPCI). *European Heart Journal, 33*, 1558–1563.

Habib, G., Lancelotti, P., Antunes, M. J., Bongiorni, M. G., Casalta, J. P., Del Zotti, F., et al. (2015). 2015 ESC Guidelines for the management of infective endocarditis. *European Heart Journal, 36*, 3075–3128.

James, A. H., Brancazio, L. R., & Price, T. (2008). Aspirin and reproductive outcomes. *Obstetrics Gynecology Survey, 63*, 49–57.

Jeejeebhoy, J. F. M., Zelop, C. M., Lipman, S., Carvalho, B., Joglar, J., Mhyre, J. M., et al. (2015). Cardiac arrest in pregnancy: a scientific statement from the American Heart Association. *Circulation, 132*, 1747–1773.

Kusters, D. M., Lahsinoui, H. H., van de Post, J. A., Wiegman, A., Wijburg, F. A., Kastelein, J. J., et al. (2012). Statin use during pregnancy: a systematic review and meta-analysis. *Expert Review of Cardiovascular Therapy, 10*, 363–378.

Nishimura, R. A., Otto, C. M., Bonow, R. O., Carabello, B. A., Erwin, J. P., 3rd, Guyton, R. A., et al. (2014). 2014 AHA/ACC guideline for the management of patients with valvular heart disease: a report of the American College of Cardiology/American Heart Association Task Force on Practice Guidelines. *Journal of the American College of Cardiology, 63*, e57–e185.

Regitz-Zagrosek, V., Blomstrom Lundqvist, C., Borghi, C., Cifkova, R., Ferreira, R., et al. (2011). ESC Guidelines on the management of cardiovascular diseases during pregnancy: the task force on the management of cardiovascular diseases during pregnancy of the European Society of Cardiology (ESC). *European Heart Journal, 32*(24), 3147–3197.

Reimold, S. C., & Rutherford, J. D. (2003). Clinical practice: valvular heart disease in pregnancy. *New England Journal of Medicine, 349*, 52–59.

Weiss, B. M., Zemp, L., Seifert, B., & Hess, O. M. (1998). Outcome of pulmonary vascular disease in pregnancy: a systematic overview from 1978 through 1996. *Journal of the American College of Cardiology, 31*, 1650–1657.

Yarrington, C. D., Valente, A. M., & Economy, K. E. (2015). Cardiovascular management in pregnancy; antithrombotic agents and antiplatelet agents. *Circulation, 132*, 1354–1364.

CHAPTER 52

HEART DISEASE IN WOMEN

Jaya Chandrasekhar, Roxana Mehran

1. Are there gender differences in presentation of acute coronary syndromes?

Women comprise 20% to 30% of all acute coronary syndrome (ACS) presentations. Cross-sectional US data for the year 2010 identified 625,000 unique hospitalizations for ACS, including 262,000 women.

According to the Atherosclerosis Risk in Communities (ARIC) study and National Heart Lung and Blood Institute (NHLBI) report, the average age at first myocardial infarction (MI) in men and women is 65.1 years and 72.0 years, respectively. Although the prevalence of coronary disease increases with age, prevalence is also on the rise in younger women. Women in general (young or old) have greater baseline risk factors than men, including active smoking, diabetes, chronic kidney disease, cerebrovascular disease, and depression. Women also present more often than men with sudden cardiac death as their first presentation of ACS.

Symptoms in women may include pain in the chest, neck, shoulders or arm (56%), shortness of breath (38%), nausea (18%), or fatigue (10%). A National Registry of Myocardial Infarction (NRMI) report for the period 1994–2006 showed that women were more likely than men to present without chest pain.

Late hospital presentations are observed more often in women than men, which may be due to lower awareness of heart disease, cultural issues, as well as atypical symptoms. Although women's awareness of cardiovascular disease as the leading cause of death has increased from 30% in 1997, it was still only 56% in 2012. Women are more likely to use emergency medical transport for hospital presentation than men based on data from the National cardiovascular data registry-Acute Coronary Treatment and Intervention Outcomes Network (NCDR-ACTION)—Get With the Guidelines Registry.

2. Are there gender differences in cardiovascular disease outcomes?

In both men and women, coronary artery disease (CAD) is the leading cause of death. Based on pooled data from 1995 to 2012, women have a higher rate of death within 1 year of first MI and higher rate of recurrent MI within 5 years of first MI than men. Similarly, among individuals greater than 45 years of age, women have a higher rate of heart failure within 5 years of a first MI compared with men.

Outcomes of MI have improved in both men and women, and a decreasing trend in gender differences has been observed. However, studies indicate that there has been less improvement in women compared to men. Similarly while there has been a decline in the overall rate of sudden cardiac death, the decline has been observed to be lower in women compared with men. From 1989 to 1998, women between the ages of 35 to 44 years had a 21% rise in the incidence of spontaneous coronary artery dissection (SCD), whereas men had a 2.8% decline.

Observational data indicate that women with MI undergoing coronary artery bypass surgery have higher in-hospital mortality than men, which is a function of greater baseline comorbidities in women. Analogously, studies also indicate that women have worse unadjusted outcomes than men after percutaneous coronary intervention. These differences are attenuated after adjustment for baseline comorbidities, implying that a worse risk profile rather than female gender is the reason for the higher ischemic adverse event rate.

3. Are there gender biases in the management of cardiovascular disease?

The term *Yentl syndrome* was conceived by Dr. Bernadine Healy in 1991 for the observed gender bias in the management of coronary heart disease. Prior reports indicate that women receive less guideline-directed management than men, including stress testing, cardiac catheterization and revascularization, antiplatelet therapy, beta-blockers, and lipid-lowering therapies. Although women derive the same treatment benefit from beta-blockers, statins, and antiplatelet therapy, they are underprescribed acute care therapies as well as treatments for secondary prevention compared to men.

Women are less likely to undergo stress testing than men due to perceived lower prevalence of cardiovascular disease. Further, women with an abnormal stress test are less likely to be referred for diagnostic testing. This may be due to greater false positive results compared to men. Indeed, the sensitivity and specificity of detecting CAD on stress testing in women have been shown to range from

31% to 71% and 66% to 86%, respectively. In one study, the positive predictive value of ST-segment depression in symptomatic patients undergoing angiography was 47% in women versus 77% in men.

In a Medicare study for the period 1994–1996, researchers found that fewer women than men underwent coronary catheterizations (36% vs. 47%). The Euro Heart Survey in 2005 showed that fewer women with stable angina underwent coronary angiography (odds ratio [OR] 0.59) or revascularization, and women were more likely to experience death or MI during 1-year follow-up compared to men (hazard ratio [HR] 2.09).

Despite heightened awareness on this subject, a recent prospective observational study of 1465 acute myocardial infarction (AMI) patients from 103 US centers showed that young women less than 55 years were less likely to receive reperfusion therapies compared to similarly aged young men. This discordance was more apparent in patients transferred to PCI centers and in the case of fibrinolytic therapy. Conversely, among the patients who received revascularization, there was no sex-based difference in reperfusion strategy.

Women are less likely to receive statin therapies compared to men. An observational study from 2008 to 2009 showed that women were prescribed lipid-lowering therapies less often than men with CAD (7.8% vs. 12.8%) and achieved low-density lipoprotein cholesterol goal lower than 70 mg/dL less often than men (30.6% vs. 38.4%).

4. What are the differences in anatomic disease and plaque morphology among men and women?

Women appear to have more diffuse CAD rather than focal obstructive lesions. Men and women with ACS have similar numbers of culprit lesions; however, men demonstrate more plaque rupture and thin-cap fibroatheroma (TCFA) than women. With respect to non-culprit lesions, women have fewer non-culprit lesions and less plaque rupture and necrotic core volume but similar TCFA and pathologic intimal thickening. These differences in men and women are more apparent under the age of 65 years, beyond which differences are largely attenuated.

In general men have greater coronary calcification than women. In an autopsy study of 108 patients with sudden cardiac death, women had less calcification than men until the seventh decade of life, beyond which prevalence was similar. Calcific nodules are irregular luminal protrusions that are observed in older patients in association with tortuous coronary arteries; coronary tortuosity is more commonly seen in women.

5. What is the underlying pathobiology of plaque morphology in women with coronary artery disease?

Pathology studies have shown that women are more likely to present with plaque erosion, whereas men present with plaque rupture. Studies have also shown that premenopausal women more often present with erosion, whereas postmenopausal women present with rupture. Importantly, these findings highlight that plaque erosion is not a benign entity.

6. Is fractional flow reserve testing useful in women?

Yes, fractional flow reserve (FFR) testing is useful in both men and women. The Fractional Flow Reserve Versus Angiography for Multivessel Evaluation (FAME) trial showed that both men and women derived benefit from the use of FFR to guide decisions regarding PCI. Coronary FFR is higher in women than men for any given stenosis, due to smaller body surface area, coronary vessel diameter, left ventricular mass and myocardial territory supplied in women. In a study evaluating intravascular ultrasound (IVUS) and FFR, women were more likely than men to demonstrate mismatch with angiographic diameter stenosis $> 50\%$ or IVUS minimum lumen area $< 2.5\ mm^2$ and FFR was > 0.80.

7. What is microvascular angina?

Microvascular angina (Fig. 52.1) is the occurrence of chest pain and abnormal coronary flow reserve due to microvascular disease in the absence of obstructive CAD. This condition was previously referred to as "syndrome X" and may result from endothelial dysfunction, arterial stiffness as well as due to atherosclerosis and microembolization. Microvascular angina is more common in women and often underdiagnosed.

Abnormal coronary flow reserve is diagnosed as a coronary flow reserve of less than 2.5, which requires measurement using invasive (flow wire) or noninvasive (positron emission tomography [PET], echo Doppler, or cardiac magnetic resonance imaging) techniques.

Since patients with microvascular angina cannot adequately increase coronary flow in response to increasing oxygen demands, beta-blockers are the currently recommended first-line therapy. Numerous other medications, including calcium channel blockers, nitrates, angiotensin converting enzyme inhibitors, and ranolizine have been studied, with generally modest or disappointing results.

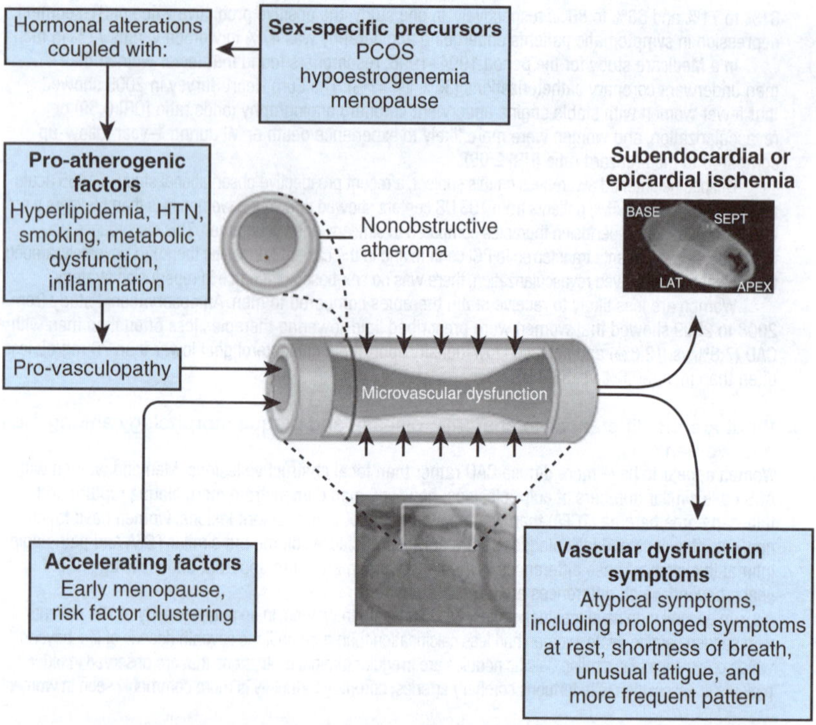

Fig. 52.1. Model of microvascular angina in women. *APEX,* Left ventricular apex; *BASE,* left ventricular base; *HTN,* hypertension; *LAT,* left ventricular lateral wall; *PCOS,* polycystic ovarian syndrome; *SEPT,* inter-ventricular septum. *(Image from Shaw, L. J., Bugiardini, R., & Merz, C. N. [2009]. Women and ischemic heart disease.* Journal of the American College of Cardiology, 54*[17], 1561–1575.)*

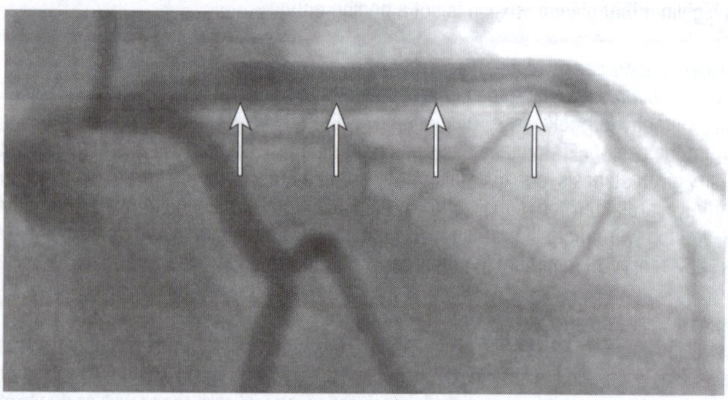

Fig. 52.2. Spontaneous coronary dissection. Note the linear dissection *(arrows)* in the proximal left anterior descending artery. *(Image from Alfonso, F., Paulo M., Lennie, V., Dutary, J., Bernardo, E., Jiménez-Quevedo, P., et al. [2012]. Spontaneous coronary artery dissection.* Journal of the American College of Cardiology, 5*[10], 1062–1070.)*

8. What is the significance of spontaneous coronary artery dissection in women?

Spontaneous coronary artery dissection (SCAD) (Figs. 52.2 and 52.3) is an unusual presentation for ACS and is more likely to present in women than in men, particularly in the postpartum period. It is defined as a nontraumatic and noniatrogenic separation of the coronary arterial walls creating a false lumen and may be associated with fibromuscular dysplasia. In one observational study, the left anterior descending

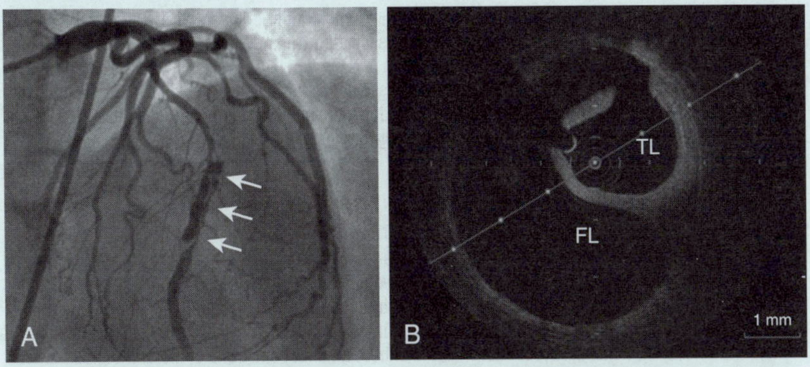

Fig. 52.3. Spontaneous coronary artery dissection in a patient with coronary fibromuscular dysplasia. **A,** Angiogram showing extensive dissection *(arrows)* of the left anterior descending artery. **B,** Optical coherence tomography (OCT) showing the dissection separating the true lumen (TL) from the false lumen (FL). *(Image from Michelis, K. C., Olin, J. W., Kadian-Dodov, D., d'Escamard, V., & Kovacic, J. C. [2014]. Coronary artery manifestations of fibromuscular dysplasia.* Journal of the American College of Cardiology, 64*[10], 1033–1046.)*

artery was the most frequently affected target vessel, and multivessel involvement was noted in 23% cases. Diagnosis may require intravascular imaging in addition to angiography. Management is conservative, and coronary stenting is not recommended for risk of propagating the dissection. Over a follow-up period of 47 months, the rate of recurrence has been observed to be 17.2%.

9. What is takotsubo cardiomyopathy?

Takotsubo or stress cardiomyopathy is an ACS presentation that is more common in post-menopausal women and is triggered by emotional or physical stress. The pathognomonic feature of this condition is left ventricular apical ballooning and absence of obstructive CAD on angiography (Fig. 52.5). Despite good in-hospital outcomes, the annual mortality rate was reported to be 5.6% per patient per year over a 10-year follow-up in the International Takotsubo Registry. Compared to women, men with Takotsubo cardiomyopathy had worse short-term (30-day mortality 12.2% vs. 5.2%, $p = 0.001$) and long-term (1-year mortality 12.9% vs. 5.0% per patient-per year, $p < 0.001$) outcomes.

10. What is coronary artery spasm? Are there sex-based differences in prevalence and outcomes?

Coronary artery spasm, also referred to as variant or Prinzmetal's angina, is characterized by severe chest pain at rest with concurrent ST-segment elevation on electrocardiography. Patients may also experience ventricular arrhythmias and complete atrioventricular block, which can occur even in the absence of chest pain.

The pathophysiology is related to vagal withdrawal and a change in sympathetic activity, smooth muscle hyper-reactivity, and endothelial dysfunction. Prior studies report a genetic role in some populations as well as an association with cigarette smoking, type A behavior patterns, anxiety or panic disorders, and use of cocaine, amphetamines, and other drugs. While some data suggest coronary artery spasm may be more common in women, other observational studies indicate a greater frequency in men. Racial differences have also been documented, with the highest occurrence in Japanese populations.

Although the rate of recurrent angina is high, the rate of MI in long-term follow-up is low. No sex-based differences in major adverse cardiac events were noted during 5-year follow-up. A history of ventricular arrhythmias and coexisting coronary disease has been shown to be a predictor of mortality. Cohort studies suggest a beneficial role of calcium channel blockers and long-acting nitrates in reducing anginal symptoms, whereas beta-blockers may be detrimental.

11. Does history of depression have an impact on cardiovascular outcomes in women?

Observational studies have indicated that the rate of depression is higher in women and in patients with cardiac disease, particularly after AMI. The INTERHEART study identified psychosocial factors as a potentially modifiable risk associated with MI. In the PREMIER MI registry, women had a higher prevalence of depression (28.9% vs. 18.8%). Women under 60 years of age had the highest depression scores (8.2) after MI. Depression was associated with adverse outcomes (1-year rehospitalization and recurrent angina) in both men and women in this registry. In the Women's Ischemia Syndrome Evaluation (WISE) study, depression was associated with 15% to 53% increase in health care costs over 5 years, suggesting that identification and treatment of depression in women may reduce cardiac care costs. In this study, depression was shown to be associated with high inflammatory markers, C-reactive protein and interleukin-6, and higher adverse cardiovascular outcomes.

12. Are there sex differences regarding the effects of antiplatelet therapies?

Yes. Berger et al. performed a gender-specific meta-analysis of aspirin for primary prevention from six trials comprising 95,456 patients. Among 51,342 women, aspirin was associated with 12% reduction in composite cardiovascular events (death, MI, or stroke) and 17% reduction in stroke, without an effect on MI or mortality. Among 44,114 men, aspirin was associated with 14% reduction in composite cardiovascular events and 32% reduction in MI without an effect on stroke or mortality. In both men and women, aspirin increased the risk of bleeding similarly.

Gender-related differences have also been noted in the relative benefit with clopidogrel therapy. In a gender-based meta-analysis of 23,533 women and 56,091 men with a spectrum of coronary disease from five randomized controlled trials, treatment with clopidogrel compared to placebo in women resulted in a nonstatistically significant lower composite endpoint of cardiovascular death, MI, or stroke (OR: 0.93), whereas in men there was a statistically significant reduction (OR: 0.84). Further, in women there was reduction in risk of MI but not in stroke or death, whereas in men there was a significant reduction in risk of MI, death, and stroke. Clopidogrel was associated with greater bleeding compared to placebo in both men and women (OR 1.43 in women, OR 1.22 in men).

No sex-related differences have been reported in the treatment effects of potent $P2Y_{12}$ platelet receptor inhibitors ticagrelor and prasugrel compared to clopidogrel.

13. How should antiplatelet and anticoagulant therapies be selected in women?

Women have higher rates of bleeding with treatment for ACS and with percutaneous coronary intervention. Several factors may contribute to greater bleeding risk in women than men, such as vascular biology, hormonal influences, lower body mass index, and lower renal function. The American College of Cardiology/American Heart Association guidelines state that although antithrombotic therapies in women should be the same as for men, they should be selected with careful attention to weight and renal function in women.

14. Is history of preeclampsia relevant in patients presenting with cardiovascular disease?

Women with history of preeclampsia are more likely to be at risk for early progression of atherosclerotic disease. Routine cardiovascular evaluation in women should therefore include detailed assessment of history of pregnancy and pregnancy-induced complications (Table 52.1).

15. What are the observed sex-based differences in patients undergoing transcatheter aortic valve replacement?

In contrast to percutaneous coronary intervention trials, men and women are equally represented in transcatheter aortic valve replacement (TAVR) studies. Women undergoing TAVR for the treatment of severe aortic stenosis have a distinctive risk profile compared to men. While women have fewer comorbidities (such as CAD, diabetes, and atrial fibrillation) than men, women also have some higher risk features such as lower BMI, lower glomerular filtration rate, and greater prevalence of porcelain aorta and higher incidence of moderate or severe mitral valve regurgitation.

Women undergoing TAVR have been shown to have a higher incidence of procedural complications, including coronary obstruction, the need for surgical conversion, vascular complications, and bleeding complications. Despite this, long-term survival after TAVR is higher in women than in men.

16. Is estrogen considered to have a role in protection from cardiovascular disease?

The Women's Ischemia Syndrome Evaluation (WISE) study found women with endogenous estrogen deficiency to be at higher risk of angiographic CAD. Prior observational studies also suggest that women with premature menopause have greater incidence of cardiac events. However, these observational findings were not confirmed by randomized controlled trials. At present, estrogen replacement therapy is not recommended for the prevention of CAD.

Table 52.1. Classification of Risk for Cardiovascular Disease in Women

RISK STATUS	CRITERIA
High risk (≥1 high-risk state)	Clinically manifested CHD Clinically manifested CVD Clinically manifested PAD Abdominal aortic aneurysm End-stage or chronic kidney disease Diabetes mellitus 10-year predicted CVD risk ≥10%
At risk (≥1 risk factor)	Cigarette smoking SBP ≥120 mm Hg, DBP ≥80 mm Hg, or treated hypertension Total cholesterol ≥200 mg/dL, HDL-C <50 mg/dL, or treated for dyslipidemia Obesity, particularly central adiposity Poor diet Physical inactivity Family history of premature CVD occurring in first-degree relatives in men <55 years of age or in women <65 years of age Metabolic syndrome Evidence of advanced subclinical atherosclerosis (e.g., coronary calcification, carotid plaque, or increased intima-media thickness) Poor exercise capacity on a treadmill test and/or abnormal heart rate recovery after stopping exercise Systemic autoimmune collagen-vascular disease (e.g., SLE, RA) History of preeclampsia, gestational diabetes, or pregnancy-induced hypertension
Ideal cardiovascular health (all of these)	Total cholesterol <200 mg/dL (untreated) BP <120/<80 mm Hg (untreated) Fasting blood glucose <100 mg/dL (untreated) BMI <25 kg/m^2 Abstinence from smoking Healthy (DASH-like) diet

BMI, Body mass index; *BP*, blood pressure; *CHD*, coronary heart disease; *CVD*, cardiovascular disease; *DASH*, Dietary Approaches to Stop Hypertension; *DBP*, diastolic BP; *PAD*, peripheral artery disease; *RA*, rheumatoid arthritis; *SBP*, systolic BP; *SLE*, systemic lupus erythematosus.

From Martha, G., & Bairey Merz, C. N. (2015). Cardiovascular disease in women. Braunwald's heart disease: a textbook of cardiovascular medicine *(chapter 77, pp. 1744–1754). Philadelphia, PA: Saunders.*

Modified from Mosca, L., Benjamin, E. J., Berra, K., Bezanson, J. L., Dolor, R. J., Lloyd-Jones, D. M., et al. (2011). Effectiveness-based guidelines for the prevention of cardiovascular disease in women—2011 update: a guideline from the American Heart Association. Circulation, 123, *1243.*

17. What is peripartum cardiomyopathy, and how can it be recognized?

Peripartum cardiomyopathy refers to dilated cardiomyopathy and heart failure in postpartum women, commonly presenting within 3 months of delivery. It can be difficult to recognize since it may be masked by the symptoms of pregnancy; thus diagnosis may be missed or delayed. The incidence is 1 in 2500 to 4000 women. Risk factors include high maternal age at pregnancy, hypertension in pregnancy, multiparity, and multi-fetal pregnancy. No clear cause has been identified, although potential causes may include nutritional deficiency and coronary artery spasm. Women who have peripartum cardiomyopathy are often advised against future pregnancy, as recurrent peripartum cardiomyopathy can occur.

18. What is fibromuscular dysplasia of the coronary arteries?

FMD of the coronary arteries (Fig. 52.4) is an uncommon condition that can present as coronary aneurysm or SCAD, resulting in ACS, sudden cardiac death, or left ventricular dysfunction. It is an arteriopathy that is distinct from vasculitis or atherosclerosis and is common in middle-aged women but may occur at any age, in both men and women. The etiology is poorly understood, and it has been suggested that FMD may be genetically mediated with an autosomal dominant trait and variable penetrance.

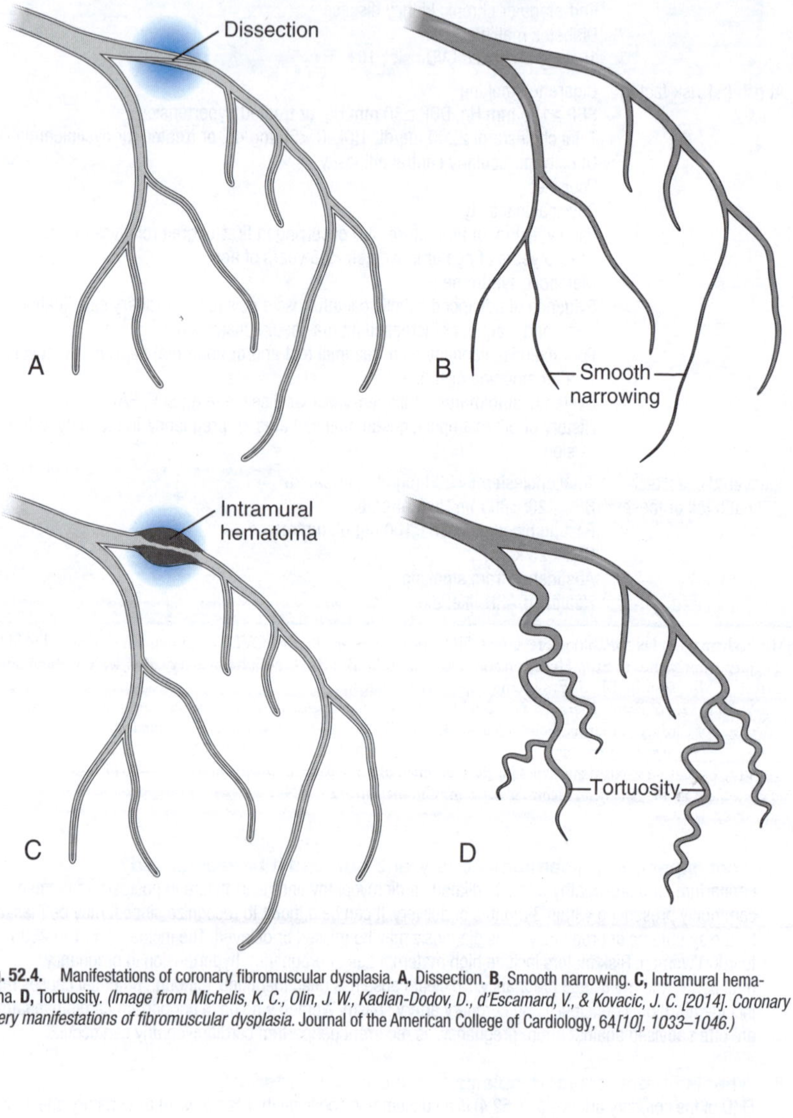

Fig. 52.4. Manifestations of coronary fibromuscular dysplasia. **A,** Dissection. **B,** Smooth narrowing. **C,** Intramural hematoma. **D,** Tortuosity. *(Image from Michelis, K. C., Olin, J. W., Kadian-Dodov, D., d'Escamard, V., & Kovacic, J. C. [2014]. Coronary artery manifestations of fibromuscular dysplasia.* Journal of the American College of Cardiology, *64[10], 1033–1046.)*

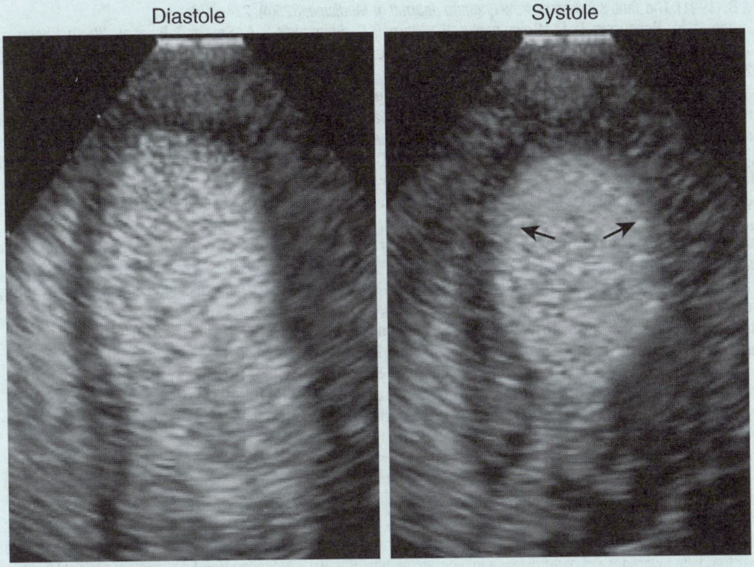

Fig. 52.5. Takotsubo cardiomyopathy. Contrast-enhanced transthoracic echocardiography demonstrating aneurysmal systolic bulging (dyskinesis) of the LV apex in a patient with takotsubo cardiomyopathy. *The* arrows *denote ballooning of the left ventricular apex relative to the left ventricular base. (Adapted from Lonnebakken, M. T., & Berdts, E. [2001]. Contrast echocardiography in coronary artery disease. In Baskot, B [Ed.].* Coronary angiography—advances in noninvasive imaging approach for evaluation of coronary artery disease. *Rijeka, Croatia: Intech. Intechweb.org.)*

The classic "string of beads" appearance noted in the renal arteries may not be observed in the coronary arteries. Intravascular ultrasound or optical coherence tomography may be used to facilitate diagnosis.

Bibliography and Suggested Readings

Ahmed, B., & Dauerman, H. L. (2013). Women, bleeding, and coronary intervention. *Circulation, 127*(5), 641–649.

Amsterdam, E. A., Wenger, N. K., Brindis, R. G., Casey, D. E., Jr., Ganiats, T. G., Holmes, D. R., Jr., et al. (2014). 2014 AHA/ACC Guideline for the Management of Patients with Non-ST-Elevation Acute Coronary Syndromes: a report of the American College of Cardiology/American Heart Association Task Force on Practice Guidelines. *Journal of the American College of Cardiology, 64*(24), e139–e228.

Bairey Merz, C. N., & Pepine, C. J. (2011). Syndrome X and microvascular coronary dysfunction. *Circulation, 124*(13), 1477–1480.

Bairey Merz, C. N., Shaw, L. J., Reis, S. E., Bittner, V., Kelsey, S. F., Olson, M., et al. (2006). Insights from the NHLBI-Sponsored Women's Ischemia Syndrome Evaluation (WISE) Study: Part II: gender differences in presentation, diagnosis, and outcome with regard to gender-based pathophysiology of atherosclerosis and macrovascular and microvascular coronary disease. *Journal of the American College of Cardiology, 47*(Suppl. 3), S21–S29.

Berger, J. S., Bhatt, D. L., Cannon, C. P., Chen, Z., Jiang, L., Jones, J. B., et al. (2009). The relative efficacy and safety of clopidogrel in women and men a sex-specific collaborative meta-analysis. *Journal of the American College of Cardiology, 54*(21), 1935–1945.

Berger, J. S., Roncaglioni, M. C., Avanzini, F., Pangrazzi, I., Tognoni, G., Brown, D. L., et al. (2006). Aspirin for the primary prevention of cardiovascular events in women and men: a sex-specific meta-analysis of randomized controlled trials. *Journal of the American Medical Association, 295*(3), 306–313.

Camici, P. G., & Crea, F. (2007). Coronary microvascular dysfunction. *New England Journal of Medicine, 356*(8), 830–840.

Chandrasekhar, J., Dangas, G., Yu, J., Vemulapalli, S., Suchindran, S., Vora, A.N., et al. (2016). *Sex based differences in outcomes with transcatheter aortic valve therapy: TVT Registry* from 2011 to 2014. *Journal of the American College of Cardiology*, in press. http://dx.doi.org/10.1016/j.jacc.2016.10.041.

Daly, C., Clemens, F., Lopez Sendon, J. L., Tavazzi, L., Boersma, E., Danchin, N., et al. (2006). Gender differences in the management and clinical outcome of stable angina. *Circulation, 113*(4), 490–498.

Gulati, M., Shaw, L. J., & Bairey Merz, C. N. (2012). Myocardial ischemia in women: lessons from the NHLBI WISE study. *Clinical Cardiology, 35*(3), 141–148.

Healy, B. (1991). The Yentl syndrome. *New England Journal of Medicine, 325*(4), 274–276.

Herrington, D. M., Reboussin, D. M., Brosnihan, K. B., Sharp, P. C., Shumaker, S. A., Snyder, T. E., et al. (2000). Effects of estrogen replacement on the progression of coronary-artery atherosclerosis. *New England Journal of Medicine, 343*(8), 522–529.

Hulley, S., Grady, D., Bush, T., Furberg, C., Herrington, D., Riggs, B., et al. (1998). Randomized trial of estrogen plus progestin for secondary prevention of coronary heart disease in postmenopausal women. Heart and Estrogen/progestin Replacement Study (HERS) Research Group. *Journal of the American Medical Association, 280*(7), 605–613.

Jani, S. M., Montoye, C., Mehta, R., Riba, A. L., DeFranco, A. C., Parrish, R., et al. (2006). Sex differences in the application of evidence-based therapies for the treatment of acute myocardial infarction: the American College of Cardiology's Guidelines Applied in Practice projects in Michigan. *Archives of Internal Medicine, 166*(11), 1164–1170.

Kang, S.J., Ahn, J.M., Han, S., Lee, J.Y., Kim, W.J., Park, D.W., et al. (2013).Sex differences in the visual-functional mismatch between coronary angiography or intravascular ultrasound versus fractional flow reserve. *JACC Cardiovasc Interv*, 6(6):p. 562–568.

Kwok, Y., Kim, C., Grady, D., Segal, M., & Redberg, R. (1999). Meta-analysis of exercise testing to detect coronary artery disease in women. *American Journal of Cardiology, 83*(5), 660–666.

Mehta, L. S., Beckie, T. M., DeVon, H. A., Grines, C. L., Krumholz, H. M., Johnson, M. N., et al. (2016). Acute myocardial infarction in women: a scientific statement from the American Heart Association. *Circulation, 133*(9), 916–947.

Michelis, K. C., Olin, J. W., Kadian-Dodov, D., d'Escamard, V., & Kovacic, J. C. (2014). Coronary artery manifestations of fibromuscular dysplasia. *Journal of the American College of Cardiology, 64*(10), 1033–1046.

Mieres, J. H., & Bonow, R. O. (2016). Ischemic heart disease in women: a need for sex-specific diagnostic algorithms. *JACC: Cardiovascular Imaging, 9*(4), 347–349.

Mosca, L., Collins, P., Herrington, D. M., Mendelsohn, M. E., Pasternak, R. C., Robertson, R. M., et al. (2001). Hormone replacement therapy and cardiovascular disease: a statement for healthcare professionals from the American Heart Association. *Circulation, 104*(4), 499–503.

Mosca, L., Hammond, G., Mochari-Greenberger, H., Towfighi, A., Albert, M. A., & American Heart Association Cardiovascular Disease and Stroke in Women and Special Populations Committee of the Council on Clinical Cardiology (2013). Fifteen-year trends in awareness of heart disease in women: results of a 2012 American Heart Association national survey. *Circulation, 127*(11), 1254–1263, e1–e29.

O'Donoghue, M., Boden, W. E., Braunwald, E., Cannon, C. P., Clayton, T. C., de Winter, R. J., et al. (2008). Early invasive vs conservative treatment strategies in women and men with unstable angina and non-ST-segment elevation myocardial infarction: a meta-analysis. *Journal of the American Medical Association, 300*(1), 71–80.

Reynolds, H. R., Srichai, M. B., Iqbal, S. N., Slater, J. N., Mancini, G. B., Feit, F., et al. (2011). Mechanisms of myocardial infarction in women without angiographically obstructive coronary artery disease. *Circulation, 124*(13), 1414–1425.

Sliwa, K., Hilfiker-Kleiner, D., Petrie, M. C., Mebazaa, A., Pieske, B., Buchmann, E., et al. (2010). Current state of knowledge on aetiology, diagnosis, management, and therapy of peripartum cardiomyopathy: a position statement from the Heart Failure Association of the European Society of Cardiology Working Group on peripartum cardiomyopathy. *European Journal of Heart Failure, 12*(8), 767–778.

Stone, N. J., Robinson, J. G., Lichtenstein, A. H., Bairey Merz, C. N., Blum, C. B., Eckel, R. H., et al. (2014). 2013 ACC/AHA guideline on the treatment of blood cholesterol to reduce atherosclerotic cardiovascular risk in adults: a report of the American College of Cardiology/American Heart Association Task Force on Practice Guidelines. *Journal of the American College of Cardiology, 63*(25 Pt B), 2889–2934.

Yu, J., Mehran, R., Grinfeld, L., Xu, K., Nikolsky, E., Brodie, B. R., et al. (2015). Sex-based differences in bleeding and long term adverse events after percutaneous coronary intervention for acute myocardial infarction: three year results from the HORIZONS-AMI trial. *Catheterization and Cardiovascular Interventions, 85*(3), 359–368.

SLEEP APNEA AND THE HEART

Ihab Hamzeh, Fidaa Shaib

CHAPTER 53

1. How much sleep is typically needed?

In general the ideal duration of sleep for an average adult is around 7.5 to 8 hours. Average sleep of less than 6 hours or more than 9 hours is associated with increased mortality risk.

2. What are the different types of sleep apneas?

There are two types of sleep apneas:

- Obstructive sleep apnea (OSA): Episodes of repetitive narrowing or complete collapse of the upper airway resulting in decreased air flow and associated with brief arousal on electroencephalogram and/or oxygen desaturation.
- Central sleep apnea (CSA): Absence of respiratory effort resulting in lack of airflow and associated with arousal on electroencephalogram and/or oxygen desaturation. Cheyne-Stokes respiration is a form of CSA characterized by crescendo-decrescendo changes in respiratory effort with an associated central apnea event.

3. What are important symptoms of obstructive sleep apnea?

The symptoms associated with OSA include snoring, excessive daytime sleepiness, and sudden arousals with choking/gasping and are important clues to suspect the diagnosis. Some OSA symptoms may be difficult to distinguish from cardiac symptoms (sudden arousals with gasping vs. paroxysmal nocturnal dyspnea), and others overlap with cardiac symptoms like fatigue or nocturia. Importantly these improve with treating OSA. Symptoms of OSA are summarized in Table 53.1.

4. What are important risk factors for sleep apnea?

- Weight gain (a 10% weight gain leads to a sixfold increase in the risk of OSA)
- Anatomic: Craniofacial abnormalities such as retrognathia, relative macroglossia, nasal obstruction, tonsillar hypertrophy, and increased pharyngeal adiposity
- Chemical: Benzodiazepines, alcohol

5. How is sleep apnea diagnosed?

The gold standard for diagnosis is polysomnography, an elaborate recording of multiple physiologic parameters during sleep. Polysomnography enables calculation of the apnea/hypopnea index (AHI), which reflects the average frequency of episodes of partial (hypopnea) or complete (apnea) airway narrowing per hour of sleep. A normal AHI is less than 5 per hour, and moderate to severe sleep

Table 53.1. Symptoms of Obstructive Sleep Apnea
Snoring
Excessive daytime sleepiness
Sudden arousals with choking/gasping
Witnessed apnea
Nonrefreshing sleep
Morning or daytime fatigue
Morning dry throat
Morning headaches
Nocturnal sweating
Insomnia (particularly in women or patients with central sleep apnea)

OSA, Obstructive sleep apnea.

apnea is present when AHI is greater than 15. Home sleep apnea testing is another option with limited monitoring and is indicated for patients with high pretest probability for obstructive sleep apnea (OSA) and without significant cardiopulmonary comorbidities.

6. What are the pathophysiologic effects of obstructive sleep apnea in cardiovascular disease?

The hypoxemia and sleep fragmentation resulting from apnea/hypopnea episodes lead to a sympathetic surge and a rise in endothelin levels with significant elevation of blood pressure (BP) at the end of apneic episodes. Vagal tone is also blunted, further increasing the heart rate. There is also evidence that sleep deprivation and repetitive hypoxemia augment oxidative stress, activate proinflammatory mediators with elevations of C-reactive protein, induce inflammatory cytokines, and promote endothelial dysfunction. Furthermore, high negative intrathoracic pressure is generated during apnea/hypopnea episodes from vigorous inspiratory effort occurring against the collapsed airway. This leads to increased transmural pressure and wall stress in the cardiac chambers and great vessels, thus further increasing myocardial afterload (Fig. 53.1).

7. What are the cardiovascular sequelae of obstructive sleep apnea?

Cardiovascular sequelae of OSA include systemic hypertension, coronary artery disease (CAD), congestive heart failure (CHF), and pulmonary hypertension. These sequelae are summarized in Table 53.2.

8. Does obstructive sleep apnea predispose to hypertension?

Fifty percent of patients with OSA have hypertension (HTN). Animal models have shown that sleep apnea leads to elevated BP. Cross-sectional studies have revealed that OSA severity is linearly

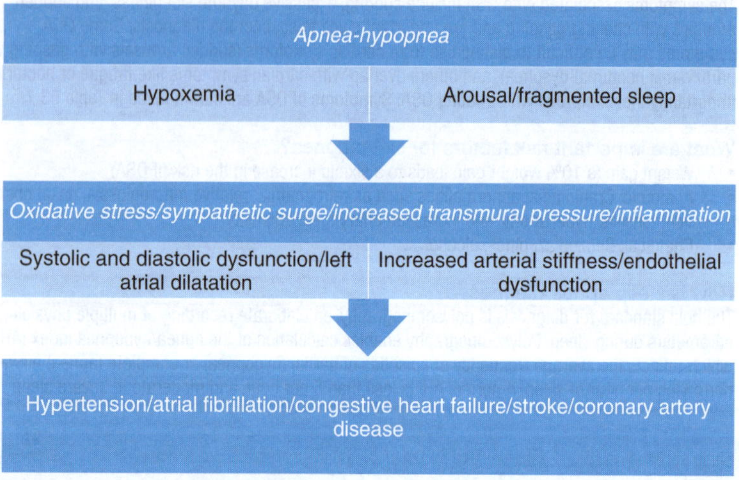

Fig. 53.1. Pathophysiologic effects of sleep apnea and the resultant cardiovascular complications. Figure created by author.

Table 53.2. Cardiovascular Sequelae of Obstructive Sleep Apnea
Systemic hypertension
Coronary artery disease
Congestive heart failure
Stroke
Pulmonary hypertension
Death
Arrhythmia

OSA, Obstructive sleep apnea.

associated with BP independent of relevant confounders. Importantly, a longitudinal cohort study of patients with OSA found an independent dose–response association between OSA severity at baseline and developing HTN 4 years later.

9. **Is obstructive sleep apnea implicated in uncontrolled hypertension?**
In two series of patients with uncontrolled HTN, OSA was found the most common associated condition (in 64% to 84% of patients). The seventh report of the Joint National Committee on prevention, detection, evaluation, and the treatment of high blood pressure (JNC VII) recognized OSA as an identifiable cause of uncontrolled HTN. In addition to the episodic repetitive BP surges from apneic episodes during sleep that disrupt the normal nocturnal dipping pattern, there is spillover of sympathetic activation into the daytime, leading to diurnal BP elevation.

10. **Does treating obstructive sleep apnea actually improve blood pressure control?**
Continuous positive airway pressure (CPAP) significantly decreases systolic and diastolic BP, albeit modestly (2 to 3 mm Hg range). However, in patients with resistant HTN, the magnitude of the systolic and diastolic BP reduction is higher (6.7 and 5.9 mm Hg, respectively). Interestingly, a recent study showed that a cluster of three plasma micro-ribonucleic acids (RNA) predicted the BP response to CPAP in patients with resistant HTN. In the absence of resistant HTN, the salutary effects of CPAP on BP may not be evident in those who do not have daytime sleepiness or those who use it for less than 4 hours per night.

11. **Other than continuous positive airway pressure, do other therapeutic modalities for obstructive sleep apnea improve blood pressure?**
Supplemental nocturnal oxygen to prevent OSA-induced hypoxemia has been shown not to improve BP. Mandibular advancement devices do appear to reduce BP reduction, similar to the reduction seen with CPAP.

12. **Is arterial stiffness affected by obstructive sleep apnea?**
Arterial stiffness is determined by several parameters, including aortic distensibility index, aortic elastance, pulse wave velocity, and aortic pressure augmentation, and has been found to be increased with OSA. This was noted even in the absence of HTN, further supporting the deleterious effects of OSA on vascular and endothelial function.

13. **Have the hemodynamic derangements that occur in obstructive sleep apnea been found to affect myocardial structure or function?**
Left ventricular (LV) posterior wall thickness and LV mass are increased in patients with OSA to the same degree as those with HTN. Left atrial (LA) volume index is increased in OSA. OSA is associated with impairment of systolic and diastolic myocardial function. Systolic and diastolic function Doppler-derived indices are reduced in OSA. Importantly, CPAP therapy was found to significantly reduce LV posterior wall thickness and LA volume and to improve systolic and diastolic function indices.

14. **Since sleep apnea is associated with increased blood pressure, arterial stiffness, and oxidative stress and may be proinflammatory, does it increase the risk of coronary artery disease?**
Sleep apnea is two times more likely to be found in patients with CAD than in those without. OSA was associated with coronary artery calcification (CAC), and the severity of OSA was associated with higher CAC scores. In a prospective cohort study, OSA was associated with CAC progression over 8 years of follow-up.

15. **Does obstructive sleep apnea increase the risk of stroke?**
In a longitudinal study, OSA was independently associated with increased risk of stroke or death during follow-up, and the risk was higher in those with more severe OSA at baseline. Patients with stroke who have OSA had worse functional impairment and length of hospitalization and decreased post-stroke survival.

16. **Do patients with obstructive sleep apnea have worse survival?**
Long-term follow-up studies have shown decreased survival in patients with OSA (particularly when severe), even after adjusting for associated comorbidities like HTN and obesity.

17. **Does sleep apnea predispose to arrhythmias?**
Ventricular pauses, second-degree atrioventricular (AV) block, premature ventricular contractions (PVCs), and nonsustained ventricular tachycardia do occur more frequently in patients with sleep apnea. Prolonged pauses up to 15 seconds have been reported during OSA in patients in whom

electrophysiologic evaluation did not reveal significant intrinsic sinus or AV nodal disease. In another study, OSA-related pauses resolved completely after 2 months of CPAP therapy. Patients with sleep apnea are at an increased risk of atrial fibrillation (AF). Importantly, compared to patients with OSA treated with CPAP, those who were untreated had double the risk of AF recurrence after cardioversion and had more AF recurrences even after pulmonary vein isolation (ablation) procedures, underscoring the importance of identifying and treating OSA in patients with AF.

18. Since sleep apnea predisposes to ventricular arrhythmias during sleep, does it increase the risk of sudden death?

A recent study has implicated OSA as risk factor for sudden cardiac death. Patients with OSA had their peak in sudden cardiac death between midnight and 6 am, which is the nadir for sudden death in those without OSA. Similarly, patients with sleep apnea with implantable defibrillators (ICD) experienced most life-threatening ventricular arrhythmic events requiring ICD therapy during sleeping hours. The risk of appropriate ICD therapy was also 50% higher among patients with sleep apnea, which occurred mainly during the vulnerable hours from 12 to 6 am.

19. How are sleep apnea and congestive heart failure related?

CSA is present in approximately 25% to 40% of patients of CHF (with higher prevalence in patients with more advanced CHF and ventricular dysfunction). The presence of CSA in CHF patients confers an increased mortality risk. CPAP was tested in a randomized control trial for patients with CHF and CSA, but despite improvement in AHI and LV ejection fraction, it failed to reduce mortality. Adaptive servo-ventilation provides servo-controlled inspiratory pressure in addition to positive expiratory pressure. It was used to treat CSA in CHF patients in the treatment of sleep-disordered breathing with predominant central sleep apnea by adaptive servo ventilation in patients with heart failure (SERVE-HF) trial but disappointingly was associated with significantly increased mortality. Beyond using guideline-directed therapy for the underlying CHF, the optimal approach to CSA in CHF has yet to be determined.

OSA is present in 26% of patients with CHF. OSA contributes to CHF by its untoward effects on myocardial structure and function, mediated by increasing BP, afterload, and sympathetic activation (which can potentiate sodium retention by activating the renin-angiotensin system). CPAP use in patients with CHF and OSA led to improved BP and LV ejection in small studies. Observational data suggest a trend to lower mortality in patients with CHF whose OSA is treated with CPAP.

20. Does sleep apnea lead to pulmonary hypertension?

OSA in general leads to mild elevation of pulmonary arterial (PA) pressures. A recent meta-analysis found that CPAP therapy is associated with significant reduction of PA pressure in patients with isolated OSA and pulmonary hypertension.

21. Which cardiac patients will benefit from having a sleep evaluation?

Most patients with AF, CHF, resistant HTN, or pulmonary hypertension should be referred. Patients with CAD or coronary risk factors who also have daytime fatigue/somnolence or have increased risk of OSA (increased body mass index) will benefit from referral for sleep study.

Bibliography and Suggested Readings

Butt, M., Dwivedi, G., Shantsila, A., Khair, O. A., & Lip, G. Y. (2012). Left ventricular systolic and diastolic function in obstructive sleep apnea: impact of continuous positive airway pressure therapy. *Circulation Heart Failure, 5*(2), 226–233. http://dx.doi.org/10.1161/CIRCHEARTFAILURE.111.964106.

Cowie, M. R., Woehrle, H., Wegscheider, K., Angermann, C., d'Ortho, M. P., Erdmann, E., et al. (2015). Adaptive servo-ventilation for central sleep apnea in systolic heart failure. *New England Journal of Medicine, 373*(12), 1095–1105. http://dx.doi.org/10.1056/NEJMoa1506459.

Floras, J. S. (2014). Sleep apnea and cardiovascular risk. *Journal of Cardiology, 63*(1), 3–8. http://dx.doi.org/10.1016/j.jjcc.2013.08.009.

Imran, T. F., Ghazipura, M., Liu, S., Hossain, T., Ashtyani, H., Kim, B., et al. (2016). Effect of continuous positive airway pressure treatment on pulmonary artery pressure in patients with isolated obstructive sleep apnea: a meta-analysis. *Heart Failure Reviews, 21*, 591–598.

Somers, V. K., White, D. P., Amin, R., Abraham, W. T., Costa, F., Culebras, A., et al. (2008). Sleep apnea and cardiovascular disease: an American Heart Association/American College of Cardiology Foundation Scientific Statement from the American Heart Association Council for High Blood Pressure Research Professional Education Committee, Council on Clinical Cardiology, Stroke Council, and Council on Cardiovascular Nursing. *Journal of the American College of Cardiology, 52*(8), 686–717. http://dx.doi.org/10.1016/j.jacc.2008.05.002.

VIII

PERIPHERAL VASCULAR AND CEREBROVASCULAR DISEASE

CHAPTER 54

PERIPHERAL ARTERIAL DISEASE

Elias Kfoury, Panos Kougias

1. **What are the key components of the vascular physical examination?**
According to the American College of Cardiology/American Heart Association (ACC/AHA) guidelines on peripheral arterial disease (PAD), the key components of the vascular physical examination include the following:
   - Blood pressure measurements in both arms
   - Carotid pulse palpation for upstroke and amplitude and auscultation for bruits
   - Auscultation of the abdomen and flank for bruits
   - Palpation of the abdomen for aortic pulsation and its maximal diameter
   - Palpation of brachial, radial, ulnar, femoral, popliteal, dorsalis pedis, and posterior tibial pulses
   - Performance of Allen test when knowledge of hand perfusion is needed
   - Auscultation of the femoral arteries for the presence of bruits
   - Inspection of the feet for color, temperature, and integrity of the skin and for ulcers
   - Observation of other findings suggestive of severe PAD, including distal hair loss, trophic skin changes, and hypertrophic nails

2. **How on pulse palpation is the intensity of the pulsation scored?**
Pulse intensity is scored on a 0 to 3 scale as follows:
   - Absent: 0
   - Diminished: 1
   - Normal: 2
   - Bounding: 3

3. **Can the location of the patient's lower extremity claudication help to localize the site of occlusive disease?**
The answer is a qualified yes. Because the pathophysiology of claudication is complex, there is not a perfect correlation between anatomic site of disease and location of symptoms. However, in general, the following statements can be made:
   - Occlusive iliac artery disease may produce hip, buttock, and thigh pain, as well as calf pain.
   - Occlusive femoral and popliteal artery disease usually produces calf pain.
   - Occlusive disease in the tibial arteries may produce calf pain or, more rarely, foot pain and numbness.

4. **What noninvasive tests are used in the assessment of lower limb claudication?**
   - **Ankle-brachial index (ABI):** The ABI is the ankle systolic pressure (as determined by Doppler) divided by the brachial systolic pressure (Fig. 54.1). An abnormal index is less than 0.90. The sensitivity is approximately 90% for diagnosis of PAD.
   - **Post-exercise ABI:** The post-exercise ABI entails measuring the ABI after treadmill walking with a slope of up to 10% at a rate of 2 mph. A recovery of at least 90% of the baseline ABI value within 3 minutes post exercise has a 94% specificity to rule out PAD. Post-exercise ABI is especially useful in patients with suspected PAD but normal ABI and in patients with atypical symptoms of claudication.
   - **Pulse volume recordings (PVRs):** PVRs measure changes in volume of toes, fingers, or parts of limbs that occur with each pulse beat as blood flows into or out of the extremity. A toe-to-brachial index of less than 0.6 is abnormal, and values of less than 0.15 are seen in patients with rest pain (toe pressures of less than 20 mm Hg).
   - **Duplex ultrasonography:** Duplex ultrasonography is a noninvasive method of evaluating arterial stenosis and blood flow. This method can localize and quantify the degree of stenosis. Ultrasonography is dependent on operator skill.

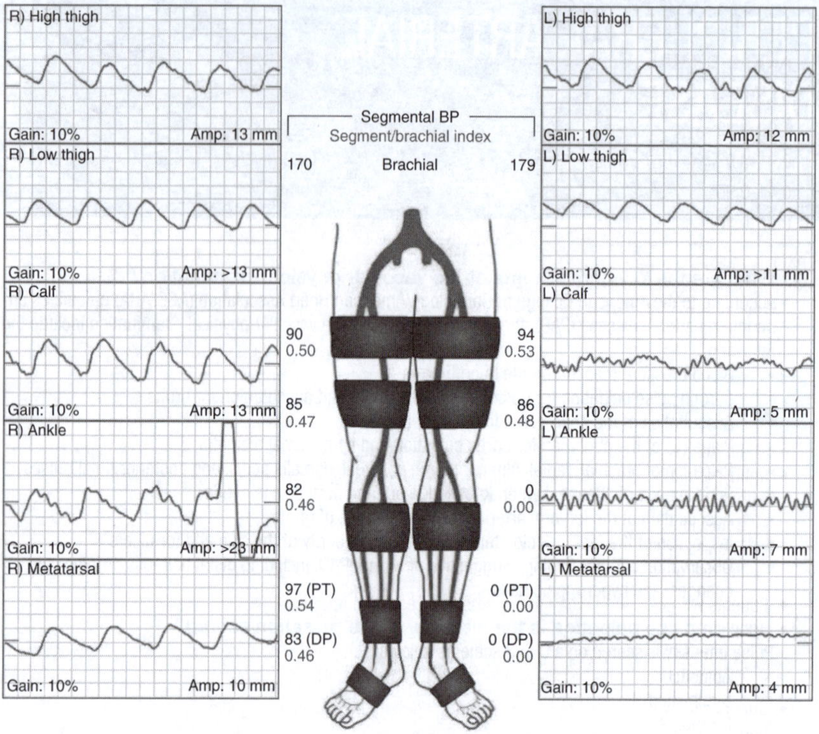

Fig. 54.1. Technique and tracings in determining the ankle-brachial index. Study demonstrates absent arterial flow in the left posterior tibial and dorsalis pedis arteries. *BP*, Blood pressure; *DP*, dorsalis pedis; *PT*, posterior tibial. *(Image from Al-Sahfie, T., & Suman, P. [2012].* Aortoiliac occlusive disease. *In D. Yamanouchi [Ed.],* Vascular surgery. *Rijeka, Croatia: InTech. Intechopen.com. http://www.intechopen.com/books/vascular-surgery. Accessed December 12, 2016.)*

- **Transcutaneous oxygen tension measurements**: These measurements are useful in assessing tissue viability for wound healing. Measurements greater than 55 mm Hg are considered normal and less than 20 mm Hg are associated with nonhealing ulcers.

5. What is the ankle-brachial index?

The ABI is the ratio of systolic blood pressure at the level of the ankle to the systolic blood pressure measured at the level of the brachial artery. More specifically, blood pressure is measured in both brachial arteries (with the higher systolic blood pressure being used) and is measured using a Doppler instrument with a blood pressure cuff on the lower calf, in both posterior tibial and dorsalis pedis arteries. Pulse wave reflections in healthy persons should result in higher blood pressures in the ankle vessel pressure (10 to 15 mm Hg higher than in the brachial arteries), and thus a normal ABI should be greater than 1.00. Using a diagnostic threshold of 0.90 to 0.91, several studies have found the sensitivity of the ABI to be 79% to 95% and the specificity to be 96% to 100% to detect stenosis of 50% or more reduction in lumen diameter. Experts emphasize that the ABI is a continuous variable below 0.90. Values of 0.41 to 0.90 are considered to be mildly to moderately diminished; values of 0.40 or less are considered to be severely decreased. An ABI of 0.40 or less is associated with an increased risk of rest pain, ischemic ulceration, or gangrene. Patients with long-standing diabetes or end-stage renal disease on dialysis and older patients may have noncompressible leg arterial segments caused by medial calcification, precluding assessment of the ABI. These patients are best evaluated using digital pressures and with assessment of the quality of the arterial waveform in the PVR studies. A system for interpretation of the ABI is given in Table 54.1.

Table 54.1. Interpretation of the Ankle-Brachial Index

ANKLE-BRACHIAL INDEX	INTERPRETATION
>1.30	Noncompressible
1.00-1.29	Normal
0.91-0.99	Borderline (equivocal)
0.41-0.90	Mild to moderate PAD
0.00-0.40	Severe PAD

PAD, Peripheral arterial disease.
Modified from Hiatt, W. R. (2001). Medical treatment of peripheral arterial disease and claudication. New England Journal of Medicine, 344, *1608–1621.*

Table 54.2. Recommended Medical Therapies and Lifestyle Interventions in Patients with Lower Extremity Peripheral Arterial Disease

- Statin treatment to lower LDL level to <70-100 mg/dL
- Antihypertensive therapy to lower blood pressure to <140/90 mm Hg (<130/80 mm Hg in patients with diabetes or those with chronic kidney disease)
  - Beta-blockers are not contraindicated in patients with PAD.
  - The use of ACE inhibitors is reasonable in symptomatic lower extremity PAD patients to reduce the risk of adverse cardiovascular events.
- Patients with PAD should be offered smoking cessation interventions.
- Antiplatelet therapy is indicated to reduce the risk of MI, stroke, or vascular death.
  - Aspirin in doses of 75-325 mg is recommended.
  - Clopidogrel can be used as an alternate therapy to aspirin.
- Supervised exercise training is the recommended initial treatment modality for intermittent claudication.
  - Exercise should be for a minimum of 30-45 min at least three times per week.
- Cilostazol (100 mg orally twice a day) is recommended to improve symptoms and increase walking distance in patients with intermittent claudication. (Cilostazol should not be used in patients with heart failure.)

ACE, Angiotensin-converting enzyme; *beta-blocker*, beta-adrenergic blocking agent; *LDL*, low-density lipoprotein; *MI*, myocardial infarction; *PAD*, peripheral arterial disease.

6. What are the recommended medical therapies and lifestyle interventions in patients with lower extremity peripheral arterial disease?

A supervised exercise regimen is recommended as the initial treatment modality for patients with intermittent claudication. Supervised exercise training is recommended instead of unsupervised exercise training. Cilostazol treatment can lead to a modest increase in exercise capacity. It is contraindicated in patients with heart failure. Cilostazol should be considered in patients with lifestyle-limiting claudication (ACCF/AHA class I recommendation). Smoking cessation must be strongly emphasized to the patient. Other measures include general secondary prevention interventions. Recommended medical therapies and lifestyle interventions in patients with lower extremity PAD are summarized in Table 54.2. An algorithm for the management of patients with suspected PAD is presented in Fig. 54.2.

7. What are the interventional treatment options for patients with claudication?

Claudication that severely interferes with quality of life or employment should be treated. Endovascular and open surgical reconstruction have both been extensively used for this purpose. Endovascular options are less invasive, typically performed on an outpatient basis, and associated with lower complication rates. Open surgical options are more durable and best suited for good risk or young patients. Outcomes of either type of intervention are vascular bed dependent. Iliac stenting has been associated with 5-year patency rates that in most cases are only slightly inferior

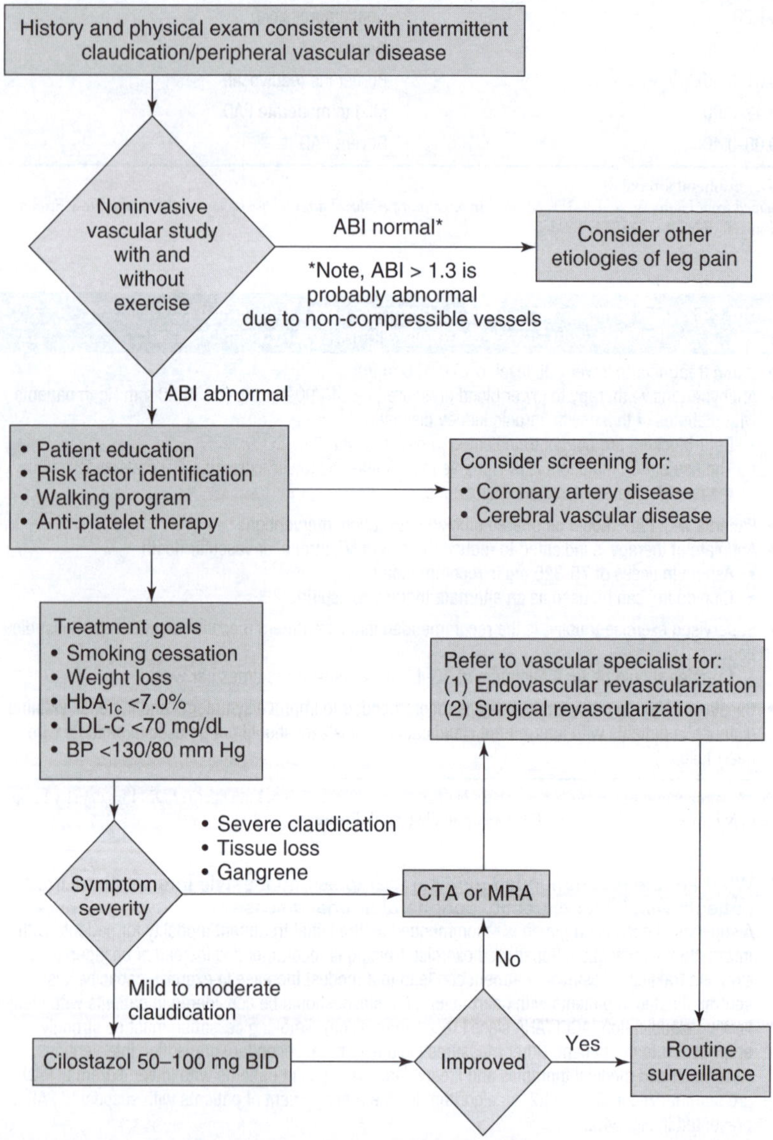

Fig. 54.2. Algorithm for the evaluation and management of patients with suspected lower extremity peripheral artery disease. *ABI*, Ankle-brachial index; *BP*, blood pressure; *CTA*, computed tomographic angiography; *Hg*, glycated hemoglobin; *LDL*, low-density lipoprotein; *MRA*, magnetic resonance angiography. *(From Toth, P. P., Shammas, N. W., Dippel, E. J., et al. [2007]. Cardiovascular disease. In R. E. Rakel [Ed.],* Textbook of family medicine *[7th ed.]. Philadelphia, PA: Saunders.)*

Table 54.3. Clinical Categories of Chronic Limb Ischemia

GRADE	CATEGORY	CLINICAL DESCRIPTION
	0	Asymptomatic, not hemodynamically correct
I	1	Mild claudication
	2	Moderate claudication
	3	Severe claudication
II	4	Ischemic rest pain
	5	Minor tissue loss: nonhealing ulcer, focal gangrene with diffuse pedal ulcer
III	6	Major tissue loss extending above transmetatarsal level, functional foot no longer salvageable

From Rutherford, R. B., Baker, J. D., Ernst, C., Johnston, K. W., Porter, J. M., Ahn, S., et al. (1997). *Recommended standards for reports dealing with lower extremity ischemia: revised version.* Journal of Vascular Surgery, 26, 517.

to that of their open counterparts. However, endovascular intervention in the infrainguinal segment is associated with inferior patency, particularly when compared with open bypass using venous conduit.

8. What is critical limb ischemia?

Whereas claudication is produced by decreased perfusion to the muscles upon increased demand, critical limb ischemia (CLI) refers to inadequate tissue perfusion at rest and is manifested as rest pain or tissue loss. Patients with CLI have multilevel disease that typically involves iliac, femoral, and tibial arteries. Because of the extent of the disease and the coexistent comorbidities, the management of the patient with CLI involves substantial judgment. Hybrid procedures that include simultaneous open and endovascular component, multiple débridements, and extensive rehabilitation therapy programs are fairly typical. Best results are achieved with multidisciplinary approaches that involve interventionalists, surgeons, internists, podiatrists, and infectious disease and endocrine specialists. Isolated vessel-based intervention in the absence of a grand plan for overall patient management should be discouraged because most of these patients benefit from coordinated treatment in centers familiar with the intricacies and issues surrounding the management of CLI.

9. How is critical limb ischemia graded clinically?

One widely used scheme for classifying limb ischemia is given in Table 54.3, based on the spectrum from asymptomatic to major tissue loss and nonsalvageable.

10. What are the main complications of open and endovascular infrainguinal interventions?

Complications of open interventions include cardiac events, respiratory complications, bleeding, wound infection, hernias, and graft failure. Complications associated with endovascular procedures include access site hematoma, bleeding or pseudoaneurysm, vessel rupture, contrast-induced nephropathy or anaphylactic reactions, recurrent stenosis or occlusion, and radiation-related patient injury. Thrombolytic treatment in particular is associated with increased risk of intracavitary, extremity, or intracranial bleeding, which is heavily dependent on the thrombolytic dose and duration of administration.

11. What are the causes of renal artery stenosis?

Approximately 90% of all renal arterial lesions are due to atherosclerosis. Atherosclerotic-related lesions usually affect the ostium and the proximal 1 cm of the main renal artery.

Fibromuscular dysplasia (FMD) is the next most common cause. Although it classically occurs in young women, it can affect both genders at any age. Less common causes of renovascular hypertension include renal artery aneurysms, Takayasu arteritis, atheroemboli, thromboemboli, William syndrome, neurofibromatosis, and spontaneous renal artery dissection.

12. What are American College of Cardiology/American Heart Association class I indications for the referral for diagnostic study to identify clinically significant renal artery stenosis?

Clinical scenarios that are recognized as class I indications for the performance of a diagnostic study to identify renal artery stenosis (RAS) include the following:

- Onset of hypertension before age 30
- Onset of hypertension after age 55
- Accelerated hypertension (sudden and persistent worsening of previously controlled hypertension), resistant hypertension (failure to achieve blood pressure goal with full adherences to full doses of an appropriate three-drug regimen that includes a diuretic), and malignant hypertension (hypertension with acute end-organ damage)
- New azotemia or worsening renal function after angiotensin-converting enzyme (ACE) inhibitor or angiotensin receptor blocker (ARB) treatment
- Unexplained atrophic kidney or discrepancy in size between the two kidneys of more than 1.5 cm
- Sudden, unexplained pulmonary edema (especially in azotemic patients)

13. What are the main indications for renal artery stenosis percutaneous revascularization?

Most ACC/AHA indications for percutaneous revascularization are class IIa recommendations, meaning the procedure is reasonable. Class I and class IIa recommendations for RAS include

- Class I (indicated)
    - Hemodynamically significant RAS and recurrent, unexplained congestive heart failure or sudden, unexplained pulmonary edema.
    - Renal artery stenting is indicated for RAS due to atherosclerosis, whereas balloon angioplasty with selective stenting is indicated for RAS secondary to FMD.
    - Surgical revascularization is recommended for complex disease involving branching/ segmental arteries, early primary branching of the main renal artery, or when aortic surgery is also indicated.
- Class IIa (reasonable)
    - Hemodynamically significant RAS and accelerated hypertension, resistant hypertension, malignant hypertension, hypertension with an unexplained unilateral small kidney, and hypertension with intolerance to medication
    - Hemodynamically significant RAS and unstable angina
    - RAS and progressive chronic kidney disease with bilateral RAS or RAS to a solitary functioning kidney

14. What are most common types of visceral artery aneurysms?

Visceral artery aneurysms are an uncommon form of vascular disease whose pathogenesis and natural history remain incompletely characterized. Their typical presentation involves rupture or erosion into an adjacent viscus, resulting in life-threatening hemorrhage. Nearly 22% of reported visceral artery aneurysms present with rupture, resulting in an 8.5% mortality rate. The distribution of aneurysms among the visceral vessels includes the splenic artery (60%), hepatic artery (20%), superior mesenteric artery (5.5%), celiac artery (4%), gastric and gastroepiploic arteries (4%), jejunal, ileal, colic (3%), pancreaticoduodenal and pancreatic arteries (2%), gastroduodenal artery (1.5%), and inferior mesenteric artery (<1%). Typical indication for open or endovascular treatment includes size greater than 2 cm and childbearing age in a female patient, because rupture is more common during pregnancy and is associated with very high maternal and fetal mortality.

15. In general, when should patients with an infrarenal or juxtarenal abdominal aortic aneurysm undergo repair?

Current recommendations are that patients with an infrarenal or juxtarenal abdominal aortic aneurysm (AAA) should undergo repair when the aneurysm measures 5.5 cm or greater (although it is also a class IIa recommendation that it can be beneficial to repair aneurysms 5.0 to 5.4 cm in diameter). Patients with infrarenal or juxtarenal AAA measuring 4.0 to 5.4 cm in diameter should be monitored by ultrasound or computed tomography (CT) scans every 6 to 12 months. In those with AAA smaller than 4.0 cm, ultrasound examination every 2 to 3 years is thought to be reasonable.

16. **What are the relative pros and cons of the treatment options for patients with infrarenal abdominal aortic aneurysm that meets size criteria for repair?**

The traditional open AAA repair has been compared with endovascular infrarenal AAA repair (EVAR) extensively with three large multicenter trials, two in Europe and one in the United States. EVAR is associated with lower perioperative mortality and complication rates, particular respiratory complications. However, it also implies the need for long-term follow-up with serial CT scans to assess the endograft and confirm the absence of endoleak or migration. The impact of this follow-up protocol in terms of impact on renal function and radiation-related injury is currently unclear. Secondary intervention rate after EVAR occurs in approximately 15% of patients and is mainly related to the presence of endoleak with continued sac expansion. The survival benefit of EVAR disappeared in all studies after 2 to 3 years of follow-up. Open AAA repair has the additional issue of postoperative late ventral hernia development, which appears to occur in approximately 15% to 20% of patients.

17. **What are the anatomic eligibility criteria for endovascular infrarenal abdominal aortic aneurysm repair?**

These include the following:

- Proximal aortic neck of at least 15 mm in length and no more than 32 mm in diameter
- Angulation of aortic neck less than 60 degrees
- Iliac vessels of adequate diameter to accommodate the delivery device

As device platforms evolve, more challenging anatomies are routinely treated today with endovascular means. In addition, fenestrated and branched devices and advanced "snorkel" techniques have enabled physicians to successfully treat juxtarenal and thoracoabdominal aneurysms in high-risk patients with endovascular means.

18. **What are the primary indications for treatment of extracranial carotid artery occlusive disease?**

In very general terms, indications for intervention are as follows:

- Symptomatic stenosis of 50% to 99% diameter if the risk of perioperative stroke or death is less than 6%
- Asymptomatic stenosis of greater than 60% diameter if the expected perioperative stroke rate is less than 3% and if life expectancy is greater than 2 years

Controversy surrounds the overall topic of interventional treatment of asymptomatic carotid artery occlusive disease. The notion that maximizing medical treatment can be as good as intervention with respect to stroke prevention has been gaining acceptance; however, high-quality data to support it are scarce.

19. **What are the relative indications for carotid endarterectomy and carotid stenting?**

Carotid stenting (CAS) indications include the following:

- High carotid lesion not approachable via neck incision using standard techniques
- Redo neck surgery, including prior carotid endarterectomy (CEA)
- History of radiation in the neck
- Presence of tracheostomy
- High physiologic risk for open CEA

CEA and CAS have been compared in four large randomized controlled trials that are listed in the references section, and the reader is encouraged to review their results. CEA has been considered the procedure of choice for carotid stenosis. CAS is an effective alternative for CEA in symptomatic and asymptomatic carotid stenosis and should be the first-line treatment for patients with the conditions listed above. CAS was found to be associated with higher perioperative stroke rate but lower myocardial event rates and no cranial nerve damage. In addition, CAS seems to have worse outcomes in older patients. Long-term (10-year) follow-up in the CREST study found no significant differences between CEA and CAS with respect to death, myocardial infarction (MI), or stroke.

20. **What are possible causes of lower limb arterial disease and ischemia or claudication in young patients?**

Atherosclerosis tends to primarily affect older persons; however, it can manifest in younger patients who have familial hyperlipidemic syndromes, Buerger disease (thromboangitis obliterans), or hypercoagulable disorders. Popliteal entrapment syndrome is an anatomic abnormality in which the popliteal artery gets compressed either by an abnormal muscle band or because it has taken an abnormal (medial) course behind the knee and is compressed by a normal gastrocnemius muscle. Popliteal adventitial cystic disease is also in the differential diagnosis of claudication in young patients; it produces a popliteal stenosis that gives a classic "scimitar sign" on angiography. Exercise-induced compartment syndrome may produce similar symptoms of leg pain with exercise that is relieved by rest.

21. What is fibromuscular dysplasia?

FMD, formerly called fibromuscular fibroplasia, is a group of nonatherosclerotic, noninflammatory arterial diseases that can affect almost any artery but most commonly involves the renal arteries (Fig. 54.3). Histologic classification discriminates three main subtypes—intimal, medial, and perimedial—which may be found in a single patient. Angiographic classification includes the following:

- Multifocal type, with multiple stenoses and the "string-of-beads" appearance that is classic for medial fibroplasias
- Focal type, which is more suggestive of intimal fibroplasia

22. What is Buerger disease?

Buerger disease, more appropriately called thromboangiitis obliterans, is a disease of small- and medium-sized arteries, as well as veins and nerves. Buerger disease is a nonatherosclerotic disease instead caused by inflammatory processes and thrombosis.

Clinically, it presents most commonly with ischemia of the digits and hand, arm, feet, or calf claudication. Ischemic ulcers may also occur. It occurs almost exclusively in tobacco users, and the only true "treatment" is smoking cessation. The presence of "corkscrew" collaterals is a pathognomonic angiographic finding.

23. What is Takayasu arteritis?

Takayasu arteritis is a vasculitis of unknown cause, primarily affecting the aorta and its primary branches. It is more common in Asian populations and predominantly affects women. Over time it can lead to narrowing or occlusion of the aorta and its branches, such as the subclavian artery. Clinically, patients most commonly manifest upper arm claudication but may also develop neurologic symptoms as a result of vertebrobasilar ischemia.

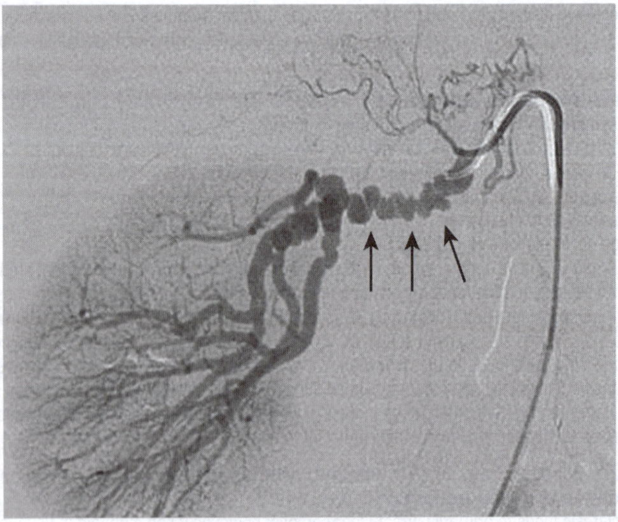

Fig. 54.3. Fibromuscular dysplasia. Digital subtraction angiography revealing changes *(arrows)* typical of the medial fibroplasia variant of fibromuscular dysplasia. *(Reproduced from Levine, G. N. [2014].* Color atlas of cardiovascular disease. *New Delhi, India: Jaypee Brothers Medical Publishers.)*

24. What is May-Thurner syndrome?

Iliocaval compression, or May-Thurner syndrome (MTS), was initially described as the development of spurs in the left iliac vein as a consequence of compression from the contralateral right common iliac artery against the lumbar vertebra. The pathogenesis of MTS is not completely understood, but it is theorized that it may be a combination of both mechanical compression and arterial pulsations by the right iliac artery that leads to the development of intimal hypertrophy within the wall of the left common iliac vein. This can lead to potential endothelial changes and thrombus formation. Patients with MTS tend to be young women in the second to fourth decade of life who develop the syndrome after periods of prolonged immobilization or pregnancy. Patients may have a history of several days or more of persistent, unexplained pain and swelling of the left thigh and calf. Duplex ultrasound characteristically may reveal left common iliac vein thrombosis. Management of symptomatic MTS in association with deep vein thrombosis may involve catheter-directed thrombolysis, anticoagulation, and potentially iliocaval stenting.

Bibliography and Suggested Readings

Aboyans, V., Criqui, M. H., Abraham, P., Allison, M. A., Creager, M. A., Diehm, C., et al. (2012). Measurement and interpretation of the ankle-brachial index: a scientific statement from the American Heart Association. *Circulation*, *126*(24), 2890–2909.

Berger, J. S., & Hiatt, W. R. (2012). Medical therapy in peripheral artery disease. *Circulation*, *126*, 491–500.

Blankensteijn, J. D., de Jong, S. E., Prinssen, M., van der Ham, A. C., Buth, J., van Sterkenburg, S. M., et al. (2005). Two-year outcomes after conventional or endovascular repair of abdominal aortic aneurysms. *New England Journal of Medicine*, *352*, 2398–2405.

Brott, T. G., Halperin, J. L., Abbara, S., Bacharach, J. M., Barr, J. D., Bush, R. L., et al. (2011). ASA/ACCF/AHA/AANN/AANS/ACR/ASNR/CNS/SAIP/SCAI/SIR/SNIS/SVM/SVS guideline on the management of patients with extracranial carotid and vertebral artery disease: executive summary. *Circulation*, *124*, 489–532. *Stroke, 42*, e420–e463. *Journal of the American College of Cardiology, 57*, 1002–1044.

Brott, T. G., Hobson, R. W., 2nd, Howard, G., Roubin, G. S., Clark, W. M., Brooks, W., et al. (2010). Stenting versus endarterectomy for treatment of carotid-artery stenosis. *New England Journal of Medicine*, *363*, 11–23.

Brott, T. G., Howard, G., Roubin, G. S., Meschia, J. F., Mackey, A., Brooks, W., et al. (2016). Long-term results of stenting versus endarterectomy for carotid-artery stenosis. *New England Journal of Medicine*, *374*(11), 1021–1031.

Eckstein, H. H., Ringleb, P., Allenberg, J. R., Berger, J., Fraedrich, G., Hacke, W., et al. (2008). Results of the stent-protected angioplasty versus carotid endarterectomy (space) study to treat symptomatic stenoses at 2 years: a multinational, prospective, randomised trial. *Lancet Neurology*, *7*, 893–902.

Greenhalgh, R. M., Brown, L. C., Kwong, G. P., Powell, J. T., & Thompson, S. G. (2004). Comparison of endovascular aneurysm repair with open repair in patients with abdominal aortic aneurysm (EVAR trial 1), 30-day operative mortality results: randomised controlled trial. *Lancet*, *364*, 843–848.

Hennion, D. R., & Siano, K. A. (2013). Diagnosis and treatment of peripheral arterial disease. *American Family Physician*, *88*(5), 306–310.

Hiatt, W. R. (2001). Medical treatment of peripheral arterial disease and claudication. *New England Journal of Medicine*, *344*(21), 1608–1621.

Hirsch, A. T., Haskal, Z. J., Hertzer, N. R., Bakal, C. W., Creager, M. A., Halperin, J. L., et al. (2006). ACC/AHA guidelines for the management of patients with peripheral arterial disease. *Journal of the American College of Cardiology*, *47*(6), 1239–1312.

Inter-Society Consensus (TASC) II Guidelines. <http://www.tasc-2-pad.org>.

Lederle, F. A., Freischlag, J. A., Kyriakides, T. C., Padberg, F. T., Jr., Matsumura, J. S., Kohler, T. R., et al. (2009). Outcomes following endovascular vs open repair of abdominal aortic aneurysm: a randomized trial. *Journal of the American Medical Association*, *302*, 1535–1542.

Mas, J. L., Trinquart, L., Leys, D., Albucher, J. F., Rousseau, H., Viguier, A., et al. (2008). Endarterectomy versus angioplasty in patients with symptomatic severe carotid stenosis (eva-3s) trial: results up to 4 years from a randomised, multicentre trial. *Lancet Neurology*, *7*, 885–892.

Mohler, E. R. Clinical features, diagnosis, and natural history of lower extremity peripheral arterial disease. <http://www.utdol.com>.

Murad, M. H., Shahrour, A., Shah, N. D., Montori, V. M., Ricotta, J. J., et al. (2011). A systematic review and meta-analysis of randomized trials of carotid endarterectomy vs stenting. *Journal of Vascular Surgery*, *53*, 792–797.

Norgren, L., Hiatt, W. R., Dormandy, J. A., Nehler, M. R., Harris, K. A., Fowkes, F. G., et al. (2007). Inter-Society Consensus for the Management of Peripheral Arterial Disease (TASC II). *European Journal of Vascular and Endovascular Surgery*, *33*(Suppl. 1), S1–S75.

Ricotta, J., AbuRahma, A., Ascher, E., Eskandari, M., Faries, P., Lal, B. K., et al. (2011). Updated Society for Vascular Surgery guidelines for management of extracranial carotid disease. *Journal of Vascular Surgery*, *54*, 832–836.

Ringleb, P. A., Allenberg, J., Bruckmann, H., Eckstein, H. H., Fraedrich, G., Hartmann, M., et al. (2006). 30 day results from the space trial of stent-protected angioplasty versus carotid endarterectomy in symptomatic patients: a randomised non-inferiority trial. *Lancet*, *368*, 1239–1247.

Rooke, T. W., Hirsch, A. T., Misra, S., Sidawy, A. N., Beckman, J. A., Findeiss, L., et al. (2013). Management of patients with peripheral artery disease (compilation of 2005 and 2011 ACCF/AHA Guideline Recommendations): a report of the American College of Cardiology Foundation/American Heart Association Task Force on Practice Guidelines. *Journal of the American College of Cardiology*, *61*(14), 1555–1570.

Rosenfield, K., Matsumura, J. S., Chaturvedi, S., Riles, T., Ansel, G. M., Metzger, D. C., et al. (2016). Randomized trial of stent versus surgery for asymptomatic carotid stenosis. *New England Journal of Medicine*, *374*(11), 1011–1020.

White, C. J., Jaff, M. R., Haskal, Z. J., Jones, D. J., Olin, J. W., Rocha-Singh, K. J., et al. (2006). Indications for renal arteriography at the time of coronary arteriography: a science advisory from the American Heart Association Committee on Diagnostic and Interventional Cardiac Catheterization, Council on Clinical Cardiology, and the Councils on Cardiovascular Radiology and Intervention and on Kidney in Cardiovascular Disease. *Circulation*, *114*(17), 1892–1895.

Yadav, J. S., Wholey, M. H., Kuntz, R. E., Fayad, P., Katzen, B. T., Mishkel, G. J., et al. (2004). Protected carotid-artery stenting versus endarterectomy in high-risk patients. *New England Journal of Medicine*, *351*, 1493–1501.

AORTIC ANEURYSM

Andrew Vekstein, Haytham Elgharably, Faisal G. Bakaeen, Eric E. Roselli

CHAPTER 55

1. **What are the common pathologies affecting the thoracic aorta?**
   Aneurysm and dissection are the most common pathologies affecting the thoracic aorta. The incidence of aneurysm is probably underestimated. A Swedish population study demonstrated an incidence of 16.3 per 100,000 per year in men and 9.1 per 100,000 per year in women and trends demonstrating an increase in diagnoses. Congenital aortic diseases that may present in adulthood include coarctation and Kommerell diverticulum (aneurysmal dilatation of an anomalous subclavian artery) often found incidentally during cross-sectional thoracic imaging for other causes. Inflammatory conditions of the aorta include autoimmune aortitis (Takayasu, giant cell, focal isolated) and infectious aortitis (with the most common pathogens being bacteria from the genera *Staphylococcus, Streptococcus, Salmonella,* and Treponema).

2. **What is the definition of aneurysm?**
   Arterial aneurysm is generally defined as greater than 50% increase in diameter compared with the normal diameter. An alternate definition of infrarenal abdominal aortic aneurysm (AAA) that has been proposed is ≥30 mm. Examples of thoracic and abdominal aneurysms are shown in Figs. 55.1 and 55.2.

3. **What is the most common pathologic cause of thoracic aortic aneurysm?**
   The pathologic processes causing aneurysm in the ascending and descending aorta are varied, reflecting the unique embryologic origins of vascular smooth muscle cells proximal and distal to

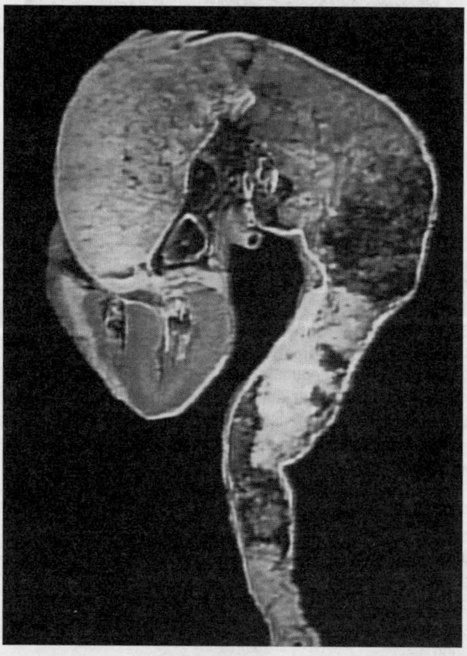

Fig. 55.1. Massive thoracic aortic aneurysm. Note that the size of the aneurysm dwarfs that of the heart. *(Image courtesy of William D. Edwards, MD, Mayo Clinic.)*

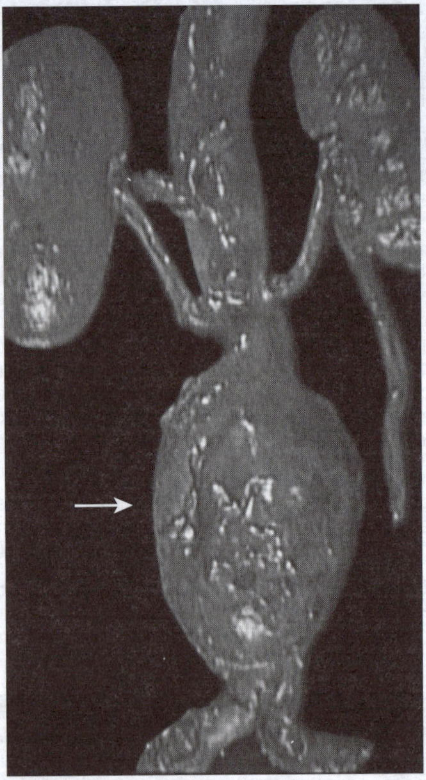

Fig. 55.2. Abdominal aortic aneurysm *(arrow). (Image from Armed Forces Institute of Pathology.)*

the ligamentum arteriosum. Aneurysm of the ascending aorta is most often attributed to cystic medial degeneration related to wall shear stress and chronic uncontrolled hypertension. Aneurysm of the descending aorta is more commonly associated with atherosclerotic disease. Cystic medial degeneration is also found in genetically triggered causes of aneurysm, such as Marfan syndrome. Risk factors for thoracic aneurysm include age, male gender, hypertension, family history of aneurysm, and other known atherosclerotic disease risks.

4. Which genetic conditions predispose patients to aortic aneurysm and dissection?

Connective tissue disorders, including Marfan syndrome, Loeys-Dietz syndrome, and vascular Ehlers-Danlos, are associated with medial degeneration, leading to increased incidence of thoracic aortic aneurysm, more rapid aneurysm growth, and dissection at smaller diameters. Bicuspid aortic valve (BAV) patients also have a higher risk of aortic dissection, especially if associated with other risk factors. Turner syndrome patients are also more prone to aneurysm and dissection, and this condition is often associated with BAV and coarctation.

5. List findings in other systems that may help to predict silent thoracic aortic aneurysm.

- Abdominal aortic aneurysm
- Simple renal cysts
- Intracranial aneurysm
- Hyperextensible joints
- Lens dislocation
- Musculoskeletal anomalies like scoliosis and pectus excavatum
- Arthritis

Table 55.1. Estimated Annual Risk of Abdominal Aortic Aneurysm Rupture

AAA DIAMETER	RUPTURE RISK (% PER YEAR)
<4	0
4-5	0.5-5
5-6	3-15
6-7	10-20
7-8	20-40
>8	30-50

AAA, Abdominal aortic aneurysm.
Adapted from Brewstera, D. C., Cronenwett, J. L., Hallett, J. W., Johnston, K. W., Krupski, W. C., & Matsumura, J. S. (2003). Guidelines for the treatment of abdominal aortic aneurysms. Journal of Vascular Surgery, *37(5), 1106–1117.*

6. How fast does an aortic aneurysm grow?

Aneurysms expand exponentially (ie, the larger the aneurysm the more rapid the growth). On average, the descending thoracic aorta grows faster than the ascending thoracic aorta (10 to 30 mm/year vs. 7 to 10 mm/year). The annual growth rates of aneurysms in patients with chronic dissections are significantly higher, ranging from 0.24 cm/year for small (4.0 cm) aneurysms to 0.48 cm/year for large (8.0 cm) aneurysms.

7. What are the survival rates for untreated thoracic aortic aneurysms?

Survival rates for thoracic aortic aneurysms not undergoing surgical repair are

- 65% at 1 year
- 36% at 3 years
- 20% at 5 years

Aneurysm rupture occurs in 32% to 68% of patients not treated surgically, with rupture accounting for 32% to 47% of all deaths. It is estimated that less than one-half of patients with rupture actually arrive to the hospital alive. The mortality rates for aneurysmal rupture are 54% at 6 hours and 76% at 24 hours. Because death is the most likely outcome after unexpected rupture, more patients should be encouraged to undergo elective repair, and those managed conservatively should have risk factors aggressively controlled.

8. List the risk factors for rupture of thoracic aortic aneurysms.

Risk factors for rupture can be divided into dimensional and nondimensional factors. The dimensional factors include size and growth rate, whereas the nondimensional factors include smoking/chronic obstructive lung disease (COPD), age, hypertension, renal failure, and pain.

9. How likely are untreated abdominal aortic aneurysms to rupture?

The eventual risk for rupture is approximately 20% for aneurysms that measure larger than 5.0 cm in diameter, 40% for those measuring at least 6.0 cm in diameter, and higher than 50% for aneurysms that exceed 7.0 cm in diameter, with annual rates of rupture in the range of 4%, 7%, and 20%, respectively. The risks of rupture for AAA are summarized in Table 55.1.

10. How does ruptured abdominal aortic aneurysm present?

Dramatically, usually with acute abdominal pain and shock. It is estimated that mortality from AAA rupture, when taking into account those who do not reach the operating room and those who die after surgery, may be as high as 90%.

11. Can a widened mediastinum suggest the presence of thoracic aortic aneurysm?

Yes. Although the specificity and sensitivity of widened mediastinum on chest x-ray (Fig. 55.3) for aortic aneurysm are not well defined, this finding should at minimum prompt consideration of aortic aneurysm.

12. What are the best imaging modalities for diagnosing and evaluating aortic aneurysm?

- Computed tomography (CT): Advances in image quality and three-dimensional (3D) CT technology have resulted more accurate assessments of aortic pathology, including measurements of aortic aneurysm (Fig. 55.4) in a plane perpendicular to axis of blood flow.

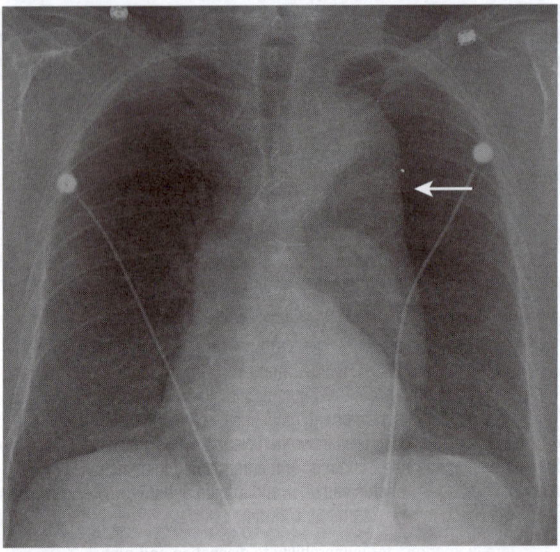

Fig. 55.3. Posteromedial chest x-ray demonstrating a widened mediastinum in a patient with thoracic aortic aneurysm. The arrow marks the lateral border of the aorta. *(Image posted by James Heilman, MD, on Wikimedia Commons.)*

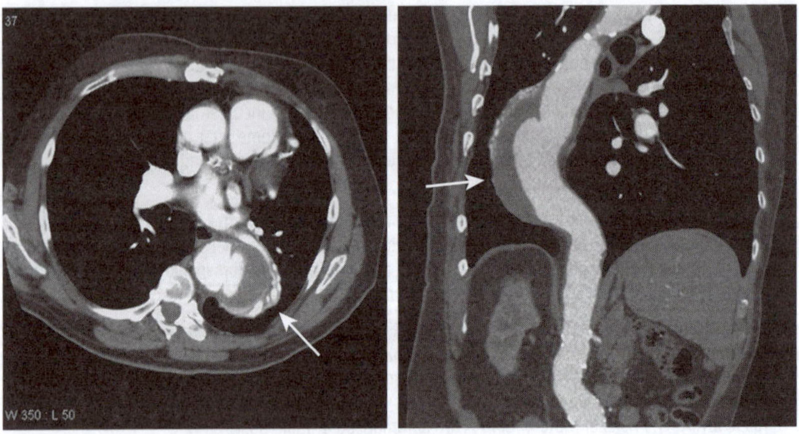

Fig. 55.4. Computed tomography scan of a thoracic aortic aneurysm (arrows). There is thrombus within the aneurysm. *(Image from Sidebotham, D., McKee, A., Gillham, M. & Levy, J. [2007].* Chapter 11: *Thoracic Aorta.* Cardiothoracic Critical Care. *Butterworth-Heinemann (an imprint of Elsevier, Inc). Philadelphia, PA.)*

- Magnetic resonance imaging (MRI): MRI's role in the evaluation of aortic pathology has expanded in recent years, due to the ability to assess flow dynamics, such as an aberrant jet directed at the aortic wall in a patient with a bicuspic aortic valve.
- Transesophageal echocardiography (TEE): TEE is most useful for diagnosis of dissection in the proximal ascending aorta, with sensitivities ranging from 88% to 98% and specificities ranging from 90% to 95%. It is the modality of choice at many institutions for patients who are intubated or are otherwise already requiring sedation.
- Conventional angiography (aortography): Not used frequently nowadays. Has low sensitivity and requires a high contrast load.

13. Should imaging of the thoracic aorta be performed in those discovered to have an abdominal aortic aneurysm?

Yes. Approximately 20% to 27% of patients with AAA will also have thoracic aortic aneurysm (TAA), either contiguous with the AAA or distinct as a second aneurysm.

14. Should imaging of the abdominal aorta be performed when thoracic aortic atheromata is detected by transesophageal echocardiography?

Perhaps. In one study, 14% of those with aortic atheromata detected by TEE were found to have AAA.

15. Can abdominal aortic aneurysm be detected during standard transthoracic echocardiography?

Yes. Imaging of the abdominal aorta has become a standard part of the transthoracic echocardiography (TTE) examination. The incidence of detected AAA ranges from 0.8% to 6.0%. In one nationwide survey from France, the prevalence of detected AAA was 3.7%.

16. Is screening for abdominal aortic aneurysm recommended?

The incidence of detected AAA in studies of older men, smokers, and those with family history of AAA is 5.5%. Screening for AAA with ultrasound examination in older (>65 years) men has been shown to decrease AAA-related mortality. In the European guidelines, screening for AAA is recommended in all men older than 65 years and may be considered in women older than 65 years of age with history of current or past smoking. In the US guidelines, screening is recommended in men older than 60 years who are either the siblings or offspring of patients with AAA and in men age 65 to 75 who have ever smoked.

17. At which diameters is elective repair of thoracic aortic aneurysm indicated?

Although research into biomarkers for vulnerability to dissection and rupture is ongoing, diameter and rate of growth are currently the most reliable tools to assess thoracic aortic aneurysm. Studies have shown that there are specific "hinge points" in terms of diameter, beyond which risk of dissection or rupture increases exponentially. This point is 6.0 cm in the ascending aorta (34% risk) and 7.0 cm in the descending aorta (43% risk). In addition, consideration of patient height can be a vital tool, with increased risk demonstrated beyond maximum aortic area: height in meters ratio greater than 10. Furthermore, all patients with aortic root or ascending aortic growth of greater than 0.5 cm per year are recommended to undergo surgery.

18. When should one operate on a patient with ascending thoracic aortic aneurysms due to aortopathy?

In patients with Marfan syndrome, surgery is generally recommended for TAA ≥"4.5 to 5.0 cm". In patients with BAVs, who also will have an aortopathy, surgery is generally recommended for TAA ≥"5.0-5.5 cm". Management of ascending aortic aneurysms is summarized in Fig. 55.5. Recommendations for repair of aortic aneurysms in general are summarized in Table 55.2.

19. When is intervention for descending TAA recommended?

In general, thoracic endovascular aortic repair (TEVAR) (Fig. 55.6) is often performed in preference to open surgical repair when possible. TEVAR should be considered in patients with descending TAA ≥5.5 cm. When TEVAR is not an option, open surgical repair should be considered when TAA is ≥6.0 cm.

In patients with Marfan syndrome, surgery is generally preferred over TEVAR. A threshold for surgery of less than 60 mm can be considered in such patients.

20. When is intervention for abdominal aortic aneurysm recommended?

Open surgical and endovascular repair are both accepted options for AAA. Endovascular aortic repair (EVAR) is associated with lower short-term mortality, though at longer term follow-up mortality is comparable. EVAR is associated with a higher incidence of need for reintervention. Intervention is recommended for AAA greater than 5.5 cm or aneurysm growth greater than 1.0 cm/year. Repair of infrarenal or juxtarenal AAA 5.0 to 5.4 cm in diameter is a class IIa recommendation in US guidelines. Patients with AAA 4.0 to 5.4 cm should be monitored with ultrasound or CT every 6 to 12 months.

21. What is the recommended frequency for surveillance imaging of known thoracic aortic dilation?

After dilation beyond 4.0 cm is discovered in the thoracic aorta, it is recommended that patients get repeat imaging 6 months later to assess rate of growth. Stable aortic dilation is typically managed with imaging yearly or every other year. Shorter intervals (3 to 6 months) may be preferred if continued growth is discovered.

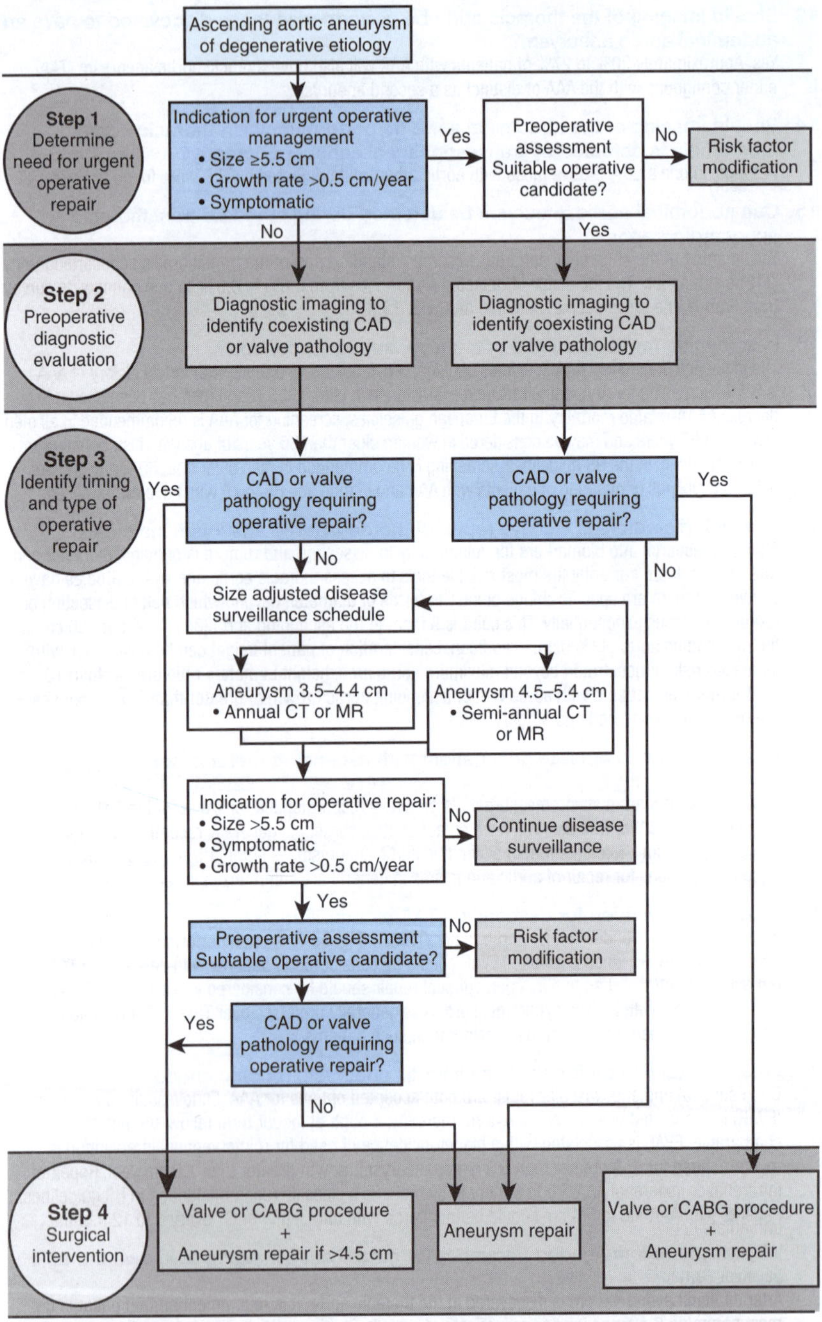

Fig. 55.5. Management algorithm for patients with ascending thoracic aneurysm of degenerative etiology (nongenetic disorders). *CABG*, Coronary artery bypass grafting; *CAD*, Coronary artery disease; *CT*, Computed tomography; *MR*, Magnetic resonance imaging. *(Image from Hiratzka, L. F., Bakris, G. L., Beckman, J. A., Bersin, R. M., Carr, V. F., Casey, D. E., Jr., et al. [2010]. 2010 ACCF/AHA/AATS/ACR/ASA/SCA/SCAI/SIR/STS/SVM guidelines for the diagnosis and management of patients with thoracic aortic disease.* Journal of the American College of Cardiology, 55, *1509–1544.)*

Table 55.2. Summary of Recommendations from the Society of Thoracic Surgeons Guidelines and American Association of Thoracic Surgeons for Repair of Thoracic Aortic Aneurysms

	GENERAL POPULATION	MARFAN OR BICUSPID AORTIC VALVE	LOEYS-DIETZ	DISSECTED
Aortic root	5.0 cm	5.0 cm	4.2 cm	Always
Ascending thoracic aorta	5.5 cm	5.0 cm	4.2 cm	Always
Descending thoracic aorta	6.0 cm or Twice the size of contiguous aorta	6.0 cm	6.0 cm	5.5 cm

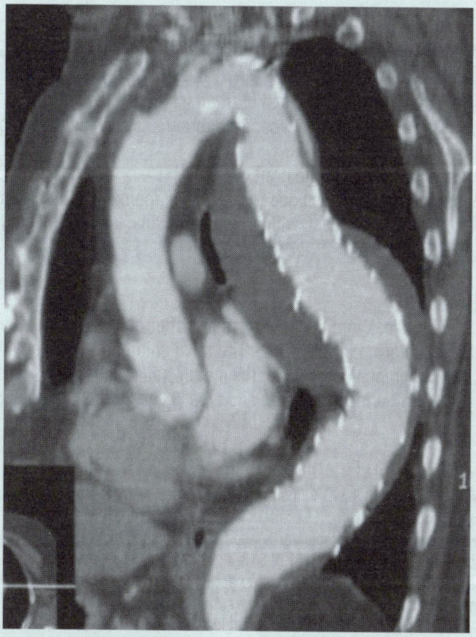

Fig. 55.6. Thoracic endovascular aortic repair. *(Image from Cheshire, N., & Bicknell, C. [2013]. Thoracic endovascular aortic repair: the basics.* Journal of Thoracic and Cardiovascular Surgery, 145*[3], S149–S153.)*

22. What are the complications of endovascular aortic repair?

Immediate conversion to an open surgical procedure occurs less than 1%. The risk of stent-graft infection is similarly less than 1%, although when this occurs it is associated with high mortality. Vascular damage and bleeding may occur with EVAR. Occlusion of branches of the aorta (mesenteric arteries, renal arteries, spinal arteries) can lead to complications of the relevant vascular bed. The most common complication is endoleak, discussed later.

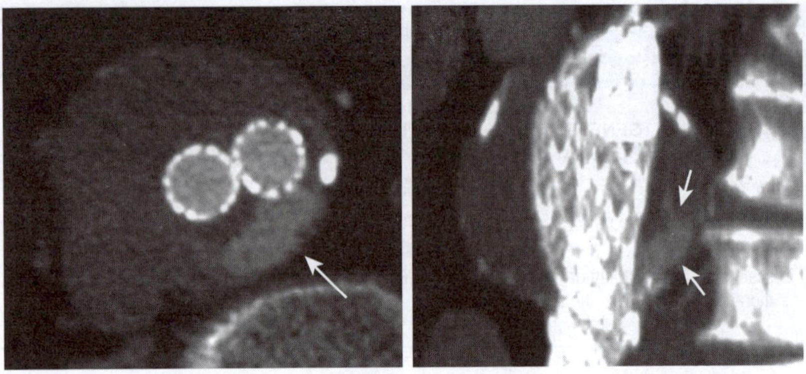

Fig. 55.7. Contrast-enhanced computed tomography studies showing endoleak *(arrows)* in patients with infrarenal abdominal aortic aneurysms treated with EVAR. *(Images courtesy of Dr. Benjamin Y. Cheong, Texas Heart Institute.)*

Table 55.3. Classification of Endoleaks

- Type I—Perigraft leakage at proximal or distal graft attachment sites
- Type II—Retrograde filling of the aneurysm sac from branches such as the lumbar and inferior mesenteric arteries
- Type III—Leakage through a defect in the graft
- Type IV—Leakage through the graft wall due to the quality (porosity) of the graft material
- Type V—Expansion of the aneurysm sac without an identifiable leak on imaging

23. What is an endoleak?

An endoleak (Fig. 55.7) is a leak into the aneurysm sac after endovascular repair (EVAR or TEVAR). The five types of endoleaks are given in Table 55.3. The most common type of endoleak is type II, in which the aneurysm sac fills via branch vessels. Approximately half of these will seal spontaneously over time. Type I (leak at the graft attachment site) and type III (leak through a defect in the graft) require intervention.

Bibliography and Suggested Readings

Brewstera, D. C., Cronenwett, J. L., Hallett, J. W., Johnston, K. W., Krupski, W. C., & Matsumura, J. S. (2003). Guidelines for the treatment of abdominal aortic aneurysms. *Journal of Vascular Surgery, 37*(5), 1106–1117.

Elefteriades, J. A. (2002). Natural history of thoracic aortic aneurysms: indications for surgery, and surgical versus nonsurgical risks. *Annals of Thoracic Surgery, 74*(5), S1877–S1880; discussion S1892–S1898.

Erbel, R., Aboyans, V., Boileau, C., Bossone, E., Di Bartolomeo, R., Eggebrecht, H., et al. (2014). 2014 ESC Guidelines on the diagnosis and treatment of aortic diseases. *European Heart Journal, 35*, 2873–2926.

Goldfinger, J. Z., Halperin, J. L., Marin, M. L., Stewart, A. S., Eagle, K. A., & Fuster, V. (2014). Thoracic aortic aneurysm and dissection. *Journal of the American College of Cardiology, 64*(16), 1725–1739.

Griepp, R. B., Ergin, M. A., Galla, J. D., Lansman, S. L., McCullough, J. N., Nguyen, K. H., et al. (1999). Natural history of descending thoracic and thoracoabdominal aneurysms. *Annals of Thoracic Surgery, 67*(6), 1927–1930; discussion 1953–1958.

Hiratzka, L. F., Bakris, G. L., Beckman, J. A., Bersin, R. M., Carr, V. F., Casey, D. E., Jr., et al. (2010). 2010 ACCF/AHA/AATS/ACR/ASA/SCA/SCAI/SIR/STS/SVM guidelines for the diagnosis and management of patients with thoracic aortic disease. *Journal of the American College of Cardiology, 55*, 1509–1544.

Hirsch, A. T., Haskal, Z. J., Hertzer, N. R., Bakal, C. W., Creager, M. A., Halperin, J. L., et al. (2006). ACC/AHA 2005 guidelines for the management of patients with peripheral arterial disease (lower extremity, renal, mesenteric, and abdominal aortic). *Journal of the American College of Cardiology, 47*(6), 1239–1312.

Khan, I. A., & Nair, C. K. (2002). Clinical, diagnostic, and management perspectives of aortic dissection. *Chest Journal, 122*(1), 311–328.

Olsson, C., Thelin, S., Ståhle, E., Ekbom, A., & Granath, F. (2006). Thoracic aortic aneurysm and dissection: increasing prevalence and improved outcomes reported in a nationwide population-based study of more than 14,000 cases from 1987 to 2002. *Circulation, 114*(24), 2611–2618.

Roselli, E. E., Idrees, J. J., Lowry, A. M., Masabni, K., Soltesz, E. G., Johnston, D. R., et al. (2016). Beyond the aortic root: staged open and endovascular repair of arch and descending aorta in patients with connective tissue disorders. *Annals of Thoracic Surgery*, *101*(3), 906–912.

Suzuki, T., Mehta, R. H., Ince, H., Nagai, R., Sakomura, Y., Weber, F., et al. (2003). Clinical profiles and outcomes of acute type B aortic dissection in the current era: lessons from the International Registry of Aortic Dissection (IRAD). *Circulation*, *108*(Suppl. 1), II312–II317.

Svensson, L. G., Kouchoukos, N. T., Miller, D. C., Bavaria, J. E., Coselli, J. S., Curi, M. A., et al. (2008). Expert consensus document on the treatment of descending thoracic aortic disease using endovascular stent-grafts. *Annals of Thoracic Surgery*, *85*(Suppl. 1), S1–S41.

CHAPTER 56

AORTIC DISSECTION

Haytham Elgharably, Andrew Vekstein, Eric E. Roselli

1. **What is the definition of a dissection?**
The essential feature of aortic dissection is a tear in the intima, which consequently allows medial disruption with formation and propagation of a subintimal hematoma, often occupying half of the aortic circumference.

2. **What is the epidemiology of aortic dissection?**
The incidence of aortic dissection is approximately 6 per 100,000 per year. Aortic dissection is more common in men than in women and increases with age.
The most important risk factor for aortic dissection is hypertension (present in approximately two-thirds of patients with aortic dissection). Other factors associated with increased risk for aortic dissection include smoking, preexisting aortic disease, history of cardiac surgery, blunt trauma, and family history of aortic dissection.

3. **Which genetic conditions predispose patients to aortic dissection?**
Connective tissue disorders, including Marfan syndrome, Loeys-Dietz syndrome, and vascular Ehlers-Danlos, are associated with medial degeneration, leading to increased incidence of thoracic aortic aneurysm, more rapid aneurysm growth, and dissection at smaller diameters. Bicuspid aortic valve (BAV) patients also have a higher risk of aortic dissection, especially if associated with other risk factors. Turner syndrome patients are also more prone to aneurysm and dissection, and this condition is often associated with BAV and coarctation.

4. **What are the best options for imaging thoracic aortic dissections?**
   - Computed tomography (CT) scan. Sensitivities of 83% to 94% and specificities of 87% to 100% have been reported with the use of CT scanning for the diagnosis of aortic dissection (Fig. 56.1), and this is increased with the use of modern helical CT scanners.
   - Magnetic resonance imaging (MRI). Both the sensitivity and the specificity of MRI are in the range of 95% to 100%. Particularly useful tools are the dynamic images of MRI, which afford the physician further information.

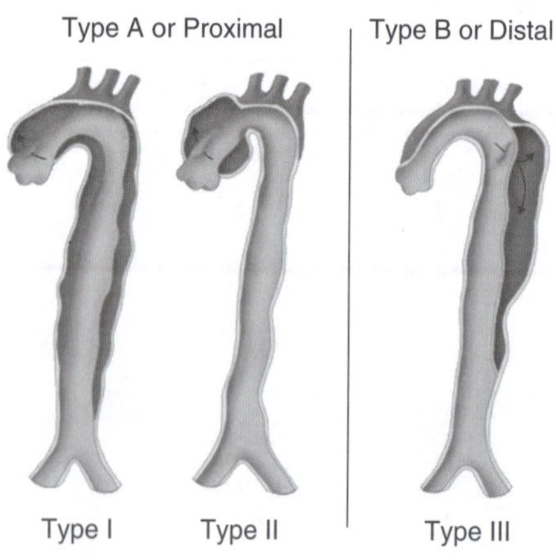

Fig. 56.1. Classification systems for aortic dissection based on the DeBakey classification system (type I, II, or III) or the Stanford system (type A or B). *Braunwald E, Zipes DP, Libby P, Bonow RO. [2004].* Braunwald's Heart Disease: *A Textbook of Cardiovascular Medicine, Ed 7, Philadelphia, PA, Saunders.*

- Transesophageal echocardiography (TEE). The sensitivity of TEE has been reported to be as high as 98%, and the specificity ranges from 63% to 96%. TEE is less sensitive in assessing the aortic arch, due to suboptimal windows.

5. **Describe the different types of acute aortic syndromes.**
   - Aortic dissection: Tear in the intimal layer, leading to formation of a false lumen in the medial layer of the aorta, potentially propagating antegrade or retrograde in the aortic wall.
   - Aortic rupture: Full-wall thickness tear, leading to cardiac tamponade among other complications. Rupture is frequently preceded by dissection.
   - Intramural hematoma (IMH): Thrombosis of a false lumen secondary to dissection or rupture of vasa vasorum, leading to intramural hemorrhage. Although risk of rupture is unclear, management of IMH is typically the same as for aortic dissection.
   - Penetrating atherosclerotic ulcer (PAU): Infiltration of the media by an atherosclerotic plaque, most commonly in localized areas in the descending aorta. This is commonly associated with IMH, and rate of rupture is high.

6. **How does acute aortic syndrome present?**
   Dramatically, usually with abrupt onset of chest, back, or abdominal pain. If the aorta is ruptured, shock soon follows. It is estimated that mortality from aortic rupture, including those who do not reach the operating room and those who die after surgery, may be as high as 90%. Results of dissection without rupture are better, but they also require emergency care. With dissection symptoms after initial presentation may vary depending on whether a vascular bed is compromised by malperfusion, which is also a risk factor for death with our without treatment.

7. **What are the most common symptoms, signs, and radiographic findings associated with dissection?**
   According to a long-term review of the international registry of aortic dissection (IRAD) database, the most common presentation is pain with abrupt onset in 89% of patients. Pain is described as tearing, sharp, and/or migrating. Type A dissection is more likely than type B to present as chest pain (85% vs. 67%), and type B is more likely than type A to cause back pain (70% vs. 43%). Additional findings include hypertension (more common in type B) and pulse loss (equally common in types A and B). Widened mediastinum on chest x-ray (CXR) is found in 52% of patients with type A dissection. Acute onset of aortic regurgitation may also produce symptoms of heart failure. Type B dissection may cause extremity, bowel, or renal malperfusion, leading, for example, to acute kidney injury.

8. **How are aortic dissections classified?**
   In general terms, most classification systems for location identify the dissection's position relative to the origin of the subclavian artery. That is, the dissections involve either the ascending aorta, descending aorta, or both. Ninety percent of thoracic dissections involve the first 10 cm of the aorta. The accepted classification systems are DeBakey and Stanford. In the DeBakey classification, type I aortic dissections involve the ascending and descending aorta, type II dissections involve the ascending aorta alone, and type III dissections are limited to the descending aorta (thoracic alone [IIIa] or with the abdominal aorta [IIIb]). The Stanford classification condenses the DeBakey classification so that type A refers to ascending dissections and type B to descending dissections. Although the Stanford classification more succinctly emphasizes a patient's need for emergent surgery (type A), it ignores what is happening in the remainder of the aorta, which is important for follow-up. These classifications are illustrated in Fig. 56.2.

9. **What is the method for classifying the timing of aortic dissection?**
   Dissection is described in terms of the time, with the onset of symptoms as time zero. Conventionally, 14 days has served as the cutoff point between acute and chronic. More recent data have demonstrated multiple phases, with the first 24 hours being hyperacute associated with the highest morbidity and mortality, 1 to 7 days as acute, 8 to 30 days as subacute, and later as chronic. Other variations on this multiphase designation based on the ability of the aorta to remodel after endovascular therapy have also been suggested. It is important to compare the current presentation to prior history and imaging to accurately assess the acuity.

10. **What are the complications of aortic dissection?**
    - Cardiac tamponade. Dissections involving the aortic root can lead to bleeding into the pericardium with resulting cardiac tamponade. Because the bleeding occurs acutely, the pericardium does not have time to gradually expand (as what occurs with gradually increasing pericardial effusions).

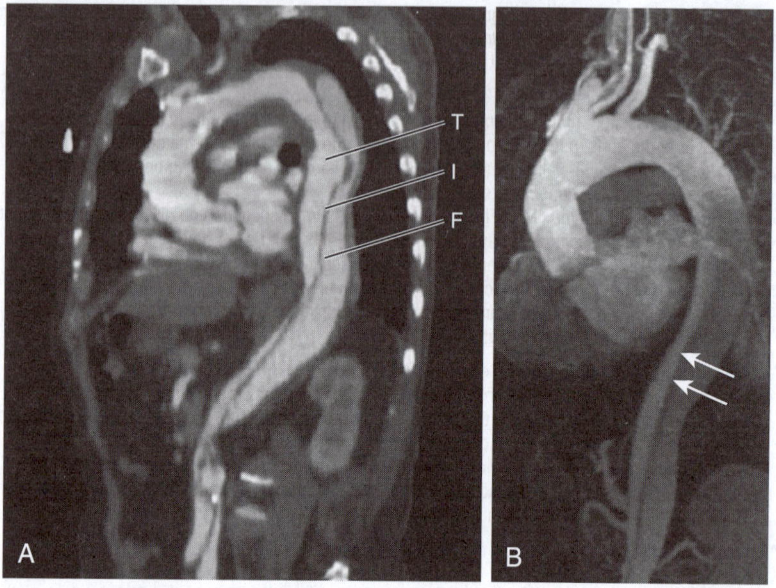

Fig. 56.2. Computed tomography (CT) and magnetic resonance images of aortic dissections. **A,** CT demonstrating aortic dissection. Shown is a contrast-enhanced spiral CT scan of the chest at the level of the pulmonary artery showing an intimal flap (I) in the descending thoracic aorta separating the two lumina in a type B aortic dissection. *F*, False lumen; *T*, true lumen. (Braunwald E, Zipes DP, Libby P, Bonow RO. [2004]. Braunwald's Heart Disease: A Textbook of Cardiovascular Medicine, *Ed 7, Ch. 56. Philadelphia, PA, Saunders.*) **B,** Gadolinium-enhanced magnetic resonance angiography of a patient with aortic dissection. The intimal flap *(arrows)* is clearly delineated.

Thus even a small amount of hemorrhage into the pericardium (on the order of one to several hundred milliliters of blood) can lead to tamponade.

- Aortic insufficiency. Dissections involving the aortic root can lead to acute, often severe, acute aortic regurgitation. As with tamponade, because the left ventricle has not gradually dilated over time (as in the case of chronic aortic insufficiency), the acute regurgitation is not well tolerated.
- Myocardial infarction. Dissection involving the sinus of Valsalva can lead to compromise of coronary artery flow. Clinically, one more commonly sees compromise of the right coronary artery.
- Proximal or distal malperfusion syndromes.
- Branch vessel compromise and effects, such as mesenteric ischemia, stroke, and renal failure
- Aortic rupture

11. What are the most reliable symptoms, signs, and radiographic findings associated with dissection?

The most reliable symptoms, signs, and radiographic findings associated with dissection include chest/back pain (86%), abrupt onset of pain (89%), hypertension (69%), any pulse loss (21%), and migrating pain (24%). Widened mediastinum is found in up to 56% of patients. Other symptoms include acute neurologic symptoms, syncope, dyspnea, and symptoms of mesenteric ischemia.

12. What is an intramural hematoma?

IMH is part of the spectrum of what is now often referred to as acute aortic syndrome (which includes aortic dissection and PAU), as illustrated in Fig. 56.3. IMH is hematoma that develops in the media of the aortic wall without an initiating intimal tear or resultant false lumen. Similar to aortic dissection, it can result in chest pain and can have lethal consequences (see later). IMH involves the ascending aorta and aortic arch in half of cases and the descending thoracic aorta in two-thirds of cases. IMH has been estimated to account for 10% to 25% of all cases of acute aortic syndrome. IMH is diagnosed by CT or MRI and can be missed if not read by a careful and experienced radiologist.

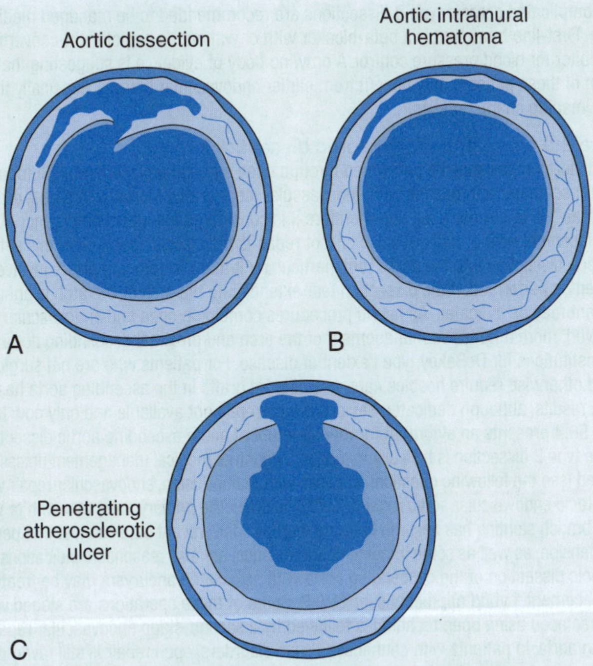

Fig. 56.3. Acute aortic syndromes. **A,** Classic aortic dissection. There is a tear in the intima with blood entering the media and a dissecting cleavage plane propagating for variable distances anterograde (and occasionally retrograde) throughout the aortic wall. **B,** Aortic intramural hematoma. A spontaneous hemorrhage of the vasa vasorum leads to bleeding within the media in the absence of an intimal tear or intimal flap. **C,** Penetrating atherosclerotic aortic ulcer. An ulcerated aortic plaque ruptures into the media leading to an outpouching or ulceration in the aortic wall. This may be associated with intramural hematoma formation, pseudoaneurysm, or a focal, thick-walled aortic dissection. *(Reproduced with permission from Braverman, A. C., Thompson, R., & Sanchez, L. [2011]. Diseases of the aorta, chapter 60. In R. O. Bonow, D. L. Mann, D. P. Zipes, & P. Libby [Eds.],* Braunwald's heart disease *[9th ed., pp. 1309–1337]. Philadelphia, PA: Elsevier.)*

13. What is a penetrating aortic ulcer?

A penetrating aortic ulcer has been defined as "ulceration of an aortic atherosclerotic plaque penetrating through the internal elastic lamina into the media." Penetrating aortic ulcers are estimated to be the cause of 2% to 7% cases of acute aortic syndrome. They are commonly found in the setting of extensive aortic atherosclerosis. Penetrating aortic ulcer most commonly occurs in the middle and lower descending thoracic aorta. Complications of penetrating aortic ulcers include progressive aortic enlargement and aneurysm formation, IMH, aortic dissection, pseudoaneurysm formation, and aortic rupture.

14. Is there a need to distinguish intramural hematoma and penetrating atherosclerotic ulcer from aortic dissection?

The diagnoses of IMH and PAU are mostly a consequence of the refined diagnostic modalities currently available. However, there are at least three reasons why IMH and PAU are of great concern:

1. The rate of rupture on initial presentation is high (45%).
2. The rate of radiographic advancement is significant (50%).
3. Delayed rupture occurs with great frequency and is fatal.

15. How should aortic dissection be managed medically?

In the acute setting the goal of medical management of aortic dissection (type A or B) is to reduce left ventricular contractility and thus shear wall stress on the aorta. Beta-blockers, including short-acting esmolol or labetalol, which has partial alpha antagonist activity, are first line. Nitroprusside or calcium channel blockers, such as nicardipine, may also be titrated to control hypertension. Direct vasodilators are contraindicated due to increased shear forces.

Uncomplicated chronic type B dissections are recommended to be managed medically in the long term. First-line treatment is a beta-blocker with or without an angiotensin-converting enzyme (ACE) inhibitor for blood pressure control. A growing body of evidence is suggesting that a large proportion of these patients may benefit from earlier endovascular therapy, especially those with high-risk imaging characteristics.

16. What are the repair options for aortic dissection?

In general, aortic repair may be performed through open surgical replacement with tubular grafts or through transcatheter approaches with endovascular stent grafts. Mortality in type A dissection can be as high as 1% to 2% per hour, and therefore it is considered a surgical emergency. Ascending aortic replacement with or without valve or root repair is the classic approach in this setting. If there is retrograde dissection into the aortic root, particularly if there is coronary artery involvement, root replacement is performed. If the dissection tear extends into the arch or the arch is aneurysmal, arch replacement may be indicated. As hybrid procedures combining open and endovascular techniques have evolved, more aggressive management of the arch and proximal descending aorta is performed at some institutions for DeBakey type I extent of disease. For patients who are not surgical candidates and would otherwise require hospice care, use of stent grafts in the ascending aorta has shown promising results, although dedicated devices are currently not available and only now beginning trials. Fig. 56.4 presents an algorithm for management of acute ascending aortic dissection.

Acute type B dissection is typically managed by optimal medical management unless it is complicated (see the following question). In cases with malperfusion, endovascular repair with stent grafts (thoracic endovascular aortic repair [TEVAR]) to cover the primary entry tear with or without additional branch stenting has become first-line therapy. More recent data suggest that persistent pain and hypertension, as well as some imaging characteristics, are also reasonable indications for TEVAR.

Chronic dissection of the descending aorta with associated aneurysm may be treated with open aortic replacement, hybrid approaches, or TEVAR. Some of these operations are staged with part of the aorta replaced using open techniques followed by a second-stage endovascular repair of the descending aorta. In patients with connective tissue disorders, open repair is still favored.

17. What are the indications for repair of type B dissection?

Surgical and endovascular management of type B dissection involve patient-specific decisions based on low/high risk profile for rupture. However, repair is indicated in "complicated" type B dissection, which is characterized by one or more of the following:

- Acute
    - End-organ malperfusion
    - Rapidly expanding false lumen
    - Impending or frank rupture (periaortic hematoma, hemorrhagic pleural effusion, refractory pain)
- Chronic
    - Dilation (>5.5-cm diameter or >5mm/year growth)
    - Malperfusion

18. What are the complications of surgical or endovascular thoracic aortic repair?

The most feared complication of thoracic aortic repair is paraplegia, due to interruption of blood flow to the spinal cord via the collateral network of perfusion. For this reason, adjunctive therapies, such as cerebrospinal fluid drainage, active cooling, and partial cardiopulmonary bypass, are usually used. In addition, it is recommended that mean arterial pressures be maintained in the 80- to 100-mm Hg mean pressure range in the postoperative period to prevent delayed onset paraplegia. Both repair techniques can also lead to renal/visceral ischemia and graft infection. Open repair may be complicated by bleeding and respiratory compromise. Complications specific to endovascular aortic repair are endoleak and graft migration. In patients treated with TEVAR, retrograde dissection of the ascending aorta requires emergency surgical repair.

19. What factors lead to the classification of a type B aortic dissection as "complicated"?

- Malperfusion
- Persistent or recurrent pain
- Uncontrolled hypertension despite maximum medical therapy
- Early aortic expansion
- Imaging features suggestive of higher risk for rupture or rapid degeneration including but not limited to: initial aortic diameter >40mm, false lumen diameter >22mm.

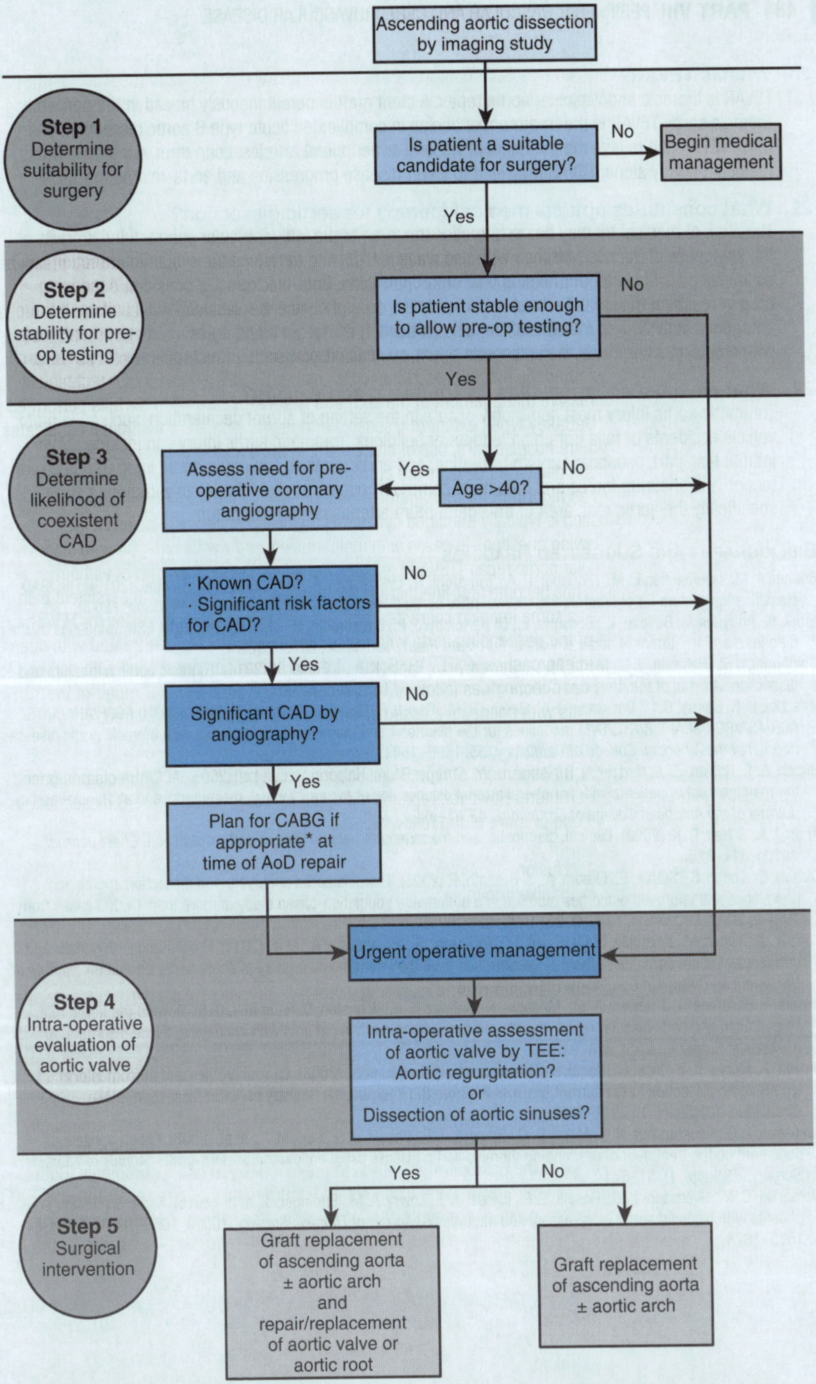

Fig. 56.4. Algorithm for the evaluation and management of ascending aortic dissection. *AoD*, aortic dissection, *CABG*, coronary artery bypass grafting, *CAD*, coronary artery disease, *TEE*, transesophageal echocardiogram *(Image from Hiratzka, L. F., Bakris, G. L., Beckman, J. A., Bersin, R. M., Carr, V. F., Casey, D. E., Jr., et al. [2010]. 2010 ACCF/AHA/AATS/ACR/ASA/SCA/SCAI/SIR/STS/SVM guidelines for the diagnosis and management of patients withthoracic aortic disease. Journal of the American College of Cardiology, 55, 1509–1544.)*

20. What is TEVAR?

TEVAR is thoracic endovascular aortic repair. A stent graft is percutaneously placed in the descending thoracic aorta. TEVAR is the treatment of choice in complicated acute type B aortic dissection. Short term, TEVAR can relieve malperfusion of visceral or peripheral arteries. Long term, compared with medical therapy alone, TEVAR may lead to lower disease progression and aorta-related mortality.

21. What constitutes optimal medical therapy for aortic dissection?

The aims of medical therapy are to decrease the force of the left ventricular contractions, to reduce the steepness of the rise of the aortic pulse wave (dP/dt), and to reduce the systemic arterial pressure as low as possible without affecting vital organ perfusion. Beta-blockers are considered the optimal drug in reaching this goal. Esmolol is generally the drug of choice, but labetalol (which also adds alpha antagonist activity) and metoprolol can also be used. If the target blood pressure cannot be achieved with a beta-blocker alone, then a second agent, such as nitroprusside or nicardipine, can be used.

22. What are most common sites for traumatic aortic injury?

Traumatic aortic injury most commonly occurs in the setting of abrupt deceleration, such as in motor vehicle accidents or falls from high ladders or buildings. Traumatic aortic injury can include aortic intimal tear, IMH, pseudoaneurysm formation, and aortic rupture. Traumatic aortic injury results from torsion and shearing forces and thus most commonly occurs at sites of relatively immobile aorta, specifically the aortic root, area of the ligamentum arteriosus, and diaphragm.

Bibliography and Suggested Readings

Booher, A. M., Isselbacher, E. M., Nienaber, C. A., Trimarchi, S., Evangelista, A., Montgomery, D. G., et al. (2013). The IRAD classification system for characterizing survival after aortic dissection. *American Journal of Medicine, 126*(8), 730.

Erbel, R., Aboyans, V., Boileau, C., Bossone, E., Di Bartolomeo, R., Eggebrecht, H., et al. (2014). 2014 ESC Guidelines on the diagnosis and treatment of aortic diseases. *European Heart Journal, 35*, 2873–2926.

Goldfinger, J. Z., Halperin, J. L., Marin, M. L., Stewart, A. S., Eagle, K. A., & Fuster, V. (2014). Thoracic aortic aneurysm and dissection. *Journal of the American College of Cardiology, 64*(16), 1725–1739.

Hiratzka, L. F., Bakris, G. L., Beckman, J. A., Bersin, R. M., Carr, V. F., Casey, D. E., Jr., et al. (2010). 2010 ACCF/AHA/AATS/ACR/ASA/SCA/SCAI/SIR/STS/SVM guidelines for the diagnosis and management of patients with thoracic aortic disease. *Journal of the American College of Cardiology, 55*, 1509–1544.

Hirsch, A. T., Haskal, Z. J., Hertzer, N. R., Bakal, C. W., Creager, M. A., Halperin, J. L., et al. (2006). ACC/AHA guidelines for the management of patients with peripheral arterial disease (lower extremity, renal, mesenteric, and abdominal aortic). *Journal of the American College of Cardiology, 47*, e1–e92.

Khan, I. A., & Nair, C. K. (2002). Clinical, diagnostic, and management perspectives of aortic dissection. *Chest Journal, 122*(1), 311–328.

Olsson, C., Thelin, S., Ståhle, E., Ekbom, A., & Granath, F. (2006). Thoracic aortic aneurysm and dissection: increasing prevalence and improved outcomes reported in a nationwide population-based study of more than 14,000 cases from 1987 to 2002. *Circulation, 114*(24), 2611–2618.

Pape, L. A., Awais, M., Woznicki, E. M., Suzuki, T., Trimarchi, S., Evangelista, A., et al. (2015). Presentation, diagnosis, and outcomes of acute aortic dissection: 17-year trends from the international registry of acute aortic dissection. *Journal of the American College of Cardiology, 66*(4), 350–358.

Roselli, E. E., Idrees, J. J., Lowry, A. M., Masabni, K., Soltesz, E. G., Johnston, D. R., et al. (2016). Beyond the aortic root: staged open and endovascular repair of arch and descending aorta in patients with connective tissue disorders. *Annals of Thoracic Surgery, 101*(3), 906–912.

Suzuki, T., Mehta, R. H., Ince, H., Nagai, R., Sakomura, Y., Weber, F., et al. (2003). Clinical profiles and outcomes of acute type B aortic dissection in the current era: lessons from the International Registry of Aortic Dissection (IRAD). *Circulation, 108*(Suppl. 1), II312–II317.

Svensson, L. G., Kouchoukos, N. T., Miller, D. C., Bavaria, J. E., Coselli, J. S., Curi, M. A., et al. (2008). Expert consensus document on the treatment of descending thoracic aortic disease using endovascular stent-grafts. *Annals of Thoracic Surgery, 85*(Suppl. 1), S1–S41.

Wojnarski, C. M., Svensson, L. G., Roselli, E. E., Idrees, J. J., Lowry, A. M., Ehrlinger, J., et al. (2015). Aortic dissection in patients with bicuspid aortic valve-associated aneurysms. *Annals of Thoracic Surgery, 100*(5), 1666–1673; discussion 1673–1674.

CHAPTER 57

CAROTID ARTERY DISEASE

Lee Joseph, Vijay Nambi, Esther S. H. Kim

1. Describe extracranial carotid artery anatomy. What are the common causes of carotid artery disease?

The carotid arteries originate as the common carotid artery (CCA) from the brachiocephalic trunk on the right side and from the aortic arch on the left side, ascend up the neck, and bifurcate into the external carotid artery (ECA) and internal carotid artery (ICA). The carotid bulb is a dilated portion at the origin of ICA. The CCA prior to its bifurcation and the extracranial ICA usually have no branch arteries.

The most common cause of carotid artery stenosis (CAS) is atherosclerosis. Fibromuscular dysplasia, dissection, radiation arteritis, and vasculitis are other causes of carotid artery disease. Atherosclerotic lesions frequently occur at the bifurcation of CCA into ECA and ICA and at the branch ostia.

Fig. 57.1 displays the carotid and vertebral artery anatomy as visualized on computed tomography (CT) scan.

2. What are the clinical manifestations of carotid artery stenosis?

Neurologic symptoms of cerebrovascular ischemia and a carotid bruit on physical examination are the most common clinical manifestations of CAS. Patients with CAS may develop cerebrovascular ischemia due to a variety of pathophysiologic mechanisms, including atherosclerotic plaque rupture leading to acute thrombotic occlusion, thromboembolism, atheroembolism, arterial dissection, and hypoperfusion in the setting of a stenotic lesion. Arterial embolism to the distal cerebrovascular circulation is the most common event leading to cerebrovascular ischemia. Although a carotid bruit has relatively poor sensitivity in detecting a hemodynamically significant carotid stenosis, it is a strong marker of systemic atherosclerosis with associated increased risk of stroke, myocardial infarction, and cardiovascular death.

Distinguishing between symptomatic and asymptomatic CAS is important for choosing appropriate therapies. Transient or permanent focal neurologic deficits in the ipsilateral retina or the cerebral hemisphere within the previous 6 months constitute symptomatic carotid artery disease. Patients without symptoms or those who develop nonfocal neurologic symptoms, such as dizziness, generalized weakness, syncope, blurry vision, or confusion in the absence of symptomatic ischemic events, are considered to have asymptomatic carotid artery disease. Though testing for CAS in patients presenting with syncope remains a common clinical practice, syncope without associated carotid bruit or focal neurologic symptoms or signs is not a typical manifestation of CAS.

The majority of CAS (>50% stenosis) is asymptomatic, more prevalent in males and older individuals, and associated with a 5% to 10% annual risk of cardiovascular events. The prevalence of hemodynamically significant carotid stenosis, usually greater than 70% stenosis, is 14% in asymptomatic patients and approaches 18% to 20% in symptomatic patients. CAS is not the most common cause of stroke and accounts for only approximately 10% to 15% of cases.

3. What is the difference between transient ischemic attack and stroke?

Transient ischemic attack (TIA) is defined as transient neurologic dysfunction from focal brain, spinal cord, or retinal ischemia, without evidence of acute infarction on neuroimaging. Symptoms due to central nervous system infarction based on neuropathology, neuroimaging, or clinical evidence of permanent injury is termed an *acute ischemic stroke.* Patients with symptomatic carotid artery disease have a 10% to 20% risk of stroke within the initial 4 weeks following a TIA or acute stroke. However, the stroke risk is low, at approximately 1% per year for those individuals with asymptomatic carotid artery disease.

4. How is carotid artery stenosis diagnosed?

Catheter angiography (Fig. 57.2) is the gold standard test for evaluating CAS, but it is invasive, requires contrast, and is not cost effective. Carotid duplex ultrasound (CDUS) is a reliable, noninvasive tool for evaluating the degree of CAS, with a sensitivity of 84% and a specificity of 89% in identifying

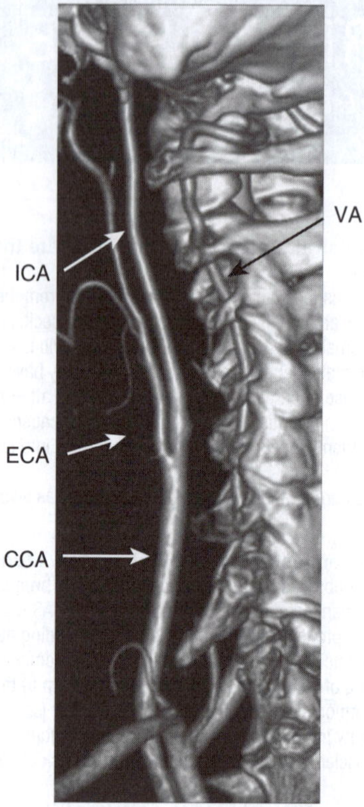

Fig. 57.1. Anatomy of the carotid artery. The carotid arteries originate as the common carotid artery (CCA) from the brachiocephalic trunk on the right side and from the aortic arch on the left side, ascend up the neck, and bifurcate into the external carotid artery (ECA) and internal carotid artery (ICA). Also visualized is the vertebral artery (VA). *(Reprinted from Standring, Susan, ed. Gray's anatomy: the anatomical basis of clinical practice. Elsevier Health Sciences, 2015. Page 455, Fig 29.9)*

hemodynamically significant lesions. Although CDUS is readily available, it is operator dependent. CDUS is increasingly becoming the only preoperative imaging study for patients with asymptomatic CAS, but computed tomographic angiography (CTA) or magnetic resonance angiography (MRA) of the neck may also be performed to confirm lesion severity. Alternatively, patients with high pretest probability could initially be assessed using MRA or CTA because these modalities can also assess intrathoracic and intracranial arteries. MRA is preferred to image patients with extensive arterial calcification.

5. How is degree of carotid stenosis determined by carotid duplex ultrasound?

CDUS has three key components: grayscale or B-mode imaging, color Doppler, and spectral Doppler analysis (Fig. 57.3). Hemodynamically significant CAS causes focal acceleration of blood flow, which can be evaluated by CDUS using velocity parameters—namely, the ICA peak systolic velocity (PSV), the ICA end-diastolic velocity (EDV), and the carotid index (ICA/CCA PSV ratio). The ICA PSV in conjunction with grayscale imaging and color Doppler imaging are the primary parameters used for determining the degree of ICA stenosis. ICA EDV and the carotid index are additional parameters for resolving any discrepancy arising between the primary parameters. A carotid index greater than 4.0 is the most accurate predictor of 70% to 99% carotid stenosis, with overall accuracy of 88%. Although CDUS is a reliable indicator of greater than 70% stenosis, it is relatively less accurate in assessing lesions with less than 70% stenosis and subtotal occlusion. In addition, significant calcification, tortuosity, access to only the cervical portion of carotid arteries, tandem lesions, in situ carotid stents, and operator dependence are other potential pitfalls of CDUS imaging.

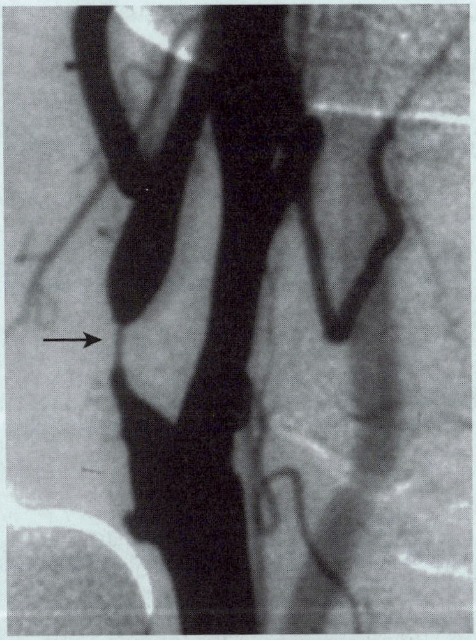

Fig. 57.2. Critical internal carotid artery stenosis (black arrow) demonstrated by angiography *(Reprinted from White, C. J. [2014]. Carotid artery stenting.* Journal of the American College of Cardiology, 64*[7], 722–731. With permission from Elsevier.)*

Velocity criteria for the determination of CAS using CDUS are not standardized. There is substantial variability in interpretation criteria among vascular laboratories. In the absence of national standards, vascular laboratories still use a wide variety of reference or internally validated criteria for diagnosing ICA stenosis. The Society of Radiologists in Ultrasound Consensus Criteria for Diagnosis of Internal Carotid Artery Stenosis is one example of diagnostic criteria vascular laboratories may use (Table 57.1).

6. Which are the appropriate clinical indications for carotid duplex ultrasound imaging?

CDUS imaging is recommended in individuals with symptoms of cerebrovascular ischemia, carotid bruit on neck auscultation, and asymptomatic individuals with atherosclerotic disease in other vascular beds. Routine surveillance duplex imaging is also recommended for patients with known moderate or severe CAS and after surgical or endovascular carotid intervention.

7. How do cardiac conditions affect the performance and interpretation of carotid duplex ultrasound?

An underlying cardiac condition must be suspected if there are abnormal spectral Doppler waveforms in carotid arteries bilaterally and/or extremes of flow velocity unexplained by focal pathology on CDUS. Several cardiac states produce characteristic carotid Doppler waveform patterns. Severe aortic stenosis is associated with a parvus et tardus pattern and usually has no effect on velocity measurements. The bisferiens waveform morphology with pandiastolic flow reversal is seen in patients with severe aortic regurgitation. In hypertrophic cardiomyopathy, carotid Doppler waveforms demonstrate the characteristic spike-and-dome pattern and a high resistance signal. A very low PSV with preserved upstroke is present in the setting of low cardiac output. Because this may mask significant carotid stenosis when only absolute velocity criteria are used, grayscale analysis and secondary parameters, such as carotid index, become important. Intra-aortic balloon pump (IABP) results in two peaks, a ventricular systolic peak and an augmented peak, due to IABP inflation followed by flow reversal. This results in inaccurate velocity measurements and an absent EDV. Most accurate velocity measurements require turning the IABP off or switching to 1:2 or 1:3 modes. Left ventricular assist devices result in a characteristic nonpulsatile, low-velocity flow with delayed upstroke.

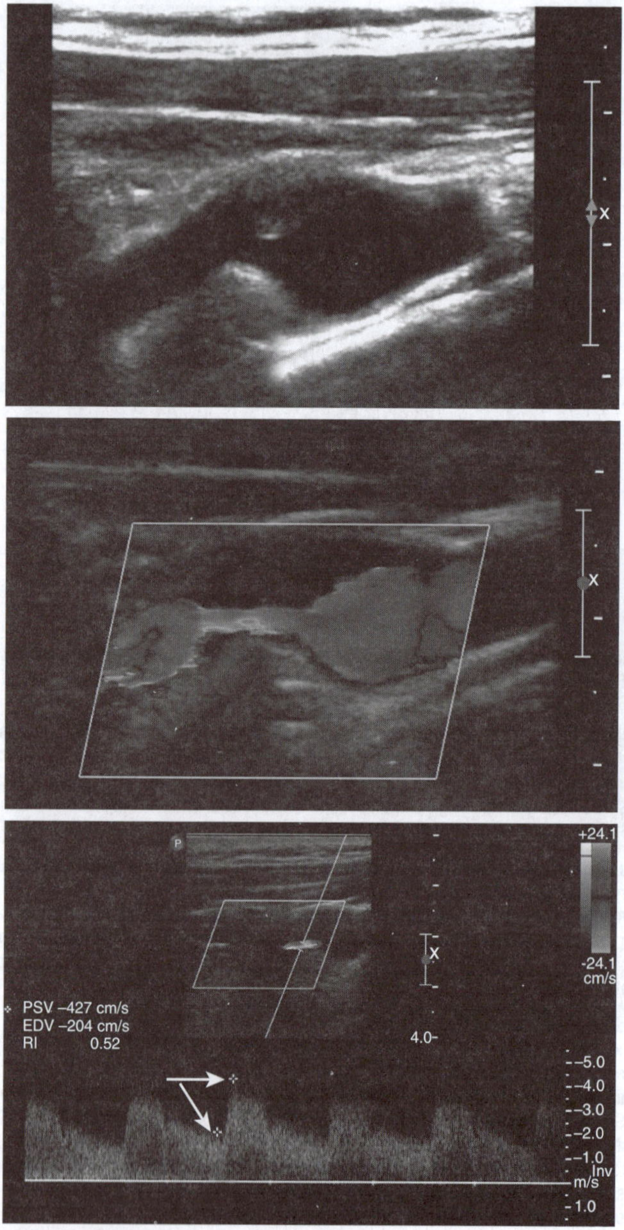

Fig. 57.3. Carotid duplex ultrasound examination (CDUS). A high-grade left internal carotid artery stenosis due to plaque *(top panel)* is visualized. Turbulent and accelerated blood flow is demonstrated using color Doppler *(middle panel)*. There is high peak systolic velocity (PSV, *horizontal arrow*) and high end-diastolic velocity (EDV, *angulated arrow*) *(lower panel)*. This lesion would be consistent with a ≥70% stenosis when using the Society of Radiologists in Ultrasound Consensus criteria (see Table 57.1).

Table 57.1. Society of Radiologists in Ultrasound Consensus Criteria for Diagnosis of Internal Carotid Artery Stenosis

	Primary Parameters		***Secondary Parameters***	
DEGREE OF STENOSIS (%)	**ICA PSV (CM/S)**	**PLAQUE ESTIMATE (%)**	**ICA/CCA PSV RATIO**	**ICA EDV (CM/S)**
Normal	<125	None	<2.0	<40
<50	<125	<50	<2.0	<40
50-69	125-230	≥50	2.0-4.0	40-100
≥70 but less than near occlusion	>230	≥50	>4.0	>100
Near occlusion	High, low, or undetectable	Visible	Variable	Variable
Total occlusion	Undetectable	Visible, no detectable lumen	Not applicable	Not applicable

CCA, Common carotid artery; *EDV*, end-diastolic velocity; *ICA*, internal carotid artery; *PSV*, peak systolic velocity.

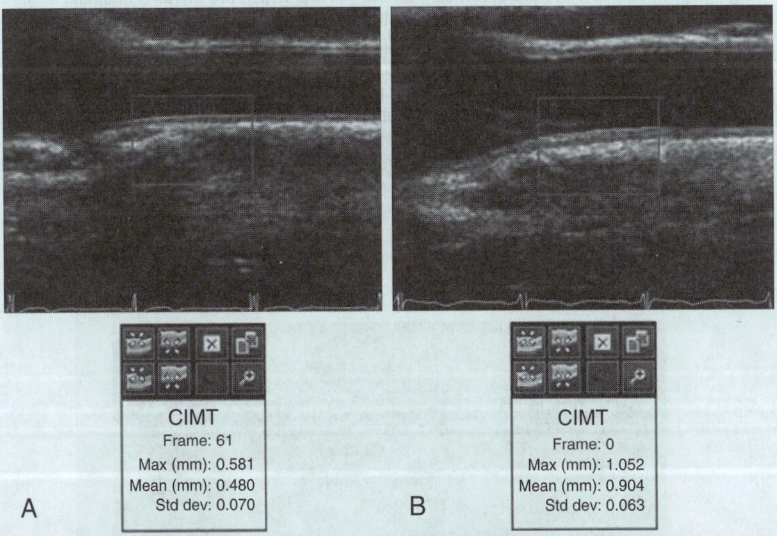

Fig. 57.4. Carotid intima media thickness. Longitudinal ultrasound images of the common carotid artery showing normal carotid intima-media thickness (<25th percentile) **(A)**, and greater than 75th percentile common carotid artery intima-media thickness **(B)**. *(Reprinted from Naqvi, T. Z., & Lee, M. S. [2014]. Carotid intima-media thickness and plaque in cardiovascular risk assessment.* JACC: Cardiovascular Imaging, *7[10], 1025–1038, with permission from Elsevier.)*

8. What is the significance of carotid intima-media thickness measurement?

Carotid intima-media thickness (CIMT) is defined as the distance from the lumen-intima interface to the media-adventitia interface and can be measured using carotid ultrasound (Fig. 57.4). CIMT is a surrogate marker of atherosclerotic risk and along with plaque information (i.e., presence or absence) can have value in improving cardiovascular disease risk prediction. Well-established protocols to measure CIMT exist and should be followed carefully because small changes in CIMT measures can result in major changes in estimated risk.

9. What constitutes medical management for treating patients with carotid artery stenosis?

As with other cardiovascular diseases, modifiable risk factors for atherosclerotic CAS are tobacco use, diabetes mellitus, hypertension, and hyperlipidemia. Risk factor modification along with antiplatelet therapy form the principal components of medical management. Patients with CAS should be prescribed antiplatelet therapy to prevent ischemic cardiovascular events. Aspirin is recommended in asymptomatic patients. Those individuals with symptomatic carotid disease should be treated with aspirin alone, clopidogrel alone, or a combination of aspirin and extended-release dipyridamole. For patients with allergy or contraindications to aspirin other than bleeding, clopidogrel or ticlopidine are alternate options. There is no role for oral or parenteral anticoagulation in the absence of concomitant indications, such as atrial fibrillation or a mechanical cardiac valve. Dual antiplatelet therapy with aspirin and clopidogrel increases bleeding risk in the first 3 months following a stroke or TIA.

10. What are the factors that affect the carotid revascularization strategy for a patient with symptomatic carotid stenosis?

Carotid revascularization options include carotid artery endarterectomy (CEA) (Fig. 57.5) and carotid artery stenting (CS) (Fig. 57.6). Presence of cerebral ischemic symptoms, severity of stenosis, surgical or procedural risk, age, gender, life expectancy, and carotid anatomy are the factors that influence the decision regarding whether to pursue carotid revascularization and whether to opt for CEA or CS.

CEA is indicated in symptomatic patients who suffered stroke or TIA within the previous 6 months, have ipsilateral carotid stenosis (>70% by noninvasive imaging or >50% by catheter angiography), and have average or low surgical risk (<6% perioperative mortality or stroke risk). For these patients, CS is a reasonable alternative option, especially if the arterial anatomy is unfavorable for CEA, the surgical risk is high, in cases of radiation-induced stenosis, or in whom a repeat CEA is being considered. Patients older than 70 years have a twofold higher risk for periprocedural stroke or death with CS compared with CEA. For patients without contraindications, CEA should be performed within 2 weeks of the index event. Carotid revascularization is contraindicated in patients with chronic total carotid occlusion, less than 50% stenosis, and severe disability due to stroke. Symptomatic patients have a reduced annual stroke risk of 1.1%, stroke-free 5-year survival of 93%, and actuarial 5-year survival of 75% after CEA.

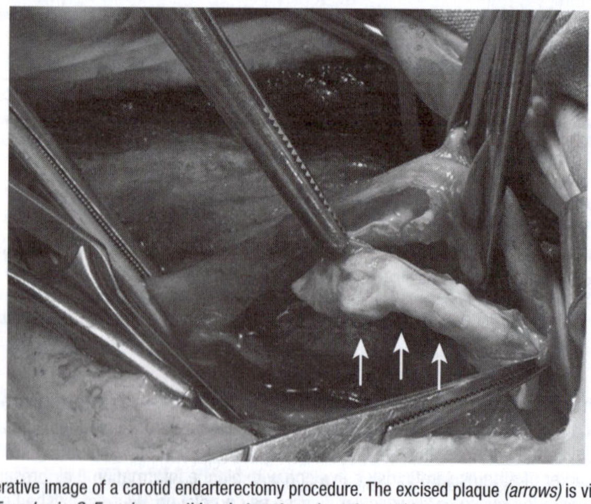

Fig. 57.5. Intraoperative image of a carotid endarterectomy procedure. The excised plaque *(arrows)* is visualized. *(Image from Radak, D., & Tanaskovic, S. Eversion carotid endarterectomy in patients with near-total internal carotid artery occlusion—diagnostic modalities, indications and surgical technique. In D. Yamanouchi [Ed.],* Vascular surgery. <http://Intechopen.com>. *Accessed 29.09.16.)*

11. When is revascularization appropriate in asymptomatic carotid stenosis?

Annual stroke risk for asymptomatic carotid stenosis patients is 0.5% to 1%. Despite the results of several large trials investigating the benefits of carotid stenting and CEA for asymptomatic CAS, the net benefits remain uncertain.

In clinical trials, CEA resulted in significant reductions in the incidence of TIA or nondisabling stroke but not in fatal or disabling stroke rates. In addition, the 30-day perioperative stroke or mortality risk was 3.1%. Asymptomatic women appear to have lower benefits than men after CEA. Thus CEA is considered reasonable in asymptomatic patients with carotid stenosis (>70% by noninvasive imaging or >50% by catheter angiography), and low procedural risk (<3%). CEA for asymptomatic patients must only be performed at experienced surgical centers with less than 3% perioperative complication rate.

Prophylactic carotid artery stenting is a reasonable noninferior alternative to CEA for carotid revascularization in highly selected patients with asymptomatic carotid stenosis (at least 60% by angiography or 70% by CDUS). Even though earlier studies showed higher perioperative stroke in carotid stenting groups and higher rates of myocardial infarction in CEA groups, more recent data from the Asymptomatic Carotid Trial (ACT) I trial showed that these outcomes are broadly similar in both groups. Notably, older patients have better outcome with CEA than with carotid stenting. In addition, the benefits of CEA or carotid stenting over modern optimal medical therapy are not established. The ongoing Carotid Revascularization Endarterectomy versus Stenting Trial (CREST)-2 trial comprising two parallel trials comparing CEA and stenting to optimal medical therapy in patients with asymptomatic high-grade CAS will help to clarify this question.

12. What are the common clinical manifestations and causes of spontaneous cervical artery dissection, and how do you manage them?

Severe headache, neck pain, cranial nerve abnormalities (such as Horner syndrome), TIA, and stroke are the common clinical manifestations of spontaneous cervical artery dissection. It is also a common presentation in patients with fibromuscular dysplasia (FMD) and other connective tissue disorders.

Patients presenting with very early acute ischemic stroke due to extracranial cervical artery dissection should be treated with standard stroke care per contemporary guidelines, including thrombolytic therapy if there are no contraindications. Aortic dissection may extend after thrombolysis. Patients with cervical artery dissection and ischemic stroke or TIA are treated using antithrombotic therapy with either antiplatelet drugs or anticoagulation with heparin or low-molecular-weight heparin followed by oral anticoagulation with warfarin for 3 to 6 months and eventually transitioned to antiplatelet therapy. Results of a recent trial and meta-analysis showed no benefit of anticoagulation

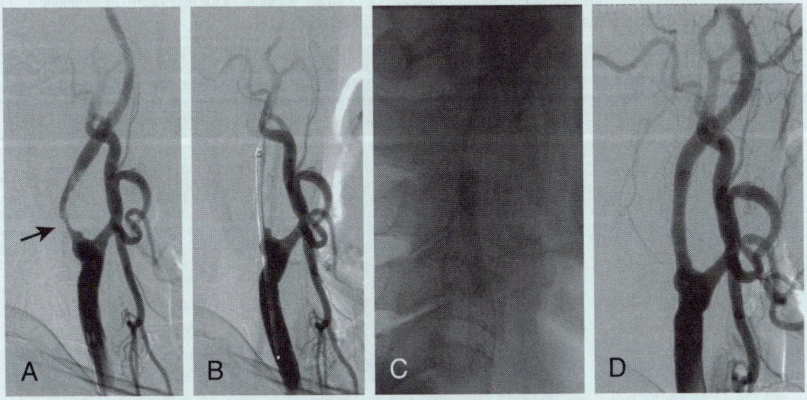

Fig. 57.6. Stenting of a proximal internal carotid artery stenosis with a self-expanding stent. **A,** Stenosis (black arrow) predilation. **B,** Placement of the self-expanding stent. **C,** Postdilation of the deployed stent. **D,** Final angiogram showing the deployed post-dilated stent. *(Image from Myouchin, K., Takayama, K., Taoka, T., Nakagawa, H., Wada, T., Sakamoto, M., et al. [2013]. Carotid Wallstent placement difficulties encountered in carotid artery stenting.* SpringerPlus, 2, *468.* <http://www.springerplus.com/content/2/1/468>. *Accessed 23.09.16.)*

over antiplatelet treatment. The optimal duration of antithrombotic therapy is not established. Tailoring antithrombotic therapy to the presence of symptoms or residual lesion on repeat vascular imaging in 3 to 6 months is an appropriate strategy. Thrombolysis or anticoagulation in the presence of intracranial dissection is controversial due to concerns about the risk of subarachnoid hemorrhage. Revascularization strategy by endovascular or surgical means is reserved for those patients with refractory ischemic symptoms or those patients with acute stroke who are not candidates for intravenous thrombolysis.

13. **What are the clinical manifestations of vertebral artery stenosis?**

The vertebral arteries arise from the first portion of the subclavian artery and have three extracranial and one intracranial segments. Vertebral artery stenosis or reduced flow due to subclavian or aortic disease can lead to vertebrobasilar or watershed ischemic symptoms, stroke/TIA, and lightheadedness or mental status changes secondary to postural changes or arm exercises in case of subclavian steal syndrome. In vertebral subclavian steal syndrome, there is hemodynamically significant ipsilateral proximal subclavian artery stenosis and retrograde flow in the vertebral artery that supplies the arm circulation at the expense of the vertebrobasilar circulation.

On duplex ultrasound (DUS), high-grade vertebral artery stenosis can result in a bidirectional flow pattern. Flow reversal pattern in the vertebral artery waveform and low resistance waveform in the subclavian artery are characteristic of vertebral subclavian steal syndrome. Due to shadowing from the vertebrae, the entire length of extracranial vertebral artery cannot be visualized using DUS. Likewise, proximal subclavian artery interrogation is also suboptimal. CTA, MRA, or catheter angiography is often required to confirm when vertebral or proximal subclavian stenosis is suspected.

Bibliography and Suggested Readings

American College of Cardiology Foundation (ACCF), American College of Radiology (ACR), American Institute of Ultrasound in Medicine (AIUM), American Society of Echocardiography (ASE), American Society of Nephrology (ASN), Intersocietal Commission for the Accreditation of Vascular Laboratories (ICAVL), et al. (2012). ACCF/ACR/AIUM/ASE/ASN/ICAVL/SCAI/SCCT/SIR/SVM/SVS/SVU [corrected] 2012 appropriate use criteria for peripheral vascular ultrasound and physiological testing part I: arterial ultrasound and physiological testing: a report of the American College of Cardiology Foundation appropriate use criteria task force, American College of Radiology, American Institute of Ultrasound in Medicine, American Society of Echocardiography, American Society of Nephrology, Intersocietal Commission for the Accreditation of Vascular Laboratories, Society for Cardiovascular Angiography and Interventions, Society of Cardiovascular Computed Tomography, Society for Interventional Radiology, Society for Vascular Medicine, Society for Vascular Surgery [corrected] and Society for Vascular Ultrasound [corrected]. *Journal of the American College of Cardiology*, *60*(3), 242–276.

Brott, T. G., Halperin, J. L., Abbara, S., Bacharach, J. M., Barr, J. D., Bush, R. L., et al. (2011). 2011 ASA/ACCF/AHA/AANN/AANS/ACR/ASNR/CNS/SAIP/SCAI/SIR/SNIS/SVM/SVS guideline on the management of patients with extracranial carotid and vertebral artery disease. *Journal of the American College of Cardiology*, *57*(8), 1002–1044.

Kernan, W. N., Ovbiagele, B., Black, H. R., Bravata, D. M., Chimowitz, M. I., Ezekowitz, M. D., et al. (2014). Guidelines for the prevention of stroke in patients with stroke and transient ischemic attack: a guideline for healthcare professionals from the American Heart Association/American Stroke Association. *Stroke*, *45*(7), 2160.

CHAPTER 58

ISCHEMIC STROKE

Sharyl R. Martini, Thomas A. Kent

1. **What is a stroke?**

   Stroke is a *focal* disturbance of blood flow into or out of the brain, either primarily ischemic (87%) or hemorrhagic (13%). Stroke is not a single disease but the end result of many different pathophysiologies leading to cerebrovascular occlusion or rupture. The key clinical feature of a stroke is *very rapid symptom onset*: "it hit me like a ton of bricks" or "like someone flipped a light switch." Although the initial onset is *sudden*, symptoms may fluctuate.

2. **What are the three basic causes of stroke?**

   The most common basic types of stroke are ischemic stroke and hemorrhagic stroke. Less commonly, cerebral venous sinus thrombosis can also lead to stroke. Ischemic stroke can be due to large vessel atherosclerosis, intrinsic small vessel disease, and cardioembolic stroke. Hemorrhagic stroke includes intracranial hemorrhage and subarachnoid hemorrhage. Ischemic stroke and transient ischemic attack (TIA) are addressed in this chapter. Hemorrhagic stroke and cerebral venous sinus thrombosis are addressed in the following chapter 59. Fig. 58.1 summarizes the causes of stroke.

3. **What is a transient ischemic attack?**

   TIA is an abrupt onset neurologic deficit due to interruption of blood flow to a portion of the brain, followed by complete symptom resolution. If the interruption continues long enough, an ischemic stroke will result. By classic definition, TIA deficits resolve within 24 hours, although most resolve

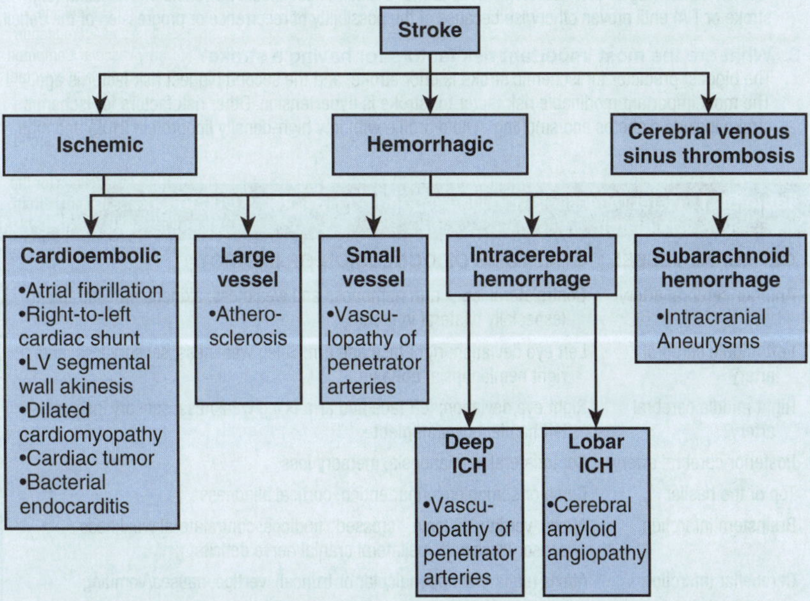

Fig. 58.1. Types and common causes of strokes. Stroke is a term encompassing arterial occlusion (ischemic), arterial rupture (hemorrhagic), and venous occlusion (cerebral venous sinus thrombosis). Major subtypes within each category are indicated, with the most common underlying etiology or etiologies listed below. *LV*, Left ventricle; *ICH*, intracerebral hemorrhage *(Adapted from Martini, S. R., Grossman, A. W., Kent, T. A. [2014]. Stroke. In G. N. Levine [Ed.],* Color atlas of cardiovascular disease. *New Delhi: Jaypee Brothers Medical Publishers.)*

within 5 to 15 minutes. Transient neurologic symptoms of unclear etiology are most appropriately referred to as spells; only those thought to be due to brain ischemia should be referred to as TIAs.

4. **Why is prompt recognition of transient ischemic attacks important?**
TIAs herald the possibility of a completed stroke: appropriate intervention may prevent strokes and thus permanent disability. Ninety-day stroke rates for patients with TIA are greater than 10% in some series, with the greatest risk within 48 hours to 7 days. Longer symptom duration and presence of large cerebral artery (e.g., carotid) stenosis are associated with higher risk of stroke following TIA. All patients with a recent TIA (within 2 weeks) need an expedited workup to determine cause and prompt intervention tailored to the cause (e.g., carotid intervention for symptomatic carotid stenosis, initiation of anticoagulation for underlying atrial fibrillation, or antiplatelet agents if the cause is under investigation while the workup is under way). Recurrent stroke from TIA has dropped dramatically with this more aggressive approach to TIA.

5. **How common are stroke and transient ischemic attack?**
According to the Centers for Disease Control and Prevention, there are more than 795,000 strokes per year in the United States, and it is the leading cause of disability. There are at least 250,000 TIAs each year in the United States, but this number is likely an underestimate because many are not reported.

6. **What types of symptoms can strokes cause?**
Focal weakness, numbness, facial asymmetry, or speech difficulties are classic presentations. Altered level of consciousness, vertigo, and cranial nerve deficits are seen with posterior circulation (vertebrobasilar/brainstem) and cerebellar strokes. Diminished level of consciousness is unusual for ischemic strokes. Table 58.1 lists common stroke symptoms associated with occlusion of specific cerebral vessels.

7. **How are stroke and transient ischemic attack diagnosed?**
Stroke and TIA are diagnosed clinically, and no imaging correlation is required for the acute diagnosis. Imaging studies are performed to rule out other causes, such as tumor, and to determine whether there is brain hemorrhage. Focal neurologic deficits with sudden onset should be considered vascular (e.g., stroke or TIA) until proven otherwise because of the possibility of recurrence or progression of the deficit.

8. **What are the most important risk factors for having a stroke?**
The biggest predictor for ischemic stroke is prior stroke, and the second biggest risk factor is age. The most important modifiable risk factor for stroke is hypertension. Other risk factors for ischemic stroke include diabetes and smoking. A lipid profile with low high-density lipoprotein (HDL) and high

Table 58.1. Cerebral Vessels and Corresponding Symptoms Due to Occlusion or Infarct

CEREBRAL VESSEL	SYMPTOMS OF OCCLUSION OR INFARCT
Anterior cerebral artery	Contralateral leg > arm numbness and weakness; akinetic mutism/abulia (especially bilateral infarcts)
Left middle cerebral artery	Left eye deviation; right face and arm > leg weakness, sensory loss, and right hemianopsia; **aphasia**
Right middle cerebral artery	Right eye deviation; left face and arm > leg weakness, sensory loss, and left hemianopsia; **neglect**
Posterior cerebral artery	Contralateral hemianopsia, memory loss
Top of the basilar	Coma or somnolence/inattention, cortical blindness
Brainstem infarction	Ataxia, vertigo, diplopia, "crossed" findings: contralateral weakness / sensory loss with ipsilateral cranial nerve deficits
Cerebellar infarction	Ataxia (unilateral appendicular or truncal), vertigo, nausea/vomiting
Vertebral artery	Loss of pain and temperature sensation from the contralateral body and ipsilateral face; dysarthria, dysphagia, ataxia, hiccups (lateral medullary [Wallenberg] syndrome)
Penetrating artery	Contralateral face = arm = leg weakness or numbness

triglycerides is also associated with ischemic stroke, whereas high low-density lipoprotein (LDL) is most closely associated with cardiac disease. Such cardiac diseases as atrial fibrillation and valvular disease are ischemic stroke risk factors. The most significant risk factor for the most common type of hemorrhagic stroke is hypertension.

9. **What stroke syndromes are associated with occlusion of the cerebral arteries?**
Stroke signs and symptoms depend on the part of the brain that is damaged. Although there is person-to-person variation in arterial supply, classic syndromes are frequently seen.

10. **What are the major etiologies of ischemic stroke?**
The major etiologies of ischemic stroke are (1) cardioembolism, (2) small vessel vasculopathy (arteriolosclerosis, lipohyalinosis) involving the penetrating arteries branching off the major intracerebral arteries, and (3) large vessel atherosclerosis due to plaque rupture involving the intracranial or extracranial cerebral arteries. Table 58.2 lists characteristics of these etiologic stroke subtypes.

11. **What cardiac conditions are considered sources of cardioembolic stroke?**
Cardiac conditions associated with stroke include atrial fibrillation or flutter, mechanical valves, cardiomyopathies, infarction of the cardiac apex, septic emboli, and marantic endocarditis. Patent foramen ovale (PFO) is prevalent and is not considered a likely cardioembolic source unless left-to-right shunting and a venous clot can be demonstrated. Figs. 58.2 and 58.3 show examples of thrombus in the left atrial appendage (LAA) in a patient with atrial fibrillation and left ventricular thrombus in a patient with anteroapical infarct.

12. **What are some less common causes of ischemic stroke?**
Dissection of the cervical vessels needs to be considered, especially if there is neck or face pain or a history of trauma. Horner syndrome may be seen with carotid injury. Illicit drug use can cause ischemic stroke (cocaine, stimulant-induced spasm). Rarer causes of stroke include hypercoagulable states (e.g., active cancer, genetic clotting disorder, or autoimmune conditions, such as lupus/antiphospholipid antibody syndrome) and genetic disorders, such as cerebral autosomal dominant arteriopathy with subcortical infarcts and leukoencephalopathy (CADASIL) and fibromuscular dysplasia. PFO remains controversial as a cause of stroke. Cases in which no specific cause is identified are called "cryptogenic."

Table 58.2. Clues to the Commonest Ischemic Stroke Etiologies

ETIOLOGY	CLINICAL FEATURES
Large vessel atherosclerosis	• Plaque rupture results in in situ large artery thrombosis or artery-to-artery thromboembolism • Often occur in early morning hours/on waking • History of TIAs in same vascular distribution • Symptoms may fluctuate
Cardioembolism	• History or clinical features of heart disease • Stroke symptoms are maximal at onset because clot is preformed • TIA symptoms are usually different from one another, representing emboli to different vascular distributions • Often occur during waking hours • Can be associated with Valsalva • Caused by embolism, usually from LAA (in setting of atrial fibrillation) or left ventricle (in case of akinetic segment) • May have strokes of different ages in different vascular territories
Small vessel vasculopathy	• Strong association with hypertension and diabetes • Diameter <1.5 cm • Occur in subcortical regions such as basal ganglia, thalamus, or brainstem • Never see cortical findings (aphasia, neglect) • Symptoms may fluctuate dramatically • May have TIAs with similar symptoms • Occlusion of small penetrating arteries is not always due to small vessel etiology—alternate etiologies must be evaluated

LAA, Left atrial appendage; *TIA*, transient ischemic attack.

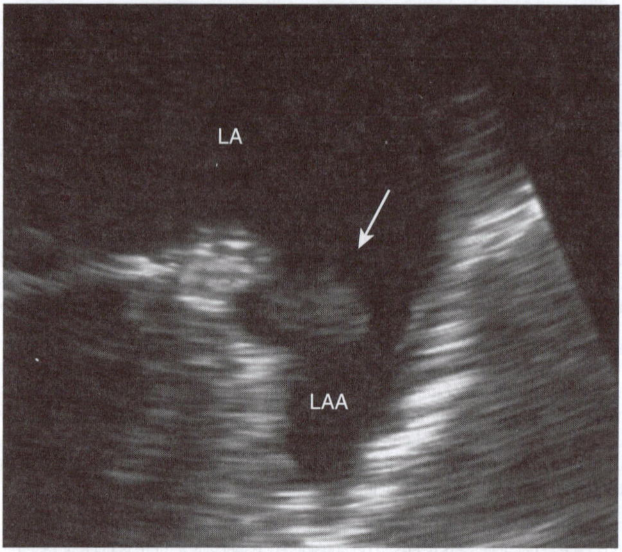

Fig. 58.2. Example of a thrombus *(arrow)* visualized in the left atrial appendage by transesophageal echocardiography. *LA,* Left atrium; *LAA,* left atrial appendage.

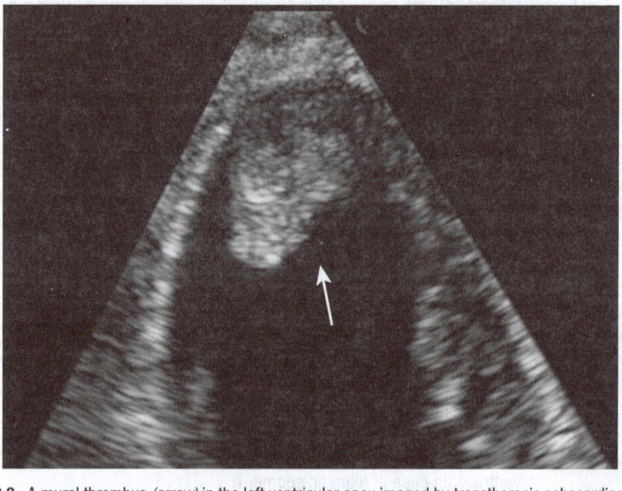

Fig. 58.3. A mural thrombus *(arrow)* in the left ventricular apex imaged by transthoracic echocardiography.

13. How do ischemic strokes appear on imaging?

On computed tomography (CT), most ischemic strokes eventually become visible as hypodensities of the brain parenchyma (Fig. 58.4), but CT is largely normal for at least 6 hours. The earliest CT signs are loss of the cortical ribbon and gyral edema. On magnetic resonance imaging (MRI), strokes will appear hyperintense on T2-weighted sequences. Diffusion-weighted imaging (DWI) detects cytotoxic edema that accompanies ischemic cell death and can appear very shortly after onset of ischemia. True diffusion positivity will appear dark on the apparent diffusion coefficient (ADC) map sequence. Onset of DWI positivity may be delayed up to 48 to 72 hours, particularly in the brainstem, and typically lasts 10 to 14 days. The ADC map normalizes more quickly, often 4 to 7 days after onset. Examples of ischemic strokes visualized by MRI are shown in Fig. 58.5.

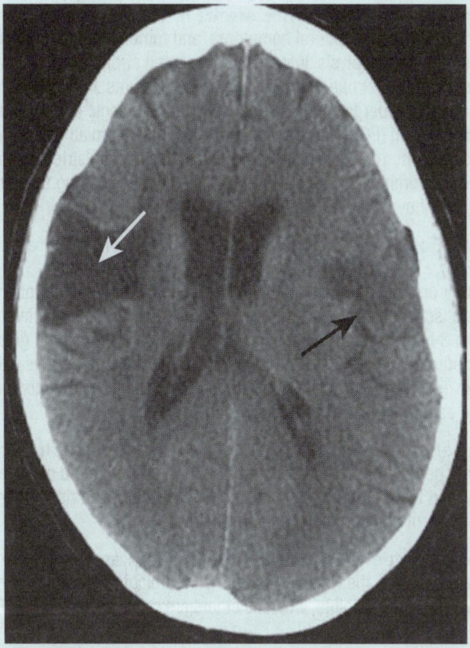

Fig. 58.4. Computed tomography scan showing a remote infarct in the right middle cerebral artery (MCA) territory *(white arrow)* and a more recent (subacute) infarct in the left MCA territory *(black arrow)*. These findings of strokes of different ages in multiple vascular territories suggest cardioembolic etiology.

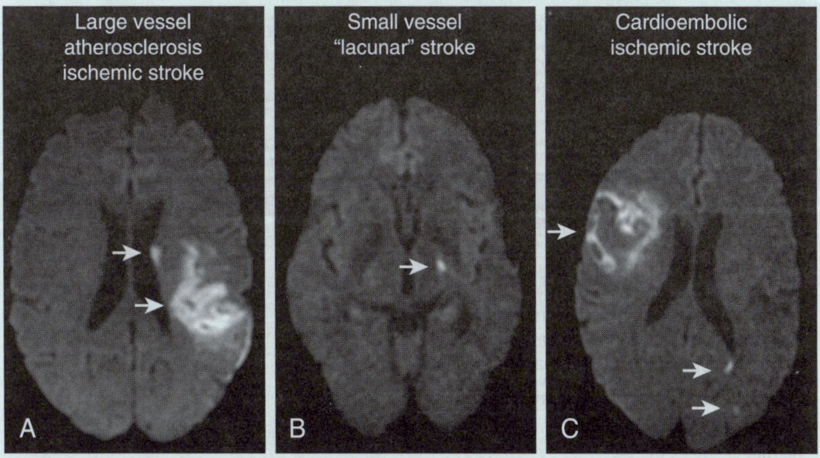

Fig. 58.5. Diffusion-weighted magnetic resonance imaging of ischemic stroke subtypes. **A,** Ischemic stroke due to large vessel atherosclerosis. **B,** Small vessel ("lacunar") ischemic stroke. **C,** Cardioembolic ischemic stroke. A large stroke with areas of hemorrhage in the right MCA distribution is seen *(single arrow)*, as well as punctate areas of infarction in the left PCA distribution *(two arrows)*. *(Images courtesy of Dr. Achala Vagal. Images reproduced from Martini, S. R., Grossman, A. W., Kent, T. A. [2014]. Stroke. In G. N. Levine [Ed.],* Color atlas of cardiovascular disease. *New Delhi: Jaypee Brothers Medical Publishers.)*

14. What are the initial steps if ischemic stroke is suspected?

Head CT rules out hemorrhage, subdural hematoma, and tumor. It is the first and most important test when evaluating for thrombolysis. In cases of suspected stroke, page the service responsible for rapidly addressing stroke (stroke team)—every minute counts. Immediately check blood glucose because hypoglycemia or hyperglycemia can cause focal neurologic deficits mimicking stroke. Also obtain an electrocardiogram (ECG) and troponin because initial cardiac workup can reveal atrial fibrillation or myocardial infarction. Coagulation studies, basic chemistries, and complete blood count should be drawn, but thrombolysis should not be delayed while awaiting these results unless there is reason to suspect that they would be abnormal.

15. What are the US Food and Drug Administration–approved treatments for acute ischemic stroke?

The only medication currently approved by the US Food and Drug Administration (FDA) to improve outcome after acute ischemic strokes is intravenous tissue plasminogen activator (IV tPA), administered within 3 hours of symptom onset. American Heart Association guidelines recommend treatment in selected patients out to 4.5 hours after symptom onset, but this extended time window was not FDA approved. The earlier IV tPA is given, the better the clinical outcome: an estimated 1 million neurons die each minute that thrombolysis is delayed.

16. How much do patients benefit from tissue plasminogen activator?

Eight stroke patients need to be treated with IV tPA to give one patient a complete or near-complete recovery, and this number takes into account the increased risk of hemorrhage after tPA administration. Patients of any age may benefit from tPA.

17. What are contraindications to intravenous tissue plasminogen activator?

Contraindications are based on the National Institute of Neurological Disorders and Stroke (NINDS) tPA trial: some are considered absolute, whereas others are relative (Table 58.3). The most frequent

Table 58.3. Contraindications to Intravenous Tissue Plasminogen Activator

Absolute Contraindications
Greater than 4.5 h from the time patient was last seen normal
Initial head CT suggests time of onset is inaccurate
Suggestion of intracranial hemorrhage on pretreatment imaging
Subarachnoid hemorrhage
Intracranial neoplasm or arteriovenous malformation
Active internal bleeding
Uncontrolled hypertension greater than 185/110 mm Hg despite antihypertensive treatment
Current bacterial endocarditis
Head trauma or intracranial/intraspinal surgery within 3 months
Known bleeding diathesis • INR >1.7 or prothrombin time >15 s • Platelets <100,000 mm^3 • Heparin within 48 h if partial thromboplastin time is elevated • PTT outside of the normal range • Dose of nonwarfarin oral anticoagulant within past 12 h
Relative Contraindications
Minor or rapidly resolving deficits
Seizure
Major surgery in the previous 2 weeks
GI or urinary hemorrhage in the previous 3 weeks
Puncture at noncompressible site within 7 days (including lumbar puncture)

GI, Gastrointestinal; *INR*, international normalized ratio.

exclusion is time from when the patient was last seen normal (not when symptoms were discovered)—a particular problem for "wake-up strokes." Patients with minor/rapidly resolving deficits (possible TIAs) and seizure at stroke onset were excluded from the NINDS trial to avoid treating conditions that would return to baseline without thrombolysis. However, patients may be left disabled by "mild" or "improving" strokes, and seizures complicate acute strokes approximately 15% of the time; however, the optimum treatment for patients with these characteristics is still being determined.

18. How are patients monitored after administration of intravenous tissue plasminogen activator?

Frequent clinical examinations are crucial, and blood pressure must be controlled to less than 180/105 mm Hg to prevent bleeding into the infarcted brain tissue. Anticoagulant (including subcutaneous heparin) and antiplatelet agents are held for 24 hours, until follow-up imaging confirms absence of hemorrhagic conversion. Any change in exam warrants a stat head CT.

19. When should intra-arterial therapy be used for acute ischemic stroke?

The role for endovascular therapy of acute ischemic stroke is rapidly evolving. After three randomized clinical trials of older endovascular devices failed to show improved clinical outcomes, four randomized clinical trials that primarily used new stent retriever devices all demonstrated improved clinical outcome. These more recent trials were mostly in patients who had received intravenous tPA, but non-tPA patients were represented and each trial used different selection criteria, mostly related to enrolling patients who had not yet demonstrated evidence of a completed stroke by imaging and some residual perfusion by vascular imaging. There is no support for skipping the administration of tPA if the patient qualifies to go directly to endovascular therapy. These trials are currently being carefully assessed by a variety of organizations, and recommendations for their appropriate use are under discussion. Currently, endovascular therapy, especially with stent-retriever devices, appears reasonable in patients whose brain imaging does not show evidence of early ischemic changes and who have a proximal large vessel occlusion accessible by these devices. Faster time to treatment appears to be associated with better outcomes, and many centers are modifying their policies and procedures to incorporate fast deployment of endovascular therapy. Given the potential dangers of device-related complications (11% to 16%) and reperfusion injury, it is important to select patients for intra-arterial therapy based on the inclusion-exclusion criteria of these trials.

20. What if the patient is not a candidate for intravenous tissue plasminogen activator?

Endovascular therapy can still be considered. In patients not treated with thrombolysis, aspirin (orally or rectally) reduces the chances of recurrent stroke when given within 48 hours. Optimal blood pressure for nonthrombolysed patients is not known but is often permitted to run high as long as there are no signs of hypertensive end-organ damage. This "permissive hypertension" is theoretically designed to increase perfusion of brain tissue at continued risk for ischemia, but it is not clear that this strategy improves outcomes.

Sudden drops in blood pressure should be avoided. Relative hypotension associated with neurologic worsening should be treated with IV fluids. Lowering the head of the bed and administering vasopressors may also be considered.

21. What are the major clinical concerns in the initial days following an ischemic stroke?

Clots may propagate, particularly those due to large artery atherosclerosis. The most life-threatening complication of stroke is herniation due to cerebral edema, which manifests 12 hours to 5 days after onset. Clinical signs include somnolence, pupillary dilation from third nerve compression, and signs of increased intracranial pressure (nausea, vomiting). Herniation may occur either upward or downward through the tentorium, or under the falx cerebri. Large hemispheric and cerebellar strokes are most likely to cause herniation. Manipulation of serum osmolarity (mannitol, hypertonic saline) or hyperventilation may be used, although definitive treatment is surgical decompression.

22. When is hemicraniectomy recommended?

Patients with malignant middle cerebral artery occlusion are at risk of death from cerebral edema and herniation. Removal of the overlying skull has been shown to reduce mortality, with a number needed to treat of two: fewer die, but less than 10% achieve functional independence. Surgical decompression is often suggested for large strokes within the cerebellar hemispheres because patients tend to recover well from these strokes if they survive the acute period. Early consultation with neurosurgeons is suggested.

23. **What is hemorrhagic transformation (hemorrhagic conversion)?**
Ischemic strokes can develop a hemorrhagic component, especially if they are large or if the degree of ischemia is severe. This hemorrhagic transformation occurs because all tissue (brain and vasculature) downstream of an ischemic stroke becomes ischemic. In many cases, blood flow to the ischemic area is reestablished too late to benefit the brain and returns via weakened, damaged vessels. These vessels may leak, resulting in petechial hemorrhage, or burst, resulting in a hematoma. Hemorrhagic transformation is most likely in the first days to a week after stroke. This is why clinical worsening in an ischemic stroke patient should be immediately evaluated with noncontrast head CT.

24. **What are the goals of hospitalization for an ischemic stroke?**
The goals of hospitalization for a stroke patient are to (1) prevent complications, such as stroke progression, aspiration pneumonia, and pulmonary embolism, (2) develop a plan for functional recovery with the help of physical, occupational, and speech therapies, and (3) determine stroke mechanism to design an optimal secondary stroke prevention strategy.

25. **How can systemic complications of stroke be prevented?**
In all cases of stroke, ensure adequate deep vein thrombosis (DVT) prophylaxis to prevent pulmonary emboli. Keep patients nothing per os (NPO) until safe swallowing can be confirmed to prevent aspiration and subsequent pneumonia. Frequent turning prevents skin breakdown. Catheters should be removed as soon as possible. Patients should be mobilized as soon as safely possible, although many are at high risk of falls and may need constant supervision—particularly those with neglect because they are unaware of their deficits.

26. **What is considered a complete ischemic stroke workup?**
Patients with anterior circulation strokes need urgent carotid imaging. Intracranial and extracranial imaging is performed in most cases. MRI is useful for detecting strokes not apparent on head CT. Additional small strokes in different vascular distributions point to a cardioembolic source. In patients with suspected cardioembolism, echocardiogram is indicated. All patients should have telemetry for atrial fibrillation identification—ECGs are inadequate for detection of this important risk factor. Implantable event monitors reveal subclinical atrial fibrillation in a substantial proportion of patients with cryptogenic stroke and are warranted in cases in which clinical suspicion is high.

27. **How would stroke workup differ for a young person or someone without usual stroke risk factors?**
Stroke workup in a young patient begins with a detailed history, including personal or family history of clotting, autoimmune disease, trauma, and cardiac disease. Careful examination of eyes and skin may provide clues to neurofibromatosis, Fabry disease, connective tissue diseases, or endocarditis. Because young stroke patients are more likely to have cardiac abnormalities, a detailed cardiac evaluation including transesophageal echocardiography should be performed. MRI of the brain, vessel imaging, and hypercoagulable workup are standard, as are toxicology, autoimmune, and vasculitis labs erythrocyte sedimentation rate, c-reactive protein, anti-nuclear antibody, anti-neutrophil cytoplasmic antibody rheumatoid factor, complement). Syphilis and human immunodeficiency virus testing are obtained. Lumbar puncture may reveal additional infectious or inflammatory conditions.

28. **What is a hypercoagulable workup?**
Family history of clotting, miscarriages, or a paucity of vascular risk factors should raise suspicion for a hypercoagulable state. Hormone use (oral contraceptives, testosterone replacement, hormone replacement) is associated with an increased thrombotic risk and should be specifically sought from history. Laboratory tests include antithrombin III, protein C, protein S, activated protein C resistance/factor V Leiden mutation, and prothrombin mutation. Lupus anticoagulant and anticardiolipin or beta-2 glycoprotein antibodies point to antiphospholipid antibody syndrome. Cancer produces a hypercoagulable state, so malignancy evaluation should be considered.

29. **What is the best strategy to prevent additional strokes?**
The best strategy depends on the causative etiology: options for the treatment of carotid stenosis, intracranial stenosis, and atrial fibrillation are presented below. Prevention of secondary stroke from small vessel disease relies solely on aggressive risk factor management. Goals for secondary stroke prevention include a target blood pressure less than 140/90, antiplatelet or anticoagulant as appropriate, statin therapy,

hemoglobin A1C less than 7 to 8, smoking cessation, regular exercise, and weight loss to a body mass index less than 25. Obstructive sleep apnea is associated with increased stroke risk, independent of its association with hypertension, so treatment seems prudent.

30. What options exist for evaluating cerebral vessels?

Carotid duplex ultrasound is cost effective but inadequate for evaluation of intracranial vessels or the posterior circulation. Transcranial Doppler ultrasound evaluates intracranial vessels but is operator-dependent and not widely available. CT angiogram is fast, readily available, and provides detailed information from the aortic arch to the intracranial vessels. Disadvantages include radiation exposure and the need for iodinated contrast. Magnetic resonance (MR) angiogram also evaluates the entire cerebrovascular tree, although motion artifacts can obscure the arch and great vessel origins. MR angiography's major disadvantage is the need for the patient to lie still for 30 to 45 minutes.

31. How should carotid stenosis be managed?

Patients with symptomatic carotid stenosis greater than 70% should be treated with carotid endarterectomy (CEA) or carotid stenting within 2 weeks of a TIA or nondisabling stroke: risk of recurrent stroke is 15% per year, and CEA cuts it in half. Patients with 50% to 70% symptomatic stenosis benefit less from carotid intervention and have the same upfront procedure risk. If procedural risk is low at the patient's institution, intervention is still often recommended for this group. Stenosis less than 50% may still be responsible for the patient's symptoms, but intervention does not appear to be beneficial relative to lower recurrence risk and periprocedure complication risk. The Carotid Revascularization Endarterectomy versus Stenting Trial (CREST) showed higher stroke and death rates in the stenting group but higher myocardial infarction rates with CEA; overall rates of the combined endpoint were not different. Older patients fared better with CEA than carotid stenting, and quality of life was better in those with myocardial infarction than those with stroke.

32. How should intracranial stenosis be managed?

In the Stenting vs. Aggressive Medical Management for Preventing Recurrent Stroke in Intracranial Stenosis (SAMMPRIS) trial, patients with recent mild stroke or TIA due to 70% to 99% intracranial stenosis were randomized to stenting plus aggressive medical management versus aggressive medical management alone. All subjects received aspirin plus clopidogrel for 90 days, followed by aspirin alone. In addition to blood pressure and lipid goals, lifestyle coaches developed goals for weight loss, regular exercise, and smoking cessation with each participant. The trial was stopped early because 14.7% of patients in the stenting arm had a stroke within 30 days (most within 1 day of stenting) compared with 5.8% in the medical management group; 1-year stroke rates were 20% and 12.2%, respectively. As such, intracranial atherosclerosis is now managed medically.

33. What if the patient has a patent foramen ovale?

PFOs are present in up to 25% of the population and, in most cases, confer little if any stroke risk. Large PFOs with a right-to-left shunt and those with atrial septal aneurysms are of greater concern. In a patient with stroke and concerning PFO, a venous source for thromboembolism should be investigated. Pelvic vein MRI may identify DVTs not apparent by standard vascular ultrasound techniques. PFO closure has been hotly debated: CLOSURE I (Closure or medical therapy for cryptogenic stroke with patent foramen ovale) compared PFO closure to best medical management in subjects with cryptogenic stroke and did not find a benefit of PFO closure after 2 years of follow-up. Most subjects with recurrent stroke had evidence of a mechanism other than paradoxic embolism. At this point, PFO closure is best done in the setting of a randomized controlled trial.

34. How well do anticoagulants work to prevent stroke in the setting of atrial fibrillation?

All patients with stroke and atrial fibrillation merit consideration for long-term anticoagulation because it reduces ischemic stroke by more than 60%. The CHA2DS2-VASc risk stratification scheme integrates risk factors to assist in the decision for anticoagulation therapy. Factors in this risk score include older age, hypertension, diabetes, female gender, poor left ventricular function or recent heart failure, and prior stroke. The greater the number of risk factors, the higher the risk of stroke. Stroke or TIA automatically places a patient in the high-risk category, so secondary prevention of stroke in patients with atrial fibrillation should involve oral anticoagulation unless there is a contraindication.

35. Do patients who have percutaneous or surgical procedures to treat atrial fibrillation still need anticoagulation?

Restoring sinus rhythm via pulmonary vein ablation, resecting the left atrial appendage (LAA) and transcatheter closure of the LAA opening have thus far not demonstrated a sufficient reduction of stroke risk to warrant discontinuing anticoagulation. The Atrial Fibrillation Follow-up Investigation of Rhythm Management

(AFFIRM) trial found that restoring sinus rhythm did not reduce stroke risk. The WATCHMAN trial (WATCHMAN Left Atrial Appendage System for Embolic PROTECTion in Patients With Atrial Fibrillation) similarly did not find a reduction in stroke risk; additional device trials are ongoing. The LAA Occlusion Study II is an ongoing phase III trial comparing surgical excision of the LAA with best medical therapy. At this time, anticoagulation is the only intervention proven to reduce stroke in the setting of atrial fibrillation.

36. What about anticoagulation in patients at high risk for bleeding?

Although older patients are at high risk for bleeding, they are also at high risk for stroke from atrial fibrillation; thus age is not a contraindication to anticoagulation. Contraindications include history of severe gastrointestinal (GI) bleeding, history of falls, or an extremely high fall risk. The Hypertension, Abnormal renal/liver function, Stroke, Bleeding, Labile INR, Elderly, Drugs or alcohol use (HAS-BLED) score is a simple method for assessing bleeding risk. After stroke, many patients are at risk for falls: as they recover, reconsider anticoagulation. The decision for anticoagulation should be an ongoing collaborative discussion of the risks, benefits, and monitoring schedule so that the patient can make an informed decision.

37. How soon after a stroke should anticoagulation be started?

Large strokes and those due to cardioembolism are most likely to bleed. As such, it is common practice to wait 3 to 4 weeks after a large stroke before initiating anticoagulation for atrial fibrillation. Patients with very small cardioembolic strokes may be started on anticoagulation within 1 to 2 days. In patients with large strokes at high risk for embolization (mechanical valves, cardiac thrombus), anticoagulation may be started cautiously after 5 to 15 days. Retrospective data suggest that bridging with heparin or low-molecular-weight heparin causes more bleeding, but this has not been confirmed prospectively. In the case of use of warfarin, in the absence of a hypercoagulable state, it is acceptable to start warfarin at low doses to achieve therapeutic anticoagulation slowly. Some clinicians suggest aspirin until an international normalized ratio (INR) of 2 is achieved.

38. How are antiplatelet agents used after stroke?

Patients who do not meet criteria for anticoagulation should receive antiplatelet therapy: aspirin, clopidogrel, or extended-release dipyridamole plus aspirin. All are similarly efficacious, decreasing stroke risk 14% to 18%. Ensuring adherence is probably more important than the agent used, so choice should be guided by comorbidities, tolerability, and cost. Antiplatelet therapy should be initiated immediately in patients who are not tPA candidates and do not have any hemorrhagic component. Wait 24 hours after tPA to start antiplatelet medications.

39. Should aspirin and clopidogrel be used together for stroke prevention?

Aspirin should not be combined with clopidogrel for long-term secondary stroke prevention, due to unacceptably high bleeding risk without additional protection from strokes (Secondary Prevention of Small Subcortical Strokes and Management of ATherothrombosis with Clopidogrel in High-risk patients trials). The Clopidogrel with Aspirin in Acute Minor Stroke or Transient Ischemic Attack trial found that aspirin plus clopidogrel for the 21 days after stroke reduced the odds of a second stroke within 90 days. Most participants were from China, where blood pressure control is less frequently achieved. In the absence of definitive data, either *short-term* dual antiplatelet therapy or a single antiplatelet agent may be used for secondary stroke prevention. Patients on dual antiplatelet therapy for other indications may be continued on this combination after stroke, with the understanding that bleeding risk may be elevated.

40. Should aspirin be added to anticoagulation?

In patients requiring anticoagulation, bleeding risk increases with the addition of antiplatelet agents. Except in cases of unstable coronary disease or mechanical valves, this increased bleeding risk is not offset by a decrease in thrombotic events. Because ischemic stroke and intracerebral hemorrhage increase dramatically with age, patients presenting with stroke are quite different from those presenting with acute coronary syndromes. As such, it is not valid to extrapolate stroke secondary prevention from cardiac studies, as the MATCH trial exemplified. The decision to add aspirin to anticoagulation is a difficult one, best made collaboratively among patient, neurologist, and cardiologist.

41. What if a patient has a stroke while taking an antiplatelet agent?

The notion of treatment "failure" has been proposed if a patient has a stroke or TIA while on a specific antiplatelet agent. Genetic variation in antiplatelet response has been demonstrated for clopidogrel and suggested for aspirin, but genetic testing is not routinely used in the selection of antiplatelet agents. Currently, only limited retrospective data support changing to a different antiplatelet agent

Table 58.4. Key Points in the Evaluation and Management of Ischemic Stroke

Basics Key Points
- The main clinical feature of stroke is sudden onset of a focal neurologic deficit.
- TIA serves as a warning for a completed stroke, with the greatest risk for stroke in the first 72 h to 2 weeks following the TIA.
- The biggest predictor of ischemic stroke is a prior stroke.
- The most important modifiable risk factor for stroke is hypertension.

Ischemic Stroke Causes
- Determining stroke etiology is key to proper acute management and secondary prevention.
- Major ischemic stroke subtypes include (1) large artery stroke due to atherosclerotic plaque rupture; (2) cardioembolism, usually due to atrial fibrillation; and (3) small vessel vasculopathy.
- Other causes of stroke include arterial dissection, hypercoaguable state, substance abuse, and infectious/inflammatory conditions.

Ischemic Stroke Acute Management
- Noncontrast CT is used acutely to rule out hemorrhage or tumor (not to diagnose stroke).
- For IV tPA eligibility, stroke onset is defined as the time the patient was **last seen normal**, not when he or she was discovered to have symptoms.
- Clinical deterioration in the acute period following stroke may be due to clot propagation (large vessel subtype), cerebral edema/herniation, or hemorrhagic transformation.

Ischemic Stroke Workup and Management
- Diffusion-weighted MRI can identify cytotoxic edema from ischemic strokes but may be negative in small strokes or TIAs.
- CT angiogram or MR angiogram can suggest stroke etiology by identifying arterial thrombus, dissection, or atherosclerotic stenosis.
- Symptomatic carotid stenosis requires urgent intervention; asymptomatic carotid stenosis does not.
- For strokes due to atrial fibrillation, anticoagulation decreases risk of a subsequent stroke by 60%.

IV tPA, Intravenous tissue plasminogen activator; *MRI*, magnetic resonance imaging; *TIA*, transient ischemic attack.

after stroke. In the absence of definitive data, it may be more fruitful to address risk factor reduction strategies and medication adherence. The role of laboratory platelet inhibition measures in choice of antiplatelet agent remains to be established.

42. How well do patients recover following ischemic stroke?

Younger patients and those with smaller strokes tend to recover better, but there is remarkable person-to-person variation. The best predictor of how a person will recover is the initial stroke severity and the trajectory of their recovery within the first weeks following the stroke. Much of the recovery occurs within the first month, and the majority of recovery is complete by 3 months. Recovery occurs after 3 months, especially for higher cortical function, such as language, but at a slower pace.

In cases of motor weakness, recovery usually begins proximally and moves distally as recovery progresses. The Fluoxetine for motor recovery after acute ischaemic stroke (FLAME) study found that fluoxetine initiated within 5 to 10 days of ischemic stroke was associated with lower rates of depression and improved motor recovery.

43. What are additional considerations when stroke patients return for follow-up?

Stroke follow-up visits should address new neurologic symptoms, stroke risk factors, depression, and recovery. New neurologic symptoms may represent stroke, TIA, or seizure. Those with ongoing paralysis should be assessed for conditions that may adversely affect their recovery, including depression, spasticity, shoulder subluxation or frozen shoulder, and post-stroke pain. Complex regional pain syndrome is characterized by intermittent symptoms (cold feeling, purplish mottled skin, swelling) in the areas affected by the stroke.

The key points in the evaluation and management of ischemic stroke are summarized in Table 58.4.

Bibliography and Suggested Reading

NINDS rt-PA Stroke Study Group. (1995). Tissue plasminogen activator for acute ischemic stroke. *New England Journal of Medicine, 333*, 1581–1587.

Brott, T. G., Howard, G., Roubin, G. S., Meschia, J. F., Mackey, A., Brooks, W., et al. (2016). Long-term results of stenting versus endarterectomy for carotid-artery stenosis. *New England Journal of Medicine, 374*, 1021–1031.

Chimowitz, M. I., Lynn, M. J., Derdeyn, C. P., Turan, T. N., Fiorella, D., Lane, B. F., et al. (2011). Stenting versus aggressive medical therapy for intracranial arterial stenosis. *New England Journal of Medicine, 365*, 993–1003.

Grise, E. M., & Adeoye, O. (2012). Blood pressure control for acute ischemic and hemorrhagic stroke. *Current Opinion in Critical Care, 18*(2), 132–138. http://dx.doi.org/10.1097/MCC.0b013e3283513279.

Hacke, W., Kaste, M., Bluhmki, E., Brozman, M., Dávalos, A., Guidetti, D., et al. (2008). Thrombolysis with alteplase 3 to 4.5 hours after acute ischemic stroke. *New England Journal of Medicine, 359*, 1317–1329.

Martini, S. R., Grossman, A. W., & Kent, T. A. (2014). Stroke. In G. N. Levine (Ed.), *Color atlas of cardiovascular disease*. New Delhi: Jaypee Brothers Medical Publishers.

HEMORRHAGIC STROKE AND CEREBRAL VENOUS SINUS THROMBOSIS

CHAPTER 59

Sharyl R. Martini, Thomas A. Kent

1. **What are the most common types of stroke?**
   The most common types of stroke are ischemic and hemorrhagic; less commonly, cerebral venous sinus thrombosis (CVST) can also lead to stroke. Ischemic stroke can be due to large-vessel atherosclerosis, intrinsic small-vessel disease, and cardioembolism. The causes of hemorrhagic stroke include intracranial hemorrhage and subarachnoid hemorrhage (SAH). Hemorrhagic stroke and CVST are addressed in this chapter. Ischemic stroke and transient ischemic attack (TIA) are addressed in Chapter 58.

2. **What are the major types of hemorrhagic stroke?**
   Hemorrhagic strokes include SAH (usually due to the rupture of an aneurysm) and parenchymal intracerebral hemorrhage (ICH). Overall, approximately 6% of strokes are due to deep ICH, 3% are due to lobar ICH, and 3% are due to SAH. Although ischemic strokes are more frequent, hemorrhagic strokes have a higher morbidity and mortality. Because subdural and epidural hematomas are extra-axial, these bleeds are not considered strokes.

3. **How can you distinguish hemorrhagic from ischemic strokes?**
   Clinical clues pointing to a hemorrhagic etiology include an early diminished level of consciousness and worsening of symptoms over minutes to hours. Headache is more common in hemorrhagic stroke and is the cardinal feature of SAH. Computed tomography (CT) of the head is the most reliable way to distinguish ischemic and hemorrhagic strokes, with acute hemorrhage appearing hyperdense (Fig. 59.1).

4. **Why is the location of an intraparenchymal hemorrhage important?**
   Intraparenchymal ICHs are classified by their location: deep or subcortical ICHs are associated with uncontrolled hypertension in 60% of cases; lobar or cortical ICHs are more concerning for underlying mass, arteriovenous malformation (AVM), or cerebral amyloid angiopathy (CAA).

5. **What is the typical clinical profile of a patient with a hypertensive hemorrhage?**
   Hypertensive hemorrhages occur most frequently in patients with a history of poorly controlled hypertension. They are associated with small-vessel ischemic changes and microbleeds of the basal ganglia, deep white matter, brainstem and cerebellum. These hemorrhages can occur in the young and old and arise more frequently and at younger ages in black and Hispanic individuals.

6. **What is the typical clinical profile of a patient with cerebral amyloid angiopathy?**
   CAA is most common in elderly Caucasian individuals. It is associated with Alzheimer disease, particularly in those carrying the APOE4 allele. CAA hemorrhages have a predilection for the occipital cortex but can occur in any cortical region.

7. **How is intracerebral hemorrhage managed?**
   ICHs are managed by reversing coagulopathy, including reversal agents if the ICH is related to an anticoagulant drug. Clot evacuation for lobar ICHs and ventriculostomy in cases with hydrocephalus or intraventricular blood may be considered. Intraventricular clot lysis with tissue plasminogen activator (tPA) is being studied but has not yet proven its efficacy. High blood pressure (BP) is associated with hematoma expansion and rebleeding, so systolic BP is generally maintained below 180 mm Hg if there is no clinical deterioration. The Intensive Blood Pressure Reduction in Acute Cerebral Hemorrhage Trial (INTERACT) and Antihypertensive Treatment of Acute Cerebral Hemorrhage (ATACH) trials have found that a further lowering of systolic BP to 140 mm Hg does not improve clinical outcomes, and rapid BP lowering may be associated with kidney injury. Deep venous thrombosis (DVT) is common following

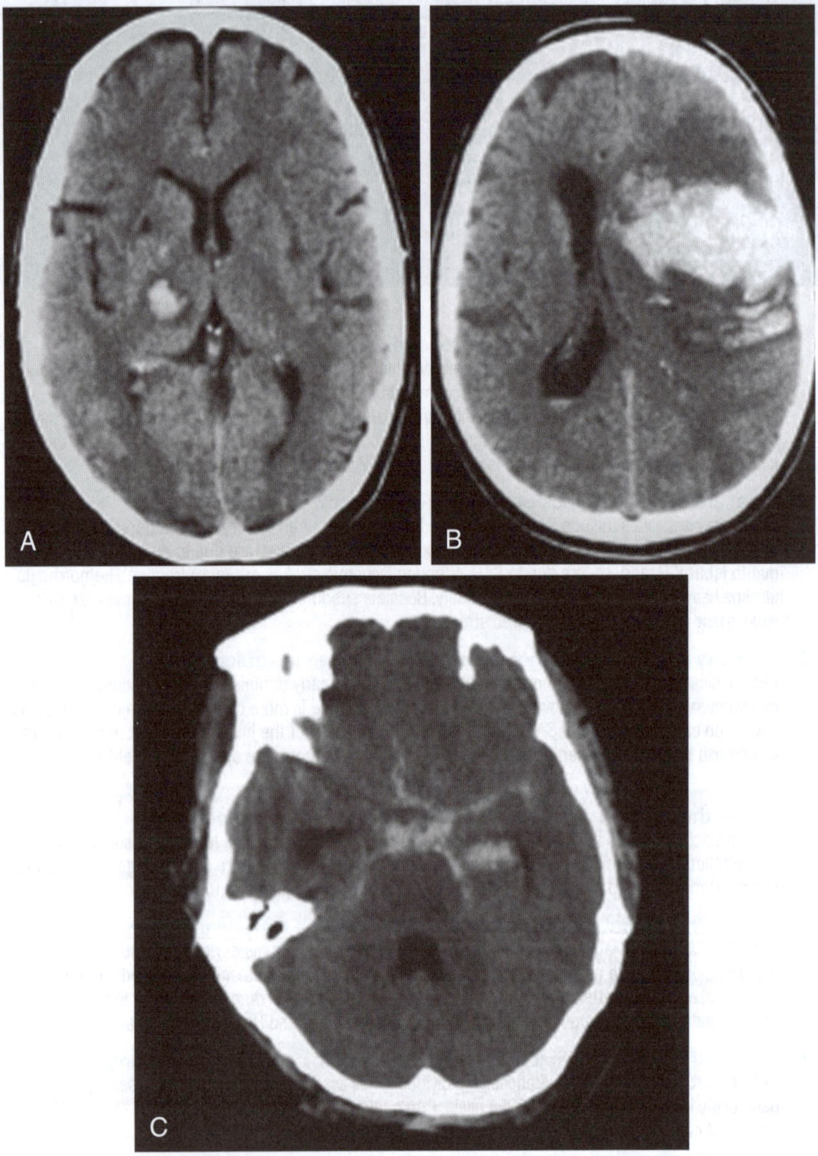

Fig. 59.1. Computed tomography (CT) of the head showing different types of hemorrhagic strokes, with the acute hemorrhage appearing hyperdense. **(A)**, small deep parenchymal intracerebral hemorrhage (ICH) typically seen with uncontrolled hyptension; **(B)**, Lobar ICH typically seen with tumor or vascular malformation; **(C)**, subarachnoid hemorrhage typically seen with ruptured berry aneurysm.

ICH with hemiplegia or bed rest; therapy with a pneumatic compression device is more effective than compression stockings alone. Some practitioners add subcutaneous heparin after 48 hours.

8. What is considered a complete workup for intracerebral hemorrhage?

The urgency and possibly extent of workup will depend on the clinical scenario: an octogenarian with Alzheimer disease and an occipital ICH may require a less etiologic workup, as would a 65-year-old

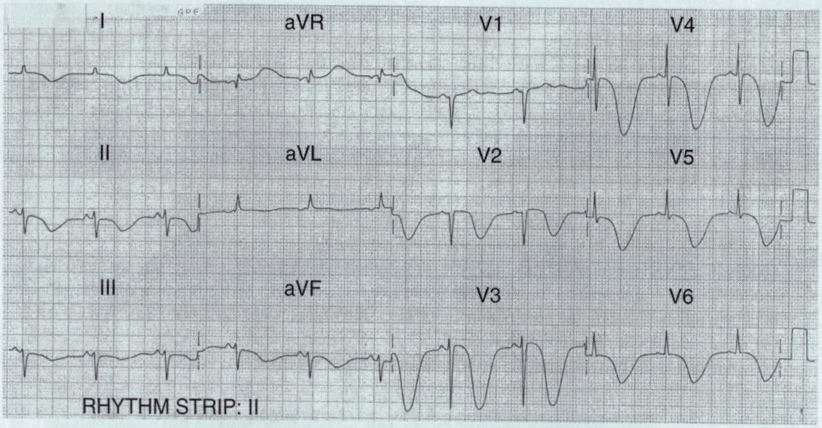

Fig. 59.2. Unusual electrocardiographic (ECG) findings (diffuse deep T-wave inversions, often with prolongation of the QT interval) in patients with hemorrhagic stroke.

with basal ganglia ICH and decades of poorly controlled hypertension. Patients who do not fit these profiles require vessel imaging to evaluate for AVMs or aneurysms and magnetic resonance imaging (MRI) with contrast to evaluate for tumors. Aneurysmal rupture can cause intraparenchymal hemorrhage; therefore it is important to consider SAH as well as CVST (see below). If the initial workup is unrevealing, repeat studies after the hematoma has resolved (2 to 3 months) may be useful.

9. What causes subarachnoid hemorrhage?

SAH is typically caused by a ruptured berry aneurysm, although subarachnoid blood may also be seen with trauma. Hypertension, larger size (especially >7 mm), and location in the posterior circulation are associated with aneurysmal rupture. Hypertension and smoking contribute to aneurysmal growth. Polycystic kidney disease and inherited connective tissue defects are also associated with intracranial aneurysms.

10. How is subarachnoid hemorrhage diagnosed?

SAH due to aneurysmal rupture classically presents with the worst headache ever; loss of consciousness, nausea/vomiting, nuchal rigidity, and focal neurologic signs are also common. Although large amounts of subarachnoid blood are readily apparent on CT, even small amounts can provoke symptoms. Detection of these small "sentinel bleeds" is vital, as they herald aneurysmal rupture. The sensitivity of CT declines over time from symptom onset, so spinal fluid should be examined for red blood cells or xanthochromia if head CT is negative and clinical suspicion high. Because of its ready availability, CT angiography for surgical planning is often performed acutely in lieu of conventional angiography.

11. How is subarachnoid hemorrhage managed?

SAH is managed by securing the aneurysm as soon as possible and monitoring for vasospasm in an intensive care unit (ICU) setting for up to 2 weeks. Vasospasm can be evaluated by transcranial Doppler or CT angiography. Cardiac arrhythmias are common following SAH. Pneumatic compression devices and a subcutaneous heparinoid (once the aneurysm is secure) are used for DVT prophylaxis.

12. What unusual electrocardiographic findings may be seen in patients with hemorrhagic stroke?

An unusual electrocardiographic (ECG) finding in such cases (as in other intracerebral processes) is cerebral t waves: diffuse deep T-wave inversions, often with prolongation of the QT interval (Fig. 59.2). This finding is likely caused by abnormalities of cardiac repolarization due to dysfunctional cerebral control of the autonomic nervous system. Importantly, the T-wave inversions should not be seen as indicative of cardiac ischemia.

13. What causes cerebral venous sinus thrombosis?

CVST is caused by clot formation in large draining veins or dural sinuses. Congenital or acquired hypercoagulable states, dehydration, and oral contraceptive use are associated with CVST.

14. How is cerebral venous sinus thrombosis diagnosed?

CVSTs usually present with continuous headache, worse in the morning or after lying down. If intracranial pressure is elevated, patients may experience impaired consciousness or blurry vision due to cerebral edema, and subsequent papilledema. Venous infarctions are frequently hemorrhagic and can result in focal neurologic signs and symptoms that do not respect typical arterial distributions. Seizures are common and may be a presenting symptom. A high index of suspicion is needed to diagnose and appropriately treat CVST, since cases may easily be missed during the course of a standard ischemic or hemorrhagic stroke workup. CVST is diagnosed with CT (Fig. 59.3) or magnetic resonance (MR) venography.

15. How is cerebral venous sinus thrombosis managed?

Venous sinus thrombosis is most commonly managed by anticoagulation, which may be counterintuitive in cases of venous infarction with hemorrhage. Other options include mechanical thrombectomy and intrasinus thrombolysis, especially if the patient's status is worsening despite anticoagulation. This is a fairly uncommon condition, so no randomized controlled trials have been performed to compare treatment strategies.

Key points for hemorrhagic stroke and CVST are given in Table 59.1.

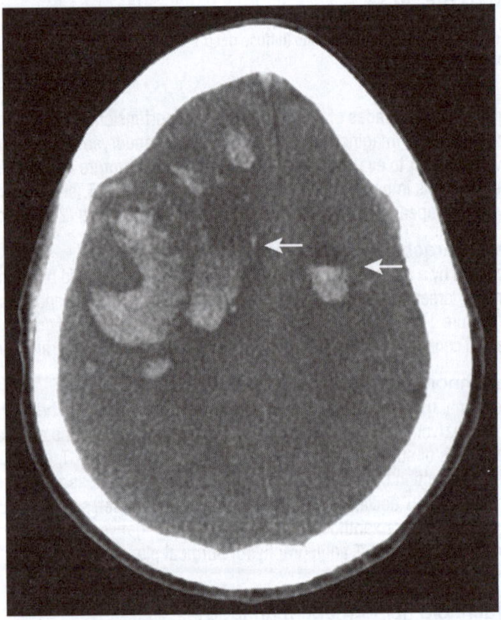

Fig. 59.3. CT scan of hemorrhages due to cerebral venous sinus thrombosis. Arrows indicate layering of red blood cells in regions where the blood has not yet clotted.

Table 59.1. Key Points for Hemorrhagic Stroke and Cerebral Venous Sinus Thrombosis

- Hemorrhagic strokes are more likely to be fatal than ischemic strokes.
- The location of a hemorrhagic stroke suggests its etiology.
  - Deep: Hypertensive etiology
  - Lobar: CAA, AVM, or tumor
  - SAH: Aneurysm rupture or trauma
- Clinically, hemorrhagic strokes present with headache, a diminished level of consciousness, and (in the case of SAH) meningeal signs.
- CVST may cause venous infarction—often hemorrhagic—which is treated with anticoagulation.

AVM, Arteriovenous malformation; *CAA*, cerebral amyloid angiopathy; *CVST*, cerebral venous sinus thrombosis; *SAH*, subarachnoid hemorrhage.

Bibliography and Suggested Readings

Caceres, J. A., & Joshua, N. Goldstein (2012). Intracranial hemorrhage. *Emergency Medicine Clinics of North America, 30*(3), 771–794.

Grise, E. M., & Adeoye, O. (2012). Blood pressure control for acute ischemic and hemorrhagic stroke. *Current Opinion in Critical Care, 18*(2), 132–138. http://dx.doi.org/10.1097/MCC.0b013e3283513279.

Martini, S. R., Grossman, A. W., & Kent, T. A. (2014). Stroke. In G. N. Levine (Ed.), *Color atlas of cardiovascular disease.* New Delhi: Jaypee Brothers Medical Publishers.

Sahni, R., & Weinberger, J. (2007). Management of intracerebral hemorrhage. *Vascular Health and Risk Management, 3*(5), 701–709.

Smith, S. D., & Eskey, C. J. (2011). Hemorrhagic stroke. *Radiologic Clinics of North America, 49*(1), 27–45. http://dx.doi.org/10.1016/j.rcl.2010.07.011.

Zaheer, A., Ozsunar, Y., & Schaefer, P. W. (2000). Magnetic resonance imaging of cerebral hemorrhagic stroke. *Topics in Magnetic Resonance Imaging, 11*(5), 288–299.

IX
Venous Thromboembolic Disease

CHAPTER 60

DEEP VEIN THROMBOSIS: PROPHYLAXIS AND TREATMENT

Geno J. Merli

1. **What three primary factors promote venous thromboembolic disease?**
   Development of venous thrombosis is promoted by the following (Virchow's triad):
   - Venous blood stasis
   - Injury to the intimal layer of the venous vasculature
   - Abnormalities in coagulation or fibrinolysis

2. **List the risk factors for thromboembolic disease.**
   The numerous risk factors for thromboembolic disease include surgery, trauma, immobility, cancer, pregnancy, prolonged immobilization, estrogen-containing oral contraceptives or hormone replacement therapy, and acute medical illnesses. A more complete listing of these risk factors is given in Table 60.1.

3. **What is the natural history of venous thrombosis?**
   Resolution of fresh thrombi occurs by endogenous fibrinolysis and organization. *Fibrinolysis* results in actual clot dissolution. *Organization* reestablishes venous blood flow by reendothelializing and incorporating into the venous wall residual clot not dissolved by fibrinolysis.

4. **Can patients with deep venous thrombosis be accurately diagnosed clinically?**
   No. The clinical diagnosis of deep venous thrombosis is neither sensitive nor specific. Less than 50% of patients with confirmed deep venous thrombosis present with the classic symptoms and signs of deep vein thrombosis (DVT), which include pain, tenderness, redness, swelling, and *Homan's sign* (calf pain with dorsiflexion of the foot). This sole use of clinical findings is artificial because clinicians

Table 60.1. Risk Factors for Deep Venous Thromboembolism

- Surgery
- Trauma (major or lower extremity)
- Immobility, lower extremity paresis
- Cancer (active or occult)
- Cancer therapy (hormonal, chemotherapy, angiogenesis inhibitors, or radiotherapy)
- Venous compression (tumor, hematoma, arterial abnormality)
- Previous history of thromboembolic disease
- Obesity
- Pregnancy and postpartum period
- Prolonged immobilization
- Lower extremity or pelvic trauma or surgery
- Surgery with greater than 30 min of general anesthesia
- Congestive heart failure
- Nephrotic syndrome
- Estrogen-containing oral contraceptives or hormone replacement therapy
- Selective estrogen receptor modulators
- Inflammatory bowel disease
- Acute medical illness
- Myeloproliferative disorders
- Paroxysmal nocturnal hemoglobinuria
- Central venous catheter
- Inherited or acquired thrombophilia
- Increasing age

couple the medical and surgical history, concomitant medical problems, medications, and risk factors to decide on further testing to confirm DVT.

5. **Where is the most common origin for thrombi that result in pulmonary emboli?**
Thrombosis in the deep veins of the lower extremities accounts for 90% to 95% of pulmonary emboli. Less common sites of origin include thrombosis in the right ventricle; in the upper extremity, prostatic, uterine, and renal veins; and, rarely, in superficial veins (Fig. 60.1).

6. **How is the diagnosis of lower extremity deep vein thrombosis confirmed?**
Diagnostic evaluation of suspected DVT includes a clear correlation among clinical probability, test selection, and test interpretation.

Contrast venography is no longer appropriate as the initial diagnostic test in patients exhibiting DVT symptoms, although it remains the gold standard for confirmatory diagnosis of DVT. It is nearly 100% sensitive and specific and provides the ability to investigate the distal and proximal venous system for thrombosis. Venography is still warranted when noninvasive testing is inconclusive or impossible to perform, but its use is no longer widespread because of the need to administer a contrast medium and the increased availability of noninvasive diagnostic strategies.

Ultrasound is safe and noninvasive and has a higher specificity than impedance plethysmography for the evaluation of suspected DVT. With color-flow Doppler and compression ultrasound, DVT is diagnosed based on the inability to compress the common femoral and popliteal veins. In patients with lower extremity symptoms, the sensitivity is 95% and specificity 96%. The diagnostic accuracy of ultrasound in asymptomatic patients, those with recurrent DVT, or those with isolated calf DVT is less reliable. The sensitivity of ultrasound improves with serial testing in untreated patients. Repeat testing at 5 to 7 days will identify another 2% of patients with clots not apparent on the first ultrasound. Serial testing can be particularly valuable in ruling out proximal extension of a possible calf DVT. Because the accuracy of ultrasound in diagnosing calf DVT is acknowledged to be lower (81% for DVT below the knee vs. 99% for proximal DVT), follow-up ultrasounds at 5 to 7 days

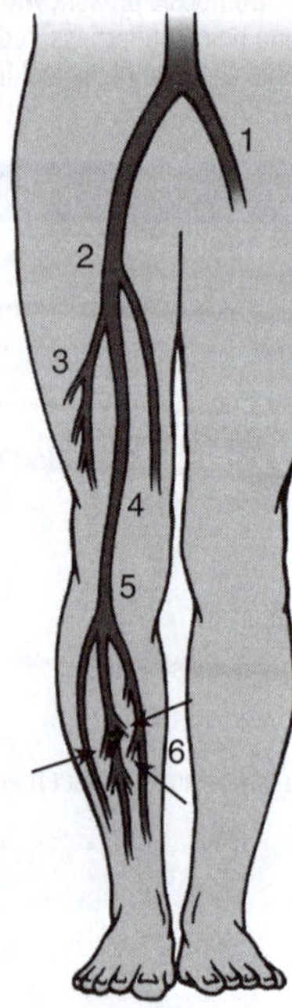

Fig. 60.1. Common sites of deep vein thrombosis (DVT) in the lower body. *1,* Left iliac vein; *2,* common femoral vein; *3,* termination of deep femoral vein (profunda femoris); *4,* femoral vein; *5,* popliteal vein at adductor canal; *6,* posterior tibial vein; *7,* intramuscular veins of calf. *(From Pfenninger, J. L., & Fowler, G. C. [2010].* Pfenninger and Fowler's procedures of primary care *[3rd ed.]. Philadelphia, PA: Saunders.)*

are reasonable, because most calf DVTs that extend proximally will do so within days of the initial presentation (Fig. 60.2).

7. When should prophylaxis of deep venous thrombosis be considered?

Two factors must be weighed in deciding to initiate prophylaxis of deep venous thrombosis: the degree of risk for thrombosis and the risk of prophylaxis. The risk factors for deep venous thrombosis are cumulative. The primary risk of pharmacologic prophylaxis is hemorrhage, which is generally uncommon if no coagulation defects or lesions with bleeding potential exist.

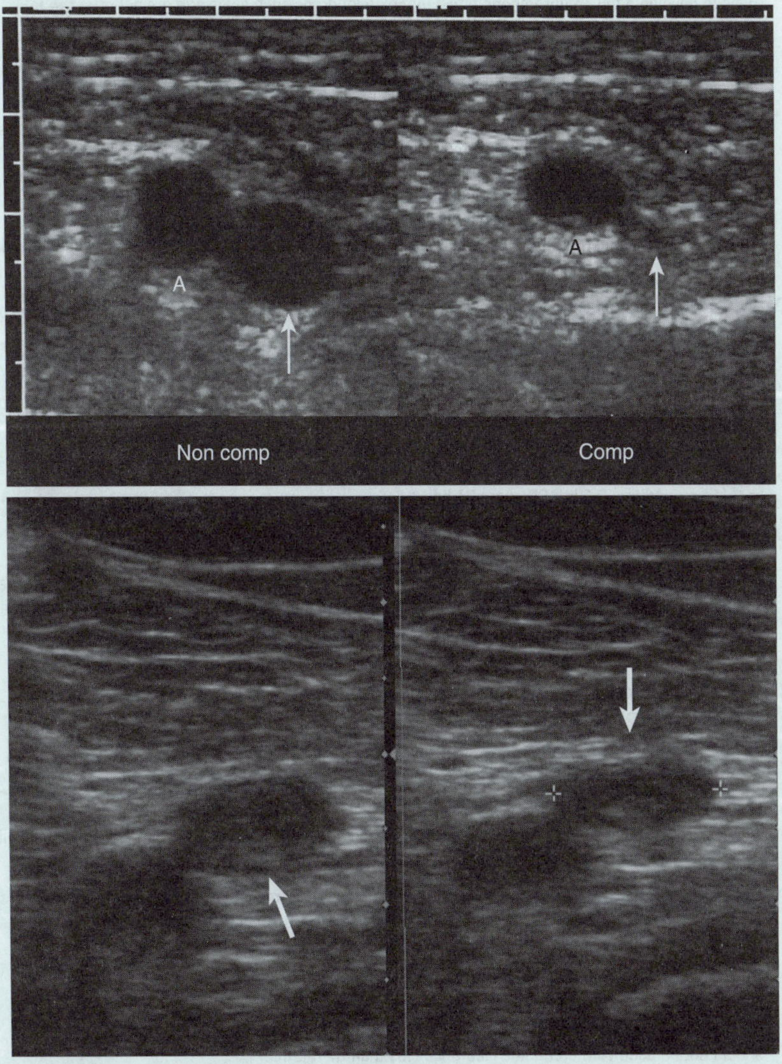

Fig. 60.2. Normal and abnormal compression of the femoral vein with ultrasound examination. *Top images:* Transverse image of the femoral artery (A) and vein *(thin white arrow)* before *(Non Comp)* and after *(Comp)* compression with the sonographic transducer, demonstrated normal vein collapse with compression. *Bottom images:* There is minimal compression of the common femoral vein *(thick white arrow)* in this patient with DVT. *(Top images from Rumack, C. M., Wilson, S. R., Charboneau, J. W., & Levine, D. [2010].* Diagnostic ultrasound *[4th ed.]. Philadelphia, PA: Mosby. Bottom images from Mason, R. J., Broaddus, V. C., Martin, T., King, T. E., Schraufnagel, D., Murray, J. F., et al. [2010].* Murray and Nadel's textbook of respiratory medicine *[5th ed.]. Philadelphia, PA: Saunders.)*

8. What prophylactic measures are available?

Approaches to prophylaxis of DVT include antithrombotic drugs and pneumatic-compressive devices. Heparin, low-molecular-weight heparin (LMWH), fondaparinux, and warfarin are effective in preventing DVT. Subcutaneous heparin has been the mainstay of DVT prophylaxis with efficacy in multiple surgical and medical scenarios. The LMWHs have been shown to be as effective or superior to unfractionated heparin in different clinical circumstances. Warfarin dosing to maintain an international normalized ratio (INR) between 2 and 3 also poses a low risk of bleeding and is effective in patients with total hip arthroplasty, total knee arthroplasty, and hip fracture surgery. However, warfarin takes several days to develop a full antithrombotic effect. Antiplatelet drugs such as aspirin are not effective in DVT prophylaxis in the general medical population, but aspirin has been used with efficacy in the orthopedic surgery population.

The two factor Xa inhibitors, rivaroxaban and apixaban, have been approved for venous thromboembolic (VTE) prophylaxis in total hip and knee arthroplasty, while the factor IIa inhibitor dabigatran has received approval only for VTE prophylaxis in total hip arthroplasty.

Intermittent pneumatic-compressive devices effect prophylaxis by maintaining venous flow in the lower extremities and are especially efficacious in patients who cannot receive anticoagulant medications. Modalities available include compressive devices applied to the feet alone, covering the calves, or extending to the thighs. No version has been shown to provide superior prophylaxis. There has been concern that compression stockings used for prophylaxis may cause unintended skin trauma without substantial benefit.

9. What is the approach to deep vein thrombosis prophylaxis in the hospitalized, medically ill patient?

The acutely ill medical patient admitted to the hospital with congestive heart failure or severe respiratory disease or who is confined to bed and has one or more additional risk factors (including active cancer, previous VTE, sepsis, acute neurologic disease, or inflammatory bowel disease) should receive DVT prophylaxis with the following agents:

- Unfractionated heparin: 5000 U subcutaneously (SC) every 8 or 12 hours
- LMWH: Dalteparin 5000 IU SC every 24 hours or enoxaparin 40 mg SC every 24 hours
- Fondaparinux: 2.5 mg SC every 24 hours

10. Should patients undergoing surgery receive deep vein thrombosis prophylaxis based on specific recommendations for each respective procedure?

Yes. Most surgical procedures have defined recommendations for preventing DVT in the postoperative period if age and other clinical comorbidities demonstrate an elevated risk based upon risk assessment models such as that of the Rogers or Caprini score. The various prophylaxis regimens for different surgical procedures are listed in Table 60.2.

11. Are there specific surgical groups that require extended deep vein thrombosis prophylaxis following hospital discharge?

- For a patient undergoing total hip replacement, total knee replacement, and hip fracture surgery, extended DVT prophylaxis is recommended for up to 35 days after surgery with LMWH, unfractionated heparin, fondaparinux, warfarin, rivaroxaban, apixaban, dabigatran, or acetylsalicylic acid (ASA).
- For selected high-risk general surgery patients undergoing major cancer surgery or who have previously had venous thromboembolism, it is recommended that DVT prophylaxis be continued with LMWH: enoxaparin 40 mg SC every 24 hours or dalteparin 5000 IU SC every 24 hours for 35 days.

12. What treatment regimens are available for the treatment of deep vein thrombosis?

Several treatment regimens using unfractionated heparin (UFH), an LMWH, or a direct oral anticoagulant (DOAC) are available for the treatment of DVT. These are listed in Table 60.3.

13. Which low-molecular-weight heparins are renally excreted?

All the LMWHs are renally excreted. Enoxaparin is the only LMWH that has a recommended dose for creatinine clearance less than 30 mL/min (1 mg/kg SC every 24 hours). All other LMWHs listed here should not be used with creatinine clearance less than 30 mL/min.

14. When should warfarin be started in the treatment regimens for deep vein thrombosis listed earlier?

Older dosing protocols proposed a delay in warfarin administration, but this only prolongs the therapeutic onset of warfarin and may extend the hospitalization. Given the long period until therapeutic benefit, warfarin should be given on the first day of treatment with UFH or an LMWH

Table 60.2. Deep Vein Thrombosis Prophylaxis Regimens for Various Surgeries

General/Urologic/Gastrointestinal/Gynecologic/Bariatric/Vascular/Plastic/ Reconstructive Surgery

The following regimens are for patients undergoing major surgical procedures for benign or malignant disease and associated DVT risk factors:

- Unfractionated heparin: 5000 U SC q8h
- LMWH: Enoxaparin 40 mg SC q24h, dalteparin 5000 IU SC q24h
- External pneumatic compression sleeves plus one of the above regimens
- Fondaparinux 2.5 mg SC q24h can be considered for patients with a history of heparin-associated thrombocytopenia.
- Roux-en-Y gastric bypass: BMI <50 kg/m^2 40 mg SC q12h,BMI >50 kg/m^2 60 mg SC q12h

Orthopedic Surgery

The following regimens are for patients undergoing orthopedic surgery:

Total Hip/Knee Surgery

- LMWH: Enoxaparin SC 40 mg qday as dose option, enoxaparin 30 mg SC q12h, dalteparin 5000 IU SC q24h
- Unfractionated heparin: 5000 U SC q8h
- Fondaparinux 2.5 mg SC q24h
- Rivaroxaban 10 mg q24h

Dabigatran 220 mg every 24 h (initiation of first dose 24 h postoperatively)—approved in the United States only for total hip arthroplasty

- Aspirin (optimal dosing not universally agreed upon)
- Warfarin 5 mg on the evening of surgery, then adjust dose to achieve an INR of 2 to 3
- Intermittent pneumatic compression devices

Hip Fracture

- LMWH: Enoxaparin 40 mg SC qday as dose option, enoxaparin 30 mg SC q12h, dalteparin 5000 IU SC q24h
- Unfractionated heparin: 5000 U SC q8h
- Fondaparinux 2.5 mg SC q24h
- Aspirin (optimal dosing not universally agreed upon)
- Warfarin 5 mg on the evening of surgery, then adjust dose to achieve an INR of 2 to 3
- Intermittent pneumatic compression devices

Neurosurgery

The following regimens are for patients undergoing neurosurgery:

- External pneumatic compression sleeves are the prophylaxis of choice.
- Combination therapy with either unfractionated heparin (5000 U SC q8h or q12h) or LMWH (enoxaparin 40 mg SC q24h) can be used,

Coronary Artery Bypass Surgery

The following regimens are for patients undergoing coronary artery bypass surgery:

- LMWH (preferred over unfractionated heparin): enoxaparin 40 mg SC q24h or dalteparin 5000 IU SC q24h
- Unfractionated heparin: 5000 U SC q8h
- Fondaparinux 2.5 mg SC q24h for patients with history of heparin-induced thrombocytopenia
- External pneumatic compression sleeves for high-bleeding-risk patients

DVT, Deep vein thrombosis; *INR*, international normalized ratio; *LMWH*, low-molecular-weight heparin.

to minimize the period of bridging anticoagulation. Warfarin dosing need not wait until the day of discharge, as this may mean costly bridging therapy for the patient as an outpatient. The usual dose is 5 to 10 mg daily.

15. **Can the international normalized ratio in patients treated with warfarin be influenced by food and drug intake?**

Yes. Warfarin is influenced by numerous medications and dietary components. INR monitoring must be vigilant when medication and dietary changes occur. Foods rich in vitamin K, such as leafy green

Table 60.3. Regimens for the Treatment of Deep Vein Thrombosis

Unfractionated Heparin
• Administer intravenous bolus of UFH (80 U/kg or 5000 U) followed by continuous infusion of 18 U/kg per hour or 1300 U/h. The activated partial thromboplastin time (APTT) is checked q6h to adjust the infusion to achieve the therapeutic aPTT of the hospital laboratory.
• Subcutaneous UFH at 333 U/kg is the initial dose, followed in 12 h by 250 U/kg SC q12h. Monitoring of the APTT is not necessary.
Low-Molecular-Weight Heparin
• Enoxaparin 1 mg/kg SC q12 h or 1.5 mg/kg SC q24h
• Dalteparin 200 IU/kg SC q24h
• Tinzaparin 175 IU/kg SC q24h
Fondaparinux
• Fondaparinux dosed by weight range: Less than 50 kg, 5 mg SC; 50 to 100 kg, 7.5 mg SC q24h; more than 100 kg, 10 mg SC q24h
Oral Anti-Xa Inhibitors
• Rivaroxaban 15 mg q12h for 21 days; then 20 mg/d to complete 3 or 6 months of treatment
• Apixaban 10 mg q12h for 7 days; then 5 mg q12h to complete 3 to 6 months of treatment
• Edoxaban: This agent is initiated only after 5 to 10 days of therapeutic LMWH or IV UFH at the following schedule: 60 mg q24h for 3 to 6 months. Do not use this agent if the creatinine clearance is greater than 95 mL/min.
Oral Anti-IIa Inhibitor
• Dabigatran 150 mg q12h for 3 to 6 months. This agent is initiated only after 5 to 10 days of therapeutic LMWH or IV UFH at the following schedule: 150 mg q12h for 3 to 6 months.

aPTT, Activated partial thromboplastin time.

vegetables, will lower the INR level and diminish the anticoagulant effect of warfarin. Medications such as erythromycin and phenytoin may increase the serum concentration of warfarin, which can increase bleeding risk. Substances such as ginkgo biloba and cranberry juice may also increase the risk of bleeding in combination with warfarin. A full medication inventory including that of supplements is essential to reducing complications associated with the use of vitamin K antagonists (VKAs). Antiplatelet agents have an anticoagulant effect that enhances the bleeding risk associated with warfarin use.

16. When should these therapeutic regimens for treating deep vein thrombosis be discontinued and warfarin remain as the sole therapy?

These therapies must be used for at least 5 days and until the INR is between 2 and 3 for 2 consecutive days.

17. What is the target international normalized ratio for treating patients with deep vein thrombosis?

The target INR for the treatment of DVT to prevent recurrent disease is 2 to 3.

18. How long should patients with acute deep vein thrombosis be treated with warfarin?

For patients with DVT secondary to a transient risk factor, 3 months of warfarin is appropriate. Unprovoked (previously called "idiopathic") proximal DVT in patients without risk factors for bleeding should receive long-term warfarin therapy with a target INR of 2 to 3. Patients with DVT and cancer should receive LMWH for 3 to 6 months as the initial approach to management and long-term treatment with either warfarin or LMWH until the cancer is resolved or in remission.

19. Does thrombosis of the great saphenous vein usually require full-dose anticoagulation?

The great saphenous vein is a superficial vein, not a deep vein. Full-dose anticoagulation is usually not required if the area of superficial phlebitis is not near the common femoral junction. The American College of Chest Physicians (ACCP) has recommended that greater saphenous vein thrombosis that is greater than 5 cm in length should receive treatment with fondaparinux 2.5 mg daily, enoxaparin 40 mg daily, or dalteparin 5000 U daily for 6 weeks.

20. What is the currently preferred name for the superficial femoral vein?

The *femoral vein.* The superficial femoral vein has been reclassified as the femoral vein because of how often with its former name it was mistakenly thought to be a superficial vein.

21. When can patients with acute deep vein thrombosis ambulate?

Patients can ambulate with acute DVT and should not be placed on bed rest unless the lower extremity is painful and cannot bear weight.

22. Can patients with acute deep vein thrombosis be treated as outpatients?

Yes. The LMWH and DOAC regimens listed here can be used to treat patients in the outpatient setting. The same principles of management should be followed using these agents as with inpatient treatment.

23. When should catheter-directed thrombolysis be used to treat acute deep vein thrombosis?

In selected patients with extensive acute proximal iliofemoral DVT where symptoms have been present for less than 14 days—patients who are functionally active and who have a low bleeding risk—the use of pharmacomechanical thrombolysis is recommended if the appropriate expertise and resources are available.

24. Are inferior vena caval filters indicated for the initial treatment of acute deep vein thrombosis?

No. Vena caval filters are indicated when the patient cannot receive anticoagulation for the treatment of acute DVT. In certain cases (temporary contraindication to anticoagulant therapy), retrievable vena caval filters have been placed, with the intention of removing them within a defined time (based on the specific filter), after which anticoagulation therapy could be reinstituted.

25. When are gradient elastic stockings recommended as part of the treatment of acute deep vein thrombosis?

For patients with symptomatic DVT the use of gradient elastic stockings with an ankle pressure of 30 to 40 mm Hg is recommended. The pressure may not be tolerated because of the degree of lower extremity edema. Elastic bandages may be used because they can be adjusted to control swelling and the pain associated with increased external pressure. The elastic bandages can be used initially, but as the swelling recedes, gradient elastic stockings at 20 to 30 or 30 to 40 mm Hg may be applied.

26. When is a low-intensity international normalized ratio indicated for the treatment of deep vein thrombosis?

For patients with idiopathic (unprovoked) DVT who have a strong preference for less frequent INR testing to monitor their therapy, it is recommended that after the first 3 months of therapy low-intensity therapy at an INR of 1.5 to 1.9 with less frequent INR monitoring be employed instead of stopping warfarin anticoagulation.

27. Can direct oral anticoagulants be used for extended treatment of deep vein thrombosis?

Yes. The following DOACs have been approved for extended treatment of DVT after the initial 3 to 6 months of therapy:

- Rivaroxaban 20 mg every day
- Apixaban 2.5 mg every 12 hours
- Dabigatran 150 mg every 12 hours

Recommendations on short- and long-term DVT treatment from the ACCP are summarized in Table 60.4.

28. Should compression ultrasound be used at the time of discharge as routine screening in the patient who has undergone total joint replacement surgery?

Asymptomatic patients who have undergone joint replacement surgery should not have compression ultrasound on discharge as a screening test for DVT because the ultrasound is not as sensitive and specific in asymptomatic patients. Appropriate DVT prophylaxis should be the approach to management.

Table 60.4. Summary of the 2016 American College of Clinical Pharmacy Recommendations on Antithrombotic Therapy for Venous Thromboembolism

Choice of Long-Term (First 3 Months) and Extended (No Scheduled Stop Date) Anticoagulant Treatment

- In patients with proximal DVT or PE, we recommend long-term (3-month) anticoagulant therapy over no such therapy.
- In patients with DVT of the leg and no cancer, we suggest dabigatran, rivaroxaban, apixaban, or edoxaban as long-term (first 3 months) anticoagulant therapy over VKA therapy.
- For patients with DVT of the leg or PE and no cancer who are not treated with dabigatran, rivaroxaban, apixaban, or edoxaban, we suggest VKA therapy over LMWH.
- In patients with DVT of the leg or PE and cancer ("cancer-associated thrombosis"), we suggest LMWH as long-term (first 3 months) anticoagulant therapy over VKA therapy, dabigatran, rivaroxaban, apixaban, or edoxaban.
- In patients with DVT of the leg or PE who receive extended therapy, we suggest that there is no need to change the choice of anticoagulant after the first 3 months.

Duration of Anticoagulant Therapy

- In patients with a proximal DVT of the leg or PE provoked by surgery, we recommend treatment with anticoagulation for 3 months over (i) treatment for a shorter period (grade 1B), (ii) treatment for a longer time-limited period (e.g., 6, 12, or 24 months), or (iii) extended therapy (no scheduled stop date).
- In patients with a proximal DVT of the leg or PE provoked by a nonsurgical transient risk factor, we recommend treatment with anticoagulation for 3 months over (i) treatment for a shorter period (grade 1B) or (ii) treatment for a longer time-limited period (e.g., 6, 12, or 24 months) (grade 1B). We suggest treatment with anticoagulation for 3 months over extended therapy if there is a low or moderate bleeding risk (grade 2B) and recommend treatment for 3 months over extended therapy if there is a high risk of bleeding.
- In patients with an isolated distal DVT of the leg provoked by surgery or by a nonsurgical transient risk factor, we suggest treatment with anticoagulation for 3 months over treatment for a shorter period (grade 2C). We recommend treatment with anticoagulation for 3 months over treatment for a longer time-limited period (e.g., 6, 12, or 24 months) (grade 1B), and we recommend treatment with anticoagulation for 3 months over extended therapy (no scheduled stop date).
- In patients with an unprovoked DVT of the leg (isolated distal or proximal) or PE, we recommend treatment with anticoagulation for at least 3 months over treatment for a shorter period (grade 1B), and we recommend treatment with anticoagulation for 3 months over treatment of a longer time-limited period (e.g., 6, 12, or 24 months).
- In patients with a first VTE that is an unprovoked proximal DVT of the leg or PE and who have a (i) low or moderate bleeding risk (see the text), we suggest extended anticoagulant therapy (no scheduled stop date) for 3 months (grade 2B). For patients with a (ii) high bleeding risk (see the text), we recommend 3 months of anticoagulant therapy over extended therapy (no scheduled stop date).
- For patients with a second unprovoked VTE who have a (i) low bleeding risk (see the text), we recommend extended anticoagulant therapy (no scheduled stop date) for 3 months (grade 1B); for those with a (ii) moderate bleeding risk (see the text), we suggest extended anticoagulant therapy for 3 months (grade 2B); and for patients with a (iii) high bleeding risk (see the text), we suggest 3 months of anticoagulant therapy over extended therapy (no scheduled stop date).
- For patients with DVT of the leg or PE and active cancer ("cancer-associated thrombosis") who (i) do not have a high bleeding risk, we recommend extended anticoagulant therapy (no scheduled stop date) over 3 months (grade 1B) or those who (ii) have a high bleeding risk, we suggest extended anticoagulant therapy (no scheduled stop date) for 3 months.

DVT, Deep vein thrombosis; *LMWH*, low-molecular-weight heparin; *PE*, pulmonary embolism; *VKA*, vitamin K antagonist; *VTE*, venous thromboembolic.

Adapted from Kearon, C., Akl, E. A., Ornelas, J., Blaivas, A., Jimenez, D., Bounameaux, H., et al. (2016). Antithrombotic therapy for VTE disease CHEST guideline and expert panel report. Chest, *149(2),315–352.*

Bibliography, Suggested Readings, and Websites

British Thoracic Society Standards of Care Committee Pulmonary Embolism Guideline Development Group. (2003). British Thoracic Society guidelines for the management of suspected acute pulmonary embolism. *Thorax*, *58*(6), 470–483.

Decousus, H., Leizorovicz, A., Parent, F., Page, Y., Tardy, B., Girard, P., et al. (1998). A clinical trial of vena caval filters in the prevention of pulmonary embolism in patients with proximal deep-vein thrombosis. *New England Journal of Medicine*, *338*, 409–415.

Falck-Ytter, Y., Francis, C. W., Johanson, N. A., Curley, C., Dahl, O. E., Schulman, S., et al. (2012). Prevention of VTE in orthopedic surgery patients: antithrombotic therapy and prevention of thrombosis, 9th ed: American College of Chest Physicians evidence-based clinical practice guidelines. *Chest*, *141*(Suppl. 2), e278S–e325S.

Gould, M. K., Garcia, D. A., Wren, S. M., Karanicolas, P. J., Arcelus, J. I., Heit, J. A., et al. (2012). Prevention of VTE in non-orthopedic surgical patients: antithrombotic therapy and prevention of thrombosis, 9th ed: American College of Chest Physicians evidence-based clinical practice guidelines. *Chest*, *141*(Suppl. 2), e227S–e277S.

Kahn, S. R., Lim, W., Dunn, A. S., Cushman, M., Dentali, F., Akl, E. A., et al. (2012). Prevention of VTE in nonsurgical patients: antithrombotic therapy and prevention of thrombosis, 9th ed: American College of Chest Physicians evidence-based clinical practice guidelines. *Chest*, *141*(Suppl. 2), e195S–e226S.

Kearon, C., Akl, E. A., Ornelas, J., Blaivas, A., Jimenez, D., Bounameaux, H., et al. (2016). Antithrombotic therapy for VTE disease CHEST guideline and expert panel report. *Chest*, *149*(2), 315–352.

Kearon, C., Ginsberg, J. S., Julian, J. A., Douketis, J., Solymoss, S., Ockelford, P., et al. (2006). Comparison of fixed-dose weight adjusted unfractionated heparin and low-molecular-weight heparin for acute treatment of venous thromboembolism. *Journal of the American Medical Association*, *296*, 935–942.

Koopman, M. M., Prandoni, P., Piovella, F., Ockelford, P. A., Brandjes, D. P., van der Meer, J., et al. (1996). Treatment of venous thrombosis with intravenous unfractionated heparin administered in the hospital as compared with subcutaneous low-molecular-weight heparin administered at home. *New England Journal of Medicine*, *334*, 682–687.

Levine, M., Gent, M., Hirsh, J., Leclerc, J., Anderson, D., Weitz, J., et al. (1996). A comparison of low-molecular-weight heparin administered primarily at home with unfractionated heparin administered in the hospital for proximal deep vein thrombosis. *New England Journal of Medicine*, *334*, 677–681.

Mechanick, J. I., Youdim, A., Jones, D., et al. (2013). Clinical practice guidelines for the perioperative nutritional, metabolic, and nonsurgical support of the bariatric patient—2013 update. *Obesity, 21*(Suppl.), S1–S27.

Merli, G. J. (2008). Pathophysiology of venous thrombosis and the diagnosis of deep vein thrombosis-pulmonary embolism in the elderly. *Cardiology Clinics*, *26*, 203–219.

Merli, G., Spiro, T., Olsson, C. G., Abildgaard, U., Davidson, B. L., Eldor, A., et al. (2001). Subcutaneous enoxaparin once or twice daily compared with intravenous unfractionated heparin for treatment of venous thromboembolic disease. *Annals of Internal Medicine*, *134*, 191–202.

Nicolaides, A. N., Fareed, J., Kakkar, A. K., & Breddin, H. K. (2006). Prevention and treatment of venous thromboembolism. International consensus statement (guidelines according to scientific evidence). *International Angiology*, *25*(2), 101–161.

Snow, V., Qaseem, A., Barry, P., Hornbake, E. R., Rodnick, J. E., Tobolic, T., et al. (2007). Management of venous thromboembolism: a clinical practice guideline from the American College of Physicians and the American Academy of Family Physicians. *Annals of Internal Medicine*, *146*(3), 204–210.

The Matisse Investigators. (2003). Subcutaneous fondaparinux versus intravenous unfractionated heparin in the initial treatment of pulmonary embolism. *New England Journal of Medicine*, *349*, 1695–1702.

Wells, P. S., Anderson, D. R., Rodger, M. A., Forgie, M. A., Florack, P., Touchie, D., et al. (2005). A randomized trial comparing two low-molecular-weight heparins for the outpatient treatment of deep vein thrombosis and pulmonary embolism. *Archives of Internal Medicine*, *165*, 733–738.

CHAPTER 61

PULMONARY EMBOLISM

A. Weinberg, V. F. Tapson

1. **Who first described pulmonary embolism?**
Pulmonary embolism (PE) was probably first reported in the early 1800s clinically, but Rudolf Virchow elucidated the mechanism by describing the connection between venous thrombosis and PE in the late 1800s. He also coined the term *embolism*.

2. **How common are pulmonary emboli, and what is the mortality rate?**
Venous thromboembolic (VTE) disease is a common condition with an estimated incidence of 900,000 individuals in the United States and over 700,000 cases in France, Italy, Germany, Spain, Sweden, and the United Kingdom combined each year. Pulmonary emboli are associated with substantial mortality, resulting in at least 100,000 annual deaths in the United States per year, with 10% to 30% of patients dying within the first month of diagnosis.

3. **What is Virchow's triad?**
These are the three broad categories of risk factors that contribute to thrombosis:
   - Endothelial injury
   - Stasis or turbulence of blood flow
   - Blood hypercoagulability

4. **What percentage of patients with acute pulmonary embolism have clinical evidence of deep venous thrombosis in a lower extremity?**
In the Prospective Investigation of Pulmonary Embolism Diagnosis (PIOPED II) study of 192 patients with angiographically documented PE, 47% had evidence of deep venous thrombosis (DVT) by physical examination. The majority of patients with proven PE do have residual DVT present as proven by imaging. More than 90% of emboli originate in the deep veins of the legs and thighs.

5. **What percentage of patients with proximal deep venous thrombosis will develop pulmonary embolism?**
Approximately 50%.

6. **What is the usual cause of death in patients with pulmonary embolism?**
It is well established that right ventricular (RV) failure is the cause of cardiovascular collapse and death in acute massive PE. Registry data have also suggested that patients with RV dysfunction on echocardiography are at increased risk of all-cause mortality at 3 months.

7. **What are the major risk factors for venous thromboembolism?**
Risk factors are crucial in raising suspicion for acute VTE, although the disease may be idiopathic. Previous thromboembolism, immobility, cancer, advanced age, major surgery, trauma, acute medical illness, and certain thrombophilias impart significant risk. A list of risk factors is shown in Table 61.1.

8. **What are the symptoms and signs of acute pulmonary embolism?**
The symptoms and signs of PE are generally nonspecific but most commonly include dyspnea and chest pain. The most common symptoms were identified from the PIOPED II study. These symptoms and their frequency are given in Table 61.2.

9. **If pulmonary embolism is associated with the development of pulmonary hypertension, what additional physical findings may be noted?**
If PE is associated with pulmonary hypertension, elevated neck veins in addition to the physical findings rarely, one or more bruits may be heard over the lung fields.(Table 61.2)

Table 61.1. Risk Factors for Venous Thromboembolism

HEREDITARY	ACQUIRED	PROBABLE OR UNCERTAIN
• Antithrombin deficiency • Protein C deficiency • Protein S deficiency • Factor V Leiden • Activated protein C resistance without factor V Leiden • Prothrombin gene mutation • Dysfibrinogenemia • Plasminogen deficiency • Elevated factor VIII level	• Reduced mobility • Advanced age • Active cancer • Acute medical illness • Nephrotic syndrome • Major surgery • Trauma • Spinal cord injury • Pregnancy/postpartum period • Myeloproliferative disorders: polycythemia vera • Antiphospholipid antibody syndrome • Oral contraceptives • Hormonal replacement therapy • Chemotherapy • Obesity • Central venous catheters • Immobilizer/cast	• Low tissue factor pathway inhibitor levels • Elevated levels of the following: ◦ Homocysteine ◦ Factors VIII, IX, XI ◦ Fibrinogen ◦ Thrombin-activatable fibrinolysis inhibitor ◦ Lipoprotein (a)

The hereditary versus acquired nature of some disorders listed remains unclear, and causes may involve both genetic and environmental factors.

Table 61.2. Frequency of Symptoms and Physical Findings in Pulmonary Embolism

SYMPTOM/PHYSICAL FINDING	FREQUENCY
Dyspnea with rest or exertion (either sudden in onset or evolving over days)	73%
Chest pain (often pleuritic)	44%
Cough	37%
Hemoptysis	13%
Palpitations	*
Lightheadedness	*
Orthopnea	28%
Syncope	<10%
Tachypnea	54%
Tachycardia	24%
Pleural rub	<10%
Fever	3%
Wheezing	21%
Rales	18%

Data derived from the Prospective Investigation of Pulmonary Embolism Diagnosis II (PIOPED II) study.

*First PIOPED study data palpitations = 10%, lightheadedness = 15% (from PIOPED I study). *From the PIOPED Investigators [1990]. Value of the ventilation/perfusion scan in acute pulmonary embolism: results of the Prospective Investigation of Pulmonary Embolism Diagnosis [PIOPED].* Journal of the American Medical Association, 263, *2753–2759.*

10. What are four clinical syndromes sometimes (or that can be) seen with acute pulmonary embolism?

- **Massive pulmonary/acute cor pulmonale:** Not all patients with acute cor pulmonale will go on to develop hypotension (which defines massive PE), but such a presentation should raise concern.
- **Submassive PE:** This is defined as acute PE that causes RV dysfunction and can be suggested by either elevated troponin, elevated B-type natriuretic peptide (BNP), or direct visualization using echocardiography. Of note, based on the Pulmonary Embolism Severity Index, low- and intermediate-risk categories have been referred to as "nonmassive PE."
- **Pulmonary infarction/pulmonary hemorrhage:** Because of the dual blood supply and free anastomoses between the pulmonary capillaries, emboli usually do not cause infarction in a healthy lung. Pulmonary infarction is uncommon when emboli obstruct central arteries but much more common when distal arteries are occluded. Obstruction of distal arteries can result in pulmonary hemorrhage as a result of an influx of bronchial arterial blood at systemic pressure. Hemorrhage causes symptoms and radiographic changes usually attributed to pulmonary infarction.
- **Acute unexplained dyspnea:** A diagnosis of PE should be considered in patients with dyspnea of unclear cause and may merit consideration even when there is another potential explanation, as in the case of patients with chronic obstructive pulmonary disease (COPD).

11. What is the Wells score for suspected acute pulmonary embolism?

First described in 1998, the Wells score is a clinical prediction score based on simple noninvasive clinical parameters. It has evolved over the years, has been validated, and is useful in determining the pretest probability of suspected acute PE. Pretest probability can be defined based on the calculated score from the modified Wells score (Table 61.3). PE has ultimately been classified as "unlikely" if the

Table 61.3. The Modified Wells Pretest Probability Scoring of Pulmonary Embolism—Point Score

Score Assignment	
VARIABLE	**SCORE**
• PE is likely or more likely than alternate diagnosis	3.0
• Clinical signs or symptoms of DVT	3.0
• Heart rate 100 beats per minute	1.5
• Prior DVT or PE	1.5
• Immobilization, limited to bed rest for >3 days	1.5
• Surgery within the past 4 weeks	1.5
• Hemoptysis	1.0
• Active malignancy	1.0
Modified Wells Pretest Probability Assessment (Use with V/Q Study)	
SCORE	**PRETEST PROBABILITY**
Score <2	Low probability
Score 2-6	Intermediate probability
Score ≥6	High probability
Dichotomized Wells Pretest Probability Assessment (Use with CT Angiography)	
SCORE	**PRETEST PROBABILITY**
Score ≤4	PE unlikely
Score >4	PE likely

CT, Computed tomography; *DVT*, deep venous thrombosis; *PE*, pulmonary embolism; *V/Q*, ventilation/perfusion.

clinical decision score was 4 or less and "likely" with a score of more than 4 points. This cutoff was chosen because it has been shown to give an acceptable VTE diagnostic failure rate of 1.7% to 2.2% in combination with a normal D-dimer test. Moreover, with a score of 4 or less and a negative D-dimer test, no further testing appears to be necessary. A score greater than 4 requires further evaluation, and computed tomographic angiography (CTA) is usually performed. High clinical suspicion, however, should always take precedence, even if the Wells score is low.

12. What are the most common findings on electrocardiography in acute pulmonary embolism?

Sinus tachycardia is commonly present in acute PE. The "classic" S1Q3T3 pattern (Fig. 61.1) is seen in a minority of patients. Other ECG findings include the following:

- Arrhythmias (premature atrial and ventricular beats)
- First-degree atrioventricular block
- Supraventricular tachycardia
- RV strain (right axis deviation)
- RV hypertrophy
- Right bundle branch block
- Depression, elevation, or inversion of ST segments and T waves

ST-T changes, when present, are often most marked in the right precordial leads. Although the ECG may be suggestive of PE, it cannot diagnose or rule out acute PE.

13. What are the common chest radiographic findings in patients with acute pulmonary embolism?

The chest radiograph is commonly abnormal in acute PE, although a significant minority of patients have a normal film. When it is abnormal, however, the findings are nonspecific and include an elevated hemidiaphragm, focal or multifocal infiltrates, pleural effusion, plate-like atelectasis, enlarged pulmonary arteries, focal oligemia (Westermark's sign), and RV enlargement.

Hampton and Castleman described in detail the radiographic findings in PE and pulmonary infarction in 1940, having assembled 370 cases of PE and infarction. In pulmonary infarction, they suggested that the cardiac margin of the opacity of a pulmonary infarction on chest radiograph is rounded or *hump*-shaped (i.e., Hampton's hump).

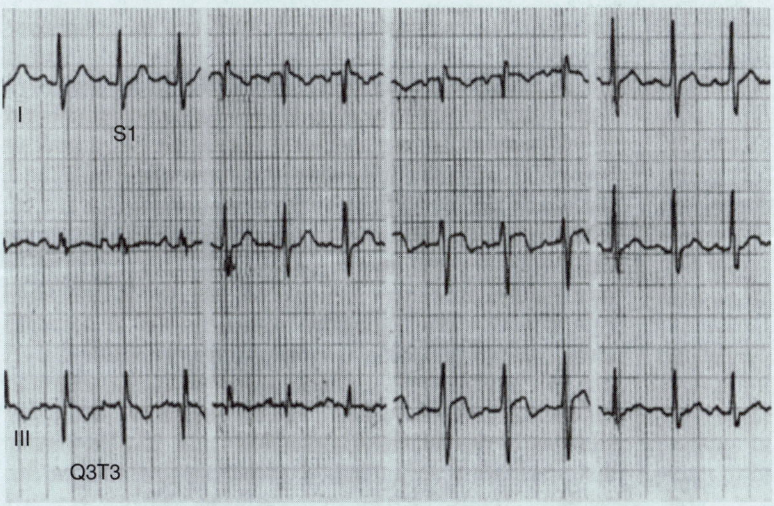

Fig. 61.1. A large embolism *(long arrow)* in the right main pulmonary artery, and smaller emboli *(short arrows)* are shown in the left lung by computed tomographic arteriography. Sinus tachycardia, the most common ECG finding in PE, is present. In addition, there is an S1Q3T3 pattern present, with an S wave in lead I and Q and T waves in lead III. The S1Q3T3 pattern finding is an uncommon in PE, but its presence in the appropriate clinical context should raise suspicion for PE.

14. What are typical arterial blood gas findings in patients with pulmonary embolism?

The common findings are a low PaO_2, low $PaCO_2$, and a high alveolar-arterial oxygen difference. Although nonspecific, one of these findings is likely to be present in up to 97% of cases. A normal arterial blood gas (ABG) reading does not absolutely exclude PE.

15. When should a ventilation/perfusion scan be performed?

The ventilation/perfusion (V/Q) scan is most useful when the chest radiograph is normal and there is no cardiopulmonary disease. In this setting, it has the highest likelihood of being either normal or of high probability. Diagnostic tests (especially those for PE) must be interpreted in light of the clinician's pretest probability. It is crucial to remember that commonly the V/Q scan is of low or intermediate probability even when PE is present. V/Q scanning may also be useful in patients with acute or chronic kidney disease (CKD), in whom a CTA using iodinated contrast may be contraindicated.

16. Does a negative computed tomographic angiogram indicate with *certainty* that pulmonary embolism is not present?

No, but a good-quality CTA is extremely sensitive. We learned from the PIOPED II, published in 2006, that clinical probability is extremely important in considering CTA results. Approximately 60% (9 of 15) of patients who had a high clinical pretest probability but a negative CTA were ultimately diagnosed with PE. Similarly, 16 of 38 (42%) patients with a low clinical pretest probability and a positive CTA did not have PE. A recent study by the Christopher Investigators of more than 3000 patients with suspected acute PE suggested that if CTA is negative, outcome at 3 months is excellent without therapy. Nonetheless it is prudent to consider additional imaging when a negative CTA is accompanied by high clinical suspicion. Furthermore, imaging quality is not uniformly high in all clinical settings. Finally, CT scanning has evolved such that modern-day multislice scanners are more sensitive than their predecessors. A large PE, documented by CTA, is shown in Fig. 61.2. A diagnostic algorithm that can be used as a guide is offered in Fig. 61.3.

17. How does echocardiography aid in the diagnosis of pulmonary embolism?

Transthoracic echocardiography can detect RV strain and dilation and offer guidance in the risk stratification and treatment of PE. McConnell's sign, a normally contracting RV apex associated with severe hypokinesis of the mid-free wall, is an echocardiographic pattern that suggests but is *not* diagnostic of acute PE. Furthermore, occasionally, "clot-in-transit" may be seen on echocardiography which offers additional diagnostic certainty.

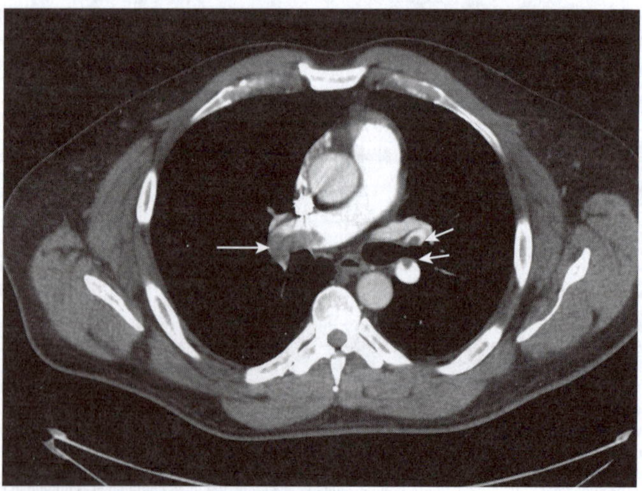

Fig. 61.2. A large embolism *(arrow)* in the left pulmonary artery is shown by computed tomographic arteriography.

18. What are some of the late complications of pulmonary embolism?

Late complications of PE include the development of chronic thromboembolic pulmonary hypertension (approximately 5% of patients) as well as complications from therapy itself, such as bleeding, skin necrosis (warfarin), osteoporosis, thrombocytopenia, and device migration in the case of inferior vena cava (IVC) filters. Patients who have had a PE also have an increased overall lifetime risk of a recurrent thrombotic event. In those who do not have a clear provoking event for the initial PE, the embolus may be a consequence of an underlying and not yet uncovered malignancy or inherited thrombotic disorder.

19. What is the most appropriate initial therapy for patients with documented acute pulmonary embolism?

Anticoagulation improves survival in patients with acute symptomatic PE. In patients with acute PE, a therapeutic level of anticoagulation should ideally be achieved within 24 hours because this reduces the risk of recurrence. If clinical suspicion is deemed high, the 9th American College of Chest Physicians Evidence-Based Clinical Practice (ACCP) Guidelines from February 2012 recommended initiation of treatment while awaiting diagnostic tests. The 10th set of ACCP Guidelines (February 2016) have maintained this recommendation.

Direct oral anticoagulants (DOACs) (such as rivaroxaban, apixaban, edoxaban, and dabigatran) can now be considered as initial treatment modalities without the need for parenteral or subcutaneous therapies in stable patients based on the EINSTEIN, RELY, and AMPLIFY studies. The 2016 ACCP guidelines recommend their use over warfarin (grade 2B).

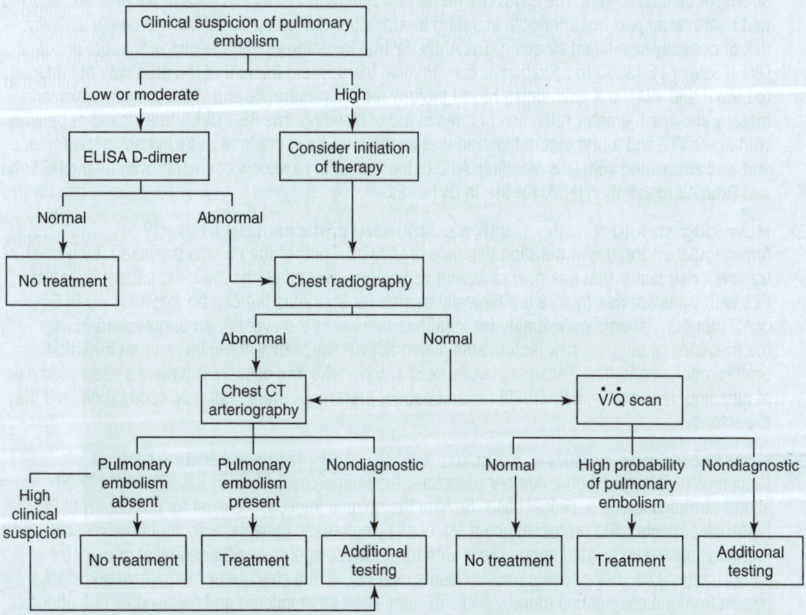

Fig. 61.3. A diagnostic strategy for suspected acute pulmonary embolism (PE). The use of a clinical prediction score and D-dimer testing may reduce the need for imaging. If suspicion for acute PE is high and the bleeding risk deemed low, initiation for anticoagulant therapy should be considered. The V/Q scan is most useful when the chest radiograph is normal or minimally abnormal. When significant renal insufficiency is present, computed tomographic arteriography (CTA) is contraindicated and the V/Q scan may be useful. Finally, when chest CTA is nondiagnostic, V/Q scanning can be considered; a negative V/Q scan is highly sensitive and a high-probability scan is quite sensitive. However, V/Q scans are often nondiagnostic, particularly when underlying lung disease is present. When the V/Q scan is nondiagnostic, and CTA cannot be done, ultrasound of the legs or magnetic resonance imaging of the legs and/or lungs can be considered. A *negative* leg study, does not, however, rule out PE. *CT*, Computed tomography; *ELISA*, enzyme-linked immunosorbent assay; *V/Q*, ventilation/perfusion. *(Modified from Tapson, V. F. [2008]. Acute pulmonary embolism.* New England Journal of Medicine, 358, *1037–1052.)*

Alternatively treatment could include low-molecular-weight heparin (LMWH), unfractionated heparin (UFH), or fondaparinux, followed by the initiation of oral anticoagulant therapy with either DOACs, which are now commonly used, or warfarin (i.e., if there is a contraindication to DOAC use such as renal dysfunction). One convenient advantage is that DOACs do not require bridging with a second agent, nor do they need lab monitoring. If warfarin is used, it should be started on the first day of treatment and must be overlapped with either LMWH, UFH, or fondaparinux until the international normalized ratio (INR) is 2.0 or more for at least 24 hours.

The ACCP also recommends that in patients with acute nonmassive PE, initial treatment with LMWH rather than intravenous UFH be used, if feasible, based on advantages of LMWH, including subcutaneous rather than intravenous delivery, much less need for monitoring, and a lower rate of heparin-induced thrombocytopenia. The LMWH heparin preparations are also more bioavailable and thus more predictable than standard UFH in terms of degree of anticoagulation. There are certain contraindications/cautions for its use in those with poor renal function or patients with severely elevated body mass index (BMI). In patients with underlying malignancy, LMWH has also shown some superiority as the primary agent for anticoagulation.

20. Are the newer oral anticoagulation medications safe and effective?

Several new oral anticoagulant drugs have been developed; these include direct inhibitors of factor Xa (e.g., rivaroxaban, edoxaban, apixaban) or thrombin (e.g., dabigatran). These agents avoid many of the drawbacks of heparin and vitamin K antagonists. They are administered in fixed doses, do not need laboratory monitoring, do not require bridging therapy with a second agent, and have few drug-drug or drug-food interactions. The EINSTEIN-PE Clinical Trial randomized some 4832 patients and showed that rivaroxaban was not inferior to standard treatment of warfarin plus LMWH and posed a similar risk of clinically significant bleeding. The AMPLIFY trial randomized 5395 adults with acute proximal DVT (65%) or PE (35%) to apixaban or conventional therapy and found that the drug was not inferior to LMWH and vitamin K antagonist–based therapy for VTE recurrence and VTE mortality. Apixaban therapy showed a greater reduction in rates of major bleeding. The RE-COVER trial looked at patients with acute VTE and found that dabigatran was as effective as warfarin at reducing risk of recurrence and was associated with less bleeding. All 3 of these agents have now been approved by the US Food and Drug Administration (FDA) for use in DVTs/PEs.

21. How long should a patient with a pulmonary embolism be treated?

Anticoagulation treatment duration depends greatly on whether the PE was provoked (by a clear transient risk factor that has now resolved) versus unprovoked (without a clear cause). Provoked PEs with transient risk factors are typically treated for 3 months but can be extended up to 6 or 12 months. Patients may qualify for indefinite therapy in the event of an unprovoked PE, or the presence of ongoing risk factors such as an active malignancy, immobility, or an inherited prothrombotic condition. These decisions must always take into account a patient's estimated risk of bleeding, recurrence, comorbidities, and patient preferences (e.g., fall risk, occupation, and life expectancy).

22. How should one stratify patient risk with acute pulmonary embolism?

Outcomes of PE depend on a number of factors. The Pulmonary Embolism Severity Index (PESI) allows stratification on a clinical basis. Several therapeutic implications exist for patients with PE. High-risk patients (who represent about 5% of all symptomatic patients, with about a 15% short-term mortality) should be treated aggressively with thrombolytic agents or either surgical or catheter embolectomy. Low-risk patients (most patients with PE), with a short-term mortality of about 1%, benefit from anticoagulation therapy and can sometimes be monitored and followed as outpatients. Intermediate-risk patients (who represent about 30% of all symptomatic patients) should be admitted to the hospital, anticoagulated, and considered for thrombolytic therapy if indicated. Low-risk and intermediate-risk categories can be said to have nonmassive PE. The Pulmonary Embolism Severity Index for Prognosis (sPESI) has been simplified (Table 61.4) to ease clinical application. The 305 of 995 patients (30.7%) who were classified as being at low risk by the sPESI had a 30-day mortality of 1.0% (95% CI, 0.0% to 2.1%) compared with a mortality rate of 10.9% (8.5% to 13.2%) in the high-risk group.

23. Are there any laboratory investigations that may help in determining the prognosis of patients with pulmonary embolism?

NT-proBNP and BNP levels and cardiac biomarkers such as troponin T or I may help to identify the severity of PE as a surrogate for right heart strain/dysfunction. These two tests, either together or

Table 61.4. Original and Simplified Pulmonary Embolism Severity Index

VARIABLE	ORIGINAL PULMONARY EMBOLISM SEVERITY INDEX*	SIMPLIFIED PULMONARY EMBOLISM SEVERITY INDEX†
Age >80 years	Age in years	+1
Male sex	+10	
History of cancer	+30	+1
History of heart failure‡	+10‡	+1‡
History of chronic lung disease‡	+10‡	
Heart rate ≥110 beats per min	+20	+1
Systolic blood pressure <100 mm Hg	+30	+1
Respiratory rate ≥30 breaths per minute	+20	
Temperature <36°C	+20	
Altered mental status	+60	
Arterial oxygen saturation <90%	+20	+1

Patients classified as being at low risk by the simplified PESI had a 30-day mortality of 1.0% (95% CI, 0.0-2.1%) compared with 10.9% (8.5-13.2%) in the high-risk group.

*For the original index, the total point score is reached by adding the total points plus the patient's age in years: Class 1 = ≤65 points; class 2 = 66-85; class 3 = 86-105; class 4 = 106-125; class 5 = >125. (Classes 1 and 2 are considered low risk and classes 3-5 high risk).

†For the simplified index, the total points are added. 0 = low risk, 1 = high risk. Empty cells imply that the variable is not included.

‡For the simplified index, history of heart failure and of chronic lung disease are combined as cardiopulmonary disease for 1 point.

individually are not sufficiently sensitive nor specific to serve as a basis for clinical decisions; they should be used together with other information.

24. **What is the primary indication for thrombolytic therapy?**
Proven PE with cardiogenic shock is the clearest indication. The ACCP Guidelines also note that in selected high-risk patients without hypotension who are judged to have a low risk of bleeding, thrombolytic therapy can be considered. This received a grade 2C recommendation—that is, a decision made based on limited data and expert opinion to support the suggestion. An example would be in a patient with submassive PE (RV dilation and hypokinesis without hypotension) who is deteriorating but not yet hypotensive. The decision to use thrombolytic therapy depends on the clinician's assessment of PE severity, prognosis, and risk of bleeding. Thus it is often considered in patients with hypotension without shock. Table 61.5 summarizes recommendations with regard to thrombolytic therapy in PE.

25. **What are some complications and contraindications of thrombolytic therapy?**
Intracranial hemorrhage is the most devastating complication of thrombolytic therapy and has been reported in approximately 1% of patients in clinical trials but in about 3% of patients in data from the International Cooperative Pulmonary Embolism Registry (ICOPER), which represents a more "real world" patient population. Other complications include retroperitoneal and gastrointestinal bleeding and bleeding from surgical wounds or from sites of recent invasive procedures. Contraindications to thrombolytic therapy are divided into major and relative contraindications and are listed in Table 61.6.

26. **Has thrombolytic therapy been shown to improve mortality from pulmonary embolism?**
No. Thrombolytic therapy has never been shown to improve mortality from PE in a randomized controlled clinical trial. It has been shown to improve hemodynamics and lung scans with a suggestion that younger (less than 50 years old) patients, patients with new emboli (less than 48 hours old), and those with larger emboli respond better.

Table 61.5. Synopsis of Recommendations from the 10th American College of Chest Physicians Evidence-Based Clinical Practice Consensus for Systemic Thrombolytic Therapy and for Catheter-Based Thrombus Removal for the Initial Treatment of Pulmonary Embolism*

Systemic Thrombolytic Therapy

1. In patients with acute PE associated with hypotension (e.g., systolic BP <90 mm Hg) who do not have a high bleeding risk, we suggest systemically administered thrombolytic therapy over no such therapy (grade 2B).
2. In most patients with acute PE not associated with hypotension, we recommend against systemically administered thrombolytic therapy (grade 1B).
3. In selected patients with acute PE who deteriorate after starting anticoagulant therapy but have yet to develop hypotension and who have a low bleeding risk, we suggest systemically administered thrombolytic therapy over no such therapy (grade 2C). (It is noted that patients with PE and without hypotension who have severe symptoms or marked cardiopulmonary impairment should be monitored closely for deterioration.

Catheter-Based Thrombus Removal for the Initial Treatment of PE

1. In patients with acute PE who are treated with a thrombolytic agent, we suggest systemic thrombolytic therapy using a peripheral vein over catheter-directed therapy (CDT) (grade 2C). *It is noted by the ACCP that the higher risk of bleeding with systemic thrombolytics, available resources, and expertise will play a role in the decision process.*
2. In patients with acute PE associated with hypotension and who have (i) a high bleeding risk, (ii) failed systemic thrombolysis, or (iii) shock that is likely to cause death before systemic thrombolysis can take effect (e.g., within hours), if appropriate expertise and resources are available, we suggest catheter-assisted thrombus removal (with or without catheter-directed thrombolysis) over no such intervention (grade 2C).

It should be noted that the ACCP recommendations do not elaborate on different clot extraction techniques or catheter-directed thrombolysis regimens, as the number of randomized trials precludes this. The ULTIMA study (EKOS technique) is the only randomized trial. Furthermore, it should be recognized that systemic (intravenous) *thrombolysis is generally faster than catheter-directed thrombolysis*, based upon transport to the cardiac or intervention radiology lab, and obtaining access and performing the procedure.

*Recommendations are graded based on the evidence. Grade 1 indicates that benefit appears to outweigh potential harm, whereas with grade 2, this is less certain. The lettered recommendation indicates the quality of the methodology used to make the recommendation. "A" recommendations are the strongest and are based on data from very good quality prospective, randomized trials, whereas grade "C" recommendations indicate that the data are from uncontrolled, observational studies.

Recommendations adapted from Kearon, C., Akl, E. A., Ornelas, J., Blaivas, A., Jimenez, D., Bounameaux, H., et al. (2016). Antithrombotic therapy for VTE disease CHEST guideline and expert panel report. Chest, *149(2), 315–352. http://dx.doi.org/10.1016/j.chest.2015.11.026.*

The Thrombolysis for Pulmonary Embolism and Risk of All-Cause Mortality, Major Bleeding, and Intracranial Hemorrhage study was a 2014 meta-analysis appearing in *JAMA* that looked at 16 trials comprising 2115 individuals with PE, including those with submassive PE, and suggested that thrombolytic therapy compared with anticoagulation alone was associated with a lower all-cause mortality (2.17% vs. 3.89%; number needed to treat [NNT] = 59) and recurrent PE risk. However those receiving thrombolytic therapy had a greater risk of major bleeding (number needed to harm [NNH] = 18) or intracranial hemorrhage (ICH) (NNH = 78). The major bleeding risk was not significantly increased in patients younger than 65 years of age. Interpretation of this information must be within the context of the inherent limitations of a meta-analysis, which can include bias in terms of the selection of studies, heterogeneity of results, analysis of selected studies, and information available.

27. What is the role of embolectomy, catheter-directed thrombolytic therapy, and catheter-based clot retrieval?

Embolectomy is a procedure to remove a proximal PE either surgically or by using a percutaneous endovascular clot-retrieving catheter. The procedure may be considered in patients with hemodynamically unstable PE and a contraindication to thrombolytic therapy. It can also be considered in those who fail systemic thrombolysis, those with submassive PE and poor hemodynamic reserve, or clot in transit with potentially dire consequences.

Table 61.6. Major and Relative Contraindications to Thrombolytic Therapy

Major Contraindications

- Structural intracranial disease
- Previous intracranial hemorrhage
- Ischemic stroke within 3 months
- Active bleeding
- Recent brain or spinal surgery
- Recent head trauma with fracture or brain injury
- Bleeding diathesis

Relative Contraindications

- Systolic blood pressure above or equal to 180 mm Hg
- Diastolic blood pressure above or equal to 110 mm Hg
- Recent bleeding (nonintracranial)
- Recent surgery
- Recent significant head trauma without fracture or obvious brain injury
- Recent invasive procedure
- Ischemic stroke more than 3 months previously
- Traumatic cardiopulmonary resuscitation
- Pericarditis or pericardial fluid
- Diabetic retinopathy
- Pregnancy
- Age 75 years or above
- Female sex
- Black race

Catheter-directed thrombolysis can be used for patients with persistent hemodynamic instability despite systemic thrombolysis. Catheter-based thrombolysis can also potentially be used for those with submassive PE to help improve cardiac function and reduce long-term sequelae from residual clot. Catheter-based thrombolysis may pose a lower risk of bleeding complications than systemic thrombolysis.

The ULTIMA study randomized patients with submassive PE to the catheter-based "EKOS (EkoSonic® Endovascular system) technique" using low-dose tPA or to anticoagulation alone. Significant improvement in RV/LV ratio was shown by echocardiography with the catheter-based approach. A second large single-arm study (SEATTLE II) included patients with submassive as well as massive PE and also demonstrated improvement of RV/LV ratio using the EKOS technique.

These modalities should be considered on a case-by-case basis in consultation with a specialist and based on the expertise of the performing center.

28. What are the indications for the placement of an inferior vena cava filter?

The most widely recognized indications for placement of an IVC filter include contraindications to anticoagulation, major bleeding complications during anticoagulation, and recurrent PE despite adequate anticoagulation. Although there are no firm trial data, some experts suggest filter placement in the case of massive PE when it is believed that additional emboli might be lethal, particularly if thrombolytic therapy is contraindicated. The recent PREPIC (Prévention du Risque d'Embolie Pulmonaire par Interruption Cave Study Group) 2 trial did not find a difference in 90-day outcome when 400 patients with acute PE were anticoagulated and randomized to IVC filter placement versus no filter. Although the population enrolled was "enriched" in an attempt to find patients who would be expected to have a high recurrence rate, some experts argue that it was not adequately enriched. Perhaps patients with very extensive residual DVT should be the only ones to be included. Nonetheless, IVC filters may well be overused and appear to be removed too infrequently. The earlier PREPIC trial suggested that IVC filters increase the subsequent incidence of DVT (in about 20% of patients) and have not been shown to increase overall survival.

29. What are some complications of the placement of inferior vena cava filters?

Complications of IVC filters include procedure-related insertion site thrombosis (8%), pneumothorax, air embolism, or hematoma and late complications of IVC thrombosis (2% to 10%), postthrombotic syndrome, IVC penetration, aortic penetration, and filter migration. Most models of IVC filters are retrievable, typically within several months of insertion. Although this may alleviate some of the late complications of IVC filter placement, complications can also occur with retrieval.

30. Can PE be treated on an outpatient basis?

Although the use of LMWH and newer oral agents as outpatient therapy for DVT has been established, the data for outpatient treatment of acute PE are less robust. Recent data suggest that outpatient therapy or early discharge in acute PE can be done safely if patients are carefully screened. Several clinical trials and a 2013 meta-analysis found no increased rates of recurrent VTE, mortality, or major bleeding events in those who were believed to be at lower risk and treated as outpatients.

Factors that may make outpatient treatment relatively safe include incidental segmental/ subsegmental PE, a low predicted risk of a poor outcome (PESI class I or II), normal blood pressure, good home support, and absence of supplemental oxygen, respiratory distress, bleeding risk factors, serious comorbidities, and concomitant DVT. When there is concern, a short hospital stay with direct observation may still be the prudent course even in lower risk patients until further risk stratification is clearer. The MERCURY PE study may add additional useful data on the topic of outpatient PE management.

Bibliography and Suggested Readings

Agnelli, G., Buller, H. R., Cohen, A., Curto, M., Gallus, A. S., Johnson, M., et al. (2013). Oral apixaban for the treatment of acute venous thromboembolism. *New England Journal of Medicine, 369*(9), 799–808.

Beckman, M. G., Hooper, W. C., Critchley, S. E., & Ortel, T. L. (2010). Venous thromboembolism: 2010 a public health concern. *American Journal of Preventive Medicine, 38*, S495–S501.

Christopher Study Investigators. (2006). Effectiveness of managing suspected pulmonary embolism using an algorithm combining clinical probability, D-dimer testing, and computed tomography. *Journal of the American Medical Association, 295*, 172–179.

Chunilal, S. D., Eikelboom, J. W., Attia, J., Miniati, M., Panju, A. A., Simel, D. L., et al. (2003). Does this patient have pulmonary embolism? *Journal of the American Medical Association, 290*(21), 2849–2858.

Cohen, A. T., Agnelli, G., Anderson, F. A., Arcelus, J. I., Bergqvist, D., Brecht, J. G., et al. (2007). Venous thromboembolism (VTE) in Europe. *Journal of Thrombosis and Haemostasis, 98*, 756–764.

Cohen, A. T., Tapson, V. F., Bergmann, J. F., Goldhaber, S. Z., Kakkar, A. K., Deslandes, B., et al. (2008). Venous thromboembolism risk and prophylaxis in the acute hospital care setting (ENDORSE study): a multinational cross-sectional study. *Lancet, 371*, 387–394.

Dalen, J. E. (2002). Pulmonary embolism: what have we learned since Virchow? Natural history, pathophysiology, and diagnosis. *Chest, 122*, 1440–1456.

Dalen, J. E. (2002). Pulmonary embolism: what have we learned since Virchow? Treatment and prevention. *Chest, 122*, 1801–1817.

Dong, B., Jirong, Y., Liu, G., Wang, Q., & Wu, T. (2006). Thrombolytic therapy for pulmonary embolism. *Cochrane Database of Systematic Reviews, 2*, CD004437. http://dx.doi.org/10.1002/14651858.CD004437.pub2.

Goldhaber, S. Z., Visani, L., & De Rosa, M. (1999). Acute pulmonary embolism: clinical outcomes in the International Cooperative Pulmonary Embolism Registry (ICOPER). *Lancet, 353*, 1386–1389.

Goldhaber, S., & Bounameaux, H. (2012). Pulmonary embolism and deep vein thrombosis. *Lancet, 379*, 1835–1846.

Hanna, C. L., Michael, B., & Streiff, M. B. (2005). The role of vena caval filters in the management of venous thromboembolism. *Blood Reviews, 19*, 179–202.

Jiménez, D., Aujesky, D., Moores, L., Gómez, V., Lobo, J. L., Uresandi, F., et al. (2010). Simplification of the pulmonary embolism severity index for prognostication in patients with acute symptomatic PE. *Archives of Internal Medicine, 170*, 1383–1389.

Kearon, C., Aki, E. A., Ornelas, J., Blaivas, A., Jimenez, D., Bounameaux, H., et al. (2016). Antithrombotic therapy for VTE disease: chest guideline and expert panel report. *Chest, 149*(2), 315–352.

Kucher, N., Boekstegers, P., Müller, O. J., Kupatt, C., Beyer-Westendorf, J., Heitzer, T., et al. (2014). Randomized, controlled trial of ultrasound-assisted catheter-directed thrombolysis for acute intermediate-risk pulmonary embolism. *Circulation, 129*, 479–486.

Kurzyna, M., Torbicki, A., & Pruszczyk, P. (2002). Disturbed right ventricular ejection pattern as a new Doppler echocardiographic sign of acute pulmonary embolism. *American Journal of Cardiology, 90*, 507–511.

Mismetti, P., Laporte, S., Pellerin, O., Ennezat, P. V., Couturaud, F., Elias, A., et al. (2015). Effect of a retrievable inferior vena caval filter plus anticoagulation versus anticoagulation alone on risk of recurrent acute pulmonary embolism. *Journal of the American Medical Association, 313*, 1627–1635.

Piazza, G., & Goldhaber, S. Z. (2010). Fibrinolysis for acute pulmonary embolism. *Vascular Medicine, 15*, 419.

Piazza, G., Hohlfelder, B., Jaff, M. R., Ouriel, K., Engelhardt, T. C., Sterling, K. M., et al. (2015). A prospective, single-arm, multicenter trial of ultrasound-facilitated, catheter-directed, low-dose fibrinolysis for acute massive and submassive pulmonary embolism: the SEATTLE II study. *JACC Cardiovascular Interventions, 24*, 1382–1392.

PIOPED Investigators. (1990). Value of the ventilation/perfusion scan in acute pulmonary embolism. *Journal of the American Medical Association, 263*(20), 2753–2759.

Roger, V. L., Go, A. S., Lloyd-Jones, D. M., Benjamin, E. J., Berry, J. D., Borden, W. B., et al. (2012). Heart disease and stroke statistics—2012 update: a report from the American Heart Association. *Circulation, 125*, e2–e220.

Schulman, S., Kearon, C., Kakkar, A. K., Mismetti, P., Schellong, S., Eriksson, H., et al. (2009). Dabigatran versus warfarin in the treatment of acute venous thromboembolism. *New England Journal of Medicine, 361*(24), 2342–2352.

Simonneau, G., Sors, H., Charbonnier, B., Page, Y., Laaban, J. P., Azarian, R., et al. (1997). A comparison of low-molecular weight heparin with unfractionated heparin for acute pulmonary embolism. *New England Journal of Medicine, 337*, 663–669.

Skaf, E., Beemath, A., Siddiqui, T., Janjua, M., Patel, N. R., & Stein, P. D. (2007). Catheter-tip embolectomy in the management of acute massive pulmonary embolism. *American Journal of Cardiology, 99*, 415–420.

Stein, P. D., Alnas, M., Skaf, E., Kayali, F., Siddiqui, T., Olson, R. E., et al. (2004). Outcomes and complications of retrievable inferior vena cava filters. *American Journal of Cardiology, 94*, 1090.

Stein, P. D., Fowler, S. E., Goodman, L. R., Gottschalk, A., Hales, C. A., Hull, R. D., et al. (2006). Multidetector computed tomography for acute pulmonary embolism (PIOPED II). *New England Journal of Medicine, 354*(22), 2317–2327.

Tapson, V. F. (2008). Acute pulmonary embolism. *New England Journal of Medicine, 358*, 1037–1052.

The EINSTEIN–PE Investigators. (2012). Oral rivaroxaban for the treatment of symptomatic pulmonary embolism. *New England Journal of Medicine, 366*, 1287–1297.

Venous thromboembolism: impact of blood clots on the United States. (2015). Atlanta: Centers for Disease Control and Prevention. http://www.cdc.gov/ncbddd/dvt/infographic-impact.html. Accessed 12.15.16.

Zondag, W., Kooiman, J., Klok, F. A., Dekkers, O. M., & Huisman, M. V. (2013). Outpatient versus inpatient treatment in patients with pulmonary embolism: a meta-analysis. *European Respiratory Journal, 42*(1), 134–144.

CHAPTER 62

HYPERCOAGULABLE STATES

Yamin Sun, Michael H. Kroll

1. What is hypercoagulability?

Hypercoagulability is a state of increased risk for thrombosis. The risk is often presented as a relative risk, hazard ratio, or annual incidence. Increased risk may relate to venous, arterial, and microvascular thrombosis, and thrombosis risk is measured (and usually different) for both initial and recurrent events. Hypercoagulability is also designated "thrombophilia," and there are inherited and acquired hypercoagulable states. Most patients with thrombosis are found to have predispositions and triggers, and the challenge is to identify and rank them with an eye toward optimizing therapy to prevent recurrent thrombosis. In most cases of thrombosis, "hypercoagulability" is considered to be a predisposing factor separate from other risk factors for atherothrombotic disease (such as smoking and hypercholesterolemia) and venous thrombosis (such as hormonal therapy and immobility). Hypercoagulability is also typically considered to represent a pathologic condition (so that pregnancy, although associated with increased risk of venous thromboembolism [VTE], is usually not considered a hypercoagulable state).

2. What are the inherited hypercoagulable disorders?

The common inherited hypercoagulable states are *factor V Leiden* and *prothrombin G20210A*, which are due to mutations in the genes for factor V and prothrombin. Factor V Leiden is a point mutation in factor V that renders factor V resistant to breakdown by activated protein C (R506Q), and prothrombin G20210A is a mutation in the noncoding region of the prothrombin gene that results in increased protein synthesis (prothrombin levels of 110% to 120%).

Less common inherited hypercoagulable states are due to deficiencies of the natural anticoagulant proteins *antithrombin*, *protein C*, and *protein S*. Mutations in the folate-metabolizing enzyme methylene tetrahydrofolate reductase (MTHFR) leading to elevated blood homocysteine levels are sometimes mistakenly designated an inherited hypercoagulable state. Table 62.1, Fig. 62.1 summarizes the inherited hypercoagulable states.

3. What are the acquired hypercoagulable states?

The antiphospholipid syndrome is the most important cause of acquired hypercoagulability. It develops de novo or secondary to lymphoproliferative or rheumatologic conditions. Other acquired hypercoagulable states are heparin-induced thrombocytopenia, myeloproliferative neoplasms (MPNs), paroxysmal nocturnal hemoglobinuria (PNH), and cancer. The prevalence of cancer-associated VTE varies with the type of malignancy and its treatment. It is associated with an average relative risk of a first VTE of approximately 6, with an absolute 6-month incidence of recurrence—on anticoagulation—of at least 10%. Table 62.2 summarizes the acquired hypercoagulable states.

4. What is the antiphospholipid syndrome?

The antiphospholipid syndrome is the combination of venous thrombosis, arterial thrombosis, microvascular thrombosis (such as livedo reticularis), miscarriage, preeclampsia, migraine, and/or thrombocytopenia associated with either a lupus anticoagulant (LA), an antiphospholipid antibody (APA), or an antibody to beta-2 glycoprotein-1. An LA is an APA that interferes with an in vitro clotting assay. The assay used is the "dilute Russell viper venom time," which measures fibrin generation following the phospholipid-dependent activation of factor X by the venom. All LAs are due to APAs, but only approximately one-third of APAs are an LA. The actual pathogenetic element is the antibody to beta-2 glycoprotein-1, which is a phospholipid-binding protein that protects the vascular endothelium from complement-mediated injury. The antibody eliminates this protective function, resulting in a prothrombotic vascular response.

5. What types of thromboses are due to hypercoagulable states?

The inherited thrombophilias are caused by increased activity of procoagulant proteins (factor V and prothrombin) or decreased activity of natural anticoagulant proteins (antithrombin, protein C, and protein S). These proteins are all part of the soluble coagulation system, which operates to generate

Table 62.1. Inherited Hypercoagulable States

INHERITED THROMBOPHILIA	EPIDEMIOLOGY	LABORATORY TESTING	RELATIVE RISK OF FIRST VENOUS THROMBOEMBOLISM	RECURRENCE RELATIVE RISK
Factor V Leiden	Heterozygote ~5/100	PCR	3-10	<1.5
	Homozygous ~2/1000	PCR	80	~3
Prothrombin G210210A	Heterozygote ~2/100	PCR	6-10	<1.7
	Homozygous ~0.4/1000	PCR	Unknown (but perhaps not much higher)	Unknown
Compound heterozygotes	~1/1000	PCR	6-10	~7
Antithrombin deficiency	~ 0.5-2/1000	Antigen and activity	5	3
Protein C deficiency	~1.5-5/1000	Antigen and activity	3	2
Protein S deficiency	<1/1000	Antigen (total and free) and activity	2	1

PCR, Polymerase chain reaction.

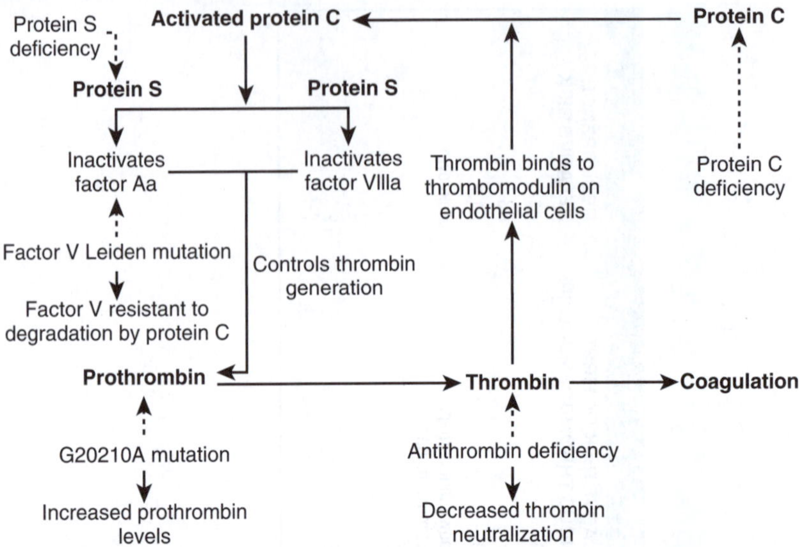

Fig. 62.1. Effects of inherited thrombophilia on the coagulation pathway. The inherited hypercoagulable states affect the enzymatic reactions leading to fibrin production. Factor V Leiden results from a point mutation in factor V that prevents its breakdown by activated protein C and its cofactor protein S. Prothrombin G20210A is a point mutation in a regulatory element of the prothrombin (factor II) gene that increases its synthesis, so that prothrombin levels are increased by 10% to 20%. Deficiencies of antithrombin decrease its effect on keeping the brakes on factor X activation. Deficiencies on protein C or its essential cofactor protein S increase fibrin deposition by decreasing the breakdown of the procoagulant cofactors V and VIII. *(Image from Oner, G. [2011]. Thrombophilia and recurrent pregnancy loss. In A. L. Trandquilli [Ed.],* Thrombophilia. *Rijeka, Croatia: InTech.)*

insoluble fibrin. Fibrin deposition resulting in thrombosis can develop only in low-flow vascular systems. Accordingly, the inherited hypercoagulable states result only in venous thrombosis. These thromboses can occur in any venous compartment but are typically deep vein thromboses (of legs is greater than that of arms), pulmonary emboli, splanchnic vein thrombosis, and cerebral vein thrombosis.

The acquired thrombophilias lead to widespread vascular perturbation and are associated with both venous thromboembolic and arterial thromboses, such as coronary, cerebral, and peripheral arterial ischemia and infarction. Arterial thromboses are rarely de novo, and hypercoagulability-induced arterial thromboses are most frequent in patients who are known to have atherothrombotic arterial occlusive disease.

6. When does one suspect that a patient has a hypercoagulable state?

A hypercoagulable state should be suspected when a patient has any of the following:

- Idiopathic thrombosis at any age
- Family history of venous thromboembolism
- Thrombosis at unusual sites, such as cerebral, hepatic, mesenteric, renal, or portal veins
- Recurrent unprovoked or unexplained thromboses
- Recurrent unexplained fetal loss
- Warfarin-induced skin necrosis
- Purpura fulminans
- Recurrent superficial thrombophlebitis

7. When should hypercoagulability be tested for?

Hypercoagulability should be tested for in any individual with a single unprovoked venous thromboembolic event. In the absence of a family history, testing is limited to the antiphospholipid syndrome. In the presence of a history of a first-degree relative with VTE,

Table 62.2. Acquired Hypercoagulable States

ACQUIRED THROMBOPHILIA	EPIDEMIOLOGY	LABORATORY TESTING	RISK OF FIRST VENOUS THROMBOEMBOLISM	RECURRENCE RELATIVE RISK
Antiphospholipid antibody syndrome	10% of women with recurrent miscarriage 16% of patients with lupus 14% of patients with first VTE	Always three tests Lupus anticoagulant Anti-phospholipid antibody testing Anti-beta-2-glycoprotein-1 antibody testing	Relative risk ~9	~3
Heparin-induced thrombocytopenia	<2% of heparin-treated patients	Anti-heparin/platelet factor 4 antibody Serotonin release assay	Incidence up to 50%	Unknown
MPN (polycythemia vera, essential thrombocytosis, and myelofibrosis)	50% of hepatic vein thrombosis (Budd-Chiari syndrome) 10% of all splanchnic vein thromboses Up to 4% of all MPN patients suffer thrombosis Rate of arterial thromboses 3 times greater than VTE rate	Janus kinase 2 (JAK2) and calreticulin gene analyses	Annual incidence up to 4%	Unknown
Paroxysmal nocturnal hemoglobinuria	15% prevalence, most of which are splanchnic vein thrombosis 50% of all pregnancies are complicated by preterm delivery Up to 20% of all women suffer postpartum VTE	Blood flow cytometry for blood cells deficient in CD55 and CD59	Relative risk ~60	Unknown

MPN, Myeloproliferative neoplasm; *VTE*, venous thromboembolism.

testing for the five inherited thrombophilias should be undertaken. Any patient with a personal *and* family history of venous thrombosis should be tested for an inherited hypercoagulable state. No testing of any type should be done for a patient with provoked VTE, unless there is a family history. Asymptomatic blood relatives of patients with inherited thrombophilia may be screened to provide counseling about VTE symptoms and signs and to optimize prophylaxis in high-risk situations.

There is no reason to test for any of the inherited thrombophilias in adult patients with myocardial infarction, stroke, or peripheral occlusive arterial disease. The antiphospholipid syndrome is often tested for in young patients with myocardial infarction or stroke without arterial occlusive disease or any obvious cardiac source of arterial thromboembolism, but evidence for this is ambiguous. Less ambiguous are data that one must test for the antiphospholipid syndrome in every woman who has suffered recurrent first trimester or a single second or third trimester miscarriage and test for an inherited hypercoagulable state in any woman who has suffered miscarriage and has a family history of thrombosis.

8. **When should occult malignancy or myeloproliferative neoplasm be considered?**
At least 5% of patients with idiopathic VTE will have a cancer diagnosed within the next 12 months. There is no standard US approach to evaluating these patients, but in the United Kingdom all unprovoked VTEs trigger an evaluation that includes complete history and examination, complete blood count (CBC), liver function tests (LFTs), calcium, urinalysis, and chest x-ray (CXR), and we recommend appropriate imaging to evaluate any abnormality, particularly to look for occult digestive, gynecologic, or thoracic malignancies. One must also look for MPN in patients with splanchnic vein thromboses, because at least 10% of such patients will have undiagnosed MPN. More than half of those with hepatic vein thrombosis (Budd-Chiari syndrome) will be diagnosed with Janus kinase 2 (JAK2) V617F-positive MPN or PNH. Women with recurrent fetal loss and signs of a blood disorder (hemolysis or cytopenias) should be tested for PNH.

9. **When does one test for hypercoagulability?**
Testing for factor V Leiden, prothrombin G210210A, APAs, and anti-beta-2 glycoprotein-1 antibodies can be done at any time. Testing for antithrombin, protein C, protein S, and the LA should be done at least 3 weeks after anticoagulation has been discontinued, with repeat testing after 3 months. Note that the direct factor Xa inhibiting anticoagulants (rivaroxaban, apixaban, and edoxaban) give a false-positive LA screen.

10. **How does the presence of a hypercoagulable state affect treatment decisions?**
In most cases of VTE it has no bearing. If a patient suffers a provoked VTE and the provocation is eliminated, therapeutic anticoagulation for 3 months is used, and this treatment program is unaltered by the presence of an associated inherited or familial thrombophilia. Conversely, all patients with idiopathic VTE, without or with associated hypercoagulability, require long-term anticoagulation unless they can be stratified low risk by D-dimer or residual venous thrombosis testing. Only the presence of a LA, APA, or anti-beta-2 glycoprotein-1 antibody would direct *indefinite* anticoagulation in *all* patients with unprovoked VTE, including those with low risk stratification. Indefinite anticoagulation is also recommended for all patients with VTE plus active cancer or who are receiving cancer treatment, although there is evidence that recurrence is uncommon after completing 6 months of anticoagulation among cancer patients with deep vein thrombosis (DVT) and residual venous thrombosis less than 40%.

11. **What is the recommended target international normalized ratio in patients with arterial thrombosis associated with the antiphospholipid syndrome?**
In patients with arterial thrombosis associated with the antiphospholipid syndrome, treatment with anticoagulation (e.g., warfarin targeting a slightly higher INR of 2.5 to 3.5) rather than antiplatelet therapy is recommended, although warfarin may not be better than aspirin when it is being used for antiphospholipid syndrome patients with transient ischemic attacks (TIAs) or stroke.

12. **Why is it important to identify an underlying hypercoagulable state in women who have suffered a miscarriage?**
Identifying an underlying hypercoagulable state in women who have suffered a miscarriage will have a huge bearing on their management. The presence of an LA, APA, or anti-beta-2 glycoprotein-1 antibody would direct beginning baby aspirin preconception and prophylactic enoxaparin as soon as a fetal heartbeat is recognized; this regimen results in greater than 80% successful pregnancies.

In contrast, testing for an inherited thrombophilia in these cases is discouraged as most data indicate that anticoagulation is not effective at protecting against miscarriage in woman with inherited thrombophilia or no thrombophilia.

It is also important to note that, because hypercoagulability synergizes with pregnancy to effect VTE risk, specific VTE prevention measures for hypercoagulable women during pregnancy and post parturition are suggested:

- Pregnant women with homozygous factor V Leiden or prothrombin G20210A *plus* a family history of VTE should receive prophylactic anticoagulation during the entire pregnancy and for 6 weeks postpartum.
- Pregnant women with any other inherited hypercoagulable state *plus* a family history of VTE or pregnant women with homozygous factor V Leiden or prothrombin G20210A *without* a family history of VTE should receive prophylactic anticoagulation for 6 weeks postpartum.

13. Does mutant methylene tetrahydrofolate reductase cause an inherited thrombophilia?

Although elevated homocysteine probably carries a significant thrombotic risk, including increased coronary artery disease and VTE, there is good evidence that homocysteine-lowering therapy has no effect on arterial or venous thrombosis, and that the homozygous C677T mutation of MTHFR is *not* a risk factor for VTE and probably is not a risk factor for coronary and cerebrovascular disease.

Bibliography and Suggested Readings

Dalen, J. E. (2008). Should patients with venous thromboembolism be screened for thrombophilia? *American Journal of Medicine*, *121*(6), 458–463. http://dx.doi.org/10.1016/j.amjmed.2007.10.042.

Garcia, D., Akl, E. A., Carr, R., & Kearon, C. (2013). Antiphospholipid antibodies and the risk of recurrence after a first episode of venous thromboembolism: a systematic review. *Blood*, *122*(5), 817–824. http://dx.doi.org/10.1182/blood-2013-04-496257.

Kroll, M. H., Michaelis, L. C., & Verstovsek, S. (2015). Mechanisms of thrombogenesis in polycythemia vera. *Blood Reviews*, *29*(4), 215–221. http://dx.doi.org/10.1016/j.blre.2014.12.002.

Lijfering, W. M., Brouwer, J. L., Veeger, N. J., Bank, I., Coppens, M., Middeldorp, S., et al. (2009). Selective testing for thrombophilia in patients with first venous thrombosis: results from a retrospective family cohort study on absolute thrombotic risk for currently known thrombophilic defects in 2479 relatives. *Blood*, *113*(21), 5314–5322. http://dx.doi.org/10.1182/blood-2008-10-184879.

Martí-Carvajal, A. J., Solà, I., & Lathyris, D. (2015). Homocysteine-lowering interventions for preventing cardiovascular events. *The Cochrane Database of Systematic Reviews*, *1*, CD006612. http://dx.doi.org/10.1002/14651858.CD006612.pub4.

Martinelli, I., De Stefano, V., & Mannucci, P. M. (2014). Inherited risk factors for venous thromboembolism. *National Reviews Cardiology*, *11*(3), 140–156. http://dx.doi.org/10.1038/nrcardio.2013.211.

Ruiz-Irastorza, G., Crowther, M., Branch, W., & Khamashta, M. A. (2010). Antiphospholipid syndrome. *Lancet*, *376*(9751), 1498–1509. http://dx.doi.org/10.1016/S0140-6736(10)60709-X.

Segal, J. B., Brotman, D. J., Necochea, A. J., Emadi, A., Samal, L., Wilson, L. M., et al. (2009). Predictive value of factor V Leiden and prothrombin G20210A in adults with venous thromboembolism and in family members of those with a mutation: a systematic review. *Journal of the American Medical Association*, *301*(23), 2472–2485. http://dx.doi.org/10.1001/jama.2009.853.

X

Additional Topics in Cardiology

ADULT CONGENITAL HEART DISEASE

Luc M. Beauchesne

CHAPTER 63

1. What are the three main types of atrial septal defects, and what are their associated anomalies?

The three main types of atrial septal defects (ASDs) are secundum (70%), primum (20%), and sinus venosus (10%). The secundum ASD is a defect involving the floor of the fossa ovalis of the atrial septum. It usually presents as an isolated anomaly. The primum ASD is a defect at the base of the atrial septum adjacent to the atrioventricular valves. It is invariably part of an atrioventricular septal defect (endocardial cushion defect), and a cleft mitral valve is almost always present. The sinus venosus ASD is a defect of the posterior part of the septum, usually located in the superior part. In the majority of cases a sinus venosus ASD is associated with anomalous connections or drainage of the right-sided pulmonary veins (Fig. 63.1).

2. When should an atrial septal defect be closed? Which atrial septal defects cannot be closed by a percutaneous device?

ASDs vary in size. If the ASD is large enough, the associated left-to-right shunt will lead to right-sided volume overload and pulmonary overcirculation. Chronic right-sided volume overload leads to pulmonary hypertension, right ventricular dysfunction, tricuspid regurgitation, and right atrial dilation. Patients with ASDs also often develop atrial arrhythmias. Hemodynamically significant ASDs are usually 10 mm or larger, have a shunt ratio greater than 1.5, and are associated with right ventricular enlargement on imaging. It is recommended that only hemodynamically significant ASDs be closed. Most secundum ASDs can be closed percutaneously. Primum and sinus venosus ASDs *cannot* be closed percutaneously and require surgical closure.

Guideline recommendations on closure of ASDs are summarized in Table 63.1.

3. List the four types of ventricular septal defects.

Different classifications for ventricular septal defects (VSDs) have been used; one common approach divides VSDs into four types:

- Membranous or perimembranous VSDs involve the membranous ventricular septum, a small localized area of the normal ventricular septum that is fibrous. This is the most common type of VSD seen in the adult.
- Muscular VSDs involve the trabecular portion of the septum.
- Inlet VSDs involve the part of the ventricular septum that is adjacent to the tricuspid and mitral valves. Inlet VSDs are always associated with atrioventricular septal defects.
- Outlet VSDs (also known as supracristal VSDs) involve the portion of the ventricular septum that is just below the aortic and pulmonary valve (Fig. 63.2).

4. What are the long-term complications of a small ventricular septal defect in the adult patient?

In the adult, there are two groups of patients with unrepaired VSDs. The smallest group consists of patients with a large VSD that has been complicated by severe pulmonary hypertension (Eisenmenger's syndrome). However, the vast majority of adult patients with VSDs have small defects that are hemodynamically insignificant (i.e., do not cause left ventricular dilation or pulmonary hypertension). As a rule, these patients have a benign natural history. Rarely, some patients develop complications, such as endocarditis, atrial arrhythmias, tricuspid regurgitation, aortic regurgitation, and double-chambered right ventricle.

5. When should a ventricular septal defect be closed?

Guideline recommendations on closure of a VSD are predicated primarily on the Qp/Qs ratio ("shunt ratio"), which in essence is flow through the pulmonary artery divided by flow through the aorta. This

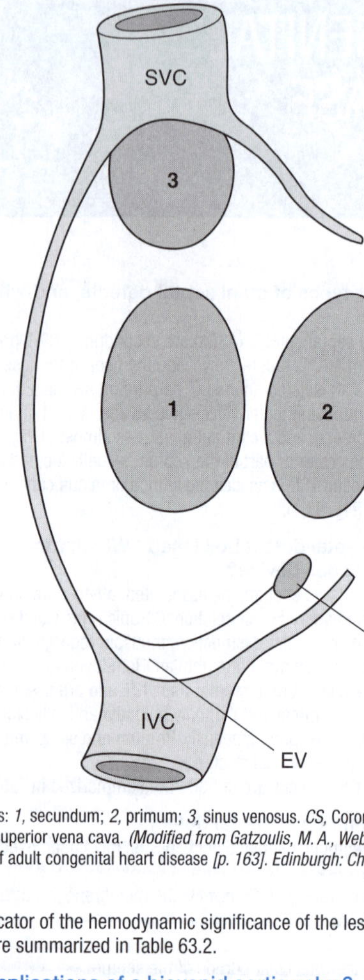

Fig. 63.1. Atrial septal defects: *1*, secundum; *2*, primum; *3*, sinus venosus. *CS*, Coronary sinus; *EV*, eustachian valve; *IVC*, inferior vena cava; *SVC*, superior vena cava. *(Modified from Gatzoulis, M. A., Webb, G. D., & Daubeney, P. E. F. [2003]. Diagnosis and management of adult congenital heart disease [p. 163]. Edinburgh: Churchill Livingstone.)*

is one important indicator of the hemodynamic significance of the lesion. Guideline recommendations on closure of VSDs are summarized in Table 63.2.

6. **What are the complications of a bicuspid aortic valve?**

A bicuspid aortic valve is present in 0.5% to 1% of the population. The main complications are progressive aortic stenosis, aortic regurgitation, or a combination of both (Fig. 63.3). Other complications include aortopathy and endocarditis. Although infrequent (<10%), aortic coarctation is also a well-described association and must be ruled out in these patients. Patients in whom the bicuspid valve demonstrates signs of valve degeneration on echocardiography are at an increased risk of cardiovascular events and need close regular follow-up.

7. **How is hemodynamic severity of coarctation of the aorta assessed in the adult patient?**

In coarctation of the aorta the narrowing is typically in the proximal portion of the descending aorta just distal to the left subclavian artery (Fig. 63.4). Adult patients can be divided into two groups: those with *native* (i.e., unrepaired) coarctation and those who are post repair (some of whom have residual stenosis). Some coarctations are mild and not hemodynamically significant. Findings suggestive of a hemodynamically significant coarctation include small luminal diameter (less than 10 mm or less than 50% of reference normal descending aorta at the diaphragm), presence of collaterals, and elevated gradient (more than 20 mm Hg clinically or by catheterization). The clinical gradient can be measured by comparing the highest arm systolic pressure (left or right) to the systolic pressure in the

Table 63.1. Indications for Interventional and Surgical Therapy for Atrial Septal Defects

Class I (is recommended)
• Closure of an ASD either percutaneously or surgically is indicated for right atrial and RV enlargement with or without symptoms.
• A sinus venous, coronary sinus, or primum ASD should be repaired surgically rather than by percutaneous closure.
• Surgeons with training and expertise in CHD should perform operations for various ASD closures.
Class II (is reasonable)
• Surgical closure of secundum ASD is reasonable when concomitant surgical repair/replacement of a tricuspid valve is considered or when the anatomy of the defect precludes the use of a percutaneous device.
• Closure of an ASD, either percutaneously or surgically, is reasonable in the presence of a. Paradoxic embolism b. Documented orthodeoxia-platypnea
Class IIb (may be reasonable)
• Closure of an ASD, either percutaneously or surgically, may be considered in the presence of net left-to-right shunting, pulmonary artery pressure less than two-thirds systemic vascular resistance, or when responsive to either pulmonary vasodilator therapy or test occlusion of the defect (patients should be treated in conjunction with providers who have expertise in the management of pulmonary hypertensive syndromes).
• Concomitant maze procedure may be considered for intermittent or chronic atrial tachyarrhythmias in adults with ASDs.
Class III (not recommended)
• Patients with severe irreversible PAH and no evidence of a left-to-right shunt should not undergo ASD closure.

ASD, Atrial septal defect; *CHD*, congenital heart disease; *PAH*, pulmonary arterial hypertension; *RV*, right ventricle.

Adapted from Warnes, C. A., Williams, R. G., Bashore, T. M., Child, J. S., Connolly, H. M., Dearani, J. A., et al. (2008). ACC/AHA 2008 guidelines for the management of adults with congenital heart disease: a report of the American College of Cardiology/American Heart Association Task Force on Practice Guidelines (Writing Committee to Develop Guidelines for the Management of Adults With Congenital Heart Disease). Journal of the American College of Cardiology, *52*, e143–e263.

leg (typically measured by palpation of the pedal pulses while inflating a cuff at the calf level). Patients with hemodynamically significant coarctations are at risk of a number of complications, including refractory hypertension, accelerated atherosclerosis, cerebrovascular disease, and aortopathy.

8. In coarctation of the aorta in the adult patient, when should percutaneous stenting be considered?

Most clinicians think that adult patients with hemodynamically significant coarctation of the aorta should be considered for intervention. Although surgery has been available for several decades, percutaneous dilation with stenting has evolved as an alternative. In the adult patient with residual stenosis after repair, stenting has become the first-line therapy at most centers. For adults with native coarctation, stenting has also become the first-line therapy at many centers. In patients who undergo percutaneous stenting, the anatomy needs to be suitable (i.e., no significant arch hypoplasia). In adult patients who undergo surgery, the usual procedure is placement of an interposition graft that is done through a left-sided thoracotomy approach.

9. Which adult patients with patent ductus arteriosus require percutaneous device closure?

A patent ductus arteriosus (PDA) connects the proximal part of the left pulmonary artery to the proximal descending aorta, just distal to the left subclavian artery (Fig. 63.5). The unrepaired ductus in an adult is usually small in diameter, and the resultant left-to-right shunt is hemodynamically insignificant. However, in some patients the ductus diameter is large and results in severe pulmonary hypertension (Eisenmenger's syndrome) if not repaired in childhood. Occasionally, some adults have

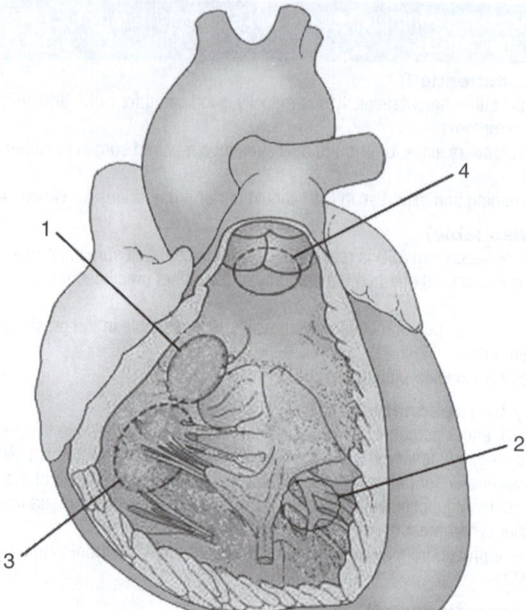

Fig. 63.2. Ventricular septal defects: *1*, perimembranous; *2*, muscular; *3*, inlet; *4*, outlet. *(Modified from Gatzoulis, M. A., Webb, G. D., & Daubeney, P. E. F. [2003].* Diagnosis and management of adult congenital heart disease *[p. 171]. Edinburgh: Churchill Livingstone.)*

Table 63.2. Recommendations for Surgical Ventricular Septal Defect Closure

Class I

- Surgeons with training and expertise in CHD should perform VSD closure operations.
- Closure of a VSD is indicated when there is a Qp/Qs (pulmonary to systemic blood flow ratio) of 2.0 or more and clinical evidence of LV volume overload.
- Closure of a VSD is indicated when the patient has a history of IE.

Class IIa

- Closure of a VSD is reasonable when net left-to-right shunting is present at a Qp/Qs greater than 1.5 with pulmonary artery pressure less than two-thirds of systemic pressure and PVR less than two-thirds of systemic vascular resistance.
- Closure of a VSD is reasonable when net left-to-right shunting is present at a Qp/Qs greater than 1.5 in the presence of LV systolic or diastolic failure.

Class III

- VSD closure is not recommended in patients with severe irreversible PAH.

CHD, Congenital heart disease; *IE*, infective endocarditis, *LV*, left ventricle; *PAH*, pulmonary arterial hypertension; *PVR*, pulmonary valve replacement; *VSD*, ventricular septal defect.

Adapted from Warnes, C. A., Williams, R. G., Bashore, T. M., Child, J. S., Connolly, H. M., Dearani, J. A., et al. (2008). ACC/AHA 2008 guidelines for the management of adults with congenital heart disease: a report of the American College of Cardiology/American Heart Association Task Force on Practice Guidelines (Writing Committee to Develop Guidelines for the Management of Adults With Congenital Heart Disease). Journal of the American College of Cardiology, 52, *e143–e263.*

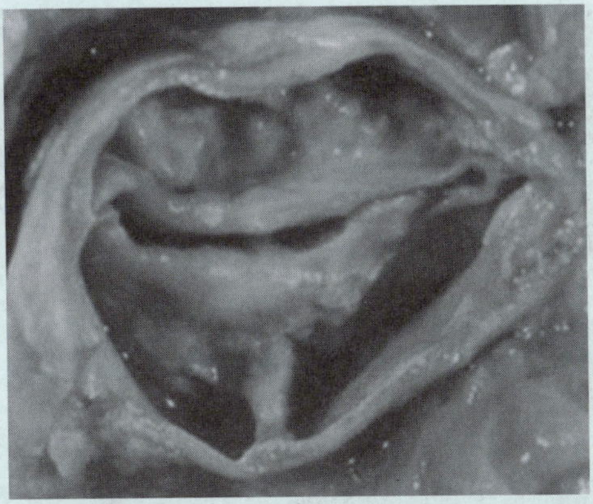

Fig. 63.3. Aortic stenosis that has developed in a bicuspid aortic valve. *(Image from Libby, P., Bonow, R. O., Mann, D. L., & Zipes, D. P. [2008].* Braunwald's heart disease: a textbook of cardiovascular medicine *(8th ed.). Philadelphia: Saunders.)*

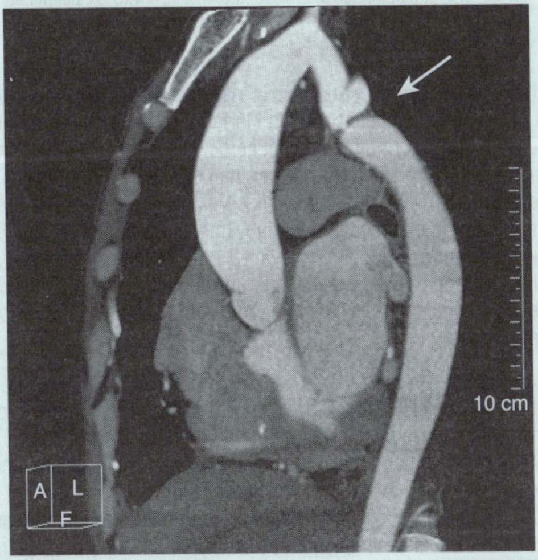

Fig. 63.4. Computed tomography scan demonstrating severe aortic coarctation *(arrow). AAo,* Ascending aorta; *DDo,* descending aorta. *(Image courtesy of Dr. Cafer Zorkun.)*

moderate-size ducts resulting in shunting that is not hemodynamically negligible but not significant enough to cause severe pulmonary hypertension. In these patients the left ventricle will be dilated and the pulmonary pressure may be mildly elevated. Clinically they will have a continuous murmur, a large pulse pressure, and signs of left ventricular dilation. This latter group should undergo percutaneous closure in an attempt to prevent long-term complications. Although controversial, some centers advocate routine closure of small PDAs to prevent endarteritis.

10. How is Marfan syndrome diagnosed?

The criteria for the diagnosis of Marfan syndrome have evolved over the years. The latest iteration was published in 2010 and has put more emphasis on gene testing, presence of aortic dilation, and abnormalities of the corneal lens. The main role of the cardiologist is to carefully assess the patient for aortic abnormalities. This usually consists of performing an echocardiogram and magnetic resonance imaging (MRI) of the thoracic aorta. Patients with suspected Marfan syndrome should be referred to a geneticist because the clinical phenotype overlaps with multiple other systemic disorders, and the role of genetic testing is continuously evolving.

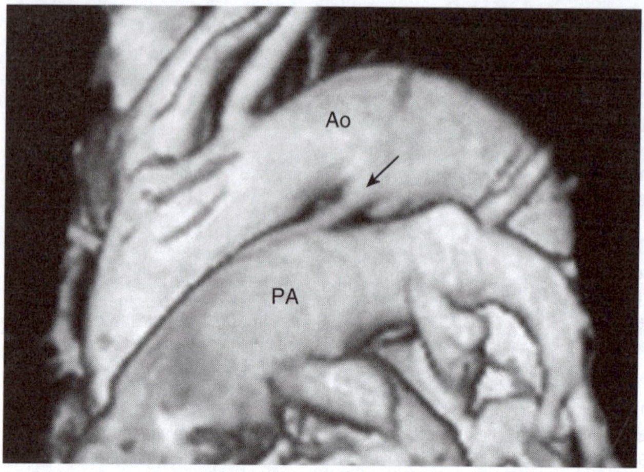

Fig. 63.5. A small patent ductus arteriosus *(arrow). Ao,* Aorta; *PA,* pulmonary artery.

11. When should Marfan patients with aortic root dilation be referred for surgery?

Although any part of the aorta can be involved in Marfan syndrome, the root is usually affected. Surgery (for root dilation) is performed to prevent aortic dissection or rupture and is generally recommended when the aortic diameter is greater than or equal to 50 mm. For patients with rapid progression (more than 5 mm/year) or a family history of dissection, intervention is recommended by some specialists at greater than or equal to 45 mm. Traditionally a Bentall procedure was performed in which the native aortic valve and root are replaced with a composite conduit (a tube graft attached to a prosthetic valve). If technically possible, the preferred first-line approach now consists of a valve-sparing procedure (David procedure) in which the root is replaced by a prosthetic conduit and the native valve is kept in place.

12. What is tetralogy of Fallot, and what is the main complication seen in the adult?

Tetralogy of Fallot (TOF) consists of four features: right ventricular outflow tract (RVOT) obstruction, a large VSD, an overriding ascending aorta, and right ventricular hypertrophy. The RVOT obstruction is the clinically important lesion and may be subvalvular, valvular, or supravalvular or may be at multiple levels. Repair, done in infancy, involves closing the VSD and relieving the RVOT obstruction. In many patients, to relieve the RVOT obstruction, surgery on the pulmonary annulus and valve leaflets is required and is usually complicated by severe residual pulmonary insufficiency. In the adult, over time, chronic severe pulmonary insufficiency often leads to right ventricular dysfunction and exercise intolerance, for which a pulmonary valve replacement (PVR) may be necessary. When PVR is performed, a tissue prosthesis is usually placed (homograft or porcine/bovine prosthesis). The problem with tissue prostheses in young adults is that they require replacement at 10- to 15-year intervals. A percutaneous pulmonary valve prosthesis approach is increasingly being used to manage these patients with severe pulmonary insufficiency. Other complications in TOF include residual RVOT obstruction, residual VSD leak, right ventricular dysfunction, aortic root dilation, and arrhythmias.

13. What are the three *d*s of Ebstein anomaly?

Ebstein anomaly is characterized by an apically *displaced* tricuspid valve that is *dysplastic*, with a right ventricle that may be *dysfunctional.* The displacement affects predominantly the septal and posterior leaflets of the valve. The leaflets are usually diminutive and tethered to the ventricular wall. Typically the anterior leaflet is unusually elongated. The right ventricle is often thin and can have both diastolic and systolic dysfunction. Half of patients have an interatrial communication, either patent foramen ovale (PFO) or ASD. Fifteen percent of patients have accessory pathways, which will manifest clinically as Wolf-Parkinson-White syndrome. The primary complication of Ebstein anomaly is tricuspid regurgitation and right-sided heart failure. If significant enough, placement of a tissue prosthesis or valve repair (if the valve anatomy is suitable) is indicated.

14. What drug therapy should now be considered in all patients with Eisenmenger's syndrome?

Eisenmenger's syndrome refers to markedly elevated pulmonary pressures caused by a long-standing left-to-right shunt between the systemic and pulmonary artery circulations because of a congenital defect. *Left-to-right* shunting initially leads to increased pulmonary vascular flow, which over time induces changes in the pulmonary vasculature leading to increased pulmonary vascular resistance. When the pulmonary vascular resistance is near, or exceeds, the systemic vascular resistance, the shunt reverses. The resultant *right-to-left* shunting results in hypoxia and cyanosis. The most common defect causing Eisenmenger's syndrome is a VSD. Other causes include PDAs, atrioventricular septal defects, and ASDs. Traditionally these patients have been treated with supportive measures. However, studies have shown the beneficial use of pulmonary vasodilators, such as bosentan (an endothelin blocker), sildenafil (a nitric oxide promoter), and various prostacyclins. These agents decrease pulmonary artery pressure, improve functional capacity, and have a mortality benefit. All Eisenmenger's patients should be assessed by an appropriate specialist regarding the use of pulmonary vasodilators.

15. When should an Eisenmenger's patient be phlebotomized?

In Eisenmenger's syndrome, hypoxia resulting from the right-to-left shunt stimulates marrow production of red blood cells and leads to an elevated hematocrit. Historically, Eisenmenger's patients were phlebotomized routinely because an elevated hematocrit was thought to predispose to a thrombotic event, as with patients with the hematologic condition polycythemia vera. However, contemporary data suggest that prophylactic phlebotomy in Eisenmenger's patients is more harmful than beneficial (i.e., it causes iron deficiency, decreases exercise tolerance, potentially increases the risk of stroke). As such, the use of phlebotomy is now more restrictive and should be considered only in patients with symptoms of hyperviscosity (headaches, dizziness, fatigue, achiness), who have a hematocrit greater than 65%, with no evidence of iron deficiency; in modern practice, only a minority of Eisenmenger's patients should undergo phlebotomy.

16. Which types of congenital heart disease lesions have particularly poor outcomes in pregnancy?

Very high-risk congenital heart disease lesions include the following:

- Unrepaired cyanotic heart disease
- Eisenmenger's syndrome
- Severe aortic stenosis
- Marfan syndrome with a dilated aortic root (>40 to 45 mm)
- Mechanical valve prosthesis
- Significant systemic ventricular dysfunction (ejection fraction [EF] 40% or less)

These patients should be counseled accordingly about the significant maternal risks and poor fetal outcomes that are associated with pregnancy.

17. What are the two types of transpositions?

Transposition complexes can be divided into two groups. In complete transposition of the great arteries (D-TGA), the anomaly can be simplistically conceptualized as an *inversion of the great vessels* (Fig. 63.6A). The aorta comes out of the right ventricle, and the pulmonary artery comes out of the left ventricle. Desaturated blood is pumped into the systemic circulation, whereas oxygenated blood is pumped into the pulmonary circulation. Without intervention, this condition is associated with very poor outcomes and usually demise in early infancy.

Congenitally corrected transposition of the great arteries (L-TGA) can be conceptualized as an *inversion of the ventricles* (see Fig. 63.6B). Desaturated blood and oxygenated blood are thus pumped in the appropriate arterial circulations. In many cases, associated anomalies, such as a VSD, pulmonary stenosis, an abnormal tricuspid valve, and heart block, are present. These patients can survive or present de novo in adulthood without surgical intervention.

18. What is meant by a *systemic* right ventricle?

A *systemic right ventricle* refers to a heart anomaly in which the *morphologic* right ventricle pumps blood into the aorta. Ventricular morphology is determined by anatomic features typical to each ventricle. For example, the morphologic right ventricle has a tricuspid atrioventricular valve (with attachments to the septum and apical displacement compared with the mitral valve) and coarse apical trabeculations. L-TGA is a congenital heart defect in which there is a systemic right ventricle. In the first few decades of life, the right ventricle is able to handle pumping into the high-pressure systemic circulation; however, in adulthood, the right ventricular function begins to deteriorate in the majority of patients. This is usually associated with tricuspid regurgitation and manifests clinically as heart failure.

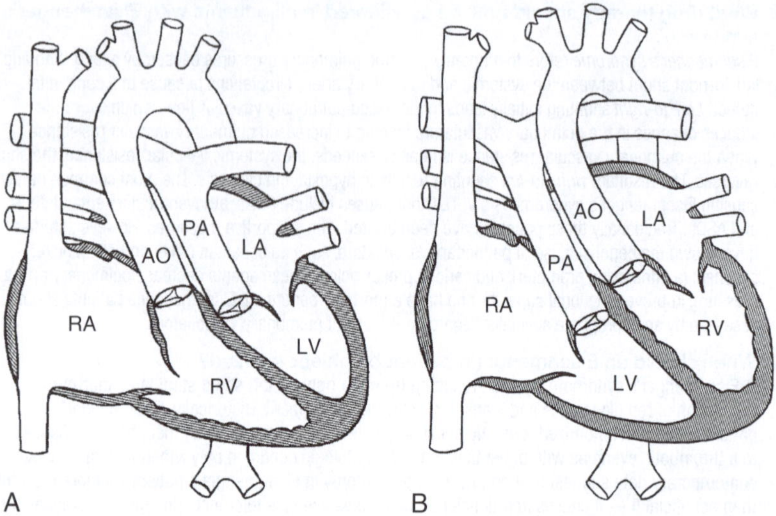

Fig. 63.6. **A,** D-TGA. **B,** L-TGA. *AO,* Aorta, *LA,* left atrium; *LV,* left ventricle; *PA,* pulmonary artery, *RA,* right atrium; *RV,* right ventricle. *(Modified from Mullins, C. E., & Mayer, D. C. [1988].* Congenital heart disease, a diagrammatic atlas *[pp. 164, 182]. New York, NY: Wiley-Liss.)*

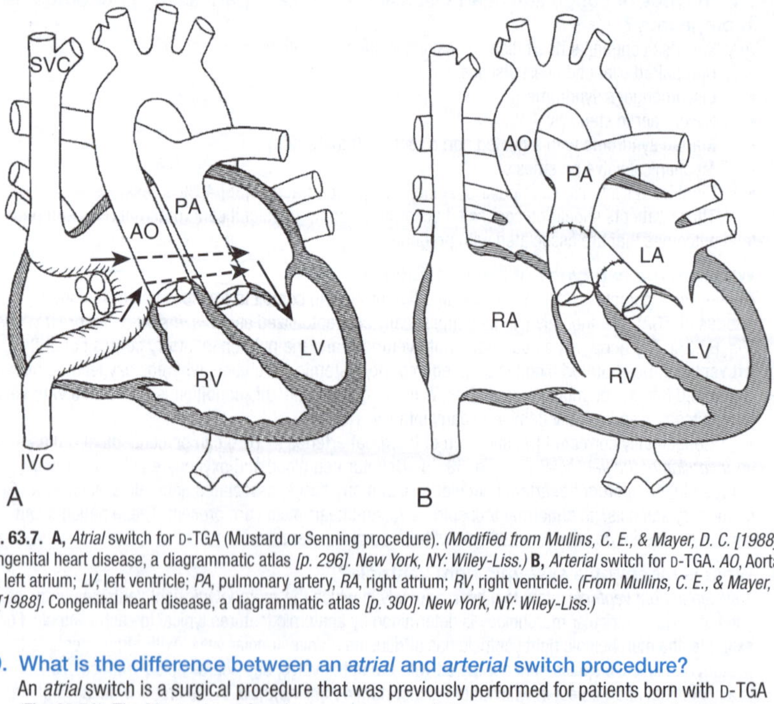

Fig. 63.7. **A,** *Atrial* switch for D-TGA (Mustard or Senning procedure). *(Modified from Mullins, C. E., & Mayer, D. C. [1988].* Congenital heart disease, a diagrammatic atlas *[p. 296]. New York, NY: Wiley-Liss.)* **B,** *Arterial* switch for D-TGA. *AO,* Aorta, *LA,* left atrium; *LV,* left ventricle; *PA,* pulmonary artery, *RA,* right atrium; *RV,* right ventricle. *(From Mullins, C. E., & Mayer, D. C. [1988].* Congenital heart disease, a diagrammatic atlas *[p. 300]. New York, NY: Wiley-Liss.)*

19. What is the difference between an *atrial* and *arterial* switch procedure?

An *atrial* switch is a surgical procedure that was previously performed for patients born with D-TGA (Fig. 63.7A). The Mustard and Senning procedures are both examples of an atrial switch and involve rerouting systemic and pulmonary venous flow to the respective pulmonary and systemic ventricles. This procedure was replaced by the *arterial* switch, which consists of "switching" the great arteries and reimplanting the coronary arteries to the *new* aorta (see Fig. 63.7B). The arterial switch is performed in the first few weeks after birth and has been the standard of care since the mid 1980s for patients born with D-TGA.

20. **Which patients with adult congenital heart disease require antibiotic prophylaxis?**
In the last iteration of the American Heart Association guidelines for antibiotic prophylaxis for endocarditis, a more restricted use of antibiotic prophylaxis in congenital heart disease was proposed, with increased emphasis on oral health. Prophylaxis is now suggested only in the following circumstances:
- Unrepaired cyanotic heart disease
- Prosthetic valves
- Residual defects after repair in the setting of prosthetic material
- The first 6 months after repair with a device or prosthesis
- Patients with a history of prior endocarditis

Bibliography and Suggested Readings

Baumgartner, H., Bonhoeffer, P., De Groot, N. M., de Haan, F., Deanfield, J. E., Galie, N., et al. (2010). ESC guidelines for the management of grown-up congenital heart disease. *European Heart Journal, 31*(23), 2915–2957.

Broberg, C. S. (2016). Challenges and management issues in adults with cyanotic congenital heart disease. *Heart, 102*, 720–725.

Dimopoulos, K., Inuzuka, R., Goletto, S., Giannakoulas, G., Swan, L., Wort, S. J., et al. (2010). Improved survival among patients with Eisenmenger syndrome receiving advanced therapy for pulmonary arterial hypertension. *Circulation, 121*, 20–25.

Gatzoulis, M. A., Webb, G. D., & Daubeney, P. E. F. (2011). *Diagnosis and management of adult congenital heart disease* (2nd ed.). Philadelphia, PA: Churchill Livingstone.

Regitz-Zagrosek, V., Blomstrom Lundqvist, C., Borghi, C., Cifkova, R., Ferreira, R., Foidart, J. M., et al. (2011). ESC Guidelines on the management of cardiovascular diseases during pregnancy. *European Heart Journal, 32*, 3147–3197.

Silversides, C. K., Marelli, A., Beauchesne, L., Dore, A., Kiess, M., Salehian, O., et al. (2010). Canadian Cardiovascular Society 2009 Consensus Conference on the management of adults with congenital heart disease: executive summary. *Canadian Journal of Cardiology, 26*(3), 143–150.

Warnes, C. A., Williams, R. G., Bashore, T. M., Child, J. S., Connolly, H. M., Dearani, J. A., et al. (2008). ACC/AHA 2008 guidelines for the management of adults with congenital heart disease: a report of the American College of Cardiology/American Heart Association Task Force on Practice Guidelines (Writing Committee to Develop Guidelines for the Management of Adults With Congenital Heart Disease). *Journal of the American College of Cardiology, 52*, e143–e263.

CHAPTER 64

CARDIAC TUMORS

David Aguilar, Glenn N. Levine

1. Which are more common, primary cardiac tumors or metastatic tumors to the heart?

Metastatic tumors to the heart are markedly more common than primary cardiac tumors, with one source reporting metastatic involvement of the heart to be 20 to 40 times more prevalent than primary cardiac tumors. Primary cardiac tumors are extremely rare, occurring in one autopsy series in less than 0.1% of subjects.

2. What are the most common tumors that metastasize to the heart?

The most common tumors that spread to the heart are lung (bronchogenic) cancer, breast cancer, melanoma, thyroid cancer, esophageal cancer, lymphoma, and leukemia. Malignant melanoma has the greatest propensity to spread to the heart, with 50% to 65% of patients with malignant melanoma having cardiac metastases. Tumors may spread to the heart via direct extension, the circulatory system, or via lymphatics. Renal cell carcinoma may extend up the inferior vena cava all the way into the heart.

3. Are most primary cardiac tumors benign or malignant?

Most primary cardiac tumors are benign. In adults, 75% of all primary cardiac tumors are benign. In children, 90% of primary cardiac tumors are benign.

4. What are the most common primary cardiac tumors?

The most common benign cardiac tumors in adults are myxomas, accounting for approximately half of all primary cardiac neoplasms; other common benign cardiac tumors are lipomas and papillary fibroelastomas. Rhabdomyomas are the most common benign tumor occurring in infants and children. Interestingly, rhabdomyomas usually regress over time and do not require specific treatment in asymptomatic individuals (Table 64.1).

5. In what chamber do most myxomas occur?

Approximately 75% to 80% of myxomas occur in the left atrium (LA) (Fig. 64.1), with 15% to 20% occurring in the right atrium. Only 3% to 4% of myxomas arise in the left ventricle (LV), and 3% to 4% arise in the right ventricle (RV). Myxomas are usually pedunculated and typically arise from the interatrial septum via a stalk. They are described on gross pathologic examination as gelatinous in consistency. The majority of myxomas are solitary. They most commonly occur between the third and sixth decades of life and more frequently occur in women.

The clinical manifestations of myxomas often include one or more of the three classic symptoms: (1) embolism, (2) intracardiac obstruction, and (3) constitutional symptoms. Systemic embolism occurs in 30% to 40% of patients. Myxomas can cause effective obstruction of filling of the LV or RV, leading to left or right heart failure symptoms and findings, mimicking the symptoms and findings

Table 64.1. Primary and Secondary (Metastatic) Tumors Involving the Heart

PRIMARY TUMORS	SECONDARY (METASTATIC) TUMORS
Myxoma	Lung (bronchogenic) cancer
Lipoma	Breast cancer
Papillary fibroelastoma	Esophageal cancer
Rhabdomyoma	Thyroid cancer
Fibroma	Melanoma
Angiosarcoma	Lymphoma
Rhabdomyosarcoma	Leukemia
Lymphoma	Renal cell carcinoma
Lipomatous hypertrophy	

of mitral or tricuspid valve stenosis. Constitutional symptoms and findings are also common. The systemic symptoms include anemia, leukocytosis, elevated erythrocyte sedimentation rate, fevers, arthralgias, myalgias, rash, and fatigue. These systemic symptoms, which may be seen in 25% to 40% of individuals with myxomas, are thought to be due to the tumor secretion of interleukin-6. Most myxomas occur sporadically, but approximately 7% to 10% may be familial.

6. What are the most common primary malignant tumors?

The most common primary malignant tumors are sarcomas (Figs. 64.2 and 64.3). Such sarcomas include angiosarcomas (the most common), rhabdomyosarcomas, fibrosarcomas, and leiomyosarcomas. Upon imaging, sarcomas often appear as large, heterogeneous, infiltrative masses that frequently occupy most of the affected chamber (Fig. 64.4). The results of surgery or chemotherapy in the treatment of cardiac sarcomas have been generally poor, with mean survival of only 6 to 12 months.

7. What symptoms do cardiac tumors cause?

Symptoms of tumors often depend on the size and location of the tumor, as well the histology of the tumor itself. Left-sided cardiac tumors may manifest with cardioembolic features, such as stroke, visceral infarction, or peripheral emboli. Large cardiac tumors may also present with symptoms attributed to obstruction of flow or valvular dysfunction. Left atrial myxomas may cause effective mitral valve stenosis (or regurgitation). Tumors may also cause hemodynamic effects via compression or mass effects. Tumors may lead to atrial or ventricular arrhythmias. Tumors involving the pericardium can cause pericardial effusion and tamponade. Constitutional symptoms (fatigue, weight loss, fever) occur not infrequently, as well as anemia, elevated erythrocyte sedimentation rate, elevated C-reactive protein, and other nonspecific laboratory findings. In patients with known noncardiac cancer, the development of arrhythmias (particularly atrial fibrillation) or development of findings suggesting pericardial

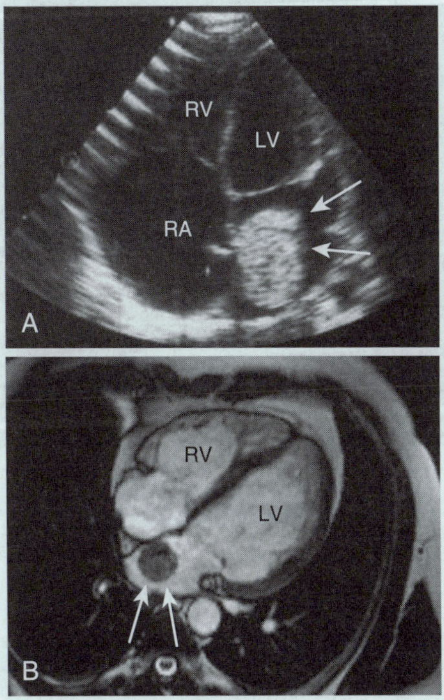

Fig. 64.1. Left atrial myxoma, as visualized **(A)** on transthoracic echocardiogram and **(B)** on cardiac magnetic resonance imaging. *LV,* Left ventricle; *RV,* right ventricle. *(A—modified from Erdol, C., Ozturk, C., Ocal, A., Bozat, T., Koca, V., Ozdemir, A. [2001]. Contralateral recurrence of atrial myxoma—case report and review of the literature,* Images in Paediatric Cardiology, 8, *3–9.)*

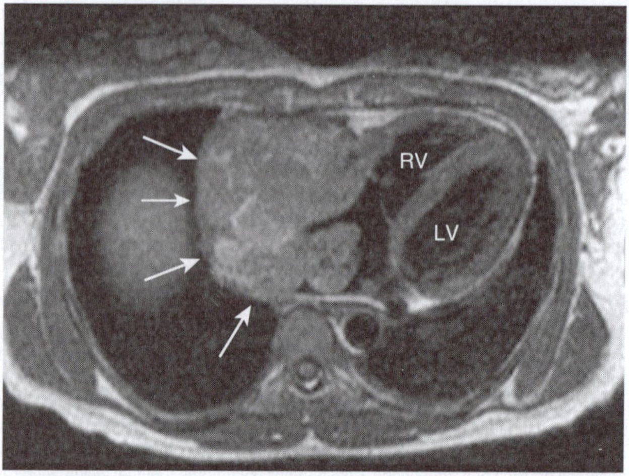

Fig. 64.2. Massive angiosarcoma *(arrows)* arising from the right atrium, as visualized by magnetic resonance imaging. *LV,* Left ventricle; *RV,* right ventricle. *(Modified from Sparrow, P. J., Kurian, J. B., Jones, T. R., Sivananthan, M. U. [2005]. MR imaging of cardiac tumors,* Radiographics, *25[5], 1255–1276.)*

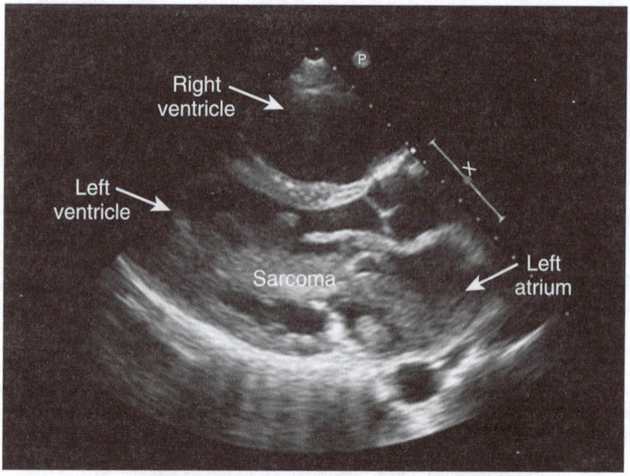

Fig. 64.3. Large undifferentiated sarcoma in the left atrium (LA) visualized by echocardiography.

effusion/tamponade (distended neck veins, hypotension, pulsus paradoxus, new low voltage on the electrocardiogram [ECG]) should prompt immediate evaluation for cardiac/pericardial metastasis.

8. **What is the workup for suspected cardiac tumors?**
The initial workup is a transthoracic echocardiogram (echo). Many tumors will also be discovered incidentally or surreptitiously by cardiac echo. Tumors may be further evaluated with transesophageal echo (TEE), cardiac magnetic resonance imaging (MRI), or cardiac computed tomography (CT). The role of positron emission tomography (PET) in the evaluation of cardiac tumors is in evolution. Transvenous endomyocardial biopsy is generally not warranted for diagnosis but could be considered if the diagnosis cannot be established by noninvasive modalities (such as cardiac MRI) or less invasive (noncardiac) biopsy. Cytologic analyses of pericardial effusion or pericardial biopsy may provide diagnostic information regarding metastatic cardiac tumors.

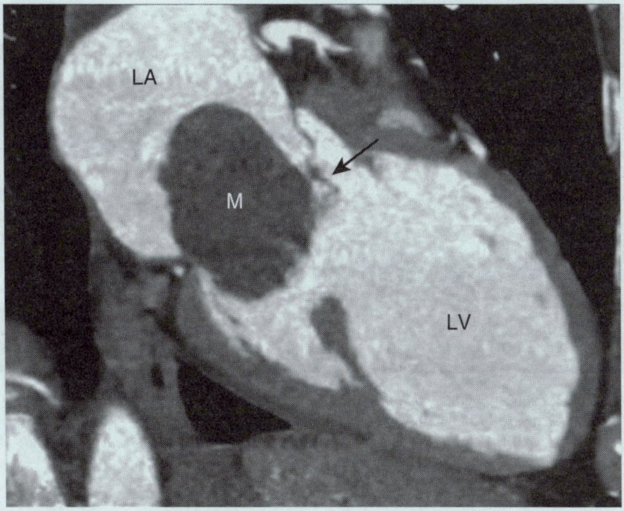

Fig. 64.4. A left atrial myxoma *(M)* transiting across the mitral valve *(black arrow)* into the LV. This may cause an audible *tumor plop. LA,* Left atrium; *LV,* left ventricle.

9. What are the most common tumors affecting the pericardium?

Primary tumors of the pericardium are rare. Benign pericardial tumors and lesions include cysts, lipoma teratoma, fibroma, and angioma. Malignant pericardial tumors include mesothelioma and sarcoma. More common is secondary involvement of the pericardium. This may occur through direct extension, retrograde lymphangitic spread, or hematogenous dissemination. Tumor involvement of the pericardium most commonly manifests as pericardial effusion or, occasionally, pericardial tamponade.

10. What is a tumor plop?

A tumor plop is a sound heard in early diastole during auscultation produced when a left atrial myxoma prolapses into the LV during diastole (see Fig. 64.4). The sound may be due to the tumor striking the left ventricular wall or to tension created on the tumor stalk.

11. What is lipomatous hypertrophy of the interatrial septum?

Lipomatous hypertrophy is an abnormal, exaggerated growth of normal fat cells. It occurs in the interatrial septum, resulting in the appearance of a thickened atrial septum. Lipomatous hypertrophy of the interatrial septum involves the limbus of the fossa ovalis and spares the fossa ovalis membrane, giving the atrial septum a “dumbbell shape.” The finding itself is benign.

12. What is the most common valvular tumor?

The most common valvular tumor is papillary fibroelastoma. Papillary fibroelastomas are the second most common primary benign cardiac tumors and comprise 75% of valvular tumors. Echocardiographic and pathologic databases suggest that the diagnosis is increasing in frequency. More than 70% of papillary fibroelastomas occur on cardiac valves, and more than 80% to 90% of papillary fibroelastomas are solitary. The most usual location is on the mitral and aortic valves, although they can occur on right-sided valves. Papillary fibroelastomas are often small (<1 cm) and appear flower-like or frond-like with a narrow stalk. Most common symptoms related to papillary fibroelastomas are related to embolic events, such as stroke or transient ischemic attacks. The optimal treatment of papillary fibroelastomas has not been well defined. Surgical resection may be recommended in individuals who have had an embolic event. In asymptomatic individuals, surgical resection may be considered in those with mobile, left-sided papillary fibroelastomas in whom the risk of surgery is low (Fig. 64.5).

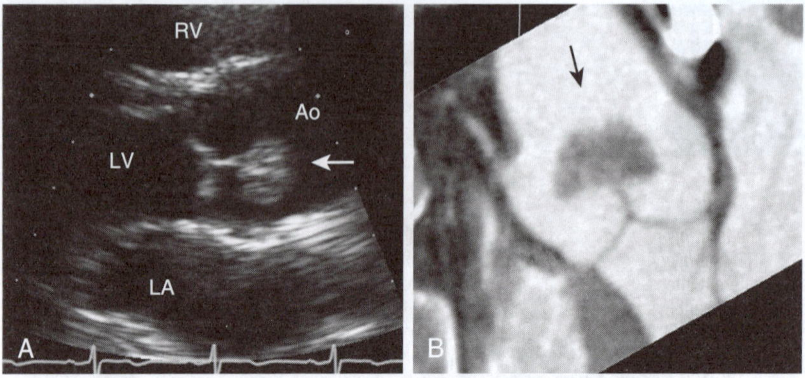

Fig. 64.5. Fibroelastoma. Echocardiography *(left panel)* and cardiac computed tomography *(right panel)* images of a papillary fibroelastoma *(arrows)* attached to the aortic valve. *Ao,* Aorta; *LA,* left atrium; *LV,* left ventricle; *RV,* right ventricle. *(Images from Levine, G. N. [2014].* Color atlas of cardiovascular disease. *New Delhi, India: Jaypee Brothers Medical Publishers.)*

13. What is the Carney complex?

Known by various names and acronyms, the Carney complex is an autosomal dominant syndrome consisting of cardiac myxomas, cutaneous myxomas, spotty pigmentation of the skin, endocrinopathy, and other tumors. Myxomas occurring as part of the Carney complex are reported to account for 7% of all cardiac myxomas. Myxomas occurring as part of the Carney complex often present earlier in life, tend to be located in atypical locations, are often multiple, and often have a higher rate of recurrence after surgical resection than sporadic myxomas. Linkage studies of the Carney complex have revealed two genetic susceptibility loci.

Bibliography and Suggested Readings

Basso, C., Rizzo, S., Valente, M., & Thiene, G. (2012). Prevalence and pathology of primary cardiac tumours. *Cardiovascular Medicine, 15*(1), 18–29.

Bruce, C. J. (2011). Cardiac tumours: diagnosis and management. *Heart, 97*(2), 151–160.

Carney, J. A., Gordon, H., Carpenter, P. C., Shenoy, B. V., & Go, V. L. (1985). The complex of myxomas, spotty pigmentation, and endocrine overactivity. *Medicine (Baltimore), 64*(4), 270–283.

Hudzik, B., Miszalski-Jamka, K., Glowacki, J., Lekston, A., Gierlotka, M., Zembala, M., et al. (2015). Malignant tumors of the heart. *Cancer Epidemiology, 39*(5), 665–672.

Kassop, D., Donovan, M. S., Cheezum, M. K., Nguyen, B. T., Gambill, N. B., Blankstein, R., et al. (2014). Cardiac masses on cardiac CT: a review. *Current Cardiovascular Imaging Reports, 7*, 9281.

O'Donnell, D. H., Abbara, S., Chaithiraphan, V., Yared, K., Killeen, R. P., Cury, R. C., et al. (2009). Cardiac tumors: optimal cardiac MR sequences and spectrum of imaging appearances. *AJR American Journal of Roentgenology, 193*(2), 377–387.

Paraskevaidis, I. A., Michalakeas, C. A., Papadopoulos, C. H., & Anastasiou-Nana, M. (2011). Cardiac tumors. *ISRN Oncology, 2011.* Article ID 208929. <http://www.hindawi.com/journals/isrn/2011/208929/> Accessed April 16, 2016.

Reardon, M. J., Walkes, J. C., & Benjamin, R. (2006). Therapy insight: malignant primary cardiac tumors. *Nature Clinical Practice. Cardiovascular Medicine, 3*(10), 548–553.

Reynen, K. (1995). Cardiac myxomas. *New England Journal of Medicine, 333*, 1610–1617.

Reynen, K., Kockeritz, U., & Strasser, R. H. (2004). Metastases to the heart. *Annals of Oncology, 15*(3), 375–381.

Tamin, S. S., Maleszewski, J. J., Scott, C. G., Khan, S. K., Edwards, W. D., Bruce, C. J., et al. (2015). Prognostic and bioepidemiologic implications of papillary fibroelastomas. *Journal of the American College of Cardiology, 65*(22), 2420–2429.

HYPERTENSIVE CRISIS

Nicholas Governatori, Charles V. Pollack Jr.

CHAPTER 65

1. **What is a hypertensive crisis?**
   The term *hypertensive crisis* generally is inclusive of two different diagnoses, *hypertensive emergency* (HE) and *hypertensive urgency*. Distinguishing between the two is important because they require different intensities of therapy. It should be noted that older and less specific terminology, such as "malignant hypertension" and "accelerated hypertension," should no longer be used. The Seventh Report of the Joint National Committee on Prevention, Detection, Evaluation, and Treatment of High Blood Pressure (JNC-7) defines HE as being "characterized by severe elevations in blood pressure (BP) (>180/120 mm Hg), complicated by evidence of impending or progressive target organ dysfunction." JNC-7 defines hypertensive urgency as "those situations associated with severe elevations in blood pressure without progressive target organ dysfunction." The updated JNC-8 did not change these definitions. The important thing to remember is that there is no absolute value of BP that separates the two syndromes. Instead, the most important distinction is whether there is evidence of impending or progressive end-organ damage, which defines an emergency, or other symptoms that are felt referable to the BP.

2. **How commonly do these situations occur?**
   It is estimated that 50 to 75 million people have hypertension and more than half of them are unaware of having this condition. Overall, hypertension accounts for 110 million emergency department (ED) visits per year, with an estimated 0.5% of all ED visits attributed to hypertensive crises.

3. **What are the causes of hypertensive crisis?**
   The most common cause of HE is an abrupt increase in BP in patients with chronic hypertension. Medication noncompliance is a frequent cause of such changes. BP control rates for patients diagnosed with hypertension are less than 50%. Older adults and African Americans are at increased risk of developing an HE. Other causes of HEs include stimulant intoxication (cocaine, methamphetamine, and phencyclidine), withdrawal syndromes (clonidine, beta-adrenergic blockers), pheochromocytoma, physiologic stress in the postoperative period (following cardiothoracic, vascular, or neurosurgical procedures), and adverse drug interactions with monoamine oxidase (MAO) inhibitors.

4. **What are the common clinical presentations of hypertensive crisis?**
   Typical presentations include severe headache, shortness of breath, epistaxis, faintness, or severe anxiety. Clinical syndromes typically associated with HE include hypertensive encephalopathy, intracerebral hemorrhage, acute myocardial infarction (MI), acute heart failure, pulmonary edema, unstable angina, dissecting aortic aneurysm, or preeclampsia/eclampsia (Fig. 65.1). Note that in HE presentations, there is evidence of impending or progressive target organ dysfunction and that the absolute value of the BP is not pathognomonic.

5. **What historical information should be obtained?**
   A thorough history, especially as it relates to prior hypertension, is important to obtain and document because most patients with an HE carry a diagnosis of hypertension and are either inadequately treated or are noncompliant with treatment.

   A thorough medication history is also essential. The patient's current medications need to be reviewed and updated to include timing, dosages, recent changes in therapy, last doses taken, and compliance. Patients should also be questioned about over-the-counter medication usage and recreational drug use because these agents may also affect BP.

6. **How should the physical examination be focused?**
   Physical examination should start with recording the BP in both arms with an appropriately sized BP cuff. Direct ophthalmoscopy should be performed with attention to evaluating for papilledema and hypertensive exudates. A brief, focused neurologic examination to assess mental status and the presence or absence of focal neurologic deficits should be performed. The cardiopulmonary examination should focus on signs of pulmonary edema and aortic dissection, such as rales, elevated

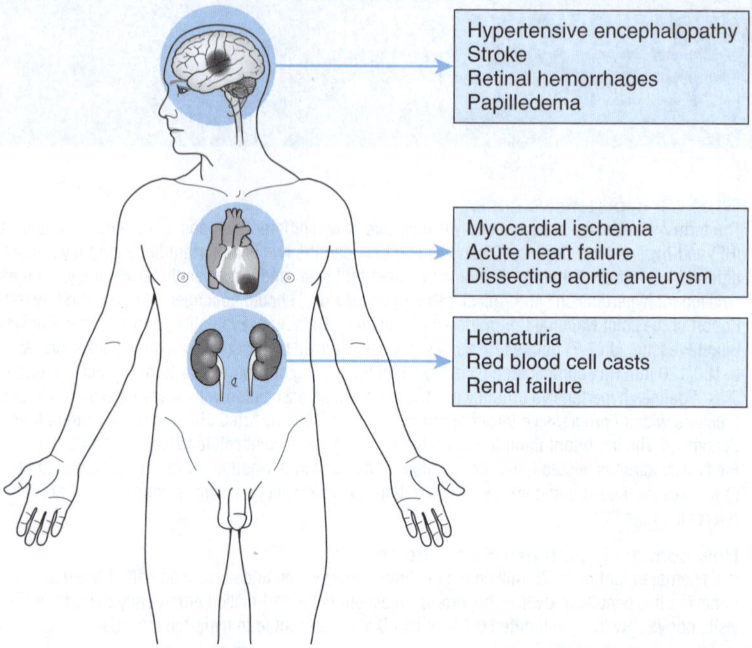

Fig. 65.1. End-organ failure in hypertensive emergency. *(Image from Zanotti-Cavazzoni, S. L. [2014]. Hypertensive crises. In J. E. Parrillo, & R. P. Dellinger (Eds.),* Critical care medicine: principles of diagnosis and management in the adult *[chapter 34, pp. 585–593.e2]. Philadelphia, PA: Saunders.)*

jugular venous pressure, cardiac gallops, or new aortic insufficiency murmur. Peripheral pulses should be palpated and assessed. Abdominal examination should include palpation for abdominal masses and tenderness and auscultation for abdominal bruits.

7. **What laboratory and ancillary data should be obtained?**
All patients should have an electrocardiogram (ECG) performed to assess for left ventricular hypertrophy, acute ischemia or infarction, and arrhythmias. Urinalysis (UA) should be performed to evaluate for hematuria and proteinuria as signs of acute renal failure. Women of child-bearing age should have a urine pregnancy test performed. Laboratory studies should include a basic metabolic profile with blood urea nitrogen (BUN) and creatinine, a urine or serum toxicology screen, and a complete blood count (CBC) with a peripheral smear to evaluate for signs of microangiopathic hemolytic anemia. If acute coronary syndrome is suspected, cardiac biomarkers should be assessed. Choice of radiographic studies, if any, should be based on the presentation and diagnostic considerations. A chest radiograph is often ordered to evaluate for pulmonary edema, cardiomegaly, and mediastinal widening. If there are any focal neurologic findings, a computed tomography (CT) scan of the brain should be performed to evaluate for hemorrhage.

8. **What are the cardiac manifestations of hypertensive emergencies?**
Cardiac manifestations of HE include acute coronary syndromes, acute cardiogenic pulmonary edema, and aortic dissection. The latter deserves special attention because it has much higher short-term morbidity and mortality, requires more urgent and rapid reduction in BP, and also requires specific inhibition of the reflex tachycardia often associated with BP-lowering agents. It is recommended that patients with aortic dissection have their systolic BP (SBP) reduced to at least 120 mm Hg within 20 minutes, a much more rapid decrease than is recommended for other syndromes associated with HE.

9. **What are the central nervous system manifestations of hypertensive emergency?**
Neurologic emergencies associated with HE include subarachnoid hemorrhage, cerebral infarction, intraparenchymal hemorrhage, and hypertensive encephalopathy. Patients with hemorrhage and

infarction usually have focal neurologic findings and may have corresponding findings on head CT or magnetic resonance imaging (MRI) of the brain. Hypertensive encephalopathy is more difficult to diagnose; symptoms may include severe headache, vomiting, drowsiness, confusion, visual disturbances, and seizures; coma may ensue. Papilledema is often present on physical examination.

10. What are the renal manifestations of hypertensive emergencies?

Renal failure can both cause and be caused by HE. Hypertensive renal failure typically presents as nonoliguric renal failure, often with hematuria.

11. What are the pregnancy-related issues with hypertensive emergency?

Preeclampsia is a syndrome that includes hypertension, peripheral edema, and proteinuria in women after the 20th week of gestation. Eclampsia is the more severe form of the syndrome, with severe hypertension, edema, proteinuria, and seizures. Unlike other forms of acute hypertension, intravenous magnesium is a key component of BP management in eclampsia.

12. What are general issues in the treatment of hypertensive urgency?

Patients with hypertensive urgencies often have elevated BP and nonspecific symptoms but no evidence of progressive end-organ damage. These patients do not often require urgent treatment with parenteral antihypertensives. There is no evidence to suggest that urgent treatment of patients with hypertensive urgencies in an ED setting reduces morbidity or mortality. Indeed, there is evidence that too-rapid treatment of asymptomatic hypertension has adverse effects. Rapidly lowering BP below the autoregulatory range of an organ system (most importantly the cerebral, renal, or coronary beds) can result in reduced perfusion, leading to ischemia and infarction. It is usually appropriate in these situations instead to gradually reduce BP over 24 to 48 hours. Most patients with hypertensive urgency can be treated as outpatients, but some may need to be admitted, as dictated by symptoms and situation and to ensure close follow-up and compliance. The most important intervention for hypertensive urgency is to ensure good follow-up, which helps to promote ongoing, long-term control of BP. No guidelines and no evidence support a specific BP *target* number that must be achieved to safely discharge a patient with hypertensive urgency.

13. What are general issues in treating hypertensive emergencies?

Different scientific societies have repeatedly produced up-to-date guidelines. As discussed previously, acute and overzealous treatment of hypertensive *urgencies* is deemed inappropriate. However, patients with HE should be treated as inpatients in an intensive care setting with an initial goal of reducing mean arterial BP by 10% to 15%, but no more than 25%, in the first hour and then, if stable, to a goal of 160/100 to 110 mm Hg within the next 2 to 6 hours. This requires parenteral agents. Aortic dissection is a special situation that requires reduction of the SBP to at least 120 mm Hg within 20 minutes. Treatment is also required to help to blunt the reflex tachycardia associated with most antihypertensive agents. Ischemic stroke and intracranial hemorrhage are also special situations, and guidelines exist for the treatment of hypertension in these settings from multiple expert societies, including guidelines from the American Stroke Association/American Heart Association (ASA/AHA). These guidelines state that "there is little scientific evidence and no clinically established benefit for rapid lowering of BP among persons with acute ischemic stroke." Too rapid a decline in BP during the first 24 hours after presentation of an intracranial hemorrhage has been independently associated with increased mortality. The overall weight of evidence currently supports only judicious use of antihypertensive agents in the treatment of acute ischemic or hemorrhagic stroke. Expert guidance is recommended, especially if fibrinolytic therapy is being considered for acute ischemic stroke.

An algorithm for evaluation and management of patients with severely elevated BP is given in Fig. 65.2.

14. What specific agents are used for treating patients with hypertensive emergencies?

Intravenous agents recommended for treatment of HE include nitroprusside, nicardipine, enalaprilat, labetalol, and several other agents. Each agent has specific pharmacokinetics, advantages, and disadvantages. Table 65.1 reviews specific agents available for use.

15. Are different agents more helpful for different clinical situations?

Yes. Depending on the specific syndrome (e.g., aortic dissection, eclampsia, pulmonary edema) certain specific agents are suggested. Table 65.2 reviews specific agents recommended for specific situations.

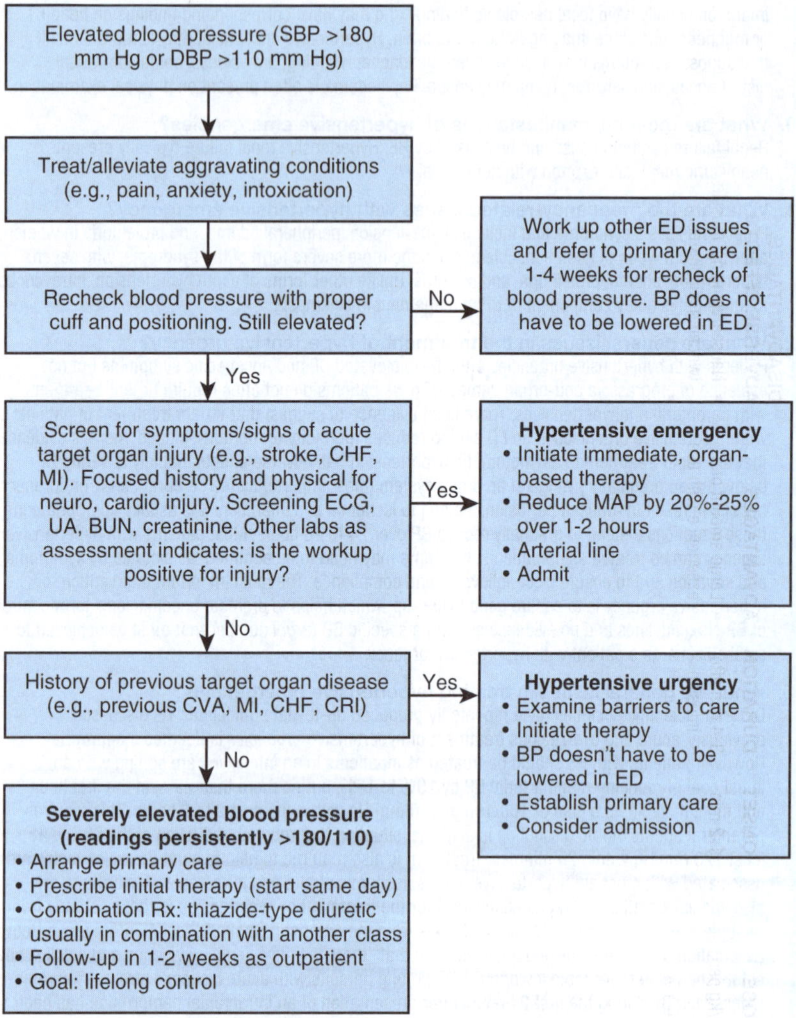

Fig. 65.2. Evaluation and management of patients with severely elevated blood pressure (BP). *BUN,* Blood urea nitrogen; *CHF,* congestive heart failure; *CRI,* chronic renal insufficiency; *CVA,* cerebrovascular accident; *DBP,* diastolic BP; *ECG,* electrocardiogram; *ED,* emergency department; *MAP,* mean arterial pressure; *MI,* myocardial infarction; *Rx,* therapy; *SBP,* systolic BP; *UA,* urinalysis. *(Image from Shayne, P., Lynch, C. A. [2013]. Hypertensive crisis.* Emergency Medicine, 69, *592–601.e1.)*

Table 65.1. Parenteral Agents for Use in Hypertensive Emergencies

DRUG	CLASS/ MECHANISM	USUAL DOSE	ONSET	DURATION	ADVANTAGES	DISADVANTAGES/ ADVERSE EFFECTS	COMMON USES
Sodium nitro-prusside	Direct arterial and venous vasodilator via cGMP	0.25-10 μg/kg per minute Average effective dose 3 μg/kg per minute	1-2 min	3-4 min after infusion stopped	• Large amount of experience with use	• Nausea/vomiting, muscle twitching, diaphoresis • Cyanide toxicity, especially with renal insufficiency and prolonged infusions (>48 h) • Inactivated by light • Requires invasive intra-arterial BP monitoring • Use cautiously with ↑ICP as can worsen • Careful with ACS as can cause coronary steal	Has been used in all syndromes of HE
Clevidipine	Ultra-short-acting dihydropyridine calcium channel blocker. Vasodilator	1-2 mg/hr (2-4 mL/hr), double dose q90sec initially; as blood pressure approaches goal, increase dose by less than doubling, and increase time between adjustments to q5-10min Maintenance: 4-6 mg/hr; not to exceed 21 mg/hr (1000 mL within 24 hour period)	1-5 min	$T_{1/2}$ = 1 min, effect lasts 5-10 min after stopping	• Ultra-short acting with rapid onset, offset of effect • Mild/no reflex tachycardia • Metabolism independent of renal and hepatic function • Arterial line not required • Can give peripherally	• Reduced mortality when compared with sodium nitroprusside	Studied in post-operative HTN, post cardiac surgery, and ED treatment of HE. Useful for all types of HEs
Fenoldo-pam	Peripheral, dopamine-1 receptor agonist, causes vasodilation especially in renal, cardiac, splanchnic beds	0.1 μg/kg per minute to maximum 1.6 μg/kg per minute. Titrate in 0.05- to 0.1- μg/kg per minute increments	10 min Maximum effect in 30 min	1 h after stopping	• Increases renal blood flow, improving CrCl especially in setting of impaired renal function • Used without invasive BP monitoring	• Reflex tachycardia • HA, dizziness, flushing, nausea • Worsening angina • Atrial fibrillation • Tachyphylaxis after 48 h • Contraindicated in glaucoma as causes dose-related increase in IOP	Especially useful in HE syndromes complicated by renal insufficiency or failure

Continued on following page

Table 65.1. Parenteral Agents for Use in Hypertensive Emergencies *(Continued)*

DRUG	CLASS/ MECHANISM	USUAL DOSE	ONSET	DURATION	ADVANTAGES	DISADVANTAGES/ ADVERSE EFFECTS	COMMON USES
Nicardipine	Dihydropyridine calcium channel blocker. Vasodilator	5 mg/h can ↑ by 2.5 mg/h to max 15 mg/h	Within 10 min	2-6 h after stopping	• Dilates coronary vessels, can use with known CAD • Used without invasive BP monitoring	• HA, flushing, dizziness, hypotension, digital dysesthesias • Abrupt withdrawal can cause or worsen angina or hypertension • Metabolized in liver, caution in cirrhotics	Has been used extensively in postoperative HTN, especially post CT surgery
Nitroglycerin	Direct venous vasodilator	5 µg/kg/min to max 200 µg/kg/min	2-5 min	5-10 min	• Dilates coronary vessels	• Ineffective arterial vasodilator • HA, hypotension, tachycardia	Reserved for ACS and cardiogenic pulmonary edema
Enalaprilat	ACE-I	1.25 mg IVP at 4-6 h intervals, max 5 mg in 6 h	15 min-4 h	12-24 h	—	• BP response variable, unpredictable, and not dose related • May not peak for 4 h • Contraindicated in pregnancy	Not generally useful for HE syndromes
Hydralazine	Direct arterial vasodilator	10-20 mg IV	10-20 min	1-4 h	• Increases uterine blood flow	• Flushing, HA, nausea • Significant reflex tachycardia • Has precipitated MI • Use cautiously in CKD, CAD, CVD	Used only for eclampsia/ preeclampsia

ACS, Acute coronary syndrome; *BP*, blood pressure; *CAD*, cardiovascular disease; *cGMP*, cyclic guanosine monophosphate; *CKD*, chronic kidney disease; *CT*, computed tomography; *CVD*, cardiovascular disease, *ED*, emergency department; *HA*, headache; *HE*, hypertensive emergency. *HTN*, hypertension; *ICP*, inductively coupled plasma; *IV*, intravenous.

Table 65.2. Specific Antihypertensive Agents Suggested for Specific Hypertensive Emergency Syndromes

SYNDROME	SUGGESTED ANTIHYPERTENSIVE AGENTS	
Aortic dissection	• Nitroprusside, often in combination with (esmolol, labetalol) • Nicardipine with beta-blocker • Beta-blocker alone	
Acute pulmonary edema	• Nitroglycerin preferred • Fenoldopam	• Nicardipine • Clevidipine
Acute coronary syndrome	• Beta-blocker • Nitroglycerin • Clevidipine	
HE with acute or chronic renal failure	• Labetalol • Fenoldopam	• Nicardipine • Clevidipine
Eclampsia	• Labetalol • Nicardipine • Hydralazine (all in conjunction with magnesium sulfate)	
Acute ischemic stroke or ICH (if expert guidance deems BP control necessary)	• Nicardipine • Labetalol • Clevidipine	
Hypertensive encephalopathy	• Clevidipine • Labetalol • Esmolol	• Nicardipine • Fenoldopam • Nitroprusside
Adrenergic crisis with HE	• Phentolamine • Nitroprusside • Beta-blocker	

BP, Blood pressure; *HE*, hypertensive emergency, *ICH*, intracranial hemorrhage.

Bibliography and Suggested Readings

Alexander, J. M., & Wilson, K. L. (2013). Hypertensive emergencies of pregnancy. *Obstetrics and Gynecology Clinics of North America*, *40*(1), 89–101.

Amin, A. (2005). Parenteral medication for hypertension with symptoms. *Annals of Emergency Medicine*, *1*(3), S1–S15.

Anderson, C. S., Heeley, E., Huang, Y., Wang, J., Stapf, C., Delcourt, C., et al. (2013). Rapid blood-pressure lowering in patients with acute intracerebral hemorrhage. *New England Journal of Medicine*, *368*(25), 2355–2365.

Chobanian, A. V., Bakris, G. L., Black, H. R., Cushman, W. C., Green, L. A., Izzo, J. L., Jr., et al. (2003). The seventh report of the joint national committee on prevention, detection, evaluation, and treatment of high blood pressure: the JNC 7 report. *Journal of the American Medical Association*, *289*(19), 2560–2571.

De Gaudio, A. R., Chelazzi, C., Villa, G., & Cavaliere, F. (2009). Acute severe arterial hypertension: therapeutic options. *Current Drug Targets*, *10*(8), 788–798.

Hebert, C. J., & Vidt, D. G. (2008). Hypertensive crises. *Primary Care: Clinics in Office Practice*, *35*, 475–487.

James, P. A., Oparil, S., Carter, B. L., Cushman, W. C., Dennison-Himmelfarb, C., Handler, J., et al. (2014). 2014 evidence-based guideline for the management of high blood pressure in adults: report from the panel members appointed to the Eighth Joint National Committee (JNC 8). *Journal of the American Medical Association*, *311*(5), 507–520.

Kessler, C. S., & Joudeh, Y. (2010). Evaluation and treatment of severe asymptomatic hypertension. *American Family Physician*, *81*(4), 470–476.

Marik, P. E., & Varon, J. (2007). Hypertensive crises: challenges and management. *Chest Journal*, *131*(6), 1949–1962.

Muiesan, M. L., Salvetti, M., Amadoro, V., di Somma, S., Perlini, S., Semplicini, A., et al. (2015). An update on hypertensive emergencies and urgencies. *Journal of Cardiovascular Medicine*, *16*(5), 372–382.

Peacock, W. F., 4th, Hilleman, D. E., Levy, P. D., Rhoney, D. H., & Varon, J. (2012). A systematic review of nicardipine vs. labetalol for the management of hypertensive crises. *American Journal of Emergency Medicine*, *30*(6), 981–993.

Sarafidis, P. A., Georgianos, P. I., Malindretos, P., & Liakopoulos, V. (2012). Pharmacological management of hypertensive emergencies and urgencies: focus on newer agents. *Expert Opinion on Investigational Drugs*, *21*(8), 1089–1106.

Shayne, P., & Lynch, C. A. (2013). Hypertensive crisis. *Emergency Medicine*, *69*, 592–601 e1.

Tulman, D. B., Stawicki, S. P., Papadimos, T. J., Murphy, C. V., & Bergese, S. D. (2012). Advances in management of acute hypertension: a concise review. *Discovery Medicine*, *13*(72), 375.

Wood, S. (2013). JNC 8 at last! Guidelines ease up on BP thresholds, drug choices. *Heartwire*.

Zanotti-Cavazzoni, S. L. (2014). Hypertensive crises. In J. E. Parrillo, & R. P. Dellinger (Eds.), *Critical care medicine: principles of diagnosis and management in the adult* (chapter 34) (pp. 585–593.e2). Philadelphia, PA: Saunders.

CHAPTER 66

ORAL ANTICOAGULATION THERAPY

Sarah A. Spinler

1. How does warfarin work?

Warfarin (and related coumarin compounds) inhibit the activity of hepatic vitamin K-2,3 epoxide, which is used to recycle the *active* form of vitamin K, vitamin K hydroquinone. Without sufficient vitamin K hydroquinone, clotting factors II, VII, IX, and X fail to be carboxylated, leaving them in an inactive state. The onset of warfarin anticoagulation (AC) is gradual and related to the elimination half-lives of the already synthesized active forms of these procoagulation factors.

In addition to inhibiting the formation of active factors II, VII, IX, and X, warfarin also inhibits the vitamin K–dependent formation of two coagulation inhibitors, proteins C and S, which may temporarily create a relative procoagulant state until full AC is achieved.

Warfarin is a racemic mixture of S and R isomers. The S isomer has more inhibitory activity and is metabolized primarily by cytochrome P450 (CYP) 2C9, which is the major source of drug interactions with warfarin. The R isomer is metabolized primarily by CYP3A4 and CYP1A2, resulting in additional drug interactions.

2. What are the clinical situations in which warfarin is used and at what anticoagulation intensity?

The intensity of AC with warfarin depends primarily on the indication for AC. These are given in Table 66.1.

3. What is the role of warfarin in preventing transient ischemic attack/stroke in a patient with a history of ischemic stroke?

For most patients with noncardioembolic ischemic stroke, the underlying pathophysiology is similar to that of acute coronary syndromes—that is, arterial atherothrombosis. Therefore antiplatelet drugs either alone or in combination have been slightly superior to warfarin in comparative trials for stroke prevention. In addition, despite no clinical advantage, the warfarin patients experience much more major and minor bleeding. Thus warfarin has a limited role added to antiplatelet therapy in selected patients with stroke or transient ischemic attack (TIA) (see Table 66.1).

4. How should unfractionated heparin, low-molecular-weight heparin, or fondaparinux and warfarin be overlapped for acute treatment of venous thromboembolism?

Regardless of the parenteral agent chosen for initial AC, warfarin should be initiated on day 1 of treatment. Choice of dose must be individualized based on patient-specific factors (age, concurrent medications, nutrition status, and comorbidities). However, for most patients, 5 mg daily is an adequate starting dose. According to the 2016 AC Forum Guidance document, the initial dose of warfarin should be 5 mg or 10 mg for most patients. Lower doses may be considered for patients with heart failure, those taking interacting drugs that inhibit warfarin metabolism, malnourished patients, those with liver disease, and for patients older than 75 years of age. Initial doses higher than 10 mg should be avoided.

The INR should be measured daily starting at day 3 of treatment, and the dose should be adjusted to achieve an INR of at least 2.0 by day 5. Unfractionated heparin (UFH), low-molecular-weight heparin (LMWH), or fondaparinux should be overlapped with warfarin for a minimum of 4 to 5 days and until the international normalized ratio (INR) is therapeutic (INR more than 2.5 for 1 day or more than 2.0 for two consecutive days). Switching between warfarin and the direct oral anticoagulants (DOACs) is reviewed later in this chapter.

5. What are some of the common drug interactions with warfarin?

Because of its complex metabolism and relatively narrow therapeutic index, drug interactions involving warfarin are both common and clinically significant. The majority of the interactions occurs at the level of CYP metabolism, although other mechanisms may be possible. Table 66.2 lists some of the more common interactions.

Table 66.1. Indications for Anticoagulation With Warfarin and Recommended International Normalized Ratio Intensity

INDICATION	CLASS AND SOURCE OF RECOMMENDATION	INTERNATIONAL NORMALIZED RATIO INTENSITY
Stroke prevention in AF	2014 AHA/ACC/HRS Guideline for the Management of Patients with AF • Class Ia recommendation • Preferred over DOACs for patients with valvular AF defined as presence of prosthetic (either bioprosthetic or mechanical) heart valve or rheumatic mitral valve disease (e.g., mitral stenosis)	• 2.0-3.0
Post-MI or LV thrombus	2013 ACC/AHA STEMI guideline • Class IIa level of evidence C for asymptomatic LV thrombus • Class IIb, level of evidence C for anterior apical akinesis or dyskinesis on echocardiogram	2013 ACC/AHA STEMI guideline • Class IIb, level of evidence C: with 81 mg aspirin and/or a P2Y12 inhibitor, 2.0-2.5
DVT/PE Treatment in the absence of active malignancy	2016 Anticoagulation Forum Guidance • Preferred over DOACs for patients with CrCl <30 mL/min • Preferred over DOACs for patients with a history of poor medication adherence • Preferred over DOACs for patients with unavoidable major drug-drug interactions • Preferred over DOACs for patients with APLA syndrome 2016 CHEST Guideline and Expert Panel Report • Preferred over DOACs for patients with CrCl <30 mL/min • Option (along with rivaroxaban and edoxaban) when once daily oral therapy is preferred • Option (along with apixaban) when dyspepsia or a history of GI bleeding • Preferred over DOACs if poor compliance • Preferred when reversal agent needed	2016 Anticoagulation Forum: • Target INR 2.0-3.0 • Target INR 2.0-3.0 for APLA syndrome 2016 CHEST Guideline and Expert Panel Report • Target 2.0-3.0 for 3 months following provoked VTE and for a duration of anticoagulation determined by risk/benefit for unprovoked VTE
Ischemic stroke or TIA	2014 AHA/ASA Stroke and TIA Guidelines: • Class IIb, level of evidence C. The combination of anticoagulation plus antiplatelet agents is not routinely recommended following stroke or TIA. • Class IIB, level of evidence C recommendation for warfarin plus antiplatelet therapy for patients with stroke or TIA and clinically apparent CAD (such as ACS or PCI/stent placement) • Class IIB, level of evidence C recommendation for warfarin instead of antiplatelet agent for patients with rheumatic mitral valve disease without AF or another cause of their symptoms (such as carotid artery stenosis)	

Table 66.1. Indications for Anticoagulation With Warfarin and Recommended International Normalized Ratio Intensity *(Continued)*

INDICATION	CLASS AND SOURCE OF RECOMMENDATION	INTERNATIONAL NORMALIZED RATIO INTENSITY
	• Class IIB, level of evidence C recommendation to add aspirin to warfarin for patients with ischemic stroke or TIA while receiving adequate anticoagulation • Class IIa, level of evidence B to initiate anticoagulation 14 days after the onset of neurologic symptoms in patients with atrial fibrillation and stroke or TIA • Class IIA, level of evidence B to delay anticoagulation initiation beyond 14 days in patients at high risk of hemorrhagic conversion (e.g., large infarct, hemorrhagic transformation on initial imaging, uncontrolled hypertension or hemorrhagic tendency)	
Mechanical heart valves	2014 ACC/AHA Valvular Heart Disease Guidelines: • Class 1B recommendation for mechanical aortic valves without additional risk factors for thromboembolism* • Class IB recommendation for all patients with mechanical mitral valves • Class IA recommendation to add aspirin 75 mg-100 mg/day to warfarin	• Target 2.5 (range 2.0-3.0) for 3 months for bioprosthetic mitral valve • Target 2.5 (range 2.0-3.0) for all mechanical aortic heart valves and no risk factors for thromboembolism* • Target 3.0 (range 2.5-3.5) for all mechanical mitral valves and for mechanical aortic valves in the presence of additional risk factors for thromboembolism*

ACC, American College of Cardiology; *AF*, atrial fibrillation; *AHA*, American Heart Association; *CAD*, coronary artery disease; *CHEST*, American College of Chest Physicians; *CrCl*, creatinine clearance; *DOACs*, direct-acting oral anticoagulants; *DVT*, deep vein thrombosis; *GI*, gastrointestinal; *HRS*, Heart Rhythm Society; *INR*, international normalized ratio; *PCI*, percutaneous coronary intervention; *PE*, pulmonary embolism; *TIA*, transient ischemic attack.

*Risk factors for thromboembolism: atrial fibrillation, previous thromboembolism, left ventricular dysfunction, hypercoagulable conditions or older generation mechanical valves (such as ball-in-cage).

For interactions listed as the causation being probable or highly probable, the strength of the clinical evidence is sufficient to expect a change in INR, requiring either adjusting the warfarin dose up or down by 25% to 50% in anticipation of the resulting change in INR or frequent INR monitoring to determine the dose adjustment necessary.

Foods and supplements may also alter the INR. Foods that increase the INR include garlic, mango, ginseng, grapefruit juice, and possibly cranberry juice. Ginger and fish oil have additive antithrombotic effects. Foods and supplements that reduce the INR include high vitamin K–content foods, enteral feeds, and soy milk.

6. What is the role of pharmacogenomics in warfarin dosing?

Warfarin dosing is challenging, in part, because of the varied response and the wide range of doses required to achieve a therapeutic INR in an individual patient. Contributors to this variability are polymorphisms in the CYP 2C9, metabolizing enzyme responsible for the majority of warfarin

Table 66.2. Commonly Encountered Medications That Increase or Decrease Warfarin International Normalized Ratio

MEDICATIONS THAT INCREASE INTERNATIONAL NORMALIZED RATIO	PROPOSED MECHANISM	MEDICATIONS THAT DECREASE INTERNATIONAL NORMALIZED RATIO	PROPOSED MECHANISM
Amiodarone	CYP3A4, CYP1A2, and CYP2C9 inhibitor	Carbamazepine	Induces CYP3A4
Cimetidine	CYP3A4 and CYP1A2 inhibitor	Methimazole	Unknown
Ciprofloxacin	CYP1A2 inhibitor	Nelfinavir	Unknown
Clarithromycin	CYP3A4 inhibitor	Nevirapine	CYP3A4 inducer
Corticosteroids	CYP3A4 substrate (unknown)	Phenobarbital	Induces CYP3A4
Cyclosporine	CYP3A4 substrate	Phenytoin	Induces CYP3A4
Efavirenz	CYP2C9 inhibitor	Rifampin	Induces CYP3A4 and CYP2C9
Erythromycin	CYP3A4 inhibitor	Ritonavir, ritonavir/ lopinavir	CYP3A4 and CYP2C9 inducer
Fenofibric acid	CYP2C9 inhibitor	—	—
Fluconazole	CYP3A4 and CYP2C9 inhibitor	—	—
Fluvastatin	CYP2C9 inhibitor	—	—
Fluvoxamine	CYP1A2 inhibitor	—	—
Itraconazole	CYP3A4 inhibitor	—	—
Ketoconazole	CYP3A4 inhibitor	—	—
Levofloxacin	CYP1A2 inhibitor	—	—
Lovastatin	CYP3A4 substrate	—	—
Metronidazole	CYP3A4 inhibitor	—	—
Miconazole	CYP3A4 inhibitor	—	—
Nelfinavir	CYP3A4 inhibitor	—	—
Phenytoin	CYP2C9 substrate	—	—
Prednisone	CYP3A4 inhibitor	—	—
Rosuvastatin	Unknown	—	—
Saquinavir	CYP3A4 substrate and inhibitor	—	—
Simvastatin	CYP3A4 substrate	—	—
Sulfamethoxazole	CYP3A4 substrate	—	—
Tamoxifen	CYP2C9 substrate	—	—
Voriconazole	CYP3A4 and CYP2C9 inhibitor	—	—

metabolism and, in the target enzyme for warfarin, vitamin K epoxide reductase. Patients with either or both of these genetic polymorphisms tend to be more sensitive to warfarin and require lower doses. Three large randomized clinical trials have failed to demonstrate the clinical utility of routine pharmacogenomic testing. At present, such testing is neither inexpensive nor readily acceptable. For these reasons, the 2012 American College of Chest Physicians (ACCP) Guidelines and the 2016 AC Forum Guidance document recommend against pharmacogenetic testing for most patients initiating warfarin at this time.

7. How should warfarin be managed in patients with underlying chronic liver disease?

Management of warfarin in patients with underlying significant liver disease can be difficult. In addition to elevated baseline INRs, these patients often have low protein stores, thrombocytopenia, and reduced hepatic clearance, making them especially sensitive to effects of warfarin and more likely to have significant bleeding issues. Recommendations include lower starting doses and more frequent laboratory and clinical monitoring.

8. How should warfarin be managed in patients who need surgery or invasive procedures?

For electrophysiology procedures such as pacemaker or defibrillator implantation or for atrial fibrillation (AF) ablation, continuing warfarin uninterrupted at a therapeutic INR is associated with similar thrombotic risk and lower bleeding risk than bridging with LMWH.

For patients who need INR normalized before surgery, warfarin should be stopped at least 5 days before the procedure. Depending on the reason for AC, bridging may be necessary. The most common indications for bridging therapy are patients with mechanical valves and recent deep vein thrombosis/pulmonary embolism (DVT/PE). A systematic review of LMWH used for warfarin bridging found increased bleeding and no decrease in thromboembolic events. The BRIDGE trial was a large randomized, double-blind, placebo-controlled trial evaluating LMWH for periprocedural bridging in patients with AF in mostly lower thromboembolic risk patients. The study found no bridging to be noninferior to and have a lower bleeding risk than bridging.

For patients with venous thromboembolism (VTE), the 2016 AC Forum Guidance in VTE Treatment suggests that warfarin is continued in patients undergoing dental work, minor dermatologic procedures, cataract surgery, and other procedures posing minimal bleeding risk rather than interruption/bridging. For procedures that have a high risk of bleeding, warfarin should be stopped at least 4 to 5 days prior to the procedures and the INR rechecked to make sure it is near normal. For most patients, warfarin, without bridging, should be resumed. Those that should be considered for bridging include VTE within the past month, prior history of recurrent VTE during therapy interruption, and those undergoing a procedure that has an inherently high VTE risk such as orthopedic surgery or major abdominal surgery for cancer resection.

For patients with AF, the 2016 North American Thrombosis Forum (NATF) recommend no AC interruption for procedures with minor bleeding risk, such as tooth extraction or cataract surgery. For other procedures requiring temporary interruption, patients at low risk for thromboembolism with a CHADS2 score of ≤1 should hold warfarin for 4 to 5 days before the procedure and resume following the procedure without bridging with a parenteral anticoagulant. The BRIDGE trial published in 2013 demonstrated that temporary interruption without bridging was noninferior in terms of thromboembolism and had a lower frequency of major bleeding compared with parenteral bridging with LMWH for patients with a moderate stroke risk (62% had CHADS2 scores of 2 or 3).

For patients with mechanical heart valves, the 2014 American College of Cardiology (ACC)/American Heart Association (AHA) Guideline for the Management of Patients with Valvular Heart Disease recommends no interruption/bridging for dental extractions or cataract surgery or where bleeding can be easily controlled. Temporary interruption without bridging is recommended for patients with bileaflet mechanical aortic valve without additional risk factors for thromboembolism (see Table 66.1). Bridging with either LMWH or UFH is recommended for patients with mechanical aortic valves with one or more risk factors for thromboembolism, for patients with older generation mechanical aortic valves, and for patients with mechanical heart valves.

Patients treated with LMWH for bridging should receive full-dose (therapeutic dose) SC LMWH during the bridging period. The last dose of LMWH should be given no later than 24 hours before the procedure. (The 2014 AHA/ACC Valvular Heart Disease guidelines recommend 12 hours.) LMWH should be resumed 24 to 48 hours (the next evening) after the procedure, depending on bleeding and thrombotic risks of the patient. (The 2014 AHA/ACC Valvular Heart Disease Guidelines recommend 12 hours for LMWH.) Warfarin should be restarted within 12 to 24 hours after the procedure (evening of or next morning). The reader should be aware that, as with many drugs, although LMWH is not approved for bridging, it is often used for this purpose. Different practitioners will have different thresholds of confidence for the use of LMWH as a bridging agent.

For patients who need urgent surgery, it is recommended to give intravenous vitamin K 5 to 10 mg. Fresh frozen plasma will give a more rapid (albeit temporary) reversal of AC therapy and can be combined with vitamin K. For patients with warfarin-associated major bleeding, prothrombin complex concentrate (PCC), rather than plasma, is recommended for reversal, in combination with intravenous vitamin K.

A general approach to management of periprocedural anticoagulation as described in the 2016 ACC Clinical Decision Pathway on Peri-procedural Management of AC in patients with nonvalvular atrial fibrillation (NVAF) is given in Fig. 66.1.

9. How should elevated INRs and significant bleeding in patients taking warfarin be managed?

Management of patients depends on the INR and presence, absence, and severity of bleeding.

- If there is no overt evidence of bleeding and rapid reversal is not necessary, the 2012 ACCP guidelines recommend against routine vitamin K administration unless the INR is greater than 10.
- When the INR is greater than 10 without overbleeding, the 2012 ACCP guidelines recommend low-dose (5 mg or less) oral vitamin K.
- For INRs less than 4.5 without bleeding, the guidelines recommend lowering the dose or holding the next dose with frequent INR monitoring until the INR is within the therapeutic range and then resuming a lower dose.
- For INRs 4.5 to 10 without bleeding, the 2012 ACCP guidelines recommend omitting one to two doses, frequent INR monitoring, and resuming a lower warfarin dose when the INR is within the therapeutic range.
- For patients experiencing minor bleeding with an elevated INR, oral vitamin K is recommended at a dose of 2.5 to 5 mg, repeated at 24-hour intervals until INR is within the therapeutic range, and then resuming a lower dose of warfarin.
- For patients experiencing major bleeding, such as those with intracranial hemorrhage (ICH) or who require urgent reversal for emergent surgery, intravenous vitamin K 10 mg as well as intravenous PCC are recommended, and a dose in factor IX units is determined based upon the predose INR and patient's body weight.

10. What are important patient counseling points for warfarin?

A patient medication guide is mandated to be dispensed by pharmacists to patients receiving prescriptions for warfarin. Important counseling points are as follows:

- Explain to patients the reason for warfarin therapy.
- Explain the meaning and significance of the INR.
- Identify the patient's warfarin prescriber, current INR, and date of next scheduled INR.
- Explain the need for frequent INR testing and the target INR for the patient's medical condition(s).
- Explain the importance of compliance with therapy and related laboratory work (INR checks).
- Describe common sites and signs of bleeding and what to do if they occur. Explain that bleeding and bruising are more likely to occur and that common sites of bleeding include the gums, urinary tract, and nose. Patients should be counseled to make note of any changes in stool color and to report dark, tarry stools to the health care provider immediately. Patients should also report any blood in the urine or stool to a health care provider immediately and contact a health care provider for nosebleeds or bleeding from a cut or scrape that will not stop.
- Patients should be told to go to the emergency department immediately if they experience shortness of breath, chest pain, slurred speech, or sudden onset of a severe headache or are coughing up or vomiting up blood.
- Counsel patients to avoid alcohol and activities/sports that may result in a fall or injury.
- Explain how consuming foods containing vitamin K may impact the effectiveness of warfarin therapy and that the most important thing concerning the diet is not to make any significant changes without talking to the health care provider.
- Explain to patients the importance of telling all health care providers that warfarin is being taken and that the health care provider prescribing warfarin needs to be informed of all scenarios where warfarin might need to be held (dental work, surgery, and other invasive procedures).
- Explain to patients the importance of contacting the pharmacy if the color of the warfarin tablet is different.
- Explain that warfarin should be taken at the same time each day and that if a dose is missed and it is within 12 hours of when the dose was supposed to be taken, it is OK to take the dose. Otherwise, the dose should be skipped and resumed the next day. The dose should not be doubled.

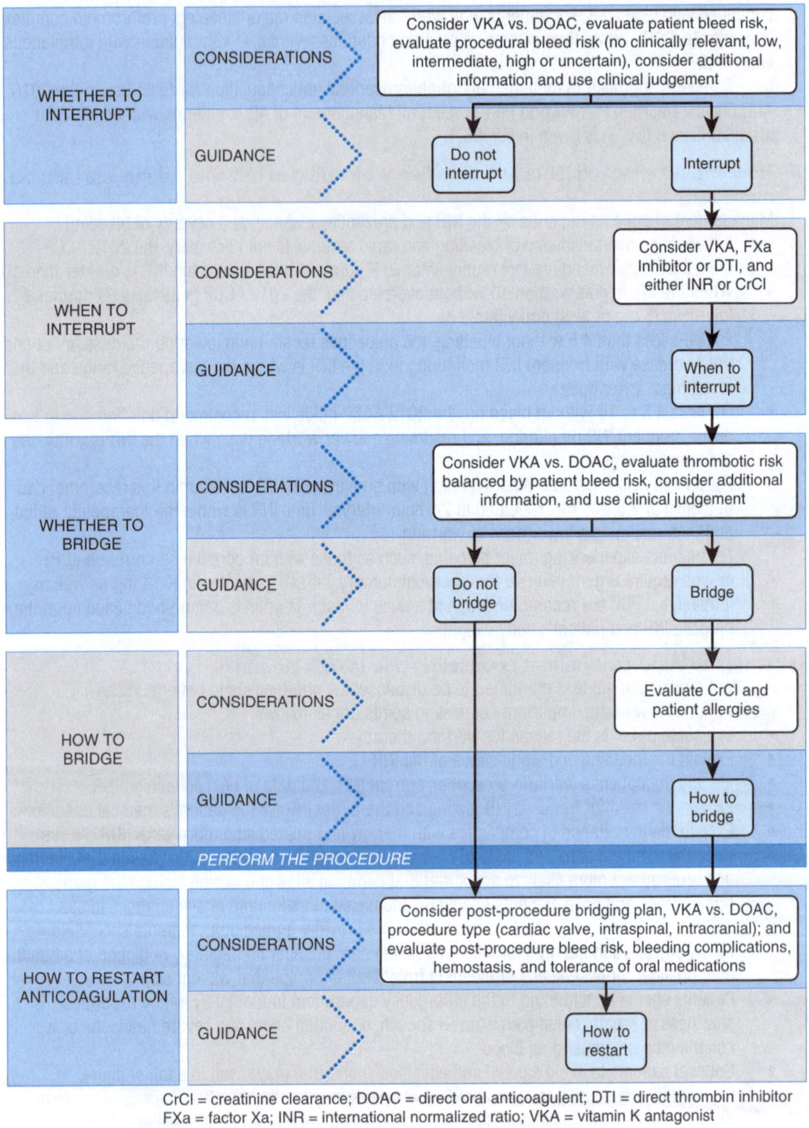

Fig. 66.1. The American College of Cardiology's clinical decision pathway on periprocedural management of anticoagulation in patients with NVAF. Adapted with permission from: 2016 ACC Expert Consensus Decision Pathway for Periprocedureal Management of Anticoagulation in Patients with Non-valvular Atrial Fibrillation. J Am Coll Cardiol. 2017;69(1):(In Press).

- Discuss potential drug interactions. Explain that patients should contact their warfarin prescriber before taking any over-the-counter medications (including herbal supplements) or if a different health care provider starts them on a new medication (especially antibiotics).
- Explain that women of childbearing age must use birth control measures and notify their health care provider immediately if they become pregnant.

- Advise patients to carry identification noting that they are taking warfarin.
- Depending on the indication for warfarin, counsel patients on signs of clot formation (such as calf pain, redness, swelling, shortness of breath, stroke symptoms, etc.).
- Document that the patient education session has occurred.

11. What are potential advantages and disadvantages of the direct-acting oral anticoagulants apixaban, dabigatran, edoxaban, and rivaroxaban?

Dabigatran is an oral direct thrombin inhibitor, and apixaban, edoxaban, and rivaroxaban are direct-acting factor Xa inhibitor anticoagulants. Potential advantages of DOACs over warfarin include quick onset of anticoagulant effects (hours not days), no need for bridging, fewer drug interactions, and no routine AC monitoring. A disadvantage of the direct-acting factor Xa inhibitors is that there is no antidote to reverse major bleeding. Dabigatran's anticoagulant effect may be reversed for major bleeding and urgent/emergent invasive procedures using idarucizumab (as discussed later).

Dabigatran is primarily eliminated renally (80%). Rivaroxaban is both metabolized (primarily by CYP3A4/5) and renally eliminated (36% of the absorbed dose). Apixaban is metabolized (25%) by CYP3A4, with 27% excreted renally. Renal clearance is about 50% of total clearance for edoxaban, and there is minimal metabolism. All agents are substrates of P-glycoprotein.

Indications and dosing recommendations are described in Table 66.3. DOACs should be avoided in patients with moderate to severe hepatic impairment.

No specific studies have been conducted with apixaban, edoxaban, or rivaroxaban for stroke prevention in AF in patients with either bioprosthetic or mechanical heart valves and AF, and therefore their use is not recommended in such patients. The presence of rheumatic mitral stenosis was an exclusion criterion for DOAC stroke prevention in NVAF clinical trials. A study comparing warfarin and dabigatran in patients with mechanical heart valves was stopped early for increased thrombotic and bleeding risk with dabigatran, and its use has not been studied in patients with bioprosthetic heart valves. Small numbers of patients in the NVAF pivotal trials with apixaban and edoxaban had bioprosthetic heart valves. Therefore, at this time, warfarin is the preferred oral anticoagulant in patients with bioprosthetic or mechanical heart valves. Currently FDA labeling regarding use in patients with valvular heart disease for the DOACs is presented in Table 66.4.

Table 66.3. Dosing Recommendations for Direct-Acting Oral Anticoagulants

AGENT	INDICATION	DOSE
Apixaban	Stroke prevention in NVAF	5 mg PO BID Reduce dose from 5 mg PO BID to 2.5 mg BID if ≥2 of the following: age ≥80 years, weight ≤60 kg, or SCr ≥1.5 mg/dL
	Acute treatment of VTE	10 mg PO BID for the first 7 days, then 5 mg PO BID
	Secondary prevention of VTE	2.5 mg PO BID after at least 6 months of treatment
	Prophylaxis of VTE following hip or knee replacement surgery	2.5 mg PO BID starting 12 to 24 h after surgery; 35 days for hip replacement and 12 days for knee replacement
	For all indications	Concomitant P-gp and strong CYP3A4 inhibitor: reduce dose from 5 mg PO BID to 2.5 mg PO BID 2.5 mg PO BID and concomitant P-gp and strong CYP3A4 inhibitor: avoid use Concomitant combined P-gp and CYP3A4 inducer: avoid use Patients with ESRD on hemodialysis: no adjustment of doses described above
	Can be crushed and administered via an oral nasogastric feeding tube?	Yes

Continued on following page

Table 66.3. Dosing Recommendations for Direct-Acting Oral Anticoagulants *(Continued)*

AGENT	INDICATION	DOSE
Dabigatran etexilate	Stroke prevention in NVAF	CrCl >30 mL/min: 150 mg PO BID CrCl 15-30 mL/min or with dronedarone or ketoconazole: 75 mg PO BID CrCl <15 mL/min or on dialysis: no dosing recommendations can be provided
	Acute VTE treatment (after 5-10 days of parenteral therapy) and secondary prevention	CrCl >30 mL/min: 150 mg PO BID CrCl ≤30 mL/min or on dialysis: no dosage recommendations can be provided CrCl <50 mL/min: avoid coadministration of P-gp inhibitors
	Prophylaxis of VTE following hip replacement surgery	CrCl >30 mL/min: 110 mg PO 1-4 hours after surgery and after hemostasis has been achieved on first day, then 220 mg PO daily for 28-35 days CrCl ≤30 mL/min or on dialysis: no dosage recommendations can be provided
	All indications	P-gp inducers: avoid use
	Can be crushed and administered via an oral nasogastric feeding tube?	No
Edoxaban	Stroke prevention in NVAF	CrCl >95 mL/min: avoid use CrCl 51-95 mL/min: 60 mg PO daily CrCl 15-50 mL/min: 30 mg PO daily
	Acute treatment of VTE (following 5-10 days of parenteral therapy)	CrCl >50 mL/min: 60 mg PO daily CrCl 15-50 mL/min or ≤60 kg or taking verapamil, quinidine, or dronedarone: 30 mg PO daily
	All indications	CrCl <15 mL/min: avoid use Rifampin: avoid use
	Can it be crushed and administered via an oral nasogastric feeding tube?	Yes
Rivaroxaban	Stroke prevention in NVAF	CrCl >50 mL/min: 20 mg PO daily with the evening meal CrCl 15-50 mL/min; ESRD on dialysis: 15 mg PO daily with the evening meal Combined P-gp inhibitors and strong CYP3A4 inhibitors: avoid use
	Acute VTE treatment and secondary prevention	15 mg PO BID with food for the first 21 days of initial treatment period, then 20 mg PO daily with food for remaining treatment
	Prophylaxis of DVT following hip or knee replacement surgery	CrCl ≥30 mL/min: 10 mg PO daily with or without food started at least 6 h following surgery and once hemostasis has been achieved; 35 days for hip replacement and 12 days for knee replacement CrCl <30 mL/min: avoid use
	Can it be crushed and administered via an oral nasogastric feeding tube?	Yes

CrCl, Creatinine clearance; *DVT*, deep vein thrombosis; *ESRD*, end-stage renal disease; *NVAF*, nonvalvular atrial fibrillation; *VTE*, venous thromboembolism.

Table 66.4. FDA Labeling of Direct-Acting Oral Anticoagulants in Valvular Heart Disease

DABIGATRAN	RIVAROXABAN	APIXABAN	EDOXABAN
Mechanical heart valves: contraindicated Bioprosthetic heart valves: not studied/use not recommended	Prosthetic heart valves: not studied/use not recommended	Prosthetic heart valves: not studied/use not recommended	Mechanical heart valves: not studied/use not recommended Moderate-severe mitral stenosis: use not recommended

12. What are the current US guideline recommendations for direct-acting oral anticoagulants for stroke prevention in nonvalvular atrial fibrillation?

The two most pertinent guidelines that address AC for stroke prevention in NVAF are the 2014 AHA/ACC/Heart Rhythm Society (HRS) guidelines and the 2016 NATF AF Action Initiative Consensus Document. In the 2014 AHA/ACC/HRSA guidelines, either warfarin or a DOAC is recommended for patients with a CHA2DS2-VASc score of ≥2, with warfarin preferred over a DOAC when a patient has a creatinine clearance (CrCl) less than 15 mL/min or is on dialysis. The 2016 NATF document is an excellent resource that reviews selecting between strategies of AC versus no AC, bleeding risk estimation, and periprocedural management.

In general, clinical trials of each DOAC compared with warfarin have found similar or better efficacy for prevention of stroke or systemic embolism, with a reduction in the rate of ICH. Major bleeding was less frequent with apixaban and edoxaban compared with warfarin and similar with rivaroxaban and dabigatran compared with warfarin.

13. What are the current US guideline recommendations for direct-acting oral anticoagulants for acute treatment and secondary prevention of venous thromboembolism?

Two current practice guidelines are available for management of acute DVT and PE, the 2016 Chest AT10 guidelines and the 2016 AC Forum Guidance on VTE Treatment. Both guidelines recommend DOACs over warfarin for initial and long-term treatment of VTE in patients without cancer. Few patients with malignancies were enrolled in pivotal trials to draw definitive conclusions regarding efficacy and safety in that patient population, where LMWHs are preferred over warfarin for acute and secondary prevention. Ongoing trials will continue to explore that question. Based upon study design and approved indications, 5 to 10 days of parenteral therapy should precede treatment with either dabigatran or edoxaban, while therapy with a higher intensity dosing scheme is used for initial therapy for apixaban and rivaroxaban without parenteral therapy.

Clinical trials comparing LMWH/warfarin with either LMWH/DOAC (dabigatran or edoxaban) or DOAC alone rivaroxaban or apixaban have generally found similar efficacy in preventing recurrent VTE with a lower or similar rate of major bleeding.

14. What are some of the common drug interactions with direct-acting oral anticoagulants?

Labeled drug interactions resulting in dosing adjustments are described in Table 66.3. Because all DOACs are P-gp substrates and rivaroxaban and apixaban are substrates for CYP3A4/5, serum concentrations may be increased by P-gp inhibitors and rivaroxaban and apixaban concentrations increased by CYP3A4/5 inhibitors. Potential drug interactions to consider, especially in patients with reduced renal function, are listed in Table 66.5.

15. How should patients taking direct-acting oral anticoagulants be transitioned to and from other anticoagulants?

One of the major advantages of the newer oral anticoagulants is their rapid onset and offset of effect. Peak concentrations, and thus the complete anticoagulant effects, of dabigatran are achieved in 1 hour in the fasting state and by 2 hours following a meal, while peak concentrations of rivaroxaban are reached in 2 to 4 hours following rivaroxaban administered with food. Peak concentrations are seen 3 to 4 hours following apixaban and in 1 to 2 hours following edoxaban administration. Recommendations for switching between oral and injectable anticoagulants are described in Table 66.6.

Table 66.5. Potential Drug Interactions With Apixaban, Dabigatran Etexilate, Edoxaban, and Rivaroxaban That Increase or Decrease Their Concentrations

Apixaban and Rivaroxaban			
POTENTIAL TO DECREASE CONCENTRATION		**POTENTIAL TO INCREASE CONCENTRATION**	
Strong CYP3A4 Inducers	P-gp Inducers	Strong CYP3A4 Inhibitors	P-gp Inhibitors
Carbamazepine	Carbamazepine	Clarithromycin	Amiodarone
Phenytoin	Phenytoin	Conivaptan	Conivaptan
Rifampin	Rifampin	Grapefruit juice (high-dose, double strength)	Clarithromycin
St. John's wort	Tipranavir/Ritonavir	Indinavir	Cyclosporine
—	St. John's wort	Itraconazole	Dronedarone
—	—	Ketoconazole	Erythromycin
—	—	Lopinavir/Ritonavir	Indinavir/Ritonavir
—	—	Nefazodone	Lopinavir/Ritonavir
—	—	Nelfinavir	Itraconazole
—	—	Posaconazole	Ketoconazole
—	—	Ritonavir	Quinidine
—	—	Saquinavir	Ritonavir
—	—	Telaprevir	Verapamil
—	—	Telithromycin	—
—	—	Voriconazole	—
Dabigatran Etexilate and Edoxaban			
POTENTIAL TO DECREASE CONCENTRATION		**POTENTIAL TO INCREASE CONCENTRATION**	
	P-gp Inducers		P-gp Inhibitors
	Carbamazepine		Amiodarone
	Phenytoin		Conivaptan
	Rifampin		Clarithromycin
	Tipranavir/Ritonavir		Cyclosporine
	St. John's wort		Dronedarone
	—		Erythromycin
	—		Indinavir/Ritonavir
	—		Lopinavir/Ritonavir
	—		Itraconazole
	—		Ketoconazole
	—		Quinidine
	—		Ritonavir
	—		Verapamil

Table 66.6. Converting From or to Parenteral Anticoagulants and Warfarin With Dabigatran Etexilate and Rivaroxaban

SWITCHING FROM	SWITCHING TO	RECOMMENDATION
Unfractionated heparin	Apixaban	• Administer first dose of apixaban at time UFH is discontinued.
	Dabigatran etexilate	• Administer first dose of dabigatran at time UFH is discontinued.
	Edoxaban	• Administer first dose of edoxaban 4 hours after UFH is discontinued.
	Rivaroxaban	• Administer first dose of rivaroxaban with a meal at time UFH is discontinued.
LMWH	Apixaban	• Administer first dose of apixaban at time next LMWH dose due.
	Dabigatran etexilate	• Administer first dose of dabigatran at time next LMWH dose due
	Edoxaban	• Administer first dose of edoxaban at time next LMWH dose due
	Rivaroxaban	• Administer first dose of rivaroxaban with a meal, at time the next LMWH dose due
Warfarin	Apixaban	• Monitor INR; start apixaban when INR <2.0.
	Dabigatran etexilate	• Monitor INR; start dabigatran when INR <2.0.
	Edoxaban	• Monitor INR; start edoxaban when INR ≤2.5.
	Rivaroxaban	• Monitor INR; start rivaroxaban when INR <3.0.
Apixaban	Unfractionated heparin	• Start UFH at time next apixaban dose due.
	LMWH	• Give first LMWH injection at time next apixaban dose due.
	Warfarin	• Stop apixaban and start a parenteral anticoagulant as noted previously with warfarin, then overlap parenteral agent with warfarin until INR ≥2.0. Or • Start warfarin, continue apixaban, measure INR 12 hours post apixaban daily (just prior to the next dose) starting on day 3 of warfarin therapy; then discontinue apixaban when INR ≥2.0.
	Different DOAC	• Stop apixaban and start DOAC at time next apixaban dose due.
Dabigatran etexilate	Unfractionated heparin	• For CrCl ≥30 mL/min, start UFH 12 hours after last dose of dabigatran. • For CrCl <30 mL/min, start UFH and start UFH 24 hours after last dose of dabigatran.
	LMWH	• For CrCl ≥30 mL/min, give first LMWH injection 12 hours after last dose of dabigatran. • For CrCl <30 mL/min, give first LMWH injection 24 hours after last dose of dabigatran.
	Warfarin	• For CrCl ≥50 mL/min, start warfarin 3 days before discontinuing dabigatran. • For CrCl 30-50 mL/min, start warfarin 2 days before discontinuing dabigatran. • For CrCl 15-30 mL/min, start warfarin 1 day before discontinuing dabigatran.
	Different DOAC	• Stop dabigatran and start DOAC at time next dabigatran dose due.

Continued on following page

Table 66.6. Converting From or to Parenteral Anticoagulants and Warfarin With Dabigatran Etexilate and Rivaroxaban *(Continued)*

SWITCHING FROM	SWITCHING TO	RECOMMENDATION
Edoxaban	Unfractionated heparin	• Start UFH at time next edoxaban dose due.
	LMWH	• Give first LMWH injection at the time next edoxaban dose due.
	Warfarin	• Stop edoxaban and start a parenteral anticoagulant as above with warfarin, then overlap parenteral agent with warfarin until INR ≥2.0. Or • For patients taking 60 mg of edoxaban, reduce edoxaban dose to 30 mg and begin warfarin concomitantly. For patients taking 30 mg of edoxaban, reduce edoxaban dose to 15 mg and begin warfarin concomitantly. Measure INR dose at least weekly just prior to the edoxaban dose and discontinue edoxaban when INR ≥2.0. Or • Start warfarin, continue edoxaban at usual dose, measure INR 24 hours postedoxaban dose daily (just prior to the next dose) starting on day 3 of warfarin therapy, then discontinue edoxaban when INR ≥2.0.
	Different DOAC	• Stop edoxaban and start DOAC at time next edoxaban dose due.
Rivaroxaban	Unfractionated heparin	• Start UFH at time next rivaroxaban dose due.
	LMWH	• Give first LMWH injection at the time next rivaroxaban dose due.
	Warfarin	• Use parenteral anticoagulant bridge.
	Different DOAC	• Stop rivaroxaban and start DOAC at time next rivaroxaban dose due.

CrCl, Creatinine clearance; *DOAC*, direct-acting oral anticoagulant; *INR*, international normalized ratio; *LMWH*, Low-molecular-weight heparin; *UFH*, unfractionated heparin.

In general the offset of DOACs is much more rapid than warfarin (which requires at least 4 to 5 days following discontinuation to restore levels of functional clotting factors). Of the DOACs, dabigatran has the greatest dependence on renal clearance, with the time to restore normal coagulation longer for patients with lower CrCl.

16. What is the effect of direct-acting oral anticoagulants on coagulation tests, and can they be monitored?

DOACs have predictable AC effects following fixed-dose administration, and therefore routine coagulation monitoring is not recommended at this time in any patient population.

DOACs may affect several common coagulation tests. Unlike warfarin, which impacts the formation of clotting factors and therefore has long-lasting effects, DOACs impact the coagulation tests in a concentration-time manner—that is, peak effects on coagulation tests occur at the time of peak drug concentration and then diminish over time. Therefore the degree of abnormality of the coagulation test depends on the time the test was drawn after the patient took his or her last dose. Following dabigatran administration, more than twofold prolongations in activated partial thromboplastin time (aPTT) may be observed.

Both dabigatran and rivaroxaban increase the prothrombin time (PT), with the PT being more sensitive to rivaroxaban than dabigatran at concentrations achieved in vivo. Edoxaban and apixaban have less effect on the PT. The INR is not interpretable following DOAC administration, and its elevation cannot be interpreted as a risk factor for bleeding as is the case with warfarin. Differences in effects are also observed among different brands of reagents for the different

Table 66.7. Suggested Management of Triple Antiplatelet/Anticoagulant Therapy Following Percutaneous Coronary Intervention/Stenting in a Patient With Nonvalvular Atrial Fibrillation

STROKE RISK	BLEEDING RISK	CLINICAL SETTING	RECOMMENDATION
Moderate (CHA2DS2-VASc score = 1 in males)	HAS-BLED score 0-2 (low or moderate)	ACS	Months 1-6: Triple therapy: OAC + aspirin 81 mg/day + clopidogrel: 6 months Months 6-12: Double therapy: OAC + clopidogrel or aspirin 81 mg/day Months 12+: OAC alone lifelong
	HAS-BLED score ≥3 (high)	ACS	Month 1: Triple therapy: OAC + aspirin 81 mg/day + clopidogrel Months 2-12: Double therapy: OAC + clopidogrel or aspirin 81 mg/day Months 12+: OAC alone lifelong
	HAS-BLED score 0-2 (low or moderate)	Stable CAD	Month 1: Triple therapy: OAC + aspirin 81 mg/day + clopidogrel Months 2-12: Double therapy: OAC + clopidogrel or aspirin 81 mg/day Months 12+: OAC alone lifelong
	HAS-BLED score ≥3 (high)	Stable CAD	Months 1-12: Double therapy OAC + aspirin 81 mg/day Months 12+: OAC lifelong
High (CHA2DS2-VASc score ≥2)	HAS-BLED score 0-2 (low or moderate)	ACS	Months 1-6: Triple therapy: OAC + aspirin 81 mg/day + clopidogrel: 6 months Months 6-12: Double therapy: OAC + clopidogrel or aspirin 81 mg/day Months 12+: OAC alone lifelong
	HAS-BLED score ≥3 (high)	ACS	1 month: Triple therapy: OAC + aspirin 81 mg/day + clopidogrel Months 2-12: Double therapy: OAC + clopidogrel or aspirin 81 mg/day Months 12+: OAC alone lifelong
	HAS-BLED score 0-2 (low or moderate)	Stable CAD	Months 1 (no longer than up to 6 months): Triple therapy: OAC + aspirin 81 mg/day + clopidogrel: 6 months Months 2 (or 6)-12: Double therapy: OAC + clopidogrel or aspirin 81 mg/day Months 12+: OAC alone lifelong
	HAS-BLED score ≥3 (high)	Stable CAD	Month 1: Triple therapy: OAC + aspirin 81 mg/day + clopidogrel Months 2-12: Double therapy: OAC + clopidogrel or aspirin 81 mg/day Months 12+: OAC alone lifelong

CAD, Coronary artery disease; *OAC*, oral anticoagulant.
CHA2DS2-VASc score, see Reference 27; HAS-BLED score, see Reference 28.

coagulation tests. Therefore elevations in either aPTT or PT or INR above baseline (control) should be interpreted as indicating presence of drug, but the risk of bleeding cannot be assessed. Values within the normal range for aPTT and INR should *not* be interpreted as the patient having normal coagulation.

There is early research suggesting that the preferred coagulation test for determining accumulation of dabigatran concentrations may be the dilute thrombin time (dTT), with trough dTT concentrations greater than 200 ng/mL suggesting increased bleeding risk.

Because apixaban, rivaroxaban and edoxaban are factor Xa inhibitors the preferred monitoring test will be antifactor Xa activity levels, but tests are not readily available and there is no guidance on interpretation of their results at this time.

When evaluating a bleeding patient, normal anti-Xa activity likely excludes clinically relevant drug levels of apixaban, edoxaban, and rivaroxaban. The 2016 Thrombosis Canada reversal guidelines state that a calibrated DOAC anti-Xa level of less than 30 ng/mL likely indicates no significant anticoagulant effect. Normal TT and aPTT likely exclude relevant dabigatran levels.

17. Can the anticoagulant effect of direct-acting oral anticoagulants be reversed?

At this time, dabigatran is the only DOAC with an available antidote, idarucizumab. Other antidotes for reversing the Xa inhibitors apixaban, edoxaban, and rivaroxaban are under clinical development.

18. What are the steps in managing a direct-acting oral anticoagulant-treated patient who is bleeding?

Three guidelines describe methods to reverse serious bleeding with DOACs: Thrombosis Canada, the 2016 AC Forum Guidance on VTE Treatment, and the 2016 guidelines on how to use antidotes and reversal agents from the International Society of Thrombosis and Haemostasis (ISTH).

Steps to manage a patient prescribed a DOAC who is bleeding include

1. Evaluate the patient for signs of shock and treat hemodynamic instability.
2. Identify the site of bleeding and treat accordingly.
3. Classify the bleeding as minor, moderate, or major. Examples of minor bleeding that do not require reversal are anterior epistaxis, hemorrhoid bleeding, subconjunctival bleeding, and ecchymosis. Examples of moderate bleeding are hemodynamically stable upper or lower gastrointestinal bleeding, major epistaxis, and hematuria. Examples of major and life-threatening bleeding are ICH, bleeding into a critical organ, intraspinal, intraocular, and pericardial bleeding.
4. Evaluate the patient's coagulation tests to confirm presence of anticoagulant activity (qualification and not quantification) if such testing is available (see Question 15).
5. Evaluate the time of the last dose, next scheduled dose, and renal function. Estimate the drug's half-life based on renal function and determine the duration of anticoagulant effect to be between four and five drug half-lives.
    - Apixaban: CrCl ≥30 mL/min: half-life 12 to 17 hours; CrCl 15 to 30 mL/min: half-life 17 hours; end-stage renal disease (ESRD) on hemodialysis: half-life 10 hours
    - Dabigatran: CrCl ≥80 mL/min half-life 13 hours; CrCl 50 to 80 mL/min: half-life 15 hours; CrCl 30 to 50 mL/min: half-life 18 hours; CrCl 15 to 30 mL/min: half-life 27 hours; ESRD on hemodialysis: half-life 2 to 3 hours
    - Edoxaban: CrCl greater than 30 mL/min: half-life 9 to 14 hours; CrCl 15 to 30 mL/min half-life 17 hours; ESRD on peritoneal dialysis: half-life 12 hours
    - Rivaroxaban: CrCl ≥15: half-life 5 to 9 hours; ESRD on or off hemodialysis: 12 to 13 hours
6. For minor bleeding, consider holding one dose. For moderate and major or life-threatening bleeding, discontinue the DOAC, monitor vital signs, and consider activated charcoal if the time of last ingestion was within 2 hours.
7. According to the 2016 Thrombosis Canada guidelines and the ISTH reversal guidelines: for major and life-threatening bleeding with dabigatran, administer idarucizumab (discussed later). For major and life-threatening bleeding with apixaban, edoxaban, and rivaroxaban, administer PCC (discussed later).
8. Administration of fresh frozen plasma alone is ineffective and not recommended. The free drug in plasma far exceeds the coagulation factor replenished with plasma, and therefore it is ineffective. Implement transfusion therapy with red blood cells if symptomatic anemia is present or platelet transfusion if platelets are less than 50,000/L or if patient is taking antiplatelet drugs.
9. Monitor abnormal coagulation tests to assess efficacy of reversal.
10. Evaluate precipitating causes such as acute kidney injury, concomitant aspirin, P2Y12 inhibitors, NSAIDs, or selective serotonin reuptake inhibitors (SSRIs), and discontinue agents affecting coagulation/platelet function if appropriate.
11. Reinitiate AC if still indicated and monitor for bleeding. Prolonged interruption results in increased thrombosis risk.

19. What is idarucizumab?

Idarucizumab is a humanized Fab fragment with a binding affinity to thrombin that is more than 350 times higher than dabigatran's binding affinity to thrombin. It has an immediate onset of action and does not activate platelets or convert fibrinogen to fibrin. Idarucizumab is available as a

2.5-mg vial for injection that does not require refrigeration. The dose is two 2.5-g vials (5-g dose) administered consecutively no more than 15 minutes apart. The aPTT and TT should be rechecked within 2 hours and should have normalized. These coagulation tests should be monitored throughout the duration of four to five estimated dabigatran half-lives (discussed previously). In patients with re-elevation of coagulation tests or if the patient continues to bleed, a second dose of 5 g may be administered.

20. What is prothrombin complex concentrate?

PCC is a four-factor PCC containing clotting factors II, VII, IX, and X. Administration of PCC has been shown to reverse prolonged PTs in healthy volunteers given factor Xa inhibitors. A dose of four-factor PCC for major and life-threatening bleeding with apixaban, edoxaban, and rivaroxaban is 50 units/kg (maximum 3000 units). Hematology should be consulted for assistance in managing patients with DOAC-associated severe and life-threatening bleeding.

21. How should direct-acting oral anticoagulants be managed in patients who need surgery or invasive procedures?

There are several observational trials and one randomized trials suggesting that DOACs may be continued without interruption or by just holding one dose for electrophysiology procedures such as pacemaker or defibrillator implantation and AF ablation.

Both the 2016 NATF AF Action Guidelines and the 2016 AC Forum Guidance on VTE Treatment recommend that for patients where interruption is necessary, DOACs be held for two to three half-lives for low-bleeding risk procedures and four to five drug half-lives for high bleeding risk procedures based on the patient's renal function. DOACS can be resumed within 24 hours for low-bleeding risk procedures and at 2 to 3 days following major surgery or procedures with high bleeding risk.

22. What are the important counseling points for patients taking direct-acting oral anticoagulants?

1. Explain to patients the reason the DOAC is being taken.
2. Advise patients taking DOACs to carry a card with them in their purse/wallet listing their medications. See http://www.afib4ward.com/resources for an example.
3. Explain that dabigatran may cause gastrointestinal upset and that, if it occurs, patients may take the medication with food to minimize effect.
4. For patients with a prior history of taking warfarin, explain that the DOAC may affect the INR blood test but it is not used for monitoring the level of AC.
5. Explain the importance of adherence with therapy and that, for patients with NVAF, abrupt discontinuation may increase stroke risk.
6. Describe common sites and signs of bleeding and what to do if they occur. Common sites of bleeding include the gums, urinary tract, and nose. Explain to patients that they should be aware of any changes in stool color and report dark, tarry stools to the health care provider immediately. Patients should also be told to report any uncontrolled bleeding to the health care provider.
7. Counsel patients to avoid alcohol and activities/sports that may result in a fall or injury.
8. Explain to patients the importance of telling all health care providers (e.g., doctors, dentists) that the DOAC is being taken and that the health care provider prescribing the DOAC needs to be informed of all scenarios where the anticoagulant might need to be held (dental work, surgery, and other invasive procedures).
9. Explain that dabigatran and apixaban should be taken at the same time each day and that if a dose is missed and it is within 6 hours of when the dose was supposed to be taken, it is OK to take the dose. Otherwise, the dose should be skipped. The dose should not be doubled.
10. Explain that rivaroxaban 20 mg, 15 mg, or 10 mg once daily and edoxaban should be taken at the same time each day and that if a dose is missed, it may be taken on the same day as soon as it is remembered; otherwise the patient can resume the medication the next day. The dose should not be doubled. If a patient is taking 15 mg twice daily rivaroxaban for VTE treatment, the patient should take the second dose immediately and may take 30 mg (both 15-mg doses) at one time and then resume twice-daily administration the next day.
11. Discuss potential drug interactions. Explain that patients should contact their anticoagulant prescriber before taking any over-the-counter medications (including herbal supplements) or if a different health care provider starts them on a new medication. Avoid taking nonsteroidal anti-inflammatory drugs, including aspirin, with dabigatran unless it is discussed with their AC prescriber.

12. Discuss the need for periodic monitoring of blood tests for kidney function.
13. Women of childbearing age must notify their health care provider immediately if they become pregnant.
14. Dabigatran cannot be placed in a pill box and must be kept in the original container. Advise the patient to date the bottle label of dabigatran when opening and discard any unused capsules after 4 months.
15. Counsel patients on signs of stroke or VTE symptoms.
16. Document that the patient education session has occurred.
17. What are the current options for combination antiplatelets and anticoagulants in patients with acute coronary syndrome or undergoing percutaneous coronary intervention?

    Adding antiplatelet therapy to warfarin or DOAC AC increases the bleeding risk up to threefold. Therefore the combined use of triple therapy—antiplatelet agents, such as P2Y12 inhibitors (clopidogrel, ticagrelor, and clopidogrel), aspirin, and AC—must be undertaken cautiously. The most common reason for triple therapy is for the prevention of CV death, MI, or stroke in a patient with NVAF who undergoes percutaneous coronary intervention (PCI)/stent placement.

    Recommended methods to reduce the risk of bleeding include the following:

- Use of 81 mg of aspirin in preference to higher doses
- Use of clopidogrel instead of prasugrel or ticagrelor
- Warfarin instead of a DOAC (able to monitor intensity of AC and potentially easier to reverse)
- Target INR of 2.0 to 2.5 with warfarin
- More frequent INR measurements
- Use of a proton pump inhibitor
- Avoidance of other NSAIDs
- Optimal control of blood pressure (to avoid ICH)

Bibliography and Suggested Readings

Burnett, A. E., Mahan, C. E., Vasquez, S. R., Oertel, L. B., Garcia, D. A., & Ansell, J. (2016). Guidance for the practical management of the direct oral anticoagulants (DOACs) in the treatment of venous thromboembolism. *Journal of Thrombosis and Thrombolysis, 41*, 206–232.

CHA2DS2-*VASc calculator for calculating stroke risk in nonvalvular atrial fibrillation.* <http://www.mdcalc.com/cha2ds2-vasc-score-for-atrial-fibrillation-stroke-risk/>. Accessed 24.06.16.

Chang, M., Yu, Z., Shenker, A., Wang, J., Pursley, J., Byon, W., et al. (2016). Effect of renal impairment on the pharmacokinetics, pharmacodynamics, and safety of apixaban. *Journal of Clinical Pharmacology, 56*, 637–645.

Dias, C., Moore, K. T., Murphy, J., Ariyawansa, J., Smith, W., Mills, R. M., et al. (2016). Pharmacokinetics, pharmacodynamics, and safety of single-dose rivaroxaban in chronic hemodialysis. *American Journal of Nephrology, 43*, 229–236.

Douketis, J. D., Spyropoulos, A. C., Kaatz, S., Becker, R. C., Caprini, J. A., Dunn, A. S., et al. (2015). Perioperative bridging anticoagulation in patients with atrial fibrillation. *New England Journal of Medicine, 373*, 823–833.

HAS-BLED *score for major bleeding risk.* <http://www.mdcalc.com/has-bled-score-for-major-bleeding-risk/>. Accessed 24.06.16.

January, C. T., Wann, L. S., & Alpert, J. S. (2014). 2014 ACC/AHA/HRSA guideline for the management of patients with atrial fibrillation: a Report of the American College of Cardiology/American Heart Association Task Force on Practice Guidelines and the Heart Rhythm Society. *Circulation, 130*, e199–e267.

Johnson, J. A., Gong, L., Whirl-Carillo, M., Gage, B. F., Scott, S. A., Stein, C. M., et al. (2011). Clinical Pharmacogenetics Implementation Consortium Guidelines for CYP2C9 and VKORC1 genotypes and warfarin dosing. *Clinical Pharmacology and Therapeutics, 90*(4), 625–629.

Kearon, C., Akl, E. A., Ornelas, J., Blaivas, A., Jimenez, D., Bounameaux, H., et al. (2016). Antithrombotic therapy for VTE disease: CHEST guideline and expert panel report. *Chest, 149*, 315–352.

Kubitza, D., Becka, M., Mueck, W., Halabi, A., Maatouk, H., Klause, N., et al. (2010). Effects of renal impairment on the pharmacokinetics, pharmacodynamics and safety of rivaroxaban, an oral, direct factor Xa inhibitor. *British Journal of Clinical Pharmacology, 70*, 703–712.

Levy, J. H., Ageno, W., Chan, N. C., Crowther, M., Verhamme, P., & Weitz, J. I. (2016). When and how to use antidotes for the reversal of direct oral anticoagulants: guidance from the SCC of the ISTH. *Journal of Thrombosis and Haemostasis, 14*, 623–627.

Nishimura, R. A., Otto, C. M., Bonow, R. O., Carabello, B. A., Erwin, J. P., Guyton, R. A., et al. (2014). 2014 AHA/ACC guideline for the management of valvular heart disease: a report of the American College of Cardiology/American Heart Association Task Force on Practice Guidelines. *Journal of the American College of Cardiology, 63*, e57–e185.

Nutescu, E. A., Burnett, A., Fanikos, J., Spinler, S., & Wittkowsky, A. (2016). Pharmacology of anticoagulants used in the treatment of venous thromboembolism. *Journal of Thrombosis and Thrombolysis, 42*, 296–311.

Parasrampuria, D. A., Marbury, T., Matsushima, M., Chen, S., Wickremasingha, P. K., He, L., et al. (2015). Pharmacokinetics, safety, and tolerability of edoxaban in end-stage renal disease subjects undergoing haemodialysis. *Thrombosis and Haemostasis, 113*, 719–727.

Picard, F., Tadros, V. X., & Asgar, A. W. (2015). Triple antithrombotic therapy in patients with atrial fibrillation with an indication for oral anticoagulation undergoing percutaneous coronary intervention: a case-based review of the current evidence. *Circulation Cardiovascular Intervention, 8*(12), e003217.

Ridout, G., de la Motte, S., Niemczyk, S., Sramck, P., Johnson, L., Jin, J., et al. (2009a). Effect of renal function on edoxaban pharmacokinetics (PK) and on population PK/PK-PD model. *Journal of Clinical Pharmacology, 49*(9), 1124.

Ruff, C. T., Ansell, J. E., Becker, R. C., Benjamin, E. J., Deicicchi, D. J., Estes, N. M., et al. (2016). North American Thrombosis Forum, AF Action Initiative consensus document. *American Journal of Medicine, 129*, S1–S29.

Smythe, M. A., Priziola, J., Dobesh, P. P., Wirth, D., Cuker, A., & Wittkowsky, A. K. (2016). Guidance for the practical management of the heparin anticoagulants in the management of venous thromboembolism. *Journal of Thrombosis and Thrombolysis, 41*, 165–186.

Streiff, M. B., Agnelli, G., Connors, J. M., Crowther, M., Eichinger, S., Lopes, R., et al. (2016). Guidance for the treatment of venous thromboembolism. *Journal of Thrombosis and Thrombolysis, 41*, 32–67.

Thrombosis Canada. *Anticoagulant-related bleeding patient order sets.* <http://thrombosiscanada.ca/wp-content/uploads/2016/05/Anticoagulant-relatedBleedMgmntOSv.12.pdf>. Accessed 24.06.16.

Thrombosis Canada. *Novel Oral Anticoagulants (NOACs) Management of Bleeding.* <http://thrombosiscanada.ca/?p=1861>. Accessed 24.06.16.

U.S. Food and Drug Administration Drug Development and Drug Interactions: Table of Substrates, Inhibitors and Inducers. <http://www.fda.gov/Drugs/DevelopmentApprovalProcess/DevelopmentResources/DrugInteractionsLabeling/ucm093664.htm>. Accessed 24.06.16.

Witt, D. M., Clark, N. P., Kaatz, S. M., Schnurr, T., & Ansell, J. E. (2016). Guidance for the practical management of warfarin therapy in the treatment of venous thromboembolism. *Journal of Thrombosis and Thrombolysis, 41*, 187–205.

Coumadin (warfarin sodium) (prescribing information). (2015). Princeton, NJ: Bristol-Myers Squibb Co.

Eliquis (apixaban) (prescribing information). (2015). Princeton, NJ: Bristol-Myers Squibb Co.

Pradaxa (dabigatran etexilate) (prescribing information). (2015). Ridgefield, CT: Boehringer Ingelheim Pharmaceuticals Inc.

Savaysa (edoxaban) (prescribing information). (2015). Parsippany, NJ: Daiichi Sankyo, Inc.

Xarelto (rivaroxaban) (prescribing information). (2016). Titusville, NJ: Janssen Pharmaceuticals, Inc.

CHAPTER 67

PERICARDITIS, PERICARDIAL CONSTRICTION, AND PERICARDIAL TAMPONADE

Rahul Thomas, Brian D. Hoit

1. **The pericardium is not necessary for life. What does it do? Why is it important?**
The pericardium serves many important but subtle functions. It limits distention and facilitates interaction of the cardiac chambers, influences ventricular filling, prevents excessive torsion and displacement of the heart, minimizes friction with surrounding structures, prevents the spread of infection from contiguous structures, and equalizes gravitational, hydrostatic, and inertial forces over the surface of the heart. The pericardium also has immunologic, vasomotor, fibrinolytic, and metabolic activities. Therapeutically the pericardial space can be used for drug delivery.

2. **What diseases affect the pericardium?**
The pericardium is affected by virtually every category of disease (Box 67.1), including idiopathic, infectious, neoplastic, immune/inflammatory, metabolic, iatrogenic, traumatic, and congenital.

3. **What is pericarditis? What are the clinical manifestations? What are the causes?**
Acute pericarditis is a syndrome of pericardial inflammation characterized by typical chest pain (sharp, retrosternal pain that radiates to the trapezius ridge, often aggravated by lying down and relieved by sitting up), a pathognomonic pericardial friction rub (characterized as superficial, *scratchy, crunchy*, and evanescent), and specific electrocardiographic changes (diffuse ST-T wave changes [Fig. 67.1] with characteristic evolutionary changes and PR segment depression). These manifestations vary in terms of presentation (chest pain >85% to 90%, pericardial friction rub ≤33%, electrocardiogram [ECG] changes 60%). The 2015 European Society of Cardiology (ESC) Guidelines suggest that at least two of four of the following criteria are needed to make the diagnosis: pericardial pain, pericardial rub, ECG changes, and pericardial effusion. Additional supporting findings include elevation in inflammatory markers (erythrocyte sedimentation rate [ESR], C-reactive protein [CRP], white blood cell [WBC]) count and evidence of pericardial inflammation by computed tomography (CT) or magnetic resonance imaging (MRI).

Causes of pericarditis include infection (viral, bacterial, fungal, mycobacterial, human immunodeficiency virus [HIV] associated), neoplasm (usually metastatic from lung or breast; melanoma, lymphoma, or acute leukemia), myocardial infarction, injury (post pericardiotomy,

Box 67.1. Causes of Pericardial Heart Disease

- **Idiopathic**

Infectious Bacterial, viral, mycobacterial, fungal, protozoal, HIV associated

- **Neoplastic**
- **Metastatic** (breast, lung, melanoma, lymphoma, leukemia), primary (mesothelioma, fibrosarcoma)
- **Immune/inflammatory** Connective tissue disease, arteritis, acute myocardial infarction, postpericardial injury syndrome
- **Metabolic** Nephrogenic, myxedema, amyloidosis, aortic dissection
- **Iatrogenic** Drugs, radiation therapy, device/instrumentation, cardiac resuscitation
- **Traumatic** Blunt, penetrating, surgical
- **Congenital** Pericardial cysts, congenital absence of pericardium, mulibrey nanism

Modified from Hoit, B. D. (2008). Diseases of the pericardium. In V. Fuster, R. A. O'Rourke, R. A. Walsh, & P. Poole-Wilson (Eds.), *Hurst's the heart* (12th ed.). New York: McGraw-Hill.

traumatic), radiation, myxedema, and connective tissue disease. In the developed world the most common cause remains viral etiologies, whereas tuberculosis is the most frequent cause in developing countries.

4. **Should patients presenting with acute pericarditis be hospitalized? Why?**
Hospitalization is warranted for high-risk patients with an initial episode of acute pericarditis to determine a cause and to observe for the development of cardiac tamponade; close, early follow-up is critically important for the remainder of patients not hospitalized. Features indicative of high-risk pericarditis include fever greater than 38°C, subacute onset, an immunosuppressed state, trauma, oral anticoagulant therapy, myopericarditis, a moderate or large pericardial effusion, cardiac tamponade, and failure of initial outpatient medical therapy.

5. **What is the treatment for acute pericarditis?**
Acute pericarditis usually responds to oral nonsteroidal anti-inflammatory drugs (NSAIDs), such as aspirin (650-1000 mg every 4-6 hours) or ibuprofen (600-800 mg every 6-8 hours). Colchicine (1 mg/day) may be used to supplement the NSAIDs because it may reduce symptoms and decrease the rate of recurrences. Chest pain is usually alleviated in 1 to 2 days, and the friction rub and ST-segment elevation resolve shortly thereafter. Most mild cases of idiopathic and viral pericarditis are adequately treated within a week or two of treatment, but the duration of therapy is variable and patients should be treated until inflammation or an effusion, if present, has resolved. The intensity of therapy is dictated by the distress of the patient, and narcotics may be required for severe pain. Corticosteroids should be avoided unless there is a specific indication (such as connective tissue disease or uremic pericarditis) because they enhance viral multiplication and may result in recurrences when the dosage is tapered.

Based on the colchicine for acute pericarditis (COPE) trial the ESC Guidelines recommend a weight-adjusted colchicine dose of 0.5 mg once daily for patients less than 70 kg or 0.5 mg BID for those ≥70 kg for at least 3 months to improve response to medical therapy and prevent recurrences.

6. **What is recurrent pericarditis? How is it treated?**
Recurrences of pericarditis (with or without pericardial effusion) occur in up to one-third of patients, usually within 18 months of the acute attack and may follow a course of many years. Although they may be spontaneous, occurring at varying intervals after discontinuation of drug, they are more commonly associated with either discontinuation or tapering of anti-inflammatory drugs. A poor initial response to therapy with NSAIDs and the use of corticosteroids predict recurrences. Two randomized placebo-controlled trials of colchicine for recurrent pericarditis (CORE, CORP) reported marked and significant reductions in symptom persistence at 72 hours and recurrence at 18 months when colchicine was added to conventional therapy. Although painful recurrences of pericarditis may require corticosteroids (preferably at low to moderate doses with slow tapering), once administered, dependency and the development of steroid-induced abnormalities are potential perils.

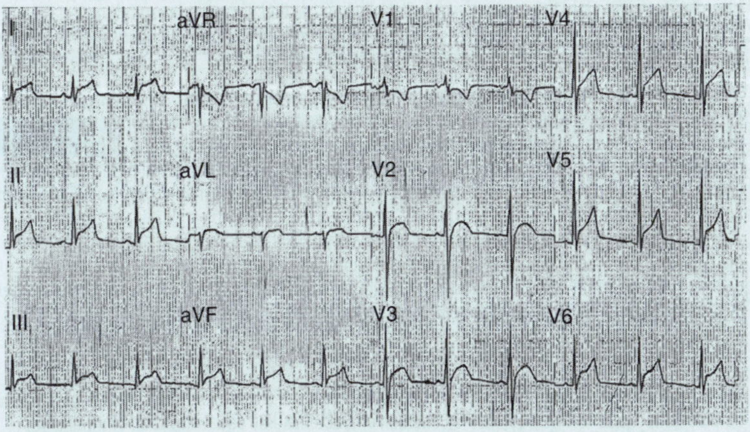

Fig. 67.1. The diffuse ST-segment elevations seen in pericarditis.

Tapering of therapy should be done gradually, with tapering of a single class of drug at a time before colchicine is discontinued. For patients who require high-dose, long-term steroids or who do not respond to anti-inflammatory therapies, several drugs (azathioprine, intravenous immunoglobulin (IVIG), and anakinra, a recombinant interleukin IL- 1) have been used; however, strong evidence-based data supporting these therapies are lacking. Pericardiectomy should be considered only when repeated attempts at medical treatment have clearly failed.

7. What is postcardiac injury syndrome?

Postcardiac injury syndrome (PCIS) refers to pericarditis or pericardial effusion that results from injury of the pericardium. The principal conditions considered under these headings include postmyocardial infarction syndrome, postpericardiotomy syndrome, and traumatic (blunt, sharp, or iatrogenic) pericarditis. Clinical features include the following:

- Prior injury of the pericardium, myocardium, or both
- A latent period between the injury and development of pericarditis or pericardial effusion
- A tendency for recurrence
- Responsiveness to NSAIDs and corticosteroids
- Fever, leukocytosis, and elevated ESR (and other markers of inflammation)
- Pericardial and sometimes pleural effusion, with or without a pulmonary infiltrate
- Alterations in the populations of lymphocytes in peripheral blood

When the PCIS occurs after an acute myocardial infarction, it is also known as Dressler syndrome, which is now much less common than in the past. In the randomized multicenter Colchicine for the Prevention of Post-pericardiotomy Syndrome (COPPS) study, prophylactically administered colchicine reduced the incidence of postpericardiotomy syndrome after cardiac surgery. According to the 2015 ESC Guidelines on Pericardial Disease, colchicine should be considered (class IIa) after cardiac surgery, using weight-based doses, for a 1-month duration as prevention.

8. What are the pericardial compressive syndromes? What are their variants?

The complications of acute pericarditis include cardiac tamponade, constrictive pericarditis, and effusive-constrictive pericarditis. Cardiac tamponade is characterized by the accumulation of pericardial fluid under pressure and may be acute, subacute, low pressure (occult), or regional. Constrictive pericarditis is the result of thickening, calcification, and loss of elasticity of the pericardial sac. Pericardial constriction is typically chronic but may be subacute, transient, and occult. Effusive-constrictive pericarditis is characterized by constrictive physiology with a coexisting pericardial effusion, usually with tamponade. Elevation of the right atrial and pulmonary wedge pressures persists after drainage of the pericardial fluid.

9. What are the similarities between tamponade and constrictive pericarditis?

Characteristic of both tamponade and constrictive pericarditis is greatly enhanced ventricular interaction (interdependence), in which the hemodynamics of the left and right heart chambers are directly influenced by each other to a much greater degree than normal. Other similarities include diastolic dysfunction and preserved ventricular ejection fraction; increased respiratory variation of ventricular inflow and outflow; equally elevated central venous, pulmonary venous, and ventricular diastolic pressures; and mild pulmonary hypertension.

10. What are the differences between tamponade and constrictive pericarditis?

In tamponade the pericardial space is open and transmits the respiratory variation in thoracic pressure to the heart, whereas in constrictive pericarditis the cavity is obliterated and the pericardium does not transmit these pressure changes. The dissociation of intrathoracic and intracardiac pressures (along with ventricular interaction) is the basis for the physical, hemodynamic, and echocardiographic findings of constriction.

In tamponade, systemic venous return increases with inspiration, enlarging the right side of the heart and encroaching on the left, whereas in constrictive pericarditis, systemic venous return does not increase with inspiration. The mechanism of diminished left ventricular and increased right ventricular volume in constrictive pericarditis is impaired left ventricular filling because of a lesser pressure gradient from the pulmonary veins.

In tamponade, early ventricular filling is impaired, whereas it is enhanced in constriction.

11. What are the physical findings of tamponade?

Cardiac tamponade is a hemodynamic condition characterized by equal elevation of atrial and pericardial pressures, an exaggerated inspiratory decrease in arterial systolic pressure (pulsus paradoxus), and arterial hypotension. The physical findings are dictated by both the severity of cardiac tamponade and the time course of its development. Inspection of the jugular venous pulse waveform reveals elevated venous pressure with a loss of the Y descent (because of the decrease in intrapericardial pressure that occurs during ventricular ejection, the systolic atrial filling wave and the X descent are maintained). Pulsus paradoxus is an inspiratory decline of systolic arterial pressure exceeding 10 mm Hg, which is measured by subtracting the pressure at which Korotkoff sounds are heard only during expiration from the pressure at which sounds are heard throughout the respiratory cycle. Tachycardia and tachypnea are usually present.

12. **What are the physical findings of constrictive pericarditis?**
Constrictive pericarditis resembles the congestive states caused by myocardial disease and chronic liver disease. Physical findings include ascites, hepatosplenomegaly, edema, and, in long-standing cases, severe wasting. The venous pressure is elevated and displays deep Y and often deep X descents. The venous pressure fails to decrease with inspiration (Kussmaul sign). A pericardial knock that is similar in timing to the third heart sound is pathognomonic but occurs infrequently. Except in severe cases, the arterial blood pressure is normal.

13. **What is the role of echocardiography in tamponade?**
Although tamponade is a clinical diagnosis, echocardiography plays major roles in the identification of pericardial effusion and in the assessment of its hemodynamic significance (Fig. 67.2). The use of echocardiography for the evaluation of all patients with suspected pericardial disease was given a class I recommendation by a 2003 task force of the American College of Cardiology (ACC), the American Heart Association (AHA), and the American Society of Echocardiography (ASE). This recommendation was supported by a 2013 ASE Expert Consensus Statement and the 2015 ESC Guidelines. Except in hyperacute cases, a moderate to large effusion is usually present, and swinging of the heart within the effusion may be seen. Reciprocal changes in left and right ventricular volumes occur with respiration. Echocardiographic findings suggesting hemodynamic compromise (atrial and ventricular diastolic collapses) are the result of transiently reversed right atrial and right ventricular diastolic transmural pressures and typically occur before hemodynamic embarrassment. The respiratory variation of mitral and tricuspid flow velocities is greatly increased and out of phase, reflecting the increased ventricular interaction. Less than a 50% inspiratory reduction in the diameter of a dilated inferior vena cava reflects a marked elevation in central venous pressure, and abnormal right-sided venous flows (systolic predominance and expiratory diastolic reversal) are diagnostic. In patients who do not have tamponade on first assessment, repeat echocardiography during clinical follow-up was given a class IIa recommendation by the 2003 ACC/AHA/ASE task force.

14. **What is the role of echocardiography in constrictive pericarditis?**
Echocardiography is an essential adjunctive procedure in patients with suspected pericardial constriction. The use of echocardiography for the evaluation of all patients with suspected pericardial disease is a class I ACC/AHA/ASE task force recommendation. Echocardiography findings to be sought include increased pericardial thickness (best with transesophageal echocardiography), abrupt inspiratory posterior motion of the ventricular septum in early diastole, plethora of the inferior vena cava and hepatic veins, enlarged atria, and an abnormal contour between the posterior left ventricular the left atrial posterior walls. Although no sign or combination of signs on M-mode is diagnostic of constrictive pericarditis, a normal study virtually rules out the diagnosis. Doppler is particularly useful, showing a high *E* velocity of right and left ventricular inflow and rapid deceleration, a normal or increased tissue Doppler *E*′, and a 25% to 40% fall in transmitral flow and marked increase of tricuspid velocity in the first beat after inspiration. Increased respiratory variation of mitral inflow may be missing in patients with markedly elevated left atrial pressure but may be brought out by preload reduction (e.g., head-up tilt). Hepatic vein flow reversals increase with expiration, reflecting the ventricular interaction and the dissociation of intracardiac and intrathoracic pressures, and pulmonary venous flow shows marked respiratory variation.

15. **Are other imaging modalities useful in pericardial disease?**
Other imaging techniques, such as CT and cardiovascular magnetic resonance (CMR), are not necessary if two-dimensional and Doppler echocardiography are available. However, pericardial effusion may be detected, quantified, and characterized by CT and CMR. CT scanning of the heart is extremely useful in the diagnosis of constrictive pericarditis; findings include increased pericardial thickness (>4 mm) and calcification. CMR provides direct visualization of the normal pericardium, which is composed of fibrous tissue and has a low MRI signal intensity. CMR is claimed by some

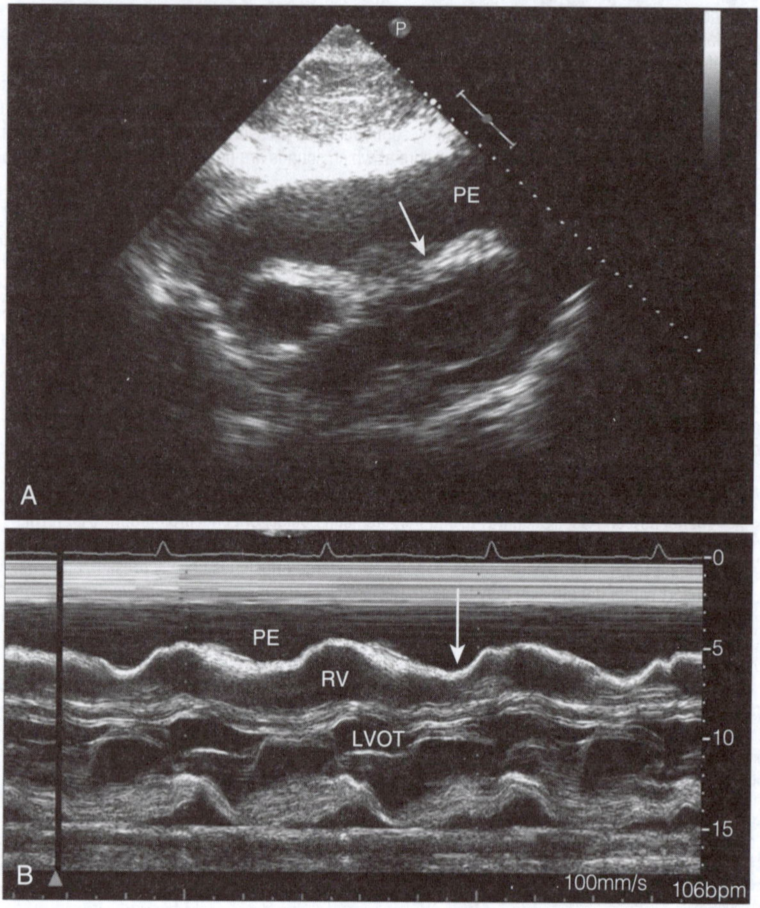

Fig. 67.2. Echocardiography in cardiac tamponade. **A,** Subcostal two-dimensional echocardiogram. A large pericardial effusion with marked compression of the right ventricle *(arrow)* is seen. **B,** M-mode of the parasternal long axis. Note the right ventricular *(long arrow)* collapse. *LVOT,* Left ventricular outflow tract; *PE,* pericardial effusion; *RV,* right ventricle.

to be the diagnostic procedure of choice for the detection of constrictive pericarditis (Fig. 67.3). Late gadolinium enhancement of the pericardium may predict reversibility of transitory constrictive pericarditis (see later) following treatment with anti-inflammatory agents. The 2015 ESC Guidelines recommend CT and/or CMR as second-level testing in the diagnostic workup of pericarditis.

16. What is the role for medical therapy in constrictive pericarditis?

Constrictive pericarditis is a surgical disease, except in cases of very early constriction or in severe, advanced disease. Medical therapy of constrictive pericarditis plays a small but important role. Medical therapy of specific etiologies (e.g., tuberculosis pericarditis) may significantly reduce progression to constriction. Medical therapy with anti-inflammatory drugs may resolve constriction (transitory constriction). Finally, medical therapy may be supportive therapy to control symptoms in patients not candidates for pericardiectomy due to their surgical risk. Diuretics and digoxin (in the presence of atrial fibrillation) are useful in these patients.

Preoperative, before pericardiectomy, diuretics should be used sparingly with the goal of reducing, not eliminating, elevated jugular pressure, edema, and ascites. Postoperatively, diuretics

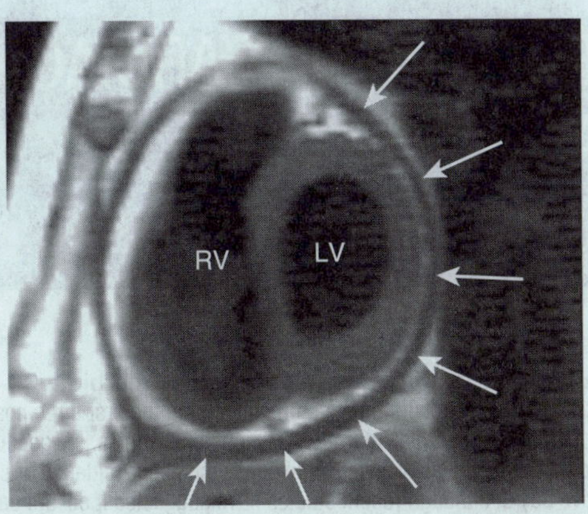

Fig. 67.3. Magnetic resonance imaging demonstrating thickened pericardium encasing the heart *(arrows)*. *LV*, Left ventricle; *RV*, right ventricle. *(Reproduced with permission from Pennell, D. [2008]. Cardiovascular magnetic resonance. In P. Libby, R. Bonow, D. Mann, & D. Zipes. [Eds.],* Braunwald's heart disease: a textbook of cardiovascular medicine *(8th ed.). Philadelphia, PA: Saunders.)*

should be given if spontaneous diuresis does not occur; the central venous pressure may take weeks to months to return to normal after pericardiectomy. In some patients, constrictive pericarditis resolves either spontaneously or in response to various combinations of NSAIDs, steroids, and antibiotics (transitory constriction). Therefore, before pericardiectomy is recommended, conservative management for 2 to 3 months in hemodynamically stable patients with subacute constrictive pericarditis is recommended.

Bibliography and Suggested Readings

Adler, Y., Charron, P., Imazio, M., Badano, L., Barón-Esquivias, G., Bogaert, J., et al. (2015). 2015 ESC Guidelines for the diagnosis and management of pericardial diseases. *European Heart Journal*, *36*, 2921–2964.

Cheitlin, M. D., Armstrong, W. F., Aurigemma, G. P., Beller, G. A., Bierman, F. Z., Davis, J. L., et al. ACC/AHA/ASE 2003 guideline update for the clinical application of echocardiography: summary article: a report of the American College of Cardiology/American Heart Association Task Force on Practice Guidelines (ACC/AHA/ASE Committee to Update the 1997 Guidelines for the Clinical Application of Echocardiography). *Circulation*, *108*, 1146–1162.

Hoit, B. D. (2002). Management of effusive and constrictive pericardial heart disease. *Circulation*, *105*, 2939–2942.

Hoit, B. D. (2011a). Diseases of the pericardium. In V. Fuster & R. A. Walsh (Eds.), *Hurst's the reart* (13th ed.). New York: McGraw-Hill.

Hoit, B. D. (2011b). Treatment of pericardial disease. In E. Antman & M. S. Sabatine (Eds.), *Cardiovascular therapeutics. A companion to Braunwald's heart disease* (4th ed.). Philadelphia, PA: Elsevier.

Klein, A. L., Abbara, S., Agler, D. A., Appleton, C. P., Asher, C. R., Hoit, B. A., et al. (2013). American Society of Echocardiography clinical recommendations for multimodality cardiovascular imaging of patients with pericardial disease. *Journal of the American Society of Echocardiography*, *26*, 965–1012.

Little, W. C., & Freeman, G. L. (2006). Pericardial disease. *Circulation*, *113*, 1622.

CHAPTER 68

PREOPERATIVE CARDIAC EVALUATION

Lee A. Fleisher

1. **What is the natural history of perioperative cardiac morbidity?**
   Perioperative cardiac morbidity occurs most commonly during the first three postoperative days and includes perioperative myocardial infarction (MI), unstable angina, congestive heart failure, cardiac death, and nonfatal cardiac arrests. Traditionally the peak incidence of perioperative MI was during postoperative day 3, although recent studies have suggested it occurs earlier and may arise most commonly in the first 48 hours. In addition, the mortality from a perioperative cardiac MI has decreased from previous rates of 30% to 50% to approximately 12%. A large number of patients also demonstrate isolated biomarker elevations, which are predictive of worse long-term but not short-term survival.

2. **What is the cause of perioperative cardiac morbidity?**
   The cause of perioperative MI is multifactorial. The postoperative period is associated with a stress response, which includes the release of catecholamines and cortisol, resulting in tachycardia and hypertension. The tachycardia can lead to supply and demand mismatches distal to a critical coronary stenosis, causing myocardial ischemia, and, if prolonged, to perioperative MI. Tissue injury, tachycardia, and the hypercoagulable state also lead to plaque rupture and acute thrombosis, potentially resulting in a perioperative MI. Therefore, many perioperative events will not be predicted by identifying critical stenoses or preoperative imaging. In addition, perioperative strategies to reduce cardiac morbidity require a multimodal approach of both reducing supply and demand mismatches and reducing the risk of acute thrombosis. Patients with coronary stents are particularly vulnerable to this prothrombotic state.

3. **What are the strongest predictors of perioperative cardiac events?**
   For some specific patients, surgery represents a very high risk of cardiac complications, and either therapy should be initiated preoperatively or the benefits of surgery must significantly outweigh the risks if the decision is to proceed to surgery. According to the 2014 American College of Cardiology/American Heart Association (ACC/AHA) Guidelines on Perioperative Cardiovascular Evaluation, active cardiac conditions for which the patient should undergo evaluation and treatment before noncardiac surgery include unstable coronary symptoms syndromes, and a recent myocardial infarction. Based upon analyses of administrative data, elevated risk related to a recent MI continues for at least the first 60 days, for the purposes of preoperative evaluation. Additional important risk factors include active heart failure, severe valvular disease, and severe arrhythmias. A summary of active cardiac conditions for which the patient should undergo evaluation and treatment before elective noncardiac surgery is given in Table 68.1.

4. **What is the American College of Surgeons National Surgical Quality Improvement Project risk calculator, and how should it be used clinically?**
   The American College of Surgeons National Surgical Quality Improvement Project (ACS- NSQIP) risk calculator was developed based on 1,414,006 patients encompassing 1557 unique Current Procedural Terminology (CPT) codes. Risk factors are shown in Table 68.2 and include clinical factors and surgical CPT. Regression models were developed to predict eight outcomes, including cardiovascular morbidity, based on the preoperative risk factors. This overall rate of cardiac morbidity and mortality can then be used in the algorithm proposed by the guidelines.

5. **What is the revised cardiac risk index, and how is it used clinically?**
   Cardiac risk indices for perioperative risk stratification have been used in clinical practice for more than 30 years. These indices do not inform clinicians on how to modify perioperative care specifically, but they do provide a baseline assessment of risk and the value of different intervention strategies.

Table 68.1. Active Cardiac Conditions for Which the Patient Should Undergo Evaluation and Treatment Before Noncardiac Surgery (Class I, Level of Evidence B)

CONDITION	EXAMPLES
Unstable coronary syndromes	Unstable or severe angina* (CCS class III or IV)† Recent MI‡ Decompensated HF (NYHA functional class IV; worsening or new-onset HF)
Significant arrhythmias	High-grade atrioventricular block Mobitz II atrioventricular block Third-degree atrioventricular heart block Symptomatic ventricular arrhythmias Supraventricular arrhythmias (including atrial fibrillation) with uncontrolled ventricular rate (HR >100 beats/min at rest) Symptomatic bradycardia Newly recognized ventricular tachycardia
Severe valvular disease	Severe aortic stenosis (mean pressure gradient >40 mm Hg, aortic valve area <1.0 cm^2, or symptomatic) Symptomatic mitral stenosis (progressive dyspnea on exertion, exertional presyncope, or HF)

CCS, Canadian Cardiovascular Society; *HF*, heart failure; *HR*, heart rate; *MI*, myocardial infarction; *NYHA*, New York Heart Association.

*According to Campeau, L. Grading of angina pectoris [letter]. *Circulation, 54*, 522–523.

†May include *stable* angina in patients who are unusually sedentary.

‡The American College of Cardiology National Database Library defines recent MI as more than 7 days but less than or equal to 1 month (within 30 days).

Modified from Fleisher, L. A., Beckman, J. A., Brown, K. A., Calkins, H., Chaikof, E. L., Fleischmann, K. E., et al. (2007). ACC/AHA guidelines on perioperative cardiovascular evaluation and care for noncardiac surgery: executive summary. Journal of the American College of Cardiology, 50, *1716*.

Calculation of an index is not a substitute for providing detailed information of the underlying heart disease, its stability, and ventricular function. The Revised Cardiac Risk Index (RCRI) was developed by studying more than 5000 patients and identifying six risk factors, including the following:

- High-risk surgery
- Ischemic heart disease
- History of congestive heart failure
- History of cerebrovascular disease
- Preoperative treatment with insulin
- Preoperative serum creatinine greater than 2 mg/dL

In determining the need and value of preoperative testing and interventions, the ACC/AHA guidelines incorporate the number of risk factors from the RCRI, other than high-risk surgery, which is incorporated elsewhere. Importantly, diabetes (without regard to type of treatment) is considered one of the risk factors, as opposed to insulin treatment.

6. What is the importance of exercise capacity?

Numerous studies have demonstrated the importance of exercise capacity on overall perioperative morbidity and mortality. Based on several of these studies, patients can be dichotomized into poor functional capacity (<4 METS) versus moderate or excellent exercise capacity. Patients with moderate to excellent exercise capacity rarely need further testing before noncardiac surgery.

7. What is the influence of the surgical procedure on the decision to perform further diagnostic testing?

In all patients, regardless of the type of surgery, determination of the presence of active cardiac conditions is first and foremost because proceeding to surgery should be done only after assessing and potentially treating these conditions. Prior guidelines have identified three levels of surgical risk.

Table 68.2. American College of Surgeons National Surgical Quality Improvement Project Variables Used in Universal Surgical Risk Calculators

VARIABLE	CATEGORIES
Age group, year	<65, 65-74, 75-84, ≥85
Gender	Male, female
Functional status	Independent, partially dependent, totally dependent
Emergency case	Yes, no
ASA class	1 or 2, 3, 4, or 5
Steroid use for chronic condition	Yes, no
Ascites within 30 days preoperatively	Yes, no
System sepsis within 48 h preoperatively	None, SIRS, sepsis, septic shock
Ventilator dependent	Yes, no
Disseminated cancer	Yes, no
Diabetes	No, oral, insulin
Hypertension requiring medication	Yes, no
Previous cardiac event	Yes, no
Congestive heart failure in 30 days preoperatively	Yes, no
Dyspnea	Yes, no
Current smoker within 1 year	Yes, no
History of COPD	Yes, no
Dialysis	Yes, no
Acute renal failure	Yes, no
BMI class	Underweight, normal, overweight, obese 1, obese 2, obese 3

ASA, American Society of Anesthesiologists; *BMI*, body mass index; *COPD*, chronic obstructive pulmonary disease; *SIRS*, systemic inflammatory response syndrome.

Modified from Bilimoria, K. Y., Liu, Y., Paruch, J. L., Zhou, L., Kmiecik, T. E., Ko, C. Y., et al. (2013). Development and evaluation of the universal ACS NSQIP surgical risk calculator: a decision aid and informed consent tool for patients and surgeons. Journal of the American College of Surgeons, 217, 833–842.

Low-risk surgeries, those associated with a perioperative cardiac morbidity and mortality less than 1%, rarely, if ever, require a change in management based on the results of a diagnostic test. The most common such procedures are those performed on an outpatient basis.

In the intermediate group of procedures, a gradation of risk is based on the specific surgical procedures, and the institution-specific risk is critical to determine if further diagnostic testing would add value. For example, increased surgical volume is associated with lower perioperative risk, and preoperative testing may not lead to changes in management in such institutions.

Multiple studies have focused on patients undergoing vascular surgery, particularly open aortic and lower extremity revascularization. Therefore these patients are treated uniquely in the assessment of the need to perform diagnostic testing based on the extensive evidence and the high perioperative cardiac morbidity and mortality, often in the range of 5% or greater.

The 2014 guidelines combine clinical and surgical risk into one overall assessment of low and elevated risk (combining the previous intermediate and high risk). As noted previously, the ACS-NSQIP Risk Calculator incorporates individual CPT codes into the assessment.

8. How do the American College of Cardiology/American Heart Association Guidelines suggest an approach to preoperative evaluation?

The algorithm from the 2014 guidelines can be found in Fig. 68.1. Importantly, any decision to perform diagnostic testing based on the algorithm must incorporate the value of the information to change perioperative management. Changes in management can include the decision to undergo coronary

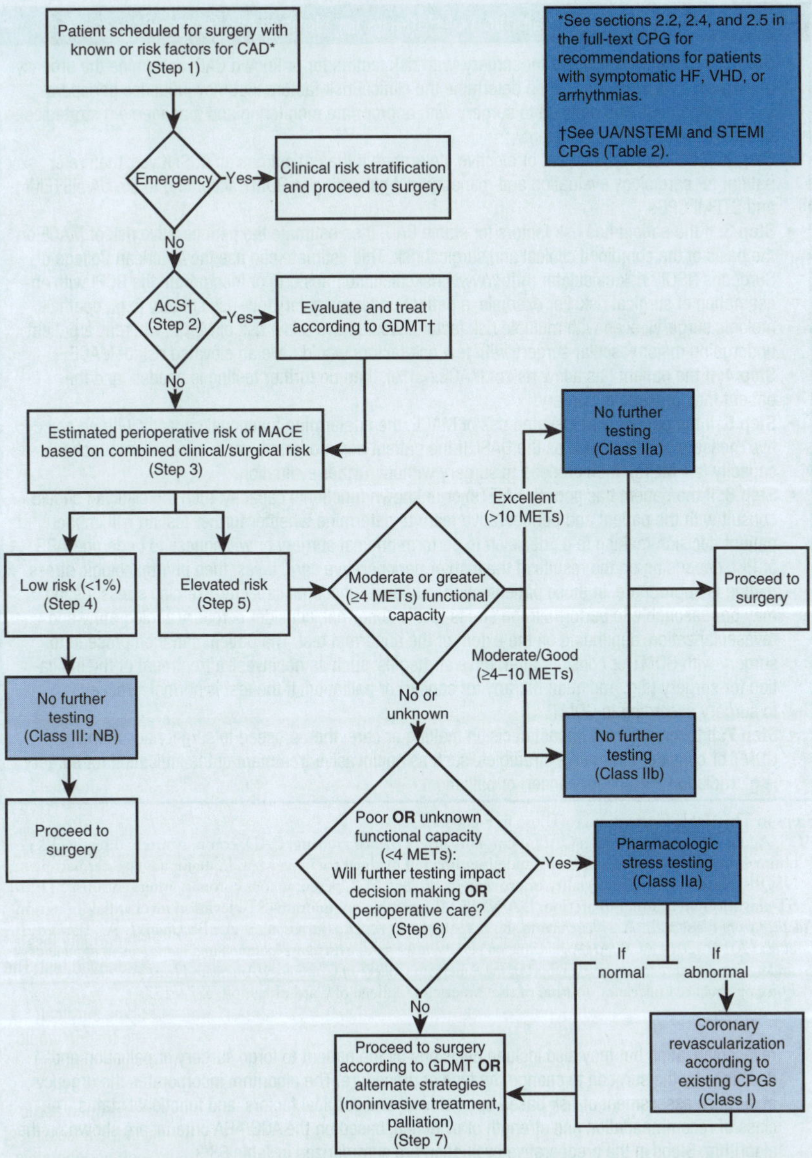

Fig. 68.1. Stepwise approach to perioperative cardiac assessment for coronary artery disease. *ACS*, Acute coronary syndrome; *CAD*, coronary artery disease; *CPG*, clinical practice guideline; *GDMT*, guideline-directed medical therapy; *HF*, heart failure; *MACE*, major adverse cardiac event; *METs*, metabolic equivalents; *NB*, no benefit; *PCI*, percutaneous coronary intervention; *STEMI*, ST-elevation myocardial infarction; *UA/NSTEMI*, unstable angina/non–ST-elevation myocardial infarction; *VHD*, valvular heart disease. *(From Fleisher, L. A., Fleischmann, K. E., Auerbach, A. D., Barnason, S. A., Beckman, J. A., Bozkurt, B., et al. [2014]. 2014 ACC/AHA guideline on perioperative cardiovascular evaluation and management of patients undergoing noncardiac surgery: a report of the American College of Cardiology/American Heart Association Task Force on Practice Guidelines.* Journal of the American College of Cardiology, 64, *e77–e137.)*

Table 68.3. Steps in the Evaluation of Patients for Noncardiac Surgery.

- **Step 1:** In patients scheduled for surgery, with risk factors for or known CAD, determine the urgency of surgery. If an emergency, then determine the clinical risk factors that may influence perioperative management, and proceed to surgery with appropriate monitoring and management strategies based on the clinical assessment.
- **Step 2:** If the surgery is urgent or elective, determine if the patient has an ACS. If yes, then refer patient for cardiology evaluation and management according to GDMT according to the UA/NSTEMI and STEMI CPGs.
- **Step 3:** If the patient has risk factors for stable CAD, then estimate the perioperative risk of MACE on the basis of the combined clinical and surgical risk. This estimate can use the American College of Surgeons NSQIP risk calculator (http://www.riskcalculator.facs.org) or incorporate the RCRI with an estimation of surgical risk. For example, a patient undergoing very low-risk surgery (e.g., ophthalmologic surgery), even with multiple risk factors, would have a low risk of MACE, whereas a patient undergoing major vascular surgery with few risk factors would have an elevated risk of MACE.
- **Step 4:** If the patient has a low risk of MACE (<1%), then no further testing is needed, and the patient may proceed to surgery.
- **Step 5:** If the patient is at elevated risk of MACE, then determine functional capacity with an objective measure or scale, such as the DASI. If the patient has moderate, good, or excellent functional capacity (≥4 METs), then proceed to surgery without further evaluation.
- **Step 6:** If the patient has poor (<4 METs) or unknown functional capacity, then the clinician should consult with the patient and perioperative team to determine whether further testing will impact patient decision making (e.g., decision to perform original surgery or willingness to undergo CABG or PCI, depending on the results of the test) or perioperative care. If yes, then pharmacologic stress testing is appropriate. In those patients with unknown functional capacity, exercise stress testing may be reasonable to perform. If the stress test is abnormal, consider coronary angiography and revascularization, depending on the extent of the abnormal test. The patient can then proceed to surgery with GDMT or consider alternative strategies, such as noninvasive treatment of the indication for surgery (e.g., radiation therapy for cancer) or palliation. If the test is normal, proceed to surgery according to GDMT.
- **Step 7:** If testing will not impact decision making or care, then proceed to surgery according to GDMT or consider alternative strategies, such as noninvasive treatment of the indication for surgery (e.g., radiation therapy for cancer) or palliation.

Steps in This Table Correspond to Those in Fig. 68.1.

ACS, Acute coronary syndrome; *CABG*, coronary artery bypass grafting; *CAD*, coronary artery disease; *CPG*, clinical practice guideline; *GDMT*, guideline-directed medical therapy; *MACE*, major adverse cardiac event; *NSQIP*, National Surgical Quality Improvement Project; *PCI*, percutaneous coronary interventions; *STEMI*, ST-elevation myocardial infarction; *UA/NSTEMI*, unstable angina/non–ST-elevation myocardial infarction.

Adapted from Fleisher, L. A., Fleischmann, K. E., Auerbach, A. D., Barnason, S. A., Beckman, J. A., Bozkurt, B., et al. (2014). 2014 ACC/AHA guideline on perioperative cardiovascular evaluation and management of patients undergoing noncardiac surgery: a report of the American College of Cardiology/American Heart Association Task Force on Practice Guidelines. Journal of the American College of Cardiology, *64, e77–e137.*

revascularization but may also include decisions by the patient to forgo surgery or palliation and decisions by the surgeon to change the type of procedure. The algorithm incorporates the urgency of surgery, assessment of risk based upon clinical and surgical factors, and functional status. The class of recommendation and strength of evidence, based on the ACC/AHA criteria, are shown on the algorithm. Steps in the preoperative evaluation are summarized in Table 68.3.

9. What is the value of coronary revascularization before noncardiac surgery?

Traditionally it was thought that patients who had undergone prior coronary artery bypass grafting (CABG) had a lower rate of perioperative cardiac morbidity compared with patients with a similar extent of coronary disease who had not undergone revascularization. Several randomized trials have questioned the value of acute revascularization before noncardiac surgery, although the integrity of the Dutch Echocardiographic Cardiac Risk Evaluation (DECREASE) trials by the Poldermans group has been questioned and therefore were not used by the AHA/ACC Committee to make recommendations. In the Coronary Artery Revascularization Prophylaxis (CARP) trial, 500 patients were randomized to coronary revascularization versus medical therapy and followed for up to 6 years. Importantly, patients with left main disease, severe triple-vessel disease with depressed ejection fraction, and severe comorbidities were excluded. Two-thirds of the patients who underwent coronary revascularization had percutaneous coronary interventions (PCIs). There was no difference in either perioperative or long-term morbidity and mortality. The analysis of the nonrandomized patients in the CARP database demonstrated improved perioperative outcomes in the subset of patients with left main disease who underwent coronary revascularization. Therefore current high-quality evidence suggests that coronary revascularization before major noncardiac surgery is of limited or no benefit in stable patients and in those with only 1 to 2 risk factors; however, there may be benefit to CABG in patients with left main or severe triple-vessel disease. Guideline recommendations for preoperative evaluation and management of patients undergoing noncardiac surgery are summarized in Table 68.4.

10. What is the concern regarding surgery in patients with a previous percutaneous coronary interventions?

Patients who have previously undergone PCI have not been shown to have a significant difference in perioperative outcomes compared with case-matched controls. Importantly, the risk of thrombosis after PCI is high, and the hypercoagulable perioperative state increases the probability of this occurring. Multiple cohort studies and case reports have reported the occurrence of acute thrombosis and perioperative MI at the site of coronary stents. In patients with bare metal stents, this most commonly occurs in patients who have undergone noncardiac surgery within 30 days. In patients with first-generation drug-eluting stents, the higher rates of acute thrombosis were initially seen for at least 1 year, and there were data to suggest it continues after this period. More recent data with newer generation drug-eluting stents have suggested that the period of highest risk has shortened to between 3 and 6 months. The current recommendation is to delay elective surgery for at least 14 days after balloon angioplasty (without stenting). The 2016 Update on Dual Antiplatelet Therapy recommends delaying at least 30 days after placement of bare metal stents and until 6 months after placement of drug-eluting stents. Importantly, elective noncardiac surgery after drug-eluting stent implantation in patients for whom P_2Y_{12} inhibitor therapy will need to be discontinued may be considered after 3 months if the risk of further delay of surgery on DAPT is greater than the expected risks of stent thrombosis.

11. How should antiplatelet agents be managed in the perioperative period?

The 2016 ACC/AHA Guideline Focused Update on Duration of Dual Antiplatelet Therapy advocates continuing aspirin in all patients who have had a previous PCI. In patients currently taking a $P2Y_{12}$ inhibitor, particularly those within 30 days of placement of a bare metal stent or 6 months for drug-eluting stents, the agent should either be continued or discontinued for a short period, if possible, and restarted as quickly as possible in the postoperative period. As noted previously, the $P2Y_{12}$ inhibitor may be discontinued after 3 months in certain high-risk situations. In patients who require a brief discontinuation of the $P2Y_{12}$ inhibitor, some authors suggest performing surgery approximately 5 days after discontinuation, given the theoretical risks of increased thrombotic tendency given longer periods. The timing of elective noncardiac surgery in patients treated with PCI and Dual anti-platelet therapy (DAPT) is summarized in Fig. 68.2, based on the 2016 ACC/AHA Guideline Focused Update on Duration of DAPT in patients with coronary artery disease (CAD).

12. How should beta-blockers be managed in the perioperative period?

Based on cohort studies and consensus opinion, patients who are receiving chronic beta-blocker therapy at the time of surgery should be continued on these agents to avoid the risk of beta-blocker withdrawal, which is associated with tachycardia and an increased incidence of perioperative MI. Currently, controversy exists regarding the acute administration of beta-blocker therapy for those patients at high risk of perioperative event but not currently taking these agents. The strongest evidence in support of acute beta-blocker administration are the DECREASE trials and subsequent cohort studies from the Erasmus group, but the Guideline Committee decided that no recommendation can be based solely on these results. In the Perioperative Ischemic Evaluation (POISE) study, 8351 patients were randomized to high-dose metoprolol succinate, a long-acting agent, compared with placebo. Although nonfatal perioperative MIs were reduced, the incidence of death and stroke was significantly increased and was associated with higher rates of hypotension. Therefore initiating high-dose beta-blocker therapy in the perioperative period without titration to heart rate and blood pressure could lead to greater harm than benefit and should not be considered, as demonstrated by a systematic review completed as part of the guideline process. However, heart rate control remains a critical approach to reducing perioperative cardiac morbidity, and initial treatment should focus on

Table 68.4. Summary of Recommendations for the Preoperative Evaluation of Patients Undergoing Noncardiac Surgery

RECOMMENDATIONS	COR	LOE
The 12-lead ECG		B
Preoperative resting 12-lead ECG is reasonable for patients with known coronary heart disease or other significant structural heart disease, except for low-risk surgery	IIa	
Preoperative resting 12-lead ECG may be considered for asymptomatic patients, except for low-risk surgery	IIb	B
Routine preoperative resting 12-lead ECG is not useful for asymptomatic patients undergoing low-risk surgical procedures	III: No Benefit	B
Assessment of LV function		C
It is reasonable for patients with dyspnea of unknown origin to undergo preoperative evaluation of LV function	IIa	C
It is reasonable for patients with HF with worsening dyspnea or other change in clinical status to undergo preoperative evaluation of LV function	IIa	C B
Reassessment of LV function in clinically stable patients may be considered	IIb	
Routine preoperative evaluation of LV function is not recommended	III: No Benefit	
Exercise stress testing for myocardial ischemia and functional capacity		
For patients with elevated risk and excellent functional capacity, it is reasonable to forgo further exercise testing and proceed to surgery	IIa	B B
For patients with elevated risk and unknown functional capacity, it may be reasonable to perform exercise testing to assess for functional capacity if it will change management	IIb	B
For patients with elevated risk and moderate to good functional capacity, it may be reasonable to forgo further exercise testing and proceed to surgery	IIb	C
For patients with elevated risk and poor or unknown functional capacity, it may be reasonable to perform exercise testing with cardiac imaging to assess for myocardial ischemia	IIb	B
Routine screening with noninvasive stress testing is not useful for low-risk noncardiac surgery	III: No Benefit	
Cardiopulmonary exercise testing		B
Cardiopulmonary exercise testing may be considered for patients undergoing elevated risk procedures	IIb	
Noninvasive pharmacologic stress test before noncardiac surgery		
It is reasonable for patients at elevated risk for noncardiac surgery with poor functional capacity to undergo either DSE or MPI if it will change management	IIa	B
Routine screening with noninvasive stress testing is not useful for low-risk noncardiac surgery	III: No Benefit	B
Preoperative coronary angiography		C
Routine preoperative coronary angiography is not recommended	III: No Benefit	

COR, Class of recommendation; *DSE*, dobutamine stress echocardiogram; *ECG*, electrocardiogram; *HF*, heart failure; *LOE*, level of evidence; *LV*, left ventricular; *MPI*, myocardial perfusion imaging.

Reproduced from Fleisher, L. A., Fleischmann, K. E., Auerbach, A. D., Barnason, S. A., Beckman, J. A., Bozkurt, B., et al. (2014). 2014 ACC/AHA guideline on perioperative cardiovascular evaluation and management of patients undergoing noncardiac surgery: a report of the American College of Cardiology/American Heart Association Task Force on Practice Guidelines. Journal of the American College of Cardiology, *64, e77–e137.*

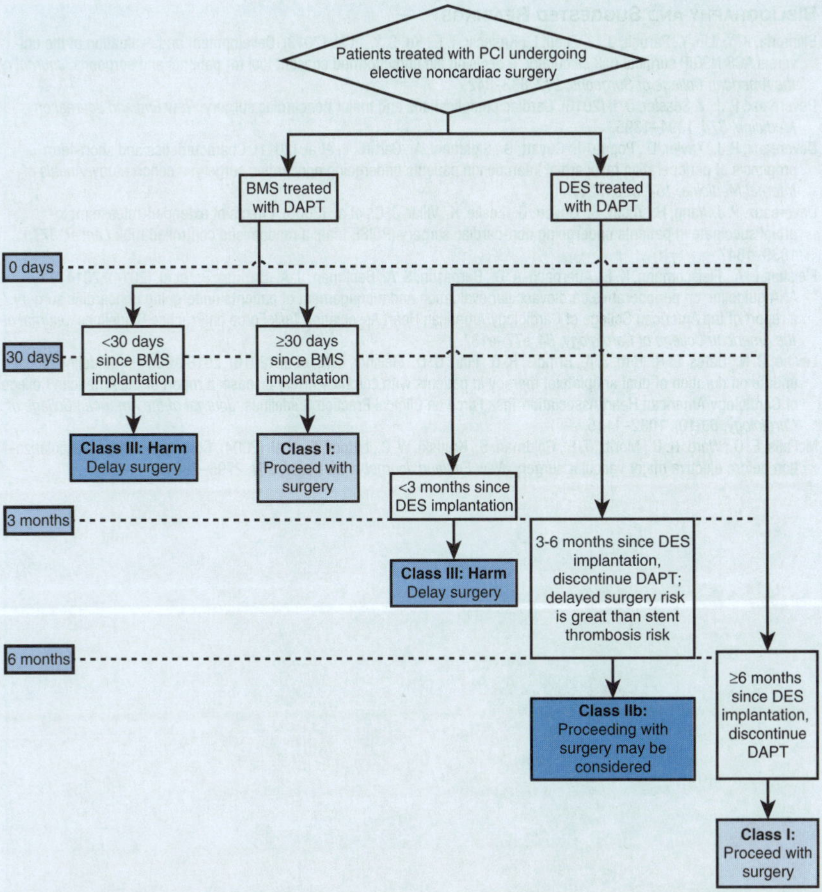

Fig. 68.2. Treatment algorithm for the timing of elective noncardiac surgery in patients with coronary stents. *BMS*, Bare metal stent; *DAPT*, dual antiplatelet therapy; *DES*, drug-eluting stent; *PCI*, percutaneous coronary intervention. *(Reproduced from Levine, G. N., Bates, E. R., Bittl, J. A., Brindis, R. G., Fihn, S. D., Fleisher, L. A., et al. [2016]. 2016 ACC/AHA guideline focused update on duration of dual antiplatelet therapy in patients with coronary artery disease: a report of the American College of Cardiology/American Heart Association Task Force on Clinical Practice Guidelines.* Journal of the American College of Cardiology, 68*[10], 1082–1115.)*

treating the cause of tachycardia, including pain management, after which careful titration of beta-blockers is appropriate. In patients who should be taking beta-blockers independent of noncardiac surgery for underlying coronary artery disease, initiation and titration a week or more in advance has been advocated based upon data by some authors, but what the safest protocol is remains controversial.

13. How should statins be managed in the perioperative period?

Traditionally, there was concern that continuation of statins in the perioperative period could lead to an increased incidence of rhabdomyolysis, and most clinicians discontinued these agents before surgery. Evidence has accumulated that statin therapy is protective and that withdrawal is harmful. There are randomized data to suggest that starting statin therapy at least 7 days in advance in high-risk patients is associated with improved outcome. In the 2014 Perioperative Guidelines, the committee advocated continuing statins in all patients currently taking these agents.

Bibliography and Suggested Readings

Bilimoria, K. Y., Liu, Y., Paruch, J. L., Zhou, L., Kmiecik, T. E., Ko, C. Y., et al. (2013). Development and evaluation of the universal ACS NSQIP surgical risk calculator: a decision aid and informed consent tool for patients and surgeons. *Journal of the American College of Surgeons, 217*, 833–842.

Devereaux, P. J., & Sessler, D. I. (2016). Cardiac complications and major noncardiac surgery. *New England Journal of Medicine, 374*, 1394–1395.

Devereaux, P. J., Xavier, D., Pogue, J., Guyatt, G., Sigamani, A., Garutti, I., et al. (2011). Characteristics and short-term prognosis of perioperative myocardial infarction in patients undergoing noncardiac surgery: a cohort study. *Annals of Internal Medicine, 154*, 523–528.

Devereaux, P. J., Yang, H., Yusuf, S., Guyatt, G., Leslie, K., Villar, J. C., et al. (2008). Effects of extended-release metoprolol succinate in patients undergoing non-cardiac surgery (POISE trial): a randomised controlled trial. *Lancet, 371*, 1839–1847.

Fleisher, L. A., Fleischmann, K. E., Auerbach, A. D., Barnason, S. A., Beckman, J. A., Bozkurt, B., et al. (2014). 2014 ACC/AHA guideline on perioperative cardiovascular evaluation and management of patients undergoing noncardiac surgery: a report of the American College of Cardiology/American Heart Association Task Force on Practice Guidelines. *Journal of the American College of Cardiology, 64*, e77–e137.

Levine, G. N., Bates, E. R., Bittl, J. A., Brindis, R. G., Fihn, S. D., Fleisher, L. A., et al. (2016). 2016 ACC/AHA guideline focused update on duration of dual antiplatelet therapy in patients with coronary artery disease: a report of the American College of Cardiology/American Heart Association Task Force on Clinical Practice Guidelines. *Journal of the American College of Cardiology, 68*(10), 1082–1115.

McFalls, E. O., Ward, H. B., Moritz, T. E., Goldman, S., Krupski, W. C., Littooy, F., et al. (2004). Coronary-artery revascularization before elective major vascular surgery. *New England Journal of Medicine, 351*, 2795–2804.

PULMONARY HYPERTENSION

Lavannya M. Pandit, Zeenat Safdar

CHAPTER 69

1. **What are the definitions of pulmonary hypertension and pulmonary arterial hypertension?**
   At the Fifth World Symposium on Pulmonary Hypertension held in Nice, France, in 2013, a consensus expert panel reestablished the definition of pulmonary hypertension (PH) as a mean pulmonary arterial pressure of ≥25 mm Hg or more as measured during invasive hemodynamic testing. The exercise and pulmonary vascular resistance criteria were removed from this updated definition owing to the poor availability of evidence. The subgroup of PH known as pulmonary arterial hypertension (PAH) is a clinical condition characterized by a mean pulmonary arterial pressure of 25 mm Hg or more and the presence of precapillary PH (pulmonary arterial occlusion pressure of 15 mm Hg or less) and a pulmonary vascular resistance >3 Wood units, in the absence of other causes of precapillary PH, such as PH due to lung diseases, chronic thromboembolic PH, or other rare diseases (Table 69.1).

2. **How and why is pulmonary hypertension classified?**
   The concept supporting the most recent 2013 classification is to group patients with PH with similar pathologic findings, hemodynamic profiles, and management. The five different categories in the updated classification for PH, derived from the last world symposium, are presented in Table 69.2. PH is classified as (PAH, group 1), PH owing to left heart disease (group 2), PH owing to lung diseases and/or hypoxia (group 3), chronic thromboembolic pulmonary hypertension (CTEPH) (group 4), and PH with unclear multifactorial mechanisms (group 5).

3. **How do patients with pulmonary hypertension present?**
   Because the earliest symptoms in patients with PH are manifest with activity, PH can have an insidious presentation but usually includes dyspnea on exertion. With the onset of right ventricular (RV) failure, characteristic complaints include lower extremity edema and/or abdominal distention or early satiety secondary to venous congestion. Angina is also common, likely reflecting demand ischemia from impaired coronary blood flow to a marked right ventricular hypertrophy (RVH). As cardiac output becomes fixed and eventually falls, patients may have episodes of syncope or near syncope. Patients with PH are also categorized in classes based on functional status and symptom presentation. Establishing a functional class in PH is important as this determines the type of therapy (Table 69.3).

Table 69.1. Hemodynamic Definition of Pulmonary Hypertension

PULMONARY HYPERTENSION TYPE	HEMODYNAMICS	GROUP(S)
Pulmonary hypertension	• Mean PAP >25 mm Hg	• *Groups 1-4*
Precapillary pulmonary hypertension	• Mean PAP >25 mm Hg • PCWP <15 mm Hg • Cardiac output normal or reduced	• *Group 1—PAH* • *Group 3—PH due to lung disease* • *Group 4—CTEPH* • *Group 5—PH multifactorial etiology*
Postcapillary pulmonary hypertension	• Mean PAP >25 mm Hg • PCWP >15 mm Hg • Cardiac output normal or reduced/increased	• *Group 2—PH due to left heart disease (PH-LHD)*

CTEPH, Chronic thromboembolic pulmonary hypertension; *PAH*, pulmonary arterial hypertension; *PAP*, pulmonary artery pressure; *PCWP*, pulmonary capillary wedge pressure; *PH*, pulmonary hypertension; *PH-LHD*, pulmonary hypertension-left sided heart disease.

Table 69.2. Updated Classification of Pulmonary Hypertension (Nice, 2013)

Group 1—Pulmonary Arterial Hypertension
1.1 Idiopathic PAH
1.2 Heritable—BMPR2, Alk1, ENG, SMAD9, CAV1, KCNK3, unknown
1.3 Drug- and toxin-induced
1.4 PAH associated with
  Collagen vascular disease
  Congenital heart disease
  HIV
  Schistosomiasis
  Portal hypertension
1″ Persistent pulmonary hypertension of newborn
1′ Pulmonary veno-occlusive disease and/or pulmonary capillary hemangiomatosis

Group 2—Pulmonary Hypertension Due to Left Heart Disease
2.1 Systolic dysfunction
2.2 Diastolic dysfunction
2.3, 4 Valvular disease, congenital/acquired left ventricular outflow tract obstruction and congenital cardiomyopathies

Group 3—Pulmonary Hypertension Due to Lung Disease and/or Hypoxemia
3.1 Chronic obstructive pulmonary disease
3.2 Interstitial lung disease
3.3 Other pulmonary disease with mixed restrictive and obstructive pattern
3.4 Sleep-disordered breathing
3.5 Alveolar hypoventilation disorders
3.6 Chronic exposure to high altitude
3.7 Developmental abnormalities

Group 4—Chronic Thromboembolic Pulmonary Hypertension (CTEPH)

Group 5—Pulmonary Hypertension with Unclear Multifactorial Mechanisms
5.1 Hematological disorders: myeloproliferative disorders, chronic hemolytic anemia, splenectomy
5.2 Systemic disorders: sarcoidosis, pulmonary Langerhans cell histiocytosis, lymphangioleiomyomatosis, neurofibromatosis, vasculitis
5.3 Metabolic disorders: glycogen storage disease, Gaucher disease, thyroid disorders
5.4 Others: tumoral obstruction, fibrosing mediastinitis, chronic renal failure requiring dialysis

BMPR, Bone morphogenic protein receptor type II; *CAV1*, caveolin-1; *CTEPH*, chronic thromboembolic pulmonary hypertension; *ENG*, endoglin; *HIV*, human immunodeficiency virus; *PAH*, pulmonary arterial hypertension.

Table 69.3. World Health Organization Classification of Functional Status of Patients with Pulmonary Hypertension

CLASS	DESCRIPTION
I	Patients with PH but without resulting limitation of physical activity. Ordinary physical activity does not cause undue dyspnea or fatigue, chest pain, or near syncope.
II	Patients with PH resulting in slight limitation of physical activity. They are comfortable at rest. Ordinary physical activity causes undue dyspnea or fatigue, chest pain, or near syncope.
III	Patients with PH resulting in marked limitation of physical activity. They are comfortable at rest. Less than ordinary activity causes undue dyspnea or fatigue, chest pain, or near syncope.
IV	Patients with PH with inability to carry out any physical activity without symptoms. These patients manifest signs of right-sided heart failure. Dyspnea or fatigue may be present even at rest. Discomfort is increased by any physical activity.

PH, Pulmonary hypertension.
Modified from Rubin, L. J. (2004). Diagnosis and management of pulmonary arterial hypertension: ACCP evidence-based clinical practice guidelines. Chest, 126, 7S–10S.

4. How is pulmonary hypertension diagnosed?

Right heart catheterization (RHC) remains the gold standard for diagnosing PH, assessing disease severity, and determining prognosis and response to therapy. The most critical aspects of RHC are that it must be performed appropriately and the data are interpreted accurately. Since end-expiratory intrathoracic pressure most closely correlates with atmospheric pressure, it is important that all RV, pulmonary artery (PA), PA occlusion pressure (PAOP), and left ventricular (LV) pressures be measured at end expiration (particularly in obese patients and patients with intrinsic lung disease, in whom there can be significant variation between inspiration and end-expiratory vascular pressures). Importantly, the current drugs approved for PH (see Question 12) are generally approved only for group 1 PAH or group 4 PH. Thus establishing a diagnosis of PH through RHC and classifying the type of PH are critical prior to initiating any specific PH therapy.

5. What is considered a favorable response to acutely administered vasodilators?

Prior to the initiation of advanced therapy at the time of RHC, it is recommended that patients with group 1 PAH undergo acute vasoreactivity testing with a vasodilator. Vasoreactivity testing is essential in idiopathic PAH, heritable PAH, and anorexigen-induced PAH, since these are the groups of patients most likely to respond. Other PH patients can undergo vasoreactivity testing on a case-by-case basis. Vasoreactivity testing facilitates agent selection by identifying those who may respond to calcium channel blockers (CCBs), which are less expensive and have fewer side effects than other forms of advanced therapy. A positive vasodilator response is defined as a fall in mean PA pressure of at least 10 mm Hg to 40 mm Hg or less with an increase or unchanged cardiac output. Approximately 6% to 10% of PAH patients will have an acute positive response; however, only half of these patients will have a sustained response to CCBs. The vasodilator agents used to determine vasoreactivity include intravenous epoprostenol, adenosine, and inhaled nitric oxide (NO).

6. What population group is most commonly affected by pulmonary arterial hypertension?

Although PAH occurs in both genders and virtually all age groups, it has a tendency to affect females in particular. Considerable changes in the PAH phenotype with regard to age, gender, comorbidities, and survival have been observed over time. Although the mean age of patients with IPAH in the first registry, created in 1981 (US-National Institutes of Health), was 36 ± 15 years, PH is now more frequently diagnosed in elderly patients, resulting in a mean age at diagnosis between 50 ± 14 and 65 ± 15 years in current registries. Furthermore, female predominance is quite variable among registries and may not be present in elderly patients. A potential explanation for the change in phenotype may be the increased awareness of PH in the modern management era as more effective therapies have become available.

According to 4 separate registries (Registry to Evaluate Early And Long-term PAH Disease (US-REVEAL), Pulmonary Hypertension Connection (US-PHC), French, and UK), factors associated with increased mortality from PH included (1) male gender, particularly those greater than 65 years of age, (2) hereditary PAH (HPAH), (3) higher PVR (>32 Wood units), higher mean right atrial pressures, (4) associated portopulmonary hypertension, (5) New York Heart Association (NYHA) or World Health Organization (WHO) functional class IV, and (6) elevated B-type natriuretic peptide (BNP) or NT-proBNP levels (Table 69.4).

7. Is pulmonary hypertension a genetic disease?

Between 6% and 16% of patients with PAH have HPAH, a familial disease transmitted in an autosomal dominant manner. Most heritable PAH (75%) is caused by a pathogenic variant in *BMPR2*; pathogenic variants in other genes (i.e., *ACVRL1, KCNK3, CAV1, SMAD9, BMPR1B*) are considerably less common (1% to 3%). HPAH has identical symptoms, signs, and histology as PAH of unknown cause. The time from onset of symptoms to diagnosis may be shorter in individuals with heritable PAH, possibly because of familial awareness of the disease. Owing to incomplete penetrance, most patients with an HPAH-associated genetic mutation never develop the disease. A subject with a mutation has a 10% to 20% estimated lifetime risk of acquiring HPAH. Genetic testing for known mutations in PAH-associated autosomal dominant genes is available in North America and Europe for the *BMPR2, ALK1, ENG, SMAD9, CAV1*, and *KCNK3* genes.

8. What should the clinical evaluation for possible pulmonary hypertension include?

Evaluation should begin with a thorough history and physical examination. In addition, travel to or residence in an area endemic for schistosomiasis should be considered. All patients should receive a basic initial screening evaluation consisting of collagen vascular disease serologic testing, human immunodeficiency

Table 69.4. Multivariate Predictors of Survival in Pulmonary Hypertension

CATEGORY	INCREASE RISK	DECREASE RISK
Demographics	• Gender (male) and age interaction (>65 years) • Age • Male gender Etiology: CTD, PoPH, HPAH, PVOD	—
Functional capacity	• Higher NYHA/WHO class • Lower 6MWD	• Lower NYHA/WHO class Higher 6MWD
Laboratory and biomarkers	• Higher BNP or NT-proBNP Higher creatinine	• Lower BNP or NT-proBNP
Imaging	• Echo: Pericardial effusion	—
Lung function studies	• Lower predicted DLCO	• Higher predicted DLCO
Hemodynamics	• Higher mRAP • Lower CO or CI Higher PVR or PVRI	• Higher CO or CI

BNP, B-type natriuretic peptide; *CI*, cardiac index; *CO*, cardiac output; *DLCO*, diffusing capacity of the lung for carbon monoxide; *Echo*, echocardiography; *HPAH*, heritable pulmonary arterial hypertension; *mRAP*, mean right atrial pressure; *NT-proBNP*, N-terminal pro–B-type natriuretic peptide; *NYHA*, New York Heart Association; *PoPH*, portopulmonary hypertension; *PVOD*, portopulmonary hypertension; *PVR*, pulmonary vascular resistance; *PVRI*, pulmonary vascular resistance index; *6MWD*, 6-minute walk distance.

Adapted from McGoon, M. D., Benza, R. L., Escribano-Subias, P., Jiang, X., Miller, D. P., Peacock, A. J., et al. (2013). Pulmonary arterial hypertension: epidemiology and registries. Journal of the American College of Cardiology, *62(25 Suppl.), D51–D59.*

virus (HIV) testing, hepatitis panel, chest radiograph, pulmonary function testing, ventilation-perfusion (V/Q) scan to assess for chronic thromboembolic pulmonary disease, hypercoagulable workup (if indicated), electrocardiogram, and echocardiogram. Conditions and symptoms associated with PH are listed in Table 69.5. The diagnostic approach to a patient with suspected PH is summarized in Fig. 69.1.

9. What treatment for pulmonary hypertension is deemed secondary to left-sided heart disease (group 2 PH)?

Left heart disease is the most common cause of PH and occurs in patients with heart failure with reduced ejection fraction (HFrEF), heart failure with preserved ejection fraction (HFpEF), and valvular heart disease (Fig. 69.2). The presence of PH in patients with left heart disease (PH-LHD) is associated with reduced exercise tolerance and shorter survival, especially following heart transplantation. The usual hemodynamic findings in a patient with PH due to left heart disease are mPAP at 25 mm Hg or above in combination with elevated left heart filling pressures, defined as a pulmonary artery wedge pressure (PAWP) greater than 15 mm Hg or LV end-diastolic pressure (LVEDP) greater than 15 mm Hg.

The first postulated event in the development of PH in patients with left-sided heart disease is increasing left heart filling pressures and pulmonary venous hypertension. Even with preserved LV systolic function, diastolic filling abnormalities can result in increased pulmonary arterial pressures. Additionally, elevated LV filling pressures will reduce compliance of the pulmonary vasculature and increase RV afterload by enhancing PA wave reflections. Recently the Fifth World Symposium Task Force on PH and Left Heart Disease published a proposal for the hemodynamic definition, classification, and nomenclature for PH and left heart disease. These guidelines recommend using the descriptive term *isolated post-capillary PH* (Ipc-PH) for PH caused by the transmission of elevated left heart filling pressures due to pulmonary venous hypertension or "passive" PH. In other patients the elevated pulmonary pressures cannot be fully accounted for by passive transmission of elevated left heart pressures, such that the elevated PA pressures result in part due to intrinsic remodeling of the pulmonary arterioles. It is important to differentiate this *combined postcapillary and precapillary PH* (Cpc-PH) from *Ipc-PH*, since patients with *Cpc-PH* have more severe hemodynamic impairment and a worse prognosis. *Cpc-PH* replaces the previous *out-of-proportion PH* terminology.

In patients presenting with PH-LHD, there is currently no role for treatment with PAH-specific therapies and, with few exceptions, they should not be administered because they are costly, lack

Table 69.5. Conditions and Symptoms/Presentations Associated with Pulmonary Hypertension

CONDITION	SYMPTOMS AND PRESENTATION
Heart failure (systolic/diastolic)	Dyspnea, exercise intolerance, angina, prior myocardial infarction, systemic hypertension, valvular heart disease
Obstructive sleep apnea	Snoring, excessive somnolence, witnessed apneic episodes
Chronic Lung Diseases • Chronic obstructive pulmonary disease • Interstitial lung disease	Worsening dyspnea and hypoxemia, dry cough, occupational exposures, reduced DLCO on pulmonary function testing
Autoimmune Diseases • Systemic sclerosis (especially CREST syndrome) • Mixed connective tissue disease • Systemic lupus erythematosus • Rheumatoid arthritis • Dermatomyositis and polymyositis • Sjögren syndrome	History of skin changes, arthritis, gastrointestinal problems, and renal disease
Chronic thromboembolic disease	Prior history of PE, deep venous thrombosis and genetic or acquired hypercoagulable conditions
Drug history	Illicit drug abuse, prior use of anorexiants and herbal products
Chronic liver disease	Jaundice, ascites, chronic viral hepatitis, and alcohol abuse; symptoms of portal hypertension including abdominal distention and gastrointestinal bleed
HIV infection	High-risk sexual behavior, intravenous drug abuse and needle sharing
Congenital diseases	History of congenital heart disease and intracardiac shunts, family history of sickle cell disease

CREST, Calcinosis, Raynaud phenomenon, esophageal dysmotility, sclerodactyly, and telangiectasia; *DLCO*, diffusing capacity of the lung for carbon monoxide; *HIV*, human immunodeficiency virus; *PE*, pulmonary embolism.

efficacy, and in some cases are known to increase morbidity and mortality. Treatment for PH-LHD centers around optimization of heart failure therapy and referral for heart transplantation as needed.

10. What treatment for pulmonary hypertension is deemed secondary to lung disease and/or alveolar hypoxia (group 3 PH)?

PH in the setting of parenchymal lung disease and conditions associated with chronic hypoxemia is commonly encountered in clinical practice and is known to adversely affect patients' function and mortality. Diagnosis of this subgroup of PH has evolved but still requires RHC for confirmation. The primary treatment goal of group 3 PH is optimization of the underlying lung or hypoxemia-associated condition prior to consideration of pharmacologic therapy. Limited published data have shown minor benefits in symptom relief from treating group 3 PH with vasodilator therapy; however, the potential for worsening V/Q matching exists in these cases, and any such therapy must be used with caution. Although hypoxic pulmonary vasoconstriction is postulated to be the mechanism behind group 3 PH, there is little knowledge of the mechanism in this disease, and it is unclear why some hypoxemic patients are affected more than others. At this time lung transplantation is the only potential treatment option.

11. Is surgical therapy now an option for patients with pulmonary hypertension secondary to chronic recurrent thromboembolism (group 4 PH/CTEPH)?

A patient with confirmed PAH and a V/Q scan suggestive of CTEPH (group 4 PH) should undergo pulmonary angiography for accurate diagnosis and assessment of resectability of the thrombi, since

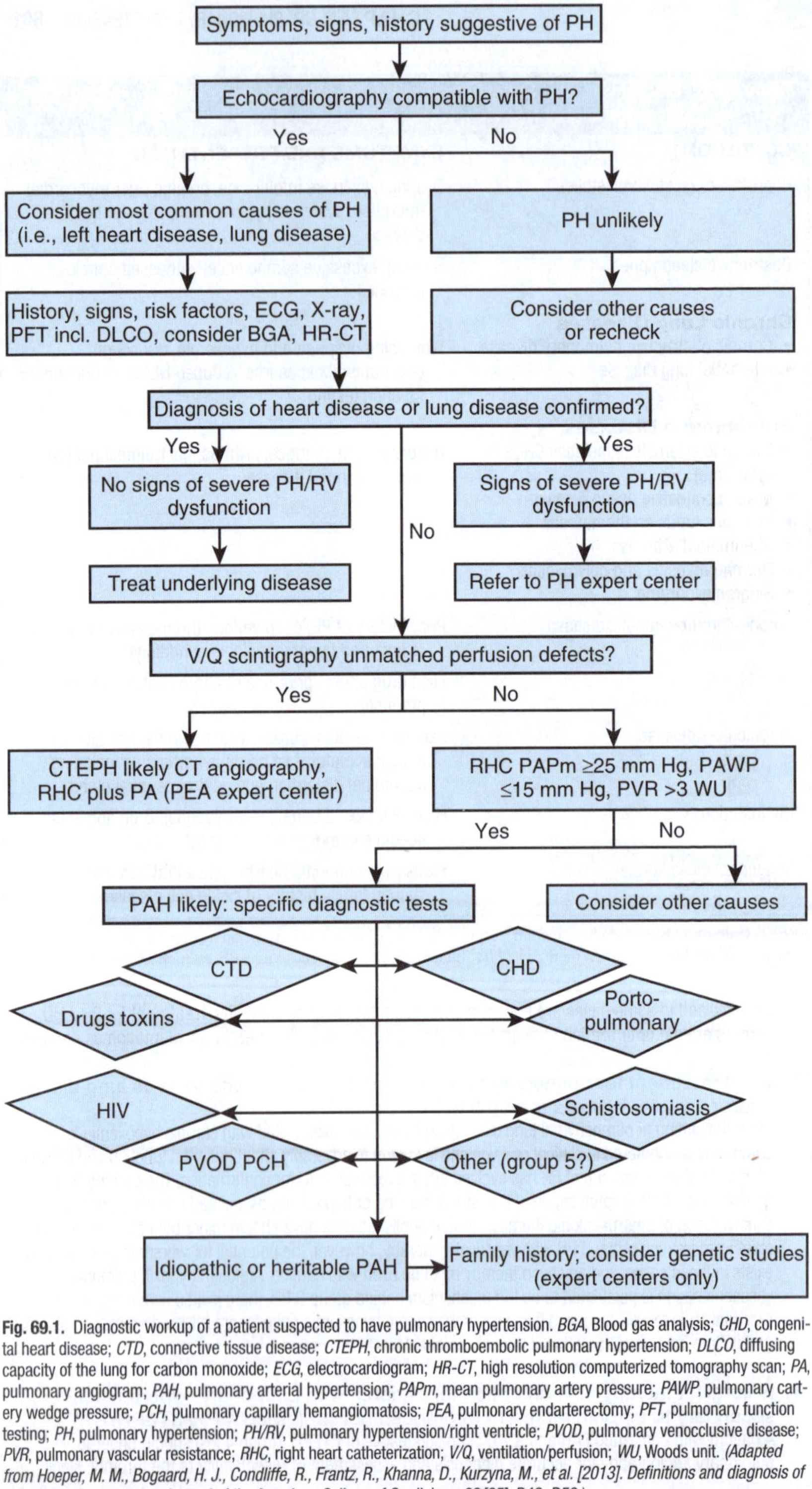

Fig. 69.1. Diagnostic workup of a patient suspected to have pulmonary hypertension. *BGA*, Blood gas analysis; *CHD*, congenital heart disease; *CTD*, connective tissue disease; *CTEPH*, chronic thromboembolic pulmonary hypertension; *DLCO*, diffusing capacity of the lung for carbon monoxide; *ECG*, electrocardiogram; *HR-CT*, high resolution computerized tomography scan; *PA*, pulmonary angiogram; *PAH*, pulmonary arterial hypertension; *PAPm*, mean pulmonary artery pressure; *PAWP*, pulmonary cartery wedge pressure; *PCH*, pulmonary capillary hemangiomatosis; *PEA*, pulmonary endarterectomy; *PFT*, pulmonary function testing; *PH*, pulmonary hypertension; *PH/RV*, pulmonary hypertension/right ventricle; *PVOD*, pulmonary venocclusive disease; *PVR*, pulmonary vascular resistance; *RHC*, right heart catheterization; *V/Q*, ventilation/perfusion; *WU*, Woods unit. *(Adapted from Hoeper, M. M., Bogaard, H. J., Condliffe, R., Frantz, R., Khanna, D., Kurzyna, M., et al. [2013]. Definitions and diagnosis of pulmonary hypertension.* Journal of the American College of Cardiology, 62*[25], D42–D50.)*

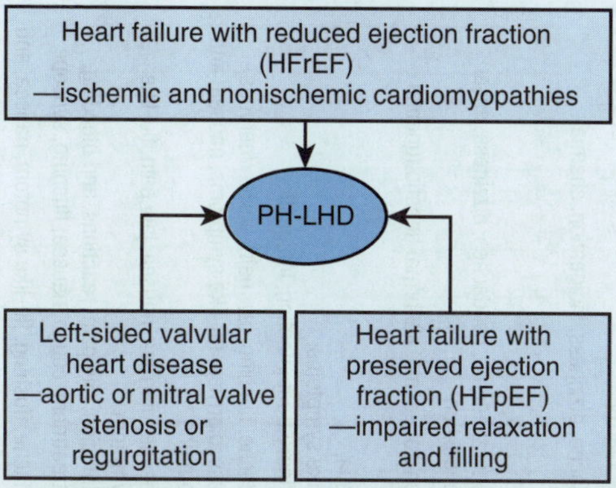

Fig. 69.2. Classification of group 2 PH or PH due to left heart disease (PH-LHD). *HFpEF*, Heart failure with preserved ejection fraction; *HFrEF*, heart failure with reduced ejection fraction. *(Adapted from Barnett, C. F., & Selby V. N. [2015]. Overview of WHO group 2 pulmonary hypertension due to left heart disease.* Advances in Pulmonary Hypertension, *14[2], 70–78.)*

pulmonary thromboendarterectomy is the only potentially curative therapy for group 4 PH/CTEPH. Operative mortality is low in most experienced centers, and both lifelong anticoagulation and inferior vena cava (IVC) filter placement are essential for such patients. The US Food and Drug Administration (FDA) recently approved the pulmonary vasodilator riociguat (see Question 12) as the first medical alternative for CTEPH patients who are not operative candidates or who have persistent PAH following pulmonary thromboendarterectomy. Riociguat can also be administered to patients as a bridge to surgery. Importantly, up to half of all patients with CTEPH do not have a history of pulmonary embolism (PE) or deep venous thromboembolism (DVT). In 2008, the World Council on Pulmonary Embolism reported that approximately 2% to 4% of people with PE develop CTEPH. Given that a large proportion of CTEPH patients have no history of PE or DVT, a diagnosis of CTEPH can be overlooked or not suspected.

12. What is considered conventional therapy for patients with pulmonary hypertension?

- Supplemental oxygen as needed to maintain an oxygen saturation of at least 91%
- Treatment of underlying conditions including obstructive sleep apnea, emphysema, heart failure, and autoimmune diseases
- Diuretics if the patient has clinically significant edema or ascites
- Anticoagulation in the absence of contraindications for some group 1 and all group 4 patients
- Digoxin, which is occasionally used to improve RV function
- Pulmonary vasodilators if indicated by RHC vasoreactivity testing

13. Are calcium channel blockers used in the treatment of pulmonary arterial hypertension?

CCBs are used only in patients with a documented vasodilator response at the time of a RHC. This comprises 6% of all PAH patients; of these, 50% turn out to be sustained responders. CCBs should not be used empirically without the demonstration of vasoreactivity. If patients have a favorable response to acutely administered vasodilators, this predicts a response to CCBs. The 1-, 3-, and 5-year survival in patients on CCBs was 94%, 94%, and 94%, respectively, as compared with 68%, 47%, and 38% of those classified as nonresponders.

14. What are the approved therapies to treat pulmonary arterial hypertension?

Therapy with approved PAH drugs (Table 69.6) must be initiated in PAH patients who are not vasoreactive or are vasoreactive but not responding appropriately to CCBs. Currently FDA-approved therapies target the four identified pathways involved in the pathogenesis of PAH:

- **Endothelin receptor antagonist pathway.** Endothelin-1, a potent vasoconstrictor, exerts its effects through the activation of ET_A and ET_B receptors. Differential activation of ET_A and ET_B receptors leads to the vasoconstrictive and vascular proliferative actions of endothelin-1. Bosentan and macitentan are dual endothelin receptor blockers, whereas ambrisentan is an ET_A blocker.

Table 69.6. FDA approved drugs to treat pulmonary arterial hypertension

CLASS	MODE OF ACTION	INDIVIDUAL DRUGS	ROUTE OF ADMINISTRATION	SIDE EFFECTS
PDE-5 inhibitors	Blocks degradation of cGMP	Tadalafil	Oral	Headache, myalgia, back/extremity pain, flushing, dyspepsia, diarrhea nausea,
		Sildenafil	Oral	Headache, myalgia, back pain, flushing, dyspepsia, diarrhea
Guanylate Cyclase Stimulants	stimulate the sGC receptor to mimic the action of NO	Riociguat	Oral	headache, dizziness, indigestion, anemia
Endothelin Receptor Antangonists	Competitive antagonists of endothelin receptor	Ambrisentan	Oral	Peripheral edema, headaches, dizziness, nasal congestion
		Bosentan	Oral	Peripheral edema, abnormal hepatic function
		*Macitentan	Oral	Anemia, Flu-like symptoms, urinary tract infection, indigestion
Prostacyclins	Enhances action of prostacyclins through exogenous increase or binding to receptor	*Epoprostenol	I.V.	headache, flushing, jaw pain, anxiety/nervousness, diarrhea, flu-like symptoms, nausea, and vomiting
		Treprostinil	I.V., S.C., INH	Headache, diarrhea, nausea, jaw pain, flu-like symptom S.C infusion: site pain, reactions, and bleeding. INH treatment: cough, nausea, flushing, syncope
		Iloprost	INH	headache, flushing, flu-like symptom, nausea, and vomiting, jaw muscle spasm, cough, tongue pain, and syncope
		Selexipag *(receptor agonist)*	Oral	headache,diarrhea, jaw pain, nausea, muscle pain, flushing

INH, inhalation treatment; *I.V.*, intravenous infusion; *NO*, nitric oxide; *PDE-5*, phosphodiesterase 5; *S.C.*, subcutaneous infusion; *sGC*, soluble guanylate cyclase; * morbidity and mortality as primary endpoint in randomized controlled study or reduction in all-cause mortality (prospectively defined).

- **Prostacyclin pathway.** Prostacyclin is the main product of arachidonic acid in the vascular endothelium. It promotes pulmonary vascular relaxation, inhibits the growth of smooth muscle cells, and is a powerful inhibitor of platelet aggregation. Epoprostenol, treprostinil, iloprost, and selexipag (a selective nonprostanoid prostacyclin receptor agonist) are the current FDA-approved drugs utilizing the prostacyclin pathway.
- **Phosphodiesterase-5 (PDE-5) inhibitor pathway.** PDE-5 inhibitors block the breakdown of cyclic guanosine monophosphate (cGMP) in the vascular endothelium, resulting in increased activity of endogenous NO, which enhances pulmonary vasodilation. Sildenafil and tadalafil are the PDE-5 inhibitors approved in the United States for the treatment of PAH.
- **Guanylate cyclase stimulant pathway.** These stimulators of the NO receptor, termed *soluble guanylate cyclase* (sGC), have a dual mode of action. This class increases the sensitivity of sGC to endogenous NO, a pulmonary vasodilator, and also directly stimulates the receptor to mimic the action of NO. Riociguat is an oral sGC stimulant that has reported benefit in patients with inoperable and persistent CTEPH (group 4 PH).

15. What is the average survival for a patient with pulmonary arterial hypertension?

In general, survival in registry populations has improved as treatment options have increased. Data from the US-REVEAL registry suggest that current median survival is 7 years for patients with PAH, compared with 2.8 years for patients with primary PH in the previous US-NIH registry.

16. Is transplantation possible in patients with pulmonary arterial hypertension?

Yes. Double lung transplantation is an option in carefully selected patients, especially those who do not respond to aggressive PAH treatment. A combined heart-lung transplant is no longer believed to be required because the RV appears to recover function after lung transplantation. Occasionally heart-lung transplantation is required in patients with uncorrectable congenital heart defects, such as those who have Eisenmenger syndrome, or in those whom right ventricular recovery is less likely.

Bibliography, Suggested Readings, and Websites

Austin, E. D., & Loyd, J. E. (2014). The genetics of pulmonary arterial hypertension. *Circulation Research, 115*, 189–202.

Badesch, D. B., Raskob, G. E., Elliott, C. G., Krichman, A. M., Farber, H. W., Frost, A. E., et al. (2010). Pulmonary arterial hypertension: baseline characteristics from the REVEAL Registry. *Chest, 137*(2), 376–387.

Barnett, C., & Selby, V. N. (2015). Overview of WHO Group 2 pulmonary hypertension due to left heart disease. *Advances in Pulmonary Hypertension, 14*(2), 70–78.

Benza, R. L., Miller, D. P., Gomberg-Maitland, M., Frantz, R. P., Foreman, A. J., Coffey, C. S., et al. (2010). Predicting survival in pulmonary arterial hypertension: insights from the Registry to Evaluate Early and Long-Term Pulmonary Arterial Hypertension Disease Management (REVEAL). *Circulation, 122*(2), 164–172.

Cogswell, R., Kobashigawa, E., McGlothlin, D., Shaw, R., & De Marco, T. (2012). Validation of the Registry to Evaluate Early and Long-Term Pulmonary Arterial Hypertension Disease Management (REVEAL) pulmonary hypertension prediction model in a unique population and utility in the prediction of long-term survival. *Journal of Heart and Lung Transplantation, 31*(11), 1165–1170.

Fang, J. C., DeMarco, T., Givertz, M. M., Borlaug, B. A., Lewis, G. D., Rame, J. E., et al. (2012). World Health Organization Pulmonary Hypertension group 2: pulmonary hypertension due to left heart disease in the adult—a summary statement from the Pulmonary Hypertension Council of the International Society for Heart and Lung Transplantation. *Journal of Heart and Lung Transplantation, 31*(9), 913–933.

Galiè, N., & Simonneau, G. (2013). The Fifth World Symposium on Pulmonary Hypertension. *Journal of the American College of Cardiology, 62*(Suppl. 25), D1–D3.

Galiè, N., Hoeper, M. M., Humbert, M., Torbicki, A., Vachiery, J. L., Barbera, J. A., et al. (2009). Guidelines for the diagnosis and treatment of pulmonary hypertension: the Task Force for the Diagnosis and Treatment of Pulmonary Hypertension of the European Society of Cardiology (ESC) and the European Respiratory Society (ERS), endorsed by the International Society of Heart and Lung Transplantation (ISHLT). *European Heart Journal, 30*(20), 2493–2537.

Ghofrani, H. A., Galiè, N., Grimminger, F., Grünig, E., Humbert, M., Jing, Z. C., et al. (2013). Riociguat for the treatment of pulmonary arterial hypertension. *New England Journal of Medicine, 369*(4), 330–340.

Hoeper, M. M., Bogaard, H. J., Condliffe, R., Frantz, R., Khanna, D., Kurzyna, M., et al. (2013). Definitions and diagnosis of pulmonary hypertension. *Journal of the American College of Cardiology, 62*(25), D42–D50.

Humbert, M., Sitbon, O., Chaouat, A., Bertocchi, M., Habib, G., Gressin, V., et al. (2010). Survival in patients with idiopathic, familial, and anorexigen-associated pulmonary arterial hypertension in the modern management era. *Circulation, 122*(2), 156–163.

McGoon, M. D., Benza, R. L., Escribano-Subias, P., Jiang, X., Miller, D. P., Peacock, A. J., et al. (2013). Pulmonary arterial hypertension: epidemiology and registries. *Journal of the American College of Cardiology, 62*(Suppl. 25), D51–D59.

McGoon, M., Gutterman, M., Steen, V., Barst, R., McCrory, D. C., Fortin, T. A., et al. (2004). Screening, early detection, and diagnosis of pulmonary arterial hypertension: ACCP evidence-based clinical practice guidelines. *Chest, 126*, 14S–34S.

McLaughlin, V. V., Archer, S. L., Badesch, D. B., Barst, R. J., Farber, H. W., Lindner, J. R., et al. (2009). ACCF/AHA 2009 expert consensus document on pulmonary hypertension: a report of the American College of Cardiology Foundation Task Force on Expert Consensus Documents and the American Heart Association developed in collaboration with the American College of Chest Physicians; American Thoracic Society, Inc.; and the Pulmonary Hypertension Association. *Journal of the American College of Cardiology, 53*(17), 1573–1619.

Poor, H. D., Girgis, R., & Studer, S. M. (2012). World Health Organization group III pulmonary hypertension. *Progress in Cardiovascular Diseases, 55*(2), 119–127.

Pulido, T., Adzerikho, I., Channick, R. N., Delcroix, M., Galiè, N., Ghofrani, H. A., et al. (2013). Macitentan and morbidity and mortality in pulmonary arterial hypertension. *New England Journal of Medicine, 369*(9), 809–818.

Rubin, L. J., & Hopkins, W. (2016 Aug). Overview of Pulmonary Hypertension. http://www.utdol.com.

Simonneau, G., Gatzoulis, M. A., Adatia, I., Celermajer, D., Denton, C., Ghofrani, A., et al. (2013). Updated clinical classification of pulmonary hypertension. *Journal of the American College of Cardiology, 62*(Suppl. 25), D34–D41.

Simonneau, G., Robbins, I. M., Beghetti, M., Channick, R. N., Delcroix, M., Denton, C. P., et al. (2009). Updated clinical classification of pulmonary hypertension. *Journal of the American College of Cardiology, 54*(Suppl. 1), S43–S54.

Simonneau, G., Torbicki, A., Hoeper, M. M., Delcroix, M., Karlócai, K., Galiè, N., et al. (2012). Selexipag: an oral, selective prostacyclin receptor agonist for the treatment of pulmonary arterial hypertension. *European Respiratory Journal, 40*(4), 874–880.

Sitbon, O., Channick, R., Chin, K. M., Frey, A., Gaine, S., Galiè, N., et al. (2015). Selexipag for the treatment of pulmonary arterial hypertension. *New England Journal of Medicine, 373*, 2522–2533.

Sitbon, O., Humbert, M., Nunes, H., Parent, F., Garcia, G., Hervé, P., et al. (2002). Long-term intravenous epoprostenol infusion in primary pulmonary hypertension: prognostic factors and survival. *Journal of the American College of Cardiology, 40*, 2522–2533.

Souza, R., & Jardim, C. (2009). Trends in pulmonary arterial hypertension. *European Respiratory Review, 18*(111), 7–12.

Taichman, D. B., Ornelas, J., Chung, L., Klinger, J. R., Lewis, S., Mandel, J., et al. (2014). Pharmacologic therapy for pulmonary arterial hypertension in adults: CHEST guideline and expert panel report. *Chest, 146*(2), 449–475.

Tapson, V. F., Torres, F., Kermeen, F., Keogh, A. M., Allen, R. P., Frantz, R. P., et al. (2012). Oral treprostinil for the treatment of pulmonary arterial hypertension in patients on background endothelin receptor antagonist and/or phosphodiesterase type 5 inhibitor therapy (the FREEDOM-C study): a randomized controlled trial. *Chest, 142*(6), 1383–1390.

Tedford, R. J., Hassoun, P. M., Mathai, S. C., Girgis, R. E., Russell, S. D., Thiemann, D. R., et al. (2012). Pulmonary capillary wedge pressure augments RV pulsatile loading. *Circulation, 125*(2), 289–297.

CHAPTER 70

SYNCOPE

Glenn N. Levine

1. What is the derivation of the word *syncope*?

According to text in the European Society of Cardiology (ESC) Guidelines on the Management of Syncope, the word *syncope* is derived from the Greek words *syn*, meaning "with," and the verb *kopto*, meaning "I cut" or "I interrupt."

2. What is the underlying mechanism causing syncope?

This mechanism is transient global cerebral hypoperfusion. Other conditions that do not cause transient global cerebral hypoperfusion can cause a transient loss of consciousness; some experts believe that these conditions should be referred to as *transient loss of consciousness* instead of syncope.

3. Cessation of cerebral blood flow of what duration causes syncope?

Cessation of cerebral blood flow for as short a period as 6 to 8 seconds can precipitate syncope.

4. What is the most common type of syncope in the general population?

Neurocardiogenic syncope is the most common type of syncope in the general population. This is also variably referred to in the literature as *vasovagal syncope, neurally mediated syncope*, and *vasodepressor syncope.*

5. What are the common causes of syncope?

- **Neurocardiogenic disturbance:** This is the most common cause of syncope in otherwise healthy persons, particularly younger persons. It is often precipitated by fear, anxiety, or other types of emotional distress. Its course is usually benign.
- **Orthostatic hypotension:** Orthostatic hypotension results from venous pooling and decreased cardiac output as well as a fall in blood pressure. It may be due to volume depletion, anemia, or acute bleeding, peripheral vasodilators (most notoriously the alpha-receptor blockers used to treat benign prostatic hypertrophy), or autonomic dysfunction (e.g., diabetic neuropathy, dysautonomia caused by central nervous system [CNS] disease).
- **Carotid sinus hypersensitivity:** This condition is suggested by syncope precipitated by neck movement or by tight collars or ties. The diagnosis is made by carotid sinus massage.
- **Tachyarrhythmias:** Ventricular tachycardia (VT) and torsades de pointes are the most ominous causes of syncope. In patients with a history of prior myocardial infarction (MI) or those with significantly depressed left ventricular (LV) ejection fraction (EF; >30% to 35%), the presumptive cause of syncope is VT until proven otherwise. Polymorphic VT and torsades de pointes are the presumptive causes of syncope in those with prolonged QT intervals because of drugs or congenital long QT syndrome and in those with Brugada syndrome (see Question 14). Supraventricular tachycardia (SVT) can produce presyncope but does not usually produce overt syncope.
- **Bradyarrhythmias:** Syncope may be caused by intermittent complete heart block. *Sick sinus syndrome* is a general term covering multiple disorders of the conduction system. *Tachy-brady syndrome* is the more appropriate term to describe patients with intermittent atrial fibrillation who, when the atrial fibrillation terminates, then have another or several more periods of asystole before normal sinus rhythm and ventricular depolarization resume.
- **Structural/Functional:** Aortic stenosis is the most common structural cause of syncope in older patients. The dynamic obstruction that occurs in hypertrophic cardiomyopathy (HCM) (see Chapter 24) is the most common cause of structurally/functionally mediated syncope in younger patients. Left atrial myxoma, causing functional mitral stenosis, is an extremely rare cause of syncope. Syncope can also occur with massive pulmonary embolism, which obstructs the pulmonary artery to such an extent that it compromises blood flow to the LV. The causes of syncope are summarized in Table 70.1.

Table 70.1. Causes of Syncope and Loss of Consciousness

Cardiac Syncope

1. Structural/functional
   - Aortic stenosis
   - HCM
   - Left atrial myxoma
   - Pulmonary embolism
2. Arrhythmic
   a. Bradyarrhythmia
      - Profound (sinus) bradycardia
      - Sick sinus syndrome/tachy-brady syndrome
      - Heart block
      - Pacemaker malfunction

   b. Tachyarrhythmia
      1. VT
         - Coronary artery disease/ischemia/MI
         - HCM
         - Dilated cardiomyopathy/depressed LV systolic function
         - Brugada syndrome
         - ARVD/C
      2. Torsades de pointes
         - Drug-induced QT prolongation
         - Congenital QT prolongation

Noncardiac Syncope

- Neurocardiogenic
- Carotid sinus hypersensitivity
- Situational (e.g., micturition, defecation, cough, swallowing)
- Orthostatic hypotension (volume depletion, anemia/bleeding, drugs, autonomic dysfunction)
- Subclavian steal
- Vertebrobasilar disease (very rarely severe bilateral carotid disease)

Nonsyncope "Loss of Consciousness"

- Seizures
- Hypoglycemia
- Hypoxemia
- Psychogenic

ARVD/C, Arrhythmogenic right ventricular dysplasia/cardiomyopathy; *HCM*, hypertrophic cardiomyopathy; *VT*, ventricular tachycardia.

6. **What are the most common causes of syncope in pediatric and young patients?**
   According to the scientific statement on syncope from the 2006 American Heart Association/American College of Cardiology (AHA/ACC) Foundation, the most common causes of syncope in pediatric and young patients are neurocardiogenic syncope, conversion reactions (psychiatric causes), and primary arrhythmic causes (e.g., long QT syndrome, Wolff-Parkinson-White syndrome). In contrast, elderly patients have a higher frequency of syncope caused by obstructions to cardiac output (e.g., aortic stenosis, pulmonary embolism) and by arrhythmias resulting from underlying heart disease.

7. **What is the most common cause of sudden cardiac death in young athletes?**
   HCM, followed by anomalous origin of a coronary artery. Other causes of sudden cardiac death in younger persons in general include long QT syndrome, Brugada syndrome, and arrhythmogenic right ventricular (RV) dysplasia/cardiomyopathy (ARVD/C), as well as pulmonary embolism.

8. **What are the important causes of ventricular tachyarrhythmias?**
   Important causes of ventricular tachyarrhythmias in patients with syncope include the following:
   - Coronary artery disease (CAD): Acute ischemia or myocardial infarction (MI) can cause VT. VT may also develop as a reentrant circuit around an old myocardial scar or ventricular aneurysm.

- Depressed left ventricular (LV) ejection fraction (EF): Whether due to CAD or nonischemic causes, cardiomyopathy with depressed ejection fraction (EF <30% to 35%) predisposes to VT.
- HCM: Patients with HCM are at increased risk of VT, particularly if there is a history of syncope, familial history of sudden cardiac death, or markedly thickened ventricular septum (>30 mm).
- Prolonged QT interval: The QT interval may be prolonged due to drugs or may be seen in congenital QT prolongation. A prolonged QT interval predisposes to torsades de pointes.
- Brugada syndrome: Discussed below, this condition predisposes to polymorphic VT.
- ARVD/C: A rare condition in which there is fatty and fibrotic infiltration of the RV.
- RV ventricular outflow tract (RVOT) VT: VT may originate from the RVOT. VT in this condition less commonly leads to death.

9. What is the approach to the patient with syncope?

The goals of the evaluation of patients with syncope are not only to identify the cause of syncope but also to determine if the cause is cardiac or noncardiac. Noncardiac causes of syncope generally have a relatively benign course (overall 1-year mortality rates of 0% to 12% and an approximately 0% mortality rate with neurally mediated syncope). Unexplained/undiagnosed causes have an intermediate 1-year mortality rate of 5% to 6%. Cardiac causes, in contrast, are associated with a 1-year mortality risk of 18.5% to 33%. Thus there is a premium on excluding a cardiac cause of syncope even if the exact cause of syncope cannot be determined.

A detailed history and physical examination, along with electrocardiogram (ECG) examination, can identify the presumptive cause of syncope in 40% to 50% of cases. Premonitory symptoms such as nausea or diaphoresis, especially in a younger person, or symptoms caused by anxiety, pain, or emotional distress, suggest neurocardiogenic syncope. Syncope during or immediately after urination, defecation, or certain other activities suggests situational syncope. Recent initiation of certain blood pressure–lowering medications, particularly alpha-receptor blockers (such as used to treat benign prostatic hypertrophy), raise suspicion for orthostatic hypotension, which can be confirmed on examination. A history of prior MI or depressed EF raises concern for VT. Cardiac systolic murmurs suggest aortic stenosis or HCM. Table 70.2 gives the factors on history, physical examination, and ECG that may suggest a specific cause for the patient's syncope. An algorithm for the approach to the patient with syncope is given in Fig. 70.1.

10. How does one properly test for orthostatic hypotension?

Recommendations vary, but according to the ESC Guidelines on the Management of Syncope, one first has the patient lie supine for 5 minutes. Blood pressure is then measured 3 minutes after the patient stands, with subsequent blood pressure measurements each minute thereafter if the blood pressure falls and continues to fall compared with supine values. Orthostatic hypotension is defined as a drop of 20 mm Hg or greater in systolic blood pressure or systolic blood pressure falling to less than 90 mm Hg. Other experts also consider a drop in diastolic blood pressure of 10 mm Hg or more or an increase in heart rate of 20 beats/minute or more as criteria for the diagnosis of orthostatic hypotension.

11. When the etiology of syncope remains unclear, what other testing can be performed?

When the diagnosis is still not clear, echocardiography can be obtained, looking for unsuspected depressed LVEF or RV dysfunction, HCM (which may predispose to VT), or obstructive heart disease (aortic stenosis, HCM, rare left atrial myxoma). Although echocardiography has become part of the "shotgun" evaluation of syncope for many practitioners, and both the AHA/ACC and ESC recommended it as a diagnostic test, its yield in patients whose cardiac histories, physical examinations, and ECGs are unremarkable is low. In cases in which neurocardiogenic syncope is suspected and further testing is desired, a tilt-table test can be obtained. Exercise stress testing has been suggested by some to assess for cardiac ischemia or exercise-induced arrhythmias in appropriately selected patients. In patients in whom a bradyarrhythmia or tachyarrhythmia is suspected, a Holter monitor, event monitor, or implantable loop recorder can be considered or, under certain circumstances, electrophysiologic testing can be performed.

12. During carotid sinus massage, what is considered a diagnostic response?

According to the ESC Guidelines, a ventricular pause lasting 3 seconds or longer (Fig. 70.2) or a fall in systolic blood pressure of 50 mm Hg or more is considered abnormal and defines carotid sinus hypersensitivity. Carotid sinus massage should not be performed in patients with a recent transient ischemic attack (TIA) or stroke or those with carotid bruits.

Table 70.2. Symptoms and Findings Obtained on the History, Physical Diagnosis, and Electrocardiogram, and the Etiology for Syncope That They Suggest

SYMPTOMS/FINDINGS	SUGGESTED ETIOLOGY
History	
Postepisode fatigue or weakness	Suggests neurocardiogenic syncope
Syncope precipitated by anxiety, pain, or emotional distress	Suggests neurocardiogenic syncope
Auras, postictal confusion, focal neurologic signs/symptoms	Favors a neurologic cause
History of MI, depressed EF, or repaired congenital heart disease	Raises concern of a ventricular arrhythmia
Syncope precipitated by neck turning	Suggests carotid sinus hypersensitivity
Sudden-onset shortness of breath and/or chest pain	Suggests pulmonary embolism or arrhythmia
Syncope related to micturition, coughing, swallowing, or defecation	Suggests "situational syncope"
Arm movement and use precipitating syncope	Suggests subclavian steal
Palpitations	Suggests cardiac tachyarrhythmia
Family history of sudden cardiac death	Suggests HCM, long QT syndrome, or Brugada syndrome
Physical Exam	
Orthostatic changes	Suggests orthostatic hypotension due to dehydration, drugs, or autonomic dysfunction
Carotid sinus hypersensitivity	Suggests carotid sinus hypersensitivity
Carotid bruit	Suggests underlying coronary artery disease as well as possible carotid stenosis
Systolic ejection murmur	Suggests aortic stenosis or HCM
Unequal blood pressures, bruit over subclavian area	Suggests subclavian steal
ECG	
Prolonged PR interval ± bundle branch block	Suggests heart block as cause
Marked sinus bradycardia	Raises the possibility of sick sinus syndrome
Prolonged QT interval	Raises the possibility of torsades de pointes due to congenital long QT syndrome or drugs
Marked left ventricular hypertrophy	Raises possibility of HCM
Q waves	Suggests old myocardial infarction and the possibility of VT
Unusual ST-segment elevation in V1-V2	Suggests Brugada syndrome and polymorphic VT

ECG, Electrocardiogram; *HCM*, hypertrophic cardiomyopathy; *VT*, ventricular tachycardia.

13. What is a tilt-table test?

Tilt-table testing is most commonly performed on patients with neurally mediated syncope (e.g., neurocardiogenic syncope). The patient first lies supine on a board with a foot support. The table is then rotated to a tilt angle of 60 to 80 degrees, so that the patient is almost in the standing position. This maneuver leads to venous pooling and later loss of plasma volume as a result of movement into interstitial spaces. Overall, there is an approximate 15% to 20% (700-mL) decrease of plasma volume. The normal neuroregulatory mechanisms of the body will usually compensate for this, maintaining blood pressure. Vasovagal reactions can occur during monitoring, leading to a decrease

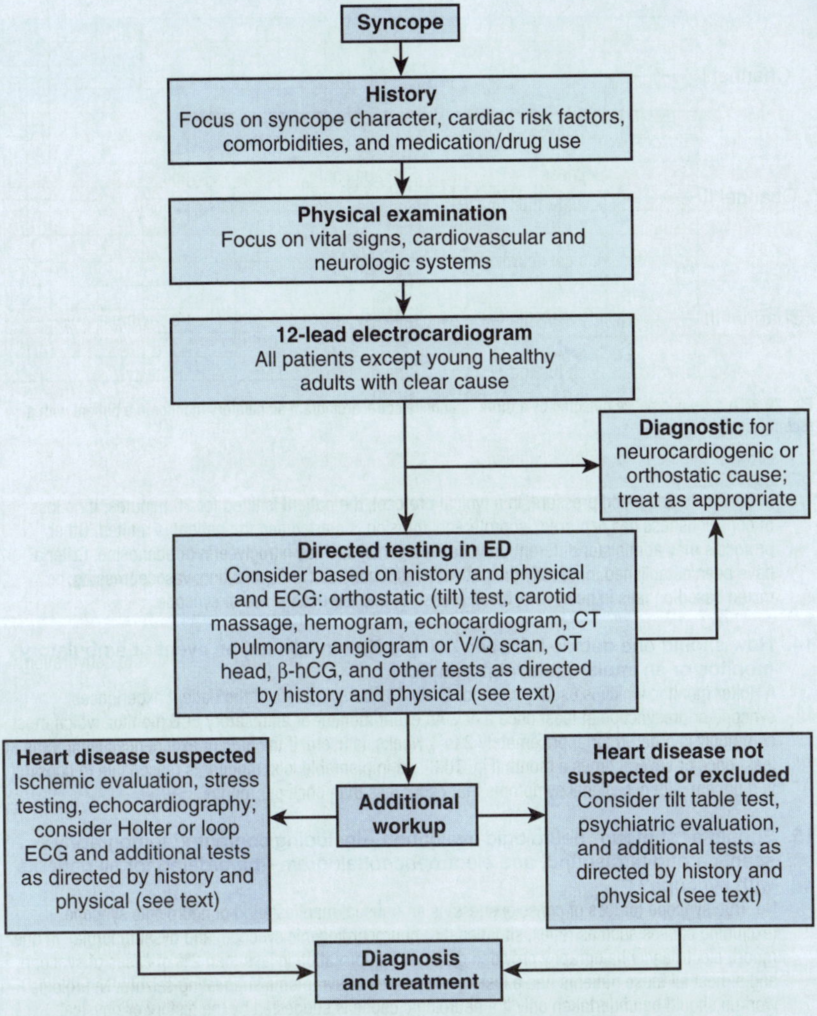

Fig. 70.1. Diagnostic algorithm for the evaluation of syncope. *CT*, Computed tomography; *ECG*, electrocardiogram; *ED*, emergency department; *V/Q*, ventilation/perfusion; *β-hCG*, Beta-Human Chorionic Gonadotropin. *(From De Lorenzo, R. A. [2013]. Syncope. In J. Marx, R. Hockberger, R. Walls (Eds.), Rosen's emergency medicine (pp. 135–141.e1), Chapter 15. Philadelphia: Saunders, Fig. 15.2.)*

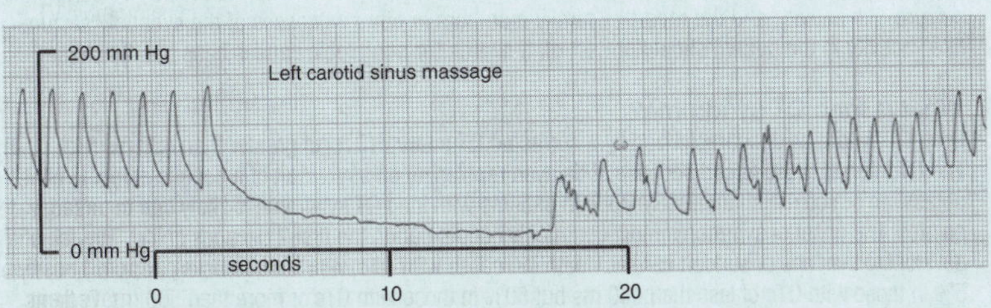

Fig. 70.2. Arterial tracing in a patient with syncope who was found to have carotid hypersensitivity. Note the greater than 10 seconds of asystole, as evidenced by the complete absence of pulsatile blood flow. *(Image courtesy of Dr. Addison Taylor. Image from Levine, G. N. [2014].* Color atlas of cardiovascular disease. *New Delhi, India: Jaypee Brothers Medical Publishers.)*

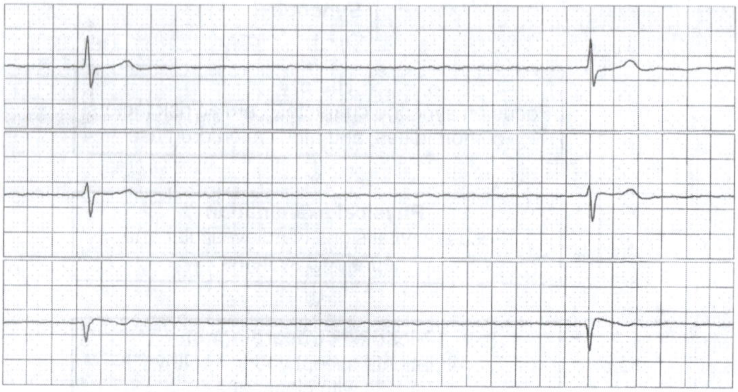

Fig. 70.3. A 4-second pause detected by a three-channel electrocardiogram ambulatory monitor in a patient with a recent history of syncope.

in heart rate and blood pressure. In a typical protocol, the patient is tilted for 30 minutes; if no loss of consciousness has occurred, isoproterenol infusion is started and the patient is retilted. Other protocols may administer different provocative agents, such as nitroglycerin or adenosine. Criteria have been established to classify the patient's responses as cardioinhibiting, vasodepressing, or mixed based on falls in heart rate, blood pressure, and the occurrence of syncope.

14. How should one decide between using a Holter monitor, an event or ambulatory monitor, or an implantable loop monitor?

A Holter monitor, which is usually worn for 24 to 48 hours, is useful if the patient experiences syncope or presyncope at least once a day. An event monitor or ambulatory ECG monitor, which most commonly is ordered for approximately 2 to 4 weeks, is useful if the patient experiences symptoms at least once or several times a month (Fig. 70.3). An implantable loop monitor is reasonable to consider in a patient with occasional symptoms that occur less than once per month.

15. Should a "shotgun" neurologic evaluation—including computed tomography scan, carotid ultrasound, and electroencephalogram—be ordered for all patients with syncope?

No. True syncope (or loss of consciousness) is an unusual manifestation of neurologic syncope (excluding causes such as reflex, situational or neurocardiogenic syncope, and dysautonomia). In one report, electroencephalography provided diagnostic information in less than 2% of cases of syncope, and almost all those patients had a history of seizures or symptoms suggesting seizure. Neurologic workup should be undertaken only if a neurologic cause is suggested by the history or physical examination. TIAs usually do not cause syncope. Carotid disease and stroke more likely lead to focal neurologic deficits than global neurologic ischemia and syncope (the rare exception being severe bilateral carotid artery disease). Severe bilateral vertebrobasilar disease can cause syncope but is not easily diagnosed by screening studies. Importantly, cerebral hypoperfusion caused by VT can result in seizure-like activity, and the report by family members or other witnesses of the event of "seizure-like" activity in the patient should not set off a search for neurologic causes based on this alone.

16. What is long QT syndrome?

Long QT syndrome is characterized by a corrected QT interval (QTc) of greater than 450 ms (Fig. 70.4). The QT interval is prolonged because of delayed repolarization as a result of a genetic defect in either potassium or sodium channels. Syncope in patients with long QT syndrome is likely due to torsades de pointes. The onset of symptoms most commonly occurs during the first 2 decades of life. The risk of developing syncope or sudden cardiac death increases with QTc, with lifetime risks of approximately 5% in those with QTc of less than 440 ms but 50% in those with QTc of more than 500 ms. Patients with long QT syndrome should be referred to an electrophysiologist for further evaluation and treatment, which may include medicines or placement of an implantable cardioverter defibrillator (ICD).

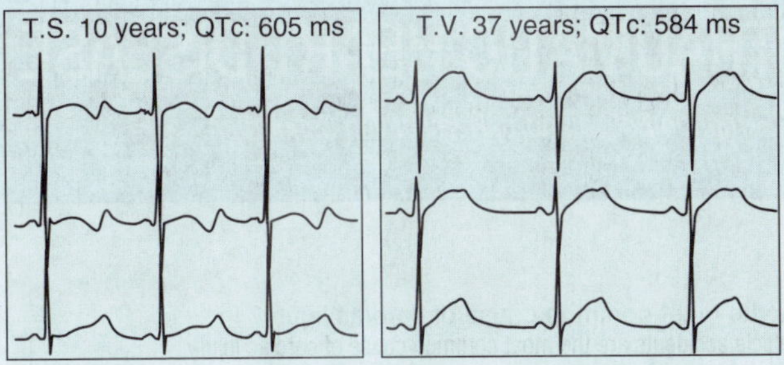

Fig. 70.4. Typical electrocardiogram of two patients with long QT syndrome showing QT-interval prolongation and T-wave morphologic abnormalities. *(From Libby, P. P., Bonow, R. O., Mann, D. L., & Zipes, D. P. [2007].* Braunwald's heart disease: a textbook of cardiovascular medicine *(8th ed.). Philadelphia, PA: Elsevier Saunders.)*

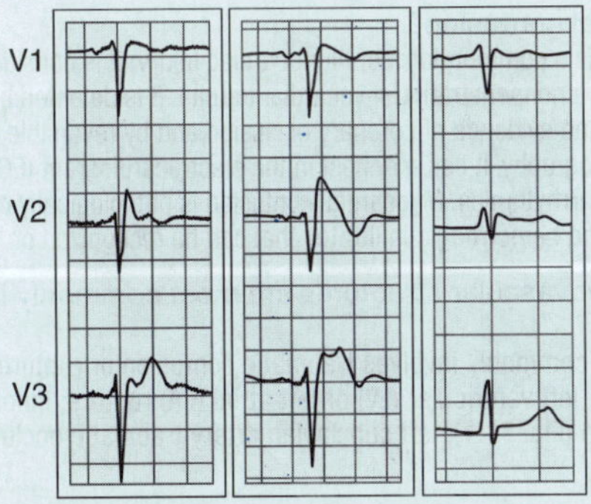

Fig. 70.5. Example of the ST-segment elevations in leads V1 to V3 seen in patients with Brugada syndrome. *(From Libby, P. P., Bonow, R. O., Mann, D. L., & Zipes, D. P. [2007].* Braunwald's heart disease: a textbook of cardiovascular medicine *(8th ed.). Philadelphia, PA: Elsevier Saunders.)*

17. What is Brugada syndrome?

Brugada syndrome is a disorder of sodium channels resulting in sometimes intermittent, unusual ST-segment elevation in leads V1 to V3 as well as a right bundle branch block–like pattern (Fig. 70.5). Such patients are susceptible to developing polymorphic VT. Patients with suspected Brugada syndrome should be referred for specialized cardiac evaluation and a probable ICD.

Bibliography and Suggested Readings

Brignole, M., & Hamdan, M. H. (2012). New concepts in the assessment of syncope. *Journal of the American College of Cardiology, 59*(18), 1583–1591. http://dx.doi.org/10.1016/j.jacc.2011.11.056.

De Lorenzo, R. A. (2013). Syncope. In J. Marx, R. Hockberger, R. Walls (Eds.), *Rosen's emergency medicine* (pp. 135–141.e1), Chapter 15. Philadelphia: Saunders.

Fogel, R. I., & Varma, J. (2000). Approach to the patient with syncope. In G. N. Levine & D. L. Mann (Eds.), *Primary care provider's guide to cardiology.* Philadelphia, PA: Lippincott Williams & Wilkins.

Moya, A. Sutton, R., & Ammirati, F. (2009). Guidelines for the diagnosis and management of syncope (version 2009): the Task Force for the Diagnosis and Management of Syncope of the European Society of Cardiology (ESC). *European Heart Journal, 30,* 2631–2671.

Saklani, P. S., Krahn, A., & Klein, G. (2013). Syncope. Contemporary reviews in cardiovascular medicine. *Circulation, 127,* 1330–1339.

Sheldon, R., Morillo, C., Krahn, A., O'Neill, B., Thiruganasambandamoorthy, V., Parkash, R., et al. (2011). Standardized approaches to the investigation of syncope—a position paper of the Canadian Cardiovascular Society. *Canadian Journal of Cardiology, 27,* 246–253.

Strickberger, S. A., Benson, D. W., Biaggioni, I., Callans, D. J., Cohen, M. I., Ellenbogen, K. A., et al. (2006). AHA/ACCF scientific statement on the evaluation of syncope. *Journal of the American College of Cardiology, 47*(2), 473–484.

CHAPTER 71

TRAUMATIC HEART DISEASE

Fernando Boccalandro, Hercilia Von Schoettler

1. **What is the most common cause of cardiac injury?**
   Motor vehicle accidents are the most common cause of cardiac injury.

2. **List the physical mechanisms of injury in cardiac trauma.**
   The physical mechanisms of injury include penetrating trauma (i.e., ribs, foreign bodies, sternum), nonpenetrating trauma (or blunt cardiac injury), massive chest compression (or crush injury), deceleration, traction, torsion of the heart or vascular structures, and a sudden rise in blood pressure caused by acute abdominal compression.

3. **What is myocardial contusion?**
   Myocardial contusion is a common form of blunt cardiac injury; it is considered a reversible insult and is the consequence of a nonpenetrating myocardial trauma. It is detected by elevations of specific cardiac enzymes with no evidence of coronary occlusion and by reversible wall-motion abnormalities detected by echocardiography. It can mânifest in the electrocardiogram (ECG) by ST segment and/or T wave changes or arrhythmias. Myocardial contusion is pathologically characterized by areas of myocardial necrosis and hemorrhagic infiltrates that can be recognized on autopsy.

4. **Which major cardiovascular structures are most commonly involved in cardiac trauma?**
   Cardiac trauma most commonly involves traumatic contusion or rupture of the right ventricle (RV), aortic valve tear, left ventricular (LV) or left atrial (LA) rupture, innominate artery avulsion, aortic isthmus rupture (Fig. 71.1), left subclavian artery traumatic occlusion, and tricuspid valve tear.

5. **What bedside findings can be seen in patients with suspected major cardiovascular trauma?**
   Obvious clinical signs in patients with nonpenetrating trauma are rare. However, a bedside evaluation by an astute clinician to detect possible life-threatening cardiovascular and thoracic complications can reveal important signs in just a few minutes (Table 71.1).

6. **Can an acute myocardial infarction complicate cardiac trauma?**
   Myocardial infarction (MI) is an unusual complication in patients with chest trauma. Chest trauma can injure a coronary artery, leading to MI due to coronary spasm, thrombosis, laceration, or dissection of the arterial wall (Fig. 71.2). Patients with underlying coronary artery disease have pathophysiologic conditions conducive to an acute coronary syndrome during trauma as a result of limited coronary flow reserve, excess of circulating catecholamines, hypoxia, blood loss, and hypotension. It may be relevant in the appropriate clinical scenario to consider the possibility of cardiac syncope as the primary cause of a traumatic event due to ventricular arrhythmias in a patient with an acute MI and concomitant trauma. Chest trauma can elevate cardiac-specific enzymes without significant coronary stenosis; therefore careful interpretation of these indicators in a trauma victim is warranted.

7. **What is the most common type of myocardial infarction suffered by trauma victims?**
   According to the universal definition of MI, patients who have myocardial necrosis during trauma usually suffer a type 2 MI. This type of myocardial necrosis is secondary to direct trauma or ischemia as a result of a relative imbalance of either increased myocardial oxygen demand and/or decreased myocardial oxygen supply (e.g., coronary artery spasm, coronary embolism, anemia, arrhythmias, hypertension, anemia, or hypotension), rather than coronary occlusion caused by advanced atherosclerosis or an acute coronary thrombotic event (type 1 MI), and is characterized by a variable increase in cardiac biomarkers with no ischemic symptoms or ECG changes.

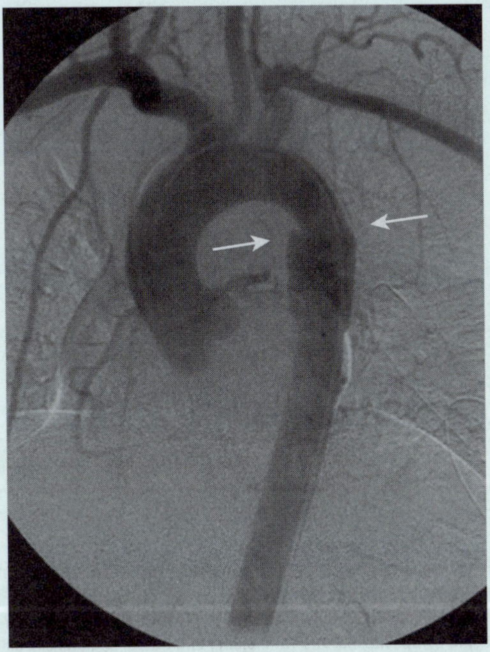

Fig. 71.1. Traumatic rupture of the descending thoracic aorta *(arrows)* at the aortic isthmus. *(Modified from Valji, K. [2006]. Vascular and interventional radiology [2nd ed.]. Philadelphia, PA: Saunders.)*

Table 71.1. Important Signs of Cardiovascular and Thoracic Trauma

FINDING	SUGGESTED LESIONS
Pale skin color, conjunctiva, palms, and oral mucosa	Suggests important blood loss
Decreased blood pressure in the left arm	Seen in patients with traumatic rupture of the aortic isthmus, pseudocoarctation, or traumatic thrombosis of the left subclavian artery
Decreased blood pressure in the right arm	Consider innominate artery avulsion
Subcutaneous emphysema and tracheal deviation	Consider pneumothorax
Elevated jugular venous pulse with inspiratory increase (i.e., the Kussmaul sign)	Suggests cardiac tamponade or tension pneumothorax
Prominent systolic V wave in the venous pulse examination	Suggests tricuspid insufficiency as a result of tricuspid valve tear
Nonpalpable apex or distant heart sounds	Suspect cardiac tamponade
Pericardial rub	Diagnostic for pericarditis
Pulsus paradoxus	Seen in patients with cardiac tamponade, massive pulmonary embolism, or tension pneumothorax
Continuous murmurs or thrills	Consider traumatic arteriovenous fistula or rupture of the sinus of Valsalva
Harsh holosystolic murmurs	Suspect traumatic ventricular septal defect
Early diastolic murmur and widened pulse pressure	Suspect aortic valve injury
Cervical and supraclavicular hematomas	Seen in traumatic carotid rupture
New focal neurologic symptoms	Traumatic carotid, aortic, or great vessel dissection

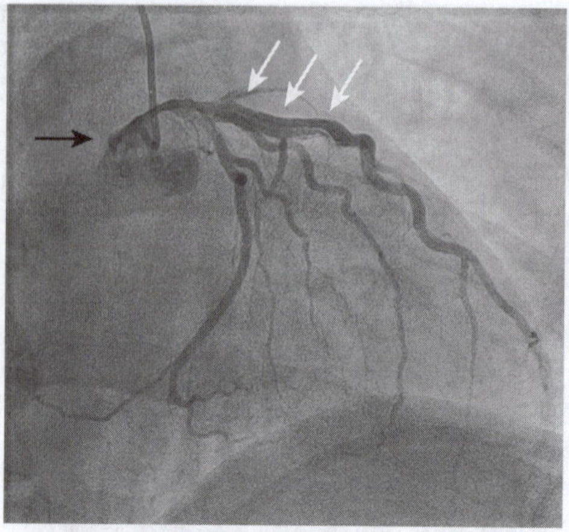

Fig. 71.2. Traumatic coronary dissection showing a double lumen in the left anterior descending artery *(white arrows)*, extending retrograde and narrowing the lumen of the left main coronary artery *(black arrow)* in a patient involved in a high-speed motor vehicle accident.

8. **What is the preferred treatment for ST segment elevation acute myocardial infarction in the event of chest trauma?**
   The treatment of choice is emergent coronary angiography. Thrombolytic therapy is associated with a high risk of bleeding complications. The withholding of nitrates, angiotensin-converting enzyme (ACE) inhibitors, and beta-blockers should be considered until it is established that the patient is hemodynamically stable. Aspirin can be used in patients with no evidence of severe bleeding. Aortic balloon counterpulsation is contraindicated in patients with acute MI and cardiogenic shock with acute traumatic aortic regurgitation or any suspected aortic lesions. If a coronary intervention is needed, balloon angioplasty without stenting is preferred. If stenting is needed, bare metal stents should be considered in case early withdrawal of antiplatelet therapy is necessary.

9. **What are the causes of shock in patients with cardiac trauma?**
   The first cause to address is always hypovolemic shock due to acute blood loss, usually from an abdominal source. If the shock persists despite fluid resuscitation or the degree of hemodynamic compromise is not in proportion to the degree of blood loss, consider cardiogenic causes or tension pneumothorax. The three main cardiac causes of cardiogenic shock are cardiac tamponade, acute valvular dysfunction, and ventricular akinesia or hypokinesia. Rupture of any intrapericardial vessel or cardiac structure (e.g., coronary arteries, proximal aorta, great veins, ventricle) can produce a rapid state of shock because of cardiac tamponade unless there is a concomitant pericardial tear (Fig. 71.3). Acute valvular dysfunction due to mechanical disruption of the valvular apparatus can lead to acute valvular regurgitation and shock; it is usually associated with the presence of a new murmur on physical examination. Cardiac akinesia or severe hypokinesia with temporary myocardial stunning can be a consequence of cardiac trauma and can lead to cardiogenic shock or acute heart failure. Cardiac akinesia or severe hypokinesia requires volume resuscitation to increase the cardiac preload and inotropic support until contractile recovery is achieved.

10. **What workup should be considered in a patient with suspected cardiac trauma?**
    Workup for suspected cardiac trauma should include the following:
    - **Laboratory testing:** Hemoglobin, hematocrit, chemistries, blood typing, and coagulation panel
    - **Chest radiography:** Radiographs are used to evaluate the cardiac silhouette, mediastinum, and lung fields.
    - **Electrocardiography:** Not a sensitive or specific test, but this may reveal nonspecific ST segment and/or T wave changes, conduction abnormalities, sinus tachycardia, premature atrial contractions, ventricular premature beats, or more complex arrhythmias suggestive of myocardial contusion. Low voltage is suggestive of pericardial effusion, whereas electrical alternans may point to impending cardiac tamponade.

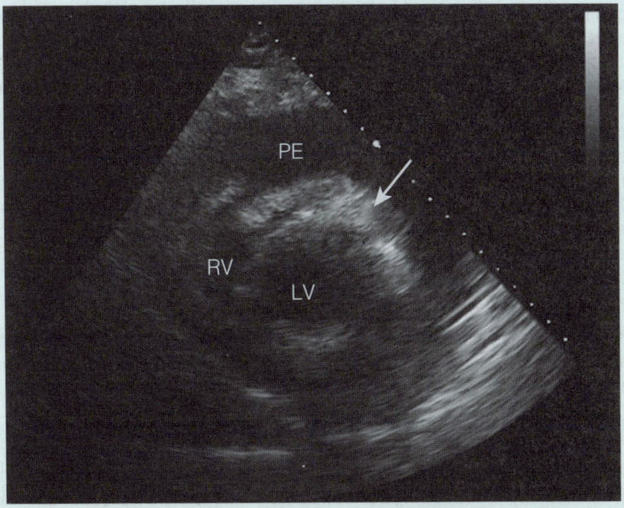

Fig. 71.3. Bedside ultrasound in a patient with cardiac tamponade due to a penetrating stab wound to the heart showing a large pericardial effusion (PE), an intrapericardial hematoma *(white arrow)*, the left ventricle (LV), and collapse of the right ventricle (RV).

- **Bedside ultrasound:** A focused assessment with sonography in trauma victims (or FAST) is encouraged since it is an accurate screening tool for pericardial tamponade and hemopericardium, allowing timely management of a life-threatening condition and identifying those patients at risk for complications.

If the patient is stable from the cardiovascular standpoint, no further workup may be required. Routine use of cardiac biomarkers does not appear to improve the management of patients with blunt chest trauma. However, in patients above 60 years of age with ischemic symptoms or new ECG ischemic changes, cardiac biomarkers and serial ECGs may be appropriate. If more complex heart lesions are suspected, a complete echocardiogram (echo) with color and spectral Doppler imaging is the test of choice. This test is fast, inexpensive, and readily available to provide information regarding the pericardial space, wall motion, valvular function, myocardium, and proximal aorta. Special attention to the RV is warranted because its anterior location close to the sternum makes it vulnerable to myocardial contusion and the development of RV thrombus. Transthoracic echo may have important limitations in patients with complicated trauma (e.g., unstable chest, ventilated patients, chest tube drainages) because of limited echocardiographic windows. Echo contrast agents and transesophageal echocardiograph can play important roles in this group of patients. Transesophageal echo may not be possible in those with an unstable neck or facial trauma. In suspected aortic involvement and in patients who are not candidates for transesophageal echo, contrast computed tomography (CT) is the test of choice.

11. What are the signs of cardiac tamponade?

Three classic signs of cardiac tamponade are known as *Beck's triad*: hypotension caused by decreased stroke volume, jugular-venous distention as a result of impaired venous return to the heart, and muffled heart sounds due to fluid inside the pericardial sac. Other signs of tamponade include pulsus paradoxus and general signs of shock, such as tachycardia, tachypnea, and decreasing level of consciousness.

12. Can a patient suffering from traumatic cardiac tamponade have a normal jugular venous pulse?

In hypovolemic patients, jugular-venous distention may be difficult to interpret even in the presence of cardiac tamponade. Thus attention to volume status is important while examining the venous pulse in trauma victims.

13. How can one confirm the diagnosis in a patient with suspected pericardial tamponade?

A large cardiac silhouette by radiography of the chest and low-voltage QRS complexes or electrical alternans in the ECG can suggest the presence of cardiac tamponade. CT can identify the size of an effusion but cannot confirm the diagnosis. Echocardiography can confirm the diagnosis of tamponade and is the test of choice. If cardiac tamponade is suspected, an echocardiogram (with respirometry) should be ordered promptly. Echocardiography can assess the amount and localization of the pericardial effusion and identify signs of elevated intrapericardial pressure suggesting a tamponade physiology (i.e., right atrial [RA] and RV collapse, LA collapse). Respirometry is a very simple technique that can be performed during the echocardiographic examination; it allows timing of the respiratory cycle with the mitral and tricuspid inflow. It assesses the hemodynamic effect of the pericardial effusion in ventricular filling using spectral Doppler analysis and can confirm the presence of cardiac tamponade.

14. How is a patient with pericardial tamponade treated?

Pericardial tamponade requires immediate treatment with either a surgical subxiphoid approach (pericardial window) or a percutaneous approach using bedside echocardiography or fluoroscopic guidance.

15. What interventions during the resuscitation and management of an unstable trauma patient with a pericardial effusion can precipitate cardiac tamponade?

In a patient with a moderate to large effusion, cardiac tamponade can be precipitated by hypovolemia or positive-pressure ventilation during trauma management. Therefore meticulous attention to the patient's hemodynamics is needed in these circumstances to avoid hemodynamic collapse.

16. What are the mechanisms of injury to the thoracic great vessels?

Deceleration and traction are the most common mechanisms of injury to the thoracic arteries. Sudden horizontal deceleration creates marked shearing stress at the aortic isthmus (i.e., the junction between the mobile aortic arch and the fixed descending aorta) (see Fig. 71.1), whereas vertical deceleration displaces the heart caudally and pulls the ascending aorta and the innominate artery. Rapid extension of the neck or traction on the shoulder can also overstretch the arch vessels and produce tears of the intima, disruption of the media, or complete rupture of the vessel wall, leading to bleeding, dissection, thrombosis, or pseudoaneurysm formation. Aortic rupture leads to immediate hypovolemic shock and death in the vast majority of cases.

17. How are thoracic arterial lesions managed?

Most arterial lesions require surgical or endovascular repair. Thoracic aortic lesions such as limited traumatic dissections are increasingly being managed using thoracic endovascular repair (TEVAR), with thoracic stent graft placement; this is associated with reduced perioperative mortality and morbidity in comparison with open surgical repair. For all traumatic arterial lesions, an effort should be made to control the blood pressure with beta-blockers if the patient is hemodynamically stable. Venous lesions usually do not lead to a rapid hemodynamic compromise unless the implicated vessel drains to the pericardium, possibly leading to cardiac tamponade.

18. What are potential late complications of heart trauma?

Late complications can include fistulas between different structures, constrictive pericarditis as a late consequence of hemopericardium, embolization from a mural thrombus, ventricular aneurysm formation, valvular insufficiency, and postpericardiotomy syndrome.

19. What is commotio cordis?

Sudden death after blunt chest trauma is a rare phenomenon known as *commotio cordis*. It is theorized that commotio cordis is caused by ventricular fibrillation secondary to an impact-induced energy transmission via the chest wall to the myocardium during the vulnerable repolarization period. This can cause lethal arrhythmias resulting in sudden death.

20. What are the cardiac complications of electrical or lightning injuries?

Patients in whom an electric current has a vertical pathway are at high risk for cardiac injury. Arrhythmias are frequently seen. Damage to the myocardium is uncommon and occurs mainly because of heat injury or coronary spasm, causing myocardial ischemia. Direct current (DC) and high-tension alternate current (AC) are more likely to cause ventricular asystole, whereas low-tension AC produces ventricular fibrillation. The most common ECG abnormalities are sinus tachycardia and nonspecific ST-T–wave changes.

The effect of lightning on the heart has been called *cosmic cardioversion* and results in ventricular standstill and, in some reports, ventricular fibrillation. Standstill usually returns to sinus rhythm, but often the patient has a persistent respiratory arrest that causes deterioration of the rhythm. If initial ECG changes are not seen, it is unlikely that significant arrhythmias will occur later.

21. Can a patient develop a trauma-related cardiomyopathy?

Takotsubo cardiomyopathy—also known as *transient apical ballooning, stress-induced cardiomyopathy,* and simply *stress cardiomyopathy*—is a nonischemic cardiomyopathy in which there is sudden temporary LV systolic dysfunction. The cause is debated; it appears to involve high circulating levels of catecholamines and is not specific for mechanical trauma but can be seen in patients after both emotional and physical trauma. Because this finding is associated with emotional stress, this condition is also known as *broken heart syndrome.* The typical presentation of someone with takotsubo cardiomyopathy is a sudden onset of congestive heart failure or chest pain associated with ECG changes suggestive of anterior wall myocardial ischemia after a major trauma; this may initially be indistinguishable from an acute coronary syndrome. During the course of evaluation, dilation of the LV apex with a hypercontractile base of the LV is often noted by echocardiography or angiography (Fig. 71.4). It is this finding that earned the syndrome its name *takotsubo*, or "octopus trap," in Japan, where it was first described. Evaluation of individuals with takotsubo cardiomyopathy may include coronary angiography, which generally does not reveal any significant coronary artery disease. Provided that the individual survives the initial presentation, LV function usually improves over several months with medical therapy.

22. How can the extent of cardiac injury be classified in a trauma patient?

The American Association for the Surgery of Trauma (AAST) heart injury scale (Table 71.2) can be used to grade the spectrum of cardiac injury in trauma patients, with higher grades associated with worse outcomes.

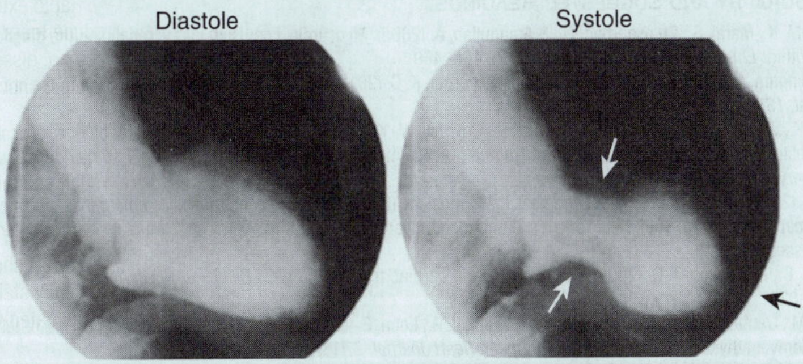

Fig. 71.4. Left ventriculography in a patient who developed a takotsubo cardiomyopathy following a crush injury, showing the classic apical ballooning of the left ventricle. There is systolic contraction of the base of the heart *(white arrows)* but apical ballooning of the left ventricular apex *(black arrow). (Modified from Daroff, R., Fenichel, G., Jankovic, J., & Mazziotta, J. [2012].* Bradley's neurology in clinical practice *(6th ed.). Edinburgh: Saunders.)*

Table 71.2. The American Association for the Surgery of Trauma Heart Injury Scale

Grade I	Blunt cardiac injury with minor ECG abnormality (nonspecific ST or T wave changes, premature atrial or ventricular contraction, or persistent sinus tachycardia Blunt or penetrating pericardial wound without cardiac injury, cardiac tamponade, or cardiac herniation
Grade II	Blunt cardiac injury with heart block or ischemic changes without cardiac failure Penetrating tangential cardiac wound, up to but not extending through endocardium, without tamponade

Continued

Table 71.2. The American Association for the Surgery of Trauma Heart Injury Scale *(Continued)*

Grade III	Blunt cardiac injury with sustained or multifocal ventricular contractions Blunt or penetrating cardiac injury with septal rupture, pulmonary or tricuspid incompetence, papillary muscle dysfunction, or distal coronary artery occlusion without cardiac failure Blunt pericardial laceration with cardiac herniation Blunt cardiac injury with cardiac failure Penetrating tangential myocardial wound, up to but not through endocardium with tamponade
Grade IV	Blunt or penetrating cardiac injury with septal rupture, pulmonary or tricuspid incompetence, papillary muscle dysfunction or distal coronary artery occlusion producing cardiac failure Blunt or penetrating cardiac injury with aortic or mitral incompetence Blunt or penetrating cardiac injury of the right ventricle, right or left atrium
Grade V	Blunt or penetrating cardiac injury with proximal coronary artery occlusion Blunt or penetrating left ventricular perforation Stellate injuries <50% tissue loss of the right ventricle, right of left atrium
Grade VI	Blunt avulsion of the heart Penetrating wound >50% tissue loss of chamber

ECG, Electrocardiogram.

Bibliography and Suggested Readings

Bansal, M. K., Maraj, S., Chewaproug, D., & Amanullah, A. (2005). Myocardial contusion injury: redefining the diagnostic algorithm. *Emergency Medicine Journal, 22*(7), 465–469.

Chockalingam, A., Mehra, A., Dorairajan, S., & Dellsperger, K. C. (2010). Acute left ventricular dysfunction in the critically ill. *Chest, 138*(1), 198–207.

Clancy, K., Velopulos, C., Bilaniuk, J. W., Collier, B., Crowley, W., Kurek, S., et al. (2012). Screening for blunt cardiac injury: an Eastern Association for the Surgery of Trauma practice management guideline. *Journal for Trauma Acute Care Surgery, 73*(5 Suppl. 4), 301.

Conn, A. (2011). Chest trauma. In E. Legome & L. W. Shockley (Eds.), *Trauma: a comprehensive emergency medicine approach* (1st ed.) (p. 190). New York, NY: Cambridge University Press. <http://www.aast.org/blunt-cardiac-injury>. Accessed 26.09.16.

Cook, C. C., & Gleason, T. G. (2009). Great vessel and cardiac trauma. *Surgical Clinics of North America, 89*(4), 797–820.

Gianni, M., Dentali, F., Grandi, A. M., Sumner, G., Hiralal, R., Lonn, E., et al. (2006). Apical ballooning syndrome or takotsubo cardiomyopathy: a systematic review. *European Heart Journal, 27*(13), 1523–1529.

Holanda, M. S., Domínguez, M. J., López-Espadas, F., López, M., Díaz-Regañón, J., & Rodríguez-Borregán, J. C. (2006). Cardiac contusion following blunt chest trauma. *European Journal of Emergency Medicine, 13*(6), 373–376.

Kapoor, D., & Bybee, K. A. (2009). Stress cardiomyopathy syndrome: a contemporary review. *Current Heart Failure Reports, 6*(4), 265–271.

Karmy-Jones, R., & Jurkovich, G. J. (2004). Blunt chest trauma. *Current Problems in Surgery, 41*(3), 211–380.

Khandhar, S. J., Johnson, S. B., & Calhoon, J. H. (2007). Overview of thoracic trauma in the United States. *Thoracic Surgery Clinics, 17*(1), 1–9.

Labovitz, A. J., Noble, V. E., Bierig, M., Goldstein, S. A., Jones, R., Kort, S., et al. (2010). Focused cardiac ultrasound in the emergent setting: a consensus statement of the American Society of Echocardiography and American College of Emergency Physicians. *Journal of the American Society for Echocardiography, 23*, 1225.

Madias, C., Maron, B. J., Weinstock, J., Estes, N. A., 3rd, & Link, M. S. (2007). Commotio cordis—sudden cardiac death with chest wall impact. *Journal of Cardiovascular Electrophysiology, 18*(1), 115–122.

Mandavia, D. P., & Joseph, A. (2004). Bedside echocardiography in chest trauma. *Emergency Medicine Clinics of North America, 22*(3), 601–619.

McGillicuddy, D., & Rosen, P. (2007). Diagnostic dilemmas and current controversies in blunt chest trauma. *Emergency Medicine Clinics of North America, 25*(3), 695–711.

Moore, E. E., Malangoni, M. A., Cogbill, T. H., Shackford, S. R., Champion, H. R., Jurkovich, G. J., et al. (1994). Organ injury scaling. IV: thoracic vascular, lung, cardiac, and diaphragm. *Journal of Trauma, 36*(3), 299–300.

Reissig, A., Copetti, R., & Kroegel, C. (2011). Current role of emergency ultrasound of the chest. *Critical Care Medicine, 39*(4), 839–845.

Ritenour, A. E., Morton, M. J., McManus, J. G., Barillo, D. J., & Cancio, L. C. (2008). Lightning injury: a review. *Burns*, *34*(5), 585–594.

Schultz, J. M., & Trunkey, D. D. (2004). Blunt cardiac injury. *Critical Care Clinic*, *20*(1), 57–70.

Thygesen, K., Alpert, J. S., Jaffe, A. S., Simoons, M. L., Chaitman, B. R., & White, H. D. (2012). Joint ESC/ACCF/AHA/WHF Task Force for the Universal Definition of Myocardial Infarction. *Journal of the American College of Cardiology*, *60*(16), 1581–1598.

Wolf, S. J., Bebarta, V. S., Bonnett, C. J., Pons, P. T., & Cantrill, S. V. (2009). Blast injuries. *Lancet*, *374*(9687), 405–415.

INDEX

A

Note: Page numbers followed by "*b*", "*t*", and "*f*" refer to boxes, tables, and figures respectively.

I

N

Q

R

S